FIELD MANUAL

NO. 8–2

HEADQUARTERS
DEPARTMENT OF THE ARMY
WASHINGTON, DC, *2 June 1988*

Fundamentals of
AEROSPACE MEDICINE

This manual is the PROPERTY OF THE US GOVERNMENT, distributed under the provisions of a controlled mode to ensure that each Flight Surgeon's Office, the School of Aviation Medicine and Aeromedical Center have copy(s) for those authorized flight surgeon positions.

The Field Manual *will not* be considered a personal use text, to be lifted and taken during transfers, retirement, or personnel change of flight surgeon offices. This reference is provided as a tool of the flight surgeon aerospace specialty to meet the vigors of today as well as the challenges of tomorrow.

Distribution methodology and issuance of this field manual to each office are made to limit printing costs, be cost effective, and disseminate the latest aerospace medical doctrine.

By Order of the Secretary of the Army:

CARL E. VUONO
General, United States Army
Chief of Staff

Official:

R. L. DILWORTH
Brigadier General, United States Army
The Adjutant General

DISTRIBUTION:
    To be distributed in accordance with Controlled distribution list.

Fundamentals of
Aerospace Medicine

Fundamentals of
Aerospace Medicine

Edited by

ROY L. DeHART, M.D., M.P.H., M.S.I.A.
President, The Industrial Medicine
Employer's Service (TIMES) of
Oklahoma, Inc.

Medical Director
Hillcrest Occupational
Medicine Services

Professor and Director
Occupational Medicine
Department of Family Practice
University of Oklahoma
College of Medicine

Former Commander, United States Air Force
School of Aerospace Medicine,
Brooks Air Force Base, Texas

Lea & Febiger   Philadelphia

Lea & Febiger
600 Washington Square
Philadelphia, PA 19106-4198
U.S.A.
(215) 922-1330

Library of Congress Cataloging in Publication Data
Main entry under title:
Fundamentals of aerospace medicine.
Includes index.
1. Aviation medicine. 2. Space medicine.
I. DeHart, Roy L. [DNLM: 1. Aerospace Medicine. WD 700 F981]
RC1062.F86   1985   616.9'80213   84-19359
ISBN 0-8121-0880-9

Printed in the United States of America

Print Number: 5   4   3   2

Julia
Evelyn
John

Foreword

This textbook reflects the dynamic and progressive nature of the specialty of aerospace medicine. The aviation industry has been explosive in development since the early 1900s, and the rapid advances in powered flight in military and civilian aviation have demanded the development of parallel medical systems to serve those who fly. The technologic advances that have occurred and continue to occur make it possible to move crews, passengers, troops, patients, and cargo far beyond all earlier expectations of time, size, weight, and distance. Although aviation has proven to be an important and increasingly rapid mode of transportation, it also has provided new methods of warfare and manned exploration beyond our planet.

Over the years, as the aviation industry grew, the stresses associated with flight, such as acceleration, speed, and altitude, became increasingly apparent. Historic events resulting from the progressive expansion of the flight environment were steadily being catalogued. The necessity for research to study and explore the physiologic effects imposed on man were recognized and vigorously pursued. Although research into the effects of unpowered balloon flights was important, the frequency and magnitude of the stresses associated with powered flight increased the urgency and sophistication of research efforts.

World War I provided the impetus for concerted educational and investigative efforts in the field of aviation medicine. Early in that war, human factors problems were strongly suspected as being the cause of many aircraft accidents and deaths. A school to train physicians to care for flyers and a medical research laboratory to consider urgent problems were established by the United States Army Air Service at Hazelhurst Field, Mineola, New York in 1917. Initial efforts to reduce the number of accidents and the loss of human life centered on good health and the application of more rigid physical standards for pilots and other aircrew members. The first class of "flight surgeons" graduated in 1918. A precipitous decrease in accidents and deaths was the direct result of these dedicated efforts. Since that time, flight surgeons have been intimately associated with flyers and their health and safety. As the list of medical responsibilities expanded, the industrial hygiene aspects of the developing industry included ground operations as well as the aerial mission. The school and laboratory at Hazelhurst Field moved a number of times and in 1959 finally arrived at its present location at Brooks Air Force Base, San Antonio, Texas. The institution is now known as the United States Air Force School of Aerospace Medicine.

Almost from the beginning of aviation medicine as a career field, it became apparent that a team effort was necessary so that an organized, multidisciplinary approach could be best applied to the problems associated with flight. Physicians, physiologists, psychologists, veterinarians, nurses, dentists, and other scientists covering many diverse skills and interests now contribute much time and effort to the men and women associated with flying.

Although much of the emphasis initially was of a military nature, the civilian aspects of aviation grew by leaps and bounds, and today there is a dedicated, cooperative, worldwide military-civilian career field. Additional schools and laboratories are now devoted to the collection of scientific data and the dissemination of vital information.

Typical of those involved in aviation or aerospace medicine has been the need and response to share openly the wealth of information being gathered. The complex and diverse data have been discussed by medical scientists of many nations at meetings and conferences. Periodicals and textbooks also have been very helpful in documenting and disseminating the knowledge that has accumulated. This text is a collection of the literary contributions of more than 40 authors representing the broad spectrum of aerospace medicine. Each contributor is a recognized expert among the many who practice within the specialty. These contributors are continuing a tradition begun over 50 years ago by Dr. Louis H. Bauer, who laid the first foundation stones with his text, *Aviation Medicine*. Dr. Bauer's work has been expanded by the contributions of Dr. Harry Armstrong and, most recently, by Dr. Hugh W. Randal. Thus, this text holds to the tradition of enumerating the basic principles of the challenging field of aerospace medicine. This book will be both a practical text for the student and most valuable reference source for the practitioner of aerospace medicine.

Howard W. Unger, M.D.
Major General, USAF, MC (retired)
Past President of the Aerospace Medical
    Association
Former Trustee of the American Board of
    Preventive Medicine

Preface

Historically, classic medicine has considered the patient with an abnormal physiology or illness in the normal, or terrestrial, environment. Since the inception of aviation, however, and continuing with the advent of space operations, aerospace medicine has been concerned primarily with the crewman and his normal, adaptive physiology in the abnormal environment of flight. This juxtaposition of classic medicine concerning illness and environment is fundamental to aerospace medicine. The phenomenon of flight has the potential to expose man to stressors beyond his ability to adapt. Decreased available oxygen, lowered barometric pressure, temperature extremes, confused sensory input, and biodynamic accelerative forces represent only a part of the unusual stressors to be experienced in flight. Thus, man finds himself in an environment filled with challenges that are not experienced when both feet are planted firmly on terra firma.

The demands of flight are such that occasionally they can be met only by individuals who are themselves free of infirmity or disability and who possess superior psychomotor skills. Such individuals reflect the normal population group with which the physician practicing aerospace medicine is concerned.

This text has been prepared for the physician providing professional care and advice to the general aviation pilot; for the specialist in aerospace medicine supporting the airline industry, the Department of Defense, and the National Aeronautics and Space Administration; and for the student, resident, or intellectually curious. The text is not intended to be a treatise on every subject introduced but rather a general review of the major facets forming the fundamentals of the practice of aerospace medicine. The reader who desires additional information is encouraged to pursue the recommended readings found at the conclusion of each section introduction.

For ease of study and to facilitate the use of the text as a reference source, the content's have been arranged into five sections.

Section I reviews the history of the field, transitioning into the state of aerospace medicine today. The section concludes with a projection of the contributions required of aerospace medicine as we approach the turn of the century with regard both to aeronautic and space systems.

Section II defines the environmental challenges of aviation and discusses the impact of flight on human physiology. The state of the art in protecting man as an operator or passenger in this stressful environment is explored.

Section III introduces the medical factors to be considered in the selection of crewmembers. Health maintenance of the crewmember is addressed from the standpoint of the primary physician and the consulting specialist. Emphasis is given to concern for the passenger in the flight environment and the patient facing aeromedical evaluation.

Section IV addresses the unique and, at times, sophisticated requirements of specific flight operations. Aviation medicine of the three military services (Army, Navy, and Air Force) airline aeromedical programs, medical support to general aviation, and professional involvement in manned spaceflight operations are discussed.

The final section (V) approaches the medical impact of the aerospace industry on the broader community. The international health concern for the aircraft as a disease vector, the occupational hazards associated with the aviation industry, and the potential impact of aerospace activity on the environment are examined.

The contributors to this text are among the most respected and authoritative experts in their respective fields. Many contributors not only are specialists in aerospace medicine but also hold credentials in a second medical specialty or are recipients of postgraduate degrees in an engineering or scientific discipline. They represent a multidisciplinary resource from industry, academia, government, and the military. Academic appointments are the norm, and most of these contributors serve on national or international advisory bodies affecting policy at the highest levels of government.

Roy L. DeHart, M.D., M.P.H.

Acknowledgements

The moment the concept for a textbook begins to take form, it necessitates the involvement of others. In the milieu of modern medical science, the universal man is an endangered species. Consequently, it is necessary to turn to others who are experts in their respective fields for aid, assistance, and contributions to scientific disciplines as diverse as aerospace medicine. We are fortunate that experts by virtue of experience, professional education, and talent, with diverse scientific backgrounds, have agreed to contribute toward this endeavor. I am indebted not only to the written word they provided, but their patience, forbearance, and many words of encouragement. In addition to the distinguished contributors to this text, other professionals in the field of aerospace medicine provided constructive criticism and invaluable assistance in its preparation.

Once the original drafts were received from the contributors, they were reviewed by an expert in medical-text editing. Essentially every word of this text has been scrutinized by Marion E. Green, for whom I will be eternally grateful. Providing library research assistance and other editing activities have been Bonnie Fridley and Elsie Wagener. Once it was time to prepare the final draft, members of the word processing team at the United States Air Force School of Aerospace Medicine under the supervision of Joyce Wilson were of great assistance. Other assistance in text preparation was provided by Mary Ellis and Leticia Solis. Sharing an undue burden were my secretaries Mary Young and Debra Mordecai. Mary, in coordination with Darwin Gordon, provided a considerable degree of executive oversight of the extensive coordination and information exchange necessary for the preparation of this text. Rolling up her sleeves and assisting me in many ways, including proofreading, text layout, and a sounding board for my ideas was Julia DeHart.

The creative talents and artistic ideas of a group of photographers and artists are specifically recognized. Each section of this text is preceded by a line drawing created by Melvan Jordan. The illustrations attempt to present on a single page the summation of the scientific contents of that section. Both Sharon Tice and Albert Young have original illustrations appearing throughout this text. Some are line drawings, others are figures. The photographic department of the United States Air Force of Aerospace Medicine provided a significant portion of the photographic copy contributing to the value of this textbook.

This has been a work of love and of commitment and I deeply appreciate and thank the many named and unnamed persons for their assistance, their contributions and their good will in bringing a concept to reality.

Roy L. DeHart, M.D., M.P.H.
Editor

Major Contributors

Kenneth N. Beers, M.D., M.P.H.
Associate Professor, Departments of
  Community Medicine and Family
  Practice
Wright State University
Dayton, Ohio

James W. Brinkley, B.S.
Chief, Biomechanical Protection Branch
Biodynamics and Bioengineering Division
Air Force Aerospace Medical Research
  Laboratory
Wright-Patterson AFB, Ohio

R. Paul Caudill, Jr., M.D., M.P.H.
Commander, Naval Aerospace Medical
  Institute
Naval Air Station, Pensacola, Florida

N. Bruce Chase, M.D., M.P.H.
Director, Medical Research, Office of the
  Surgeon General
Washington, D.C.

Robert T.P. deTreville, M.D., Sc.D.
Occupational Health Consultant to the
  Commander
United States Air Force Occupational
  and Environmental Health Laboratory
Brooks AFB, Texas

Roy L. DeHart, M.D., M.P.H., M.S.I.A.
President, The Industrial Medicine
  Employer's Service (TIMES) of
  Oklahoma, Inc.
Director, Hillcrest Occupational
  Medicine Services
Tulsa, Oklahoma

J. Robert Dille, M.D., M.I.H.
Manager, Civil Aeromedical Institute
Federal Aviation Administration
Oklahoma City, Oklahoma

Kent K. Gillingham, M.D., Ph.D.
Research Medical Officer
Crew Technology Division
United States Air Force School of
  Aerospace Medicine
Brooks AFB, Texas

Charles C. Gullett, M.D.
Vice President, Medical Services
Harvey W. Watt and Company
Former Director, Medical Services
Trans World Airlines, Inc.
Atlanta, Georgia

H. H. Hanna, M.D.
Former Chief Otolaryngology Branch
Clinical Sciences Division, United States
  Air Force School of Aerospace
  Medicine
Brooks AFB, Texas

Richard D. Heimbach, M.D., Ph.D.
Graduate School Visiting Faculty
Texas A and M University
Former Chief of Hyperbaric Medicine
  Division
United States Air Force School of
  Aerospace Medicine
Southwest Texas Methodist Hospital
Hyperbaric and Aerospace Medicine
San Antonio, Texas

James R. Hickman, Jr., M.D., M.P.H.
Deputy, Clinical Sciences Division
United States Air Force School of
  Aerospace Medicine
Brooks AFB, Texas

David R. Jones, M.D., M.P.H.
Clinical Assistant Professor of Psychiatry
University of Texas Health Science
  Center
Clinical Associate Professor of
  Psychiatry
Uniformed Services University of the
  Health Sciences
United States Air Force School of
  Aerospace Medicine
Brooks AFB, Texas

Robert J. Kreutzmann, M.D.
Commander, United States Army
  Aeromedical Center
Fort Rucker, Alabama

George D. Lathrop, M.D., M.P.H., Ph.D.
Chief, Epidemiology Division
United States Air Force School of
  Aerospace Medicine
Brooks AFB, Texas

Sidney D. Leverett, Jr., Ph.D.
Editor in Chief
*Aviation, Space and Environmental
  Medicine*
Aerospace Physiology Consultant
San Antonio, Texas

Richard L. Masters, M.D., M.P.H.
Aeromedical Advisor, Airline Pilots
  Association
Clinical Associate Professor
Preventive Medicine
University of Colorado School of
  Medicine
Denver, Colorado

George M. McGranahan, Jr., M.D.
Chief, Internal Medicine Branch
United States Air Force School of
  Aerospace Medicine
Brooks AFB, Texas

Robert R. McMeekin, M.D., J.D.
Director, Armed Forces Institute of
  Pathology
Washington, D.C.

Stanley R. Mohler, M.D., M.A.
Professor and Vice Chairman
Department of Community Medicine
Director, Aerospace Medicine
Wright State University
Dayton, Ohio

George C. Mohr, M.D., M.P.H.
Commander, Air Force Aerospace
  Medical Research Laboratory
Wright-Patterson AFB, Ohio

Royce Moser, Jr., Colonel, M.D., M.P.H.
Commander, United States Air Force
  School of Aerospace Medicine
Associate Professor
Uniformed Services University of the
  Health Sciences
Clinical Associate Professor
Family Practice
University of Texas Health Science
  Center
Adjunct Associate Professor
Department of Environmental Sciences
University of Texas School of Public
  Health
Brooks AFB, Texas

Spurgeon Neel, M.D., M.P.H.
Professor, Occupational and Aerospace
  Medicine
University of Texas Health Science
  Center
San Antonio, Texas

Arnauld E. Nicogossian, M.D.
Director, Division of Life Sciences
National Aeronautics and Space
  Administration
Assistant Professor
Department of Preventive and Military
  Medicine
Uniformed Services University of Health
  Sciences
Washington, D.C.

Charles W. Nixon, Ph.D.
Chief, Bioacoustics Branch
Biodynamics and Bioengineering
  Division
Air Force Aerospace Medical Research
  Laboratory
Wright-Patterson AFB, Ohio

John W. Ord, M.D.
Commander, Aerospace Medical
  Division
United States Air Force
Brooks AFB, Texas

James F. Parker, Jr., Ph.D.
Vice President
Biotechnology, Inc.
Annandale, Virginia

James L. Perrien, M.D.
Chief, Neurology Function,
  Neuropsychiatry Branch
United States Air Force School of
  Aerospace Medicine
Brooks AFB, Texas

James H. Raddin, Jr., M.D., M.B.A.
Aerospace Medical Division
Alfred P. Sloan Fellow
MIT Sloan School of Management,
  1982–83
Assistant Clinical Professor
Department of Community Medicine
Wright State University
Dayton, Ohio

Russell B. Rayman, M.D., M.P.H.
Commander
United States Air Force Regional
  Hospital
Langley AFB, Virginia

Paul J. Sheffield, Ph.D.
Deputy Division Chief, Hyperbaric
  Medicine Division
United States Air Force School of
  Aerospace Medicine
Brooks AFB, Texas

Thomas B. Sheridan, Sc.D.
Professor of Engineering and Applied
  Psychology
Mechanical Engineering Department
Massachusetts Institute of Technology
Boston, Massachusetts

Daniel H. Spoor, M.D., M.P.H.
Command Surgeon, United States Air
  Force Space Command
Colorado Springs, Colorado

Thomas J. Tredici, M.D.
Chief, Ophthalmology Branch
USAF School of Aerospace Medicine
Clinical Professor
University of Texas Health Science
  Center
Preventive Medicine/Biometrics Adjunct
  Associate Professor
Uniformed Services University of the
  Health Sciences School of Medicine
Brooks AFB, Texas

Henning E. von Gierke, DR., ENG.
Director, Biodynamics and
  Bioengineering Division
Air Force Aerospace Medical Research
  Laboratory
Wright-Patterson AFB, Ohio

B.E. Welch, Ph.D.
Chief Scientist, Aerospace Medical
  Division
Brooks AFB, Texas

James E. Whinnery, M.D., Ph.D.
Research Physician
Crew Systems Division (VNB)
USAF School of Aerospace Medicine
Brooks AFB, Texas

James W. Wolfe, Ph.D.
Chief, Neurosciences Function
United States Air Force School of
  Aerospace Medicine
Brooks AFB, Texas

William H. Wolfe, M.D., M.P.H.
Chief, Epidemiology Branch
United States Air Force School of
  Aerospace Medicine
Brooks AFB, Texas

C. Thomas Yarington, Jr., M.D.
Clinical Professor
University of Washington College of
  Medicine
Chief, Otolaryngology, Plastic and
  Reconstructive Surgery
The Mason Clinic
Seattle, Washington

Laurence R. Young, Sc.D.
Professor of Aeronautics and
  Astronautics
Faculty of Harvard-M.I.T. Program in
  Health Sciences and Technology
Massachusetts Institute of Technology
Boston, Massachusetts

Other Contributors

Nicholas E. Barreca, M.D., M.P.H.
Paul V. Celio, M.D.
Clarence R. Collins, B.S.
Paul H. Grundy, M.D., M.P.H.
John R. Herbold, D.V.M., M.P.H., Ph.D.
Elray Jenkins, M.D., M.P.H.
Thomas McNish, M.D., M.P.H.
Gwynne K. Neufield, M.D.

Bennett G. Owens, Jr. M.D., M.P.H.
Samuel B. Parker, II, M.D.
Dennis D. Pinkousky, Ph.D.
Dudley R. Price, M.D., M.P.H.
Ronald R. Rossing, M.D., M.P.H.
David J. Wehrly, M.D., M.P.H.
William C. Wood, M.D.

Contents

Section *I*

Aerospace Medicine in Perspective

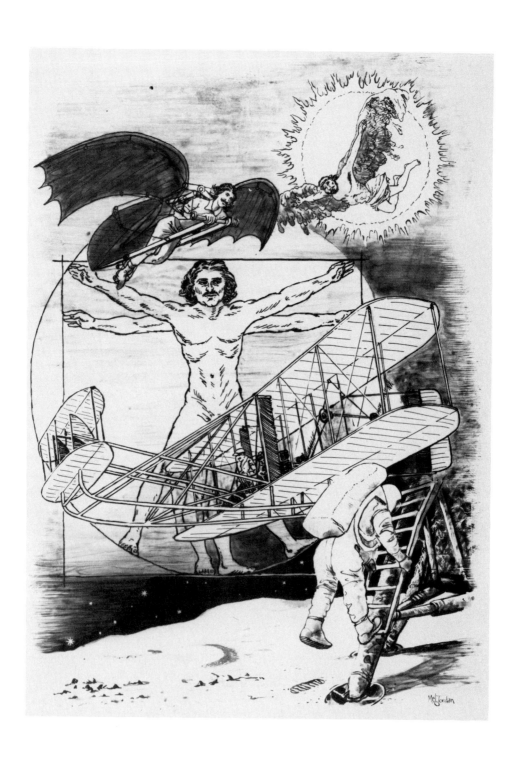

Section *I*

Aerospace Medicine in Perspective

Medicine's contribution to aviation and space flight began with an untethered hot air balloon carrying men aloft and continues with concept development for new aeronautic and astronautic systems. The historical development and transition of aviation to space flight provides the perspective for viewing the maturation of aerospace medicine.

Icarus' flight too near the sun, Leonardo da Vinci's drawings of man-powered aircraft, powered flight by the Wrights' biwing, and man's first step on the moon illustrate the progression of manned flight from dream to design to development to destiny. This progress in technologic achievement parallels the development of aerospace medicine.

Many of the fundamentals that form the foundation for the practice of aerospace medicine become evident as the perspectives of past, modern, and future activities are discussed. From the historical per-

spective, one can view the triumphs and tragedies as man probes the ocean of air. The modern perspective reviews man's ingenuity in meeting the environmental challenges of flight. The future perspective offers an opportunity to consider the possibilities and the difficulties of tomorrow and beyond. As in each branch of medical science and practice, the fundamentals of aerospace medicine must be understood in the perspective of the dynamic dimension of time.

SUGGESTED READING LIST

1. Anderson, H.G.: The Medical and Surgical Aspects of Aviation. London, Oxford University Press, 1919.
2. Armstrong, H.G.: Principles and Practice of Aviation Medicine. 3rd Ed. Baltimore, Williams & Wilkins Co., 1952.
3. Benford, R.J.: Doctors in the Sky. Springfield, Illinois, Charles C Thomas, 1955.
4. Caidin, M., and Caidin, G.: Aviation and Space Medicine. New York, E.P. Dutton, 1962.
5. Combs, H.: Kill Devil Hill. Boston, Houghton Mifflin Co., 1979.

3

6. DeHart, R.L.: Biomedical Aspects of Soviet Manned Space Flight. Washington, D.C., Defense Intelligence Agency, 1975.
7. Dhenin, G. (ed.): Aviation Medicine. London, Tri-Med Books Ltd., 1978.
8. Engle, E., and Lott, A.S.: Man in Flight. Annapolis, Maryland, Leeward Publications, Inc., 1979.
9. Gillies, J.A. (ed.): A Textbook of Aviation Physiology. London, Pergamon Press Ltd., 1965.
10. Josephy, A.M.: The American Heritage History of Flight. New York, American Heritage, 1962.
11. McFarland, R.A.: Human Factors in Air Transport Design. New York, McGraw-Hill Book Co., 1946.
12. National Aeronautics and Space Administration: Foundations of Space Biology and Medicine. Washington, D.C., United States Government Printing Office, 1975.
13. Randel, H.W. (ed.): Aerospace Medicine. Baltimore, Williams & Wilkins Co., 1971.
14. Rolt, L.T.C.: The Aeronauts. New York, Walker and Company, 1966.

Chapter *1*

The Historical Perspective

Roy L. DeHart

Lend me the stone strength of the past, and I will lend you the wings of the future.

ROBINSON JEFFERS

The building blocks of an institution are laid upon a foundation of events past. Aerospace medicine's foundation was laid by those who discovered, designed, and developed the means for man to take his first steps toward the heavens.

DREAMS, LEGENDS, AND RELIGION

In prehistoric times, man turned his face skyward and followed the majesty of birds in flight, observed the beauty of billowing clouds coursing across the sky, and was in awe of the grandeur of the celestial heavens evident in the night sky. His desire to soar above the earth took form in dreams, fantasies, legends, and religion. The desire to fly, although not to be fulfilled for untold centuries, received expression in numerous ways. The Chinese have provided the earliest recorded story of man in flight. The Emperor Shun escaped from the clutches of his captors, when only a boy, by "donning the work clothes of a bird" and flying to freedom. The legends and folklore of early civilizations all had their flying deities, heroes, and creations of the imagination.

Among those associated with aviation, perhaps the best known of the flying legends is the story of Daedalus and his son, Icarus. Held captive on the isle of Crete by King Minos, the two set to work to fashion wings of feathers attached to their bodies by hardened wax. From their site of imprisonment, Daedalus watched the soaring gulls as they flew on the updrafts rising from the steep cliffs about the island. Anticipating the dangerous heat from the sun, Daedalus warned Icarus not to soar too close to that fiery body, lest the wax become softened and the feathers detached. The moment for the escape arrived and the two captives flung themselves from their prison onto the updrafts and soared skyward. Icarus, being younger and perhaps somewhat foolhardy, surrendered to the ecstasy of the moment and soared ever higher, ignoring both advice and warning, with predictable results. As many were to learn in years to come, flying can be an unforgiving pursuit. The story goes that, with reason ruling emotion and wisdom supplanting enthusiasm, Daedalus made successful his escape.

In most cultures, similar stories are found of gods riding the winds in aerial chariots and angels with wings of eagles soaring to the music of the spheres. The ancient poets wrote wonderful descriptive odes of man flying through the air, and their contemporary artists portrayed these dreams on stone and parchment. Elijah, the Hebrew prophet, was transported alive to the heavens. For the Greeks, Apollo carried the sun in a flying chariot across the heavens on his daily obligation to the people of earth. The Romans created Mercury to serve as the rapid courier of messages between the deities. In the western hemisphere, Ayar Utso, a chief of the early Peruvian Incas, grew wings and flew away to escape imprisonment, and, even today, we turn to tradition as on Christmas Eve we await the arrival of Santa Claus, drawn across the heavens in his sleigh by his eight reindeer.

THINGS THAT FLY

Occasionally, it has been found that legends are based on fact, or may, at the very least, stimulate a discovery. The concept that the propeller was understood and used in ancient Rome is best appreciated when described as a windmill. Over 2000 years ago, the Chinese invented the kite, and it is reported to have been used in military signaling. A contemporary of Confucius, Kungsuhu Tse, built a wooden and bamboo magpie that flew for 3 days. This flying contraption was most probably a kite. In southern Italy before the Christian era, there is a report of a mysterious wooden pigeon. This dove, or pigeon, developed by Archytas, is believed to have been a model of a bird suspended by wires from a revolving arm operated by a type of steam reaction device.

Another flying toy invented by the Chinese used the helicopter principle. It apparently consisted of a lightweight spindle of wood with feathers inserted at one end. When thrown or dropped, it rapidly rotated and slowly descended to earth.

The notebooks of Leonardo da Vinci, the "universal man" of the Renaissance, were filled with material related to flight. He designed a model helicopter with a helix, or spiral screw, driven by a spring mechanism. The suggestion is that he actually flew this model. Tradition also identifies da Vinci with experiments involving hot air balloons; however, these were more likely small kites, although he was certainly aware of the physical fact that hot air rises. Among his sketches is a pyramid-shaped parachute, consisting of a tent made of linen, with the measurements provided to allow construction of a device that would enable a man to "throw himself down from any great height without sustaining any injury." Da Vinci's fascination with the flight of birds took practical form in the dozens of drawings he made of ornithopters with the operator located in various positions. Within the 5000 manuscript pages left by Leonardo da Vinci, were some 150 separate sketches of flying machines.

A Venetian mathematician, Giovanni Danti, constructed gliders composed of "wings in proportion to the gravity of his body," which were flown from the roofs of houses in Perugia. It would appear that these were models launched from the rooftops because there is no documentation of manned flight associated with these launches. For his efforts, Danti was exiled as a sorcerer.

Although Renaissance history is rife with tales and legends of rooftop, hill, and tower jumpers, few have been chronicled in such a way as to establish their authenticity. One such report may be accurate. It is documented that the Marquis de Bacqueville leaped from the roof of his Paris house in 1742 assisted by a glider-like device. He displayed more discretion than most potential aviators by aiming his flight path toward the Seine. Although his flight path was well established, the flight was short-lived due to some minor structural failure, causing him to fall upon the deck of a washerwoman's barge. Although described as a humiliating landing, it nevertheless was survivable, and the Marquis escaped with only a broken leg.

Wings of feathers, paper, and linen or strange mechanical devices combined with intestinal fortitude were tried and all failed in man's attempt for sustained flight. The physical principles of gas displacement and density would first allow man the privilege of soaring with the birds and introduce to him a new and potentially hazardous environment.

Balloons

The climb to free flight began with the thirteenth century scientist, Roger Bacon, who prepared an elaborate treatise on the navigation of air. He suggested that flying machines built of large, hollow, metal spheres or globes be constructed light enough to be supported by the density of the atmosphere. His major thesis was that air was capable of supporting a craft in the same manner that water supports a ship.

The next step upward was achieved by the English chemist, Henry Cavendish, who read a paper before the Royal Society in 1766 describing the weight of hydrogen, a gas. He called this gas "inflammable air" and announced that it was considerably lighter than ordinary air. The aeronautic significance of this finding was not realized by Cavendish. Although others recognized this potential, the immediate proof of this "lighter than air" property and the realization of flight was not to be. The intellectual curiosity and the inquiring minds of two French brothers led them to combine principle and practicality and attain sustained manned flight.

The Montgolfiers

Joseph Priestly's treatise, *Experiments and Observations on Different Kinds of*

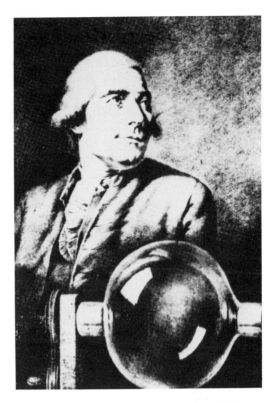

Fig. 1–1. Joseph Montgolfier, the designer of the large-capacity hot air balloon (Library of Congress).

Air, served as the stimulus for experimentation by Joseph Montgolfier (Fig. 1–1). The legends and stories surrounding the beginnings of Joseph's interest are both fanciful and interesting. One story has it that Madame Montgolfier's chemise took off when placed before the fire to air; a second story maintains that it was Joseph's own shirt which was raised in this way; and yet a third story tells of Madame Montgolfier placing a conical paper wrapping from a sugar loaf into the fire, whereupon Joseph observed it filling with hot air and flying up the chimney without igniting.[1]

Montgolfier learned the chemistry behind the production of hydrogen and used the hydrogen to fill small paper balloons or globes. He discovered, as had others before him, that the gas passes through the paper as fast as the container is filled. Silk was tried but was abandoned when it was no more successful at holding the gas. Montgolfier then turned to heated air, or what he referred to as "rarified air," as the lifting agent. Joseph was joined by his younger brother, Jacques, in the further pursuit of sustained aerial flight. The family's fortune had been made in the papermaking industry. The experience of these two brothers in paper manufacturing was essential as the size and volume of their "rarified air" balloons expanded. The Montgolfier family name was prophetic in the annals of aeronauts because it means "master of the mountain."

In November, 1782, Joseph began his first small-scale experiments with hot air balloons. A paralellepiped was made of fine silk with an open throat that, when held over an open flame, caused the envelope to inflate and to fly about the ceiling of his apartment. In the next experiment, Jacques joined his brother outdoors, where a small balloon was inflated and rose to a height of approximately 21 m.

The brothers then constructed a much larger experimental balloon with a capacity of 18 m³. This device rose successfully to a height of 183 m. In April, 1783, a balloon was constructed of a combination of paper and cloth that had a calculated lifting capacity of 204 kg. The balloon made a perfect ascent to 305 m, traveling a distance on the wind in excess of 1.2 km (Fig. 1–2).

J.A.C. Charles

While the Montgolfiers experimented with larger-capacity hot air balloons, the members of the Paris Academy of Science were pursuing another alternative by supporting a young physicist by the name of J.A.C. Charles (Fig. 1–3). It was Charles' intent to use the "inflammable air" as the lifting agent in his experiments. To this end, he constructed a perfect sphere that was 3.65 m in diameter and had a capacity of 27 m³. To generate sufficient hydrogen required nearly 226 kg of sulfuric acid and

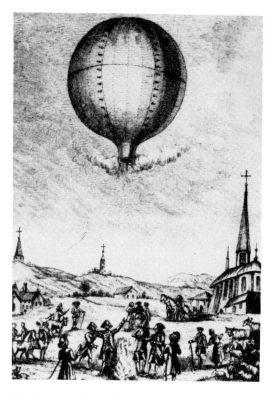

Fig. 1–2. First hot air balloon ascent, June, 1783 (courtesy of The Aeronauts, L.T.C. Rolt, Walker & Co., 1966.)

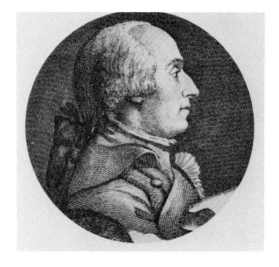

Fig. 1–3. J.A.C. Charles, the young physicist who harnessed hydrogen as a lifting agent (Library of Congress).

over 450 kg of iron filings. Repeated complications and delays in the gassing process occurred, but on August 27, 1783, Charles' hydrogen-filled balloon soared from the heart of Paris to a height of 1000 m.

Among the spectators for Charles' "inflammable air" balloon was Benjamin Franklin, who heard a skeptic in the crowd remark, "interesting, but what use is it?" The envoy from the United States growled, "What use is a newborn baby?"

Nearly an hour later and 24 km from Paris, the balloon returned to earth in a field near the village of Genesse; however, because frightened villagers attacked the balloon with pitchforks, muskets, and whatever other weapons were available, little of the balloon was left to recover.

Pilatre de Rozier

The Montgolfier brothers' experience with large hot air balloons had reached the ear of the monarch of France. King Louis XVI and Queen Marie Antoinette requested that a command performance be conducted at Versailles. A colorfully decorated balloon was constructed that measured 17 m high and 13 m in diameter, with a capacity of 1080 m³. Although rumors were rampant that this would be a manned flight, the King had directed otherwise, considering such a venture too perilous. The flight would indeed be special, however, because, as often the case in aerospace medicine today, animals were to precede man in flight. A large wicker cage was attached to the balloon and contained a sheep, a cock, and a duck. The first aeronautic instrument was attached to the cage—a barometer. The similarity to some events of today's aerospace achievements is remarkable. On this occasion, a dramatic countdown of three cannon shots took place, and with the echo of the third firing still resounding about the walls of the palace, the balloon took flight. The balloon is estimated to have achieved a height of 518 m before it began a gradual descent.

One of the first to reach the downed balloon, a young scientist and physician from Metz, Pilatre de Rozier, observed that the sheep had become free and was quietly grazing, the duck appeared no worse for the experience, and the cock had suffered a damaged wing. Much as now, an investigation was conducted into the mishap that caused the cock's injured wing. Ten witnesses testified that the sheep had kicked the cock prior to takeoff, thus explaining the injury and alleviating concern for the perils of flight.

MANNED FLIGHT. The Montgolfiers began the construction of a third giant balloon. This one was designed to carry a brazier below its throat and a two-man crew to stoke it. The young physician de Rozier volunteered persistently to crew this next historic flight (Fig. 1–4). During October, he made several tethered flights to acquaint himself with the criticality of balance and the difficulties inherent in feeding a fire attached to a paper and linen structure. De Rozier was born in Lorraine, was a member of the Academy of Sciences, and proved his scientific brilliance very early by developing a breathing apparatus, that was the forerunner of the gas mask.

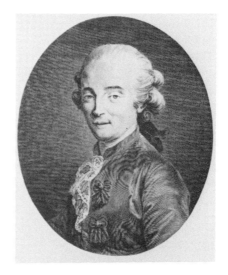

Fig. 1–4. The physician, Pilatre de Rozier, one of the first to fly in free ascent (Library of Congress).

He had a theatrical sense about him; one of his favorite lecture demonstrations was to inhale hydrogen and ignite the gas as he exhaled.

The first manned balloon was 23 m by 15 m with a neck 5 m in diameter. A 1-m broad circular gallery was suspended beneath the balloon by cords sewn into the fabric. Beneath the gallery hung a fire basket made of wrought iron wire. When completed, the balloon weighed 725 kg with a capacity of 2250 m³ and an estimated lift, or payload, of 770 kg.

On October 15, 1783, the balloon was ready for its first trial flight. De Rozier stepped into the gallery and, after only a few feet of rope had been released, the importance of balance became self-evident, and it was necessary to add ballasts to offset his weight. Further tethered flights were made, and de Rozier learned to regulate vertical movement and to extinguish the small fires that occurred on the balloon. Becoming confident in controlling his vertical ascent, de Rozier accepted single passengers. The Marquis d'Arlandes was such a passenger and was to join de Rozier in the first free ascent. At 13:54 on November 21, 1783, de Rozier and the Marquis ascended in free flight to a height of 85 m. Recognizing the significant danger, the two aeronauts each carried a pail of water and a sponge as major safety equipment. The fire suspended below them occasionally sent a shower of sparks onto the fragile fabric of painted cloth and paper. The two men had little opportunity for boredom because they were frequently involved in self-preservation by extinguishing the many little fires that were burning holes in their balloon. In all, the journey lasted some 25 minutes and took them more than 8 km across the city of Paris. This first sustained, free flight was made by a physician and a military officer.

Ten days later, on December 1, J.A.C. Charles manned the first free ascent in a hydrogen balloon with a passenger and a gondola equipped with food, extra cloth-

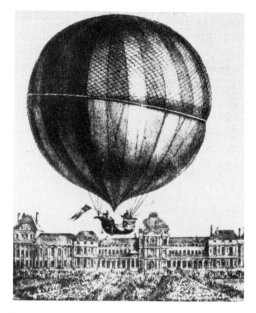

Fig. 1–5. The first manned hydrogen balloon ascent, December, 1783 (courtesy of The Aeronauts, L.T.C. Rolt, Walker & Co., 1966.)

ing, scientific instruments, including a thermometer and barometer, and bags of sand for ballast (Fig. 1–5). The two men lifted off from the Tuileries Gardens in midafternoon. After flying on the winds for 2 hours and covering some 43 km, the balloon landed and the passenger departed. Charles decided to make a solo ascent and rapidly ascended to 2750 m, where he began to experience physiologically some of the realities of this new environment. He complained of the penetrating cold at this altitude and a sharp pressure pain in one ear as he descended. Not only did this represent the first solo flight, but Charles described clearly some of the physiologic perils that can best be managed by those combining interests in aeronautics and medicine.

Once the trail was broken to sustained aerial flight, many an aeronaut followed on both sides of the English channel. In 1785, the next major, dynamic event occurred in balloon flight, and a major contributor to the event was an American physician.

John Jeffries

Dr. John Jeffries (Fig. 1–6), although an American, was a loyalist during the Revolutionary War and thus found it advantageous to practice medicine in England for a while. He was intrigued and fascinated by aerial flight and sought out a Frenchman, Jean-Pierre François Blanchard, who was in England demonstrating ballooning. A flight was agreed to, and Jeffries proceeded to assemble a collection of scientific paraphernalia to take aloft. This paraphernalia included vacuum flasks that were prepared by Cavendish for collecting upper air samples. In addition to the quality of the air, Jeffries measured air currents and temperature changes during the flight. After the successful ascent, Jeffries learned of Blanchard's plans to attempt a crossing of the English channel. Determined to crew on the flight, Jeffries organized the adventure, provided the funds, and even agreed to get out of the

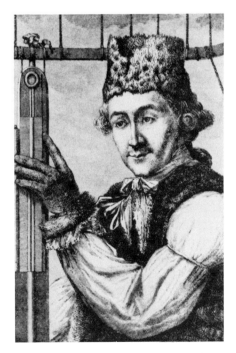

Fig. 1–6. Dr. John Jeffries, an American physician. readying for his flight across the English channel (courtesy of the National Air and Space Museum).

gondola at any point if lightening the craft became necessary. Despite numerous personality conflicts between the two men, the flight was launched on January 7, 1785. Before successfully reaching Calais, it was necessary to strip the gondola of everything movable, including all outer garments and, according to Jeffries' own estimate, some 6 lb of urine.

The First Fatality

The first 2 years of aerial flight were miraculously free of fatal accidents, but this safety record was not to be sustained. Pilatre de Rozier, one of the first men to achieve sustained flight, was to achieve notoriety with yet another first. Ignoring the advice of many, de Rozier created a hybrid balloon, combining Charles' "inflammable air" with a hot air Montgolfier design. The concept was pitifully simple—the pilot would be able to vary the lift simply by controlling the fire. The results were tragically predictable. In the summer of 1785, observers noticed de Rozier, while airborne at an altitude of 1000 m, doing something to the fire basket when a blue flame appeared, a muffled explosion occurred, and the gondola, trailing smoke and shreds of silk, plummeted to the earth. Both de Rozier and his passenger died.

American Ballooning

A 13-year-old boy by the name of Edward Warren made the first balloon ascent in the United States on June 24, 1784. Mr. Peter Carnes had constructed the balloon in Baltimore, Maryland. The youth was playing around, apparently in the basket, when the balloon became untethered and began an unplanned ascent. A month later, Mr. Carnes attempted an ascent in Philadelphia from the Walnut Street prison yard. The balloon rose 3 m, struck the prison wall severely, and knocked Carnes from the basket. The flight ended spectacularly as the lightened balloon shot skyward and caught on fire.

BENJAMIN RUSH. The Frenchman Jean-Pierre François Blanchard, the greatest balloonist of the time, having completed 44 ascents in Europe, arrived in the United States to make his forty-fifth ascent. Being an entrepreneur and exhibitionist, Blanchard advertised his plans widely in Philadelphia, attempting to raise sufficient funds to cover the cost. The Walnut Street prison yard was again designated the launch site, and the date was set for January 9, 1793. Dr. Benjamin Rush made the acquaintance of Blanchard and was on hand for the flight. Dr. Rush reported: "I went to Mr. Blanchard and requested him to examine the state of his pulse in his aerial voyage which he was to undertake the next day. He promised to do so and accepted the use of my pulse glass for that purpose." Blanchard himself noted in his journal of the event: "I passed on the observation which Dr. Rush had requested me to make upon the pulsation of the artery when I should be arrived at my greatest height. I found it impossible to make use of the quarter minute glass which he had provided for that purpose, but I supplied its place by an excellent second watch; and the result of my observations gave me 92 pulsations in the minute, the average of four observations made at the place of my highest elevation, whereas, on the ground, I had experienced no more than 84 in the same given time." This marked the first recorded contribution made in America to that branch of science that was to become known as aerospace medicine.[2]

Rush continued his inquiries of Blanchard and, upon meeting him 15 days later, inquired of discomforts he may have experienced at altitude. Blanchard related that at an altitude of 9 km blood came into his mouth and that he experienced great thirst and sleepiness from the lightness of the air. This journal entry is questionable because it is extremely doubtful that Blanchard attained an altitude as high as 9 km. As balloon ascents became more frequent,

both in Europe and the United States, and the scientific knowledge gained was made known to the public, Rush incorporated this new data in his medical lectures. His manuscripts recorded comments regarding suffering from severe cold, discomfort from an enlarged chest, and reports of epistaxis and rapid pulse rates.

Physiology at Altitude

In 1804, the hazards of high altitude flight became graphically demonstrated when three Italians, Andreoli, Brasette, and Zambeccari, attained an altitude well in excess of 6000 m, received frostbite of both their hands and feet, experienced vomiting, and each man lost consciousness. While still conscious, Andreoli had difficulty in reading the barometer because as they ascended in altitude, the candle in the lantern grew dimmer and finally went out. The flight ended with the balloon's descent into the Adriatic Sea, but, fortunately, the men were rescued.

ACOSTA. Prior to the first balloon ascent, the effects of altitude on physiology were beginning to be understood. In 1590, the Jesuit father, Acosta, may have been the first to suspect that the physical distress caused by altitude was associated with the rarefaction of air. He stated, "There is no doubt that the cause of this distress and strange affliction is the wind or air current there . . . I am convinced that the element of the air is in this place so thin and so delicate that it is not proportioned to human breathing which requires extensive and more temperate air . . . ." For over 150 years, no similar ideas were reported, but, unfortunately, Acosta's observations went unheeded. It is evident from other reports that the natives of the South American Andes were well aware of particular illnesses they associated with mountain climbs and referred to these afflictions by terms such as Veta, Soroche, la Puna, or Moreo de la Cordillera. Typical of explanations for the unknown, the Indians frequently attributed these illnesses to evil spirits.

GLAISHER AND COXWELL. The first detailed attempt to describe altered physiology at altitude was accomplished by two Englishmen, Glaisher and Coxwell, on their ascent to 9450 m (Fig. 1–7). The diary recording their flight in 1862 reports that at 5640 m their pulses had quickened to 100 beats/min. At 5850 m, breathing was affected, and palpitations were experienced. Their hands and lips had turned bluish, and they were having difficulty in reading the onboard instruments. At 6510 m, Glaisher experienced seasickness, although there was no rolling or pitching motion to the balloon. At 8700 m, the men experienced extreme muscle fatigue. Glaisher wrote, "I seem to have no limbs." And then he fell back, insensible for 7 minutes. Coxwell was likewise weak and

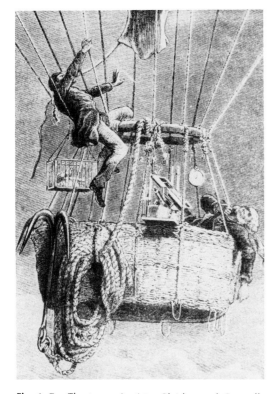

Fig. 1–7. The two scientists, Glaisher and Coxwell, nearly unconscious at 8833 m as Coxwell seizes the valve cord with his teeth (courtesy of the United States Air Force School of Aerospace Medicine).

had little control of his arms or hands because of the extreme cold; however, realizing the enormity of their predicament, he was able to raise his head sufficiently to grab the valve cord with his teeth, releasing hydrogen. The ascent of the balloon ceased. Glaisher made significant contributions to the science of meteorology and was one of the founders of the Royal Aeronautical Society.

PAUL BERT. The experiences and reports of Glaisher and Coxwell served as a strong stimulus to the physiologist-physician, Paul Bert. He would be identified by many in the years to come as the "Father of Aviation Medicine" and by all as the father of altitude physiology.[3] Bert, a Frenchman, received his Doctor of Medicine degree in 1864. He continued his education and was awarded a Doctor of Natural Sciences degree in 1866, followed by an appointment as professor of zoology at the University of Bordeaux. In many respects, Bert was a reincarnation of the universal man of the Renaissance. He was not only a physician but a naturalist, a zoologist, an anatomist, and, perhaps most importantly, a physiologist. His classic treatise, which was a major contribution to the field of physiology, was entitled *Barometric Pressure— Researches in Experimental Physiology.* The book consisted of both an historical review of earlier work in the field and Bert's own experiments. The contents included chapters concerning the effects of decreased and increased pressure on blood gases and the effect of changes in barometric pressure on a variety of biologic specimens. One of his important conclusions was that, regardless of the barometric pressure, air cannot support life when the partial pressure of oxygen reaches a certain low level. Based on experimentation, that level was determined to be 45 mm Hg. His significant conclusions influencing the field of aerospace medicine included the observations that "the diminution of barometric pressure acts upon the living being only by lowering the oxygen tension in the air, in the breath, and in the blood which supplies their tissues . . . . ". "The increase in barometric pressure acts only by increasing oxygen tension in the air and blood . . . "; and that "Sudden decompression beginning with several atmospheres has an effect . . . only by allowing to return to a free state the nitrogen which had become dissolved in the blood and the tissues under the influence of this pressure."

It is clear from the review of his experiments that Paul Bert was the first to elucidate the causes of altitude sickness, oxygen poisoning, and the bends.

ALTITUDE CHAMBER. In his review of Paul Bert's contributions to aviation medicine, Dr. Fred Hitchock[4]" identifies Bert as the first practicing flight surgeon. Two of Bert's friends who were aeronauts, Croce-Spinelli and Sivel, were anxious to pursue and, if possible, exceed the altitude record established by Glaisher and Coxwell in 1862. Bert had constructed a chamber that would reproduce the barometric pressure of altitude (Fig. 1-8). He used this chamber in a number of experiments and was to employ it for the first time as a physiologic training chamber. In this decompression or altitude chamber, he demonstrated to Croce-Spinelli and Sivel the effects of decreased oxygen partial pressure and the beneficial effects of breathing oxygen at altitude. This instruction convinced the two aeronauts of the value and importance of oxygen, and they carried this life-giving gas with them on future flights.

In March, 1874, Croce-Spinelli and Sivel carried supplemental oxygen with them on their high-altitude flight. They discovered, however, that Bert's chamber did not reproduce all the effects of altitude; the temperature at altitude was much lower than that in the chamber, far more physical activity was required on the flight than was needed in the chamber, and the exposure to altitude was longer than the chamber training session. Never-

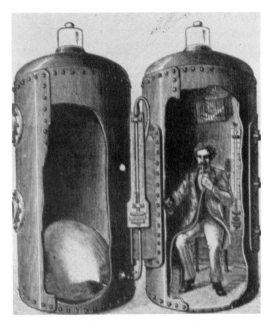

Fig. 1–8. The physician Paul Bert breathing oxygen-enriched air in his altitude chamber, (1878) (courtesy of the United States Air Force School of Aerospace Medicine).

theless, the successful use of oxygen encouraged these two adventurers to attempt a flight to an even greater altitude.

FATALITIES AT ALTITUDE. On their next flight, Croce-Spinelli and Sivel were joined by the scientist, Gaston Tissandier. The balloon was equipped with three gas bags containing 72% oxygen, the total amount available for the three men equaling 440 L. A letter was written to Bert outlining the preparations for this high-altitude flight. Bert immediately responded, warning that the supply of oxygen was entirely inadequate for the flight as planned. Not anticipating the consequences of their decision, the aeronauts chose to make the flight in any case, waiting until the absolute last moment before using their vital and short supply of oxygen. The flight was launched on April 15, 1875, and when the balloon was recovered, only one of the three men had survived. Both Croce-Spinelli and Sivel died of hypoxia. Tissandier, upon his recovery, wrote a classic description of the physiologic effects of hypoxia and is quoted in Bert's text.[5] Although many aeronauts had died in descent, these two men were the first to succumb while ascending.

The frailty of man was only second to the frailty of the large, flimsy gas-filled spheres that carried him aloft. These lighter-than-air balloons were shortly to be supplemented by the frail, unstable, heavier-than-air machines that aeronautic science and engineering were about to produce.

Machines

The historic event that occurred at Kill Devil Hill 4 miles south of Kitty Hawk, North Carolina, at 10:35 a.m. on December 17, 1903 was only a spike on an endless graph of events.

Models and Gliders

Early in the nineteenth century, George Cayley was conducting research and publishing his works while laying the foundation for modern aerodynamics. In 1809, he wrote regarding the principle of powered flight: " . . . make a surface support a given weight by the application of power to the resistance of air." His designs included a wing set at a slight dihedral, a fuselage, a tail assembly, including vertical and horizontal stabilizers, and a power source that he recognized was not then technologically available. Cayley did build monoplane and triplane gliders. It is reported that in 1849, a small 10-year-old boy was lifted off the ground and flew for several yards downhill on one such glider.

Another Englishman, Samuel Henson, further developed the work of Cayley. In 1842, he patented plans for the design for an "aerial steam carriage." The design described a monoplane with a wingspan of 50 m, a tail plane as a stabilizer, a vertical rudder, and tricycle landing gear. Power was to be provided by two steam-driven pusher propellers. The design was never converted to reality.

A colleague, Stringfellow, following a Henson design, constructed a small flying monoplane model that used a miniature steam engine. Throughout the mid-nineteenth century, numerous powered models were constructed, and several of these models are reported to have raised themselves unaided from the ground, thus achieving flight.

Two events are worth noting. The first event occurred around 1874 when a full-scale flying machine with a tractor propeller driven by a hot air engine, designed and built by DuTemple, may have departed the ground from an incline ramp under full power while carrying a young man onboard. The second event occurred in Russia in 1884. A steam-driven airplane, built by Mozhaiski, was launched down a long incline ramp and may have attained flight. Neither of these claims, however, are considered to represent sustained self-powered flight.

Toward the end of the nineteenth century, many names were associated with heavier-than-air machine flight and include engineers, scientists, inventors, and wealthy adventurers. Among this group were Sir Hiram Maxim, Clement Ader, Louis-Pierre Mouillard, and Otto Lilienthal.

OTTO LILIENTHAL. Otto Lilienthal was the nineteeth century's major contributor to the art of gliding and directly influenced Wilbur and Orville Wright. Lilienthal's enthusiasm for gliding was motivated by two factors: first, his desire to discover, to design, and to build, and second, his need to master the art of flying so that he was prepared when adequate propulsion technology became available.

Many of Lilienthal's gliders were monoplanes in which the pilot was supported in a system that resembled the trapeze system used on today's hang gliders (Figs. 1–9 and 1–10). Flight control was thus achieved by shifting the body's weight forward or back and side to side. Beginning in 1891 and continuing for 5 years, Lilienthal made over 2000 glides, occasionally

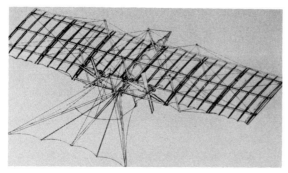

Fig. 1–9. An early engineering drawing of a cambered wing flying machine conceived in 1842 (courtesy of the National Air and Space Museum).

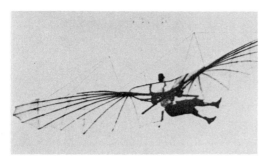

Fig. 1–10. Otto Lilienthal flying his Type 2 monoplane hang glider in Germany in 1894 (courtesy of Wright State University).

achieving flight distances in excess of several hundred feet. While testing a glider, the craft stalled and crashed to earth, and Lilienthal received injuries from which he succumbed the following day. Lilienthal was one of many who lost their lives while pursuing flight. During this period, little consideration was given to body or head protection or to any form of restraint system. The exhilaration experienced by these adventurers risking so much can, in part, be appreciated by reading the following report from Lilienthal: "I often reach positions in the air which are much higher than my starting point. At the climax of such a line of flight, I sometimes come to a standstill for some time, so that I am enabled whilst floating to speak with the gentlemen who wish to photograph me regarding the best position for the photographee."

Samuel Pierpont Langley. Samuel Pierpont Langley was simply unlucky. For over a decade, extending into the twentieth century, Langley pursued aviation with a passion. He convinced the United States War Department of the military potential of a controllable, power-driven airplane. He received from Congress a grant of $50,000 to fund his pursuit of the concept. He constructed his "aerodrome," a monoplane with two main wings in tandem, a horizontal stabilizer, and a vertical fin, which was powered by a relatively lightweight, radial, gasoline engine capable of 53 hp.

Two launches of this aircraft were conducted from a catapult mounted aboard a houseboat floating in the Potomac River. On October 7, 1903 and again on December 8, 1903, launchings were attempted, but in each case, the catapult apparently fouled and the aircraft crashed into the river. Only 9 days later, those two mechanics from Ohio, the Wright brothers, would cross the threshold of self-powered, sustained, heavier-than-air flight.

Powered Flight

The Wrights. The two Dayton, Ohio, bicycle manufacturers, Wilbur and Orville Wright, had been fascinated by Lilienthal's gliding experiences (Fig. 1–11). They were also well aware of Langley's interest in powered flight using steam-driven models. Their appetites whetted, the Wrights used some of their business capital to finance their growing interest in aviation.

From the beginning, the Wrights identified three central problems for controlled power flight: the importance of the wing shape in producing lift, three-dimensional dynamic control in the air, and the application of adequate power to drive wind over the wing.

Two major contributions to aeronautics were engineered by the Wrights.[6] The first, and most important, resulting in a patent, was "wing warping," as used by large birds

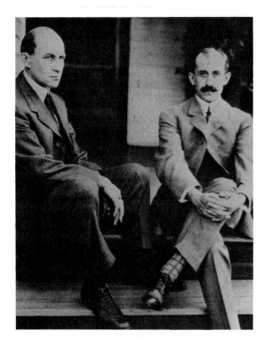

Fig. 1–11. Wilbur and Orville Wright on the back porch of their home in Dayton, Ohio (courtesy of Wright State University).

to maintain direction and stability while soaring. The technique was first proven in the glider the Wrights developed and ultimately applied to the airplane. After reviewing the work of Maxim and Langley and other aeronautic pioneers, the Wrights abandoned the concept of "automatic equilibrium," where the aircraft seeks straight and level flight, for an intentionally unstable but more flyable aircraft in which the aviator had to control direction. The Wright brothers' second major contribution was a single control system that simultaneously warped the wings and interconnected the rudder controls, thus automatically counteracting the drag produced by the downwarped wing.

Realizing the need for strong, steady, and predictable winds for their gliding test, the Wrights requested information from the National Weather Bureau. They were advised to try the beaches of North Carolina, where winds from the sea were strong and steady and the open space for

gliding was plentiful. In October, 1900, they made the first of their periodic pilgrimages to Kitty Hawk, North Carolina (Fig. 1–12).

Through trial and error, ingenuity and engineering, persistence and daring, these two brothers solved the aeronautic riddle of directional stability and control in the air. One major problem remained—the power plant. A simple 12 hp, water-cooled, gasoline engine was developed to drive two counter-rotating propellers. After an initial unsuccessful trial, the stage was set, the photographer that was so important for documenting this historic event was in place, and at 10:35 a.m. on December 17, 1903, man lifted into the air and for 12 seconds was airborne over a distance of 40 m. Three more flights were conducted that morning, the final one lasting nearly 1 minute. The legends, fantasies, and dreams of man were realized as he attained sustained, controlled, powered flight.

By the time man had experienced powered flight, he had already been exposed to low temperatures, hypoxia, pressure changes, motion sickness, crash injuries, and death. Powered flight would further broaden the horizons and increase the hazards of the aeronautic environment.

Within a decade of that flight at Kitty

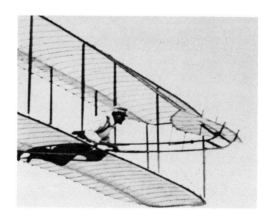

Fig. 1–12. Wilbur Wright flying a sophisticated biwing glider during early trials at Kitty Hawk, North Carolina in October, 1902 (Library of Congress).

Hawk, every industrial nation in the world had witnessed powered flight within its own boundaries. By 1918, thousands of flying machines would be swarming over the continent of Europe, engaged in the "great war."

AVIATION MEDICINE—THE FLEDGLING

Frequently, tragedy begets solution. During a demonstration of one of the Wright flying machines, Lieutenant Thomas Selfridge of the United States Army became the first fatal airplane accident victim. The lieutenant suffered massive and fatal head injuries. The subsequent investigation, which included input from the United States Army medical corps, recommended that head protection be developed and worn by aviators. The recommendation was not documented in the medical literature but rather was limited to the proceedings of the accident board.

One year earlier, in 1907, the first series of papers to deal with the physiologic factors associated with the airplane were published. The papers were written in France and addressed the subject of airsickness. Armstrong,[7] in his review of the world medical literature in the early twentieth century, cites a total of 32 medical publications devoted to some aspect of aviation medicine prior to the onset of World War I.

Medical Standards

As early as 1910, countries in Europe were considering the medical ramifications of aviation. Minimum medical standards were developed for military pilots in Germany. In Great Britain, with the formation of the Naval and Military wings of the Royal Flying Corps in 1912, two service medical officers were appointed. Both learned to fly and provided the rudiments of aviation medicine support to their units. The United States War Department published its first instructions on the physical examination of candidates for aviation duty in February, 1912. Several months later the United States Navy issued similar instructions.

The War Department's initial instructions provided that:

1. All candidates for aviation duty shall be subjected to a rigorous physical examination to determine their fitness for such duty.
2. The visual acuity without glasses should be normal. Any error of refraction requiring correction by glasses or any other cause diminishing acuity of vision below normal will be a cause for rejection. The candidates' ability to estimate distances should be tested. Color blindness for red, green, or violet is a cause for rejection.
3. The acuity of hearing should be carefully tested and the ears carefully examined with the aid of the speculum and mirror. Any diminution of the acuity of hearing below normal will be a cause for rejection. Any disease of the middle ear, either acute or chronic, or any sclerosed condition of the eardrum resulting from a former acute condition will be a cause for rejection. Any disease of the internal ear or of the auditory nerve will be a cause for rejection. The following tests for equilibrium to detect otherwise obscure diseased conditions of the internal ear should be made:
   a. Have the candidate stand with knees, heels, and toes touching.
   b. Have the candidate walk forward, backward, and in a circle.
   c. Have the candidate hop around the room.
   These tests should be made first with the eyes open and then closed, on both feet and then on one foot, and hopping forward and backward, the candidate trying to hop or walk in a straight line. Any deviation to the

right or left from the straight line or from the arc of the circle should be noted. Any persistent deviation, either to the right or left, is evidence of a diseased condition of the internal ear, and nystagmus is also frequently associated with such condition. These symptoms, therefore, should be regarded as cause for rejection.

4. The organs of respiration and the circulatory system should be carefully examined. Any diseased condition of the circulatory system, either of the heart or the arterial system, is a cause for rejection. Any disease of the nervous system is a cause for rejection.

5. The precision of the movements of the limbs should be especially carefully tested, following the order outlined in paragraph 17, General Order, 60, War Department, 1909.

6. Any candidate whose history may show that he is afflicted with chronic digestive disturbances, chronic constipation or indigestion, or intestinal disorders tending to produce dizziness, headache, or to impair his vision should be rejected.[7]

Rapidly expanding technology in the field of aeronautics was increasing the speed, altitude, performance, and complexity of the flying machine. Consequently, the demands on the aviator were likewise increasing. Although the aircraft's potential in a variety of commercial service and military roles was identified, this infant of heavier-than-air flight had yet to mature.

Aeronautics first received strong governmental support because of its potential military role. An Italian reconnaissance flight during the Tripolitan War in 1911 marked the first military use of the airplane. Bulgarian aviators hand-dropped small bombs over Turkish-held Adrianople during the first Balkan War of 1912 (Fig. 1–13). Prior to the outbreak of World

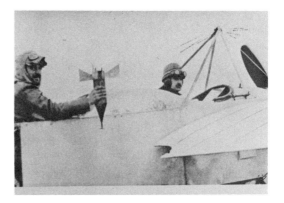

Fig. 1–13. Hand-dropped bombs used in the first Balkan War in 1912 (courtesy of the United States Air Force National Archives).

War I, Germany possessed 1200 combat aircraft, as compared with the 1000 flown by France and Britain—no small number.

The first year following the onset of hostilities, Great Britain reviewed its casualty list. Out of every 100 flyers killed, two had met their death at the hands of the enemy, eight from some defect in the airplane, and 90 deaths were ascribed to individual deficiencies, including physical defects, recklessness, and carelessness. In further refinement, it became clear that 60% of the aviation casualties were due to physical defects of the aviators. This resulted in the strongest impetus to date for the establishment of aviation medicine, and the British developed a special service for the care of the flyer. The results of this initial aviation medicine program were spectacular. Deaths due to physical defects were reduced by the end of the second year from 60% to 20%, and were down to 12% by the third year. In 1916, the Royal Flying Corps established a special medical board for the dual purpose of the medical selection of flying officers and "invalidating and disposing of those injured or broken down."

In 1914, the head of the aviation section of the United States Signal Corps requested advice of the United States Army Surgeon General as to how to determine fitness for flight. The Surgeon General's office responded promptly and prepared requirements for the examination and standards to be met by the candidates. Within a few months, the Surgeon General was requested to lower his standards because they were so high no applicant was able to pass the examination and, therefore, the aviation section was unable to obtain personnel. Standards were lowered, and Major Theodore Lyster, the father of American military aviation medicine, established physical examination units and developed realistic medical selection standards.

Rumors and gossip about the tough physical examinations were rampant. There was the so-called "needle test," during which the blindfolded applicant held a needle between his thumb and forefinger and a pistol was fired unexpectedly behind him. If the candidate was so startled by the sudden noise that he drew blood by puncturing his finger with the needle, he was disqualified because of excessive excitability. The rumors told of another test in which the applicant was hit over the head by a mallet when he least expected it. If he were coherent within the first 15 seconds after being struck, he was considered sufficiently resistant to concussion to make a good candidate. The French actually developed a test for nervous shock. They measured the changes in respiration, heart rate, and vasomotor response of a candidate when a revolver was fired near his ear.

Eventually, 67 examination centers were established in the larger cities of America. Approximately 100,000 applicants for the air service were examined. Of the cadet applicants examined, approximately 30% were disqualified for medical reasons. Table 1–1 lists the causes for those rejections.[7] Then, as now, one of the major causes for medical rejection was related to vision. Defects of vision accounted for 20% of all rejections and were frequently among the multiple defects.

Table 1–1. The Causes For Medical Rejection For All Men Who Applied as Cadet Flyers During World War I

Reason for Rejection	Percent
Disqualified on three or more tests	29
Disqualified on two tests	24
Eye	20
Equilibrium	7
Other and general subnormalities	7
Vascular system	5
Ear	4
Nose and throat	3
Urinalysis	1
Total	100

The physical standards established for aviators by Lyster and his co-workers were based on empiric grounds, and they felt the question needed further study. Following the lead of the British, an aviation medical research board was established by the United States Army. The responsibilities of this board were:

1. To investigate all conditions that affect the efficiency of pilots.
2. To institute and carry out such experiments and tests as will determine the ability of pilots to fly at high altitudes.
3. To carry out experiments and tests to provide suitable apparatus for the supply of oxygen to pilots at high altitudes.
4. To act as a standing medical board for the consideration of all matters relating to the physical fitness of pilots.

For every medical standard established, there was the anecdote of the successful hero who would not have been fit enough to pass the standard. Britain's greatest ace, Edward Mannock, had severe astigmatism and was essentially blind in one eye. Guynemer, a French ace, had pulmonary tuberculosis. The German ace, Oswald Boelcke, had periodic attacks of severe asthma. William Thaw, of "Escadrille Lafayette" fame, had good vision in only one eye. Frank Luke, the American ace, would have failed a psychiatric examination due to his moodiness and antisocial behavior. A Canadian aviator, Leeche, was a successful combat pilot despite the inconvenience of a wooden leg. In a crash that he survived, his wooden leg was broken, and he had to bear the expenses of repair himself. Nevertheless, the accident rates did improve, in large measure due to the selection of more medically qualified aviators.

The Flight Surgeon

Parallel to the establishment of the medical research board, an American medical mission to Europe revealed that the American aviator was not receiving appropriate medical support. Flying accident rates were high. Fatalities from crashes were three times the deaths due to enemy action. Accidents were occurring at the rate of one for every 241 flying hours, and a

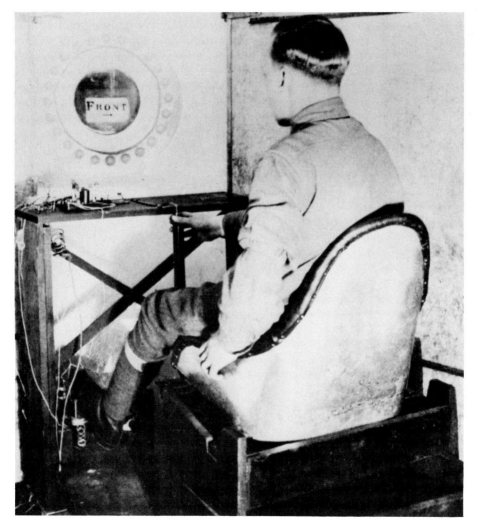

Fig. 1–14. The low-pressure chamber at the School of Aviation Medicine being used for psychologic testing at altitude in 1918 (official United States Air Force photograph).

death occurred for every 721 flight hours. Medical conditions caused or complicated by flying were not recognized or understood by the assigned medical officers. This was understandable because none of the medical officers had experience or training in aviation medicine. To add insult to injury, an aviator could not see a medical officer without the permission of his commanding officer. When these reports reached Lyster, who had by now become the first Chief Surgeon of the Aviation Section of the Signal Corps of the United States Army, he immediately undertook plans for medical officers to become trained in aviation medicine. Until a school for flight surgeons could be created, manpower was dispatched from the Air Service Medical Research Laboratory (Fig. 1–14). Among those in this cadre was Major Robert Ray Hampton who, on September 17, 1918, became the first practicing flight surgeon to the American expeditionary force.

Flight Medical Training

The informal but effective training of flight surgeons commenced immediately, and these physicians were assigned to flying fields in both the United States and Europe. By the end of the war, a complete

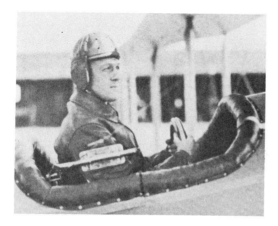

Fig. 1–15. Army flyer Benjamin Foulois wearing his own football helmet for head protection (courtesy of the United States Air Force National Archives).

medical service for the aviation arm of the United States Army was organized and functioning. This service provided for the medical selection of the aviator, for his classification, and, once on flight duty, for his health maintenance, all of which led to the formation of the new medical specialty in aviation medicine.

Simultaneously, in both the United States and Europe, operational flight medicine was being practiced and research, development, and testing conducted. The need for assessment procedures for balance, vision, cardiovascular efficiency, psychologic aptitude, and neurologic functioning were required. Solutions were needed for the problems of cold, hypoxia, disorientation, and fear of flying. Devices were needed to restrain the pilot in crash landings, to protect his head from crash injury, to protect his eyes from windblast, and to provide oxygen and warmth (Fig. 1–15). Such were the challenges to this new field of aviation medicine.

Interwar Period

During World War I, aviation medicine as a fledgling first tried its wings. A large historical volume, *Air Service Medical*, was published in 1919 by the United States War Department. In that same year, H. Graeme Anderson of the British Royal Navy authored one of the first texts on aviation medicine, a fascinating treatise entitled *The Medical and Surgical Aspects of Aviation*. The War Department was again responsible, in 1920, for publishing *Aviation Medicine in the A.E.F.* The first Commandant of the School of Aviation Medicine, Louis H. Bauer, authored the text *Aviation Medicine* in 1926.

Following the conclusion of World War I, many military pilots continued to fly, both as an avocation and a vocation. Surplus aircraft were plentiful and relatively inexpensive, and soon every city, town, and hamlet became the site for Jennies performing acrobatics, an activity that was to become known as "barnstorming."

While the American public was becoming fascinated by aviation, the development and manufacturing of new aircraft were coming to a standstill. The impetus of the war years was no longer stimulating aeronautics, and all associated programs, including military aviation medicine, were undergoing belt tightening. The possibility of aircraft carrying passengers and mail did receive support, both from the returning military pilots and from the commercial sector.

Civil Aviation Medicine

President Calvin Coolidge signed the Air Commerce Act on May 20, 1926, assigning federal responsibilities in civil aviation to the United States Department of Commerce. One of the draft proposals circulated for review that same year included a requirement for physical examinations as part of the pilot licensing procedure. It is interesting to note that up to that time no physical standards existed.

In the fall of that year, the United States Department of Commerce, recognizing the need for an expert in the field of aviation medicine, requested the Army to release Dr. Lewis Bauer so that he might serve in the civil aviation arena. He immediately set about the task of developing the first physical standards for civilian pilots and establishing a medical examination system for the United States. The physical standards were promulgated one year later in air commerce regulations, and in 1927, Dr. Bauer contacted 60 physicians, later appointing 57 as aviation medical examiners (AMEs). In addition to the AMEs, Army and Navy flight surgeons were authorized to perform civil aircrew examinations, as were several United States Public Health Service hospitals. By the third decade, over 800 AMEs had been appointed, both in the United States and overseas.

CIVIL PHYSICAL STANDARDS. Dr. Bauer proposed physical standards for three categories of pilots.

Private Pilots. The physical requirements were the absence of organic disease or defect that would interfere with the safe handling of an airplane under the conditions of private flying, visual acuity of at least 20/40 in each eye (less than 20/40 may be accepted if the pilot wears a corrective lens in his goggles and has normal judgment of distance without correction), good judgment of distance, no diplopia in any position, normal visual fields and color vision, and no organic disease of the eye or internal ear.

Industrial Pilots. The physical requirements were the absence of any organic disease or defect that would interfere with the safe handling of an airplane, visual acuity of not less than 20/30 in each eye, although in certain incidences, less than 20/30 may be accepted if the applicant wears corrective lens to 20/20 in his goggles and has good judgment of distance without correction, good judgment of distance, no diplopia in any field, normal visual fields and color vision, and no organic disease of the eye, ear, nose, or throat.

Transport Pilots. The physical requirements were a good past history, sound pulmonary, cardiovascular, gastrointestinal, central nervous, and genitourinary systems, freedom from material structural defects or limitations, freedom from disease of the ductless glands, normal central, peripheral, and color vision, normal judgment of distance, only slight defects of ocular muscle balance, freedom from ocular disease, absence of obstructive or diseased conditions of the ear, nose, and throat, and no abnormalities of equilibrium that would interfere with flying.

Medical certification rapidly grew. In 1928, the first year, 11,688 applications were processed. By 1930, nearly 44,000 certifications had been issued.

The training of designated civil aviation medical examiners was a key part of the original plan developed by Dr. Bauer. In 1930, 12 conferences were conducted for training AMEs. In addition, Dr. Bauer requested the appointment of district or regional flight surgeons to instruct and oversee the work being performed by AMEs. This did not occur until 1931, when the first district flight surgeon was assigned to Kansas City, Missouri.

Military Aviation Medicine

Throughout this interwar period, the military continued the development of newer, high-performance aircraft. Every year, records in altitude, speed, performance, endurance, and reliability were being established. Man was beginning to experience accelerated forces, or "G" forces, which were interfering dangerously with cerebral circulation. Balloon flights were reaching into the stratosphere, requiring a gondola with a sealed, pressure- and temperature-controlled environment. Aircraft were reaching altitudes where the availability of even 100% oxygen was inadequate to prevent hypoxia. Special masks were developed that were connected to a compressor system which would force oxygen into the pilot's lungs, introducing and proving the concept of positive pressure breathing. Man had reached the limit where he could safely be exposed to the elements in an open cockpit, and aircraft designers were forced to consider an enclosed cabin or cockpit for the aviator.

AEROMEDICAL RESEARCH AND DEVELOPMENT. Throughout these years, the School of Aviation Medicine continued to train military flight surgeons and served as a focal point for research regarding the selection and maintenance of aircrews. In 1934, the Aeromedical Research Laboratory was founded at Wright Field in Dayton, Ohio. The charter for this laboratory was to study the effects of flight on man and to develop methods for eliminating or neutralizing the adverse effects that would prove detrimental to mission efficiency in military aviation. Dr. Harry G. Armstrong, the laboratory's first commander, in one of his numerous technical reports, stated:

"It is concluded that sealed aircraft compartments offer the best solution for the protection of flying personnel at high altitude, and the only practical method of flight above 40,000 feet. It is recommended that projects be initiated to study, collect data, and develop aircraft incorporating the principles of pressure, oxygen, and oxygen pressure compartments." Dr. Armstrong has received credit for significant research and technology that eventually led to the pressure cabin that is so vital to both commercial and military aviation today.

On November 20, 1939, the United States Navy established its School of Aviation Medicine and Research at Pensacola, Florida. This school continues to be the premier institution conducting biomedical research in aviation medicine for the Navy.

Since World War I, the center for aviation medicine, both in education and research, for the Royal Air Force in Great Britain has been at Farnborough. This organization has supported military development, as well as satisfying British Air Ministry needs.

With the approach of the end of the fourth decade, only 35 years after the first flight at Kitty Hawk, a war was to begin in which aviation would prove decisive. Aeronautic engineering would respond with an exponential growth in technology. Larger, higher-performance aircraft, jet engines, rocket propulsion, and advances in communication and avionics would all culminate in the modern world of aerospace technology. As the handmaiden to this technology, aviation medicine would expand and change, as it made the transition to aerospace medicine in the modern era.

REFERENCES

1. Rolt, L.T.C.: The Aeronauts. New York, Walker and Company, 1966.
2. Carlson, E.T., and Heveran, B.T.: Benjamin Rush and the birth of American aviation medicine. Aerospace Med., 45:1083, 1974.

3. Engle, E., and Lott, A.: Man in Flight. Annapolis, Maryland, Leeward Publications, Inc., 1970.
4. Hitchcock, F.A.: Paul Bert and the beginnings of aviation medicine. Aerospace Med., 42:1101, 1971.
5. Gillies, J.A.: A Textbook of Aviation Physiology. London, Pergamon Press, 1965.

6. Combs, H.: Kill Devil Hill. Boston, Houghton Mifflin Co., 1979.
7. Armstrong, H.G.: Principles and Practice of Aviation Medicine. 3rd Ed. Baltimore, Williams & Wilkins Co., 1952.

Chapter 2

The Modern Perspective

Roy L. DeHart

Invention breeds invention.

RALPH WALDO EMERSON

With the advent of aviation, new professions developed, established professions evolved, and technology accelerated the demise of still other professions. The turn of the twentieth century saw the dawning of modern medicine and the birth of aerospace medicine.

The birth pains had occurred when man first was borne aloft under globes of hot air or flammable gas. Labor ensued with the onset of World War I and the need to reduce the carnage of thousands of young men who were enthusiastic but unfit to become military aviators. A product of that delivery was the flight surgeon, a title still given with pride to those physicians directly supporting our military flyers.

In the years following World War I, the medical requirements of the aviation industry caused an evolution in a small segment of the profession of medicine, led by those fledgling flight surgeons. In additon to the military practice of aviation medicine, other physicians entered the federal service or joined the expanding airlines. An association was formed and a journal established.

The technologic developments of World War II forced new efforts in aeromedical-technologic research, and the enormous increase in the numbers of aircrew resulted in a concomitant increase in physicians becoming involved in aviation medicine. Following that war, technologic advances were applied to the civil sector, resulting in an expediential growth of airline passenger miles flown.

Special training, a new vocabulary, and the peculiar trappings of the trade all gave legitimacy to the establishment of aviation medicine as a medical specialty. The evolutionary process, however, was not yet complete because technology and man were not to be limited to operations in an ocean of air. By the 1960s, it became clear that man was on his way into space and that medical support would be required to get him there. Within 10 years of the establishment of the specialty of aviation medicine, it was necessary for the science to further evolve into aerospace medicine—a specialty that extends literally "out of this world."

THE PRACTICE OF AEROSPACE MEDICINE

Classically, medicine has been concerned with the care and cure of the patient experiencing disease in his usual surroundings. Disease in this context can be considered the demonstration of disrupted or abnormal physiologic processes. The patient is considered in the environment of the home or hospital. Thus, the patient is seen as experiencing abnormal physiologic processes in a normal, terrestrial environment.

An approach to understanding the art and science of aerospace medicine is to contrast it with this classic approach to medicine. Aerospace medicine most often deals with healthy individuals; in fact, the medical selection process for aviators presupposes health. The more difficult or responsible the aviator's duty, the greater the requirement that he be free from demonstrable disease. This requirement is exemplified by the stringent health examinations given some special-mission military aircrews and, of course, the astronauts. A situation is attained where individuals selected for some aviation and space operations are not simply healthy in the general sense but, perhaps better stated, are superhealthy. Although the classic patient is comfortable in the predictable terrestrial environment, the aviator must contend with an entirely different, demanding, dynamic, and, at times, totally hostile environment.

In the practice of aerospace medicine, we may deal with the normal physiology in an abnormal environment. This reality forces a fundamental change in the physician's approach to his responsibilities toward his patient, the aviator. Health maintenance with minimal therapeutic intervention becomes the sine qua non for the practitioner of aerospace medicine. The specialist will himself often be required to assist the aviator in competing successfully in the abnormal environment of aviation. This assistance may range from simple tasks such as demonstrating how to ventilate and equilibrate the air pressure of the middle ear or sinus, demonstrating methods to improve tolerance to acceleration (G), and the management of potential airsickness to more complex tasks such as involvement in research to extend man's performance in this stressful environment. Thus, in classical medicine, one deals with abnormal physiology in a normal environment, whereas in aerospace medicine, one is concerned with normal physiology in an abnormal, or flight, environment.

In its fullest context, the practice of aerospace medicine is multidisciplinary, extending into the fields of basic science: physics, chemistry, mathematics; and the engineering disciplines: aeronautic, mechanical, electrical. Many of the health care specialties also have contributions to make in assisting the flight surgeon or aeromedical practitioner with his responsibilities in aerospace medicine.

Aviation Medicine

As was discussed in Chapter 1, aircrew medical standards were developed in a dynamic process during World War I. The concept that anyone can fly was altered so that only the most perfect human specimens were allowed to fly, then altered again to reflect the physical and psychologic health necessary to successfully meet the realistic, rather than ideal, requirements for functioning in the flight environment. Today, a flying physical examination remains one of the requirements for acquiring a pilot's license, for entering military aviation, or for fulfilling most aircrew duties aboard an aircraft.

In reflecting on those early days, Dr. H. G. Anderson, a medical officer in the Royal Air Force, described some of the factors considered with the physical requirements:

In selecting candidates for the Air Service, what is looked for is the sound constitution, free from organic disease, and a fairly strong physique in order to withstand altitude effects, such as cold, fatigue, and diminished oxygen. It is essential there should be normal hearing and good muscle and equilibration sense. As the aviator is so dependent on his eyesight, too much importance cannot be attached to this part of the examination. But next to vision, and most important of all in obtaining the best aviator, is the question of temperament. Undoubtedly, there is a particular temperament or aptitude for flying, and its distribution is peculiarly interesting, whether looked upon from its racial aspect and ethnological origin or in relation to previous health, life and habits. Unfortunately, this temperament is a difficult matter to estimate clinically, and especially so in the examining room. The ideal aviator must have good judgment, be courageous, and not upset by fear, although conscious of the perils of his work. He must be cool in emergencies, able to make careful and quick decisions and act accordingly. His reaction-times must never be delayed—he must be ever alert, as mental sluggishness in flying spells disaster.... With regard to relation of habits in this special aptitude for flying, the latter is found most commonly among those used to playing games and leading an outdoor life. The yachtsman and the horseman, with their finer sense of judgment and "lighter hands," should make the most skillful pilots.... Every now and then one meets the type with splendid physique and apparently unshakable courage and finds that he learns to fly indifferently or is unable to learn at all, and again one meets the weedy, pale type learning quickly to fly and turning out to be a first-rate pilot.[1]

Once the need for aircrew selection was firmly established, the next task became one of health maintenance. In World War I, each nation with an aviation arm independently learned of the requirements for aircrew health maintenance. Those early aviators were unable to perform and survive if suffering from minor illness, excessively fatigued, treated with medication, or under the influence of alcohol. The combat surgeon did not understand the unforgiving environment in which the aviator frequently found himself. It became necessary to train special physicians to care for the flyer and to give emphasis to the aircrew's health care maintenance. Today, the concept of the squadron flight surgeon is a principal tenet in military aerospace medicine. This concept is further represented in the Federal Aviation

Administration's (FAA) health program for air traffic controllers, in the National Aeronautics and Space Administration (NASA), and among many airlines who provide aviation medicine practitioners for the care of the cockpit and cabin crews.

As World War I continued, aircrews became ill or were injured in accidents or combat, thus creating a new question to be answered: when should a disqualified aviator be returned to aircrew duty? Today, this question poses some of the greatest challenges to the specialist. Should an individual be returned to flying following a severe head trauma, following a mild coronary infarction, following a coronary bypass, or after receiving treatment for carcinoma? Should a pilot be disqualified from flying simply because of chronologic age? Pilots see the physician as a controlling element in their careers, and this perception creates the potential for an adversary relationship. The practitioner must always remain sensitive to this perception and manage it; otherwise, his effectiveness will become compromised.

At the request of the United States Department of Commerce, the United States Army permitted Dr. Lewis Bauer to resign his commission from the medical corps to become the first medical director of the newly created aeronautics branch of the Department of Commerce (Fig. 2–1). This was in November, 1926, and many of the young men who had gained their aviator's wings in World War I were involved in the new industry of commercial aviation.[2] Dr. Bauer had two immediate tasks. One was the formulation of physical standards for licensing civilian airmen and the other was to select physicians throughout the country and qualify them to perform these new examinations. From his Army Air Corps experience, Dr. Bauer was fully familiar with the military's established physical requirements, and from this source he developed an outline of standards to be applied to the nation's civil pilots. As had been the case in the military,

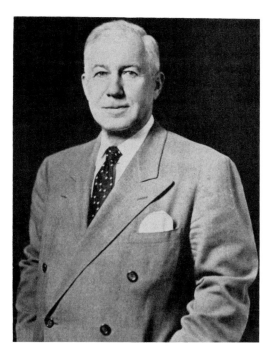

Fig. 2–1. Dr. Lewis Bauer, the founder of aviation medicine in the United States (courtesy of the Aerospace Medicine Association).

civilian physicians with impeccable credentials were not necessarily aware of the unique occupational requirements for civil flying and, thus, had little depth of understanding for the rationale embodied in the physical examination requirements. With few exceptions, these chosen physicians required further training in aviation medicine. Through these efforts, a second cadre of physicians was created that matched those in the military service.

Further maturing of the specialty of aviation medicine occurred with the extensive growth and advances of aviation during World War II. It was during this period that technology advanced from the biplane to sweptwing, from a few hundred miles an hour to supersonic flight, from the open cockpit to the pressurized cabin, and from the occasional aircraft to huge aerial armadas.

Space Medicine

The evolutionary process of space medicine began in the United States in February, 1949 when the United States Air Force School of Aviation Medicine established a department of Space Medicine.[3] This department was established under the direction of the school's commander, General Harry Armstrong. The department was interdisciplinary, with major scientific representation in the medical sciences, astronomy, engineering, and bioclimatology. Once the department of Space Medicine was organized and functioning, Dr. Hubertus Strughold was appointed Director (Fig. 2–2). To many, Dr. Strughold is recognized as the "Father of Space Medicine." The formation of this new department, so focused on the future, was anticipated by events of the previous year, when a panel was organized by the school to discuss the challenging subject, "Aeromedical Problems of Space Travel."

The dreamers and the skeptics each had their opinion and their definition of space medicine. To help bring order out of chaos, the *Journal of Aviation Medicine*, in 1950, stated in its editorial page: "Space medicine is concerned with the medical problems involved in modes of travel

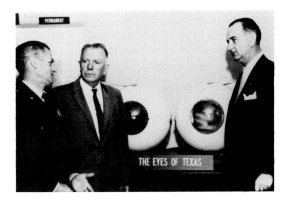

Fig. 2–2. Dr. Hubertus Strughold, the father of space medicine, second from the left with General Bensen, a pioneer in aviation and space medicine, and then Senator Lyndon Johnson in front of the "Eyes of Texas," a model used to teach flight surgeons the muscular control of the eye (official United States Air Force photo).

which are potentially capable at least of transporting us beyond the earth's gravitational field; and it is also concerned with special hazards encountered in the upper part of our atmosphere and beyond." The mood was apparently right to dream of the future, for that same year the space medicine branch of the Aviation Medicine Association was established. In 1950, Dr. Strughold presented a paper that was to become a classic, entitled "Where Does Space Begin?" which was subsequently published in 1952 as "Atmospheric Equivalence."[4] In this intellectually challenging and stimulating paper, he first proposed the now well-recognized concept that space is not a set boundary but a continuum along which, for various situations, one moves from terrestrial to celestial.

Strughold's first zone of transtion occurs at 16 km, where the pressure of the atmosphere is reduced to 87 mm Hg. At this altitude, because of water vapor and carbon dioxide offgassing, the astronaut would be unable to draw any air into the lungs, even if 100% oxygen were available. The next transition occurs at 20 km, where the atmospheric pressure drops to 47 mm Hg. Because of the astronaut's body temperature, fluids, including blood, would begin vaporizing, and the astronaut exposed to this atmosphere would experience the same desiccating process as in the farthest reaches of space. Above this altitude, the air is too rarified to be compressed effectively to support a pressurized cabin. Consequently, it is necessary to introduce the closed-cabin environment, or space cabin.

At 30 km, the astronaut moves into the ozone layer produced by the high flux of ultraviolet radiation. The space crewman is now approaching an altitude where he must be protected from the ultraviolet light itself. At 100 km, the pilot and his craft are subjected to the full impact force of meteorites. At 150 km, the astronaut witnesses the true black void of space because the atmosphere is too thin to scatter

visible light, and illumination occurs only from the direct rays of the illuminating object. Beyond 160 km, the craft reaches an orbiting altitude, and the astronaut, for the first time, experiences the weightlessness of space.

With recognition of the new frontier that was being entered, names were changing across the aeronautic world. Aerospace became a common word used in the context of aerospace industry, aerospace technology, and aerospace medicine. The Aero Medical Association became the Aerospace Medical Association, and its journal, the *Journal of Aviation Medicine*, was renamed *Aerospace Medicine*. For the time being, the transition was complete—aviation and space were integrated into aerospace. The transition from aviation to aerospace medicine was more form than function. The principles of practice are the same for both. The stressors to the crew member, whether pilot or astronaut, have many similarities, as well as occasional significant differences. The appropriately trained practitioner can function effectively in both areas.

RECENT AERONAUTIC DEVELOPMENTS

No single development or technology can describe or explain the transition that has occurred in the past several decades within the aerospace industry. As witnessed repeatedly in history, the requirements of national defense provided the needs that technology attempted to satisfy. Major developments occurred in propulsion systems, fuels, aeronautic design, structures, materials, avionics, electronics, and biotechnology.

Technology for War

In the mid- and late 1930s much was happening in the world of aviation to prepare for the war to come. The first American four-engine bomber was successfully flown in the summer of 1935 and became known in World War II as the B-17 "Flying Fortress." The aircraft could carry a full bomb load several thousand miles at an average speed of 370 kph. Without bombs, it had an altitude capability in excess of 10,000 m. Because the aircraft was unpressurized, those engaged in aviation medicine initiated major developments in oxygen systems, electrically heated thermal protective clothing, and special garments to protect against antiaircraft artillery. Although the B-17 could fly high, it in no way established an altitude record. An Italian aviator, Colonel Mario Pezzi, climbed over 18,000 m in 1938.

To support high-altitude flight, the engineers and physicians working in aviation medicine developed the novel BLB oxygen mask. The initials stood for the physicians involved with the development: Boothby, Lovelace, and Bulbulian. The mask provided a self-regulated mixture of oxygen, air exhaled from the lungs, and atmospheric air during flights to moderately high altitudes. Another hazard of high-altitude flying was pilot fatigue. Research in this area and concomitant aeromedical problems earned the coveted Collier trophy in 1940 for Boothby, Lovelace, and Armstrong. Much of this earlier research work in support of the expanding aeronautic environment was published by Armstrong in 1939 in his book, *Principles and Practices of Aviation Medicine*, which was the first inclusive text that attempted to bridge the complex and diversified engineering and medical problems encountered in modern flight of the day.

During this same period, Isaac Newton's third law of motion, "To every action there is an opposed and equal reaction," would be applied to an aeronautic propulsion system developed by Frank Whittle. In Germany, Dr. Hans von Ohain labored along similar lines to develop the engine that powered the world's first jet plane. By 1942, this technology was applied to the development of a combat-fighter aircraft, the Messerschmidt, ME-262. It was the Whittle engine, which arrived in the United States in 1941, that became the pro-

totype for America's first entry into reaction engine flight. The initial development and testing of America's first jet aircraft created a potential problem. Although test flights were flown in the Mojave Desert in California, it was still possible that some inquiring eyes might see the aircraft on the ramp while it was undergoing maintenance. The absence of a propeller might lead to some unwanted speculation. To avoid this speculation, a large balsam wood propeller was attached around a ring. The ring could be placed over the pointed nose of the airplane whenever it was outside the hangar, thus avoiding potentially embarrassing questions.

The combination of improved aeronautic structures and high-energy power plants made it possible for the airframe to withstand high acceleration, or "G." This G force acting on the pilot could exceed the compensating capacity of the cardiovascular system, rendering the pilot unconscious. A Canadian aeromedical researcher, Dr. W.M. Franks, began investigating the problems of acceleration in flight. Working at the University of Toronto, Dr. Franks developed the first operationally practical anti-G suit to be worn by pilots during combat (Fig. 2–3).

In this initial development, a fluid pressure was applied to the calves, thighs, and abdomen to prevent vascular pooling and enhance adequate return of blood to the heart. This suit successfully raised the G tolerance for the aircrew members who wore it.

With the increasing altitude capability of aircraft, there was the additional requirement for a pressure environment that was comfortable and safe for both crews and passengers. Initial work was begun at the Aeromedical Research Laboratory under the direction of its commander, Dr. Armstrong. With the use of the XC-35 in the late 1930s, the concept of a pressure cabin was proven and was later applied to passenger aircraft with the development of the Boeing 307 Stratoliner.

32 AEROSPACE MEDICINE IN PERSPECTIVE

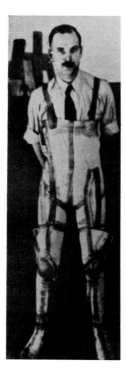

Fig. 2–3. Dr. W. M. Franks, a Canadian aeromedical researcher, in an early G protection suit of his design (courtesy of the National Air and Space Museum).

On the day the United States entered World War II, a flight surgeon made the supreme sacrifice. The first operational squadron of B-17s were being deployed to Hawaii at the time the island was under attack by the naval aircraft of the Japanese Imperial Fleet. Aboard one of the flying fortresses was the squadron's new flight surgeon, Lieutenant William R. Schick. His flight medical training had been cut short to permit him to deploy with his squadron to the Pacific. Although most of the B-17s successfully landed in Hawaii despite the ongoing Japanese attack, one plane was shot down and crashed, killing all aboard, including Dr. Schick. He was the first flight surgeon to be killed in combat and would, unfortunately, be joined by many others.

To conduct the air battles of World War II, over a million military aircraft were constructed and flown by the belligerent

forces. In the United States, tens of thousands of aircrewmen were selected to undergo aviation training. This required significant improvements in the medical selection process for aircrew personnel. Many of the techniques and examination procedures developed during the mid-1940s are still used today in the selection of military aircrew personnel. The concept of the squadron-level flight surgeon became fully ingrained into military aviation.

Postwar Aeronautic Developments

The excitement of aviation, which was so infectious during the war, spread into the postwar period. The public had lost its distrust and fear of flying. Large aircraft were now available to enter into civilian air commerce. The reliability of the Douglas DC-3 had been established, and the four-engine DC-4 had been developed, proven, and was ready to enter the civil transportation system. The Lockheed Constellation became the American flagship for a number of airlines engaged in international commerce.

In October, 1947, accompanied by his flight surgeon, Dr. John Stapp, Captain Charles Yeager was escorted to a waiting B-29, which carried under its wing the Bell X-1. On that day, Captain Yeager would be the first man in the world to accelerate past the shock wave known as the "sound barrier." To protect him from the low-pressure environment of high altitude, Yeager wore the T-1 partial-pressure suit developed by the Aeromedical Laboratory (Fig. 2–4). Thus, with each new milestone in aeronautic development, there often preceded a concomitant development in both technology and aerospace medicine.

Just as Yeager became famous as the first man to break the sound barrier, his flight surgeon, John Paul Stapp, became known as "the fastest man on earth" (Fig. 2–5). In December, 1954, while riding a rocket-propelled sled on a track nearly 7 miles in length, Dr. Stapp attained a ground speed

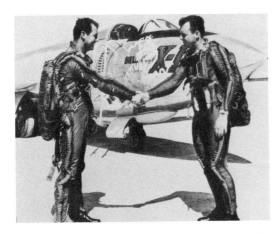

Fig. 2–4. The Aeromedical Laboratory's T-1 partial-pressure suit being worn by test pilots in front of the Bell X-1 (courtesy of Bell Aviation).

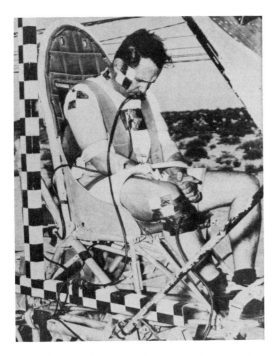

Fig. 2–5. Dr. John Stapp, "The Fastest Man on Earth," instrumented and restrained in preparation for a ride on a rocket-propelled sled (official United States Air Force photo).

of 1027.93 kph. The braking at the termination of the run was estimated to be 40 times normal earth gravity. The objective of the test was to demonstrate that a properly positioned and restrained astronaut could endure the sudden impact of his spacecraft with the atmosphere upon reentry from space.

Similarly, the high-altitude flight, Man High II, took Dr. David G. Simons in a 32-hour flight to an altitude of 34,000 m for the purpose of assaying the potential hazards from prolonged exposure to cosmic radiation (Fig. 2–6). Both the balloon flight and the sled ride were preludes to man's ventures into space.

Man's Ventures into Space

On the evening of October 4, 1957, the scientists and engineers of the Soviet Union successfully launched into orbit the earth's first artificial satellite. Sputnik I took with it into orbit more than simply a radio beacon; it also marked man's entry into the space age. A month later, on November 3, the Soviet Union launched the first biosatellite. This satellite carried aloft a female dog, Laika, but more significantly, it carried life-support systems to maintain the vital functions of this animal for a week's orbit in space. To monitor her biofunctions, automatic instruments using radiotelemetry signaled vital physiologic data back to earth-based stations.

It was clear that man would soon be voyaging in space. To prepare for the inevitable, the United States selected seven military test pilots to become America's first astronauts. Part of the selection process required an in-depth medical assessment. These extensive examinations were conducted at the Lovelace Foundation in Albuquerque, New Mexico; however, it was not one of these seven astronauts who would first fly in space but the Soviet cosmonaut, Yuri Gagarin (Fig. 2–7).

This first manned flight in space, circumnavigating the globe, was conducted on April 12, 1961 and received worldwide

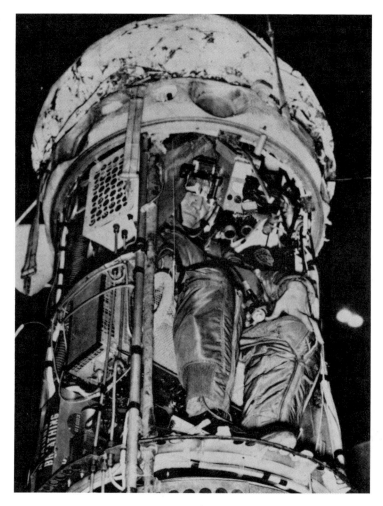

Fig. 2–6. Dr. David Simons preparing for his record altitude balloon flight in the Man High II Project (official United States Air Force photo).

acclaim. A month later an American astronaut, Alan Shepard, flew into space on a suborbital flight that lasted 15 minutes. The first American to make an orbital flight was John Glenn in the Friendship 7 in February, 1962. Supporting all of these manned flights, whether launched in the Soviet Union or in the United States, was an enormous foundation of biomedical research. The technology developed in those first days of manned space flight still has applications and provides a firm foundation for ongoing manned space programs. A major challenge to space medicine and biotechnology has been the development

of the life-support systems for the multicrewed space vehicles and laboratories: Apollo, Soyuz, Skylab, Salyut, and, to a lesser degree, the space shuttle. Just as challenging has been the development of systems permitting cosmonauts and astronauts to engage in extravehicular activity, whether in orbit or, as in the case of Apollo, on the lunar surface.

Civil Aviation

In 1952, the deHavilland Comet introduced commercial jet transportation to the flying public. Two years later, in 1954, a Comet suddenly and inexplicably disin-

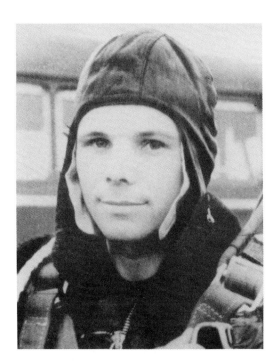

Fig. 2–7. Yuri Gagarin, the Soviet cosmonaut who was the first man into space (courtesy of the Soviet Embassy).

tegrated at an altitude of 12 km. Several months later, the accident was repeated, again over the Mediterranean and with no warning, simply a catastrophic, instantaneous failure of the aircraft. In investigating these two accidents, specialists in aviation medicine provided the vital clues for reconstructing the events of these air disasters. The investigations established metal fatigue as the culprit behind the rapid disintegration of the pressurized cabin.

A Harvard University professor, Dr. Ross MacFarland, who pioneered medical support for Pan-American Airways, published his text *Human Factors in Air Transportation* in 1953. This text became a classic in defining the human parameters that must be considered in the construction and operation of aeronautic transportation systems.

The adaptation of defense technology to civil aviation continued with the introduction of the supersonic transport. A joint effort between the British and French governments, the Concorde was built on the technologies developed for military aircraft. From the beginning, aeromedical advice was sought from specialists in aerospace medicine as the aeronautic and engineering communities began designing and developing this higher- and faster-flying commercial airliner. Designers took into consideration human factors for the cockpit crew, as well as for the passengers in the cabin. Although fraught with political and economic realities, the Anglo-French Concorde established a clear technology capability in addition to proving aeromedical feasibility.

The air transportation system in the United States is an important element in this nation's business and economic community. The aviation industry contributes over $35 billion to the gross national product and employs over a million people in a variety of jobs. Close to 80% of the free-world civilian transports are manufactured in the United States, and the sale of these aircraft has contributed significantly toward the nation's balance of trade. Today, more than 85% of long-distance travel in public carriers occurs on aircraft; domestically, over 250 million passengers will board aircraft in any one year, thus generating in excess of 250 billion revenue-passenger-miles. Internationally, 95% of travel is aboard aircraft. In any one year, approximately 25 million passengers will board international flights, generating close to 2 billion revenue-passenger-miles. During the 1980s, steady growth is expected to occur in cargo traffic carried by United States air carriers. Currently, over 6 million revenue-cargo-tons are implaned annually, and this amount is expected to increase by the end of the decade to approximately 10 million tons.

THE SPECIALTY OF AEROSPACE MEDICINE

In 1947, a motion was referred to the Executive Council of the Aero Medical Association introducing the concept of certification in aviation medicine. In supporting certification, Major General Grow, the Army Air Surgeon, stated:

> The time has come when the Aero Medical Association should adopt standards for certification in aviation medicine and proceed with the formulation with a competent board recognized by the American Medical Association and operating conjointly with the American Medical Association. We should recognize those doctors who have devoted the major portion of their professional careers to aviation, and also protect the airlines and the military services by public standards of proficiency. Certification from such a board would be evidence of recognition by a properly qualified body of an individual doctor's ability to examine flyers and to advise concerning problems in aviation medicine.[5]

In response to this resolution and additional work on the part of members of the association, a member of the association made an informal presentation of the case for the specialty of aviation medicine before the Council of Medical Education and Hospitals of the American Medical Association at its 1959 meeting in San Francisco, California.

Since the beginnings of aviation medicine in World War I, over 6000 physicians had completed postgraduate training in aviation medicine in both the United States and Canada. In addition to the 2000 medical officers serving with the aviation elements of the Armed Forces of the United States and Canada, there were 1500 medical examiners in civil aviation. Many, through experience, training, and research, had become recognized international experts in the field of aviation medicine.

Further meetings with committees of the American Medical Association led to the recommendation that the Aero Medical Association contact the American Board of Preventive Medicine and Public Health to see if some arrangements could be worked out for the possible inclusion of aviation medicine in their specialty board process. As these discussions were being conducted, the Air Force medical

service established residency training in aviation medicine at a number of its bases and coupled the program with a year of graduate training at Johns Hopkins University School of Public Health and Hygiene. Postgraduate year preceptorships were established under the sponsorship of a number of major United States airlines, and both the Mayo and Lovelace Clinics began planning for fellowships in the specialty.

In 1953, the American Board of Preventive Medicine formally appeared before the American Medical Association Council on Medical Education and Hospitals and spoke in favor of incorporating aviation medicine into their board. The day following this appearance, the council approved the decision to authorize certification in aviation medicine. In November, 1953, the American Board of Preventive Medicine officially certified the first group of physicians in the specialty of aviation medicine. As man moved into the frontiers of space, the name of the specialty became aerospace medicine.

Training in Aerospace Medicine

The physician interested in the specific requirements for becoming a candidate for board certification in aerospace medicine is referred to the current edition of the Directory of Approved Internships and Residencies. In summary, the program of education and training covers 4 postgraduate years. The candidates must have completed 1 year of clinical training, which is usually the first postgraduate year following graduation from medical school. A year of academic training is required with emphasis on biostatistics, epidemiology, health care administration, and environmental health. Most frequently, this year culminates in the award of a Master's degree in Public Health. A third year is spent concentrating on the physiologic, environmental, and clinical peculiarities of aerospace medicine. The final year is a practicum in such fields as clinical practice, research, teaching, or additional academic training.

Effective with individuals completing medical school in 1984, this formalized, structured residency program will be the only acceptable route for attaining qualification as a candidate for certification in aerospace medicine. For physicians graduating from medical school prior to 1984, options to the formalized program remain. These alternatives generally require extensive experience as a practitioner in aviation medicine or previous certification in a specialty that is parallel to aerospace medicine. It is recommended that any physician considering an alternative route to qualification communicate with the American Board of Preventive Medicine regarding current policy (Table 2–1).

Civilian Training

Training in aerospace medicine is available through a number of institutions, both governmental and academic. For the individual interested in aviation medicine as an aeromedical examiner for the Federal Aviation Administration (FAA), training programs are available in various regions throughout the United States in the form of seminars. In addition, the Civil Aviation Medicine Institute in Oklahoma City, Oklahoma provides in-resident educational programs of various durations. These educational courses are designed to meet the demanding needs of the civilian practitioner and thus are short, intense, and frequently cover weekends.

For the physician seeking a formal residency in the field, a university-based program is available at Wright State University in Dayton, Ohio. It is possible for the total residency program to be conducted at this one institution, beginning with a Master's degree in aerospace medicine and followed by practice opportunities across a broad spectrum of aeromedical interest. The university is located in the hometown of and named for Wilbur and Orville Wright, whose engineering and scientific ingenuity ushered in aviation. The site of the university is only a few miles from the farm field where the Wrights conducted much of their development and test flying. The university is also situated in the heart of the nation's major aeronautic research and development complex, the United States Air Force's Wright-Patterson installation. The

Table 2–1. Eligibility Determination for the American Board of Preventive Medicine in Aerospace Medicine

Postgraduate Year	Requirement	Equivalency
1	Clinical	None
2	An MPH or equivalent degree containing courses in the content areas of biostatistics, epidemiology, health services administration, and environmental health	An academic year whose course content includes the same major thrust areas as the MPH and deemed by the Board acceptable or certification in internal medicine, family practice, pediatrics, or similar specialty, plus 2 years full-time experience in preventive medicine. Or 4 years of full-time practice of aerospace medicine, including teaching and/or training in the core courses required of the MPH
3	Residency in aerospace medicine in an approved program	Certification in an approved alternative residency, plus 2 years of full-time practice. Or 3 years of full-time experience in aerospace medicine, including suitable periods of training or practice
4	Practicum year	A second formal academic year. Or a year in aerospace medicine residency. Or a year of full-time practice in aerospace medicine

resident has the full opportunity to make use of the technical libraries and facilities of much of the Air Force complex, including close association with the Air Force Aerospace Medical Research Laboratory.

Graduate educational and training opportunities are available with the National Aeronautics and Space Administration (NASA). Residents, usually at the third- or fourth-year level, are accepted principally at the Johnson Manned Space Center near Houston, Texas, and NASA-Ames in California for training in bioscience and operational space medicine. Because postgraduate training in aerospace medicine is a dynamic process, other institutions can be expected to offer educational, clinical, and research opportunities to residents in the field of aerospace medicine.

Air Force Programs

As would be expected, the United States Air Force has the largest training program in the field of aerospace medicine. Each year, hundreds of physicians attend the United States Air Force School of Aerospace Medicine (USAFSAM) to take an 8- to 10-week course in aerospace medicine. The course is designed to train physicians to serve as flight surgeons for operational flying units. The course is normally available only to physicians with federal affiliation in the active or reserve forces of the Department of Defense or physicians in the Coast Guard, NASA, or FAA.

To meet its mission requirements, the Air Force also conducts a residency program in aerospace medicine. Approximately 20 residents per year enter this program after first attending an academic institution to acquire a background in preventive medicine; they then spend 1 or 2 years at USAFSAM or alternate facilities for formal training and research opportunities. To maintain professional currency, each year, a 1-week seminar in advances in aviation medicine is conducted at USAFSAM for military physicians practicing in the field.

Army Programs

To support the large United States Army aviation program, physicians attend the basic course in Army aviation medicine at the Army helicopter center at Fort Rucker, Alabama. In many ways, the training program parallels that given by the Air Force. Because the Army's requirements for career aerospace medicine specialists are not as large as its sister services, Army specialty training is conducted either with the Air Force or Navy. A yearly seminar to upgrade the flight surgeon is also an important component of the Army's aeromedical educational program.

Navy Program

Pensacola Naval Air Station in Pensacola, Florida has historically been the site of Naval aviation medicine activity. The initial training of Naval flight surgeons is somewhat longer than in the Army or Air Force because their program includes practical aeronautic training and experience. The limited residency program includes 2 years at the Pensacola Aeromedical Center and 1 academic year at a school of public health. No more than five Naval flight surgeons per year receive the opportunity for residency training in aerospace medicine.

Aerospace Medicine Association

One of the major responsibilities of the Aerospace Medicine Association is to provide postgraduate continuing education in the field of aerospace medicine. This is accomplished in three ways. The Aerospace Medicine Association's major effort in continuing education is the sponsorship of the Annual Scientific Meeting held in May of each year at various locations throughout the United States. This intense 4-day program provides scientific sessions, seminars, workshops, and tutorials adequate to meet the needs of all pertinent disciplines: aerospace medicine, bioscience, and the engineering specialties.

A second effort of the Association in meeting continuing educational requirements is the publication of its journal, *Aviation, Space, and Environmental Medicine.* A feature of the journal is a continuing education question and answer program developed by a subcommittee of the Association's Education Committee. The journal contains scientific articles and clinical case reports designed to meet the needs of all specialists in the field.

Finally, the Aerospace Medicine Association sponsors regional seminars periodically that address specific topics of interest to the practitioner in aerospace medicine. The seminars are designed to provide the maximum postgraduate credit allowable for the time commitment made by the physician. The seminars provide a forum to present the most current scientific data available in areas of intense interest to the practitioner of aerospace medicine.

PROFESSIONAL OPPORTUNITIES IN AEROSPACE MEDICINE

Historically, the largest employer of physicians trained in aerospace medicine has been the United States Department of Defense. Within the three branches of the service, over 1000 flight surgeons are practicing aerospace medicine in a variety of capacities. Many of the greatest professional challenges in the field have been associated with military aviation. With few exceptions, the military aerospace medical specialist and his colleagues from other scientific and engineering disciplines first defined physiologic hazards and sought the aeromedical solutions. This has been true in the past, is true today, and is expected to remain true in the future.

Unlike their peers in civilian life, the military flight surgeon most often is a crew member flying in the aeronautic system his unit supports. This fact ensures that he becomes acquainted with the stressors of operational flying. Although recently

the military physician has been less closely associated with the nation's space activity, an inevitable change in involvement will take place as the role of military manned space missions becomes more clearly defined. For the foreseeable future, increased responsibility, new challenges, and an expanding role awaits the military flight surgeon.

Positions in both operational space mission support and research are available to the practitioner of aerospace medicine within NASA. The bioscience and aerospace research programs are broad-based and include aeronautic systems, as well as manned space activity. NASA aerospace medical physicians fulfill the classic flight surgeon role for the astronaut corps. This role includes the day-to-day medical support of the astronaut, as well as the more crucial support for actual space flight missions.

The FAA is the other major civil service employer of practitioners of aerospace medicine. Aeromedical personnel are assigned at all levels of the administration's organization and conduct clinical, administrative, and research activities.

A variety of industrial opportunities are available to the aerospace medical practitioner. Major airframe corporations in the United States employ aeromedically trained specialists not only in a clinical corporate role but also in a research and development role. These physicians serve as principal consultants on the development of new life-support systems, human factor solutions to man-machine interaction, and bioengineering requirements for new aeronautic systems. The airline industry employs aerospace medical specialists both full-time and as corporation consultants. Several of the major airlines have their own corporate aeromedical departments to support the acute and prospective health care needs of the cockpit and cabin crews. Other companies employ established clinics or private practitioners to provide aeromedical services on a fee-for-service or contractual basis.

Throughout the United States, physicians are engaged in the private practice of aerospace medicine. These clinicians meet the needs and requirements of tens of thousands of private pilots who require periodic health assessments to maintain their aeronautic rating or who require specialty care for a medical condition that could compromise their continued flying.

Since its formation, over 800 physicians have been certified by the American Board of Preventive Medicine in the specialty field of aerospace medicine. Many of these physicians continue to be actively engaged in various aspects of the field. The Board has certified approximately 4000 physicians in all fields of preventive medicine. In addition to those physicians engaged in aerospace medicine, there have been 2000 in public health, 500 in general preventive medicine, and 900 in occupational medicine. Recently, a national forum was conducted to review the availability of specialists in various fields in the future. The Graduate Medical Education National Advisory Committee (GMENAC) adopted recommendations regarding the needed number of physicians for each specialty in 1990. This forecast was made in September, 1980. The GMENAC estimated that there were 584 specialists currently practicing aerospace medicine and that by 1990 nearly 1000 will be required. In all fields of preventive medicine, there will be a need to double the number of available practitioners. It was estimated that many clinical specialties will be overmanned; however, one clear exception was in the broad field of preventive medicine, of which aerospace medicine is but one part. Few specialties in the field of medicine provide as many varied opportunities for intellectual growth and professional accomplishment and satisfaction as does aerospace medicine.

Within the United States, all are touched by the aerospace industry. The impact of aviation and space on the social fabric of the nation, on its economy, and even its political structure is scarcely appreciated; however, the impact is predictable when viewed in the context of the past. Much that has been accomplished would have been impossible without the contributions of specialists in aerospace medicine. Challenges remain as new aeronautic systems enter commercial and military service and as sustained manned space operations become a reality. Aerospace medicine will be expected to meet these challenges.

REFERENCES

1. Anderson, H.G.: The Medical and Surgical Aspects of Aviation. London, Oxford University Press, 1919.
2. Engle, E., and Lott, A.S.: Man in Flight. Annapolis, Maryland, Leeward Publications, Inc., 1979.
3. Peyton, G.: Fifty Years of Aerospace Medicine. AFSC Historical Publications. Series No. 67–180, Washington, D.C., Government Printing Office, 1967.
4. Strughold, H.: Atmospheric space equivalence. J. Aviat. Med., 25:420, 1952.
5. Benford, R.J.: Doctors in the Sky. Springfield, Illinois, Charles C Thomas, 1955.

Chapter 3

The Future Perspective

George C. Mohr

It is unwise to treat of any medical subject as if it were complete.

LATHAM

The remarkable upswing in scientific inquiry during the nineteenth and twentieth centuries provided mankind with fundamental new insights into the natural laws governing the physical environment. Armed with this new knowledge, modern society has systematically developed an interlacing set of technologies enriching the quality of life and providing additional scientific tools to acquire even more new knowledge. Consistent with this trend, the exciting advances in aviation witnessed since man's first powered flight in 1903 have literally catapulted modern aviation into the aerospace age. The initial exploration phase of aviation rapidly gave rise in less than half a century to the extensive commercial utilization of this new capability. Even while the boundaries of aviation technology were continuing to expand unabated, the first manned orbital space flight in 1961 triggered anew the cycle of exploration, expansion, and full utilization, leading once again to new discovery.

Scientific advances provide the starting point for the development of new tech-nology. Scientific investigation is basically a pioneering search for new knowledge. Technology development, on the other hand, focuses on the practical application of new knowledge to provide desired goods or services to the consumer. Transforming scientific knowledge to technology requires the combined contributions of many seemingly distinct disciplines drawn from the fields of science, engineering, and management. During the nineteenth century, the genesis of new technology was a slow evolutionary process; however, in the twentieth century, the increasing demand for new goods and services steadily narrowed the time interval between a scientific breakthrough and the availability of new technology. This progressive time compression of the technology development cycle is dramatically changing the professional demands placed on the modern technical specialist. The complexities and range of interests contributing to today's aerospace technology transcend even the wildest imaginings of the early aviation pioneers. Today's expert can no longer afford the luxury of compartmentalized thinking strictly bounded by classic disciplinary fences. As aerospace technology opens the way to the unconstrained utilization of both air and space, tomorrow's aerospace physician, like his scientist and engineering colleagues, will be challenged to contribute collectively to each exciting advance from new concept to new capability as a professional member of the aerospace team. Throughout the rest of this chapter, the nature of some of those advances that may come to be will be explored.

COMMERCIAL AVIATION

Aviation Contributions to the Transportation Industry

Modern transport aircraft provide an increasingly important means of transportation that is not only fast and reliable but also more flexible than most other forms of transportation. It is, therefore, not surprising that the volume of goods and passengers transported by air has more than doubled during the decade of the 1970s. Table 3–1 depicts the growth in international and domestic revenue air traffic between 1971 and 1980.[1]

In spite of the rapid rise in commercial air traffic, the airspace, as a whole, is still able to support continued growth in aviation. For example, in the United States in 1980, 213,700 registered aircraft, including 20,000 military aircraft, shared some 207,000,000 km^3 of regulated domestic air-

space, an average of 969 km^3 for each aircraft.[2,3] This parameter is, of course, a misleading indicator of actual air traffic congestion, which must be further analyzed in terms of specific categories of aircraft and air operations.

In the United States, the most spectacular increase in the numbers of operating aircraft has occurred in the general aviation category, up approximately 250% between 1965 and 1980. General aviation aircraft are relatively small, commonly privately owned, and usually operate in accordance with visual flight rules (VFR) at flight altitudes below 3810 m. Nonetheless, these aircraft are the principal users of commercial airfields and thus have had an increasing impact on terminal airspace and airport congestion.

The growth in the number of air carrier aircraft, while smaller in magnitude, correlates strongly with the continuing increase in passenger and air freight traffic. Air carriers uniformly operate along controlled airways, resulting in growing congestion, both enroute and in the terminal area, particularly for operations connecting major urban centers of commerce. Moreover, in recent years, airline operators have turned to aircraft with increased load-carrying capacity to remain competitive in the marketplace. The difficulties of boarding or deplaning hundreds of passengers per aircraft are causing major changes in airport design to accommodate the high-volume movement of passengers and baggage.

The most promising approach to the management of high-density enroute and terminal air traffic and increasing airport congestion is being found in the expanded use of automation. Reliance on automation is bringing about significant changes in virtually all aspects of the aerospace industry, impacting aircraft development, flight operations, air traffic control, and airport design. The human is assuming the role of a semiautonomous executive director, decision-maker, and emergency

Table 3–1. World International and Domestic Revenue Air Traffic

Year	Passenger-km × 10^10	Mail-/Freight Ton-km × 10^10
1971	49.4	1.61
1972	56.0	1.78
1973	61.8	2.04
1974	65.6	2.19
1975	69.7	2.23
1976	76.4	2.46
1977	81.8	2.68
1978	93.6	2.92
1979	105.1	3.14
1980	107.1	3.28

backup for a host of computer-managed systems in the aircraft and on the ground. This trend has raised fundamental questions about how best to integrate the human operator with high-technology automated systems to achieve optimal man-machine system performance and reliability. Finding satisfactory biomedical solutions for these questions promises to be one of the most important challenges for the aeromedical specialists who will support the development and operation of the next generation of air transports.

Technology Projections

The success of the airplane as a transportation vehicle has been due in large part to its speed and ability to interconnect virtually all urban centers worldwide. An equally important consideration is the matter of cost-effectiveness. The customer of a transportation system will always be tempted to trade off transportation time and convenience in favor of cost when the economics of the choice are grossly imbalanced. It follows, therefore, that aviation technology must continue to press for reduced cost per ton-mile transported relative to other transportation options, particularly surface modes such as the truck, train, or ship.

Shortly after the invention of powered flight, a French engineer, Louis Brequet, enunciated a principle relating the cruising range of an airplane to its cruise efficiency and fuel fraction. This principle expressed in mathematic form is called the Brequet Range Equation:

$$R = [M \times \frac{L}{D} \times I_{sp}]$$
$$\times [Ln(1 + \frac{WF}{WA})] \quad (1)$$

R is the Brequet range factor, which is usually expressed in nautical miles. The first term defines the cruise efficiency, which is equal to the product of the aircraft Mach number (M), the lift-to-drag ratio (L/D), and engine specific impulse (I_{sp}) during cruise flight. The second term is equal to the logarithm (Ln) of the quantity 1 plus the ratio of fuel weight (WF) to the combined structural and payload weight of the aircraft. It is clear from examining this equation that flight efficiency increases proportionally with overall improvements in engine design, aerodynamic performance, and cruise speed. Unfortunately, these three factors are not independent across the total speed range encompassing subsonic and supersonic flight regimes. With current technology, the reduced lift-to-drag ratio and engine specific impulse at higher Mach numbers essentially offset theoretical gains in cruise efficiency attributable to supersonic flight. Figure 3–1 illustrates that dramatic increases in cruising range, and flight efficiency are not to be expected until flight speed begins to approach hypersonic velocities above Mach 4.

Realistically, many other economic and engineering factors in addition to cruise efficiency influence the cost-effectiveness of an air transport system. Clearly, the initial capital investment, operating costs, and the revenue-producing load factor also must be considered. Nevertheless, a major challenge for the aircraft designer still remains to maximize cruise efficiency, and with this objective in mind, aviation technologists will surely continue to push toward hypersonic flight capability.

Some of the key technology areas that are critically important for achieving practical hypersonic air transportation are identified in Figure 3–2. Of particular importance is the development of advanced materials that exhibit high strength-to-weight ratios, are relatively tolerant to high-temperature conditions, and have a low susceptibility to fatigue failure. Considering future structural design, advanced composites will permit a steady reduction in structural weight, thereby in-

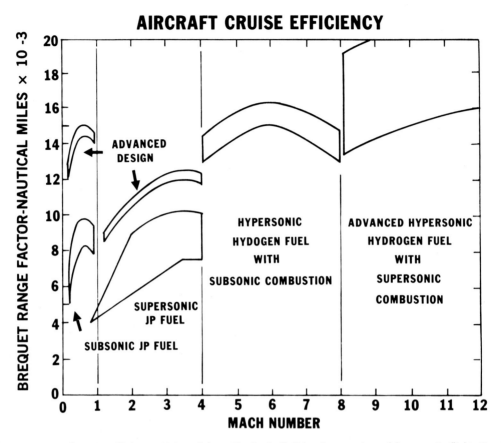

Fig. 3–1. Aircraft cruise efficiency. (Adapted from Bisplinghoff, R.L.: Supersonic and hypersonic flight. Fourth International Symposium on Bioastronautics and Exploration of Space. C.H. Roadman, et al., eds. Nov. 1968.)

TECHNOLOGY DIRECTIONS

CRUISE PERFORMANCE

AERODYNAMICS
• LIFT AUGMENTATION
• VARIABLE GEOMETRY
• SUPER-CRITICAL WING
• CONTROL CONFIGURATION

MATERIALS
• ALLOYS
• COATINGS
• REFRACTORY METALS
• CERAMICS

PROPULSION
• EXOTIC FUELS
• VARIABLE CYCLE ENGINE
• RAMJET
• SCRAMJET

Fig. 3–2. Directions of technologic development.

creasing the useful payload. High-temperature materials, including eutectic alloys and ceramics, will support the development of both heat-resistant airframe components and high-temperature exotic engines able to sustain high-Mach–number flight. Advances in computer-managed avionic systems will soon permit the exploitation of radically new designs for improving aerodynamic and propulsion efficiency. The introduction of advanced avionics integration and systems automation technologies will allow the exploitation of variable-geometry wing design and advanced stability control to optimize L over D (lift-to-drag ratio) over a wide range of airspeeds and altitudes. Similarly, computer-based propulsion control will provide for the incorporation of adaptive engine technology into future high-Mach transports. Many of the pacing technologies are already being realized in the laboratories of various governments and industries in the free world. The commercial aviation industry is being provided with an ever-expanding set of technology options for improving the performance of tomorrow's air transport system.

Aeromedical Considerations for Hypersonic Flight

The technology required to develop a practical hypersonic air transportation system will probably become available sometime after the beginning of the twenty-first century. It is important, therefore, to anticipate the potential impact of the hypersonic flight environment on passenger safety and well-being. A number of engineering considerations related to structural and propulsion limitations dictate the airspeed and altitude corridors available to air transports specifically designed for subsonic, supersonic, or hypersonic operations. Figure 3–3 depicts the major design constraints for five classes of air transports. Assuming the propulsion system is air-breathing, the upper boundary of altitude versus airspeed is primarily determined by engine performance. The lower boundary of altitude versus airspeed is driven by sonic boom restrictions for flights below 15,240 m and by structural design requirements for high-Mach–number flight above 15,240 m. By extrapolating current technology trends, a nominal cruise altitude and airspeed can be identified that is appropriate for each of the five classes of air transports shown in Figure 3–3. These projected operational environments provide a basis for examining the potential biomedical hazards peculiar to each flight regime.

High-altitude, high-Mach flight potentially exposes the passenger and crew to four types of environmental hazards over and above the risks of subsonic flight at conventional altitudes. First, cabin decompression resulting from a major leak or failure of the pressurization system could seriously incapacitate the passengers and unprotected crewmembers. Minor leaks are normally compensated for by the pressurization system; however, a major leak, such as would occur with the loss of a window, would cause rapid decompression of the crew and passenger compartment. Figure 3–4 specifies the principal factors determining the cabin decompression rate for a leak rate much larger than the compensatory capacity of the aircraft pressurization system. It is apparent that for these conditions, the decompression rate is roughly proportional

AEROSPACE VEHICLE DESIGN CONSTRAINTS

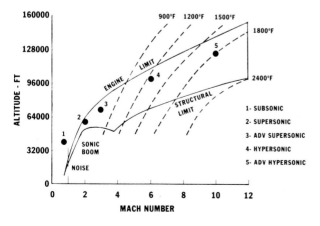

Fig. 3–3. Aerospace vehicle design constraints. (Adapted from Bisplinghoff, R.L.: Supersonic and hypersonic flight. Fourth International Symposium of Bioastronautics and Exploration of Space. C.H. Roadman, et al., eds. Nov. 1968.)

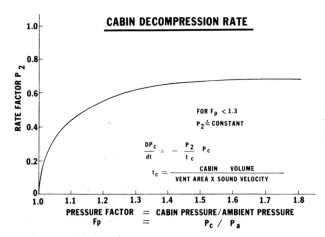

CABIN DECOMPRESSION RATE

FOR $F_p < 1.3$
$P_2 \doteq$ CONSTANT

$$\frac{DP_c}{dt} = -\frac{P_2}{t_c} P_c$$

$$t_c = \frac{CABIN \quad VOLUME}{VENT \ AREA \ X \ SOUND \ VELOCITY}$$

PRESSURE FACTOR = CABIN PRESSURE/AMBIENT PRESSURE
F_p = P_c / P_a

Fig. 3–4. Cabin decompression rate. (Adapted from Gillies, J.A.: A Textbook of Aviation Physiology. Oxford, Pergamon Press, 1965.)

to the cabin pressure when the ratio of cabin pressure to ambient pressure exceeds 1.3. For all such pressure ratios, the time to decompress to 37% (1/e) of the initial cabin pressure is roughly 1.5 times the cabin volume divided by the product of effective leak area times the velocity of sound. Basically, this means that for a situation such as a window blowout, the time to decompress to 7620 m cabin altitude is largely independent of flight altitude for aircraft operating above 10,668 m. Characteristically, this decompression time to 7620 m will be on the order of 20 to 30 seconds. Within another minute, however, an aircraft flying at 30,480 m will continue to decompress to a cabin altitude exceeding the Armstrong Line—the altitude at which the environment for the unprotected human body attains the equivalent of a vacuum (approximately 20 km). Clearly, the primary factor driving the seriousness of the decompression hazard at altitudes greater than 10,668 m is the time required to descend to 7620 m cabin altitude, where passenger supplemental oxygen systems are effective. For a hypersonic transport flying at Mach 6 at 30,480 m, the descent time would be sufficiently long to expose passengers to cabin altitudes requiring full-pressure suit protection. This clearly being impractical, the solution will necessarily require provisions for a true "space-cabin" design that

will assure a failure-proof pressurization system.

A second category of hazards peculiar to high-altitude flight pertains to the possible accumulation of toxic ozone levels in the cabin atmosphere. Ozone in the ambient atmosphere is photochemically synthesized from oxygen by the action of 100 to 200 nm ultraviolet light. Ozone is a highly reactive compound that decomposes rapidly when heated in the presence of water vapor. Consequently, the ambient ozone concentration varies widely as a function of altitude, latitude, season, and specific weather conditions. Figure 3–5 shows characteristic ozone concentrations as a function of altitude. Typical cruise altitudes for transports of various design

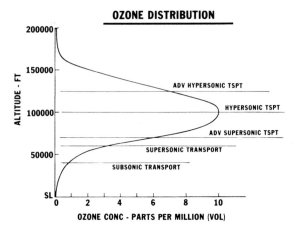

OZONE DISTRIBUTION

ADV HYPERSONIC TSPT

HYPERSONIC TSPT

ADV SUPERSONIC TSPT

SUPERSONIC TRANSPORT

SUBSONIC TRANSPORT

Fig. 3–5. Ozone concentration as a function of altitude.

are overlaid. Figure 3–6 shows representative data for the predicted and observed biologic effects of ozone. Considering the information in these two figures, it is not surprising that passenger complaints are uncommon in conventional subsonic air transport operations. If it were not for the instability of ozone, a more serious problem could be expected as flight altitudes increase. Indeed, suspected ozone-mediated respiratory complaints have been reported for intercontinental subsonic flights above 12,192 m. Fortunately, however, with increasing altitude, compressive heating of engine-bleed air used for cabin pressurization effectively decomposes much of the ozone in the ambient atmosphere. Moreover, at altitudes compatible with hypersonic flight, the air is so rarified that sealed cabin pressurization using stored gas supplies will be necessary, eliminating the ozone hazard altogether.

High thermal loading constitutes a third category of hazards that may be encountered during supersonic or hypersonic flight. Aerodynamic heating can raise the temperature of wing and fuselage surfaces to many hundreds of degrees. (See Figure 3–3.) Even higher temperatures may occur on the leading edges of wings and tail as-

semblies as a result of stagnation heating. As was previously noted, advances in high-temperature materials technology will be required to assure structural integrity in these hostile thermal environments. Excessive heating of the cabin air may occur not only by conductive heat transfer from the fuselage but also by compressive heating of the engine-bleed air used for cabin pressurization. In the rarified atmosphere above 15,240 m, very high pressure ratios are required to maintain the cabin altitude below 1829 m, which is considered safe and comfortable for passengers and crew. This means that the air exiting the compressor will be very hot and must be cooled before being used to ventilate the cabin. Figure 3–7 illustrates the relationship between flight altitude and compressor exit temperature. Clearly, failure of the cabin air-conditioning system for flight regimes above 18,288 m would quickly expose passengers and crew to dangerous cabin air temperatures unless the aircraft descended rapidly to lower altitudes.

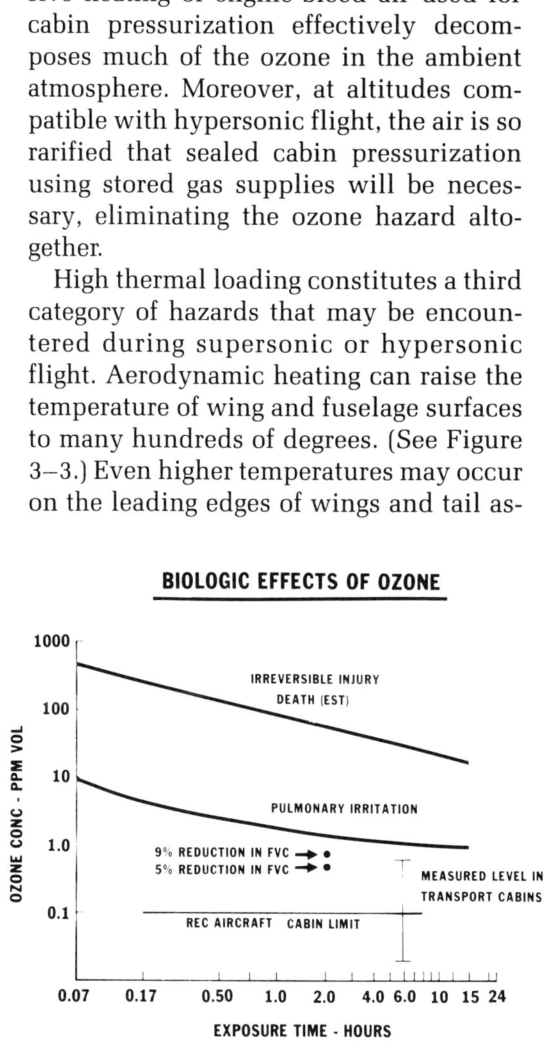

The fourth category of environmental hazards presenting a potential threat to passenger and crew safety for flights above 15,240 m is cosmic radiation. Energetic particles from solar and galactic origins interact with the earth's atmosphere to produce a complex flux of particulate and electromagnetic radiations that are considerably more intense at high altitude than near the earth's surface. The following is a summary of some of the basic characteristics of both primary and secondary cosmic radiation:

Primary cosmic radiation at 90,000 m
   Protons—85%
   Alpha particles—13%
   Heavy nuclei—2%
Interaction with upper atmosphere
   Secondary cosmic radiation at 19,500 m
      Protons
      Neutrons

BIOLOGIC EFFECTS OF OZONE

Fig. 3–6. Biologic effects of ozone.

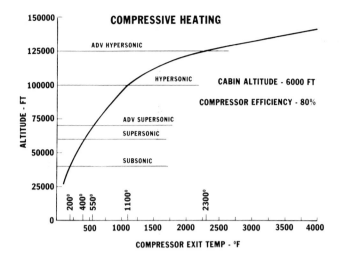

Fig. 3–7. Compressive heating. (Adapted from Gillies, J.A.: A Textbook of Aviation Physiology. Oxford, Pergamon Press, 1965.)

Pi-mesons
Gamma rays
Variable Intensity
    Altitude—7000%
    Latitude—600%
    Solar activity—75%

The atmosphere serves as a highly effective radiation shield, which accounts for the large variation in the radiation intensity encountered at various flight altitudes. A marked latitude dependence is produced by the deflecting effect of the earth's magnetic field on the solar emissions. Figure 3–8 illustrates the characteristic radiation intensities to be expected as a function of altitude and earth latitude. A hypersonic transport flying at 30,480 m or higher clearly will be exposed to much higher radiation fluxes than a conventional subsonic transport. The duration of time at cruise altitude, however, typically will be much shorter because of the high cruise speeds. Table 3–2 is a comparative analysis of the radiation dose to passengers and crew expected for several types of aircraft. This analysis indicates that, although the passengers and crew of the hypersonic transport will be exposed to relatively higher dose rates, the total cumulative dose expected actually will be considerably less than the dose received by the passengers and crew of conventional subsonic transports. It is, therefore, reasonable to conclude that cosmic radiation poses no serious threat to the passen-

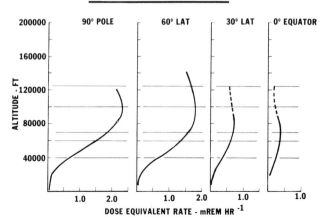

Fig. 3–8. Galactic radiation field. (Adapted from Wallace, R.W., and Sandhaus, C.A.: Cosmic radiation exposure in subsonic air transport. Aviat. Space Environ. Med., 49(4):610–623, 1978.)

Table 3–2. Comparison of Transport Radiation Exposure

Type of Aircraft	Cruise Time (hours)*	Dose Rate (mREM hr⁻¹)†	Total Dose (mREM)	Dose Ratio
Subsonic	8.4	0.50	4.2	1.00
ADV Subsonic	8.4	0.50	4.2	1.00
Supersonic	3.8	0.98	3.7	0.88
Adv Supersonic	2.5	1.11	2.8	0.67
Hypersonic	1.3	1.21	1.6	0.38
Adv Hypersonic	0.8	1.09	0.9	0.21

*Cruise range equals 8000 km.
†Flight altitude equals 13,300 m between 30° and 60° north latitude.

gers or crew of a future hypersonic transport.

GENERAL AVIATION

Growth and Complexity

Growth in the general aviation industry has been remarkable during the period since World War II. Perhaps this growth is due, in part, to the very large number of military airmen trained during the war and subsequently released to civilian life, where they exploited their flying skills for fun and profit. More likely, however, the sustaining drive to the industry resulted from the cost benefits of on-demand air mobility, providing a competitive edge for a wide variety of business enterprises from cattle ranching to international commerce. Today, owning and operating an airplane is within the economic reach of an ever-widening segment of the adult population, which portends continued growth of the general aviation industry in the future.

In 1980, approximately 210,000 general aviation aircraft were in the United States inventory. The operators of these aircraft are the major users of the nation's airports, accounting for 74% of all operations at Federal Aviation Administration (FAA) towers. The expected continued increase in the number of registered general aviation aircraft will only aggravate the congestion already occurring around major metropolitan air terminals. Trends also suggest that the operators of general aviation aircraft are more frequently using their aircraft for point-to-point transpor-tation, flying along the nation's airways. In 1980, general aviation aircraft accounted for approximately 30% of the work load at Air Traffic Control Centers. This fraction is expected to increase substantially over the next decade.

Operating an aircraft generally involves six basic kinds of activity: flight path control, vigilance to avoid other aircraft or obstacles, communication, navigation, aircraft systems operation, and ancillary housekeeping tasks. In the past, most general aviation aircraft were used for fair-weather flying in accordance with visual flight rules. With the growing popularity of privately owned aircraft to support business travel, increasing numbers of general aviation aircraft are being equipped with transponders, altitude recording equipment, and other modern communication and navigation equipment necessary for instrument flight rule operations. It is reasonable to expect that the new and emerging high-technology avionics systems which are currently radically changing the pilot-cockpit interface in air transports will, as costs come down, find increasing application in general aviation aircraft. The introduction of multipurpose displays, automated flight management systems, and sophisticated communication navigation systems will change the work load placed on the general aviation pilot in the same manner it is affecting the work load of the air transport pilot.

Medical Challenges

The future general aviation pilot will undoubtedly fly a far more complex machine than the conventional private aircraft used in the 1970s. Moreover, he will want to fly primarily in controlled airspace, operating in and out of busy urban airports. He also will be less and less constrained by weather conditions and distance. Although his routine piloting tasks will be simplified, he will need to depend on increasingly complex "black box" systems that he must thoroughly understand and be able to back up in the event of a system failure. These changes in the character of general aviation will require a concomitant reassessment of aeromedical practices. First, medical qualification standards will undoubtedly become more selective. In particular, conditions that might significantly degrade visual functions or increase the risk of in-flight incapacitation will receive increased attention. Because the general aviation pilot frequently will be competing with the transport pilot for a safe share of the same airspace, the medical selection and retention standards for both groups can be expected to converge. Second, automated medical data collection, storage, retrieval, and analysis systems will have to be developed. In the United States, over 500,000 medical certificates were in force in 1980. Over 9 million medical examination records have been entered into the FAA's data bank. To ensure an effective medical standards program capable of dealing with an enlarging and increasingly mobile population of flyers, the medical examination, review, and certification process will need to be electronically managed in near realtime. Individual medical findings will be assessed against population norms validated by operational experience data. High-risk cases will be isolated for more intensive evaluation before exceptions are granted. Finally, good human-factors engineering practice will receive greater emphasis during the design and certification of general aviation aircraft. The private aircraft of the future will be equipped to fly faster, farther, and

higher, employing today's high-technology systems that will be affordable tomorrow. The designer will need to build in "pilot friendliness and reliability" to ensure that proficiency levels attainable by the part-time pilot are sufficient for managing the aircraft safely under both nominal and degraded flight conditions. Even with optimal aircraft design, tomorrow's aeromedical provider will have to be increasingly aware and vigilant concerning the physiologic and cognitive demands of even the routine flying experience. Disturbed mental states, medications, substandard proficiency, minor illnesses, fatigue, and preoccupation will become matters of critical concern for both the flyer and the physician. In the end, the aeromedical provider serving tomorrow's general aviation community will become far more than a medical examiner. He will, in fact, become an integral part of the exciting and expanding age of flight.

MILITARY AVIATION

Technology Explosion

The unrelenting demand for increased performance in our first-line combat aircraft has required military aviation research and development to remain on the leading edge of technology. Advances in aircraft performance since World War I have followed the familiar sigmoid curve characteristic of most processes sustained by the investment of economic resources over time. Figure 3–9 illustrates an interesting phenomenon associated with technology-driven systems development. When further progress is inhibited by physical constraints, a technology breakthrough is usually found that permits further rapid advances until the next physical limitation is encountered. The impact of these often unexpected major technology advances makes it so difficult to forecast the future with confidence.

Military aviation contributes to national security in three critical areas: strategic

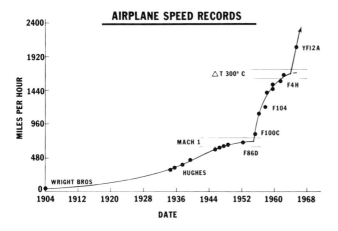

Fig. 3–9. Airplane speed records.

warfare, tactical warfare, and logistic support. To accomplish these missions, a variety of aircraft and ground-support systems are required, ranging from high-performance fighters to long-range bombers and heavy-lift transports. Whatever the design characteristics of a given aircraft system, certain basic technologies will always bound the achievable performance in the end product. The following is a list of the six key technology areas, with examples of representative technology initiatives that will likely have major impacts on next-generation military aircraft:

Propulsion
    Variable cycle engines
    Ramjets
Aerodynamics
    Drag reduction
    Adaptive wing
Flight control
    Digital flight control
    Integrated fire, flight, propulsion
        control
Structures and materials
    Composites
    High-temperature materials
Avionics
    Sensors
    Very high-speed integrated circuits
Weapons
    High accuracy standoff
    Autonomous weapons

Developing efficient propulsion sys-

tems for air vehicles capable of both subsonic and supersonic flight is a major challenge to technology. The three basic components of all jet engines employing rotating elements are the compressor, combustor, and turbine. This "core engine," being a thermodynamic system, is driven by the combustor temperature. Hence, the availability of high-strength, high-temperature materials is crucial to further engine improvements. To increase fuel efficiency for subsonic, heavy-lift aircraft, engine designers have produced the turbofan engine. This design employs a shaft-driven fan in front of the compressor to increase the momentum of a secondary stream of air bypassing the combustor. The ratio of air mass flow through the fan to the air mass flow through the core engine is defined as the bypass ratio. This parameter profoundly affects both thrust and fuel efficiency. Unfortunately, the optimum bypass ratio varies widely as a function of airspeed and engine-airframe integration. Research and development efforts may one day produce a variable-cycle engine that can be continuously optimized for all flight conditions over a broad range of airspeeds, altitudes, and thrust demands. Such an engine will require advanced electronic control systems to sense engine status and regulate gas flow, fuel flow, and internal operating pressures.

The next benchmark in advanced air-breathing engine technology will undoubtedly involve the ramjet family of propulsion systems, which are uniquely suitable for powering high supersonic and hypersonic combat aircraft. The ramjet is an exceedingly simple heat engine that consists only of an inlet, a combustor, and a nozzle. From a thermodynamic standpoint, the ramjet is extremely efficient, but, unfortunately, it operates only after high supersonic airspeeds have already been attained. To exploit ramjet power in a combat aircraft, a hybrid engine is required that is designed to operate selectively as a turbojet on takeoff, landing, and acceleration to supersonic cruise and also as a ramjet during high-Mach–number flight.

Major advances in flight control and aerodynamic design also will be needed to keep pace with aircraft performance requirements. The efficiency of an airfoil is determined by its lift-and-drag characteristics, which are commonly referred to as L/D. An airfoil optimized for high performance in subsonic regimes will normally not perform well supersonically. A number of advanced technologies are emerging that will minimize the transonic and supersonic L/D penalties while preserving superior subsonic performance. These include relaxed static stability, variable camber wing geometry, conformal weapons storage, and configuration shaping. The practical application of advanced aerodynamic designs will be possible, in large part, because of advances in computer-based, digital flight control technology. Through the extensive use of sensors, data busses, and subsystem integration, the combat aircraft of the future will be under real-time computer control, constantly adjusting flight characteristics, propulsion efficiency, and weapons delivery strategies to assure the best combat performance.

To achieve further increases in aircraft speed, maneuverability, and range, advanced structures and materials technol-ogy also will be required. New polymers and composite materials promise significant performance gains. Weight savings of as much as 50% will be possible. Moreover, composite materials are readily bonded, thus reducing the requirement for conventional fasteners, which will further improve the inherent fatigue resistance of these new materials. For other applications, advances in high-temperature materials technology will continue to be the pacing factor for the development of advanced engines and high-Mach aircraft. Superalloys, ceramics, and refractory metals technologies are expected to push the design temperature boundary out to 1550° by the year 2000.

Many forecasters believe that avionics will be the dominant technology driving the design of combat aircraft in the future. Through the magic of electromagnetic and electro-optical sensors, the pilot of the future will be able to "see" his flight environment both close at hand and beyond unaided visual range without being hindered by weather or darkness. The heart of the next-generation avionics system will be a very high-speed microcomputer. Introduction of submicron chip technology, with thousands of elements on a single 1-cm^2 chip able to perform millions of operations per second, will revolutionize aircraft and weapon systems design. Astronomic quantities of information will be gathered, processed, stored, and distributed in real-time. The number of potential applications within the grasp of future aircraft design engineers is almost unlimited. Examples of new technologies on the horizon include integrated communication, navigation, and identification systems linked to overhead satellites; integrated fire, flight, and propulsion control systems designed to deliver standoff, semiautonomous weapons on highly defended targets; automatic target detection, recognition, and tracking systems designed to operate beyond visible range; sophisticated countermeasure and counter-countermeasure systems designed for hostile electromagnetic and electro-optical environments; and advanced cockpit display systems providing three-dimensional, color, pictorial imagery obtained from stored digital data bases and processed sensor data.

Future advances in military aviation technology will not only affect what the aircraft can do but also will affect the role of the pilot and systems operator. The next section will briefly examine some of the possible impacts on the aircrewman of these new technologies as they are introduced into operational aircraft.

Aircrew Demands

The demands placed on the pilot of modern combat aircraft have become increasingly complex. The speed of battle has increased to the point where the pilot is allowed only seconds to assess the situation and take proper action. He is expected to sustain continuous operations under adverse weather conditions and at night. He must penetrate high-threat environments and strike hardened targets with pinpoint accuracy. These requirements have driven the development of "high-technology solutions" that unfortunately have added to the number and difficulty of the pilot's tasks. This increasing complexity threatens to overwhelm the pilot's capacity to cope successfully. For example, one of the front-line United States fighter aircraft has nearly 300 switches per crewmember. Similarly, a front-line British fighter has over 50 cockpit displays. When the pilot's cognitive and psychomotor performance capacities are compared with the total task demands of flying a modern combat aircraft, one must conclude that the pilot is near or at his work load saturation point.

Because of this growing complexity of military aviation systems, some forecasters believe the human pilot and systems operator will soon be removed entirely from the cockpit and be replaced by a com-

puter. In fact, computer control is already being applied to manage subsystem functions beyond the bandwidth capacity of the human sensorimotor system. A good example is the digital flight controller used to make the high-frequency control surface adjustments necessary to maintain dynamic stability of a statically unstable aircraft. The human operator, however, still has many attractive features that are advantageous to overall weapon systems effectiveness. The following list summarizes some of the more important capabilities of the human operator:

Multipurpose sensor-processor
  Large associative memory
  Multimode, multichannel sensor
    inputs
  Wide dynamic range
  High tolerance to channel noise
  Mobile platform
  Self-repairing
Multipurpose effector-manipulator
  Multimode operator
  Wide dynamic range
  Mobile platform
  Self-repairing
General Features
  Long mean-time-to-failure
  Self-programming/reprogramming
  Environmentally shielded systems
  High redundancy
  High reliability

The preferred solution to the growing operator work load problem need not be simply removing the pilot from the cockpit. The pilot contributes a level of autonomous problem-solving and executive control that will be difficult to duplicate with anything short of a computer exhibiting high-order artificial intelligence. Such a computer is not likely to be available until well into the twenty-first century. An alternative solution may be found through carefully designed hardware and software integration, permitting the aircrewman to control the total weapons system and its many subsystems simply by inputting his purpose or control objectives. With current technology, the pilot has to fuse in his mind information derived from a diverse set of unitary sources, reach a decision about a desired change in aircraft or weapons status, and then manipulate several controls in a particular sequence. In the future, through system integration, the pilot will receive processed information that is formatted to convey an accurate situational awareness, together with the control options open to him. He will only need to "command" his purpose: for example,"counter surface-to-air missile," "attack lead tank," "terrain mask on egress," or some similar intention. The computer-managed aircraft and weapons subsystems will be automatically manipulated to achieve the proper flight path, turn on countermeasures, acquire and track targets, arm and launch weapons, and safely exit the aircraft from the threat area. Although this kind of technology will likely reduce pilot work load, it will also radically change how the aircrew trains, flies, and maintains combat efficiency. A number of key crew technology initiatives are required to support the next generation of combat aircraft.

CREW TECHNOLOGY DIRECTIONS

Integrated Protection

An aircrewman flying a modern combat aircraft not only is exposed to high work load demands, but also must perform effectively in a physiologically hostile environment. The speed, range, maneuverability, and altitude capability of modern aircraft require the pilot to wear a variety of separate personal equipment assemblies. The list of such items keeps increasing with each new system. For example, protective assemblies in current use include head impact protection, flashblindness protection, noise protection, hypoxia protection, thermal burn protection, pressure protection, immersion protection, G protection, and chemical agent protection.

In addition, the pilot is seated and restrained in a powered escape system and surrounded by confining cockpit equipment and fuselage structure. The challenge today is to reverse the trend of layering on protection, which adds to the encumbrances on and discomfort of the crewman. Continuing research and development are needed to reduce the bulk, weight, and complexity of personal protective equipment through functional integration, the application of new materials, and use of microelectronics. Alternative protective approaches also must be developed such as engineering the protection into the cockpit rather than placing it on the pilot. Although a truly shirt-sleeve environment may be a long time coming, steady improvement will be essential to keep the pilot both safe and efficient.

Automation and Man-Machine Integration

When the next generation of combat aircraft enters the inventory, the extensive use of automation is expected to significantly reduce aircrew work load. At least four basic opportunities exist for the incorporation of automation into aircraft design:

1. Automation to reduce pilot work load.
2. Automation to increase operational reliability.
3. Automation to improve pilot performance.
4. Automation to add new capabilities.

Many factors contribute to pilot work load. Some of the more important sources include information saturation, divided attention, time-line compression, high bandwidth control requirements, and small-scale task demands. Many alternative automation strategies for coping with these factors are theoretically possible; however, to choose the optimum strategy, pilot work load must be measured objectively. Evidence is mounting that work load measurement using a battery of subjective, behavioral, and neurophysiologic tests is practicable. It is probable that a modular, self-contained, microcomputer-controlled test system will soon be available to assess the extent that alternative cockpit designs can reduce work load during combat operations.

The number of subsystems that must be monitored and controlled by a modern combat pilot has increased to the point that many pilots simply do not attempt to use more than a third of the available options. Moreover, a pilot, in order to accomplish his purpose, is usually required to assimilate highly abstract information portrayed by several cockpit displays while he accomplishes a sequence of time-critical switching and control tasks. Because the tasks to be performed are usually not consistent with the pilot's natural mental representation of his intent, a significant potential exists for memory overload and resulting errors of omission and commission. Automation can significantly reduce this potential for pilot error by providing displays and requiring actions that match the pilot's mental concept of the large-scale task being performed.

Modern cockpits already have been automated to a modest degree; however, the means by which the pilot interfaces with the various systems are still highly restricted. Information is generally provided by heads-up displays, panel-mounted displays, and auditory communication channels. Control inputs are made with the hands or feet via switches, levers, and pedals. To achieve the maximum benefits of automation, greater emphasis is needed on man-machine interface design. In day-to-day activities, the human frequently uses eye fixation or speech communication to interface with the world about him. Voice commands and head and eye position sensing as switching techniques may become commonplace. Such techniques have the potential to enhance performance

significantly when used in conjunction with tasks for which visual or voice modalities are "natural."

Based on current trends, the overall man-machine performance required for air combat success will soon outstrip the unaided capabilities of the pilot to perform essential tasks. For example, air-to-ground or air-to-air weapons delivery in conjunction with defensive maneuvering requires real-time solution of the equations of motion for three independent bodies. Terrain-following and terrain-masking maneuvers in night weather require the fusion of sensed data from several sources and the prediction of three-dimensional flight path trajectories optimized to avoid terrain obstacles while minimizing exposure to enemy sensors. To do these tasks at all, a high degree of automation is required. In future systems, automation strategy will become an essential part of the overall design process, when a new technology is being considered.

Modeling and the Design Process

In the most general sense, a model is an analytic description of an organized system. Because a design engineer is primarily interested in organizing a collection of components to construct a system, it is not surprising that models have found widespread application in the design process. The principal objective of man-machine modeling is to characterize the human in system terms. By capturing human behavior in a form suitable for mathematical manipulation, crew technology models provide an invaluable tool for performing man-machine analyses and for specifying human-factors design points.

Crew technology models can be classified into five general categories: inertial response models, injury response models, physiologic response models, work load models, and performance models. The models in each category are generally tailored to a common class of problems. Nevertheless, well-designed submodes often can be cascaded to provide a more global description of human behavior. Inertial response models are useful for the design of personnel seating and restraint systems, especially in conjunction with ejection seat development. When an inertial response model is cascaded with a biomechanical model defining bone, joint, and soft tissue properties, the result is an injury prediction model. Such models are used to specify injury limits for ejection seat and crash-impact protection system design. Physiologic response models provide a quantitative description of human tolerance to a variety of aviation stress environments. Models of this type are available to predict the physiologic effects of exposure to thermal extremes, hypoxia, altered atmospheres, vibration, air combat acceleration, aerobic exercise, and, in varying degrees, combinations of these stresses. Physiologic models are particularly useful in supporting personal protective equipment design and in prescribing operational safety limits.

The greatest challenge for tomorrow's model builders will be to advance the state-of-the-art in work load and performance modeling. A model is no better than the data base from which it is derived. The critical issue for work load and performance modeling is how to measure the constituent variables. Performance models have been developed to describe sensory and perceptual processes, cognitive functions, including decision-making, and motor functions, including discrete and continuous control operations. Unfortunately, a designer confronted with the task of specifying an optimal crew station usually needs a quantitative description of global human performance. With the current state of the art, available models still deal principally with human performance in a piecemeal manner. Examples of promising modeling initiatives likely to have an impact on future cockpit design are as follows:

Visual detection probability model
Manual control model
Dynamic decision model
Procedure-oriented crew model

The procedure-oriented crew model (PROCRU) is perhaps the best example of a model structure with sufficient generality to address several human functions as a single integrated system. The PROCRU model describes the human behavior that is required to achieve perceived goals by optimizing operator monitoring functions, decisions making, and control intervention in response to system dynamics and information inputs. Cascading the PROCRU model with target, threat, and weapons submodels will provide a means of predicting the impact of mission variables and system design alternatives on overall man-machine effectiveness.

Another perspective on how the human operator contributes to man-machine effectiveness is obtained through work load modeling. The concept of work load is difficult to define and has led to considerable confusion in the scientific community. Current evidence, however, suggests that work load is the complex interaction of task demands, coping capacity, coping cost, and criterion performance threshold. This relationship indicates that work load is high when the task is difficult, demanding intense effort to achieve the criterion performance required for a successful outcome. Investigations to date support the hypothesis that work load associated with combat operations can be measured and modeled using a battery of subjective, behavioral, and neurophysiologic tests. This is a critical technology that will have a profound effect on future crew technology contributions to military aviation.

As we look to the twenty-first century, the thrust of man-machine modeling will undoubtedly focus on the development of a general purpose "software pilot-assistant" equipped with a high-order level of artificial intelligence. The software pilot (embodying a mathematical description of the human operator) will be able to assume an ever-broader responsibility for accomplishing those missions that would place human health and well-being in jeopardy. The role of the human in future systems will then focus on defining goals, costs, and criteria for success, as well as disallowed options. Perhaps by that time, armed conflict itself will become a disallowed option.

THE FUTURE OF MAN IN SPACE

Exploration and Preparation

Only two decades have passed since the first human ventured into space. Man however, has already learned to live and function in this new environment for periods up to six months. This is not really surprising because space flight in many ways is a natural extension of high-Mach–number atmospheric flight. The pacing technologies are quite similar and the life-support requirements for passengers and crew tend to converge as the aircraft designer seriously contemplates flight hypersonic velocities. The nature of flight operations in true space does differ, however, in several important respects from flight operations in the sensible atmosphere. The following list describes some of the unique features of the space flight environment:

Infinitely large maneuvering volume
Sparse molecular medium
Mission duration largely independent of propulsive energy cost
Subject to the laws of orbital motion
Involves high velocities and global operations
Vehicle trajectory highly predictable
Weightless conditions
Vehicle/structure size can be quite large

Man is now on the threshold of a new era of space activity that will see extensive commercial and military utilization of space in the coming decades.

Advances in space propulsion and power are two critically important technologies required to achieve the full potential of manned operations in space. For the foreseeable future, barring a breakthrough in fusion power or antigravity technology, placing large payloads in earth orbit will depend on chemical rocketry. The two parameters that must be made large to achieve the required heavy-lift capability are the specific impulse and specific thrust of the engine. Specific impulse is directly proportional to the square root of combustion chamber temperature divided by the average molecular weight of the combustion products. Specific thrust increases in a complex manner as the product of combustion chamber temperature and the ratio of combustion chamber pressure to nozzle exit pressure increases. Figure 3–10 illustrates some of the options for future space propulsion. Clearly, with conventional fuel-oxidizer rocket engines, the relatively low achievable specific impulse is a severe constraint. With more exotic designs, such as a laser-hydrogen propulsion system, the combination of very high working temperatures and very low exhaust particle Z

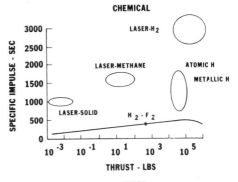

ADVANCED PROPULSION SYSTEMS

Fig. 3–10. Advanced propulsion systems.

number makes a tenfold increase in specific impulse theoretically possible. With increased propulsion performance, higher achievable payload fractions will make it economically feasible to transport into orbit sufficient material to construct large, permanent space stations.

An ability to generate substantial amounts of onboard power is the second critical requirement for operating a viable manned space station. Space vehicles in current use rely primarily on solar cells, fuel cells, and batteries. Batteries are best suited for supplying emergency power only. Fuel cells serve well as a source of power for life-support systems, communication equipment, and station-keeping services. Unfortunately, the operating lifetime of fuel cells will likely remain limited to a few months between major servicing and recharge.

For highly reliable, long-duration power generation, photovoltaic solar cells are extremely attractive. To produce significant power, however, large arrays are required. For example, a proposed design for a practical satellite solar power station with a 500-MW capacity requires two 10.4-mile^2 solar collector panels to capture the requisite amount of solar energy. Another approach for generating large quantities of power for long periods of time is to use nuclear reactors. In each case, however, many tons of material must be transported into space to build the power generation station, further underscoring the need for an efficient heavy-lift, earth-to-orbit transportation system.

Colonization and Space Enterprise

Manned space operations to date have been principally concerned with scientific investigation and lunar exploration. Unmanned satellite operations, on the other hand, have been far more extensive and are already providing profitable and essential services to the civilian and military sectors. An unmanned satellite is quite adequate to serve as a weather observatory, navigational or communications relay station, intelligence sensor platform, or even as an automated scientific laboratory. Even so, unmanned satellite systems are not well suited to carry out large-scale space operations such as earth power generation, materials processing, manufacturing, space defense, satellite repair, or complex research and development activities. For these missions, man will need to live and work in space for extended periods.

The industrialization of space has the potential to provide vast benefits to mankind. To move toward achieving this goal, a permanent orbiting research and development test center will be needed. Such a space complex initially will make possible definitive studies of human pathophysiologic responses to the space environment. Based on these studies, protective countermeasures can be identified to deal effectively with problems such as space asthenia, space sickness, and radiation hazards. Once man's physiologic capabilities are assured, assigned space test center personnel can devote their efforts to developing the special materials processing, manufacturing, and construction techniques needed to build a profitable space industry. The scientific benefits to be derived from a large manned space test center will unquestionably be great. Unique research opportunities will accrue in such areas as space physics, astronomic sciences, and earth sciences. The evolution of industry in space will become a major stimulus for developing space-adapted robots with high-order artificial intelligence. It is entirely reasonable to expect that intelligent robots will be used to perform most of the production, maintenance, and repair tasks needed to keep a space factory operating. Examples of space processing and manufacturing activities suitable for robot-managed operations include the production of ultrapure metals, flaw-free crystals, controlled-property alloys, microchips, biologic materials, and metal foam materials. The human operator will be needed, however, to supervise robot reprogramming (education), specialized robot repair and maintenance, and, of course, to intervene when anomalies occur requiring unprogrammed corrective action.

Once a significant level of space industry is established, the process of space colonization can proceed in earnest. Space mining operations to exploit mineral resources on the moon and from the asteroid belt will become practical. With the availability of both unlimited energy and virtually unlimited space material resources, the space colony could theoretically become largely self-sustaining, without needing to draw on terrestrial resources. In fact, the opposite would be more probable, with the space colony supplying power and manufactured products to the earth community. In this connection, it is not beyond reason to expect the benefits of space industry to favorably affect virtually all of the basic needs of modern society. The following is a list of the areas where space industry can enrich the quality of life:

Energy—solar power
Food production—earth resources
Education—telecommunication
Water supply—earth resources
Natural catastrophe control
   Weather prediction
   Earthquake prediction
Arms control-intelligence gathering
Pollution control—earth resources
Conservation—earth resources
Health—space processing

This chapter contains many speculations on the future of man in aerospace. How much of this speculation will become reality will only be discovered with the passage of time. The practitioner of the art and science of aerospace medicine, however, should never forget the words of Dr. Latham: "It is unwise to treat of any medical subject as if it were complete."

REFERENCES

1. Aviat. Week Space Technol., 115(19):86, Nov. 9, 1981.
2. Report of the President's Task Force on Aircraft Crew Complement. Washington, D.C., Government Printing Office, July 2, 1981.
3. Halaby, N.E.: Civilian uses of aerospace by the Federal Aviation Agency. Ann. N.Y. Acad. Sci., 134(1):5–10, Nov. 22, 1965.
4. Bisplinghoff, R.L.: Supersonic and hypersonic flight. Fourth International Symposium on Bioastronautics and Exploration of Space. Edited by C.H. Roadman, et al., Washington, D.C., Government Printing Office, Nov., 1968.
5. Gillies, J.A.: A Textbook of Aviation Physiology. Oxford, Pergamon Press, 1965.
6. Wallace, R.W., and Sandhaus, C.A.: Cosmic radiation exposure in subsonic air transport. Aviat. Space Environ. Med., 49(4):610–623, 1978.
7. Automation in Combat Aircraft. Committee on Automation in Combat Aircraft. Air Force Studies Board, Assembly of Engineering N.R.C. Washington, D.C., National Academy Press, 1982.

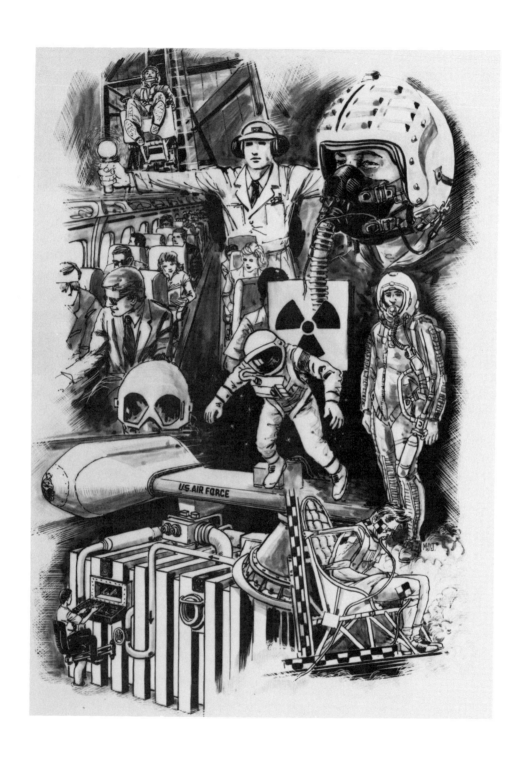

Section *II*

Physiology in the Flight Environment

The challenges to flight in the aerospace environment are many and varied. It is necessary for the aerospace physician to understand the components of that environment and the changes that occur as a result of aerospace flight activity. Man was created as a terrestrial being and must be protected as he ventures into the aerospace.

Man's demand for oxygen must be met or he becomes hypoxic. His vital physiologic functions require a pressure atmosphere. His sensory system is not adapted to rapid changes in acceleration nor, for that matter, to very gradual accelerative alterations. Mechanical forces, such as noise, vibration, and impact, can degrade the auditory sensory system or damage the musculoskeletal system. All of these stressors and more may impinge on the aviator or astronaut. Therefore, he must be protected, as must the passenger and the patient.

SUGGESTED READING LIST

1. Adler, H.F.: Dysbarism. Aeromedical Review 1–64. United States School of Aerospace Medicine, Brooks Air Force Base, Texas, 1964.
2. Benford, R.J.: Doctors in the Sky. Springfield, Illinois, Charles C. Thomas, 1955.
3. Benson, A.J., and Burchard, E.: Spatial Disorientation in Flight—A Handbook for Aircrew. AGARD-AG-170. Neuilly-sur-Seine, France, NATO/AGARD, 1973.
4. Dhenin, G. (ed.): Aviation Medicine. London, Tri-Med Books, Ltd., 1978.
5. Gillies, J.A.: A Textbook of Aviation Physiology. London, Pergamon Press, 1965.
6. Guyton, A.C.: Textbook of Medical Physiology. 6th Ed. Philadelphia, W.B. Saunders Co., 1981.
7. Harns, C.M. (ed.): Handbook of Noise Control. 2nd Ed. New York, McGraw-Hill Book Co., 1979.
8. Hanrahan, J.S., and Bushnell, D.: Space Biology: The Human Factors in Space Flight. New York, Basic Books, Inc., 1960.
9. Harris, C.M., and Crede, C.E. (eds.): Shock and Vibration Handbook. 2nd Ed. New York, McGraw-Hill Book Co., 1976.
10. Howard, I.P., and Templeton, W.B.: Human Spatial Orientation. New York, John Wiley and Sons, 1966.
11. Davis, J.C., and Hunt, T.K. (eds.): Hyperbaric Oxygen Therapy. Bethesda, Maryland, Undersea Medical Society, Inc., 1977.

61

12. Kryter, K.D.: The Effects of Noise on Man. New York, Academic Press, Inc., 1970.
13. Langham, W.L. (ed.): Radiobiological Factors in Manned Space Flight. Publication no. 1487. Washington, D.C., National Academy of Sciences, 1967.
14. National Aeronautics and Space Administration: Bioastronautics Data Book. NASA SP-3006, Washington, D.C., Government Printing Office, 1973.
15. National Aeronautics and Space Administration: Biomedical Results from Apollo. NASA SP-368, Washington, D.C., Government Printing Office, 1975.
16. National Aeronautics and Space Administration: Biomedical Results from Skylab. NASA SP-377, Washington, D.C., Government Printing Office, 1977.
17. Olsen, M.: Aviator's Breathing Oxygen Specifications. SAM-TR-76-44, Dec., 1976.
18. Payne, P.R.: The dynamics of human restraint systems. *In* Impact Acceleration Stress. National Research Council Publication no. 977, Washington, D.C., National Academy of Sciences, 1962.
19. Peters, R.A.: Dynamics of the Vestibular System and their Relation to Motion Perception, Spatial Disorientation, and Illusions. NASA CR-1309, Washington, D.C., National Aeronautics and Space Administration, 1969.
20. Bennett, P.B., and Elliott, D.H. (eds.): The Physiology and Medicine of Diving and Compressed Air Work. 2nd Ed. Baltimore, The Williams & Wilkins Co., 1975.
21. Proceedings of the Sonic Boom Symposium. Part 2. J. Acoust. Soc. Am., *31*:5, May, 1966.
22. Reason, J.R., and Brand, J.J.: Motion Sickness. New York, Academic Press, Inc., 1975.
23. Symposium of Biodynamic Models and Their Application. Aviat. Space Environ. Med., *49(1)*:109–348, 1978.
24. United States Naval Flight Surgeons Manual. Washington, D.C., Government Printing Office, 1978.
25. von Gierke, H.E., and Goldman, D.E.: Effects of shock and vibration on man. *In* Shock and Vibration Handbook. 2nd Ed. Edited by C.M. Harris and C.E. Crede. New York, McGraw-Hill Book Co., 1976.
26. Wagman, I.H., and Dong, W.K.: Principles of Biodynamics, Volume III: Physiological Mechanisms in the Mammal Underlying Posture, Locomotion, and Orientation in Space. Aeromedical Review 7–75. United States Air Force School of Aerospace Medicine, Brooks Air Force Base, Texas, 1975.
27. West, J.B.: Respiratory Physiology, 2nd Ed. Baltimore, Williams & Wilkins Co., 1979.
28. Zalesky, J., and Holden, D.: A Graphical Summary of Oxygen Regulator Performance. SAM-TR-75-12, U.S. Air Force School of Aerospace Medicine, San Antonio, TX, Apr., 1975.

Chapter 4

The Biosphere

B.E. Welch

Are virtue, courage, talent, wit, imagination—are all these qualities or faculties only a question of oxygen?

JULES VERNE

The biosphere, according to Webster's dictionary, is that part of the world in which life can exist, including parts of the lithosphere, hydrosphere, and atmosphere. This chapter will be concerned only with the atmosphere part of that definition, leaving any discussion of the lithosphere, the solid part of the earth, to that chapter dealing with accident investigation (Chapter 27) and the discussion of the hydrosphere, the aqueous part of the entire atmosphere, to those portions of the text addressing the problems of survival and thermoregulation (Chapter 30).

The atmosphere or the whole mass of air surrounding the earth serves many purposes, ranging from the aesthetics of the full moon rising over the horizon to the absorption of ultraviolet light from the sun. It is the stage on which weather plays and the milieu, at least relatively close to the surface of the earth, in which man lives. The atmosphere is both a constant and a variable, depending on the properties one is examining and the conditions and altitude limits under which that ex-

amination is made. In examining some of the properties of the atmosphere, it will be obvious that all of the atmosphere is not the biosphere, but that all of the biosphere is within and influenced by the atmosphere.

GAS LAWS

Any consideration of the atmosphere in terms of its physical properties, chemical composition, and physiologic suitability first requires an understanding of the basic and classic gas laws.

Boyle's Law

Boyle's Law, which has its origin in experiments conducted by Robert Boyle in the 1660s, states that "... when the temperature remains constant, the volume of a given mass of gas varies inversely as its pressure. . ." This law applies to all gases and may be expressed as follows:

$$\frac{V_1}{V_2} = \frac{P_2}{P_1} \tag{1}$$

where V_1 is the initial volume; V_2 is the

63

64 PHYSIOLOGY IN THE FLIGHT ENVIRONMENT

final volume; P_1 is the initial pressure; and P_2 is the final pressure.

For physiologic purposes, Boyle's Law can be considered a precise statement of facts. Under high-pressure situations, however, Boyle's Law is only an approximate statement of the facts because the attraction of the molecules for each other increases the effect of applied pressure and the space occupied by the molecules themselves, which decreases the effective volume.

It follows from Boyle's Law that ". . . at constant temperature, the density of a given mass of gas varies directly as its pressure. . . " This may be expressed as follows:

$$\frac{D_1}{D_2} = \frac{P_1}{P_2} \quad (2)$$

where D_1 is the initial density; D_2 is the final density; P_1 is the initial pressure; and P_2 is the final pressure.

Charles' Law

An additional development in the early formulation of the laws of ideal gases came from the French physicist Charles, who concluded that "When pressure is constant, the volume of a gas is very nearly proportional to its absolute temperature." This is expressed as follows:

$$\frac{V_1}{V_2} = \frac{T_1}{T_2} \quad (3)$$

where V_1 is the initial volume; V_2 is the final volume; T_1 is the initial absolute temperature; and T_2 is the final absolute temperature.

Likewise, when pressure is constant, it can be shown that density will vary inversely with temperature.

General Gas Law

Combining Boyle's and Charles' Laws to relate volume to both temperature and pressure results in the following equation:

$$\frac{P_1V_1}{T_1} = \frac{P_2V_2}{T_2} \quad (4)$$

It can be readily seen that if T_1 equals T_2, this is an expression of Boyle's Law. Likewise, if P_1 equals P_2, this is an expression of Charles' Law. Because both pressure and volume increase in proportion to the increase in temperature and these increases are equal, it is possible to express this equation as follows:

$$PV = RT \quad (5)$$

In this general gas equation, R is derived from P_2V_2, where P_2 and T_2 are standard pressure (760 mm Hg) and temperature (273°K) and V_2 is 22.4 L, the volume that a gram molecular weight (mole volume) occupies in the gaseous state under these conditions. More commonly, this equation is written as follows:

$$PV = nRT \quad (6)$$

where n is the number of moles. The typical values for R are as follows:

0.08205 L—atmosphere per degree per mole

82.05 cm³—atmosphere per degree per mole

62.36 L—mm Hg per degree per mole

8.314 × 10⁷ ergs per degree per mole

Dalton's Law

Dalton's Law deals with the pressure of a mixture of gases and states that ". . . the total pressure of a gas mixture is the sum of the individual or partial pressures of all the gases in the mixture. . . ." Thus,

$$P = P_1 + P_2 + P_3, \text{ and so forth} \quad (7)$$

where P is the total pressure of the gas mixture and P_1, P_2, and so on are the partial pressures of each gas in the mixture.

The partial pressure of each gas in the mixture is derived by the following equation:

$$P_1 = F_1 \times P \qquad (8)$$

where P_1 is the partial pressure of gas 1; F_1 is the fractional concentration of gas 1 in the mixture; and P is the total pressure of the gas mixture.

Henry's Law

Henry's Law deals with the solubility of gases in liquids and states that ". . . the quantity of gas dissolved in 1 cm^3 of a liquid is proportional to the partial pressure of the gas in contact with the liquid. . ." The absolute amount of any gas dissolved in liquid under conditions of equilibrium (i.e., the number of gas molecules entering and leaving the liquid per unit of time is equal) is dependent on the solubility of the gas in the liquid and the temperature, as well as the partial pressure of the gas. If a chemical reaction occurs between the gas and the liquid, Henry's Law does not apply.

CLASSIFICATION OF THE ATMOSPHERE

The physical and chemical properties of the atmosphere vary with altitude, although not each simultaneously nor in a consistent direction (i.e., either all increasing or decreasing). This fact has led to a system of nomenclature in which the atmosphere is considered to consist of several different groups of concentric, approximately spherical shells that are contiguous but have indistinct boundaries. The various shells within a group are normally distinguishable from each other by differences in such measurable parameters as temperature, composition, chemical reactions, and ionization phenomena. Wares and colleagues,[1] in *The Handbook of Geophysics*, have summarized these differ-

ences (Fig. 4–1) and provided a brief description of each shell (Table 4–1). The boundaries between these various shells are still being refined and, as will be pointed out in the discussion on temperature changes in the atmosphere, may vary with latitude and the season of the year. The name given to each shell within a group is composed of a root, somewhat indicative of the defining characteristic, and of the suffix *sphere*. The upper boundary of each shell has a name containing the same root but with the suffix *pause* following the root. For example, for the shell that all of us encounter on a daily basis the term troposhere is used, and for its upper boundary the term tropopause is used.

Standard Atmosphere

Because of actual atmospheric variability in the parameter being measured, as well as in the techniques being used to make the observation, numerous attempts have been made to define a standard atmosphere. The data used in this chapter have been largely obtained from information published by the United States Committee on Extension to the Standard Atmosphere and are contained in the United States Standard Atmosphere.[2,3,4] In the 1976 edition, the Committee adopted the World Meteorological Organization's (WMO) definition, as follows:

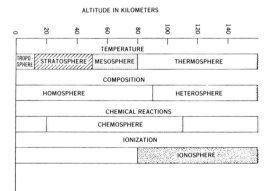

Fig. 4–1. Identification of atmospheric shells.

Table 4–1. Description of Atmospheric Shells

Name	Description
Temperature	
Troposphere	The region nearest the surface, which has a more or less uniform degree of temperature with altitude. The nominal rate of temperature decrease is 6.5°K/km, but inversions are common. The troposphere, the domain of weather, is in convective equilibrium with the sun-warmed surface of the earth. The tropopause, which occurs at altitudes between 6 and 19 km (higher and colder over the equator), is the domain of high winds and highest cirrus clouds.
Stratosphere	The region next above the troposphere, which has a nominally constant temperature. The stratosphere is thicker over the poles and thinner, or even nonexistent, over the equator. The maximum of atmospheric ozone is found near the stratopause. Rare nacreous clouds are also found near the stratopause. The stratopause is about 25 km altitude in middle latitudes. Stratospheric temperatures are in the order of arctic winter temperatures.
Mesosphere	The region of the first temperature maximum. The mesosphere lies above the stratosphere and below the major temperature minimum, which is found near 80 km altitude and constitutes the mesopause. This is a relatively warm region between two cold regions, and the region where most meteors disappear. The mesopause is found at altitudes of from 70 to 85 km. The mesosphere is in radiative equilibrium between ultraviolet ozone heating by the upper fringe of the ozone region and the infrared ozone and carbon dioxide cooling by radiation to space.
Thermosphere	The region of rising temperature above the major temperature minimum around the altitude of 80 km. There is no upper altitude limit. This is the domain of the auroras. Temperature rises at the base of the thermosphere are attributed to too infrequent collisions among molecules to maintain thermodynamic equilibrium. The potentially enormous infrared radiative cooling by carbon dioxide is not actually realized owing to inadequate collisions.
Composition	
Homosphere	The region of substantially uniform composition, in the sense of constant mean molecular weight from the surface upward. The composition changes here primarily because of the dissociation of oxygen. Mean molecular weight decreases accordingly. The ozonosphere, having its peak concentration near the stratopause altitude, does not change the mean molecular weight of the atmosphere significantly.
Heterosphere	The region of significantly varying composition above the homosphere and extending indefinitely outward. The "molecular weight" of air diminishes from 29 at about 90 km to 16 at about 500 km. Well above the level of oxygen dissociation, nitrogen begins to dissociate, and diffusive separation (lighter atoms and molecules rising to the top) sets in.
Chemical Reactions	
Chemosphere	The region where chemical activity (primarily photochemical) is predominant. The chemosphere is found within the altitude limits of about 20 to 110 km.
Ionization	
Ionosphere	The region of sufficiently large electron density to affect radio communication. However, only about one molecule in 1000 in the F_2 region to one molecule in 100,000,000 in the D region is ionized. The bottom of the ionosphere, the D region, is found at about 80 km during the day. At night the D region disappears, and the bottom of the ionosphere rises to 100 km. The top of the ionosphere is not well defined but has often been taken to be about 400 km. The upper limit has recently been extended upward to 1000 km based on satellite and rocket data.

...A hypothetical vertical distribution of atmospheric temperature, pressure and density which, by international agreement, is roughly representative of year-round midlatitude conditions. Typical usages are as a basis for pressure altimeter calibrations, aircraft performance calculations, aircraft and rocket design, ballistic tables and meteorologic diagrams. The air is assumed to obey the perfect gas law and hydrostatic equation which, taken together, relate temperature, pressure and density with geopotential. Only one standard atmosphere should be specified at a particular time and this standard atmosphere must not be subjected to amendment except at intervals of many years.

PHYSICAL AND CHEMICAL PROPERTIES OF THE ATMOSPHERE

Temperature

From a temperature point of view, the earth's atmosphere is typically divided into the troposphere, the stratosphere, the mesosphere, and the thermosphere. The troposphere, that layer closest to the ground, is complex, with that portion from ground level to approximately 2 km being significantly influenced by the earth's surface, vegetation, and water vapor. Above approximately 2 km is the advection portion of the troposphere, which is the mainstay of weather phenomena. The temperature of the troposphere decreases in a more or less linear fashion with increasing altitude until the boundary between the troposphere and the stratosphere is reached (Fig. 4–2). The boundary, or the tropopause, is reached at altitudes ranging from 8 km at high latitudes to 16 km at low latitudes. The temperature decrease, or lapse rate, although shown as a smooth line, varies not only with the latitude but also with the seasons of the year. This lapse rate is significant in that it induces rapid vertical mixing, which leads to turbulence, storms, and rainfall.

Above the tropopause is the stratosphere, an area extending to a height of about 50 km that is virtually cloudless and relatively quiescent. In contrast to the troposphere, temperatures in the stratosphere are either stable or increasing, thereby producing a permanent inversion

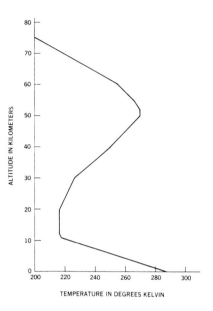

Fig. 4–2. Approximate ambient temperatures at varying altitudes at 0° latitude.

layer with greatly reduced vertical mixing. The increase in temperature in the stratosphere is largely due to the presence of ozone, which absorbs solar radiation and undergoes various chemical reactions, thereby injecting heat into the stratosphere. Although ozone is a minor constituent of the stratosphere, it is of considerable importance in terms of the overall thermal balance of the earth and because it controls the amount of ultraviolet radiation that reaches the earth's surface. The top of the stratosphere is termed the stratopause and is the transition zone to the mesosphere.

The mesosphere ranges from about 50 to 80 km above the earth's surface and is a zone of declining temperature. Above the mesosphere again is a pause zone, the mesopause, transitioning into the next layer, which is characterized thermally as the thermosphere and is a zone of increasing temperature. Although temperatures in this region are in excess of 1000°K, the density of the air in this region is so low that the general concept of temperature loses its meaning.

COMPOSITION OF THE ATMOSPHERE

The composition of the atmosphere is shown in Table 4–2.[2,3,4] These data were based on carbon[12] having an atomic weight of 12.0000; thus, the molecular weight of air is calculated to be 28.9644. This value is constant up to an altitude of approximately 90 km. Numerous photochemical reactions occur at altitudes as low as 20 km, but they do not significantly alter the molecular weight of air. From a biologic point of view, the composition also can be considered as constant, consisting naturally of a mixture of oxygen, nitrogen, argon, carbon dioxide, and several of the inert rare gases such as neon, helium, and krypton. Although the naturally occurring composition of air can be and is modified close to the surface of the earth by the products of human activity (a classic example being smog in the Los Angeles area basin), dry air is normally considered to have a composition of 20.95% oxygen, 78.08% nitrogen, 0.93% argon, and 0.03% carbon dioxide. Air in the areas of physiologic interest, that is, relatively near the earth's surface, also contains varying amounts of water vapor. As one ascends to higher altitude, the water vapor content decreases dramatically, with the stratosphere being virtually dry, having a water vapor content of a few parts per million.

Table 4–2. The Normal Composition of Clean, Dry Atmospheric Air Near Sea Level

Constituent	Content (%)*	Molecular Weight (g)†
Nitrogen	78.08	28.0134
Oxygen	20.95	31.9988
Argon	0.93	39.948
Carbon dioxide	0.03	44.00995
Neon	0.0018	20.183
Helium	0.0005	4.0026
Krypton	0.0001	83.80
Xenon	0.000009	131.30
Hydrogen	0.00005	2.01594
Methane	0.0002	16.04303

*The numbers will not add up to 100% due to rounding.
†Based on the carbon[12] isotope scale, for which C^{12} = 12.0000.

In addition to these normal constituents of the earth's atmosphere, one should also be aware of ozone and its implications on our climate.

Ozone

Ozone is produced in the upper atmosphere by the photodissociation of molecular oxygen, which is followed by the recombination of atomic oxygen with the oxygen molecule. This process is known to occur at a wavelength of approximately 200 nm, or the short ultraviolet frequencies. The normal destruction of ozone occurs as a consequence of the absorption of energy in the 210 to 290 nm range, or the long ultraviolet frequencies. This process of destruction liberates energy in the form of heat. Ozone density reaches a maximum at an altitude of some 22 km and is present in significant concentrations over a range of altitudes from about 10 to 35 km. The equilibrium of the formation and destruction of ozone has received intensive scrutiny in recent years due to concern that human activities, both on the earth's surface and in the stratosphere, could upset this balance and adversely affect our environment. Alteration of this ozone equilibrium to the negative side, resulting in an increased rate of destruction leading to lower ozone concentrations, would increase the level of ultraviolet radiation reaching the earth's surface. It is believed that relatively minor declines in the ozone concentration would lead to significant increases in the incidence of skin cancer.

PRESSURE

At sea level, the atmospheric pressure is, on the average, 760 mm Hg (760 torr), or 1013.2 millibars (mb). Sea level pressure is the pressure exerted by a 760-mm high column of mercury having a density of 13.5951 gm/cm^3 and subject to an acceleration due to gravity of 9.80665 m/sec^2. Increases in altitude result in a reduction of the barometric pressure (Table 4–3). In

Table 4–3. Altitude-Pressure-Temperature Relationships (United States Standard Atmosphere)

Altitude (m)	Pressure*		Temperature*	
	mb	torr	°K	°C
0	1013.25	760.00	288.15	15.00
100	1001.20	751.03	287.50	14.35
200	989.45	742.15	286.85	13.70
300	977.72	733.35	286.20	13.05
400	966.11	724.64	285.55	12.40
500	954.61	716.01	284.90	11.75
1000	898.76	674.12	281.65	8.50
2000	795.01	596.30	275.15	2.00
3000	701.21	525.95	268.66	−4.49
4000	616.60	462.49	262.17	−10.98
5000	540.48	405.40	255.68	−17.47
10,000	264.99	198.76	223.25	−49.90
15,000	121.11	90.85	216.65	−56.50
20,000	55.29	41.47	216.65	−56.50
25,000	25.49	19.12	221.55	−51.60
30,000	11.97	8.98	226.51	−46.64
40,000	2.87	2.15	250.35	−22.80
50,000	0.80	0.60	270.65	−2.50

*All numbers are rounded to the nearest second decimal.

addition to the effect of altitude on pressure, it should be noted that atmospheric pressure at any given altitude of interest in aviation is not constant, varying with the movement of high- and low-pressure centers, as well as with alterations in the energy absorbed by the atmosphere. This variation, although not particularly great in terms of mean monthly averages at sea level, can range from as low as 955 mb, in the case of an Icelandic low, to as high as 1055 mb, in the case of a Siberian high. At sea level, this 100-mb variation would be equivalent to approximately 853 m. The height increment, due to a 1-mb change in pressure, increases with increasing altitude. This increase has led to the use of standard pressures in aircraft flying above certain heights and the adjustment of the altimeter to airfield pressure in the preparation for landing.

Density

The density of a gas is defined as mass per unit of volume and in the Standard Atmosphere Table is expressed in kg/m³. At sea level, the density is 1.2250 kg/m³. With increasing altitude, density decreases in an exponential fashion in accordance with the perfect gas law when temperature is held constant. Thus, one would calculate that at approximately 5.5 km, the density would be one-half that at sea level, and at 11 km, the density would be one-quarter that at sea level, and so on. In actual practice, density does not decline this rapidly because the temperature is not constant from ground level up and also varies with the seasons and the location. In calculations in the United States Standard Atmosphere, the density equal to one-half that at sea level is reached at an altitude of approximately 6.65 km.

BIOSPHERIC PROPERTIES OF THE ATMOSPHERE

As noted earlier, all of the atmosphere is not the biosphere, but all of the biosphere is within the atmosphere. The unprotected human can make use of only a small portion of the atmosphere. Without clothes or some heat source for thermal protection, the thermal biosphere for man would end at an altitude of approximately 1000 m; without supplemental oxygen, the respiratory biosphere would extend (for a very small number of people and a short period of time) to the height of Mount Everest, or 8864 m. Without the pressurized aircraft cabin and even with supplemental oxygen, the biosphere would terminate at approximately 12,000 m. Thus, even though the physical aspects of the atmosphere can be described in great detail and over broad ranges, the functional limits for man in flight are reached at much lower altitudes. Beyond these functional limits, an environment is reached that Dr. Hubertus Strughold has called atmospheric space-equivalent conditions.[5]

Oxygen

As noted previously, the percentage composition of oxygen in the earth's atmosphere is virtually constant up to an altitude of about 90 km. The partial pressure (Dalton's Law) of oxygen, however, decreases with altitude as a function of decreasing total barometric pressure. The normal ambient oxygen partial pressure (P_{O_2}) of about 160 mm Hg at sea level is reduced to 80 mm Hg at 5.5 km, 40 mm Hg at 11 km, and so forth. In the alveoli, this reduction with decreasing pressure is of greater significance because of the presence of more or less constant partial pressures of both water vapor (47 mm Hg at the normal body temperature of 37°C) and carbon dioxide (40 mm Hg under normal ventilation conditions). Thus, according to the alveolar gas equation, the alveolar oxygen partial pressure $(P_{A_{O_2}})$ is about 100 mm Hg at sea level. At 523 mm Hg (3048 m), $P_{A_{O_2}}$ is around 33 mm Hg. Based on the results of various mountaineering expeditions as well as studies of people native to high-altitude regions of the world, it would appear that the limit for acclimatization or adaptation is in the range of 4572 to 5486 m. This range of total pressure breathing ambient air can, therefore, be considered as the first functional respiratory limit in the biosphere.

Breathing 100% oxygen raises this functional limit somewhat, but at an altitude of 15,240 m, or 87 mm Hg, the combined pressure of water vapor and carbon dioxide in the lung essentially equals the total barometric pressure. Physiologically, then, a point is reached where gas exchange is not possible. This point may be thought of as the dividing line between hypoxia and anoxia.

Pressure

Even if it were possible to provide respiratory support by means of pressure breathing above the 87-mm Hg limit, another functional physiologic limit would be reached at a barometric pressure of 47 mm Hg (19,202 m). At this pressure, the water vapor pressure of our body fluids equals the barometric pressure, and a phenomenon known as ebullism occurs. The manifestations of ebullism include bubble formation in the blood, mucous membranes of the mouth, and the conjunctiva of the eye, as well as a swelling of the skin due to diffuse bubble formation in the tissues. This functional limit can be circumvented only with full- or partial-pressure suits or by pressurized cabins.

Both of these solutions have finite limits. The suit solution has an altitude limit in the case of the partial-pressure suit and a time limit for wearing either of the garments. The pressurized cabin has a practical limit of 25 to 30 km due to the power required to compress the rarified atmosphere at those altitudes, as well as the difficult problem of rejecting the heat generated as a result of such compression.

Atmospheric Space-Equivalent Regions

The functional limits noted in this discussion on the biospheric properties of the atmosphere have led Strughold[5] to conclude that, although space as a physical environment reaches down to an altitude of some 200 km, as a physiologic environment it extends down as low as 20 km. One needs to be aware of these varying physiologic functional limits and recognize that support of the crewman is a complicated matter requiring a broad spectrum of responses.

REFERENCES

1. Handbook of Geophysics. Revised Edition. Edited by Campen, C.F. Jr., et al. New York, Macmillan, 1960.
2. United States Committee on Extension to the Standard Atmosphere: United States Standard Atmosphere. Washington, D.C., Government Printing Office, 1962.
3. United States Committee on Extension to the Standard Atmosphere: United States Standard Atmosphere Supplement. Washington, D.C., Government Printing Office, 1966.
4. United States Standard Atmosphere, 1976. Washington, D.C., Government Printing Office, 1976.
5. Randel, H.W. (ed.): Aerospace Medicine. 2nd Ed. Baltimore, Williams & Wilkins Co., 1971.

Chapter 5

Respiratory Physiology

Paul J. Sheffield and Richard D. Heimbach

A moralist, at least, may say, that the air which nature has provided for us is as good as we deserve.

Joseph Priestley

Man is highly adaptive and has demonstrated remarkably effective performance in a wide spectrum of aerospace and undersea environments. One of man's limitations involves respirable gases. In air, man's performance is most efficient in the environmental pressure existing between a depth of approximately 30 m of sea water, msw, to an altitude of 3048 m. A wider range of environments from deep undersea to the lunar surface, however, has been achieved by combining life-support systems, training, and human adaptation.

In both aerospace and undersea activities, life-support systems with artificial atmospheres are commonly used when breathing air is impractical. The oxygen concentration may be lower or higher than air. No inert gas may be present, or nitrogen may be replaced by helium or other gases. Barometric pressure may be subnormal in an aircraft or extremely high in a submerged diving compartment.

Deviation from the normal atmospheric environment can result in several physiologic problems involving respired gases. Hypoxia can occur when the partial pressure of oxygen (P_{O_2}) is reduced. Oxygen toxicity can occur if P_{O_2} is maintained at too high a level and breathed for too long a time. Carbon dioxide intoxication can occur in closed breathing-loop systems when CO_2 removal components fail. Decompression sickness results from bubbles in body tissues caused by inert gases that evolve from solution following decompression.

To understand the physiologic disturbances caused by these and other conditions, one must understand the physiology of respiration under both normal and abnormal environmental conditions.

THE RESPIRATORY PROCESS

Respiration is the process by which a living organism exchanges gases with its environment. The main function of respiration is to provide oxygen to and remove excess carbon dioxide from the cells of the body. The respiratory process also helps to maintain body temperature and the acid-base balance. Respiration can be divided into two processes. External respiration involves the ventilation of the lungs and the transfer of gases through the pulmonary membranes (alveolar and capillary) into the blood. Internal respiration is the process of transporting gases to and from the tissues and exchanging gases in the tissues. Gas exchange occurs in the following phases:

1. *Ventilation*—a cyclic process by which inhaled air is drawn into the alveoli and an approximately equal volume of pulmonary gas is exhaled. Some of the important conditions that interfere with the ventilation phase include exposure to reduced barometric pressure while breathing air, breathing gas mixtures with an insufficient oxygen pressure or concentration, pneumonia, atelectasis, and pneumothorax.

2. *Diffusion (lung)*—the process by which oxygen and carbon dioxide pass through the alveolar membrane and capillary walls. Examples of diffusion phase problems are emphysema, pneumonia, near-drowning, and pulmonary oxygen toxicity.

3. *Transportation*—the transfer of gases by the blood between the lungs and the tissues. Transportation problems are produced by anemia, hemorrhage, hemoglobin abnormalities, exposure to carbon monoxide, or restriction of blood flow.

4. *Diffusion (tissues)*—the process by which gases are exchanged between the blood and tissues. Examples of tissue diffusion phase problems are pH abnormalities and carbon monoxide poisoning.

5. *Utilization*—the chemical reactions within the cells that use oxygen to produce the energy needed to sustain life. This process is inhibited by carbon monoxide, ethyl alcohol, cyanide, and hydrogen sulfide.

A number of physical and physiologic conditions exist that interfere with gas exchange in the various phases of respiration and result in tissue hypoxia. These conditions are summarized in Table 5–1.

GAS EXCHANGE BETWEEN THE ATMOSPHERE AND BLOOD IN THE LUNGS

Functional Anatomy

The respiratory structure can be divided into two functional regions—the conductive airways and the gas-exchange region. The conductive airways contain the oral and nasal cavities, pharynx, larynx, trachea, and the first several branches of bronchi. The gas-exchange region contains the terminal bronchioles, respiratory bronchioles, and the alveolar ducts, which are lined with alveoli. Gas contained within the gas-exchange region is called alveolar gas. It is exchanged with blood through the alveolar-capillary membrane, which has a surface area of about 50 to 100 m². The gas-exchange region of the lung has a volume of about 2500 ml and contains most of the gas held in the lung.

Because no significant exchange of oxygen and carbon dioxide occurs in the conductive airway, the internal volume of the airway is called the anatomic dead space. The anatomic dead space, in milliliters, for an adult is about equal to his ideal weight in pounds. The anatomic dead space varies with sex and age. Measured in a reclining position, the mean anatomic dead space for young women is 104 ml; for young men, 156 ml; and for older men, 180 ml. The anatomic dead space may be reduced in asthma as a result of bronchial narrowing. It is enlarged by bronchiectasis or emphysema.

From the nasopharynx, air passes through the pharynx, where it is humidified and warmed. The air next enters the larynx and trachea and passes into two branches known as bronchi that distribute the gas to each lung. The bronchi repeatedly subdivide into smaller bronchi until

Table 5–1.　Conditions That Interfere With Gas Exchange in the Various Phases of Respiration

Phase of Respiration	Condition	Specific Cause	Type of Hypoxia
Ventilation	Reduction in alveolar P_{O_2}	Breathing air at reduced barometric pressure Strangulation/respiratory arrest/laryngospasm Severe asthma Breathholding Hypoventilation Breathing gas mixtures with insufficient P_{O_2} Malfunctioning oxygen equipment at altitude	Hypoxic hypoxia
	Reduction in gas exchange area	Pneumonia Drowning Atelectasis Emphysema (chronic lung disease) Pneumothorax Pulmonary embolism Congenital heart defects Physiologic shunting	Hypoxic hypoxia
Diffusion	Diffusion barriers	Hyaline membrane disease Pneumonia Drowning	Hypoxic hypoxia
Transportation	Reduction in oxygen-carrying capacity	Anemias Hemorrhage Hemoglobin abnormalities Drugs (sulfanilamides, nitrites) Chemicals (cyanide, carbon monoxide)	Hypemic hypoxia
	Reduction in systemic blood flow	Heart failure Shock Continuous positive pressure breathing Acceleration (G forces) Pulmonary embolism	Stagnant hypoxia
	Reduction in regional or local blood flow	Extremes of environmental temperatures Postural changes (prolonged sitting, bed rest, or weightlessness) Tourniquets (restrictive clothing, straps, and so forth) Hyperventilation Embolism by clots or gas bubbles Cerebral vascular accidents	Stagnant hypoxia
Utilization	Metabolic poisoning or dysfunction	Respiratory enzyme poisoning or degradation Carbon monoxide Cyanide Alcohol	Histotoxic hypoxia

they reach a diameter of approximately 1 mm. Cartilaginous structures of the walls disappear, and the smaller air passages are called bronchioles. The bronchioles continue to branch until they become alveolar ducts, which lead to the alveolar sacs. The septa that separate the alveoli have an excellent capillary network. Here, the air and blood meet to carry on the process of gas exchange.

In addition to the lung's role in gas exchange and metabolism, it also functions as a biologic barrier between man and the environment. The airways and lung parenchyma prevent the entry of or remove injurious particles so that the lung is sterile as the air reaches the terminal lung units. Filtration begins in the nose, where particles larger than 10 μm and smaller than 0.5 μm are removed. As the airstream changes directions sharply in the nasal pharynx, the majority of the remaining particles of about 10 μm impact on the posterior wall of the pharynx. Particles of

0.1 μm and smaller are deposited mainly as a result of Brownian motion because of their constant bombardment by gas molecules. The epithelial surface of the trachea and bronchi contains mucous-secreting goblet cells and mucous-secreting glands that distribute a layer of mucus over the surface of ciliated cells, which extend out to the terminal bronchiole, or sixteenth generation of airways. This layer of mucus is continuously moved by the action of the underlying cilia from the places of production up through the trachea, where the mucus is then swallowed or expectorated. This system, known as the mucociliary escalator, is the mechanism by which particles deposited on the airway surface down to the size of about 5.0 μm are removed.

Lungs of older individuals who have worked in dusty trades contain a residue of particles that have been deposited in the lung over several years. Autopsy findings have shown that approximately half of the particles are smaller than 0.5 μm in diameter. Of those that were larger, almost all were between 0.5 and 5.0 μm in diameter. Fibers, for the most part, were observed to be less than 50 μm long and 3 μm in diameter, although occasional fibers were as long as 200 μm. Asbestos fibers up to 300 μm long have been found in alveoli, suggesting that the aerodynamic property of asbestos fibers allows them to orient themselves parallel to the airstream and behave in a manner similar to that of particles of about 1 μm in diameter.

Composition of Respired Air

The composition of respired air varies at different sites in the respiratory process. Table 5–2 lists the gas tensions in a normal person at rest when air is breathed at sea level. Because gas molecules move by diffusion from a region of higher concentration to a region of lower concentration, the partial-pressure gradients are responsible for the entire gas exchange between the atmosphere, alveoli, blood, and tissues. No active gas-transfer mechanisms exist anywhere in the respiratory process.

At sea level, the atmospheric pressure is approximately 760 mm Hg. Excluding the rare gases of the atmosphere, air is composed principally of nitrogen, oxygen, and a small amount of carbon dioxide. The rare gases, i.e., argon and krypton, appear to have no biologic significance and are included in the values for nitrogen. As air passes through the respiratory tract, it is warmed or cooled, cleansed, and humidified by the mucous membranes. The air is saturated with water vapor by the time it reaches the trachea. At a body temperature of 37°C, water vapor exerts a pressure of 47 mm Hg. Water vapor pressure varies with the existing body temperature. In extremes of body temperature, such as fever and hypothermia, water vapor pressure is considerably altered, as shown in Table 5–3. When calculations are used for gas partial pressures, water vapor must be subtracted from the total pressure. Thus, at sea level, the total pressure of the dry gases in the alveoli is 713 mm Hg (760 mm Hg − 47 mm Hg).

Pulmonary Ventilation

Ventilation is the exchange of gases between the environment and the blood in the lungs. It primarily involves the exchange of oxygen and carbon dioxide. The lung, however, also acts as a reservoir of blood and filters certain toxic materials from the pulmonary circulation such as bubble nuclei, blood thrombi, and biologically active agents like bradykinin and serotonin.

Under normal conditions, respiration is a subconscious process that occurs at a rate of 12 to 20 breaths/min, averaging 16 breaths/min. With some conditions in aerospace operations (i.e., positive pressure breathing, sustained G forces, gastrointestinal tract distention following rapid decompression, and immersion in water to the neck), however, the breathing rate is

Table 5–2. Composition of Respired Air at Sea Level

Respiratory Gas	Gas Partial Pressure (mm Hg)				
	O_2	CO_2	N_2	H_2O	Total
Inspired ambient air	159	0.3	595	5.7	760
Tracheal air	149	0.3	563.7	47	760
Expired air	116	32	565	47	760
Alveolar air	100	40	573	47	760
Arterial blood	95	40	573	47	755
Venous blood	40	46	573	47	706
Tissues	40 or less	46 or more	573	47	706 or less

Table 5–3. Effect of Body Temperature on Water Vapor Pressure

Body Temperature (°C)	Water Vapor Pressure (P_{H_2O} in mm Hg)
40 Fever	55.3
37 Normal	47.1
35 Hypothermia	42.2
30 Hypothermia	31.8
25 Hypothermia	23.8
20 Hypothermia	17.5

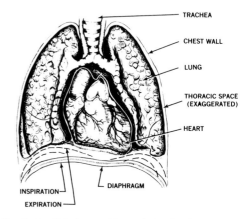

Fig. 5–1. Relative positions of the diaphragm during inhalation and exhalation.

altered, and one must make a conscious effort to breathe.

Because the lungs communicate freely with outside air and the thorax is a closed cavity, any change in thoracic volume will result in a change in lung volume. Inhalation is accomplished by contracting or lowering the diaphragm and elevating the ribs. When the diaphragm contracts, it becomes flattened and loses its dome-shaped appearance, thus increasing the top-to-bottom dimension of the thorax, as shown in Figure 5–1. Concomitantly, the external intercostal muscles contract, thereby elevating the rib cage and increasing the front-to-back dimension of the thorax. The result is an overall increase in thoracic volume and a drop in intrathoracic pressure (Boyle's Law) in the range of 4 to 9 mm Hg below atmospheric pressure. At sea level, this change would be equal to an intrathoracic pressure of 756 to 751 mm Hg during a normal inhalation. A pressure differential is thus created between the lung interior and ambient air. Because air will move from an area of higher pressure to one of lower pressure, air rushes into the lungs until the intrapulmonic pressure

again equals the ambient air pressure. When the lung reaches a certain degree of expansion, specialized stretch receptors provide inhibiting impulses via the vagus nerve to inhibit central respiratory activity (Hering-Breuer reflex). The inspiratory phase of respiration is then complete, and the lung passively recoils to its resting position.

Upon completion of inhalation, the intrapulmonic pressure is equal to the ambient pressure (760 mm Hg at sea level) and the intrathoracic pressure is about 9 mm Hg below ambient pressure (751 mm Hg at sea level).

During normal respiration, exhalation is largely passive because little muscular activity is required to assist in the process. During normal, quiet exhalation, the inflated lungs return to their original position by virtue of the elastic recoil of the tissue. Simultaneously, the diaphragm relaxes. Because of tissue recoil, the volume within the lung is decreased. Consequently, intrapulmonic pressure increases, producing a momentary pressure differential between the lung and outside air. This time, the greater pressure is within the lung (about 3 mm Hg above atmospheric pressure), and air moves from the lung to the environment.

If the expiratory muscles are needed to exhale, exhalation becomes active. This active exhalation is seen in aerospace operations when one experiences positive pressure breathing (forced, voluntary effort to exhale) or when one must use a straining maneuver during sustained G forces. Under normal conditions, however, inhalation is active and exhalation is passive.

During strenuous exercise, both rib cage and diaphragm activity are coordinated to meet the body's demand for increased lung ventilation. At rest, an individual requires 200 to 250 ml of oxygen per minute; however, this value is increased twentyfold (5500 ml) during maximal exercise. During vigorous exercise, contracting muscles depress the ribs, force the viscera up against the diaphragm, and move the diaphragm further up into the thorax. By reducing the internal volume of the lung, this action markedly increases the intrapulmonic pressure and allows a greater volume of air to be expired. The consequent increase in the rate and depth of respiration permits greater and more frequent lung ventilation to eliminate carbon dioxide and meet the increased oxygen needs of body tissues.

During heavy exercise, the muscles require about 50 times more oxygen than they need at rest. This increase is achieved by three mechanisms: a sixfold increase in cardiac output, from 5 L/min to 30 L/min; a threefold increase in circulating blood, which is diverted from the spleen and kidneys to the skin and muscles; and a threefold increase in oxygen released from

hemoglobin, due to a shift in the oxyhemoglobin dissociation curve.

Lung Measurements

For both physiologic and clinical purposes, the ventilatory function of the lung has been divided into functional volume measurements. These lung volumes are defined as follows:

1. *Tidal volume*—the volume of air inspired and expired with each normal breath (about 500 ml).

2. *Inspiratory reserve volume*—the extra volume of air that can be inspired above the normal tidal volume by a conscious, forceful inspiration (about 3100 ml).

3. *Expiratory reserve volume*—the volume of air that can be expired by a forceful expiration after the end of a normal tidal expiration (about 1200 ml).

4. *Residual volume*—the volume of air in the lungs that cannot be exhaled (about 1200 ml).

Table 5–4 lists the approximate lung volumes in healthy subjects 20 to 30 years of age. Figure 5–2 shows that the total capacity of the lungs is equal to the sum of the four volumes just defined. The capacities of the lung are important because they

Table 5–4. Lung Volumes in Healthy Subjects 20 to 30 Years of Age

Functional Measurements	Approximate Values (ml)	
	Males	Females
Tidal volume (TV)	500	450
Inspiratory reserve volume (IRV)	3100	1950
Expiratory reserve volume (ERV)	1200	800
Residual volume (RV)	1200	1000
Inspiratory capacity (IC)	3600	2400
Functional residual capacity (FRC)	2400	1800
Vital capacity (VC)	4800	3200
Total lung capacity (TLC)	6000	4200

Modified from Comroe, J.H., Jr.: Physiology of Respiration. Chicago, Yearbook Medical Publishers, Inc., 1965.

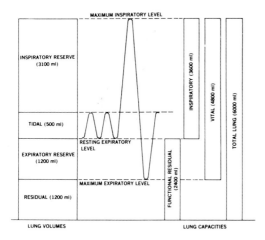

Fig. 5–2. Lung measurements.

represent the functional combinations of these volumes and are defined as follows:

1. *Inspiratory capacity*—the tidal volume plus the inspiratory reserve volume. The amount of air that one can inspire, beginning with the end of a normal expiration and forcibly inspiring to the maximum extent (about 3600 ml).
2. *Functional residual capacity*—the residual volume plus the expiratory reserve volume. The amount of air left in the lungs at the end of a normal expiration (about 2400 ml).
3. *Vital capacity*—the sum of the expiratory reserve volume, the tidal volume, and the inspiratory reserve volume. The amount of air the lungs can hold between the limits of a maximum forceful inspiration and a maximum forceful expiration (about 4800 ml).
4. *Total lung capacity*—the sum of the four lung volumes. The total capacity of the lungs to hold air (about 6000 ml).

With the exception of functional residual capacity, total lung capacity, and residual volume, measurements of all lung volumes and capacities can be made with a spirometer or similar recording device.

The values given for the lung volumes and capacities are approximations only because the values are affected by the age, sex, height, and weight of the subject. More accurate values may be calculated for individual subjects by using regression formulas that take these variables into account.

The amount of air inspired per minute is known as respiratory minute volume. It is normally about 6 to 8 L/min. The maximum breathing capacity, the largest volume of gas that can be moved into and out of the lungs in 1 minute, is about 125 to 170 L/min.

Peak inspiratory flow is an important consideration in the design of oxygen masks and regulators. As a rule of thumb, peak inspiratory flow can be determined by multiplying respiratory minute volume by a factor of 3. Thus, a respiratory minute volume in the working individual of 10 L/min would produce a peak inspiratory flow of 30 L/min.

Response to Lack of Oxygen

Table 5–5 indicates little respiratory response when hypoxic oxygen concentrations of 12 to 21% are breathed for 8 to 10 minutes but a powerful respiratory response when oxygen concentrations of 4 to 8% are breathed. At an inspired oxygen concentration of 4.2% (equivalent to breathing ambient air at 11,735 m), the respiratory rate doubles and respiratory minute volume increases by a factor of 4.

Exposure to Altitude

Table 5–6 shows the effect of acute exposure to altitude on ventilation. The threshold for increased ventilation is first seen on ascent at about 1524 m. Ventilatory changes are small until about 3658 m. Tidal volume progressively increases, but there are relatively small changes in respiratory rate until an altitude is reached where hypoxic stimulation is maximal. At 6706 m, the respiratory rate increases and minute volume is almost doubled. Hyper-

Table 5–5. Effect of Inspired Oxygen Concentration on Pulmonary Ventilation

Oxygen Concentration in Inspired Air (%)	Tidal Volume (ml)	Respiratory Rate (breaths/min)	Respiratory Minute Volume (L/min)	Alveolar Ventilation (L/min)
21	500	14	7.0	4.9
18	500	14	7.0	4.9
16	536	14	7.5	5.4
12	536	14	7.5	5.4
10	593	14	8.3	6.2
8	812	16	13.0	10.4
4.2	933	30	28.0	23.2

Modified from Comroe, J.H., Jr.: Physiology of Respiration. Chicago, Yearbook Medical Publishers, Inc., 1965.

Table 5–6. Effect of Acute Exposure to Altitude on Pulmonary Ventilation

Pulmonary Function	Altitude in Meters				
	Sea Level	3658	5486	6706	7620
Minute Volume (L/min)*	8.5	9.7	11.1	15.3	—
Respiratory Rate (per minute)*	12.0	14.0	12.0	15.0	—
Tidal Volume (L)*	0.71	0.69	0.92	1.02	—
Alveolar P_{O_2}	103.0	54.3	37.8	32.8	30.4
Alveolar P_{CO_2}	40.0	33.8	30.4	28.4	27.0

Note: The ascent was accomplished at 1372 m/min. The subjects remained at altitude for 30 to 60 minutes. Minute volume and respiratory rate are average values. The tidal volume was calculated.

*Adapted from Rahn, H., and Otis, A.B.: Alveolar air during simulated flights to high altitudes. Am. J. Physiol., 150:202,1947.

ventilation reduces the partial pressure of carbon dioxide, P_{CO_2}, causing respiratory alkalosis, and a shift of the oxyhemoglobin dissociation curve to the left, thus allowing more oxygen to bind with hemoglobin for transport to the tissues.

Alveolar Ventilation

It is estimated that at birth an infant's lungs contain about 30 million alveoli. At 8 years of age, this number increases to about 300 million. After this age, the number of alveoli do not increase, but they do continue to increase in size until the individual is mature. The diameter of the alveolus is about 0.1 to 0.4 mm, and the wall thickness is about 0.1 μm.

Alveoli resemble minute, communicating bubbles of gas in the lung fluid. The pressure (P) exerted by the surface tension of a bubble in a liquid is determined by Laplace's Law, as follows:

$$P = \frac{2T}{r} \quad (1)$$

where T is the surface tension and r is the bubble radius. As exhalation occurs and the alveolar radius decreases, the alveolus tends to collapse completely. Uncountered, this process would result in atelectasis, and respiration could not continue. To counter this problem, specialized cells lining the alveoli, type II Clara cells, secrete a lipoprotein, dipalmitoyl lecithin, which profoundly lowers the surface tension of the alveolar lining fluid and is known as pulmonary surfactant.

As the volume of an alveolus increases or decreases, so does its surface area. On exhalation there is an increase in the thickness of the surfactant film lining the alveolus. The result is a decrease in the tendency to collapse as the alveolar "bubble" becomes smaller. On inhalation, the surface area of the alveolus increases, which decreases the thickness of the surfactant film on the membrane. This process increases the surface tension and prevents overdistension of the alveolus. Thus, pulmonary surfactant reduces the tendency of small alveoli to empty into large ones during exhalation and prevents overdistension of the alveoli during inhalation. Its presence decreases the stiffness of the lung, reducing the effort required to ventilate. It also reduces the force that tends to draw fluid from the blood into the lung.

Ventilation of the alveoli occurs primarily by diffusion. Diffusion is rapid and the distance involved so small that complete mixing of gas within an alveolus occurs in less than 1 second. Dead space volume and tidal volume are important factors in determining the amount of alveolar ventilation. At the end of normal expiration, the conducting airway is filled with "alveolar gas" that has a P_{O_2} of 100 mm Hg rather than the 149 mm Hg in fresh air. Using Figure 5–3 for illustrative purposes, one can assume that the anatomic dead space is 150 ml and the volume of the next inspiration (tidal volume) is 500 ml. The alveoli receive 500 ml of gas, but its composition differs from that of fresh air entering the nose. The alveoli first receive the residual 150 ml from the conducting airway, which does not raise al-

veolar P_{O_2} or lower alveolar P_{CO_2} because it is "alveolar gas." The alveoli then receive 350 ml of fresh air. The remaining 150 ml of fresh air remains in the conducting airway at end-inspiration. Thus, the gas that is expired consists of a mixture of inspired air from the dead space and alveolar air and has a composition that is intermediate between the two.

Alveolar-Arterial Gas Exchange

The overall passage of oxygen from the alveolus to the blood involves two distinct steps in a continuous process: physical diffusion through the membrane followed by chemical combination of oxygen with hemoglobin. The amount of oxygen transferred across the alveolar-capillary membrane depends primarily on the oxygen pressure differential. Thus, the efficiency of diffusion is reduced in the presence of a low alveolar oxygen pressure. Furthermore, when the alveolar capillary membrane becomes thickened, as in pulmonary disease, gas exchange is impaired even though alveolar ventilation is normal.

The surface area of the alveolar-capillary membrane is 50 to 100 m², 40 times the surface area of the body. Its thickness is 0.1 to 0.5 µm. Resistance to gas diffusion between the lung and the blood is minimized by the large lung surface area and the thinness of the membrane. The network of capillaries around the alveoli is so dense and the capillary segments so short and narrow that there is an almost continuous sheet of blood over the alveolar wall. In the resting adult male, about 140 ml of pulmonary capillary blood is surrounded by approximately 2000 ml of alveolar air. Resistance to flow through the pulmonary bed is so low that the heart can drive 5 to 10 L of blood through the lungs with a driving pressure of less than 15 mm Hg. Pulmonary blood flow ranges from 4 L/min in a resting man to 30 to 40 L/min during heavy exercise.

Figure 5–4 illustrates four pathways

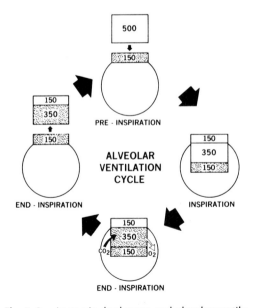

Fig. 5–3. Anatomic dead space and alveolar ventilation.

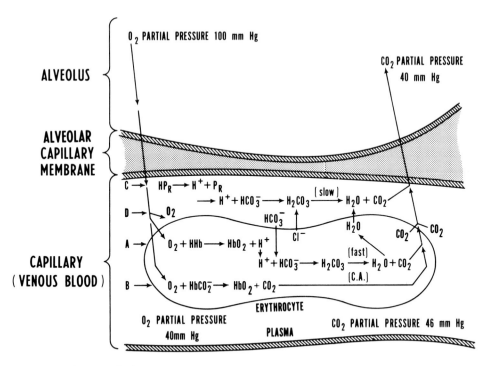

Fig. 5–4. Gas exchange in the lungs.

used to exchange oxygen and carbon dioxide in the lung. As shown in pathway A, oxygen diffuses through the plasma and into the red blood cell because of a pressure differential of 60 mm Hg. There, hemoglobin rapidly combines with oxygen to form an oxygenated compound called oxyhemoglobin (HbO_2). In the process, an ion of hydrogen ($H+$) is released. The greater the number of hydrogen ions in a solution, the more acidic the solution becomes. Rapid shifts in acidity are prevented by bicarbonate ions (HCO_3^-). HCO_3^- rapidly diffuses from the blood plasma into the red blood cell and combines with the $H+$ to form carbonic acid (H_2CO_3). This very weak acid is immediately acted on by a catalytic enzyme known as carbonic anhydrase, which breaks the H_2CO_3 molecule into molecular water and carbon dioxide. The water diffuses out into the plasma. The carbon dioxide, having a higher partial pressure than alveolar air, diffuses into the alveolus.

In pathway B, the carbon dioxide is brought from the tissues in a form called carbaminohemoglobin ($HbCO_2$). Because hemoglobin has a stronger affinity for oxygen than carbon dioxide, O_2 replaces CO_2 on the hemoglobin. Like the carbon dioxide released from H_2CO_3, it also diffuses into the alveolus.

In pathway C, plasma protein buffers, which insure a constant plasma pH, tend to release hydrogen ions due to a slight increase in the alkalinity of the plasma. When this occurs, $H+$ immediately combines with the available HCO_3^- to form H_2CO_3. This reaction is relatively slow because the catalytic enzyme, carbonic anhydrase, is not present in the plasma to speed the reaction. As in the other pathways, the carbon dioxide that is released diffuses into the alveolus because of the partial-pressure gradient. As carbon dioxide is lost, oxygen is gained.

In pathway D, oxygen enters the plasma, where it is transported in physical solution.

TRANSPORT OF GAS BY BLOOD

The red blood cell traverses the alveolus in approximately 0.75 seconds. Thus, gas transfer must occur rapidly. The transfer rate depends on both physical diffusion and the speed of chemical reactions in the blood. After diffusing through the alveolar and capillary membranes, the gas molecule must pass through plasma in the pulmonary capillary, the wall of the red blood cell, and part of the intracellular fluid of the red blood cell before entering into chemical union with hemoglobin.

Several physical factors influence the diffusion rate of a gas: differences in the partial pressure of the gas, solubility of the gas in the fluid, temperature, and the molecular weight of the gas. Under normal conditions, except for the difference in partial pressure, all of these factors remain constant for a given gas. Thus, the partial pressure of the gas determines the direction and degree of gas exchange. Diffusion, however, is greatly enhanced by four physiologic conditions: (1) the rapid circulatory renewal of blood in the gas-permeable capillaries of the lung and metabolizing tissues; (2) the rapid chemical reactions involving respiratory gases when they enter the blood; (3) the existence of specific enzymes that accelerate oxygen uptake by metabolizing cells and also accelerate the combination of carbon dioxide and water in the blood; and (4) mechanisms to adjust circulation and alveolar ventilation to meet metabolic requirements.

Inert gas (nitrogen), oxygen, and carbon dioxide are transported by the blood by various methods. Nitrogen is transported entirely in physical solution. Only 1.5% of oxygen is transported physically dissolved in the plasma, whereas 98.5% of oxygen is chemically combined with hemoglobin. About 6% of carbon dioxide is transported in physical solution, about 22% is combined with carbamino compounds such as hemoglobin, and about 72% is carried as carbonic acid or bicarbonate ions in the blood buffer system.

Nitrogen

Nitrogen is biologically inert and acts as a diluent gas. Although not involved in any known metabolic activity, it is found in solution in all body tissues and is exchanged at a constant ratio of 1:1 unless there is a pressure change on the body.

Henry's Law indicates that the degree to which a gas enters into physical solution in body fluids is directly proportional to the partial pressure of the gas to which the fluid is exposed. Thus, the partial pressure of nitrogen decreases in the alveoli during the ascent to altitude. This process reduces the quantity of nitrogen that dissolves in the plasma for transport throughout the body. The reverse of this process occurs during descent, when the partial pressure of nitrogen is less in the plasma than in the alveoli. Henry's Law defines only the relative quantity of gas entering solution as related to gas partial pressures and does not define the absolute amount of gas in physical solution. The absolute amount is determined by the solubility coefficient of the gas in a fluid. Solubility coefficients vary with different fluids and are temperature-dependent.

Nitrogen solubility in plasma at 37°C is 0.0088 ml of N_2/100 ml of plasma/mm Hg P_{AN_2}. It is five times more soluble in fat than in water. When pressure changes occur on the body, nitrogen can produce the adverse effects of decompression sickness.

Oxygen

The solubility of oxygen in plasma at 37°C is 0.0028 ml of O_2/100 ml of plasma/mm Hg P_{AO_2}. The solubility of oxygen in whole blood at 37°C is 0.0031 ml of O_2/100 ml of blood/mm Hg P_{AO_2}. When air is breathed at sea level, arterial oxygen tension is approximately 95 mm Hg, and the blood transports approximately 0.3 ml of O_2/100 ml of blood, or 0.3 vol%. The amount of dissolved oxygen can be increased to 2 vol% if 100% oxygen is breathed at sea level. Because solubility is pressure-dependent, the amount of dissolved oxygen is reduced by ascent to altitude and increased by descent below sea level.

The oxyhemoglobin dissociation curve forms a typical sigmoid curve (Fig. 5–5). The shape of the curve is ideally suited to meet human physiologic requirements. The oxygen tension normally present in the alveolar gas produces almost complete hemoglobin saturation. On the upper part of the curve, large changes in P_{O_2} have only a slight effect on hemoglobin saturation. This fact is of particular importance to the aviator who ascends to altitude. Conversely, the low P_{O_2} that exists in the tissues serves to enhance oxygen release from hemoglobin. From the slope of the oxyhemoglobin dissociation curve it can be seen that hemoglobin releases abundant oxygen to the tissues with only a small decrease in oxygen tension.

The ability of hemoglobin to combine with oxygen varies with both acidity and oxygen partial pressure. The normal physiologic curve shown in Figure 5–5 is for a pH of 7.40, which corresponds to a P_{CO_2} of 40 mm Hg. The carbon dioxide content of the blood exerts a significant influence on the oxyhemoglobin dissociation curve. An increase in P_{CO_2} shifts the dissociation curve to the right, whereas a decrease in P_{CO_2} shifts the curve to the left. This influence of carbon dioxide is largely a consequence of changes in pH, and similar changes can be produced by other acids. The influence of hydrogen ion concentration on the dissociation curve is known as the Bohr effect.

The influence of carbon dioxide on the oxyhemoglobin dissociation curve is of considerable physiologic significance. In the lung, as carbon dioxide is released, the curve is shifted to the left so that, at a given P_{O_2}, more oxygen combines with hemoglobin. In the region of the systemic capillaries, increased tissue acidity shifts the

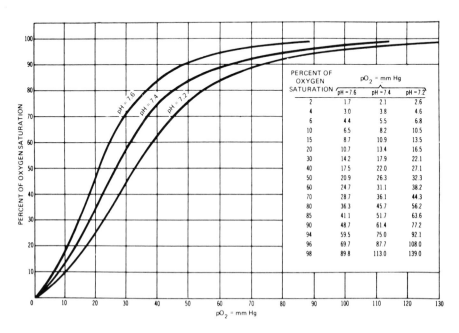

Fig. 5–5. Oxyhemoglobin dissociation curves for human blood.

curve to the right, potentiating oxygen off-loading. Tissue P_{O_2} is less than the arterial P_{O_2}, resulting in removal first of plasma (nonhemoglobin) oxygen to the tissues by simple diffusion down the pressure gradient. The loss of plasma oxygen decreases plasma P_{O_2}, and oxygen is released from hemoglobin because the association of oxygen with hemoglobin depends on the plasma P_{O_2}. Oxygen diffuses from the hemoglobin to plasma and into the tissues until a pressure gradient no longer exists.

The red blood cell contains high levels of organic phosphate 2,3-diphosphoglyceric acid (2,3-DPG). This compound combines with reduced hemoglobin and decreases the affinity of hemoglobin for oxygen over the middle range of oxygen tensions. The more 2,3-DPG present, the more oxygen will be released at a given oxygen tension. Hypoxia increases the 2,3-DPG in cells and thus increases the oxygen offloading from hemoglobin when the blood arrives at the tissues.

The oxyhemoglobin dissociation curve also is influenced by temperature. As temperature rises, the curve shifts to the right. The physiologic value of this effect is realized during exercise. As the temperature of the active muscles increases, the release of oxygen to the muscles increases. During cold exposure, when the temperature of the muscles decreases, the curve shifts to the left, and less oxygen is released from hemoglobin.

Carbon Dioxide

The solubility of carbon dioxide in plasma at 37°C is 0.0697 ml of CO_2/100 ml of plasma/mm Hg $P_{A_{CO_2}}$. Although carbon dioxide is about 20 times more soluble than oxygen, only 5 to 6% is carried as dissolved CO_2. Table 5–7 shows the distribution of carbon dioxide in arterial and mixed venous blood of individuals at rest.

Of the 492.8 ml of carbon dioxide in each liter of arterial blood, 26.9 ml (5%) is dissolved, 22.4 ml (5%) is in carbamino compounds, and 443.5 ml (90%) is in bi-carbonate. In the tissues, 40.3 ml of CO_2/L of blood is added: 2.2 ml (6%) stays in solution, 9 ml (22%) forms carbamino compounds, and 29.1 ml (72%) forms bi-carbonate. The pH of the blood drops from 7.40 to 7.37. In the lungs, the processes are reversed, and the 40.3 ml of carbon dioxide is discharged into the alveoli.

GAS EXCHANGE BETWEEN THE BLOOD AND TISSUES

When the red blood cell arrives at the tissue capillaries, it encounters an environment that is different from the one in the lung capillaries. Carbon dioxide leaves the tissues because its partial pressure is higher in the tissues than it is in the blood. As carbon dioxide diffuses from the tissues, oxygen diffuses into the tissues. As shown in Figure 5–6, the reactions that occur at tissue level are the reverse of those in the lungs. In pathway A, the carbon dioxide diffuses through the plasma into the red blood cell, where it rapidly combines with water to produce H_2CO_3, which breaks down into bicarbonate and hydrogen ions. The HCO_3^- passes back into the plasma, whereas the H+ is buffered by the red blood cell proteins. To maintain equilibrium of ions, the red blood cell must gain a negative ion in exchange for each HCO_3^- lost. To serve this purpose, the readily available chloride ion diffuses from the plasma into the red blood cell. This process is known as the chloride shift. In pathway B, carbon dioxide displaces oxygen on the hemoglobin to form carbaminohemoglobin. In pathway C, carbon dioxide slowly combines with water in the plasma to produce H_2CO_3, which breaks down into bicarbonate and hydrogen ions. The hydrogen ion is bound by plasma proteins in the blood buffer system. The remaining carbon dioxide is transported in physical solution in pathway D.

Table 5–7. Distribution of Carbon Dioxide in Arterial and Mixed Venous Blood

	ml of CO₂/L of Blood	Percent of Total
Arterial blood		
Total carbon dioxide	492.8	100
As dissolved carbon dioxide	26.9	5
As bicarbonate	443.5	90
As carbamino carbon dioxide	22.4	5
Mixed venous blood		
Total carbon dioxide	533.1	100
As dissolved carbon dioxide	29.1	5
As bicarbonate	472.6	89
As carbamino carbon dioxide	31.4	6
Arteriovenous difference		
Total carbon dioxide	40.3	100
As dissolved carbon dioxide	2.2	6
As bicarbonate	29.1	72
As carbamino carbon dioxide	9.0	22

Data from Lambertsen, C.J.: Respiration. *In* Medical Physiology. Vol. 2. 14th Ed. Edited by V.B. Mountcastle. St. Louis, C.V. Mosby Co., 1980.

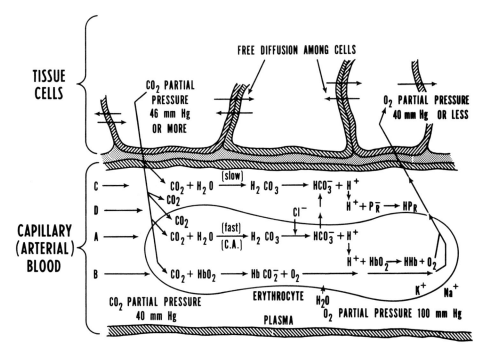

Fig. 5–6. Gas exchange in the tissues.

TISSUE RESPIRATION

Cellular Metabolism

The physical and chemical processes by which energy is made available for use by the body are called metabolism. The chemical processes that produce energy are known as catabolism. They result in the conversion of either foodstuffs or body tissue into carbon dioxide and water (and sometimes ammonia). Conversely, chemical changes that synthesize materials to be stored as a part of the body are known as anabolism. The energy required for anabolic reactions (such as the formation of protein and body fat) comes only from catabolic reactions. The energy and building blocks for the synthesis of protein and fat are acquired from one of two sources: the digestion of food or the relocation of molecules and energy from some other body tissue.

The chemical energy produced from the process of catabolism is held in the energy-rich phosphate bonds of adenosine triphosphate (ATP), which exists in the cytoplasm of the cell. The body converts this chemical energy into useful body functions such as muscle contractions, glandular secretions, chemical synthesis of protein, nerve impulses, urine formation,

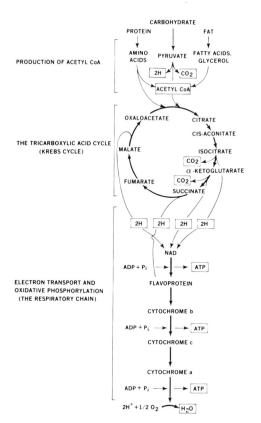

Fig. 5–7. Cellular respiration.

and body heat. This energy is made available by the hydrolysis of the ATP molecule, which releases a phosphate radical and results in the formation of adenosine diphosphate (ADP). Because the supply of ATP in the cellular cytoplasm is limited, new energy-rich bonds must be continually produced by the oxidation of carbohydrates, lipids, and amino acids. These foodstuffs are degraded in a series of consecutive enzymatic reactions to eventually produce two-carbon acetyl groups of acetyl coenzyme A (CoA). Within the mitochondria of the cell, acetyl CoA is channeled into the Krebs tricarboxylic acid cycle, which is the final common pathway of oxidative catabolism. This process is illustrated in Figure 5–7. Hydrogen atoms, or their equivalent electrons, from this process are then fed into the respiratory chain, a series of electron carriers that transport the electrons to molecular oxygen. This process produces several energy-rich ATP molecules by the oxidative phosphorylation of ADP. The production of water in the final step of the chain is catalyzed by an enzyme called cytochrome oxidase. The oxidative phosphorylation process requires a minimum oxygen tension in the mitochondria in the range of about 0.5 to 3 mm Hg. A minimum tissue oxygen value of about 30 mm Hg is required to achieve this level in the mitochondria. As the oxygen tension is increased above these minimum values in the mitochondria, oxidative phosphorylation is unaffected until levels above 250 to 300 mm Hg are reached. Above this value, the rate of oxygen consumption by the mitochondria falls sharply and oxygen toxicity occurs, presumably due to an interruption of the cytochrome oxidase enzyme system.

Tissue Oxygen Requirements

About 90% of the molecular oxygen consumed by the tissues is involved in the creation of ATP (oxidative phosphorylation); about 9% of the oxygen is used to

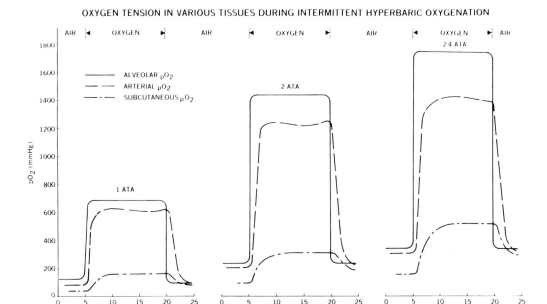

Fig. 5–8. Tissue oxygen tension during normobaric and hyperbaric oxygen breathing.

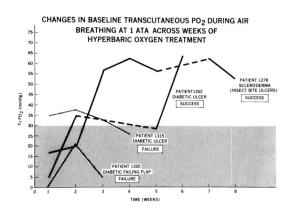

Fig. 5–9. Examples of baseline oxygen values in successful (healed) versus unsuccessful (amputees) patients treated with hyperbaric oxygen therapy.

remove hydrogen from amino acids and amines (oxidation), and about 1% is incorporated into complex organic molecules like biogenic amines and hormones (oxygenation). Varying the oxygen tension outside the tissue's normal range can profoundly affect the efficiency with which

the enzyme systems catalyze these chemical processes.

The need for maintaining minimal tissue oxygen tension is dramatically demonstrated by recent measurements in chronic, nonhealing hypoxic wounds. The tissue levels of oxygen can be increased in hyperbaric conditions, as compared with normobaric oxygen breathing (Fig. 5–8). The wounds of patients presenting for hyperbaric oxygen (HBO) therapy to aid wound healing were repeatedly measured at weekly intervals by implanting a polarographic oxygen electrode in the wound. In a series of 20 patients, all wounds were hypoxic (5 to 20 mm Hg) before HBO treatments were initiated. Daily treatments with HBO at 2.4 ATA resulted in elevating the wound oxygen tension above 30 mm Hg in all patients in whom healing occurred. Wounds that remained below 30 mm Hg oxygen tension failed to heal. Figure 5–9 shows the baseline transcutaneous oxygen values in four patients treated with hyperbaric oxygen. The two successful cases (healed) had values above 30 mm Hg, and the two unsuccessful cases (non-healing) had values that declined below 30 mm Hg.

Respiratory Quotient

The respiratory quotient (RQ) is defined as the ratio of the volume of carbon dioxide expired to the volume of oxygen consumed during the same time period. This ratio varies with the chemical composition of the food consumed. The following equations show the oxidative metabolism of carbohydrate (glucose), protein (alanine), and fat (triolein) diets:

glucose: $C_6 H_{12} O_6$ (2)

$$C_6 H_{12} O_6 + 6O_2 \rightarrow 6CO_2 + 6H_2O$$

$$RQ = \frac{6 \text{ Vol. } CO_2}{6 \text{ Vol. } O_2} = 1.00$$

alanine: $CH_3 CH (NH_2) COOH$ (3)

$$2C_3 H_7 O_2 N + 6O_2 \rightarrow (NH_2) CO + 5CO_2 + 5H_2O$$

$$RQ = \frac{5 \text{ Vol. } CO_2}{6 \text{ Vol. } O_2} = 0.83$$

triolein: $C_3 H_5 [CH_3 (CH_2)_7 CH = CH (CH_2)_7 COO]_3$ (4)

$$C_{57} H_{104} O_6 + 80O_2 \rightarrow 57CO_2 + 52H_2O$$

$$RQ = \frac{57 \text{ Vol. } CO_2}{80 \text{ Vol. } O_2} = 0.71$$

Table 5–8 lists the gas exchange, heat production, and respiratory quotients of some commonly ingested materials.

In a resting individual who has eaten a balanced diet and has a cardiac output of about 5.4 L/min, the tissues consume about 254 ml of O_2/min (4.7 ml of O_2/100 ml of blood) and produce about 210 ml of carbon dioxide (3.9 ml of CO_2/100 ml of blood) (Table 5–9). Thus, a balanced diet of carbohydrate, protein, and fat produces a respiratory quotient of about 0.83. Unfortunately, determining the respiratory quotient does not furnish exact information about the foodstuff being metabolized. Even when a subject is on a diet consisting of a chemically pure substance, oxidation of that substance to the exclusion of all others does not occur. Apparently, the cells not only oxidize a number of foodstuffs concurrently but also convert one compound to another. Thus, the gen-

Table 5–8. Gas Exchange and Respiratory Quotients (RQ) For Representative Carbohydrate, Protein, and Fat Compounds

Compound	ml of O_2 Required to Oxidize 1 g	Products of Oxidation of 1g		RQ
		CO_2 (ml)	Heat (kcal)	
Cane sugar	785.5	785.5	3.96	1.00
Protein	956.9	773.8	4.40	0.81
Animal fat	2013.2	1431.1	9.50	0.71

Data adapted from Brobeck, J.R., and Dubois, A.B.: Energy exchange. *In* Medical Physiology. 14th Ed. Edited by V.B. Mountcastle. St. Louis, C.V. Mosby Company, 1980.

Table 5–9. Gas Exchange Requirements in Body Tissues

Structure	Mass (kg)	Blood Flow/Min (ml)*	Oxygen Consumed (ml)*	Carbon Dioxide Produced (ml)*	Respiratory Quotient (RQ)
Brain	1.4	750	46.5	46.5	1.00
Heart	0.3	225	29.2	25.0	0.86
Kidney	0.3	1259	17.4	13.9	0.80
Digestive organs	2.6	1500	50.7	35.4	0.70
Skeletal muscle	31.0	837	49.3	39.6	0.80
Skin	3.6	460	11.8	9.7	0.82
Residual	24.0	380	50.0	40.3	0.81
Whole body	63.2	5411	254.9	210.4	0.83

*Mean value of data collected for 24 hours.
Modified from Lambertsen, C.J.: Respiration. *In* Medical Physiology. Vol. 2. 14th Ed. Edited by V.B. Mountcastle. St. Louis, C.V. Mosby Company, 1980.

erally accepted concept is that a "metabolic pool" exists in which compounds continually enter the pool while others leave it, either to be converted to other molecules or to be metabolized to meet the cellular energy requirements.

CONTROL OF PULMONARY VENTILATION

Normal respiratory activity is controlled by complex interactions between the brain, lungs, respiratory muscles, and chemoreceptors. Nerve impulses from each receptor are integrated with others by the respiratory control center.

Neural Control

The respiratory control center is subdivided into the inspiratory center, expiratory center, apneustic center, and pneumotaxic center. These subdivisions are found on both sides of the brain stem. The inspiratory and expiratory centers are in the medulla. The inspiratory centers excite the muscles of inspiration and cause them to contract. The expiratory centers excite the muscles of expiration. When one of these centers is stimulated, the other is automatically inhibited. Oscillation between these two centers is responsible for the respiratory rhythm. In the lower and middle pons are the apneustic centers. Stimulation of the apneustic center causes forceful inspiration but weak expirations. The pneumotaxic centers are in the upper pons. Stimulation of the

pneumotaxic center inhibits the apneustic center and accelerates the rate of breathing. Figure 5–10 illustrates the subdivisions of the respiratory center.

Located in the lungs are many stretch receptors that have a profound effect on the rhythmicity of respiration. When the lungs become stretched, impulses from the stretch receptors inhibit further inspiration and prevent overdistension of the lungs. The Hering-Breuer reflex was discussed earlier in the section entitled "Pulmonary Ventilation."

In strenuous exercise, oxygen utilization and carbon dioxide formation increase as much as twentyfold. The in-

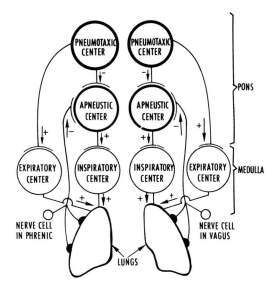

Fig. 5–10. The subdivisions of the respiratory center.

creased tidal volume and breathing rate, however, increase alveolar ventilation so that blood P_{O_2}, pH, and P_{CO_2} remain within a normal range. At least four different mechanisms may be involved: (1) as the motor cortex transmits impulses to the contracting muscles, it is believed to transmit collateral impulses to excite the respiratory center; (2) movements of the joints excite proprioceptors that transmit excitatory impulses to the respiratory center; (3) increased body temperature is believed to slightly increase respiration; and (4) apparently, a chemoreceptor reflex drive occurs even before arterial oxygen tension has been lowered by exercise.

Breathing 100% oxygen at sea level reduces the hyperpnea at a particular level of exercise. The arterial oxygen content increases by 10%, thereby reducing the degree of muscle anaerobiosis and reducing the fixed acid levels in the blood. In one study, a small decrease in ventilation of an exercising subject was reported within 10 seconds after a single breath of oxygen, which was attributed to the removal of the chemoreceptor contribution to exercise hyperpnea.[3]

Voluntary Control

Respiratory movements are under voluntary control. The decision to exert this control and the origin of the nervous impulses that produce it reside within the higher brain centers of the cerebral hemispheres. One can voluntarily breathe fast and deep enough to reduce arterial carbon dioxide tension to half its normal value and completely negate the chemoreceptor control of respiration. Loss of consciousness can result. The voluntary breath holding record (in excess of 13 minutes) was accomplished by combining hyperventilation and 100% oxygen breathing under positive pressure.

Chemical Control

Chemical control is exerted by central chemoreceptors in the respiratory center and peripheral chemoreceptors in the carotid and aortic bodies. The three most important chemical factors are carbon dioxide, hydrogen ions, and oxygen.

The respiratory center is sensitive to arterial carbon dioxide and pH. Carbon dioxide can readily diffuse across the blood-brain barrier and exert its influence on the respiratory center. Questions exist as to whether the respiratory center reacts to carbon dioxide partial pressure or pH. The weight of investigative evidence supports the view that it is pH fluctuation caused by the formation of H_2CO_3 and its subsequent dissociation to $H+$ and HCO_3^- which is of primary importance. Changes in H_2CO_3 are controlled by the net diffusion of carbon dioxide from the blood into the cells of the respiratory center. Because carbon dioxide is one of the end products of metabolism, its presence in the body fluids greatly affects the chemical reactions of the cells. Thus, the tissue P_{CO_2} must be regulated exactly. Stimulation of the respiratory center by fluctuations in carbon dioxide provides a feedback mechanism for the regulation of CO_2 throughout the body. Elevated P_{CO_2} stimulates the respiratory control center to increase alveolar ventilation, thus returning tissue P_{CO_2} to normal.

The hydrogen ion concentration appears to have the same basic effect on the respiratory center as does excess carbon dioxide. Excess hydrogen ion concentration increases the activity of the inspiratory center, thus increasing the strength of inspiratory muscle contraction. It also stimulates the expiratory center to increase the force of expiratory muscle contractions, and it excites the apneustic and pneumotaxic centers to enhance both the rate and intensity of the basic respiratory rhythm.

When the arterial carbon dioxide tension drops by as little as 5 mm Hg below normal, the drive to breathe ceases until sufficient carbon dioxide accumulates. Thus, changes in the carbon dioxide tension cause immediate compensatory changes in pulmonary ventilation.

Peripheral chemoreceptors respond to changes in oxygen, carbon dioxide, and pH. The chemoreceptors are located in the bifurcations of the common carotid arteries (carotid bodies) and in the aortic arch (aortic bodies). They are relatively insensitive to changes in carbon dioxide but are highly sensitive to hypoxia. When arterial oxygen tension falls below 45 to 50 mm Hg, the peripheral chemoreceptors stimulate the inspiratory center to increase ventilation. This process also occurs when hydrogen ion concentration is elevated.

The impulses from peripheral chemoreceptors follow two separate routes to the respiratory control center. The carotid body impulses travel to the medulla by the glossopharyngeal nerves, whereas aortic body impulses travel to the medulla by the vagus nerve. Increased hydrogen ion concentration in the arterial blood excites the chemoreceptors and indirectly increases respiratory activity. The direct effects of carbon dioxide and pH on the respiratory center are more powerful than the indirect effects of the peripheral chemoreceptors. Thus, it appears that the chemoreceptors act primarily as an accessory mechanism.

The importance of these bodies is most apparent when the oxygen content of the blood is reduced. The oxygen concentration appears to have little or no direct effect on the respiratory center. When the oxygen content of the blood declines, however, impulses from the peripheral chemoreceptors reflexly increase the respiratory activity to provide more oxygen.

Pulmonary ventilation increases twofold as arterial oxygen tension drops to 38 mm Hg (equivalent to air breathing at 5486 m). A further reduction to 35 mm Hg (equivalent to air breathing at nearly 6000 m) will increase respiration four to six times, provided carbon dioxide is maintained at its normal level, and is the compensatory mechanism for hypoxia.

HYPOXIA

The respiratory system has a wide range of flexibility to maintain normal body functions. The respiratory response to the environments to which an individual can be subjected in aerospace operations can have incapacitating results. The most common results are hypoxia, hyperventilation, and hypercapnia.

Hypoxia is a general term that describes the state of oxygen deficiency in the tissues. Hypoxia disrupts the intracellular oxidative process and impairs cellular function. Brain cells with a uniquely high oxygen demand are most susceptible to low oxygen tension. Brain impairment, deterioration of performance, reduced visual function, and unconsciousness occur as a result of hypoxia.

Causes of Hypoxia

Hypoxia from any cause can have serious ramifications and can occur at any altitude. Furthermore, hypoxic effects from varying causes are additive. A summary of the causes of hypoxia as they pertain to the various phases of respiration is given in Table 5–1. One can refer to the phases of respiration to identify those points where oxygen is prevented from fulfilling its role in cellular metabolism.

Hypoxic Hypoxia

A deficiency in alveolar oxygen exchange is referred to as hypoxic hypoxia. Oxygen deficiency may be due to a reduction in the oxygen partial pressure in inspired air or a reduction in the effective gas exchange area of the lung. The result is an inadequate oxygen supply to the arterial blood, which, in turn, decreases the amount of oxygen available to the tissues. In aircrews, hypoxic hypoxia usually is caused by exposure to low barometric pressure and is often referred to as altitude hypoxia. Hypoxic hypoxia also can occur in divers because of the low fraction of inspired oxygen in special gas mixes and the possibility of entrapment in confined spaces.

Alveolar Oxygen Pressure

The alveolar partial pressure of oxygen is the most critical factor in producing hypoxic hypoxia. It determines the plasma oxygen tension and the degree of oxygen saturation of hemoglobin. Mean alveolar oxygen pressure, P_{AO_2}, can be calculated from the alveolar gas equation, as follows:

$$P_{AO_2} = (P_B - P_{H_2O}) F_{IO_2}$$
$$- P_{ACO_2} (F_{IO_2} + \frac{1 - F_{IO_2}}{R}) \quad (5)$$

where P_B is the ambient barometric pressure; P_{H_2O} is the water vapor at body temperature (47 mm Hg at 37°C); F_{IO_2} is the fraction of inspired oxygen (1.0 for 100% oxygen, 0.21 for air); P_{ACO_2} is the mean alveolar carbon dioxide pressure (40 mm Hg at sea level); and R is the respiratory exchange ratio (RQ) (assumed to be 1.0 for 100% oxygen).

Table 5–10 shows the respiratory gas pressures and exchange ratios during exposure to altitude. Values have been measured for air-breathing exposures up to 7620 m and for 100% oxygen-breathing exposures up to 14,021 m. Above these altitudes P_{AO_2} or P_{ACO_2} cannot be measured because unconsciousness occurs so rapidly that steady-state values are not reached. The alveolar gas equation can be used to estimate the values.

Oxyhemoglobin Dissociation Curve

Figure 5–11 compares the oxyhemoglobin saturation at different altitudes. At sea level, a P_{AO_2} of 100 mm Hg results in hemoglobin saturation of 98% (example 1). Ascent to 3048 m results in a P_{AO_2} of 60 mm Hg and hemoglobin saturation of 87% (example 2). A healthy person has no difficulty at these altitudes except for a measurable reduction in night vision. With a P_{AO_2} of 38 mm Hg and oxyhemo-

globin saturation of 72%, symptoms of hypoxia would be experienced within 30 minutes of exposure to 5486 m (example 3). Any activity or exercise would reduce this time. Exposure to 6706 m results in acute hypoxia, and performance is lost within 5 to 10 minutes (example 4). Exposure to higher altitudes further decreases hemoglobin saturation and shortens the effective performance time (EPT). At altitudes above 7620 m, P_{AO_2} may actually be lower than the partial pressure of oxygen in the venous blood. This results in diffusion of oxygen from the blood back into the alveoli. The onset of hypoxia is more sudden and profound, and the EPT is correspondingly shorter.

Hypemic Hypoxia

Even with normal ventilation and diffusion, cellular hypoxia can occur if the rate of delivery of oxygen does not satisfy metabolic requirements. An oxygen deficiency due to reduction in the oxygen-carrying capacity of the blood is called hypemic hypoxia.

Oxygen is transported principally by hemoglobin. Hemoglobin has four peptide chains and four hemes. Each heme contains one atom of ferrous iron (Fe^{+2}). Because one molecule of oxygen reacts with one atom of ferrous iron, each hemoglobin molecule reacts reversibly with four oxygen molecules, as follows:

$$Hb_4 + 4O_2 \leftrightharpoons Hb_4(O_2)_4 \quad (6)$$

In the hemoglobin molecule, the iron atom remains in the Fe^{+2} state without undergoing a change in valence as oxygen is bound and lost. The iron atom can, however, be oxidized to the Fe^{+3} state by oxidizing agents, such as ferricyanide and sulfa drugs, to produce methemoglobin. If iron is oxidized to Fe^{+3}, it can no longer combine with oxygen.

Carbon monoxide is significant to aircrews because it is present in the exhaust fumes of both conventional and jet engine

Table 5–10. Respiratory Gas Pressures and Gas Exchange Ratios

Altitude		Pressure		Ambient P_{O_2} (mm Hg)	$P_{A_{O_2}}$ (mm Hg)	$P_{A_{CO_2}}$ (mm Hg)	P_{H_2O} (mm Hg)	Respiratory Exchange Ratio (R)
(m)	(ft)	(PSIA)	(mm Hg)					
				Breathing Air				
0	0	14.69	759.97	159.21	103.0	40.0	47.0	0.85
305	1000	14.17	733.04	153.57	98.2	39.4	—	—
610	2000	13.66	706.63	148.04	93.8	39.0	—	—
914	3000	13.17	681.23	142.72	89.5	38.4	—	—
1219	4000	12.69	656.34	137.50	85.1	38.0	—	—
1524	5000	12.23	632.46	132.50	81.0	37.4	47.0	0.87
1829	6000	11.77	609.09	127.60	76.8	37.0	—	—
2134	7000	11.34	586.49	122.87	72.8	36.4	—	—
2438	8000	10.91	564.64	118.29	68.9	36.0	—	—
2743	9000	10.50	543.31	113.82	65.0	35.4	—	—
3048	10,000	10.10	522.73	109.51	61.2	35.0	47.0	0.90
3353	11,000	9.72	502.92	105.36	57.8	34.4	—	—
3658	12,000	9.34	483.36	101.26	54.3	33.8	—	—
3962	13,000	8.99	464.82	97.38	51.0	33.2	—	—
4267	14,000	8.63	446.53	93.55	47.9	32.6	—	—
4572	15,000	8.29	429.01	89.88	45.0	32.0	47.0	0.95
4877	16,000	7.96	411.99	86.31	42.0	31.4	—	—
5182	17,000	7.65	395.73	84.50	40.0	31.0	—	—
5486	18,000	7.34	379.73	79.55	37.8	30.4	—	—
5791	19,000	7.05	364.49	76.36	35.9	30.0	—	—
6096	20,000	6.76	349.50	73.22	34.3	29.4	47.0	1.00
6401	21,000	6.48	335.28	70.24	33.5	29.0	—	—
6706	22,000	6.21	321.31	67.31	32.8	28.4	47.0	1.05
7010	23,000	5.95	307.85	64.49	32.0	28.0	—	—
7315	24,000	5.70	294.89	61.78	31.2	27.4	—	—
7620	25,000	5.46	282.45	59.17	30.4	27.0	47.0	—
				Breathing 100% Oxygen*				
10,058	33,000	3.81	197.10	197.10	109	40	47.0	—
10,973	36,000	3.30	170.94	170.94	85	38	47.0	—
11,887	39,000	2.86	148.08	148.08	64	36	47.0	—
12,192	40,000	2.73	141.22	141.22	—	—	—	—
12,802	42,000	2.48	128.27	128.27	48	33	47.0	—
13,716	45,000	2.15	111.25	111.25	34	30	47.0	—
14,021	46,000	2.05	105.92	105.92	30	29	47.0	—

*Data from Holmstrom, F.M.G.: Hypoxia. *In* Aerospace Medicine. Edited by H.W. Randall. Baltimore, The Williams & Wilkins Co., 1971.

aircraft, as well as in cigarette smoke. Carbon monoxide combines with hemoglobin about 200 times more readily than does oxygen and displaces oxygen to form carboxyhemoglobin. The normal carboxyhemoglobin level is less than 1% but may increase to 6 or 7% in heavy smokers. Heavy smokers may be less tolerant of increased levels of carbon monoxide in inspired air because of elevated carboxyhemoglobin and nicotine levels, which lower oxygen delivery to the tissues. Figure 5–12 illustrates that oxygen delivery to the skin of smokers is 10% below that of nonsmokers.

Carboxyhemoglobin levels of 15 to 25% produce headache and nausea. With prolonged exposures, muscular weakness, dizziness, and confusion occur. At levels above 25%, electrocardiographic changes, stupor, and eventual unconsciousness will occur.

It is interesting to note that the release of carbon monoxide from hemoglobin and from cytochrome oxidase a_3 can be accelerated by inhaling oxygen. The higher the oxygen pressure, the more rapidly carbon monoxide is eliminated. With hyperbaric oxygen, carbon monoxide is eliminated

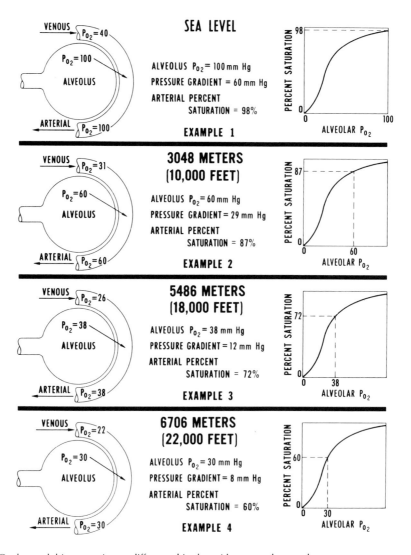

Fig. 5–11. Oxyhemoglobin saturation at different altitudes without supplemental oxygen.

much more rapidly than with air or oxygen alone.

Stagnant Hypoxia

Any condition that results in a reduction in total cardiac output, pooling of the blood, or restriction of blood flow can result in stagnant hypoxia. Heart failure, shock, continuous positive pressure breathing, and G forces sustained in flight maneuvers create stagnant hypoxia. Local cellular hypoxia can occur as a result of exposure to extreme environmental temperatures, restrictive clothing, or changes in body posture that restrict regional blood flow. Hyperventilation also can cause reduced cerebral blood flow and result in cerebral stagnant hypoxia. Blood clots or gas bubbles (as in decompression sickness) can produce pulmonary emboli and create stagnant hypoxia.

Histotoxic Hypoxia

Metabolic disorders or poisoning of the cytochrome oxidase enzyme system can result in inability of the cell to use molec-

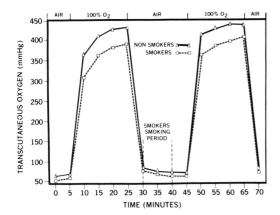

Fig. 5–12. Transcutaneous oxygen measurements in smokers and nonsmokers.

ular oxygen. This condition is called histotoxic (tissue-poisoning) hypoxia.

Unlike hemoglobin, iron atoms in the cytochromes normally undergo reversible changes between Fe^{+2} and Fe^{+3} to serve their role as electron carriers. The oxidized Fe^{+3} form of cytochrome $a + a_3$ complex can accept electrons from the reduced cytochrome c to become the Fe^{+2} form. This is reoxidized by molecular oxygen to the Fe^{+3} form. Only cytochrome a_3 molecules can transfer electrons to molecular oxygen in the final step of cellular respiration. This process is inhibited by carbon monoxide because it competes with oxygen. Ethyl alcohol, cyanide, and hydrogen sulfide also inhibit the cytochrome $a + a_3$ complex and produce histotoxic hypoxia.

Effects of Hypoxia

Hypoxia produces its effects at the cellular level and disrupts normal body functions. The highest oxygen requirements are for visual, myocardial, and nervous tissues, and these tissues are affected more readily than other tissues.

Respiratory System

One of the first respiratory effects observed in an individual who is becoming hypoxic at altitude is an increase in the depth of breathing. The next effect is an increase in the respiratory rate. These effects are caused by the aortic and carotid chemoreceptors, which sense the reduced oxygen pressure of the blood and signal the respiratory center to begin compensatory efforts. An increase in ventilation starts at 1219 m but is not significant until the arterial oxygen saturation has decreased to 93% at an altitude of 2438 m. A maximum response occurs at 6706 m, where the respiratory minute volume is almost doubled. Most of this increase is due to tidal volume rather than to respiratory rate. With the rise in pulmonary ventilation, there is a fall in the alveolar carbon dioxide tension and a concomitant increase in the alveolar oxygen tension. The reduction in carbon dioxide decreases the hydrogen ion concentration and elevates the pH. This change is detected by the chemoreceptors, which reflexly depress respiration. The effects of acute exposure to altitude on pulmonary ventilation are given in Table 5–6.

Cardiovascular System

When oxyhemoglobin saturation declines to 87%, the symptoms of hypoxia become evident. Oxyhemoglobin saturation below 65% is considered critical because the symptoms of hypoxia become severe and consciousness is maintained for only a short time.

Compared with the respiratory and nervous systems, the cardiovascular system is relatively resistant to hypoxia. Cardiovascular responses are reflexive in nature, responding to the hypoxic stimulation of several body structures: the aortic and carotid chemoreceptors, the central nervous system, and the heart. Reflex adjustments act in an integrated fashion to increase heart rate, moderately increase systolic blood pressure, and redistribute blood flow to improve circulation to the brain and heart. The heart rate progressively increases from an altitude of 1219 m and reaches a maximum rate at 6706 m. Table 5–11 shows the effect of

Table 5–11. Effect of Altitude on Heart Rate and Arterial Oxyhemoglobin Saturation

Altitude		Percent of Ground Level Value	
(m)	(ft)	Pulse (at 10 minutes)	Percent of Oxyhemoglobin Saturation (at 3 minutes)
3000	9842	—	87
3658	12,000	114	—
5000	16,404	—	76
5486	18,000	106	—
6096	20,000	124	—
6706	22,000	132	—
7000	22,966	—	71
9000	29,527	—	66

Data from Holmstrom, F.M.G.: Hypoxia. In Aerospace Medicine. Edited by H.W. Randall. Baltimore, The Williams & Wilkins Company, 1971.

altitude on heart rate and arterial oxyhemoglobin saturation.

The increase in cardiac output is significant in that it decreases the arteriovenous (AV) oxygen difference and thus elevates the mean capillary oxygen tension. It should be noted that this occurs because the intracellular utilization of oxygen does not increase with altitude. The fall in oxygen content of arteriovenous blood (AV difference) is related to the cardiac output and the oxygen consumed by the tissues. The AV oxygen difference is calculated from the Fick equation, as follows:

$$\text{AV oxygen difference (ml/L)} = \frac{\text{Oxygen consumption (ml/min)}}{\text{Cardiac output (L/min)}} \quad (7)$$

Central Nervous System

The most important alteration in the circulation during altitude exposure occurs in the brain. Upon exposure to altitude, cerebral blood flow decreases due to vasoconstriction secondary to a fall in the arterial carbon dioxide tension. This level is maintained until the arterial P_{O_2} falls to 50 to 60 mm Hg, when hypoxia, a potent vasodilator, overcomes the hypocapneic vasoconstriction and creates an increase

in the cerebral blood flow. Because the retina of the eye and the central nervous system have a great requirement for oxygen, they are the first affected by oxygen deficiency. Hypoxia decreases visual and cerebral performance. The effects are in direct proportion to the duration and severity of the exposure. If the oxygen lack becomes acute or is prolonged, cerebral activity ceases and death follows.

Once the local oxygen tension in the mitochondria falls below 1 to 3 mm Hg, the tissue in that region will convert to anaerobic metabolism and form lactic acid. Thus, the lactic acid test of cerebral tissue is used to determine the cause of death for potential altitude hypoxia victims.

Recognition of the Signs and Symptoms of Hypoxia

The following is an extract of a report filed by Captain R.W. Schroeder in which he discussed his aviation altitude record of 8809 m on September 18, 1918:

At 20,000 feet, while still climbing in large circles, my goggles became frosted, making it very difficult for me to watch my instruments. When I reached 25,000 feet I noticed the sun growing very dim. I could hardly hear my motor run, and I felt very hungry. The trend of my thoughts was that it must be getting late. . . . I went on talking to myself, and this I felt was a good sign to begin taking oxygen, so I did. I was then over 25,000 feet, and as soon as I started to inhale the oxygen the sun grew bright again, my motor began to exhaust so loud that it seemed something must be wrong with it. I was no longer hungry and the day seemed to be a most beautiful one. . . .

I kept at it until my oxygen gave out, and at that point I noticed my aneroid indicated very nearly 29,000 feet. The thermometer 32° below zero C. and the R.P.M. had dropped from 1600 to 1560. This, considered very good. But the lack of oxygen was affecting me. I was beginning to get cross, and I could not understand why I was only 29,000 feet after climbing for so long a time, I remember that the horizon seemed to be very much out of place, but I felt that I was flying correctly and that I was right and the horizon was wrong.

About this time the motor quit. I was out of gasoline, so I descended in a large spiral. When I had descended to about 20,000 feet I began to feel better. . . . I did not see the ground from the time I went up through the clouds above

Dayton, Ohio, until I came down through them again at 4000 feet above Canton, Ohio, over 200 miles from where I started.[6]

Hypoxia Characteristics

Hypoxia is particularly dangerous because its signs and symptoms do not usually cause discomfort or pain. The onset of symptoms is insidious. Individual and daily variances of tolerance occur. The effects of hypoxia begin immediately upon ascent to altitude. Below 3048 m, the deficiencies are generally so subtle that they normally go unnoticed. Decreases in night vision and drowsiness usually are the only noticeable complaints.

Judgment Impairment

Intellectual impairment is an early sign of hypoxia, making it unlikely that the individual will recognize his own disability. Thinking is slow and calculations are unreliable. Fixation, or the tendency to repeat courses of action, is common. Memory is faulty, particularly for events in the immediate past. Judgment is poor, and reaction time is delayed.

Effective Performance Time

Effective performance time (EPT) is defined as the amount of time an individual is able to perform useful flying duties in an environment of inadequate oxygen. EPT is sometimes called time of useful consciousness (TUC). The use of EPT more accurately refers to critical (functional) performance than does TUC. With the loss of effective performance in flight, the individual is no longer capable of taking proper corrective or protective action. Thus, in aerospace operations, the emphasis is on prevention instead of cure. Table 5–12 shows the EPT for healthy, resting individuals at various altitudes.

Individual variations in EPT occur, influenced by individual endurance, experience, physical exertion, and the situation under which exposure has occurred.

Two major factors that dramatically re-

Table 5–12. Effective Performance Time at Altitude

Altitude		Effective Performance Time
(m)	(ft)	
5486	18,000	20 to 30 minutes
6706	22,000	10 minutes
7620	25,000	3 to 5 minutes
8534	28,000	2.5 to 3 minutes
9144	30,000	1 to 2 minutes
10,668	35,000	0.5 to 1 minutes
12,192	40,000	15 to 20 seconds
13,106	43,000	9 to 12 seconds
15,240	50,000	9 to 12 seconds

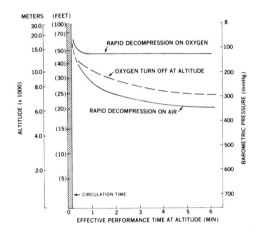

Fig. 5–13. Effective performance time (EPT) after rapid decompression.

duce EPT are rapid decompression and physical exertion. Upon decompression to altitudes above 10,058 m, there is an immediate reversal of oxygen flow in the alveoli due to a higher P_{O_2} within the pulmonary capillaries. This depletes the blood's oxygen reserve and reduces the EPT at rest by up to 50%. Exercise will reduce the EPT considerably. For example, at 7620 m, a resting individual has an EPT of 3 to 5 minutes, but after performing 10 deep knee bends, the EPT will be reduced to about 1 to 1.5 minutes. Figure 5–13 shows the effect of rapid decompression on effective performance time.

Signs and Symptoms of Hypoxia

The individual symptoms of hypoxia can be experienced and identified under safe and controlled conditions in an altitude chamber. Once experienced, these symptoms do not vary dramatically from time to time. Hypoxia can be classified by either objective signs (i.e., perceived by an observer) or by subjective symptoms (i.e., perceived by the subject). In some cases, a particular response may be noticed by both the subject and the observer.

Objective signs include increased rate and depth of breathing, cyanosis, mental confusion, poor judgment, loss of muscle coordination, slouching, and unconsciousness. Behavioral changes, such as elation or belligerence, may be noted by the hypoxic individual, as well as by the observer.

The subjective symptoms that have been reported include breathlessness, apprehension, headache, dizziness, fatigue, nausea, hot and cold flashes, blurred vision, tunnel vision, tingling, and numbness. Euphoria or anger also might be noted.

Effects on Performance

Hypoxia can be classified by stages of performance decrement. Table 5–13 shows the stages of hypoxia with respect to altitude and oxygen saturation of the blood.

In the indifferent stage, dark adaptation is adversely affected at altitudes as low as 1524 m, where visual sensitivity at night is reduced by approximately 10%. A 28% reduction in visual sensitivity occurs at 3048 m, but there are marked individual variations. Performance of new tasks may be impaired. A slight increase in heart rate and pulmonary ventilation occurs.

In the compensatory stage, cardiovascular and respiratory physiologic responses provide some protection against hypoxia. In general, these responses include increases in the respiratory minute volume, cardiac output, heart rate, and blood pressure. The effects of hypoxia on the central nervous system are perceptible after a short period of time. The most important effects of hypoxia at this altitude are drowsiness, decreased judgment and memory, and difficulty with the performance of tasks requiring mental alertness or discrete motor movements.

In the disturbance stage, the physiologic compensatory mechanisms are no longer capable of providing for adequate oxygenation of tissues. Symptoms such as headache, dizziness, somnolence, air hunger, euphoria, and fatigue may develop. Intellectual impairment may prevent the individual from properly assessing the seriousness of the condition. Thinking is slow and unreliable, memory is faulty, motor performance is severely impaired, and critical judgment is lost. The peripheral visual field may gray out to a point where only central vision remains. This is referred to as tunnel vision.

In the critical stage, mental performance deteriorates, and mental confusion or dizziness occurs within a few minutes. Total incapacitation with loss of consciousness rapidly follows with little or no warning.

Factors Influencing Symptoms

The appearance and severity of the signs and symptoms of acute hypoxia are enhanced by several factors: altitude, time spent at altitude, rapid rate of ascent, physical exertion, extreme environmental temperature, and indulgence in self-im-

Table 5–13. Stages of Hypoxia

Stage	Altitude Breathing Air (in m)	Altitude Breathing 100% Oxygen (in m)	Arterial Oxygen Saturation (%)
Indifferent	0–3048	10,363–11,887	98–87
Compensatory	3048–4572	11,887–12,954	87–80
Disturbance	4572–6092	12,954–13,655	80–65
Critical	6092–7010	13,655–13,868	65–60

posed stresses such as fatigue, alcohol consumption, tobacco products, certain medications, and inadequate nutrition.

Treatment of Hypoxia

The treatment of hypoxia is to administer 100% oxygen. If respiration has ceased, cardiopulmonary resuscitation with the simultaneous use of 100% oxygen is necessary. The type of hypoxia must be determined and treatment administered accordingly. The following steps are required:

1. *Administer supplemental oxygen under pressure.* Providing the aircrew member with adequate supplemental oxygen is the prime consideration in the treatment of hypoxia. Depending on the severity of the condition, 100% oxygen delivered under positive pressure may be required. Consideration must be given to the altitude and cause of the oxygen deficiency. Equipment malfunction or altitude exposure above 12,192 m cannot be corrected without the addition of positive pressure.
2. *Monitor breathing.* After a hypoxic episode, the resulting hyperventilation must be controlled to achieve complete recovery. Maintaining a breathing rate of 12 to 16 breaths/min or slightly lower will aid recovery.
3. *Monitor equipment.* The most frequently reported causes of hypoxia are lack of oxygen discipline and equipment malfunction. Conscientious equipment preflight checks and frequent in-flight monitoring will reduce this hazard. Inspection of oxygen equipment when hypoxia is suspected may detect its cause. Correction of the malfunction will aid in the immediate relief of the hypoxic condition. If treatment for hypoxia does not remedy the situation, oxygen contamination should be considered. Use of an alternate oxy-gen source, such as the emergency oxygen cylinder or portable assembly, should be considered. Descent should be initiated as soon as possible and the contents of the oxygen system analyzed.
4. *Descend.* Increasing ambient oxygen pressures by descent to lower altitudes, particularly below 3048 m, is also beneficial. Descent to lower altitude compensates for malfunctioning oxygen equipment that may have caused the hypoxia.

Preventing hypoxia in flying personnel is, to a great extent, a matter of indoctrination. This indoctrination is accomplished by instructing personnel in the proper use and care of oxygen equipment and ensuring that they are aware of their individual symptoms of hypoxia.

Recovery From Hypoxic (Altitude) Hypoxia

Recovery from hypoxia usually occurs within seconds after reestablishing a normal alveolar partial pressure. Nevertheless, mild symptoms, such as headache or fatigue, may persist after the hypoxic episode. The persistence of symptoms seems to have a higher degree of correlation with the duration of the episode than with its severity.

In some instances following the sudden administration of oxygen to correct the hypoxic insult, the individual develops a temporary increase in the severity of symptoms, which is known as oxygen paradox. The subject may lose consciousness or develop clonic spasms for a period lasting up to a minute. Usually, this condition is transient and may pass unnoticed. Accompanying symptoms are mental confusion, deterioration of vision, dizziness, and nausea. Initially, the arterial blood pressure falls and the rate of blood flow decreases. The hypotension produced by the sudden restoration of oxygen is probably due to vasodilatation, which occurs in the pulmonary vascular bed and is brought about by the direct action of oxygen on the pulmonary vessels. The hypocapnia produced by hypoxia and the decrease in blood pressure, which follows reoxygenation, act together to reduce cerebral blood flow. This reduction in blood flow probably intensifies the cerebral hypoxia for a short period until the cardiovascular effects have passed and the carbon dioxide tension returns to a normal range. Once the P_{CO_2} returns to a normal value, it will stimulate the respiratory center to resume ventilation and resolve the cerebral hypoxia.

Prevention of Hypoxia

Hypoxic hypoxia is prevented by ensuring that the individual has sufficient oxygen to maintain a range of alveolar P_{O_2} between 60 and 100 mm Hg. This oxygen level is achieved in aircraft by an oxygen system, cabin pressurization, or a combination of the two.

Cabin Pressurization

In most civilian and military aircraft, hypoxia is prevented by maintaining a cabin altitude below 3048 m. Supplemental oxygen is required only when cabin pressurization fails. In most military fighter and trainer aircraft, cabin altitude often exceeds this level. The cabin pressurization in such aircraft ordinarily provides a cabin altitude below 7620 m. Protection from hypoxia in these aircraft is provided by the combined application of cabin pressurization and supplemental oxygen.

Supplemental Oxygen Requirements

Table 5–14 lists the supplemental oxygen requirements for altitudes up to 10,363 m to maintain a physiologic altitude equivalent to sea level. Above this altitude, 100% oxygen must be administered along with positive pressure breathing. Without positive pressure, breathing

Table 5–14. Supplemental Oxygen Requirements at Altitude to Maintain Sea Level Air Equivalence

Altitude (m)	Altitude (ft)	Barometric Pressure (mm Hg)	Total Oxygen Requirement (%)
Sea level		760	21
1524	5000	632	25
3048	10,000	532	31
4572	15,000	429	40
6092	20,000	329	49
7620	25,000	282	62
9144	30,000	225	81
10,363	34,000	187	100

100% oxygen at 12,192 m would be equivalent to breathing air at 3048 m.

Night Requirements

Exposure to reduced oxygen tensions at altitudes below 3048 m increases dark adaptation time and decreases night vision capability. For this reason, the use of supplemental oxygen may be needed on night flights. One hundred percent oxygen is not required because the object is to maintain the blood oxygen content equivalent to exposures at altitudes of 1524 m or below.

Requirement for Pressure Breathing

Above 12,192 m, 100% oxygen must be breathed with additional pressure to achieve adequate oxygenation. Positive pressure breathing is accomplished with a pressure demand oxygen system. Oxygen regulators are designed to automatically provide positive pressure and 100% oxygen at altitudes above approximately 9144 m. Table 5–15 shows the positive pressure requirements to prevent hypoxia at altitude. Most oxygen regulators tend to maintain an alveolar oxygen partial pressure of 87 mm Hg, which is equivalent to breathing air at about 1524 m.

Figure 5–14 illustrates the decrease in hemoglobin saturation with increasing altitude. Percent saturation is plotted against altitude, and the slope of the curve is similar to the standard oxyhemoglobin dissociation curve. In the first example,

Table 5–15. Pressure Requirements For Exposure Above 10,363 Meters

Altitude		Barometric Pressure (mm Hg)	Calculated P_{AO_2} Breathing Only 100% Oxygen	Additional Oxygen Pressure Required to Provide Equivalent Altitude of	
(m)	(ft)			3048 m*	Sea Level**
10,363	34,000	187	100	None	None
12,192	40,000	141	54	6	46
13,716	45,000	111	24	36	76
15,240	50,000	87	0	60	100
19,812	65,000	43	0	104	144
Space	Space	0	0	147	187

*Equivalent altitude of 3048 m means P_{AO_2} = 60 mm Hg; P_{ACO_2} = 40 mm Hg; P_{AH_2O} = 47 mm Hg; and P total = 147 mm Hg.

**Sea level equivalent means P_{AO_2} = 100 mm Hg; P_{ACO_2} = 40 mm Hg; P_{AH_2O} = 47 mm Hg; and P total = 187 mm Hg.

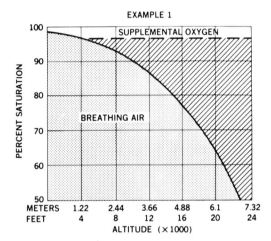

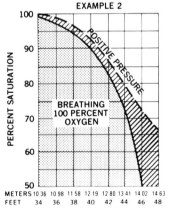

Fig. 5–14. Oxyhemoglobin saturation at different altitudes with supplemental oxygen.

the percent saturation, indicated by the dashed line, is roughly equal to that of breathing air at 1524 m. This percent saturation would remain constant up to 10,363 m, provided that the oxygen regulator delivers the percentages of oxygen shown in Table 5–15.

Figure 5–14 also illustrates the effect of breathing 100% oxygen at altitudes above 10,363 m. When positive pressure is applied to the oxygen, alveolar P_{O_2} increases. The safe ceiling is raised, as reflected by the dashed curve. This level represents the pressure output from an automatic positive pressure breathing regulator. A limit must be set with regard to the unpressurized flight altitude at which a flyer can operate and function well enough to complete the mission. This altitude limit for sustained flight without a counterpressure garment is approximately 13,106 m when using standard pressure breathing equipment that delivers 30 mm Hg pressure. Pressures greater than 30 mm Hg cannot be tolerated for long periods. Pressure breathing impedes venous return to the heart and reduces blood flow through the lungs. In the extremities and abdomen, the veins dilate to accommodate the pooled blood, resulting in a rise in venous blood pressure.

At 36 to 40 mm Hg of pressure breathing, which is required at 13,716 m, pain in the region of the eyes becomes intolerable. Subjects complain of a feeling of congestion in the region of the frontal sinuses. Overdistension may cause pain in the ears and in the posterior pharynx.

At pressures between 60 and 100 mm Hg, lung tissue damage secondary to overexpansion is likely. Loss of consciousness may occur due to decreased cardiac output and pooling of blood in the lower extremities and abdominal vessels.

Technique for Pressure Breathing

During pressure breathing, inhalation is easy and exhalation is difficult. The breathing cycle must be consciously controlled. Practice is required to become accustomed to this reversed breathing pattern. In particular, the tendency to hyperventilate must be avoided. The best technique for pressure breathing is as follows:

1. Establish mental discipline to control the breathing pattern.
2. When inhaling, maintain a conscious tension on the respiratory muscles (the intercostal muscles, diaphragm, and abdominal muscles). Control the expansion of the thorax through muscle tension. As inhalation progresses, steadily decrease muscle tension to allow inflation of the lungs.
3. Pause when the desired lung inflation has occurred.
4. When ready to exhale, positively increase muscle tension for a steady, smooth exhalation.
5. Pause and breathe at a rate slower than normal.

Requirements for a Pressure Suit

If an aviator is to survive exposures to altitudes above 15,240 m for any period of time, additional alveolar P_{O_2} must be provided. Protection is provided by counterpressure garments, commonly called pressure suits. Military directives state that flights above 15,240 m are not permissible, regardless of cabin altitude, unless the aviator is protected by a counterpressure garment.

The purpose of the pressure suit is to protect the aviator from hypoxia. This protection is achieved by applying pressure equally across the body such that a sufficiently low physiologic altitude is maintained so that positive pressure breathing is not required.

Altitude Acclimatization

Chronic exposure to altitude results in altitude acclimatization, the process by which one becomes more tolerant of an hypoxic environment. The means by which acclimatization is achieved includes the following:

1. Increased respiration and cardiac output due to the hypoxic stimulation of the carotid and aortic bodies.
2. Increased diffusion capacity of the lungs, probably achieved by a rise in the pulmonary capillary blood volume, increased lung volume, and a rise of the pulmonary arterial pressure.
3. Polycythemia, directly resulting from hypoxic stimulation of red blood cell production by the bone marrow due to an increased release of erythropoietin by the kidney. The increased hemoglobin content improves the capacity of the blood to transport oxygen. The degree of polycythemia is inversely related to the arterial oxygen saturation. This mechanism provides limited benefits within 2 to 3 weeks of exposure.
4. Increased vascularity of tissues, resulting from an increased number and size of capillaries. Like polycythemia, this response requires a long-term exposure to the hypoxic environment.
5. Cellular acclimatization, occurring as the capability of the cells to metabolize oxygen increases in spite of the low oxygen tension. This accli-

matization is probably due to changes in the cellular oxidative enzyme systems.

6. Decreased affinity of the hemoglobin for oxygen, resulting from an increased production of 2,3 diphosphoglyceric acid within the red blood cells. The result is a shift of the oxyhemoglobin dissociation curve to the right, which improves the offloading of oxygen to the tissue by as much as 10 to 20% at 4572 m. At higher altitudes, this decreased affinity for oxygen reduces the uptake of oxygen by hemoglobin in the lungs and has a detrimental effect on tissue metabolism.

7. The renal mechanism compensates for respiratory alkalosis by retaining ammonium ions and excreting large amounts of bicarbonate. Because this is a slow process, it is not detected until over an hour or more and may reach a maximum only after several days.

HYPERVENTILATION

Hyperventilation is of concern because it produces changes in cellular respiration. Although unrelated in cause, the symptoms of hyperventilation and hypoxia are similar and often result in confusion and inappropriate corrective procedures. Despite increased knowledge, training, and improved life-support equipment, both hypoxia and hyperventilation are hazards in flying and diving operations.

Hyperventilation is a condition in which ventilation is abnormally increased. As a result, a loss of carbon dioxide from the lungs occurs, lowering alveolar carbon dioxide tension below normal, a condition known as hypocapnia. The acid-base balance of the blood is disturbed, making it more alkaline, a condition known as alkalosis. Hypocapnia and alkalosis are two important results of hyperventilation.

Causes of Hyperventilation

Hyperventilation in aerospace operations is commonly caused by psychologic stress (fear, anxiety, apprehension, and anger) and environmental stress (hypoxia, pressure breathing, vibration, and heat). Certain drugs also cause or enhance hyperventilation such as salicylates and female sex hormones. In addition, any condition that creates metabolic acidosis will result in hyperventilation.

It is a common practice in diving operations for breathholding divers to voluntarily hyperventilate to extend the breathholding time. Extended breathholding after hyperventilation is an unsafe practice. During the dive, the diver consumes oxygen and produces carbon dioxide. Unfortunately, the usual carbon dioxide stimulus to breathe does not occur at depth. As the diver ascends, the carbon dioxide partial pressure in the lung drops (Dalton's Law), giving the diver the false impression that breathing is not required. Simultaneously, a drop in oxygen partial pressure occurs, causing alveolar oxygen tension to fall to a dangerously low level before the surface is reached. If the diver has remained at depth too long, unconsciousness from hypoxia may occur during the ascent.

Increased ventilation associated with exercise does not produce hyperventilation because an increase in the carbon dioxide content of the blood is maintained by the increased metabolic activity.

Effects of Hyperventilation

Hypocapnia and alkalosis produced by hyperventilation affect the respiratory (blood buffer system), circulatory (oxyhemoglobin dissociation curve), and central nervous systems.

The Respiratory System

As previously discussed, 90% of the carbon dioxide present in the blood is in the form of carbonic acid or bicarbonate. The overall reaction for bicarbonate formation occurs in two steps, as follows:

$$CO_2 + H_2O \rightleftarrows H_2CO_3 \rightleftarrows (H+)$$
$$+ (HCO_3) \quad (7)$$

The major factor that determines the direction in which this reaction proceeds is the carbon dioxide tension, P_{CO_2}. When the P_{CO_2} increases, the reaction proceeds toward the formation of more bicarbonate and hydrogen ions (acidosis). When the P_{CO_2} decreases, the reaction reverses to form carbon dioxide and water, at the expense of bicarbonate and hydrogen ions (alkalosis).

Arterial blood normally has a pH (defined as the negative logarithm of the hydrogen ion concentration) of about 7.40, a P_{CO_2} of about 40 mm Hg, and a plasma bicarbonate concentration of about 25 mmol/L. When an individual hyperventilates, the excessive elimination of carbon dioxide causes a reduction in hydrogen ion concentration that is too rapid for the blood buffers to replace it. The pH is elevated, and respiratory alkalosis occurs. Because catalytic activity of enzymes is especially sensitive to pH, there is a sharp decline in activity on either side of an optimum pH. Should the pH of the blood fall below 7.0 or rise above 7.8, irreparable damage to cellular respiration will occur. In severe cases, unconsciousness and death occur. In the less severe case, when an individual becomes unconscious, respiration slows sufficiently to allow a buildup of carbon dioxide and correct the alkalosis. Hyperventilation is always a complicating factor when hypoxic hypoxia is encountered because the effects, symptoms, degree of impairment, and EPT are so similar.

The Cardiovascular System

The cardiovascular system effects of hyperventilation are manifested by tachycardia, reduced cardiac output, declining blood pressure, and reduced peripheral vascular resistance. The combined effects of vasodilatation in the extremities and vasoconstriction of the cerebral blood vessels cause a restriction in blood flow to the brain.

The primary cardiovascular effect, however, is the Bohr effect, which causes the oxyhemoglobin dissociation curve to shift upward and to the left. This shift increases the capacity of the blood to onload oxygen in the lungs but restricts offloading of oxygen at the tissue level.

The Central Nervous System

The combined effects of restricted blood flow and oxyhemoglobin binding cause stagnant hypoxia to exist in the central nervous system, which leads to unconsciousness. Hyperventilation also causes increased neuromuscular instability with muscle spasms and tetany when the alveolar P_{CO_2} is reduced to 25 to 30 mm Hg. Tingling usually precedes muscle spasm and tetany. The hands may exhibit carpopedal spasm, a fixation of the hand wherein the fingers are flexed toward the wrist. Figure 5–15 summarizes the effects of hyperventilation.

Recognition of the Signs and Symptoms of Hyperventilation

The signs and symptoms of hyperventilation are easily confused with those of

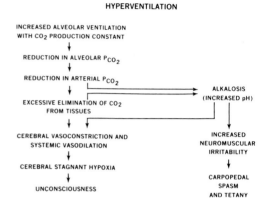

Fig. 5–15. Effects of hyperventilation.

hypoxic hypoxia. Because hyperventilation occurs as an early adaptive mechanism to hypoxia at altitude, it becomes even more difficult to differentiate between the two conditions. The objective signs that are most frequently seen in hyperventilation are increased respiratory rate and depth, muscle twitching and tightness, pallor, cold, clammy skin, muscle spasm, rigidity, and unconsciousness. Symptoms perceived by the subjects include dizziness, lightheadedness, tingling, numbness, visual disturbances, and muscle incoordination.

Table 5–16 compares the symptoms of hyperventilation and hypoxia. It should be noted that the distinguishing differences in these syndromes are few. In hyperventilation, the onset of symptoms is usually gradual, with the presence of a pale, cold, clammy appearance and the development of muscle spasm and tetany. In hypoxia, the onset of symptoms is usually rapid (depending on altitude), with the development of flaccid muscles and cyanosis.

Treatment of Hyperventilation

The treatment of hyperventilation requires a voluntary reduction in the rate and depth of ventilation. Treatment also may be accomplished by breathing into a bag that collects the exhaled carbon dioxide for rebreathing by the subject. Both breathholding and the use of a rebreathing bag are to be avoided at altitude because of the similarity of the symptoms with those of hypoxia.

Because hypoxia and hyperventilation are so similar and both can incapacitate so quickly, the recommended treatment procedures for aviators correct both problems simultaneously: (1) administer 100% oxygen under pressure; (2) reduce the rate and depth of breathing; (3) check the oxygen equipment to ensure proper functioning; and (4) descend to a lower altitude where hypoxia is unlikely to occur. A tendency to hyperventilate is apparent when one experiences positive pressure breathing. This tendency, however, can be controlled by following the positive pressure breathing procedure previously out-

Table 5–16. Comparison of Hyperventilation and Hypoxic Hypoxia Syndromes

Signs and Symptoms	Hyperventilation	Hypoxia
Onset of symptoms	Gradual	Rapid (altitude-dependent)
Muscle activity	Spasm	Flaccid
Appearance	Pale, clammy	Cyanosis
Tetany	Present	Absent
Breathlessness	X	X
Dizziness	X	X
Dullness and drowsiness	X	X
Euphoria	X	X
Fatigue	X	X
Headache	X	X
Judgment poor	X	X
Lightheadedness	X	X
Memory faulty	X	X
Muscle incoordination	X	X
Numbness	X	X
Performance deterioration	X	X
Respiratory rate increased	X	X
Reaction time delayed	X	X
Tingling	X	X
Unconsciousness	X	X
Vision blurred	X	X

X means that the sign or symptom can occur in either condition.

lined, particularly if periodically practiced in the hypobaric chamber.

Prevention of Hyperventilation

To prevent serious emergencies, the crewmembers should be able to recognize both signs and symptoms of hypoxia and hyperventilation. Recognition can only occur by experiencing one's own symptoms and observing signs in others at regular intervals in a controlled environment such as the hypobaric chamber.

HYPERCAPNIA

A person at rest will exhale about 0.8 L of carbon dioxide for each liter of oxygen consumed. Thus, in a sealed environment, an individual will gradually deplete the oxygen supply and contaminate the air with carbon dioxide. This problem would arise only if there were a failure of the life-support system that provides the oxygen and eliminates the carbon dioxide. Unlike hypoxia, in which there is a large range of variation before eliciting a respiratory drive, hypercapnia increases respiration with only a slight change in P_{CO_2}.

At sea level, the inspired partial pressure of carbon dioxide is normally less than 1 mm Hg (0.03% of 760 mm Hg). An inspired P_{CO_2} up to 40 mm Hg, about 5% carbon dioxide at sea level, can be tolerated without serious effects. When the inspired P_{CO_2} exceeds 40 mm Hg, a rise of carbon dioxide concentration occurs in the body fluids. Maximum alveolar ventilation occurs when inspired P_{CO_2} reaches about 70 mm Hg. Acidosis is produced by the inability to eliminate carbon dioxide, and the respiratory center is depressed at P_{CO_2} values above 70 mm Hg. Table 5–17 shows the effect of inhalation of carbon dioxide in air at sea level. Individuals exposed to increased carbon dioxide lose consciousness at an inspired P_{CO_2} of 150 mm Hg and die at a P_{CO_2} of 300 mm Hg.

OXYGEN TOXICITY

A common practice in both aerospace and diving operations is to provide artificial atmospheres when air breathing is not practical. Oxygen poisoning can result in either environment if the oxygen tension is maintained at too high a level and breathed for too long a time. Oxygen toxicity is related to the P_{O_2} and not to the percentage of oxygen inspired. The low oxygen partial pressures and short duration of use by flying personnel usually will not cause harm. Long-duration altitude chamber studies with pure oxygen at 250 mm Hg revealed no oxygen toxicity effects on the lung or central nervous system.

The Mercury and Gemini space flights and the pressure suits used for lunar exploration successfully used pure oxygen environments without clinical oxygen toxicity due to the low partial pressures of oxygen maintained. Reduction of red blood cell mass was identified as a physical effect of pure oxygen breathing, largely due to the absence of an inert gas. This problem was corrected by adding small amounts of nitrogen to the breathing mix.

The problem of oxygen toxicity is more significant at sea level and in hyperbaric operations where the partial pressure of oxygen is greatly increased. The toxic effect of oxygen is related to the dose (partial-pressure factor) and the duration of application (time factor). Figure 5–16 illustrates the time/oxygen partial-pressure relationships for both pulmonary and central nervous system toxicity.

Pulmonary Oxygen Toxicity

Prolonged breathing of 60 to 100% oxygen for more than 12 hours at sea level (P_{O_2} of 450 to 760 mm Hg) can irritate the respiratory passageways. Coughing, congestion, sore throat, and substernal soreness are common symptoms, known as the "Lorraine Smith effect." After about 24 hours, decreased vital capacity occurs, followed by serious pulmonary damage: lung irritation, bronchopneumonia, pulmonary edema, and atelectasis. At great oxygen pressures in the hyperbaric envi-

Table 5–17.   Effect of Inhalation of Carbon Dioxide in Air at Sea Level on Pulmonary Ventilation

P_{CO_2} (mm Hg)	$F_{I_{CO_2}}$ (%)	Tidal Volume (ml)	Frequency (breaths/min)	Respiratory Minute Volume (L/min)
0.23	0.03	440	16	7
7.6	1.0	500	16	8
15.2	2.0	560	16	9
30.4	4.0	823	17	14
38.0	5.0	1300	20	26
57.8	7.6	2100	28	52
79.0	10.4	2500	35	76

Data from Comroe, J.H., Jr.: Physiology of Respiration. Chicago, Yearbook Medical Publishers, Inc., 1965.

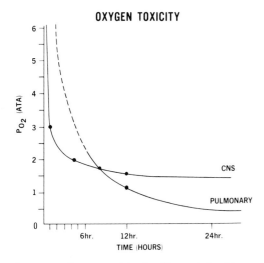

Fig. 5–16.   Oxygen toxicity time/dose relationship.

symptom was substernal distress, and the times to onset varied inversely with inspired P_{O_2}.

In animal studies involving prolonged oxygen exposures, severe pulmonary toxicity resulted in the loss of pulmonary surfactant, structural changes, pulmonary edema, extravasation of red blood cells into the airways, massive atelectasis, carbon dioxide retention, acidosis, and death from hypoxia, even in the presence of high inspired P_{O_2}. Once severe pulmonary toxicity occurs, there exists a point of no return: sustaining a high P_{O_2} will produce further pulmonary damage and death, and lowering the P_{O_2} will lead to arterial hypoxemia and death. It is imperative to prevent the damage from reaching this point by controlling the inspired oxygen pressure.

The only known pulmonary toxicity effects in aerospace operations are from the anecdotal reports of substernal awareness and cough after high sustained G maneuvers in fighter aircraft following prolonged oxygen breathing.

ronment, pulmonary toxicity can occur much more rapidly, but it is easily prevented by taking intermittent air-breathing periods between each oxygen-breathing exposure. Table 5–18 lists the time to onset of pulmonary oxygen toxicity in eight human studies at various altitudes. In these studies, the most predominant

Table 5–18.   Time to Onset of Pulmonary Oxygen Toxicity Symptoms in Man

Barometric Pressure (mm Hg)	Oxygen Partial Pressure (mm Hg)	Duration of Study (hours)	Time to Onset of Symptoms (hours)	Investigator
760	750	6–7	6–7	Behnke, 1940
760	736	24	14	Comroe, et al., 1945
760	630	57	24	Ohlsson, 1947
760	546	24	24	Comroe, et al., 1945
523	418	168	24–36	Michel, et al., 1960
760	380	24	None	Comroe, et al., 1945
258	242	336	86	Morgan, et al., 1963
190	174	408	216	Welch, et al., 1961

Central Nervous System Oxygen Toxicity

Oxygen toxicity of the central nervous system, or the "Paul Bert effect," occurs more rapidly than the pulmonary effects of oxygen toxicity. Central nervous system oxygen toxicity occurs with exposures to P_{O_2} greater than 2 ATA and is not a problem in aerospace operations. It produces convulsions much like those of grand mal epilepsy. It is of primary concern in hyperbaric chamber operations because 100% oxygen is administered at pressures of up to 2.8 ATA in the treatment of decompression sickness (see Chapter 7). Less serious symptoms related to the central nervous system may precede the convulsion: hypersensitivity, nausea, muscular twitching (particularly facial muscles), fatigue, and muscle incoordination. If such symptoms are recognized in time, the convulsion may be avoided by removing the breathing mask to reduce the inspired oxygen pressure.

The events and signs of an oxygen convulsion are usually the same for each individual. Consciousness is lost when the convulsion starts. Respiration ceases during the tonic convulsive stage, which may last for 1 to 2 minutes. If left unprotected, the convulsing person may sustain physical injuries due to striking hard objects or biting the tongue. Following the convulsion, respiration normally resumes spontaneously, but the victim may remain semiconscious, irrational, and restless for several minutes.

Treatment

If an individual displays any sign of central nervous system oxygen toxicity, the hyperoxic breathing source must be removed quickly. Ambient pressure must never be altered until the convulsion ceases and breathing resumes. Ascent with a closed glottis may lead to fatal air embolism. A padded mouthpiece (never the fingers) should be used to prevent tongue-biting. The victim should be restrained to prevent injury from flailing or falling. The victim's head should be turned to one side to prevent aspiration should vomiting occur. If the victim does not resume normal breathing following the convulsion, the airway should be checked for obstruction and immediate cardiopulmonary resuscitation begun with air.

Victims of central nervous system oxygen toxicity recover promptly and completely when the high oxygen tension is removed. There are no lasting or residual effects, and the victim will be no more susceptible to oxygen toxicity in the future.

Prevention

Breathing 100% oxygen at 2.8 ATA while at complete rest for 30 minutes is an exposure that 98% of subjects can tolerate without signs of oxygen toxicity. As depth, activity, or exposure time is increased, more individuals will display signs of toxicity. In the treatment of decompression sickness, 100% oxygen is administered to the patient at pressures up to 2.8 ATA for periods up to 285 minutes. To preclude toxicity, intermittent air-breathing is used with the oxygen. If air is breathed for short periods (5 minutes) between longer oxygen-breathing periods (20 minutes), the latent period before symptoms occur is safely extended. Pure oxygen is never breathed at pressures greater than 3 ATA. As C.J. Lambertsen has stated: "With more prolonged O_2 exposure, total failure of gas exchange is inevitable . . . and death (occurs) from hypoxia in the presence of and due to the high inspired P_{O_2}."

REFERENCES

1. Comroe, J.H., Jr.: Physiology of Respiration. Chicago, Yearbook Medical Publishers, Inc., 1965.
2. Rahn, H., and Otis, A.B.: Alveolar air during simulated flights to high altitudes. Am. J. Physiol., 150:202, 1947.
3. Lambertsen, C.J.: Respiration. In Medical Physiology. Vol. 2. 14th Ed. Edited by V.B. Mountcastle. St. Louis, C.V. Mosby Co., 1980.

4. Brobeck, J.R., and Dubois, A.B.: Energy exchange. *In* Medical Physiology. 14th Ed. Edited by V.B. Mountcastle. St. Louis, C.V. Mosby Co., 1980.

5. Holmstrom, F.M.G.: Hypoxia. *In* Aerospace Medicine. Edited by H.W. Randall. Baltimore, Williams & Wilkins Co., 1971.

6. Air Medical Service. War Department: Air Services Division of Military Aeronautics. Washington, D.C.: Government Printing Office, 1919, pp. 423–434.

Chapter 6

Protection in the Pressure Environment: Cabin Pressurization and Oxygen Equipment

Richard D. Heimbach and Paul J. Sheffield

. . . it is becoming increasingly apparent that stratosphere, or even substratosphere, flying can never be carried out as a practical routine procedure until there is a change in aircraft design which will maintain a more nearly normal pressure about the occupants.

HARRY G. ARMSTRONG, M.D.

In 1643, Evangelista Torricelli invented the barometer and first pondered the effects that lowered atmospheric pressures would have on living organisms. Man was not destined to have to deal with these effects until his dream of sustained, controlled flight became a reality in the beginning of the twentieth century. Continual striving for ever-higher flight has brought man face to face with an unchangeable truth: man is trapped within a body biologically adapted to a very narrow range of barometric pressures. In 1939, General Harry G. Armstrong, who later became the United States Air Force Surgeon General, wrote of the need for an aircraft design to pressurize the occupants during high-altitude flight.[1] Today, aircraft and spacecraft are designed to maintain a nearly normal pressure surrounding the occupant, but circumstances can cause a reduction in pressure outside the normal range of human tolerance.

This chapter focuses on the pressurization and oxygen equipment systems that protect aircraft occupants during high-altitude flight. The type of protective equipment is determined by the physiologic needs of the aviator at the peak altitude of exposure, as indicated by the physiologic zones of the pressure environment.

THE PRESSURE ENVIRONMENT

The pressure environment surrounding the earth can be divided into four zones based on physiologic effects: the physiologic zone, the physiologically deficient zone, the space-equivalent zone, and space.

The physiologic zone extends from sea level to approximately 3048 m, encompassing the pressure area to which man is well adapted. Although middle ear or sinus problems may be experienced during ascent or descent in this zone, most physiologic problems occur outside this zone if proper protective equipment is not utilized.

The physiologically deficient zone extends from altitudes of 3048 to 15,240 m. Decreased barometric pressure results in oxygen deficiency, causing altitude hypoxia. Additional problems may arise from trapped and evolved gases. Protective oxygen equipment is mandatory in this zone.

Flight between altitudes of 15,240 m and 75 km is in the space-equivalent zone. The total pressure progressively decreases from 87 to 1 mm Hg. Travel in this zone requires protection by a sealed cabin or a full-pressure suit.

Altitudes beyond 75 km constitute space. Protection is provided by a sealed cabin or a full-pressure suit. Astronaut candidates earn astronaut status after flight above 80 km. United States Air Force Major Robert M. White became the first winged aircraft pilot to be awarded astronaut status for his X-15 flight to 95 km on July 17, 1962.

Advanced technology has allowed the aircraft industry to develop commercial and military aircraft that far exceed the physiologic tolerance of man. Such advancements include the ever-increasing service ceiling of aircraft for routine operations and manned space operations (e.g., the supersonic transport and space shuttle).

In general, the most effective way of preventing physiologic problems from occurring is to provide an aircraft pressurization system so that the occupants of the aircraft are never exposed to pressures outside the physiologic zone. In those cases when ascent above the physiologic zone is required, protective oxygen equipment must be provided. At altitudes exceeding 15,240 m, counterpressure garments are required.

AIRCRAFT AND SPACECRAFT PRESSURIZATION

Methods of Pressurization

As shown in Figure 6–1, there are two principal aircraft pressurization schedules: isobaric and isobaric-differential.

Isobaric System

Isobaric control maintains a constant cabin pressure as the ambient barometric pressure decreases. Many military and civilian aircraft are equipped with isobaric pressurization systems (e.g., the United States Air Force T-39, the Lockheed L-1011, and the Boeing B-747). These aircraft cabin altitudes are maintained at 610 to 2438 m. This pressurization increases the comfort and mobility of the passengers, negates the requirement for the routine use of oxygen equipment, and minimizes fatigue.

Isobaric-Differential System

Tactical military aircraft are not equipped with isobaric pressurization systems because the added weight would severely limit the range of the aircraft, and the large pressure differential would increase the danger of a rapid decompression during combat situations. Instead, these aircraft are equipped with an isobaric-differential cabin pressurization system. Aircraft pressurization begins as the aircraft ascends through 1524 m to 2438 m. The isobaric function controls cabin altitude until a preset pressure differential is reached. With continued ascent, the preset differential is maintained. Thus, cabin altitude progressively increases as the aircraft ascends. The aircraft featured in Figure 6–1 has an isobaric-differential pressurization system of 8.6 lb/in^2 differential (psid). If the aircraft were flying at 12,192 m, ambient pressure would be 2.72 psi. Occupants of the aircraft would be exposed to a cabin pressure of 11.32 psi (8.6 psi plus 2.72 psi), a pressure equivalent to 2134 m altitude. For example, the United

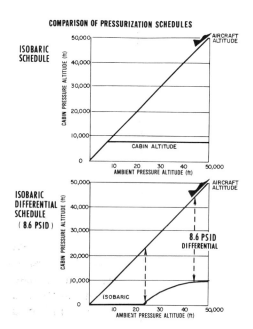

Fig. 6–1. Isobaric and isobaric-differential aircraft pressurization schedules.

States Air Force C-141 cargo aircraft is equipped with an 8.6 psi isobaric-differential pressurization system. Cabin altitude is maintained at sea level pressure until the aircraft ascends through 6401 m. Above this level, the system maintains a pressure differential of 8.6 psi up to the service ceiling of the aircraft.

In fighter aircraft, the isobaric-differential pressurization system is set at a lower pressure differential, typically 5 psid. The aircraft is unpressurized to an altitude of 2438 m, where the isobaric control starts. As the aircraft continues to ascend, cabin pressure is maintained at 2438 m until 5 psid is reached. As the flight altitude continues to increase, so does the cabin altitude but at 5 psid.

On some older fighter and bomber aircraft, an extra feature called "combat override" was incorporated in the design. The concept of this feature was to permit the combat pilot to reduce the pressure differential to reduce the adverse physiologic effects of rapid decompression while under fire. In combat situations, the pilot

could slowly reduce the pressure differential to 2.75 psid for fighters or 4.5 psid for the United States Air Force B-52. The combat override feature is not provided in newer fighter aircraft because advanced weaponry technology made this seldom-used feature impractical.

Advantages of Pressurization

Aircraft must fly at high altitudes for fuel efficiency. Because aircraft pressurization systems are so effective, aviators can participate in high-altitude flight in safety and comfort. Supplemental oxygen equipment usually is not required. In some situations, however, it may be more advantageous for the pilot to use supplemental oxygen: during night flying operations, especially on final approach, emergencies involving loss of pressurization, and emergencies involving the presence of smoke or fumes. Flight rules require one pilot to use oxygen above certain altitudes, usually 13,716 m, even though the aircraft is pressurized. With aircraft pressurization, the probability of decompression sickness is greatly reduced. Less gas expansion results in fewer gastrointestinal trapped-gas problems. Cabin humidity, temperature air-flow, and the rate of pressure change can be controlled to acceptable comfort ranges. In multiplace aircraft, passengers and crew are free to move about the cabin unhampered by oxygen masks or special high-altitude support equipment. Thus, fatigue and discomfort are minimized during prolonged passenger flights.

Disadvantages of Pressurization

The primary disadvantage of aircraft pressurization is the possibility of loss of cabin pressure. Should a decompression occur, the occupants of the aircraft are rapidly exposed to the dangers of unpressurized high-altitude flight such as hypoxia, decompression sickness, gastrointestinal gas expansion, and hypothermia. Pressurized flight requires that the aircraft structure must be strengthened to maintain structural integrity. Additional equipment and power requirements are needed to support the aircraft pressurization system. This equipment occupies space, adds weight, and increases fuel costs. The peak performance and payload of the aircraft is decreased because of the added weight, and additional manpower and maintenance costs are involved. In addition, provisions must be made for controlling cabin air contaminants such as smoke, fumes, carbon monoxide, and carbon dioxide. Nonetheless, the advantages of aircraft pressurization far outweigh the disadvantages.

Physical Limitations of Pressurization Systems

The pressurized cabin used in most conventional aircraft is shown in Figure 6–2. This system depends on air drawn from outside the aircraft being compressed and delivered to the cabin. The altitude limit is about 24,384 m on this type of system because of the inability of the compressor system to effectively pressurize the cabin in extremely low-pressure, high-altitude flight.

The mechanical ability of the compressor to provide pressure, ventilation, and air conditioning depends on the pressure ratio, $\dfrac{P \text{ cabin}}{P \text{ ambient}}$. This ratio is sometimes called the compression ratio and expresses the number of times that the am-

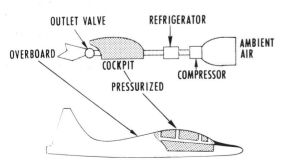

Fig. 6–2. The pressurized cabin used in most conventional aircraft.

bient air must be compressed to maintain desired cabin pressure. For example, an aircraft at 18,288 m (1.05 psi) with a cabin altitude of 3048 m (10.11 psi) has a pressure ratio of 10:1. Thus, the air in the cabin must be compressed to achieve a pressure ten times greater than ambient pressure. As flight altitude increases, the pressure ratio increases dramatically. For instance, an aircraft at 22,860 m (0.52 psi) with a cabin altitude of 3048 m (10.11 psi) has a pressure ratio of 20:1.

At very high altitudes, the heat generated in the process of compressing air causes the cabin temperature to rise. For example, an aircraft at 22,860 m with a pressure ratio of 20:1 could achieve a cabin air temperature of about 315°C due to adiabatic heating. Thus, a highly efficient cooling system is required for crew survival.

As ascent continues, a point is eventually reached where the density of ambient air is so reduced that it is impossible for the compressor to draw in enough air to pressurize the cabin. Under such conditions, a sealed cabin must be used to maintain an acceptable crew environment. A sealed cabin must be used for sustained flight at altitudes above approximately 24,384 m. As shown in Figure 6–3, pressurization is attained by the craft carrying its own supply of gases, usually oxygen and nitrogen. These gases are regulated in the proper proportion to provide the required pressure and gaseous environment within the cabin. Spacecraft and shuttlecraft are equipped with this type of system.

As with all aircraft components, the possibility of a mechanical failure of the system is always present. Failures in aircraft pressurization generally have been due to the failure of canopies, hatches, doors, and plexiglass windows.

Decompression Rates

The severity and consequences of cabin pressure loss depend on the rate of de-

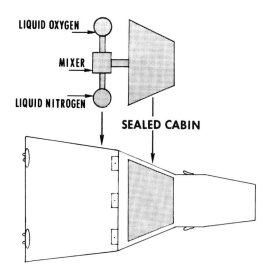

Fig. 6–3. The sealed cabin used in spacecraft and shuttlecraft.

compression and the pressure range over which it occurs. Decompressions can be divided into two categories: slow and rapid. A slow loss of cabin pressure can occur when a leak develops in a pressure seal. If unaware of the depressurization, occupants could become incapacitated by hypoxia. A rapid decompression, as will soon become evident, is easily recognized.

Several equations have been developed for estimating the time of decompression with varying degrees of accuracy. Fliegner's equation has been found to be useful as an approximation and is expressed as follows:

$$t = 0.22 \, (V/A) \, \sqrt{(P - B)/B} \qquad (1)$$

where t is the time of decompression in seconds; V is the volume of the pressurized cabin in cubic feet; A is the cross-sectional area of the opening in square inches; P is the cabin pressure in psia; and B is the actual flight pressure altitude in psia.

Thus, several physical factors determine the time of decompression:

1. *Volume of the pressurized cabin (V)*—the larger the pressurized cabin,

the slower the decompression when all other factors are equal.
2. *Size of the opening (A)*—the larger the opening, the faster the decompression. The principal factor that determines the rate and time of decompression is the ratio between the volume of the cabin and the cross-sectional area of the opening.
3. *Pressure differential (P – B)*—the initial difference between the pressure within the cabin and the ambient pressure directly influences the rate and severity of the decompression. The greater the differential, the more severe the decompression.
4. *Pressure ratio (P/B)*—the time of decompression depends on the pressure ratio between the cabin and ambient pressures. The greater the pressure ratio, the longer the time of decompression.
5. *Flight pressure altitude (B)*—The physiologic problems that occur following a loss of cabin pressure are directly related to the altitude at which the decompression occurs.

Haber and Clamann developed the general theory of rapid decompression, which offers a more complete analysis of both the decompression time and the process of a rapid decompression. In this model, the time of decompression depends essentially on two factors. One factor is the relationship between the volume of the cabin and the cross-sectional area of the opening in the cabin. Haber and Clamann define this relationship as the time-constant of the cabin (t_c) and express it as follows:

$$t_c = \frac{V}{AC} \qquad (2)$$

where V is the volume of the cabin in cubic feet; A is the area of the opening in square inches; and C is the speed of sound. A value of about 1100 ft/sec can be used for the speed of sound.

The second factor on which the time of decompression depends is a pressure-dependent factor (P_1), a complex function of the ratio P/B in which P is the cabin pressure before decompression and B is the cabin pressure after decompression. The values for P_1 for any given pressure ratio up to 30 can be obtained from Table 6–1.

The total time of decompression (T) is equal to the product of the time-constant (t_c) and the pressure factor P_1 as follows:

$$T = t_c \times P_1 \qquad (3)$$

Thus, the total time of decompression can be estimated if the volume of the cabin, the effective opening area, and the initial and final cabin pressures are known. Decompression rate calculations in Table 6–2 compare the Haber-Clamann formula with Fliegner's formula.

Table 6–1. Pressure-Dependent Factor (P_1) in Decompression

(P/B)	(P_1)	(P/B)	(P_1)
1	0	16	4.9
2	1.7	17	5.0
3	2.3	18	5.1
4	2.6	19	5.2
5	2.9	20	5.3
6	3.2	21	5.4
7	3.5	22	5.5
8	3.8	23	5.6
9	4.0	24	5.6
10	4.1	25	5.7
11	4.3	26	5.7
12	4.5	27	5.8
13	4.6	28	5.8
14	4.7	29	5.9
15	4.8	30	6.0

The relationship between the pressure-dependent factor (P_1) is seen as a ratio of cabin pressure before decompression (P) to cabin pressure at the end of decompression (B).

The pressure-dependent factor (P_1) for the total time of decompression (T) of the Haber-Clamann formula is derived from the absolute pressure ratio in the cabin before and after decompression (P/B).

Physical Characteristics of a Rapid Decompression

Noise

When two different air masses collide, a noise is heard that ranges from a "swish" to an explosive sound.

Flying Debris

Upon decompression, the rapid rush of air from a pressurized cabin causes the velocity of airflow through the cabin to increase rapidly as the air approaches the hole. Loose objects, such as maps, charts, and furnishings, will be extracted through the orifice. There have been instances of unrestrained people adjacent to and in the immediate vicinity of the opening being sucked from the aircraft. Dust and dirt will hamper vision for a short period of time.

Fogging

During a rapid decompression, both the temperature and pressure suddenly decrease. This decrease reduces the capacity of air to contain water vapor and fogging occurs. The dissipation rate of this fog is fairly rapid in fighter aircraft but considerably slower in larger, multiplace aircraft.

Physiologic Effects of Rapid Decompression

The physiologic effects of primary concern in a rapid decompression are hypothermia, gas expansion, decompression sickness, and acute hypoxia.

Hypothermia

When decompression occurs, the temperature drops to that of ambient air. Chilling and frostbite could easily occur if proper protective clothing, boots, and gloves were not worn.

Gas Expansion

The physiologic effects of gas expansion resulting from decompression occur primarily in the body cavities such as the middle ears, sinuses, gastrointestinal tract,

Table 6–2. Decompression Rate Calculations For Passenger Aircraft Following Loss of a Window

Factors	Haber-Clamann Formula	Fliegner's Formula
Cabin volume	10,000 ft³	10,000 ft³
Area of opening	0.5 ft²	72 in²
Time-constant	18.2 seconds	—
Time of decompression		
From 914 m (13.17 psi) to 7620 m (5.46 psi)	34.5 seconds	36.3 seconds
From 1524 m (12.23 psi) to 12,192 m (2.72 psi)	50.0 seconds	50.4 seconds
From 2438 m (10.91 psi) to 13,716 m (2.15 psi)	52.8 seconds	61.7 seconds

and lungs. Chapter 7 on Decompression Sickness and Pulmonary Overpressure Accidents includes a detailed discussion of these effects.

Decompression Sickness

A principal advantage of pressurized cabins is the protection they afford the aircrew against decompression sickness. In general, decompression sickness does not occur until cabin altitudes above 5486 m are reached. The incidence of decompression sickness is small unless the cabin altitude reaches at least 7620 to 9144 m. As the duration of exposure to the unpressurized environment increases, however, so does the incidence of decompression sickness.

Hypoxia

Of all the physiologic hazards associated with the loss of pressure, hypoxia is the most important. Thus, the most critical need after decompression is oxygen, especially if the cabin altitude before decompression was below 3048 m and the passengers were not breathing oxygen. The rapid reduction of ambient pressure produces a corresponding drop in the partial pressure of oxygen and reduces the alveolar oxygen tension. A twofold to threefold performance decrement occurs, regardless of altitude. The reduced tolerance to hypoxia after decompression is due to (1) a reversal in the direction of oxygen flow in the lung; (2) diminished respiratory activity at the time of decompression; and (3) decreased cardiac

activity at the time of decompression. Unless supplemental oxygen is acquired within 30 seconds after rapid decompression to 9144 m, consciousness will be lost. At 13,716 m, it is unlikely that there would be enough time to don an oxygen mask.

Rapid Decompression While Wearing an Oxygen Mask

Under certain flight conditions, it is necessary that an oxygen mask be worn securely in place at all times. During studies in which subjects were rapidly decompressed from simulated cabin pressures of 7620 to 15,240 m in less than 0.5 seconds, mask pressures reached an average peak of 62 mm Hg during the initial phase of the decompression. Immediate pressure relief occurred with leakage around the edges of the mask, regardless of how tightly the mask was secured to the face. None of the subjects showed untoward effects, and each subject continued to pressure breathe at 15,240 m for about 5 minutes without serious incapacitation.

OXYGEN EQUIPMENT

The flyer who is suffering from want of oxygen is far from normal. He may be exhilarated, he may be simply dull and sleepy, or, if he is in a position of danger he may fail to take the measures necessary for the safety of himself and those with him, even when he is well aware of the danger.

. . . [T]he aviator supplied with oxygen while flying is very much more efficient than the same man flying without oxygen, and becomes, therefore, of so much more value as a fighting force. Take, for example, two pilots of equal ability, flying machines being identical in every respect, that man supplied with oxygen will always bring down the other machine because he has retained all his judgment and rapidity of decision and movement unimpaired. He will be able to outmaneuver and outwit his opponent and fire his gun before the other has even made up his mind what to do. Not only that, when he returns to the ground after prolonged flight he will be fresh and able to start out on a new trip, while the man flying without oxygen will be tired out and unable to do any more work that day and possibly the next. The administration of oxygen must of course in no way impair the comfort or the movements of the airman, nor should he have anything further to do while flying, as he already has plenty to look after, in his machine. For this reason the apparatus used must be simple, safe, and entirely automatic; automatic in the sense that while the machine stands on the ground no oxygen is given off, but when it rises in the air the increasing deficiency in the oxygen content of the air is automatically made up for by the delivery of oxygen by the apparatus, without any personal attention from the airman.

The above quote exemplifies the recognition of the need for protective oxygen equipment early in the history of aviation. This message to the flyer was published in 1919 by the United States War Department.[2]

Historically, aircraft oxygen system development paralleled that of aircraft performance. The "pipestem" oxygen system (Fig. 6–4) was used by early aviators. Protection was limited because of the difficulty of maintaining the pipestem be-

tween the teeth, the inadequate accommodation for nose breathers, and the wasted oxygen due to continuous flow. The first practical automatic oxygen delivery system was the Dreyer apparatus (Fig. 6–5). Designed by Colonel Georges Dreyer for the British Royal Air Force, it was adapted to all United States planes flying to high altitudes by 1919, and instructions were published for its use.[2] The apparatus provided 500 L of gaseous oxygen in two steel bottles at 2200 psi. An aneroid-controlled valve delivered 100% oxygen in increasing quantities during ascent. The india rubber oronasal mask that attached to the flyer's leather helmet also contained a microphone for communication. As aircraft performance increased, so did the sophistication of the oxygen delivery system.

Oxygen Systems

An aircraft oxygen system usually consists of (1) containers for the storage of

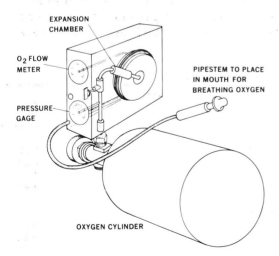

Fig. 6–4. The "pipestem" oxygen system used by early aviators.

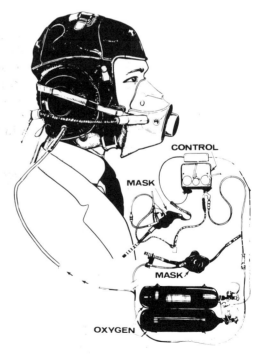

Fig. 6–5. The Dreyer oxygen apparatus, the first practical automatic oxygen delivery system.

oxygen either in a gaseous, liquid, or solid state; (2) tubing to direct the flow of oxygen from the source to a metering device or regulator; (3) regulators or metering devices that control the pressure and percentage of oxygen available to the user; and (4) a properly fitted oronasal mask, full face mask, or helmet to deliver oxygen to the user.

Gaseous Oxygen

Aviator's gaseous oxygen is classified as grade A, type I oxygen. Military systems must adhere to military specifications for oxygen, requiring 99.5% purity by volume and no more than 0.005 mg/L of water vapor at 760 mm Hg and 20°C. Limiting the water vapor content is critical because the temperature drop encountered at high altitude would freeze the system and restrict the oxygen flow. Gaseous oxygen also must be odorless and free of contaminants, including drying agents. Gaseous oxygen can be delivered either by a low-pressure or high-pressure system.

The storage system for a low-pressure gaseous oxygen system is lightweight, nonshatterable cylinders, which are color-coded yellow. When fully charged, these cylinders can hold 450 psi. Under normal conditions, they are considered full at a range of 400 to 450 psi. The major limitation of the low-pressure system is its limited volume. The system is considered empty at pressures below 100 psi. Should the pressure drop below 50 psi, the system must be purged to prevent a buildup of moisture. Table 6–3 shows the oxygen duration for the Cessna T37B aircraft.

For emergency use, most commercial aircraft rely on high-pressure gas cylinders. Most fighter, bomber, and training aircraft use high-pressure oxygen as a backup breathing system. High-pressure oxygen is contained in nonshatterable cylinders filled to a pressure of 1800 to 2200 psi. Cylinders of this type are color-coded green, are heavy, and have the advantage of storing large amounts of oxygen in a small space.

Liquid Oxygen

Aviator's liquid oxygen (LOX) is classified as grade B, type II. The boiling point of LOX is −182.8°C, and its expansion ratio is 1 to 850 ± 10 L at 760 mm Hg and 21.1°C. Thus, 1 L of liquid oxygen provides 840 to 860 L of gaseous oxygen. Liquid oxygen is produced from compressing and cooling ordinary filtered air. The liquid air produced is then warmed slowly to −195.6°C, at which point nitrogen vaporizes, leaving liquid oxygen. The entire process is repeated several times to ensure

Table 6–3. Oxygen Duration—Low-Pressure Gaseous Oxygen System

Cabin Altitude		Gauge Pressure (psi)						
		400	350	300	250	200	150	100
(m)	(ft)				Duration (hours)*			
With Regulator Diluter Lever at Normal Position								
7620	25,000	3.08	2.63	2.31	1.96	1.54	1.15	0.77
6096	20,000	3.22	2.82	2.41	2.02	1.61	1.20	0.80
4572	15,000	4.24	3.71	3.17	2.65	2.12	1.58	1.06
3048	10,000	5.63	4.95	4.21	3.52	2.80	2.10	1.41
With Regulator Diluter Lever at 100% Position								
7620	25,000	2.45	2.14	1.83	1.53	1.22	0.91	0.61
6096	20,000	1.87	1.63	1.39	1.16	0.92	0.69	0.46
4572	15,000	1.49	1.31	1.12	0.93	0.75	0.56	0.37
3048	10,000	1.20	1.05	0.89	0.75	0.60	0.45	0.29

*This oxygen duration is for two crewmembers in the Cessna T37B aircraft (double duration for one crewmember). The oxygen system is maintained at 425 ± 25 psi when fully charged. The technical directives for this system require that, when available oxygen is less than 100 psi, one descend to an altitude where oxygen is not required.

the production of nearly pure liquid oxygen. Gaseous oxygen is then produced by allowing the liquid to evaporate.

Military fighter and training aircraft usually operate with an oxygen converter pressure of 70 to 90 psi. Multiplace aircraft routinely maintain a converter pressure of 300 psi. This higher pressure is necessitated by the increased number of crew and passenger positions and by the need for a readily available oxygen source for recharging portable oxygen cylinders.

For the majority of aircraft in use today, the LOX system is superior to the gaseous oxygen system. The oxygen capacity of a single 25-L converter is equal to about 105 6.9-ft^3 bottles of high-pressure gaseous oxygen. Table 6–4 shows the oxygen duration of the General Dynamics FB111 aircraft high-pressure LOX system. Liquid oxygen has about a 3.5 to 1 weight advantage over a gaseous oxygen system and an 8 to 1 advantage in terms of space saved. A typical liquid oxygen converter flow diagram is shown in Figure 6–6.

Solid Chemical Production of Oxygen

Presently, chemical combinations, or solid-state oxygen systems, are limited to emergency use by passengers in military and civilian aircraft. The system is contained in a plastic canister and consists of a continuous flow breathing mask with lanyards connected to actuating pins of a sodium chlorate candle or some similar oxygen-producing device. Upon removal of the mask and actuation of the pins, a chemical reaction is initiated. One such candle utilizes the following chemical reaction:

$$NaClO_3 + Fe \rightarrow FeO + NaCl + O_2 \quad (3)$$

To begin the chemical process, heat is provided to an iron-enriched area by the percussion cap, or friction igniter. When the temperature of the reaction rises above 250°C, the process is self-supporting, and the reaction proceeds down the length of the candle. A harmless amount of chlorine may be detected for about 12 seconds, followed by 95% pure oxygen and 5% argon, which is provided to the mask. The amount of oxygen produced depends on the size and burning rate of the candle. The sodium chlorate candle shown in Figure 6–7 is typical.

Onboard Oxygen Generation System (OBOGS)

The concept of producing oxygen in flight has long been attractive. The OBOGS concept offers the benefits of increased operational safety and minimized logistic support of the oxygen system. Several OBOGS systems are under development and testing, including electrochemical concentration, fluomine chemical absorption, molecular sieve absorption, and permeable membrane systems.

ELECTROCHEMICAL CONCENTRATION. The early attempt at the onboard production of oxygen by the electrolysis of water met with serious drawbacks and was never fully developed. A modification called the "reversed fuel cell" offers more promise, however. In this method, the standard procedure of producing an electrical current by combining hydrogen and oxygen is reversed by providing electricity to the fuel cell, thus producing oxygen at the anode and hydrogen at the cathode. Hydrogen is then oxidized to water by combining with oxygen in the air that flows over the cathode. The equation for this process is as follows:

$$E + 2H_2O \rightarrow 2H_2 + O_2 + heat \quad (4)$$

FLUOMINE CHEMICAL ABSORPTION. This system utilizes the reversible absorption of oxygen by fluomine (Fig. 6–8). Basically, the system operates by extracting oxygen from compressed air. Air is passed over an absorbent bed that absorbs the oxygen. Oxygen is then recovered by reducing the pressure over the bed. Generally, two absorbent beds are used alternately to

Table 6–4. Oxygen Duration–High-Pressure (LOX) Oxygen System

Cabin Altitude (ft)	Consumption—Two Men (cubic feet/hr)	Duration (hours)*														
		With Regulator at 100% or EMER Position														
35,000	9.8	46.8	43.7	40.6	37.4	34.3	31.2	28.1	25.0	21.8	18.7	15.6	12.5	9.4	6.2	3.1
30,000	13.4	34.3	32.0	29.7	27.4	25.1	22.8	20.5	18.3	16.0	13.7	11.4	9.1	6.8	4.6	2.3
28,000	15.0	30.6	28.5	26.5	24.4	22.4	20.4	18.4	16.3	14.3	12.2	10.2	8.2	6.1	4.1	2.0
26,000	16.0	28.6	26.7	24.8	22.9	21.0	19.1	17.2	15.3	13.4	11.5	9.6	7.6	5.7	3.8	1.9
24,000	18.52	24.7	23.1	21.4	19.8	18.1	16.5	14.9	13.2	11.6	9.9	8.3	6.6	5.0	3.3	1.6
22,000	20.76	22.1	20.7	19.2	17.7	16.2	14.7	13.3	11.8	10.3	8.8	7.4	5.9	4.4	2.9	1.5
20,000	23.0	20.0	18.6	17.2	15.9	14.6	13.3	12.0	10.6	9.3	8.0	6.6	5.3	4.0	2.7	1.3
18,000	25.24	18.1	16.9	15.7	14.5	13.3	12.1	10.9	9.7	8.5	7.3	6.1	4.8	3.6	2.4	1.2
16,000	27.48	16.8	15.6	14.5	13.4	12.3	11.1	10.0	8.9	7.8	6.7	5.6	4.4	3.3	2.2	1.1
14,000	30.0	15.6	14.5	13.5	12.4	11.4	10.2	9.2	8.2	7.1	6.1	5.1	4.1	3.1	2.0	1.0
12,000	32.8	13.9	13.0	12.1	11.1	10.2	9.3	8.4	7.5	6.5	5.6	4.7	3.7	2.8	1.9	0.9
10,000	35.6	12.9	12.0	11.1	10.3	9.5	8.6	7.7	6.9	6.0	5.1	4.3	3.4	2.6	1.7	0.8
8,000	39.4	11.6	10.8	10.1	9.3	8.5	7.8	7.0	6.2	5.4	4.7	3.9	3.1	2.3	1.5	0.7
0	55.6	8.2	7.7	7.1	6.6	6.0	5.5	4.9	4.4	3.8	3.3	2.7	2.2	1.6	1.1	0.5
Available Oxygen	Liquid (L) Gas (cubic feet)	15 459.0	14 428.4	13 397.8	12 367.2	11 336.6	10 306.0	9 275.4	8 244.8	7 214.2	6 183.6	5 153.0	4 122.4	3 91.8	2 61.2	1 30.6
		With Regulator in NORM Position														
35,000	9.8	46.7	43.6	40.5	37.4	34.3	31.2	28.1	25.0	21.8	18.7	15.6	12.5	9.4	6.2	3.1
30,000	13.2	34.7	32.4	30.1	27.8	25.5	23.2	20.9	18.6	16.2	13.9	11.6	9.3	7.0	4.6	2.3
25,000	14.0	32.8	30.6	28.4	26.2	24.0	21.9	19.7	17.5	15.3	13.1	10.9	8.7	6.6	4.4	2.2
20,000	12.4	37.0	34.6	32.1	29.6	27.2	24.7	22.2	19.8	17.3	14.8	12.3	9.9	7.4	4.9	2.5
15,000	10.2	45.0	42.0	39.0	36.0	33.0	30.0	27.0	24.0	21.0	18.0	15.0	12.0	9.0	6.0	3.0
10,000	10.2	45.0	42.0	39.0	36.0	33.0	30.0	27.0	24.0	21.0	18.0	15.0	12.0	9.0	6.0	3.0
8,000	10.2	45.0	42.0	39.0	36.0	33.0	30.0	27.0	24.0	21.0	18.0	15.0	12.0	9.0	6.0	3.0
5,000	10.2	45.0	42.0	39.0	36.0	33.0	30.0	27.0	24.0	21.0	18.0	15.0	12.0	9.0	6.0	3.0
Sea level	10.2	45.0	42.0	39.0	36.0	33.0	30.0	27.0	24.0	21.0	18.0	15.0	12.0	9.0	6.0	3.0
Available oxygen	Liquid (L) Gas (cubic feet)	15 459.0	14 428.4	13 397.8	12 367.2	11 336.6	10 306.0	9 275.4	8 244.8	7 214.2	6 183.6	5 153.0	4 122.4	3 91.8	2 61.2	1 30.6

This oxygen duration is for two crewmembers in the General Dynamics FB111 aircraft (double duration for one crewmember). Technical directives for this system require that, when available oxygen is less than 1 L, one descend to below 3000 m MSL.

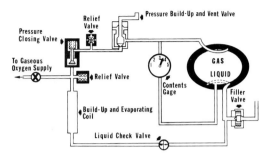

Fig. 6–6. Liquid oxygen converter flow diagram.

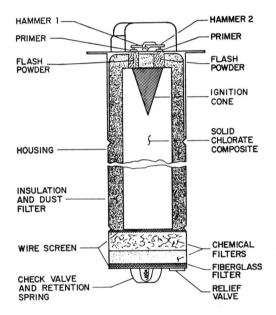

Fig. 6–7. Sodium chlorate candle.

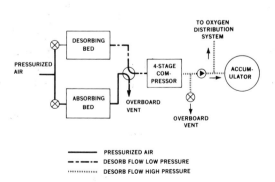

Fig. 6–8. Fluomine chemical absorption oxygen generator.

provide a continuous oxygen flow. A major drawback of this system is that the oxygen produced must be compressed before it is supplied to the oxygen breathing regulator.

MOLECULAR SIEVE. Oxygen can be produced for aircrews by a molecular sieve (Fig. 6–9). This system provides pressurized air from the turbine engine compressor stage to alternating molecular sieve beds. Each molecular sieve contains crystalline aluminosilicate compounds called Ziolites. As pressurized air is passed through the bed, the mixture is separated into its components. The oxygen-enriched portion is then separated out and temporarily stored in a plenum. From the plenum, oxygen is then provided to the breathing regulator. The major disadvantage of this system is the presence of impurities. At best, it can only provide up to 95% oxygen, with 5% argon present.

OXYGEN-PERMEABLE MEMBRANE. This system contains an oxygen-permeable membrane across which air is passed (Fig. 6–10). As the air contacts the membrane surface, the oxygen molecules present in the air dissolve in the membrane surface according to their solubility coefficients. The opposite surface of the membrane is maintained at a lower pressure and equilibrated with its gas concentration. The

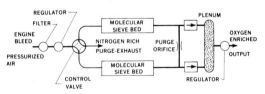

Fig. 6–9. Molecular sieve oxygen generator.

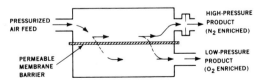

Fig. 6–10. Permeable membrane for oxygen enrichment.

high-pressure side is enriched with nitrogen, and the low-pressure side is enriched with oxygen. The nitrogen-rich high-pressure side is continuously drawn off to leave a high concentration of oxygen on the low-pressure side.

Oxygen Contaminants

Several sources of contamination are possible for aviator's breathing oxygen. In the production of liquid oxygen, the air used is 78.03% nitrogen, 20.99% oxygen, and 0.94% argon by volume. The remaining 0.04% is a composite of carbon dioxide, helium, neon, krypton, xenon, and various hydrocarbons such as methane and acetylene. Carbon monoxide, hydrogen sulfide, hydrogen cyanide, nitrous oxides, and ammonia also are found in trace amounts. In addition to trace contaminants, worn valves, pumps, and filters can contribute solid particles. Refrigerants and solvents used in the oxygen production plant also can be found. Furthermore, contaminants can be introduced during the transfer of liquid oxygen to storage facilities. When supply hoses are initially connected, atmospheric contaminants may be present and could be carried into the converter via the moving liquid. Contaminants may enter the disconnected transfer hose and enter the system in the next recharging cycle. All of these possible contaminants must be vigorously controlled to protect the aviator.

Generally speaking, breathing gas contaminants are divided into five types: solid inert contaminants, dissolved inert contaminants, toxic substances, odor-producing contaminants, and combustible contaminants. Solid inert contaminants are small, insoluble particles that do not react with liquid oxygen. These particles range from rust and metal fragments to frozen carbon dioxide and ice. Nitrogen and argon are considered dissolved inert contaminants. They are unreactive and are soluble in liquid oxygen. Toxic substances usually are found in such low concentrations that they rarely present a problem. Odor-causing contaminants are of great concern, and their presence must be kept as low as possible. Even though they may be nontoxic, they can lead to nausea, anxiety, and decreased performance. Examples of combustible contaminants are methane, ethane, acetylene, and ethylene.

Oxygen Regulators

The type of regulator used determines the overall capability of the oxygen delivery system. Three basic oxygen delivery systems are used in aircraft: continuous flow, diluter demand, and diluter demand pressure-breathing, or pressure demand.

Continuous-Flow Oxygen Systems

Although the continuous-flow oxygen system is no longer widely used in military aircraft, it is available in many civilian aircraft. Continuous-flow oxygen systems provide protection for passengers up to an operational altitude of 7620 m. It provides an emergency "get-me-down" capability for altitudes up to 9144 m. The regulators used in this system provide a continuous flow of 100% oxygen. The three major types of regulators are totally manual, automatic, and automatic with manual override.

Manual continuous-flow oxygen regulators can be adjusted to meet user requirements according to the altitude of exposure. The regulator valve is calibrated in thousands of feet and is adjusted to reflect that altitude. The primary function of the regulator is to reduce the inlet pressure to a reasonable range and to provide a flow to the breathing mask.

Automatic continuous-flow oxygen regulators are used in both military and civilian aircraft. As the altitude increases, the flow of oxygen gradually increases through the action of an aneroid. One regulator can accommodate up to 15 people, but, as a safety factor, two regulators are usually installed for 15 people. A person receives oxygen only when his breathing mask connector is plugged into one of the line outlets.

Automatic oxygen regulators with manual override offer a major advantage over other automatic continuous-flow regulators because in an emergency situation, an extra flow of oxygen can be obtained. This regulator includes a pressure gauge and a manual override selector. When the user inserts the breathing mask connector, an aneroid automatically delivers 100% oxygen at the correct flow rate. When additional oxygen is required, the manual override can be operated on three different settings to provide an increased flow.

In multiplace aircraft, portable walkaround assemblies enable personnel to move around the cabin unencumbered by long oxygen supply hoses. Most of these systems use low-pressure cylinders and regulators that complement the aircraft oxygen system. One such system is the United States Air Force A/U 265–2 assembly, which consists of a 3.0 ft³ low-pressure cylinder and a CRU-5/P automatic oxygen regulator with manual override. When fully charged (450 psi), this system will provide the user with 100% oxygen for 20 to 30 minutes. (Note: the time available until depletion of the supply depends on many factors such as altitude, respiratory rate, and activity level.) Because the system is considered to be empty at 100 psi, it should be closely monitored.

Diluter-Demand Oxygen Systems

When operational altitude increased above 7620 m, it became evident that continuous-flow oxygen systems could not provide the required physiologic protection. This requirement resulted in the development of the diluter-demand system, which allows oxygen to flow only on inspiration. The diluter feature mixes ambient air with the oxygen to achieve a gradual increase in oxygen percentage as altitude increases, until 10,363 m is reached, where the regulator provides 100% oxygen. This system has an opera-

tional altitude ceiling of 10,668 m and an emergency ceiling of 12,192 m. An example is the United States Air Force A-12A diluter-demand oxygen regulator. If the lever is placed in the 100% OXYGEN setting, 100% oxygen will be provided regardless of the altitude. When the diluter lever is placed in the NORMAL OXYGEN setting, the dilution feature is activated and air is mixed with the oxygen. For routine flying operations, the lever is placed in the NORMAL OXYGEN position. It is moved to the 100% OXYGEN setting when hypoxia is suspected, when visual acuity needs to be assisted at night, when exhaust fumes or contaminant gases are present, or when denitrogenation is required. The A-12A oxygen regulator also has an emergency valve that provides a continuous flow of 100% oxygen when activated, regardless of the altitude. Use of this feature, however, rapidly depletes the system.

Two diluter-demand portable assemblies are available. One assembly consists of a 3.8 ft³ gas cylinder and a diluter-demand oxygen regulator that provides diluted oxygen up to 10,668 m. To obtain 100% oxygen the user must manually close off the ambient air port. The oxygen duration of this system is advertised to be 20 to 30 minutes when fully charged. The cylinder should be considered empty and recharged at 100 psi. Another assembly consists of a 6.9 ft³ gas cylinder and a diluter-demand regulator that provides 100% oxygen at all times. Because of the increased size of this gas cylinder, oxygen duration is 30 to 45 minutes at altitudes of 10,668 m and above. This cylinder also should be considered empty and recharged when depleted to 100 psi.

Pressure-Demand Oxygen Systems

High-performance aircraft routinely fly above 12,192 m altitude. At altitudes above 12,192 m, even when 100% oxygen is breathed, the oxygen content of the blood is decreased below normal levels, unless positive pressure breathing is also applied, which is achieved by a pressure-demand oxygen system. The range of pressure-demand equipment is limited due to the susceptibility of lungs to damage from elevated pressures. Nonetheless, it is adequate for routine operational ceilings of 13,106 m, with an emergency ceiling of up to 15,240 m for short periods of time. The regulators used in this system are slightly different from those used in diluter-demand systems, but they function in the same manner until the positive pressure portion is activated.

MANUAL PRESSURE-DEMAND OXYGEN REGULATORS. The manual pressure-demand oxygen regulator (Fig. 6–11) functions exactly as a diluter-demand regula-

tor when the dial is on the NORMAL setting. By turning the dial in a clockwise direction, the pressure diaphragm is depressed and produces oxygen flow from the demand valve. The flow will continue until pressure in the mask and regulator is sufficient to act against the diaphragm and close the demand valve. This regulator is placed on the NORMAL setting for cabin altitudes up to 9144 m. At cabin altitudes between 9144 and 12,192 m, the regulator is dialed to the SAFETY setting, for approximately 3 mm Hg pressure. As altitudes above 12,192 m are reached, the user dials in additional pressure as indicated by an altitude setting. As an added safety factor, the user should dial to a

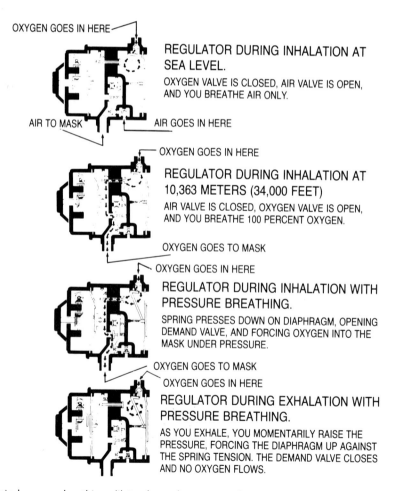

OXYGEN GOES IN HERE

REGULATOR DURING INHALATION AT SEA LEVEL.
OXYGEN VALVE IS CLOSED, AIR VALVE IS OPEN, AND YOU BREATHE AIR ONLY.

AIR TO MASK   AIR GOES IN HERE

OXYGEN GOES IN HERE

REGULATOR DURING INHALATION AT 10,363 METERS (34,000 FEET)
AIR VALVE IS CLOSED, OXYGEN VALVE IS OPEN, AND YOU BREATHE 100 PERCENT OXYGEN.

OXYGEN GOES TO MASK

OXYGEN GOES IN HERE

REGULATOR DURING INHALATION WITH PRESSURE BREATHING.
SPRING PRESSES DOWN ON DIAPHRAGM, OPENING DEMAND VALVE, AND FORCING OXYGEN INTO THE MASK UNDER PRESSURE.

OXYGEN GOES TO MASK
OXYGEN GOES IN HERE

REGULATOR DURING EXHALATION WITH PRESSURE BREATHING.
AS YOU EXHALE, YOU MOMENTARILY RAISE THE PRESSURE, FORCING THE DIAPHRAGM UP AGAINST THE SPRING TENSION. THE DEMAND VALVE CLOSES AND NO OXYGEN FLOWS.

Fig. 6–11. Typical pressure breathing, diluter-demand oxygen regulator.

higher pressure 305 m before the higher altitude is reached. For example, when the actual cabin altitude is 12,192 m, the regulator should be at the 12,497-m setting.

AUTOMATIC PRESSURE-DEMAND OXYGEN REGULATOR. The automatic pressure-demand oxygen regulator has an aneroid that automatically provides the prescribed positive pressure at a given altitude, thus replacing the manual dial. Other features include a pressure gauge, flow indicator, an oxygen on/off switch, and an emergency toggle switch.

NARROW-PANEL, AUTOMATIC PRESSURE-DEMAND OXYGEN REGULATOR. This regulator is basically the same as the previously mentioned automatic regulators but is about half the size and weight. Commonly called a "narrow-panel" regulator, it is equipped with a flow indicator, a pressure gauge, a green on/off switch, a white automix lever, and a red pressure lever.

CHEST-MOUNTED PRESSURE-DEMAND OXYGEN REGULATOR. This small pressure-demand oxygen regulator is designed to fit in the dovetail mounting block of the parachute harness or shoulder strap of the restraint system. Cabin air is automatically mixed with 100% oxygen based on cabin altitude. A manual control knob allows the user to select either 100% oxygen or an emergency pressure setting. It automatically delivers 100% oxygen at 9144 m and positive pressure at 10,666 m, however. This regulator has an operational ceiling of 13,106 m and an emergency limit of 15,240 m. It also has an antisuffocation device that warns the user when oxygen has been depleted or if he has become disconnected from the system.

PRESSURE-DEMAND PORTABLE ASSEMBLY. The pressure-demand portable assembly consists of a low-pressure gaseous cylinder coupled with a pressure-demand regulator. The system provides 100% oxygen up to 9144 m. At higher altitudes, the pressure control valve is operated manually to achieve positive pressure breathing. The duration of oxygen is similar to previously discussed low-pressure portable assemblies.

EMERGENCY OXYGEN CYLINDERS. Portable oxygen systems are used as an emergency source of oxygen during primary system failure, system depletion, or for egress from the aircraft. The assembly provides approximately 8 to 10 minutes of oxygen supply, enough oxygen to eject from an aircraft and descend in a parachute from an altitude of 15,240 m. The system can be activated manually by pulling the ball handle, or "green apple." It is automatically activated during an ejection sequence.

HIGH-PRESSURE PORTABLE SYSTEMS. Although not widely used, the high-pressure portable systems are found on some military and civilian cargo aircraft. The system consists of a high-pressure cylinder, diluter-demand regulator, oxygen pressure gauge, and flow indicator. The system is charged to 1800 to 2200 psi and provides the user with about 50 minutes of oxygen in the NORMAL setting at 7620 m and about 40 minutes of oxygen on the 100% setting at 7620 m.

Oxygen Masks

One of the most critical features in the oxygen supply system is the breathing mask. Significant reductions in oxygen delivery occur with an improperly fitted or poorly designed mask.

Continuous-Flow Masks

A multitude of masks can be used on a continuous-flow system. Most of them work on the same general principle: oxygen enters the mask from a reservoir bag, and with each inhalation from the reservoir bag, oxygen is replaced. Most of these masks mix 100% oxygen with ambient air. The most common example of a continuous-flow mask is found in commercial passenger aircraft (Fig. 6–12). These masks are usually stored in the overhead bin or in the seat back facing each passenger.

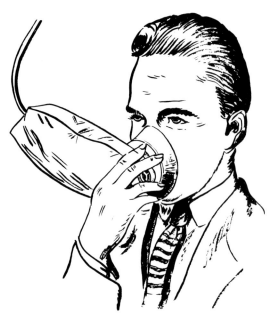

Fig. 6–12. Passenger oxygen mask with reservoir bag.

Diluter-Demand Masks

The diluter-demand mask operates with a one-way exhaust valve that opens only during exhalation. When the user inhales, the resulting slight, negative pressure seals the valve against the valve seat. An example of a diluter-demand oxygen mask is the United States Air Force MBU-4/P.

Pressure-Demand Masks

Unlike diluter-demand masks, the pressure-demand masks have the capability to hold positive pressure. A face seal allows the mask to form a pressure seal. A special inhalation/exhalation valve is located at the bottom of the mask, which allows oxygen to enter the mask upon inhalation and holds the positive pressure until exhalation pressure overrides the regulator pressure.

Pressure-Breathing Oxygen Mask

Initial pressure-breathing oxygen mask designs were distinctive because they incorporated a hard-shell body in addition to the face form. They included a combined inhalation/exhalation valve, micro-

phone, and associated harness assembly. The exhalation valve allows exhalation to take place when the internal mask pressure exceeds the pressure being supplied to the mask by 1 mm Hg.

Quick-Don Pressure-Demand Assembly

The quick-don pressure-demand assembly utilizes the standard pressure-breathing oxygen mask but adds a quick-donning harness. This system is used in multiplace aircraft where the routine use of oxygen equipment is not required. Should an emergency arise, the crew can put on the oxygen mask in a minimum amount of time, unencumbered by the need for a flight helmet.

New-Generation Pressure-Breathing Oxygen Mask

The basic functions of the new-generation pressure-breathing oxygen mask are the same as for the pressure-demand mask, but the design of the mask differs considerably. This mask has a combined lower-body hard shell and a conforming upper face-form (Fig. 6–13). The profile is lower, providing for increased visibility, and the center of gravity is more advantageous to mask retention during high accelerative forces. The face-form is wider, allowing for a comfortable fit and greater facial protection from cold or fire.

Civil and Commercial Aircraft Crew and Passenger Oxygen Systems

Pressurized or unpressurized aircraft that routinely fly at altitudes greater than 3048 m usually have a permanently installed oxygen system (Fig. 6–14). Light aircraft that fly below 3048 m usually have portable oxygen equipment. Because of the restricted size and weight of the portable system, the duration of the oxygen supply is limited.

In general and commercial aviation, there has been a dramatic increase in the number of aircraft requiring supplemental oxygen systems for flights in the range of

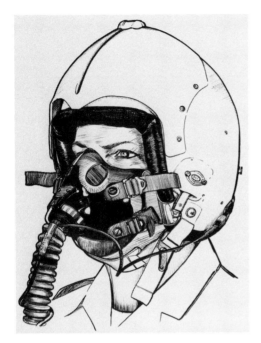

Fig. 6–13. New-generation pressure-breathing oxygen mask.

3658 to 15,240 m (Table 6–5). These aircraft are equipped with the least expensive oxygen systems available that meet minimum physiologic needs, usually a continuous-flow system.

The solid chemical generation of oxygen

is being used increasingly in private aircraft, general aviation, and commercial jumbo jets. Portable units are used primarily in private aircraft, whereas permanent units are used in commercial aircraft. Solid oxygen generators have several advantages: small storage space, limited oxygen supply lines, reduced costs, and a shelf-life of 20 years. Once activated, however, they continue to produce oxygen until the chemical agent is depleted. The location of these units varies. In the Lockheed L-1011, the units are overhead; in the Airbus Industries A-300B, the units are located in the back of the passenger seat; and in the MacDonnell-Douglas DC-10, the units may be in other locations. Each oxygen-generating unit is activated when the mask is removed from its housing or is pulled toward the face. Either action will activate a spring-loaded firing mechanism and initiate the flow of oxygen. Some units are activated by an electrical squib instead of a mechanical percussion mechanism. Masks are presented to the user when cabin altitude ascends to 4267 ± 152 m.

Some commercial air carriers use high-pressure reduction regulators and automatic aneroids set for 4267 m. Upon automatic activation, oxygen pressure in the

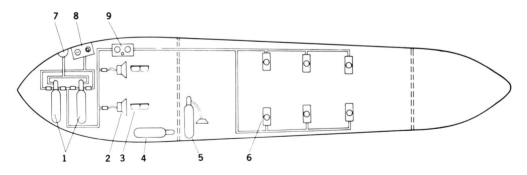

TYPICAL BREATHING OXYGEN SYSTEM FOR PASSENGER AIRCRAFT

1 - CYLINDER AND REDUCER ASSEMBLY
2 - MASK AND REGULATOR ASSEMBLY
3 - GOGGLES, SMOKE
4 - PORTABLE, CREW
5 - PORTABLE, PASSENGER
6 - MASK PRESENTATION UNIT
7 - OVERBOARD DISCHARGE INDICATOR
8 - SYSTEM FILL PANEL
9 - CONTROL PANEL

Fig. 6–14. Typical installed aircraft oxygen system.

Table 6–5.   Commercial Aircraft Oxygen Systems

Oxygen Equipment	Number of Outlets	Capacity		Hours Duration (One User)	Altitude Ceiling (above MSL)	
		Cubic feet	Liters		Meters	Feet
Puritan-Bennett						
2P 202	2	11	311	1.7	6706	22,000
2P 202	2	15	424.5	2.4	6706	22,000
2P 202	2	22	623	3.4	6706	22,000
2P 204	4	22	623	3.4	6706	22,000
2P 204	4	38	1025	5.9	6706	22,000
2P 400	4	22	623	3.86	6096	20,000
Scott Aviation						
Mark I	1	11	311	3.13	5029	16,500
Mark II	1	22	623	6.2	5029	16,500
Mark III	2	22	623	5.0	5791	19,000
Rajay Sky Ox						
Sk 9-20	2	20	566	6.2	6096	20,000
Sk 10-20	4	20	566	6.2	6096	20,000
Sk 9-35	2	35	990	7.5	6096	20,000
Sk 10-35	4	35	990	7.5	6096	20,000
Sk 9-50	2	50	1415	10.7	6096	20,000
Sk 10-50	4	50	1415	10.7	6096	20,000
Fluid Power						
Model 2500	2	10.6	300	2	7620	25,000

Data modified from Silitch, M.F.: Oxygen to go. AOPA Pilot, January, 1981.

lines opens the don latch in the mask housing compartment. Oxygen flow to the mask is initiated by removal of the mask from the compartment and pulling on the supply hose to disconnect a pin.

These continuous flow systems generally use a rebreather mask or a phase sequential type mask. Rebreather masks dilute 100% oxygen with air in the rebreather bag. Further mixing takes place upon inhalation through air inlet holes in the face piece. During exhalation, some of the air is forced back into the rebreather bag and the oxygen concentration never reaches 100%, limiting its effectiveness to about 7620 m. The rebreather mask is a low-cost, universal-fit mask, but it offers only minimal hypoxia protection. Carbon dioxide can accumulate in the rebreather bag, and the mask offers no protection against the inhalation of smoke or fumes. The phase sequential mask also has a reservoir bag, but there is a check valve between the reservoir bag and the mask. Upon inhalation, the user is provided 100% oxygen from the reservoir bag. During exhalation, the flow of oxygen fills the bag. The check valve prevents exhaled air from entering the reservoir bag, thus assuring 100% oxygen concentration for inhalation. These masks are effective up to 10,668 m and are approved for air carrier passenger use up to 12,192 m. The mask is expensive and has an inadequate suspension system, but it is effective.

PRESSURE SUITS

. . . In five minutes he was at the equivalent of 26,000 ft. In 30 minutes he was at 80,000 ft., and in 50 minutes he was at 90,000 ft. After a few minutes he was brought down none the worse for the experiment.

The above quotation came from Professor J.S. Haldane on November 27, 1933, as he described the first successful test of a high-altitude pressure suit that he had built as a modified diving suit.[4]

In 1934, Wiley Post made the world's first flight in a pressure suit. He flew approximately 25 hours on several flights up to 14,935 m in the pressure suit he designed to aid him in an attempt to break the transcontinental speed record. Although he set no records, these flights set the stage for the development of a variety of counterpressure garments and pressure suit assemblies designed to protect aviators during high-altitude and space flight.

The purpose of the counterpressure garment is as follows:

1. To protect against hypoxic hypoxia.
2. To prevent rupture of the lungs under high positive pressure breathing. The possibility of lung damage is greatly increased with breathing pressures of 60 to 100 mm Hg. This is the pressure required at 15,000 m when the individual is not protected by a counterpressure garment.
3. To prevent the undesirable effects of pressure breathing. It is undesirable to apply more than 40 mm Hg positive breathing pressure without counterpressure.

For brief exposures of approximately 2 minutes at a maximum altitude of 24,384 m, "get-me-down" counterpressure garments such as the British jerkin (Fig. 6–15) can be used. For prolonged exposures, either a partial-pressure suit (Fig. 6–16) or a full-pressure suit (Fig. 6–17) is required.

In 1947, the United States Air Force was assigned the task of developing a practical, operational, partial-pressure suit system, and the United States Navy was assigned the task of developing the full-pressure suit. Since that time, many designs from various countries have been developed, but they can all be categorized according to these two basic suit types.

Partial-Pressure Suit

The partial-pressure suit is form-fitted by adjusting laces on the sleeves, chest, back, and legs of the suit. The suit contains a torso bladder that covers the wearer completely except for the arms and lower legs. Bladders on the suit exterior, called capstans, extend down the back and along the arms and legs. The capstans are attached to the suit by means of crossing tapes sewn to the suit in a figure 8 such that when the capstans inflate, the fabric of the suit is drawn tight against the body of the wearer. When inflated, the capstan pressure must be five times the desired counterpressure. For example, should the user require a breathing pressure of 100 mm Hg (approximately 2 psi), the suit must be balanced by 2 psi of counterpressure; thus, 10 psi must be supplied to the capstan. A dual function regulator in the seat of the aircraft provides the needed oxygen breathing pressure and capstan pressure. The helmet is sealed around the neck and provides breathing oxygen and increased pressure to the entire head. The overall objective is to supply the proper amount of counterpressure to balance the breathing pressure required to prevent hypoxia at a given altitude. This protection is afforded for almost 30 minutes at 19,812 to 21,336 m and for several minutes at 30,480 m. An example is the partial-pressure suit used in U-2 aircraft flights (Fig. 6–16).

Full-Pressure Suits

The full-pressure suit is designed to provide a safe environment or counterpressure by surrounding the entire body with a pressurized gas envelope. These suits allow for better mobility, comfort, and protection of the user.

In normal operational flight, a 3.5 psi full-pressure suit is unpressurized when the aviator is exposed to altitudes below 10,668 m. If 10,668 m is exceeded by aircraft ascent or the loss of pressurization, the suit-mounted controller automatically causes the suit to inflate to a given pressure, which, when added to the atmospheric pressure at that altitude, will equal 3.5 psi. Thus, the aviator wearing a 3.5 psi full-pressure suit is never exposed to a pressure altitude greater than 10,668 m, regardless of aircraft altitude. Oxygen for breathing is supplied under a slight positive pressure directly to the helmet oronasal breathing cavity, which is separated

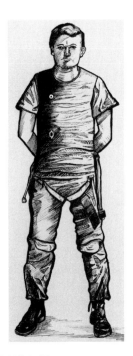

Fig. 6–15. British jerkin.

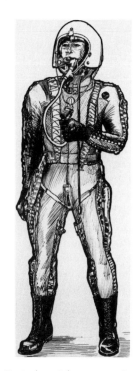

Fig. 6–16. Typical partial-pressure suit.

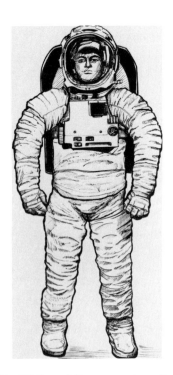

Fig. 6–17. ILC Dover full-pressure suit used to explore the lunar surface.

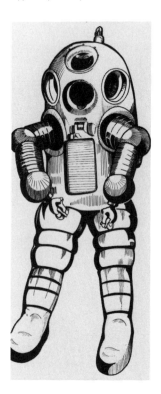

Fig. 6–18. Jims suit used to explore the ocean depths.

from the rear of the helmet by a close-fitting face barrier. The slight positive pressure is necessary to help reduce carbon dioxide pooling in the front of the helmet and to prevent the user from experiencing negative breathing pressures.

Because the suit is airtight, body heat can become a severe problem. As a result, a suit ventilation system is provided to pick up body heat and moisture to dump through the suit controller to the cabin atmosphere. Thermal regulation in some designs is achieved by a flow of air, whereas other designs use circulating fluids in the tubing network woven in the undergarment. To maintain fluid balance, the aviator can ingest liquids through a small orifice in the helmet shell. An example of a full-pressure suit is the one used to explore the lunar surface (Fig. 6–17).

Man, indeed, performs well in a very narrow range of barometric pressures. As discussed in Chapter 5 hypoxic (altitude) hypoxia is prevented by maintaining an alveolar oxygen tension range of between 60 and 100 mm Hg. In aircraft, the most logical way to provide this level of alveolar oxygenation during high-altitude flight is to use supplemental oxygen, to maintain effective cabin pressurization, or to combine the two. In many aircraft, cabin altitude is maintained below 3048 m, and supplemental oxygen equipment is read-

ily available for all occupants should the cabin pressurization system fail. In fighter-type aircraft, cabin altitude often exceeds 3048 m up to a maximum altitude of 7620 m, requiring the continuous use of supplemental oxygen equipment to prevent hypoxia. To prevent hypoxia at cabin altitudes above 3048 m, supplemental oxygen must be used. Above 10,363 m, it is necessary to breathe 100% oxygen under increasingly higher pressures. As one continues to ascend, a point is reached at about 15,240 m where the oxygen is driven into the lungs under such force that lung damage will occur unless external counterpressure is applied against the chest. Equipped with proper counterpressure garments and life-support units, man has been able to perform effectively in the extreme pressure environments extending from a complete vacuum on the lunar surface (Fig. 6–17) to an excess of 40 atm of pressure on the ocean floor (Fig. 6–18).

REFERENCES

1. Armstrong, H.G. (ed.): Principles and Practice of Aviation Medicine. Baltimore, Williams & Wilkins Co., 1939.
2. Air Medical Service. War Department: Air Services Division of Military Aeronautics. Washington, D.C., Government Printing Office, 1919, pp. 423–434.
3. Silitch, M.F.: Oxygen to go. AOPA Pilot, January 1981.
4. Wilson, C.L.: Emergency pressurization of aerospace crews. In Aerospace Medicine. 2nd Ed. Edited by H.W. Randell. Baltimore, Williams & Wilkins Co., 1971.

Chapter 7

Decompression Sickness and Pulmonary Overpressure Accidents

Richard D. Heimbach and Paul J. Sheffield

I shall add on this occasion. . . what may seem somewhat strange, what I once observed in a Viper. . . in our Exhausted Receiver, namely that it had manifestly a conspicuous Bubble moving to and fro in the waterish humour of one of its Eyes.

SIR ROBERT BOYLE, 1670

Pathologic effects can follow a significant reduction in the ambient pressure to which an individual is exposed. These effects are of two types: direct and indirect. Direct effects are the consequence of the expansion of gas within body cavities that do not have open communication with the ambient environment. Indirect effects result from the evolution of gas, which was previously dissolved in tissue fluids, when a pressure reduction occurs. This latter condition is most commonly referred to as decompression sickness.

DECOMPRESSION SICKNESS

The first human case of decompression sickness was reported in 1841 by M. Triger, a French mining engineer, who noticed symptoms of pain and muscle cramps in coal miners who had been working in an air-pressurized mine shaft. The disease was first scientifically described in 1854 by two French physicians, B. Pol

and T.J.J. Watelle, who presented a discussion with many case histories. Because the syndrome was first encountered as a result of hyperbaric exposure, the disorders are described principally using diving and caisson terminology.

Caisson Terminology

Because caisson, or tunnel, workers were the first to suffer from the syndrome now known as decompression sickness, the early terminology describing this disorder was related to that occupation, hence, the names caisson disease and compressed-air illness. The terms related to specific symptoms were devised by the caisson workers themselves. Bends was used to describe the pain in the bowels or lower extremities that caused the victim to assume a stooping posture. Chokes was the term used for victims suffering from dyspnea and a peculiar choking sensation. Other terms used by these workers included staggers (vertigo), prickles (skin sensations), and fits (convulsions).

Diving Terminology

Exhaustion and decompression sickness were common among early divers, particularly when they performed work at depths greater than 21 m. In 1869, the French physician L.R. de Mericourt published the first comprehensive medical report on diver's decompression sickness. The divers themselves added such terms as diver's bends, diver's paralysis, diver's palsy, and diver's itch to describe their symptoms. When French physiologist Paul Bert formulated the bubble theory of compressed air illness in his 1878 classic work, *Barometric Pressure,* he provided convincing evidence for the use of recompression to treat the disorder.

Aviation Terminology

As early as 1917, Yandell and Henderson predicted the possibility of decompression sickness in aviators. In the 1930s, when balloon and aircraft altitude records were set above 15,240 m, altitude decompression sickness became a common occurrence. Before 1959, among the 743 serious (type II) cases of this disorder, at least 18 aviators died from altitude decompression sickness. Variations in terminology used to describe the disorder reflected an uncertainty about its cause(s): high-altitude diver's disease, high-altitude caisson's disease, dysbarism, and aerobullosis. The term decompression sickness came from the American translation of a German term introduced by Benzinger and Hornberger in 1941. Except for the older term caisson disease, the term decompression sickness has best withstood the test of time and is now widely used to describe the disorder. The term altitude decompression sickness is now commonly used with reference to cases induced by exposure to pressures less than sea level equivalent.

THEORETICAL CONSIDERATIONS

The mechanisms involved in both altitude and diving decompression sickness are identical. Therefore, this discussion will deal primarily with the theoretical aspects of decompression sickness resulting from hyperbaric exposures. The precise causes of decompression sickness are not clearly understood. Although the conditions required to produce decompression sickness and the factors influencing bubble formation and growth are known, the relative importance of such factors as intracellular bubble formation and the release of humoral agents from the tissues by expanding gas, blood sludging, intracapillary bubble formation, and venous bubbles is unknown. Research is under way that could significantly modify the classic description presented in this chapter.

Factors Influencing Bubble Formation

Bubble Nuclei

Differential pressures between 100 and 1000 ATA are required for bubbles to form spontaneously in physical systems. Therefore, even in body fluids supersaturated with nitrogen, bubbles will not form unless bubble nuclei already exist. Bubble nuclei can be produced in areas of negative hydrostatic pressures by muscle shear forces or turbulent blood flow found at points of vessel constriction or bifurcation. Negative pressures also may exist at hydrophobic surfaces of cells or blood vessel walls. Although large microbubbles have been demonstrated in decompressed experimental animals, the actual sites for bubble formation or the sites of bubble nuclei production have not been demonstrated. Bubbles have been observed in veins, arteries, lymphatic vessels, and tissue spaces. Exactly what each compartment contributes to the syndrome of decompression sickness is difficult to interpret.

Supersaturation

During decompression from any atmospheric pressure, some quantity of inert gas in the tissues must diffuse into the blood, travel to the lungs, and leave the body in the expired air because the quantity of inert gas that can remain dissolved in tissue is directly proportional to the absolute ambient pressure. During ascent, the reduction in barometric pressure creates a condition whereby the tissue inert gas tension (P_{N_2}) is greater than the total barometric pressure (P_B). This condition is called supersaturation. Thus, if the decompression exceeds some critical rate for a given tissue, that tissue will not unload the inert gas rapidly enough and will become supersaturated.

Critical Supersaturation

Apparently, a level of supersaturation is reached that the body can tolerate without causing the inert gas to come out of solution to form bubbles. Once the critical supersaturation ratio is reached, however, bubbles develop and lead to decompression sickness. The English physiologist J.S. Haldane first described the concept of critical supersaturation in 1906. Haldane was directed by the British Admiralty to investigate and devise safe decompression procedures for Royal Navy divers, and his work demonstrated that humans could be exposed to hyperbaric pressures and subsequently decompressed without suffering decompression sickness as long as the total pressure reduction was no greater than 50%. No current decompression schedules use Haldane's 2-to-1 rule, but it is discussed here to show a mathematical concept. If Haldane's 2-to-1 relationship of allowable total pressure change is converted to a P_{N_2}-to-P_B relationship, the critical supersaturation ratio (R) would be $\frac{P_{N_2}}{P_B}$. For example,

$$R = \frac{P_{N_2} \text{ at 2 ATA}}{P_B \text{ at 1 ATA}} \quad (1)$$

$$R = \frac{(2)\ (0.79)}{1} = 1.58/1$$

In fact, there are apparently a number of critical supersaturation ratios for the various tissue compartments.

A person living at sea level and breathing atmospheric air will have a dissolved P_{N_2} of 573 mm Hg in all body tissues and fluids, assuming that P_B equals 760 mm Hg; P_{AO_2} equals 100 mm Hg; P_{ACO_2} equals 40 mm Hg; and P_{AH_2O} equals 47 mm Hg. If that person is rapidly decompressed to altitude, a state of supersaturation will be produced when an altitude is reached where the total barometric pressure is less than 573 mm Hg, a condition that occurs at an altitude of 2286 m. Thus, the altitude threshold above which an individual living at sea level would encounter supersaturation upon rapid decompression is 2286 m.

The lowest altitude where a sea-level acclimatized person has encountered symptoms of decompression sickness is approximately 5639 m. The degree of supersaturation at this altitude can be expressed as a ratio, as follows:

$$R = P_{N_2}/P_B \quad (2)$$

If the tissue P_{N_2} equals 573 mm Hg and P_B equals 372 mm Hg, then R equals 573/372, or 1.54. This value approaches the critical supersaturation ratio expressed by Haldane. The incidence of altitude decompression sickness increases markedly above 7620 m, where the supersaturation ratio is 2.03.

Symptoms can occur at much lower altitudes when "flying after diving." Many cases of decompression sickness have been documented in divers who fly too soon after surfacing. Altitudes as low as 1524 to 2286 m may be all that is necessary to induce bubble formation in a diver who has made a safe decompression to the surface. The problem involves the higher tissue P_{N_2} that exists after diving. The United States Navy has a documented case in which a diver, after making an "exceptional exposure" saturation dive, developed bends 4 days later while flying in a commercial aircraft. At present, there are no man-rated safe profiles for flying after diving, but research is currently active in this area.

Factors Influencing Bubble Growth

Gaseous Composition

Nitrogen, or another inert gas, is generally considererd to be the primary gas involved in symptomatic bubbles. If nitrogen were the only gas initially present in the newly formed bubble, an immediate gradient would be established for the diffusion of other gases into the bubble. Hence, a bubble will quickly have a gaseous composition identical to the gaseous composition present in the surrounding tissues or fluids. When bubbles are produced upon decompression from hyperbaric conditions, gases other than nitrogen represent only a small percentage of the total gas composition of the bubble. The role of other gases may be more significant in bubbles formed at altitude because they represent a much larger percentage of the total pressure within the bubble.

Hydrostatic Pressure

The tendency for gases to leave solution and enlarge a seed bubble can be expressed by the following equation:

$$\Delta P = t - Pab \qquad (3)$$

where ΔP is the differential pressure, or tendency for the gas to leave the liquid phase, in dynes/cm^2; t is the total tension of the gas in the medium, in dynes/cm^2; and Pab is the absolute pressure (that is, the total barometric pressure on the body plus the hydrostatic pressure).

Within an artery at sea level, t equals 760 mm Hg. The absolute pressure, Pab, is 760 mm Hg plus the mean arterial blood pressure (100 mm Hg), or 860 mm Hg. Therefore,

$$\Delta P = 760 - (760 + 100) \qquad (4)$$
$$\Delta P = -100 \text{ mm Hg}$$

When the value of ΔP is negative, there is no tendency toward bubble formation or growth. If the value for ΔP becomes zero or positive, bubble formation or growth is likely to occur.

Within a great vein at sea level, P_{O_2} equals 40 mm Hg, P_{CO_2} equals 46 mm Hg, and P_{H_2O} equals 47 mm Hg; thus, t equals 706 mm Hg. Absolute pressure, Pab, is 760 mm Hg plus the mean venous pressure (which in the great veins in the chest may be 0 mm Hg). Therefore,

$$\Delta P = 706 - (760 + 0) \qquad (5)$$
$$\Delta P = -54 \text{ mm Hg}$$

By suddenly exposing a person to an altitude of 5486 m without time for equilibration at the new pressure, venous ΔP would have a large positive value:

$$\Delta P = 706 - (380 + 0) \qquad (6)$$
$$\Delta P = +326 \text{ mm Hg}$$

The value for t in the above equation also can be increased in local areas by high levels of carbon dioxide production. Hence, in muscular exercise, a high local P_{CO_2} associated with a reduction in barometric pressure, P_B, causes higher positive values of ΔP than with a reduction in P_B alone. Further, because of the high solubility and rapid diffusion of carbon dioxide, locally high levels of this gas would produce the rapid growth of bubbles.

Hydrostatic pressure is, therefore, considered to be a force opposing bubble formation or bubble growth and includes not only blood pressure and cerebrospinal fluid pressure but local tissue pressure (or turgor), which varies directly with blood flow.

Boyle's Law Effects

Once a bubble is formed, its size will increase if the total pressure is decreased. During hyperbaric therapy, bubble size is reduced during compression. The surface tension of a bubble is inversely related to bubble size and opposes bubble growth. Thus, as total pressure is increased, the surface tension opposing bubble growth also is increased. Once a critically small bubble size is achieved, the surface tension is so great that the bubble can no longer exist. The bubble collapses, and its gases are redissolved.

Pathophysiology of Bubbles

Gas bubbles that form in body tissue and blood have two effects. The first is the direct mechanical effect of bubbles, which distort and disrupt tissue. This effect causes pain and blocks circulation, causing ischemia and possible infarction. The second effect results from biochemical changes occurring at the blood-bubble interface. Platelet aggregation occurs, with the release of vasoactive substances such as serotonin and epinephrine leading to vasoconstriction. The release of platelet factor 3 accelerates clotting and leads to further circulatory embarrassment. Blood viscosity increases, with a concomitant rise in capillary flow resistance and capillary pressure. This effect, coupled with an hypoxic loss of capillary wall integrity, leads to large shifts of fluid from the intravascular to the extravascular space and a further hemoconcentration. The bubble effects in decompression sickness are shown in Figure 7–1.

PROTECTION AND PREDISPOSING FACTORS

Protection against decompression sickness is based on controlling the tissue nitrogen-to-ambient pressure ratio (P_{N_2}/P_B). When an inert gas, such as nitrogen, is breathed, the tension of the gas dissolved in tissue fluids increases until equilibrium with the partial pressure of the gas in the respired medium is reached. With pressure reduction (decompression), supersaturation can occur. Some degree of supersaturation can be tolerated. The critical P_{N_2}/P_B ratio differs for each body tissue. When the safe limits of decompression are exceeded, gas separates from solution in the blood and other tissues. This process is the initiating event for decompression sickness. For diving, safe decompression limits vary with time and the depth of the dive and are published as decompression tables in a variety of diving manuals.

Even though the diver follows the decompression tables to safely decompress to sea level, he may exceed the supersaturation limits if he continues to ascend to altitude; for example, the individual who flies immediately following a scuba dive. Similarly, an individual whose body tissues are in equilibrium at sea level achieves a condition of supersaturation during decompression to altitude. Like the diver who exceeds the safe decompression limits, the aviator also can ascend to altitudes, usually above 5486 m, where gas will separate from solution to create bubbles that result in decompression sickness.

The aviator is protected from decompression sickness in two ways. Aircraft pressurization is a method of maintaining the aircraft cabin and, therefore, the physiologic altitude to which the aviator is exposed at a considerably lower pressure altitude than the actual altitude at which the aircraft is flying. With adequate aircraft pressurization, the individual is not exposed to reduced barometric pressures where bubbles can form. Protection from decompression sickness exists because the P_{N_2}/P_B ratio remains below a critical threshold as the value of P_B remains high.

Denitrogenation is a method by which one breathes 100% oxygen for the purpose of eliminating nitrogen from the body before going to altitude. This method is used to protect the individual who must ascend

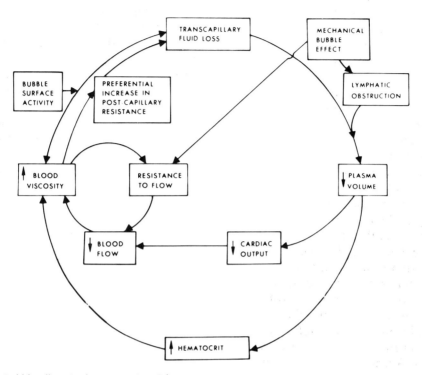

Fig. 7–1. Bubble effects in decompression sickness.

to altitudes that produce decompression sickness. With 100% oxygen breathing, oxygen replaces other tissue-dissolved gases, including nitrogen. Thus, the amount of nitrogen in each body tissue is reduced before ambient pressure reduction occurs. Again, the P_{N_2}/P_B ratio remains below a critical threshold because the value for P_{N_2} is reduced.

For example, an aviator rapidly ascends from sea level ($P_B = 760$ mm Hg) to 5486 m ($P_B = 380$ mm Hg). The aircraft pressurization system maintains pressure in the cabin at 2438 m ($P_B = 565$ mm Hg). Assuming that all tissues are saturated at sea level ($P_{N_2} = 573$ mm Hg) and that off-gassing occurring during the rapid ascent is insignificant:

$$\frac{P_{N_2}}{P_B} = \frac{573 \text{ mm Hg}}{565 \text{ mm Hg}} = 1.01 \qquad (7)$$

If the aircraft were not pressurized:

$$\frac{P_{N_2}}{P_B} = \frac{573 \text{ mm Hg}}{380 \text{ mm Hg}} = 1.51 \qquad (8)$$

If unpressurized flight occurred to 9143 m ($P_B = 226$ mm Hg):

$$\frac{P_{N_2}}{P_B} = \frac{573 \text{ mm Hg}}{226 \text{ mm Hg}} = 2.54 \qquad (9)$$

If before unpressurized flight to 9143 m the aviator had denitrogenated at sea level such that one half of the total nitrogen was eliminated from his body and state of equilibrium was reached for all body tissues:

$$\frac{P_{N_2}}{P_B} = \frac{287 \text{ mm Hg}}{226 \text{ mm Hg}} = 1.27 \qquad (10)$$

The process of denitrogenation is very effective in eliminating nitrogen from the body. When 100% oxygen is breathed using a tightly fitted mask, an alveolar nitrogen pressure of nearly zero is established and a marked pressure differential (about 573 mm Hg) between the alveoli and body tissues results. Nitrogen rapidly diffuses from the tissues into the blood, where it is transported to the alveoli and is exhaled. The amount of nitrogen eliminated is time-dependent.

Figure 7–2 shows the total amount of nitrogen washed out of the body by denitrogenation. Assuming that the average person contains 1200 cm^3 of dissolved nitrogen, slightly more than 350 cm^3 can be eliminated by prebreathing 100% oxygen for 30 minutes. Denitrogenation prior to initiating ascent to altitude significantly reduces the incidence of altitude decompression sickness. Once begun, denitrogenation should not be interrupted. Air-breathing interruptions of only a few minutes greatly decrease the efficacy of denitrogenation in the prevention of decompression sickness. If such an interruption is unavoidable, the only safe course of action is to begin denitrogenation again from time zero.

Denitrogenation eliminates nitrogen from various tissues at different rates. These rates are dependent on the solubility of nitrogen in specific tissues but, more importantly, also on the circulatory perfusion of the tissues. Thus, all body tissues come into equilibrium with each other and with respired gas at different times. As a

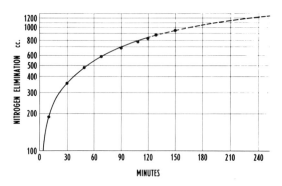

Fig. 7–2. Nitrogen elimination curve.

practical matter, then, with altitude exposure (pressure reduction), the P_{N_2}/P_B ratio of certain tissues may exceed the critical value for bubble formation while the P_{N_2}/P_B ratio of other tissues remains within a safe range. This fact may partially explain why signs and symptoms of decompression sickness occur at characteristic locations in the body.

Attempts have been made to correlate the incidence of both diving-induced and altitude-induced decompression sickness with various physical and physiologic factors. Some of these factors influence group susceptibility to decompression sickness, although none can be used to predict individual susceptibility. The association of these factors with decompression sickness is summarized in the next sections.

Altitude Attained

No reliable evidence exists for the occurrence of decompression sickness with altitude exposures of less than 5486 m unless there was a recent (within 24 hours) previous exposure to compressed gas breathing (e.g., scuba diving). With increasing altitude, the incidence of decompression sickness increases, as does the ratio of severe to mild cases. Exposures to altitudes of 7925 to 14,478 m for times varying from approximately 30 minutes to 3 hours will result in a 1.5% incidence of decompression sickness. The severity of the cases will increase with increasing altitude.

In a review of 145 cases of altitude-induced decompression sickness necessitating treatment, Davis and colleagues[1] reported that 13% of these cases occurred with altitude exposures of 7620 m or below and 79% occurred with exposures of 9144 m or greater.

Duration of Exposure

At all altitudes above 5486 m, the longer the duration of exposure, the greater the incidence of decompression sickness.

Temperature

No correlation exists between the frequency of decompression sickness and the ambient temperature in the range of 21.1 to 34.3°C. At an ambient temperature of − 23.3%C, however, the incidence of decompression sickness is twice that at 21.1°C, with a larger ratio of serious cases to mild cases.

Previous Exposures to Altitude

A second exposure to an altitude greater than 5486 m following an exposure to such an altitude in the preceding 3 hours will greatly increase the chance of decompression sickness occurring, even if the first exposure was asymptomatic. A recurrence of symptoms is almost certain if the first exposure is symptomatic.

A 2-hour exposure to an altitude of 7622 m followed in 18 hours by a rapid decompression from 2439 to 6707 m will result in detectable Doppler bubble signals over the pulmonary artery. In addition, the incidence of decompression sickness following the rapid decompression will be twice that following the initial altitude exposure.

Repeated daily exposures to altitude have been variously reported as increasing susceptibility, having no effect on susceptibility, and even decreasing susceptibility to decompression sickness. Of special interest is the series of cases reported by Davis and colleagues,[1] in which the incidence of decompression sickness in inside observers undergoing two to four altitude exposures per week accompanying students in altitude chamber training was three times greater than the incidence in students.

Flying Following Diving

If an individual breathes a gas at pressures greater than sea level before altitude exposure, his susceptibility to decompression sickness will significantly increase. Altitude decompression sickness has oc-

curred at pressure altitudes as low as 1372 m several hours following scuba diving. Any exposure to compressed gas breathing occurring within 24 hours of altitude exposure will increase the chance of altitude decompression sickness occurring.

Age

A rather striking increase in the incidence of decompression sickness occurs with increasing age. This increase occurs in both compressed air workers and aviators, with a threefold increase in incidence between the 19- to 25-year-old and 40- to 45-year-old age groups. The mechanism underlying this phenomenon is not understood but may result from changes in circulation due to aging.

Sex

A great deal of controversy exists regarding the possible differences in susceptibility to decompression sickness between men and women. The scientific resolution of this question has been hampered by emotional and political factors, and, unfortunately, no valid studies have been done. It is the clinical judgment of those most experienced in the treatment of decompression sickness, however, that women present more problems in the clinical management of this disorder than do men.

Exercise

The association between physical exertion and decompression sickness has been well established. The effect of exercise on the incidence of decompression sickness is equivalent to increasing the exposure altitude 915 to 1524 m.

Injury

No convincing evidence exists to associate previous injury with decompression sickness. Based on theoretical considerations, however, it is now thought that during the acute stages of an injury to a joint, that joint may have increased susceptibility to bends because of perfusional changes associated with the injury and/or healing mechanisms.

Body Build

For a long time, a basic tenet of diving and aerospace medicine (almost a religious dogma) has been that obesity increases the susceptibility to decompression sickness. Although it seems prudent to continue to accept this principle because of other known adverse effects of obesity, no scientific validation exists.

Other Factors

No definitive results have come from investigations of possible correlations between decompression sickness and such factors as physical fitness, hypoxia, diet, and fluid intake.

MANIFESTATIONS OF DECOMPRESSION SICKNESS

In decompression sickness, bubbles can form in all parts of the body. Various target organs, however, seem to be affected most readily, and the effects on these anatomic locations account for the signs and symptoms seen. The pathophysiology of bubbles was discussed earlier in the section so named. In this section, the clinical manifestations of bubble formation and the classic syndromes of decompression sickness will be described.

Bends

The bends, manifested by pain only, is seen in 65 to 70% of the cases of altitude-induced decompression sickness. It tends to be localized in and around the large joints of the body. Smaller joints, such as the interphalangeal areas, sometimes may be affected, particularly if these joints underwent significant active motion during altitude exposure.

Bends pain is deep and aching in character and ranges from very mild (joint awareness) to so severe that the patient does not wish to move the affected joint.

Active and passive motion of the joint tends to aggravate the discomfort, whereas local pressure, such as with an inflated blood pressure cuff, tends to relieve the pain temporarily.

The pain may occur during the altitude exposure, on descent, shortly after descent, or, in some cases, only become manifest many hours after descent. In most cases, bends occurring at altitude will be relieved by descent because of the increase in barometric pressure. In some cases, bends relieved by returning to ground level will recur at ground level. In these cases, as well as those cases where pain is not relieved by descent, hyperbaric oxygen therapy is the definitive form of treatment.

Chokes

The syndrome called chokes is rare in both diving and aviation, accounting for less than 2% of decompression sickness cases. This condition is a life-threatening disorder, however. The mechanism of chokes is multiple pulmonary gas emboli. The characterisitic clinical picture consists of substernal chest pain, dyspnea, and a dry, nonproductive cough. In most cases, the pain is made worse on inhalation. Patients with chokes feel generally and severely ill. Altitude-induced chokes will invariably progress to collapse of the individual if the altitude is maintained. The aviator whose symptoms are not completely relieved by descent to ground level must be treated in a hyperbaric chamber as quickly as possible. This treatment also is required for chokes secondary to decompression following diving.

Neurologic Decompression Sickness

Neurologic decompression sickness presents a clinical picture with signs and symptoms referable to the nervous system. In recent years, it has become apparent that one should probably limit the term neurologic decompression sickness to those cases in which there is involvement of the central nervous system. Peripheral nerve involvement with mild paresthesia is commonly associated with bends and does not increase the gravity of the disorder from a prognostic point of view. Central nervous system involvement, however, can herald significant and permanent neurologic deficits, particularly if aggressive and proper treatment is not instituted promptly.

Central nervous system involvement occurs in 5 to 7% of cases of decompression sickness, either from diving or altitude exposure. In cases of altitude decompression sickness where symptoms are not relieved totally by descent, however, the central nervous system is involved 35 to 50% of the time.

Neurologic decompression sickness presents in one of two forms: a spinal cord form and a brain form. The spinal cord form is seen almost exclusively following diving and is extremely rare following altitude exposure. The brain form of the disorder is more commonly seen following altitude exposure and is uncommon but not rare following diving exposure. The reasons for the variance in the incidence of brain and spinal cord neurologic decompression sickness in diving and altitude exposure have yet to be elucidated. The clinical manifestations of the two forms of this disorder will be discussed separately.

Spinal Cord Decompression Sickness

In many cases, the first symptom of spinal cord decompression sickness is the insidious onset of numbness or paresthesia of the feet. The sensory deficit spreads upward, accompanied by an ascending weakness or paralysis to the level of the spinal lesion. Other cases begin with girdling abdominal or thoracic pain, which precedes the onset of sensory and motor deficits. Within 30 minutes of onset, the entire clinical picture of a partial or complete transverse spinal cord lesion is manifest.

The lesion in spinal cord decompression sickness has been well documented as bubbles formed in or embolized to the paraspinal venous plexus. Poorly collateralized segmental venous drainage of the spinal cord and normally sluggish blood flow through the paraspinal venous plexus can result quickly in mechanical blockage of venous drainage by bubbles and solid elements formed at the blood-bubble interface. This blockage, in turn, results in a congestive, or "red", infarct of the spinal cord.

Brain Form of Decompression Sickness

In most cases, the clinical picture of a patient suffering from the brain form of decompression sickness is one of spotty sensory and motor signs and symptoms not attributable to a single brain locus. Headache, at times of a migrainous nature, is commonly present. Visual disturbances, consisting of scotomas, tunnel vision, diplopia, or blurring, are common. At times, extreme fatigue or personality changes that range from emotional lability to a significantly flattened affect are the presenting symptoms.

For the physician not acquainted with the clinical picture of multiple brain lesions, the diagnosis can be very difficult. A number of these patients have been misdiagnosed as hysterical and have progressed to vasomotor collapse because proper and immediate definitive treatment was not rendered.

Circulatory Manifestations

Generally, circulatory impairment is manifested as shock following the development of chokes, severe bends, or severe neurologic impairment (secondary collapse). Circulatory collapse without other symptoms preceding the development of shock (primary collapse) occurs rarely. So-called postdecompression collapse following altitude exposure, with the shock state occurring after descent to ground level, has been described as a separate type of circulatory impairment. It probably is not separate but rather represents the same sort of delay in onset sometimes seen with other types of altitude decompression sickness.

Possible mechanisms of circulatory collapse include direct involvement of the vasomotor regulatory center or massive blood vessel endothelial damage by bubbles, with a subsequent loss of intravascular volume. Extreme hemoconcentration has been documented in many cases, with hematocrits up to 70%.

Circulatory collapse is marked by its lack of response to fluid replacement, which is similar to the lack of response commonly seen in cases of severe head injury that results in a central sympathectomy.

Minor Manifestations

Skin bends is a disorder that may present as pruritus or formication only. The sensation generally passes within 20 to 30 minutes, and no treatment is necessary. Skin bends, however, may occur with the appearance of mottled or marbled skin lesions. The appearance of these lesions is evidence of a neurocirculatory effect of bubbles within the body. Up to 10% of patients with such skin lesions will experience circulatory collapse if untreated.

Pitting edema, if seen alone, is considered a minor manifestation of decompression sickness in that it will resolve spontaneously without sequelae. Pitting edema is thought to arise from lymphatic blockage by bubbles. It rarely results from altitude exposure.

Chronic Effects

Aseptic bone necrosis is a debilitating condition, common among divers and caisson workers but has only been well documented in three cases following altitude exposure. Areas of bone infarction, if located in juxta-articular locations, rapidly lead to erosion of overlying cartilage and severe osteoarthritis. The shoulders, knees, and hips are the only joints affected. Early lesions are asymptomatic and are only found on radiographic surveys. The exact relationship between aseptic bone necrosis and episodes of bends is unknown. The disease is seen when compressed air exposure occurs on a regular and frequent basis and is seldom seen in less than 1 year after beginning such exposures.

Permanent neurologic deficits result from spinal cord decompression sickness and are most feared by divers. Even with proper and rapid treatment, approximately 15% of patients who have suffered spinal cord decompression sickness will manifest some degree of permanent neurologic deficit from minor sensory and motor losses to complete paraplegia.

DIAGNOSIS AND MANAGEMENT OF DECOMPRESSION SICKNESS

Decompression sickness rarely occurs unless one of the following conditions exists:

1. A diver surfaces following a dive deeper than 10 m of sea water. In most cases, the diver will have failed to follow recognized single or repetitive dive decompression schedules.
2. Exposure to altitude greater than 5488 m. In most instances, decompression sickness will not occur (without preceding exposure to compressed gas breathing) at altitudes below 7622 m, although a few cases have been documented at altitudes of 5640 m.
3. Exposure to altitude shortly following exposure to compressed gas breathing (e.g., scuba diving or hyperbaric chamber exposure). Decompression sickness has occurred while flying in pressurized aircraft at a cabin altitude as low as 1372 m following scuba diving in the preceding 3 hours.

The following procedures should be followed in all cases of decompression sickness (including bends pain only) persisting after a dive or after a flight:

1. One hundred percent oxygen should be administered using a well-fitted aviator's mask or anesthesia mask.
2. If a hyperbaric chamber is on site, the patient should be immediately treated according to the proper treatment table. No observation period is warranted at ground level.
3. If there is no on-site hyperbaric chamber, arrangements should be made to immediately transport the patient to the nearest hyperbaric facility capable of administering proper treatment. The patient should be kept on 100% oxygen by mask while awaiting and during transportation to the chamber. If the patient has bends pain only, the symptoms of which clear completely without recurrence while awaiting transport, movement to the hyperbaric chamber can be cancelled.
4. If bends pain is relieved while awaiting transport but recurs, the patient should be transported to the hyperbaric chamber and treated even if symptoms are relieved again after recurrence.
5. Any patient with signs or symptoms of neurologic decompression sickness, chokes, or circulatory collapse should be immediately transported to the nearest hyperbaric chamber for treatment, regardless of whether the symptoms persist.
6. Transportation must be at or near the ground-level barometric pressure of the site at which the patient embarks. Aircraft used for the movement of these patients must possess this pressurization capability. In no case should the cabin pressure altitude be more than 305 m higher than the pressure altitude at the point of embarkation. If at all possible, it is best to avoid moving patients to a hyperbaric chamber located at a pressure altitude greater than 1067 m higher than the point of embarkation.

The diagnostic and treatment decision points described above are summarized in Figure 7–3.

HYPERBARIC THERAPY FOR DECOMPRESSION SICKNESS

Physiologic Basis of Hyperbaric Therapy

Hyperbaric therapy is achieved by applying two physical factors related to the pressure environment. The first factor is the mechanical compression of gas-filled entities such as bubbles. The second factor is the elevation of the partial pressure of inspired gases and the subsequent increase in the amount of the various gases that enter into physical solution in body fluids. The use of hyperbaric therapy for treating decompression sickness results in bubble size reduction, a positive nitrogen gradient to reduce the size of bubbles and resolve them, perfusion of ischemic tissues, and correction of local tissue hypoxia.

As an individual is exposed to a change in barometric pressure, a bubble deep within the body tissues responds to the pressure change. During compression, the surrounding barometric pressure is increased, producing a reduction in bubble volume in accordance with Boyle's Law. Figure 7–4 presents the expected decrease in bubble volume and diameter as a function of the total pressure applied. Figure 7–5 compares the expected decrease in bubble size of a bubble formed at sea level with those formed at altitudes of 5486 and 11,600 m. During compression, the bubble becomes smaller and the surface tension increases. Below a certain critical diameter, the surface tension becomes so great that the bubble collapses and the gas within it redissolves.

Applying hyperbaric pressure in treat-

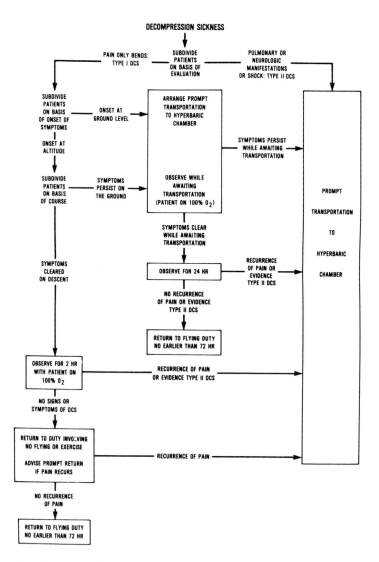

Fig. 7–3. Diagnostic and treatment decision points for decompression sickness.

ing decompression sickness will, therefore, either eliminate the bubbles entirely or reduce their size to a significant extent. The amount of size reduction will depend on the absolute bubble size at the onset of therapy. Even though some bubbles may not be eliminated completely by the initial application of pressure, their reduction in size aids in partially restoring circulation in the case of intravascular bubbles and reducing the mechanical effects of extravascular bubbles.

Bubbles that are too big to resolve upon the initial application of pressure will continue to decrease in size with the time spent at increased pressure. This gradual decrease in size is due to the diffusion of gases from the bubble to the surrounding tissues and fluids. Diffusion of gases from the bubble occurs because the partial pressure of gases within the bubble increases when the volume is reduced during compression. The elevated partial pressure of gases inside the bubble creates a

DEPTH IN FEET	PRESSURE IN ATA	RELATIVE VOLUME (PERCENT)		RELATIVE DIAMETER (PERCENT)
0	1	100		100
33	2	50		79.3
66	3	33.3		69.3
99	4	25		63
132	5	20		58.5
165	6	16.6		55
297	10	10		46.2

Fig. 7–4. Bubble volume and diameter relationships.

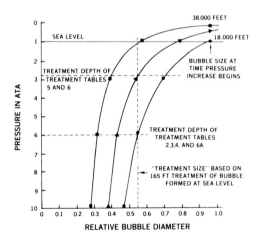

Fig. 7–5. Relative bubble diameters at sea level, 5486 m, and 11,600 m. The treatment tables referred to in this figure are the standard United States Navy treatment tables. See Table 7–1 and Figures 7–8, 7–9, 7–13, and 7–14 for more information on these tables.

the new nitrogen partial pressure. Thus, the bubble will be resolved more rapidly if the individual breathes 100% oxygen because a favorable gradient for nitrogen elimination from a bubble will improve with time, and the bubble will more rapidly diminish in size. During hyperbaric therapy, the patient intermittently breathes 100% oxygen at increased pressure. Breathing 100% oxygen provides an increased gradient for eliminating nitrogen from evolved bubbles and aids in their resorption. The increased gradient also speeds the elimination of nitrogen from supersaturated tissues and thus helps prevent further bubble formation. Therefore, if a sufficient time is spent at depth, all bubbles will resolve.

Hyperbaric oxygenation results in increased oxygen tension in the capillaries surrounding ischemic tissue. The increased oxygen tension extends the oxygen diffusion distance from functioning capillaries and corrects the local tissue hypoxia. Overcoming the tissue hypoxia tends to disrupt the vicious cycle of hypoxia-induced tissue damage that causes tissue edema and interferes with circulation and oxygenation.

Figure 7–7 shows the level of tissue P_{O_2} that can be achieved in ischemic tissue during 100% oxygen breathing at 1 ATA and 2.4 ATA. These data were collected by Sheffield and Dunn[2] using a polarographic oxygen electrode implanted in an ischemic, hypoxic, nonhealing wound and are shown to illustrate that tissue P_{O_2} can be elevated in areas with poorly functioning capillaries when hyperbaric oxygenation is applied. In this case, the baseline wound oxygen tension during air breathing at 1 ATA was 20 mm Hg, compared with 30 to 40 mm Hg in healthy skin. Wound oxygen tension increased to 200 to 300 mm Hg during 100% oxygen breathing at 1 ATA and above 1000 mm Hg during 100% oxygen breathing at 2.4 ATA. It should be noted that the higher tissue oxygen tensions achieved under hyperbaric

gradient favorable for gas elimination from the bubble, as presented in Figure 7–6. Figure 7–6 also shows that if the individual breathes air, the favorable gradient will lessen with time as the surrounding tissues and fluids approach equilibrium at

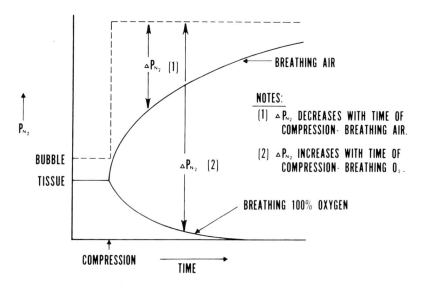

Fig. 7-6. Bubble nitrogen gradients when breathing air versus pure oxygen.

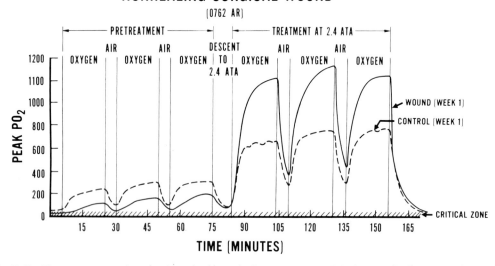

Fig. 7-7. Tissue oxygen tension after 1 week of hyperbaric oxygenation (HBO) for a nonhealing surgical wound.

conditions result in an increased oxygen diffusion distance. This phenomenon is especially important when one considers the need to deliver oxygen to an area in which flow through several capillaries may be disrupted due to bubbles or sludging.

Treatment of Altitude Decompression Sickness

Although most cases of decompression sickness occurring at altitude will be completely relieved by descent to ground level, approximately 2% of cases will persist. In addition, a significant number of patients will experience the initial onset of symptoms of decompression sickness after descent, so-called "delayed cases."

Prior to 1959, over 17,000 cases of altitude-induced decompression sickness were documented. Of these cases, 743 were reported as serious, including 17 fatalities. Davis and colleagues,[1] commenting on a review of these 17 fatalities, made the following observations. All died in irreversible shock that was unresponsive to fluid replacement and drug therapy. Almost all cases began as simple bends pain, neurologic manifestations, or chokes, which only after several hours progressed to circulatory collapse and death. It should be noted that none of the 17 fatalities were treated by hyperbaric therapy. In their review of 145 cases of altitude decompression sickness treated in hyperbaric chambers, these same authors emphasized that shock was the initial clinical picture in only one case, whereas seven other cases began with other manifestations and progressed to shock. In this series of patients, no fatalities occurred among those who were treated in hyperbaric chambers.[1]

Although as early as 1945 Behnke[3] had advocated the use of compression therapy to treat cases of altitude decompression sickness that did not resolve upon descent to ground level, it was not until 1959 that a United States Air Force aviator was successfully treated by compression.[4] In 1963, Downey and colleagues,[5] using a human serum in vitro model, demonstrated the persistence, at ground level, of bubbles formed at altitude. Upon compression to pressures greater than sea level, the bubbles cleared. In vivo confirmation of Downey's work was reported by Leverett and colleagues in 1963.[6] Much of the present-day understanding of bubble behavior and effects with changing pressures is based on this work. Present-day standards of care mandate immediate hyperbaric therapy for all cases of altitude decompression sickness persisting or recurring after descent to ground level.

Treatment Procedures

Once the diagnosis of decompression sickness has been made, hyperbaric therapy is required. It is never acceptable to continue observation of a patient with signs or symptoms of decompression sickness. The use of oxygen at 1 ATA for such patients should be restricted to the period of initial observation and examination, the time required for transportation to a hyperbaric chamber, and the time required to prepare the hyperbaric facility for use. Oxygen at 1 ATA is not a substitute for hyperbaric therapy.

Although a number of treatment tables are used successfully throughout the world, the United States Navy treatment tables are used in essentially all cases of decompression sickness in this country. Standard United States Navy treatment tables 1, 2, 3, and 4 are shown in Table 7–1. Because of the poor success rate of these air treatment tables before 1964, Goodman and Workman[7] developed the oxygen treatment tables now labeled as tables 5 and 6. The oxygen treatment tables were adopted by the United States Navy in 1967 and have proved to be highly effective in treating decompression sickness. Treatment table 5, as modified by the United States Air Force, is shown in Figure 7–8. It is 135 minutes in length and is designed for the treatment of bends pain only. Treatment table 5 can be used for bends if the patient responds completely within 10 minutes of breathing oxygen at 18.3 m (60 fsw). If the symptoms do not disappear within 10 minutes, the patient is committed to treatment table 6. Treatment table 6, as modified by the United States Air Force, is shown in Figure 7–9. It is reserved for cases involving the central nervous system or cardiopulmonary systems and for recurrences of previously treated decompression sickness. Treatment table 6 also is used to treat bends pain cases that are not relieved within 10 minutes on 100% oxygen at 18.3 m. De-

Table 7–1.   Standard United States Navy Treatment Tables 1, 2, 3, and 4

Stops	Table 1	Table 2	Table 3	Table 4
Feet of Seawater	Time at Stop (minutes)	Time at Stop (minutes)	Time at Stop (minutes)	Time at Stop (minutes)
165	—	30 (air)	30 (air)	30—120 (air)
140	—	12 (air)	12 (air)	30 (air)
120	—	12 (air)	12 (air)	30 (air)
100	30 (air)	12 (air)	12 (air)	30 (air)
80	12 (air)	12 (air)	12 (air)	30 (air)
60	30 (oxygen)	30 (oxygen)	30 (oxygen)	360 (air)
50	30 (oxygen)	30 (oxygen)	30 (oxygen)	360 (air)
40	30 (oxygen)	30 (oxygen)	30 (oxygen)	360 (air)
30		60 (oxygen)	720 (air)	660 (air)
				60 (oxygen)
20			120 (air)	60 (air)
				60 (oxygen)
10			120 (air)	60 (air)
				60 (oxygen)
	5 minute ascent on oxygen	5 minute ascent on oxygen	1 minute ascent on air	1 minute ascent on air
Surface	↓	↓	↓	↓

TABLE 5—BENDS PAIN ONLY

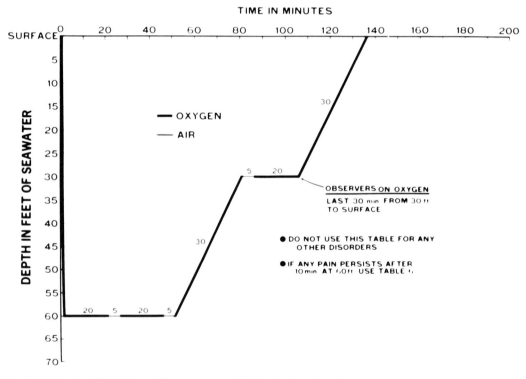

Fig. 7–8.   Standard United States Navy treatment table 5—bends pain only.

TABLE 6 — DECOMPRESSION SICKNESS

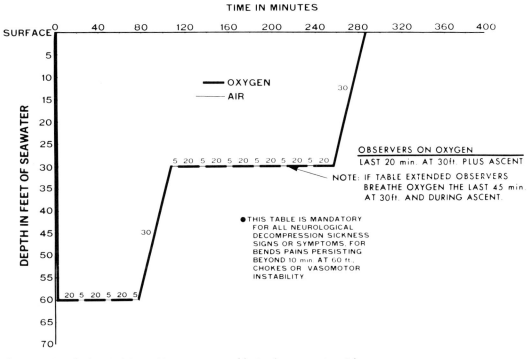

Fig. 7–9. Standard United States Navy treatment table 6—decompression sickness.

cision points for the treatment of decompression sickness are shown in Figure 7–10.

Where long delays between onset and treatment occur, the manifestations of decompression sickness become more serious. They seem to be aggravated by the development of secondary edema and vascular obstruction or impairment from thrombosis. Hyperbaric oxygenation in such circumstances probably provides more benefit than does the mechanical compression of the bubbles.

General considerations in the use of the decompression sickness treatment tables are as follows:

1. Follow the treatment tables accurately.

2. Have qualified medical attendants inside the chamber at all times.
3. Maintain the normal ascent and descent rates.
4. Examine the patient thoroughly at the depth of relief or treatment depth.
5. Treat an unconscious patient for air embolism or serious decompression sickness unless the possibility of such a condition can be ruled out.
6. Use the air tables only if oxygen cannot be used.
7. Be alert for oxygen toxicity.
8. If oxygen convulsion occurs, remove the oxygen mask and restrain the patient to prevent injury.
9. Maintain oxygen usage within the time and depth limits.
10. Check the patient's status before and

DECOMPRESSION SICKNESS TREATMENT

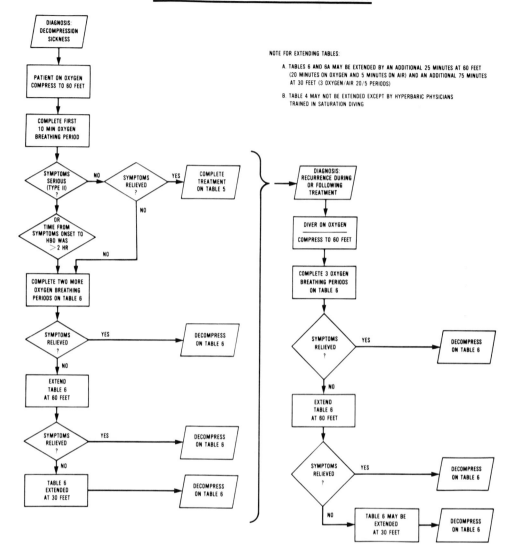

NOTE FOR EXTENDING TABLES:

A. TABLES 6 AND 6A MAY BE EXTENDED BY AN ADDITIONAL 25 MINUTES AT 60 FEET (20 MINUTES ON OXYGEN AND 5 MINUTES ON AIR) AND AN ADDITIONAL 75 MINUTES AT 30 FEET (3 OXYGEN/AIR 20/5 PERIODS)

B. TABLE 4 MAY NOT BE EXTENDED EXCEPT BY HYPERBARIC PHYSICIANS TRAINED IN SATURATION DIVING

Fig. 7–10. Decision points for the treatment of decompression sickness. See Figures 7–8 and 7–9 for Standard United States treatment tables 5 and 6.

after coming to each stop and periodically during long stops.

11. Do not let the patient sleep through changes of depth or for more than 1 hour at a time at any stop (symptoms can develop or recur during sleep).

12. Observe the patient for at least 6 hours after the treatment for a recurrence of symptoms.

13. Maintain accurate timekeeping and recording.

14. Maintain a well-stocked medical kit.

Patient Getting Worse

The following is a list of considerations if the patient's condition worsens:

1. Never continue the ascent if the patient's condition is worsening.

2. Treat the patient as a recurrence during treatment.

Recurrence of Symptoms During Treatment

The following is a list of considerations in the event of a recurrence of symptoms during treatment:

1. Recompress to 18.3 m and treat on table 6 with extensions as needed.
2. Start the intravenous infusion of low molecular weight dextran and start the following dexamethasone schedule: 20 mg intravenously immediately, then 4 mg every 6 hours intramuscularly.

Recurrence of Symptoms Following Treatment

The following is a list of considerations in the event of a recurrence of symptoms after treatment:

1. Recompress to 18.3 m and use table 6.
2. Do not hesitate to repeat table 6 if the patient becomes worse after initial treatment. In neurologic cases, continue daily hyperbaric oxygen on table 6 for as long as improvement occurs.

Using Oxygen

The following is a list of considerations for using oxygen:

1. Use oxygen as permitted by the treatment tables. Halt the use of oxygen only if the patient tolerates the oxygen poorly or if it is unsafe to use in the chamber.
2. Take all precautions against fire.
3. Attend the patient carefully, being alert for the symptoms of oxygen toxicity.

Inside Observers

The following is a list of considerations for inside observers:

1. Any team member should be qualified to serve as an inside medical attendant during treatment. A patient should never be left alone in the chamber.
2. The inside medical attendant should be alert for any change in the condition of the patient, especially during oxygen breathing.
3. The inside medical attendant who has been with a patient throughout treatment should breathe oxygen, as follows:
   a. On table 1, breathe oxygen at 12.2 m for 30 minutes.
   b. On table 2, breathe oxygen at 9.15 m for 1 hour.
   c. On table 3 or 4, breathe oxygen the last 30 minutes at 12.2 m and the last hour each at 9.15 m, 6.1 m, and 3.05 m.
   d. On tables 5 and 6, breathe oxygen during the last 30 minutes of treatment, that is, on ascent from 9.15 m to the surface.
   e. On table 6, which has been lengthened, breathe oxygen during the last 45 minutes at 9.15 m and during the 30-minute ascent to the surface.

Anyone entering or leaving the chamber before completing the treatment should be decompressed according to the standard United States Navy air or oxygen decompression tables.

Outside observers should specify and control the decompression of anyone leaving the chamber. A physician outside the chamber must review recommendations concerning the treatment or decompression made by those, including physicians, inside the chamber.

Most Frequent Errors Related to Treatment

The following is a list of the most frequent errors related to treatment:

1. Failure of the patient to report symptoms early.

2. Failure to treat doubtful cases.
3. Failure to treat promptly.
4. Failure to treat adequately.
5. Failure to recognize serious symptoms.
6. Failure to keep the patient near the chamber after treatment.
7. Failure to ensure that personnel inside the chamber avoid cramped positions that might interfere with circulation.

Adjuvants to Hyperbaric Therapy

Hyperbaric therapy is the only definitive treatment for decompression sickness. Secondary effects resulting from biochemical events at the blood-bubble interface or damage to vessel endothelia, however, must be treated appropriately. In serious cases of decompression sickness, a marked loss of intravascular volume can occur by transudation of plasma across damaged capillary walls. Hemoconcentration producing malperfusion of tissue and sludging of red blood cells should be avoided or corrected by the prompt and adequate administration of intravenous Ringer's lactate or normal saline solution. In some cases, up to 1 L/hr of intravenous crystalloid solution will be necessary to correct the hemoconcentration. Frequent checks of urinary output are the best guide to the adequacy of the intravenous fluid therapy. Urinary output should be maintained at 1 to 2 ml/kg/hr. Dextran solutions may be helpful in maintaining an adequate intravascular volume by increasing the intravascular osmotic pressure and in preventing sludging of red blood cells. The use of dextran should be limited to 500 cm³ every 12 hours for a 24-hour period. Dexamethasone, 20 mg intravenously followed by 4 mg intramuscularly every 6 hours, may be useful in the prevention or treatment of central nervous system edema. In cases of neurologic decompression sickness affecting the spinal cord, an indwelling urinary catheter should be

placed because these patients most commonly develop a neurogenic bladder.

Cases of decompression sickness following diving do not result in near-drowning as frequently as do patients suffering from cerebral air embolism; nevertheless, the possibility of near-drowning must be evaluated and treatment begun when warranted. In such cases, intensive pulmonary care is mandatory. Endotracheal intubation, assisted ventilation, and correction of acidosis by the frequent and adequate intravenous administration of bicarbonate may be necessary.

None of the above procedures should delay movement of the patient to a hyperbaric chamber except when necessary as immediate life-sustaining measures. It is just as important, however, to institute or continue such procedures after hyperbaric therapy is begun as part of the overall intensive care management of serious cases.

DIRECT EFFECTS OF PRESSURE CHANGE

Gas contained within body cavities is saturated with water vapor, the partial

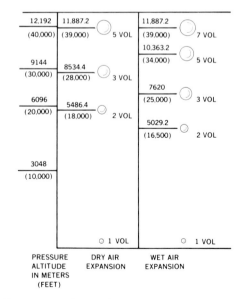

Fig. 7–11. Volumes of wet and dry gases with varying pressures.

pressure of which is related to body temperature. Because body temperature is relatively constant (37°C), the partial pressure of the water vapor is also constant at 47 mm Hg. In determining the mechanical effect of gas expansion, one must account for the noncompressibility of water vapor, which causes wet gases to respond to pressure changes differently than dry gases. Thus, the following relationship can be expressed as Boyle's Law with reference to wet gas:

$$V_i (P_i - PH_2O) = V_f (P_f - PH_2O) \quad (11)$$

where V_i is the initial volume of the gas; V_f is the final volume of the gas; P_i is the initial pressure of the gas in the cavity in mm Hg; P_f is the final pressure of the gas in the cavity in mm Hg; and PH_2O is the partial pressure of water vapor (47 mm Hg at 37°C). Over a given pressure reduction, wet gas will expand to a greater degree than dry gas. The relative gas expansion is a ratio of the final volume of the gas (V_f) to the initial volume (V_i) of the gas and is expressed in the following equation:

$$\text{Relative gas expansion} = \frac{V_f}{V_i}$$
$$= \frac{P_i - PH_2O}{P_f - PH_2O} = \frac{(P_i - 47)}{(P_f - 47)} \quad (12)$$

Figure 7–11 illustrates the increased volume of wet gases at a given pressure over that of a dry gas.

When one experiences a change in ambient pressure, a pressure differential is established between gas-containing body cavities and the external environment. To the extent that gas can move between body cavities and the external environment, this pressure differential will be relieved. It also can be relieved by a change in the volume of the body cavity (compliance). When the pressure differential is not relieved, pathologic effects on involved tissues are likely to occur. The magnitude of

the pathologic effects is related to the ratio of the pressure of the gas within the affected body cavity to the ambient pressure and not to the absolute value of the pressure differential. This is predictable from examining the pressure-volume relationships of Boyle's Law. Therefore, divers, for example, experience more difficulties with the mechanical effects of pressure change when descending from sea level to 10 m of sea water, msw (equations 13 and 14), than they do when descending from 30 to 40 msw (equations 15 and 16). Note that the pressure differential is identical for both circumstances, but the pressure ratio is considerably different.

Pressure differential: $P_f - P_i$
$$= 1520 \text{ mm Hg} - 760 \text{ mm Hg} \quad (13)$$
$$= 760 \text{ mm Hg}$$

Pressure ratio, $\frac{P_f}{P_i}$
$$= \frac{1520 \text{ mm Hg}}{760 \text{ mm Hg}} = 2 \quad (14)$$

Pressure differential: $P_f - P_i$
$$= 3800 \text{ mm Hg} \quad (15)$$
$$- 3040 \text{ mm Hg}$$
$$= 760 \text{ mm Hg}$$

Pressure ratio, $\frac{P_f}{P_i}$
$$= \frac{3800 \text{ mm Hg}}{3040 \text{ mm Hg}} = 1.25 \quad (16)$$

Medically significant pressure changes occur in both flying and diving. There is a marked difference, however, between these two operations with respect to the magnitude and rate of the pressure changes. An aviator descending to sea level from 7620 m at 1524 m/min will experience a total pressure change of 478 mm Hg at a rate of 2.3 mm Hg/sec. A diver descending from sea level to 50 msw at a rate of 18m/min will experience a total pressure change of 3800 mm Hg at a rate of 23 mm Hg/sec.

In general, one can successfully cope with the changes in barometric pressures that occur within the flying or diving envelopes. As long as the pressure in the various body cavities can equalize with the ambient pressure, one can withstand tremendous pressure changes. For example, meaningful work has been performed by aviators at pressures equivalent to 0.1 ATA (15,240 m) and by divers at pressures equivalent to 69 ATA (686 m).

If equalization of pressure is not attained, difficulties ranging from mild discomfort to severe pain, tissue damage, and complete incapacitation will be experienced. The areas of primary concern are the lungs, middle and inner ear, paranasal sinuses, teeth, and the gastrointestinal tract.

The Lungs

Unless air is continually exchanged between the lungs and the outside environment during changes in ambient pressure, severe pathologic disorders can result from the effects of Boyle's Law. Airflow during pressure change will not occur with voluntary breathholding or the apneic phase of a tonoclonic seizure.

Consider the potential problem of a breathholding descent during diving. The average total lung capacity is 5800 cm³. The residual volume (i.e., the volume to which the lungs can be reduced with forceful expiration) is 1200 cm³. If the air volume within the lungs is reduced below 1200 cm³, the actual lung volume will decrease no further due to the elastic and fibrous skeletal structure of the lung tissue. The volume deficit is made up by the leakage of plasma and whole blood into the lungs. This is the classic description of the pathologic condition called "lung squeeze" and is more common in breathhold diving than in descent from altitude. To achieve lung squeeze, the air volume within the lungs must be reduced to about 20% of the original volume. To achieve this on descent from altitude, an aviator would have to make a breathholding descent from 11,890 m to sea level. A breathholding dive to 40.23 msw, however, will result in such a fivefold decrease in the original lung volume. Such a dive is well within the capabilities of many expert divers.

In compressed-gas diving, respirable gas is supplied to the diver from the surface, from a diving bell or hyperbaric chamber, or from a self-contained underwater breathing apparatus (scuba). The gas may be supplied through regulators designed to match intrapulmonary gas pressure to the surrounding ambient pressure. The compressed-gas-supplied diver avoids lung squeeze on descent but runs an added risk on ascent. During ascent to the surface, the diver must continually equilibrate the intrapulmonary pressure to the surrounding ambient pressure. This equilibration is usually accomplished by releasing gas from the lungs by normal breathing or, in the event of the loss of gas supply at depth, by slow continual exhalation. Failure to do so results in intrapulmonary gas expansion according to Boyle's Law and, after the elastic limit of the thorax is reached, a relative rise of intra-alveolar pressure. A rise of intra-alveolar pressure to 50 to 100 mm Hg above ambient pressure is sufficient to force gas into extra-alveolar compartments, resulting in one or more of the clinical conditions grouped under the term pulmonary overpressure accidents.

Pressure differentials sufficient to cause a pulmonary overpressure accident in the compressed-gas–supplied diver can occur on ascents as shallow as from 2 m to the surface. Moreover, a pulmonary overpressure accident is a distinct risk to an aviator whose aircraft suffers a sudden loss of cabin pressure at high altitude.

Autopsies of fatalities following pulmonary overpressure accidents have demonstrated extra-alveolar gas in essentially every tissue examined. Following such an accident, however, the clinical picture seen will be that of arterial gas embolism, mediastinal and subcutaneous emphysema, and/or pneumothorax. The latter two manifestations are recognized by physical and radiographic examination and are managed by conventional measures. The manifestations of arterial gas embolism have an immediate onset following the rapid pressure reduction and may include loss of consciousness, local or generalized seizures, visual field loss or blindness, weakness, paralysis, hypoesthesia, or confusion. A patient presenting with any of these signs or symptoms within 15 minutes following exposure to a rapid pressure reduction must be assumed to have suffered an arterial gas embolism and be treated for such.

Predisposing Factors

In addition to breathholding during ascent, pulmonary overpressure accidents also can occur as a consequence of preexisting disease that limits the egress of gas from the lungs. Thus, the risk is increased by asthma, chronic bronchitis, air-containing pulmonary cysts, and other obstructive airway diseases. Some pulmonary overpressure accidents have occurred without demonstrable cause in patients who exhaled during ascent and had no subsequent lung disorders. In these cases, local pulmonary air trapping is thought to have occurred by redundant tissue, mucous plugs, or similar mechanisms establishing a one-way valve in a small air passage, which allowed gas to pass during compression but not during decompression.

An increasing number of cases of gas embolism are caused by the introduction of air or other gas into the arterial or venous system during surgical procedures or following the establishment of indwelling arterial catheters. With the increasing use of indwelling catheters and surgical procedures involving invasion of the cardio-vascular system, the number of gas embolism cases also has increased. Stoney and colleagues[8] have estimated that the accidental introduction of air through arterial lines occurs in more than 1 in 1000 cases.

Diagnosis

The most difficult differential diagnosis is between gas embolism and neurologic decompression sickness when decompression is involved. This diagnosis is important because of the need to select a proper treatment table. The key factor in reaching a proper diagnosis is the time before the onset of symptoms. The onset is immediate with gas embolism, with symptoms usually occurring within 1 to 2 minutes of reaching the surface. This fact is of critical importance if the person is diving alone because drowning may obscure the underlying gas embolism.

The symptoms and signs elicited in a United States Air Force series of 13 patients treated for gas embolism as a result of sport scuba diving are listed in Table 7–2. The most common presenting sign was coma, noted in 70% of patients, followed by paralysis, which occurred in 54% of patients. These signs may clear rapidly, and, by the time the patient is first seen by a physician, the clinical picture may be quite similar to a mild stroke or transient ischemic attack. This should not,

Table 7–2. Signs and Symptoms in Scuba-Related Gas Embolism—13 Cases

Sign/symptom	Number of Cases	Percent
Loss of consciousness	9	70
Loss of movement—extremity	7	54
Seizure	5	38
Loss of sensation—extremity	4	31
Vertigo	4	31
Mediastinal emphysema	3	23
Nausea and vomiting	3	23
Chest pain (unilateral)	2	15
Subcutaneous emphysema	2	15
Aphasia	1	8
Blindness	1	8
"Spaced-out" aura	1	8

however, interfere with the diagnosis of a probable gas embolism if the patient has been exposed to a rapid pressure change.

The diagnosis of surgical gas embolism should be considered in any patient with indwelling arterial or venous lines (particularly a central line). The sudden onset of seizure or coma is frequently the presenting sign. Venous gas embolism is more common and much less of a problem due to the well-known microfiltration capability of the lung. Nonetheless, it may present as a systemic embolism in the presence of a patent foramen ovale with right to left shunting.

In surgical cases, general anesthesia may mask the usual symptoms; however, failure of the patient to awaken normally or the presentation of an unexplained neurologic deficit should alert one to the diagnosis of possible intraoperative gas embolism. A brief neurologic examination may reveal a myriad of central nervous system findings depending on the location of the gas. Funduscopic examination may reveal arteriolar bubbles in some instances. Computerized tomographic (CT) scanning of the head may be used diagnostically when it is immediately available.

In the diagnosis and treatment of gas embolism, it is critically important to remember that time is of the essence. Although some patients may survive a delay of up to 24 hours, their prognosis worsens with time. The United States Air Force treatment experience, with a 21% mortality in 24 cases, seems to indicate that time is a most important factor.

Treatment

To provide effective therapy for gas embolism, it is important to remember the basic difference between decompression sickness (air or gas bubbles evolving from solution) and gas embolism (gas bubbles that enter the arterial or venous circulation directly). Although the manifestations of decompression sickness are diverse, they

are rarely fatal when treated by proper hyperbaric therapy within hours to days of occurrence. Conversely, the onset of gas embolism is sudden, dramatic, and life-threatening. Bubbles obstruct the systemic or pulmonary arterial circulation. As decompression continues, they expand to produce local endothelial cell damage and herniation into the vessel walls. In addition, plasma proteins react to the invading bubbles by denaturization and attachment to the bubble wall. Activation and agglutination of platelets to the bubbles occur, with release of very potent vasoactive amines and prostaglandins, which produce immediate hypoxia symptoms that may appear as neurologic deficits.

The rationale for hyperbaric therapy for decompression sickness also applies to the management of gas embolism: mechanical compression of bubbles and hyperbaric oxygenation of tissues. Because of the massive amounts of air that are often introduced into the cerebral circulation of gas embolism victims, it is usually necessary to mechanically compress the entrapped air maximally. The volume of air can be reduced by 83% by compressing to 6 ATA (50.33m) (see Figure 7–4). The volume is further reduced by placing the victim in the Trendelenburg (30° head-low) position. This position increases cerebral hydrostatic pressure and, in some cases, forces small bubbles from the arterial circulation across the cerebral capillary bed into the venous circulation, where it produces less potential harm to the victim. It must be emphasized that 100% oxygen breathing cannot be administered at 6 ATA due to the extremely short time to central nervous system oxygen toxicity. Convulsive seizures would occur in less than 5 minutes. Elevated oxygen percentages, however, can be administered in the form of 50/50 Nitrox (a mixture of 50% oxygen and 50% nitrogen). This mixture will assist in correcting tissue hypoxia and ischemia because of the improved oxygen diffusion distance.

When it has been determined that maximum benefit has been attained from the mechanical compression of the entrapped air, the patient must be brought to shallower depths so that 100% oxygen can be administered.

A summary of the decision points in the treatment of gas embolism is presented in Figure 7–12. Hyperbaric therapy is the only definitive treatment for arterial gas embolism. All other methods are adjunctive in nature. As soon as the diagnosis is made, the patient should be placed in the chamber and rapidly compressed with air to 6 ATA according to Table 6A (Fig. 7–13). The patient's condition and progress will determine the duration of time at 6 ATA. If the patient's condition does not improve within 30 minutes at 6 ATA, the time can be extended up to a maximum of 2 hours with decompression on the modified treatment table 6A shown in Figure 7–14.

Variation from the standard Table 6A is potentially harmful to both the patient and inside observers and should not be done without prior consultation with experts in diving medicine.

Adjunctive measures that should be used are intravenous fluids and steroids in pharmacologic doses. Hemoconcentration is frequently seen in gas embolism and may be related to tissue hypoxia and edema. Divers also are commonly dehydrated secondary to pressure diuresis and lack of normal oral fluid intake. Vigorous hydration is important to minimize sludging and obstruction of microvascular blood flow caused by the elevated hematocrit. Balanced saline solution (Ringer's lactate) or isotonic saline without dextrose should be administered intravenously at the rate of 1 L/hr until the patient voids or is catheterized for at least 500 cm³. Sugar (glucose) is specifically not given to prevent further dehydration secondary to glycosuria and a resultant osmotic diuresis. Once adequate hydration is achieved, the rate is slowed to 150 to 200 cm³/hr for the remainder of the treatment.

As soon as possible, dexamethasone is administered intravenously in a dose of 20 mg followed by 4 mg intramuscularly every 6 hours for 24 to 48 hours. There is no supportive evidence for the idea that steroids may increase an individual's susceptibility to oxygen toxicity. Anticoagulant or antiplatelet medications are not currently recommended for treating gas embolism.

Transport of Patients

One hundred percent oxygen should be started as soon as possible, using a tightly fitted aviator's or anesthesia-type mask. The patient should be placed in a Trendelenburg (30° head-low) position while awaiting and during transport to the hyperbaric chamber. If transport is required, it is of utmost importance to maintain near sea-level pressure. The use of "low-flying" helicopters is contraindicated if ground transportation is available. Even slight decreases in pressure cause bubble enlargement and may significantly alter the clinical course of the patient.

During transport, intravenous fluids should be administered using balanced saline solutions or normal saline. Patients suffering from the more serious forms of decompression sickness or from cerebral gas embolism should be accompanied during transport by personnel capable of giving respiratory and cardiac life-support care.

Immediate hyperbaric therapy is essential. Good response, however, has been seen in some cases after long delays before reaching the chamber. This makes it mandatory to give the patient the benefit of a trial of compression and hyperbaric oxygen even in the late case. Of course, every minute that elapses before the start of compression makes the prognosis more guarded.

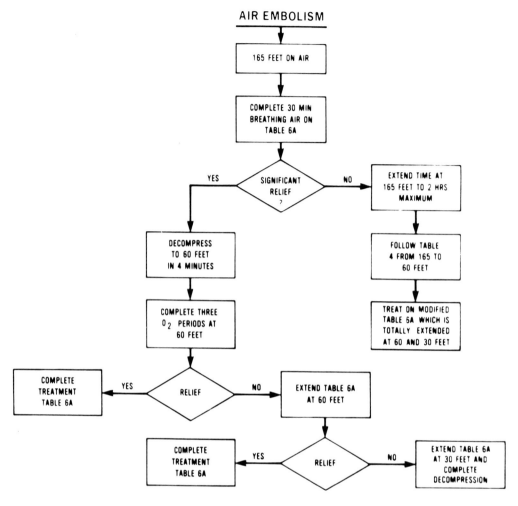

Fig. 7–12. Decision points for the treatment of air embolism. See Table 7–1 and Figures 7–13 and 7–14 for Standard United States treatment tables 4 and 6A.

Other Gas-Containing Cavities

Direct effects of pressure change on the ear, paranasal sinuses, and teeth are described in Chapter 16, Otolaryngology in Aerospace Medicine. This section addresses these effects on the gastrointestinal system and on medical equipment.

The Gastrointestinal Tract

Gas is normally contained in the stomach and the large bowel. As previously discussed, wet gases expand to a greater extent than do dry gases. Expansion within the closed confines of the gastrointestinal tract during ascent can cause stretching of the enclosing organ and produce abdom-

TABLE 6A — AIR EMBOLISM

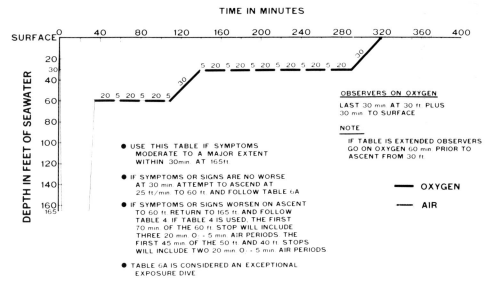

Fig. 7–13. Standard United States Navy treatment table 6A—air embolism.

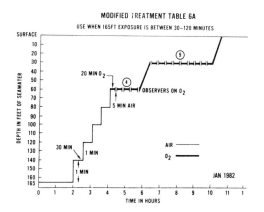

Fig. 7–14. Standard United States Navy treatment table 6A (modified)—air embolism.

inal pain. In addition to pain, respiration also can be compromised by expansion, forcing the diaphragm upward. If pain is allowed to proceed and relief is not obtained by belching or the passing of flatus, flight operations will be jeopardized. Severe pain may cause a vasovagal reaction with hypotension, tachycardia, and fainting. The best treatment of gastrointestinal tract discomfort due to gas expansion is the avoidance of gas-producing foods.

Chewing gum may promote air swallowing and should be avoided at least during ascent. The crewmember should be instructed to pass gas when discomfort occurs. Abdominal massage and physical activity may promote the passage of gas. If this is unsuccessful, a descent should be initiated to an altitude at which comfort is achieved.

Effects of Pressure Change on Medical Equipment

Varying volumes of gas may be trapped in medical equipment being used in the aerospace or hyperbaric environment. Examples of such equipment include drip chambers for intravenous fluids, endotracheal cuffs, water traps used with chest tubes, and sphygmomanometer cuffs.

During ascent, an unvented sphygmomanometer cuff will inflate and tighten around a patient's arm. If air is used to inflate an endotracheal cuff, significant ambient pressure reductions, particularly as seen with ascents from hyperbaric environments, can cause tracheal mucosal sloughing if allowed to persist. A wise precaution is to inflate endotracheal cuffs with normal saline rather than air in such environments. Water levels in water traps should be checked often or opened to ambient pressure when significant changes in pressure occur. The airspace in intravenous line drip chambers will decrease in volume with increased pressure in hyperbaric chambers. Additional air will have to be added to the drip chamber to monitor the drip rate. On ascent, the volume of air will increase, and if added air is not replaced with fluid, intravenous air will inadvertently be administered.

The possible effects of changes in pressure on all medical equipment should be considered before such equipment is used either in a hyperbaric chamber or in flight. When possible, the equipment should be functionally tested in the pressure environment in which it is to be used before it is used with patients.

The quest to fly ever higher and dive ever deeper has expanded man's pressure environmental envelope well beyond that to which he is physiologically adapted. Pathologic changes resulting from exposure to these environments have defined new sets of clinical syndromes specifically related causally to pressure changes. Studies of the pathophysiology underlying these syndromes have unmasked two separate categories of disorders: indirect effects of pressure change resulting from the evolution of gas from solution and direct effects of pressure change on gas-containing body cavities. In addition, it is now recognized that the pressure environment represents a physiologic continuum from the increased pressures encountered by divers to the decreased pressures encountered by aviators and astronauts. This continuum is dramatically exemplified by the diver who surfaces safely only to experience decompression sickness a few hours later while flying at low altitude.

As we have learned more about the physiologic changes that occur with changes in pressure, we have been able to

develop rational treatment methods to cope with the medical disorders they bring about. Thus, hyperbaric therapy, with specific treatment profiles for mild and severe decompression sickness and for gas embolism, has lessened mortality and the incidence of permanent residual deficits. Adjuvants to hyperbaric therapy are increasing our ability to deal with these disorders. Further refinements in therapeutic techniques are necessary, however, as evidenced by a 15% failure rate in the treatment of serious forms of decompression sickness and cerebral gas embolism.

Advances in technology have allowed for the development of systems capable of transporting man into increasingly more severe pressure environments. Similar technologic advances have made possible the development of the life-support equipment necessary to prevent the pathophysiologic consequences of exposure to these environments. Unfortunately, the development of practical, effective life-support systems tends to lag behind the development of transport systems. Historically, this lag resulted from a lack of knowledge about the physiologic consequences of exposure to hostile environments. Today, however, these consequences are much more predictable. The effective and safe use of advanced flying and diving systems depends on parallel developments in biotechnology. The compatible marriage of man to machine presents an ongoing challenge now and in the foreseeable future.

REFERENCES

1. Davis, J.C., Sheffield, P.J., Schuknecht, L., Heimbach, R.D., et al.: Altitude decompression sickness: Hyperbaric therapy results in 145 cases. Aviat. Space Environ. Med., 48:722, 1977.
2. Sheffield, P.J., and Dunn, J.M.: Continuous monitoring of tissue oxygen tension during hyperbaric oxygen therapy—a preliminary report. Proceedings of the Sixth International Congress of Hyperbaric Medicine. Edited by G. Smith. Aberdeen, Scotland, Aberdeen University Press, 1979.
3. Behnke, A.R.: Decompression sickness incident

to deep sea diving and high altitude ascent. Medicine, 24:381, 1945.

4. Donnell, A.M., Jr., and Morgan, C.P.: Successful use of the recompression chamber in severe decompression sickness with neurocirculatory collapse. Aerospace Med., 31:1004, 1960.

5. Downey, V.M., Worley, T.W., Hackworth, R., and Whitley, J.L.: Studies on bubbles in human serum under increased and decreased atmospheric pressures. Aerospace Med., 35:116, 1963.

6. Leverett, S.D., Bitter, H.L., and McIver, R.G.: Studies in decompression sickness: Circulatory and respiratory changes associated with decompression sickness in anesthetized dogs. SAM-TDR-63-7, United States Air Force School of Aerospace Medicine, Brooks Air Force Base, Texas, 1963.

7. Goodman, M.W., and Workman, R.D.: Minimal-recompression oxygen-breathing approach to treatment of decompression sickness in divers and aviators. Research Report 8–65, United States Navy Experimental Diving Unit, Washington, D.C., Government Printing Office, 1965.

8. Stoney, W.S., Alford, W.C., Jr., Burrus, G.R., Glassford, D.M. Jr., et al.: Air embolism and other accidents using pump oxygenators. Ann. Thorac. Surg., 29:336, 1980.

Chapter 8

Biodynamics: Transitory Acceleration

James W. Brinkley and James H. Raddin, Jr.

Real science exists, then, only from the moment when a phenomenon is accurately defined as to its nature and rigorously determined in relation to its material conditions, that is, when its law is known. Before that, we have only groping and empiricism.

CLAUDE BERNARD

From the dawn of time, man has had a problem with transitory acceleration. Pedestrian existence was fraught with a wide range of hazards, from falls onto hard surfaces to hard surfaces falling. The equestrian age led to new respect for the low but sturdy tree limb. Surface vehicles increased the potential for relative velocities and their rapid diminishment. The greatest relative velocities could always be produced through the use of two such vehicles. The advent of powered flight provided the potential for establishing even larger relative velocities between man and his accustomed environment. Well-laid plans have usually been made to allow the gradual elimination of these velocities and a benign termination of the experience. This chapter recognizes the inadequacy of some of those plans.

HISTORY OF THE SCIENCE

In 1908, when man had little experience in powered flight, United States Army Lieutenant Frank Selfridge died of injuries

sustained in the crash of the airplane in which he was riding. The pilot, Orville Wright, also was injured. Attention was drawn to the problem of minimizing the adverse effects of sudden changes in velocity. At first, little was done. After all, aviation presented a multiplicity of challenges that were encountered on every flight. Crashes did not occur with each flight, and if you planned to crash, some would suggest that you shouldn't go up. Eventually, the necessity for transitory acceleration protection became more clearly recognized.

The seat belt was probably introduced in 1910. Its initial function was simply to hold the occupant in the seat during vibration, turbulence, or maneuvers. The seat belt, however, was eventually refined to act as an impact protection device. A double shoulder harness was added to the belt in 1939.

The protective helmet was adapted from sports following Selfridge's accident but did not come into general military use until much later. Early helmet tests were performed by volunteer subjects who dashed their heads against stone walls and then described the experience. Refinements, such as accelerometer measurement and a heavy pendulum for controlled impacts, were added later.

Rigid parachutes apparently were used to jump from high places by the Chinese around 1100. The parachute, as an alternate means of descending from flight, dates to around 1793 for descent from a balloon and as early as 1911 for descent from a conventional powered aircraft. The 1911 jump was said to have taken place from a Wright model B aircraft over Venice, California. The 54-year-old parachutist, Grant Morton, apparently jumped with the parachute canopy folded in his arms and then threw it. As aircraft speeds increased and the motion of the aircraft became more violent when control was lost, bailing out over the side became more and more difficult. Some mechanism was, therefore, sought to facilitate escape from a disabled aircraft.

The work on ejection seats was done by the Germans, Swedish, British, and Americans during and after World War II. The primary stimulus for most early developments was the use of centered, aft-mounted pusher propellers. The Germans apparently had an operational ejection seat in the Heinkel 162 in 1944. The Swedish conducted dummy ejections from a B-3 bomber using compressed air in January, 1942 and from a B-17 using a ballistic catapult in February, 1944. The first Swedish emergency ejection took place on July 29, 1946 from a J-21A with a pusher propeller, saving the life of the pilot. Sir James Martin conducted the British developments, achieving an experimental ejection of a volunteer subject on July 24, 1946 from a modified Meteor III. The first British emergency ejection took place on May 30, 1949 from a prototype flying wing. United States researchers at Wright-Patterson AFB, Dayton, Ohio, conducted an experimental airborne ejection in August, 1946. The first emergency ejection in the United States Air Force took place on August 29, 1949 from an F-86.

Developments in protecting humans from the adverse effects of transitory acceleration have been pursued along many lines. Definition of man's ability to withstand brief acceleration has proceeded hand-in-hand with the search for more efficient and less injurious ways to apply the forces necessary to produce it. Vehicle designers have improved structural designs to decrease the potential for collapse or intrusions into the occupant's living space. The means have been devised to provide supplemental protection when the need arises and to adapt the performance of the protection system to the challenge being encountered.

At the same time, advances in aerospace technology and new applications of existing technology have been accompanied by the potential for more severe acceleration environments. Moderate- and high-speed flight at very low altitude has decreased the time and distance available to accomplish ejection initiation and recovery prior to ground impact. High-speed flight at high altitude has compounded the problems of vehicle clearance during emergency egress, windblast, and parachute opening shock, as well as the necessity for simultaneous protection from other environmental extremes. Space operations may well require orbital vehicle escape systems, which will experience even greater environmental extremes, including those of atmospheric reentry.

The impact protection field is diverse, challenging, and complex. Certain fundamental underpinnings, however, provide the basis for understanding the specific techniques and applications.

DEFINITIONS AND BASIC PHYSICAL RELATIONSHIPS

Acceleration

Acceleration takes place whenever the velocity of an object changes, either in magnitude or direction. Acceleration is a vector quantity. This means that it has a direction or orientation, as well as magnitude or size. Whenever the magnitude is expressed, the direction also must be specified before the acceleration can be considered to be defined. Acceleration magnitude is expressed in terms of velocity units per unit of time. For example, if velocity magnitude is expressed in meters per second, acceleration magnitude would be expressed in meters per second per second or meters per second squared. For convenience, transitory and sustained accelerations in aerospace applications are frequently expressed in terms of "G." One G is the magnitude of the acceleration of an object when it is dropped in a vacuum at the earth's surface. The value is approximately 9.8 m/sec^2. Substantial confusion has resulted from the erroneous practice of using G as a unit of force instead of or as well as acceleration. Meters per second squared and G are always and only units of acceleration magnitude. Another source of confusion is the use of the term deceleration, as if it were physically distinct from acceleration. When used, deceleration simply refers to acceleration that tends to reduce an established velocity.

Impact Acceleration

Impact acceleration is defined as a short-term or transitory acceleration that is not sustained long enough to result in a significant steady-state component in the mechanical response by the accelerated body. Longer duration accelerations are called sustained accelerations and are treated in Chapter 9. Implicit in this response definition of impact is the requirement for an acceleration magnitude sufficiently high for some observable transitory mechanical response to occur. The accelerated body must be compressed, rearranged, or otherwise mechanically affected in an impact acceleration. A further implication of this is that various parts of the impacted body will experience somewhat different accelerations in response to impact. Sustained acceleration eventually tends to produce substantially similar acceleration responses in all the body parts.

Attempts have been made to define impact accelerations in terms of duration. For example, acceleration events having durations less than 1 or 2 seconds have been defined as impacts by various authors. The transitory versus steady-state response definition proposed in this chapter, however, will have different ranges of duration for different accelerated bodies, depending on the frequency response of the body. A fixed time duration definition is, therefore, not generally applicable over the range of acceleration profiles and accelerated bodies that are of interest in aerospace medicine. Instead, the response and the resulting stress determine the category.

Sustained acceleration protection is applied in those situations in which the stresses are primarily physiologic and sustained. Impact acceleration protection is applied in those situations in which the stresses are primarily mechanical and transitory. Extensive overlap occurs in the two forms of acceleration. Physiologic disruptions, such as unconsciousness, may be produced by impact or by sustained acceleration, but the mechanism in impact is traumatic instead of hemodynamic. Ideally, the techniques of impact protection should blend into and complement the techniques of sustained acceleration protection, just as the actual acceleration stresses often overlap the two definitions.

Coordinate Systems

The direction and magnitude of an object's velocity must always be measured with respect to some other points that establish a reference frame. For example, an aircraft flying in formation may have a low velocity with respect to a wingman and a relatively high velocity with respect to a control tower. The velocity of an object, which is a vector quantity, is simply the time rate of change of the object's position vector in the chosen reference frame. Similarly, the acceleration of an object, also a vector quantity, is simply the time rate of change of the object's velocity vector in the chosen reference frame. Velocity and acceleration values measured with respect to one reference frame are identical to those measured in another reference frame if, and only if, there is no relative motion between the reference frames. Acceleration will still be the same even when one frame is translating at constant velocity with respect to the other frame. In general, the velocity and acceleration values to be observed with respect to one frame can be computed from the values observed with respect to another frame if the relative motions between the two frames are well described.

The reason all of this is important in a discussion of impact is that experimental measurements and real-world situations frequently may be misinterpreted if the reference frames are not clearly understood. For example, a fixed motion picture camera on an impact test sled will measure the motion of a subject with respect to the sled, but the sled will generally be moving and accelerating with respect to the earth. Linear accelerometers mounted to the subject are sometimes used to deduce acceleration with respect to the earth. Rotation of the subject, and thus the accelerometers, however, can make this determination difficult at best and often impossible. Comparison of impact response data derived from a sled-fixed camera with data derived from a subject-fixed accelerometer will require additional measures of sled and subject motions, including rotations.

Reference frames used in describing impact accelerations vary with the vehicle and the measurement systems involved. For human exposures, however, it has been convenient at least to express head and chest accelerations with respect to the subject's own body parts. A convention has been established to define an orthogonal, mutually perpendicular set of three axes for the head and chest. In a forward-facing, erect position, the x-axis is oriented front to back or perpendicular to a coronal plane, the y-axis is oriented laterally or perpendicular to a sagittal plane, and the z-axis is oriented vertically or perpendicular to a horizontal plane. These axes are shown in Figure 8–1. Some attempts have been made to define these axes very precisely using radiographic landmarks, but the practical utility of these approaches has not been established because anatomic variations tend to nullify the presumed increase in accuracy. Approximate definitions have been adequate for most purposes. Other groups have defined anatomic coordinate systems for other body parts such as the pelvis, hand, and foot, but these have not found wide practical application in aerospace medicine.

Confusion has resulted from the definition of the positive directions for the

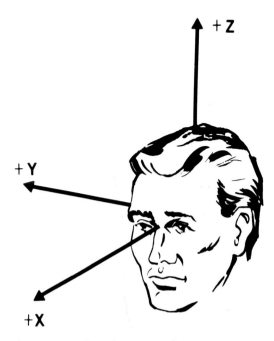

Fig. 8–1. Head acceleration coordinate system.

axes defined above. As shown in Figure 8-1, +x is anterior, +z is cephalad, and +y is to the right, by convention. This leads to a so-called left-handed system. In the more common right-handed system, the vector cross-product operation of x with y produces a result along +z. If +x is along the right index finger and +y is along the right middle finger held at a right angle, the right thumb will point along +z when held at a right angle to the other two. In the head or chest coordinate system, x cross y is along −z, which follows the finger rule when applied to the left hand. The left-handed convention, however, appears to be too well established to be reversed by this text. The convention has resulted from an early approach that defined reaction forces instead of accelerations. The reaction forces are positive in the directions opposite to the accelerations, leading to a right-handed system. If you don't believe that, turn a left-handed glove inside out and try it on.

An acceleration that tends to increase the forward velocity of the head and/or torso, then, is +x acceleration. Equivalently, +x acceleration also may decrease the rearward velocity of these structures. Reaction forces commonly have been used to visualize these motions. With this technique, +x acceleration becomes eyeballs-in acceleration. This works well and accommodates both increasing forward velocity and decreasing rearward velocity because it is easy to imagine which way you accelerate to push your eyeballs in. One still must, however, remember the sign change associated with eyeballs-in (-x reaction) for +x acceleration. Similarly, +z is eyeballs-down and +y is eyeballs-left.

Acceleration and Force

Perhaps the most basic tenet of physics is the Newtonian relationship between acceleration and force:

$$F = m\,a \qquad (1)$$

A net force (F) on a mass (m) will produce an acceleration (a) in the same direction as the force. Equivalently, the velocity of a mass cannot be altered, either in direction or magnitude, without application of a force to produce the change. Acceleration can be measured by multiple, timed observations of position, and force can be measured by the use of a spring scale, but aggregate mass is deduced from equation 1. Force may be applied mechanically, gravitationally, electrostatically, or magnetically. Mechanical force application is most common in impact situations and requires physical contact between the accelerated object and some object that applies the accelerating force. Force application, by any means, is always a mutual experience for at least two objects. When a hammer applies force to a nail, the nail applies an equal and opposite force to the hammer. An ejection seat applies force to the occupant, but the occupant applies an equal and opposite force to the seat. The force applied to the seat has been termed a reaction force. It can be seen that accelerated bodies apply reaction forces in a direction opposite to the direction of the acceleration. This is a consequence of the accelerating force being applied in the direction of acceleration. In this chapter, impact always will be an acceleration expressed in G or meters per second squared. It always will be produced by a force in the direction of acceleration expressed in newtons (kilogram-meters per second squared). It will be seen that force units are simply the product of mass units and acceleration units, which is to be expected from equation 1. Thus, the commonly used term, G-forces, is a misnomer.

Translational and Angular Motion

Motion can be described in a displacement sense, such as for a piston with respect to a cylinder, or a rotational sense, such as for a drive shaft with respect to an engine. Many displacements have an angular quality to them even when no true rotation or spinning is taking place. This occurs whenever the motion is not precisely along the radius or line connecting the object's center of mass to the chosen reference point. It is called orbital motion because none of the displacement motion of an object in a perfect circular orbit is along a radius drawn to the center of the circle. In general, motions must be characterized by three components: rotation, called spin, displacement perpendicular to the reference radius, called orbital, and displacement along the reference radius, called central. The first two are angular motions. The last two are translational motions because they always involve motion of the center of mass. It should be observed that the angular and translational definitions overlap and both apply to orbital motions. Forces applied to an object may be resolved into components along the radial reference line and perpendicular to it. The perpendicular component, multiplied by the length of the radius, is a measure of the angular force, or torque. If the chosen reference point is the center of mass of the object, the torque is a measure of a tendency to change its spin motion. The other component, radial to the center of mass, is a measure of the tendency to change its translational motion. If the chosen reference point is other than the center of mass, the force component radial to the center of mass can be further resolved into a component radial to the outside reference point and a component perpendicular to it. The perpendicular component, multiplied by the radius, is a torque with respect to the reference point and measures the tendency of the force to change the orbital motion with respect to the reference point. The radial component of the force measures the tendency to change the central motion with respect to the reference point and is termed a central force.

In general, motions of objects undergoing impact accelerations include spin, orbital, and central components with respect to commonly used frames of reference. Furthermore, the chosen reference frames frequently are accelerating and rotating during the events, leading to relatively involved computations to arrive at comparable, comprehensible, and relevant descriptions of the forces and motions involved.

Velocity Change and Momentum

Balanced forces on an object, yielding a net force of zero, do not cause acceleration, and, therefore, no velocity change takes place. Impact, being an acceleration, requires a nonzero net force application to the impacted or accelerated object. The characteristics of the force, the means of application, and the characteristics of the impacted object taken together determine the response. Impacts, in order to create a problem for human subjects, must be sustained long enough to produce some significant velocity change. Automobile crashes at 1 km/hr are not really crashes.

In situations of interest for human occupants of aerospace vehicles, impact conditions tend to be defined by velocity changes or, equivalently, by acceleration histories as a function of time instead of by applied forces. In fact, the definition is often provided by giving vehicle accelerations and/or velocities because the forces imposed on the human occupant are difficult to describe, involving curving, yielding contact surfaces for the human body and for the restraints and supports. The problem is avoided by defining a collision situation between the occupant and his own vehicle. The situation may arise from a prior collision of the vehicle with something else, such as the ground, in which the vehicle velocity is rapidly changed, or it may arise from a sudden velocity change to which the occupant must accommodate, such as that imparted to an ejection seat. In any case, the velocity change of the vehicle is specified, and the occupant's behavior in the resulting collision with his vehicle is observed.

This is where momentum comes in. Momentum is simply a measure of the authority one has in conducting the business of collisions. Newton expressed it as follows:

$$p = m \, v \qquad (2)$$

Momentum (p) equals mass (m) times velocity (v). It makes sense intuitively, too. If one has great mass, one has great authority. If one has great speed, one has great authority. If one has both great mass and great speed, one's great authority is multiplied. Momentum also is a vector quantity, with its direction determined by the velocity vector.

In many cases, the total momentum of colliding bodies is virtually unchanged, as in the contact between two billiard balls. In aerospace vehicle collisions, either the vehicle isn't affected much by the occupant or, if it is, the defined velocity change of the vehicle already includes the occupant's effects on it. In such cases, the occupant's momentum, or authority in future collisions, is changed. The currency for transacting changes in authority is called kinetic energy, or work.

$$E = 1/2 \, m \, v^2 \qquad (3)$$

Kinetic energy (E) equals 1/2 mass (m) times velocity squared (v^2).

$$W = Fx \qquad (4)$$

Work (W) equals force (F) times the distance through which the force acts (x). Units of work and energy are both kilogram-meters squared per second squared or Newton-meters. Work and energy are, therefore, equivalent. Neither is a vector quantity. Comparing equations 2 and 3 demonstrates that velocity is more important than mass in determining energy, whereas mass and velocity are equivalent in determining momentum. Less apparent is the observation that, whereas energy is a measure of the effect of force over distance (equation 4), momentum is a measure of the effect of force over time (equation 2, with the understanding that velocity is acceleration times time and with a good recall of equation 1).

$$p = m \, v = m \, a \, t = F \, t \qquad (5)$$

Equations 4 and 5 are only true for constant forces. If the forces vary with distance or time, each little distance or time increment must be multiplied by the effective force during that time and the resulting products summed up. This process will be recognized as integration. Momentum transfer becomes the integral of net force with respect to time, whereas work is the integral of net force with respect to distance. Because the relationship between distance and time is velocity, work is a function of force, velocity, and time, whereas momentum is related simply to force and time.

These concepts are presented primarily to establish a basis for an appreciation of the impact event. Specifically, peak acceleration is clearly not of significance unless it is sustained for an adequate time to lead to an appreciable velocity change. In addition, the energy transfer associated with an acceleration pulse of a given duration is greater for objects moving at higher velocity in the direction of the acceleration. Because energy or work is required to produce mechanical damage, this consideration is of no small importance but not particularly obvious without recourse to the basic equations. At least it should be apparent that peak vehicle acceleration in G does not satisfactorily describe an impact event. Instead, at the minimum, the acceleration history prior to the event, the acceleration pulse shape, magnitude, direction, and duration from which velocity change can be computed, the characteristics of the impacted subject, and the nature of the subject's contacts and attachments to the vehicle must be specified.

Angular Momentum and Torque

Angular motion can be described using a quantity analogous to linear momentum. Because there are two kinds of angular motion, two terms are in the description. Orbital motion leads to a momentum based on mass, the radius or distance to the reference point, and the velocity perpendicular to the radius. For pure, circular orbital motion about a fixed reference point, the velocity is always perpendicular to the radius. Spin motion provides the second term and is described by the moment of inertia and the angular velocity, where the moment of inertia is simply a measure of the mass and its distribution with respect to the axis of rotation of interest. Mass concentrations located well off this axis are far more significant than mass near the axis. In fact, each piece of mass is multiplied by the square of its distance from the axis of rotation to arrive at the moment of inertia, which has units of kilogram-meters squared. Angular velocity is in radians per second, where radians do not count as units because they are not mass, length, or time. The complete angular momentum definition, then, is as follows:

$$L = I\omega + mrv_\perp \qquad (6)$$

Angular momentum (L) equals moment of inertia (I) times angular velocity (ω) plus mass (m) times radius (r) times velocity perpendicular to that radius ($v_\perp$). The units of each term are kilogram-meters squared per second squared, or newton-meters, just like linear momentum. Changing angular momentum requires an expenditure of energy, just as for the linear case. Changes require the application of torque, as previously defined. Angular momentum is a vector quantity and requires torque to change its direction as well as its magnitude. In impact events, linear momentum is frequently converted to angular momentum before being dissipated. The required torque is a result of typical cantilevered structures and the proximal location of typical anchor points.

Stress-Strain

So far, relationships have been discussed which have been applied to and illustrated with rigid bodies. A rigid body is an imaginary nondeformable solid that can be completely described by its shape, mass distribution, position, orientation, and motion. It never breaks, bends, or distorts and, therefore, does not exist. Things that do exist also move under the influence of forces, but they can and do break, bend, and otherwise distort, thus making their physical description more difficult. The approach that has been taken conceptually involves the treatment of each tiny segment of the object as a rigid body, so that the summation of the behavior of the parts describes the behavior of the whole. This concept is called continuum mechanics because objects are described as continuous aggregates of tiny rigid bodies held together in various ways. In practice, since the forces cannot be measured for each little part, gross observations are made of forces and motions and the infinitesimal values deduced for purposes of description.

An example should help. In Figure 8–2, a and b show loadings of an imaginary rigid bar in tension. The situations are well described by the tension forces, as noted. Any weight could be used with easily calculable results. Similar loadings of real bars in tension are shown in c and d of Figure 8–2; if the bars don't break, the tension force descriptions are identical to those of Figure 8–2b, but the description here is inadequate. It is clear that, if the bar material is identical, the situation is more stressful for the thin bar than for the fat one. The stressfulness of the situation

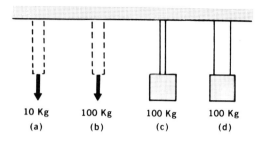

(a) 10 Kg TENSION FORCE APPLIED TO IDEALIZED BAR,

(b) 100 Kg TENSION FORCE APPLIED TO IDEALIZED BAR,

(c) FORCE APPLIED AS IN (b) TO A SMALL CROSS-SECTION BAR,

(d) FORCE APPLIED AS IN (b) TO A LARGE CROSS-SECTION BAR .

Fig. 8–2. Model of stress and strain.

must be evaluated when real materials are used. This has been formalized as follows:

$$\sigma = \frac{F}{A} \qquad (7)$$

Stress (σ) equals force (F) divided by the cross-sectional area (A). This equation works rather well because the force on each little cross-sectional portion of the bar can be deduced if its area is defined. For the same total force, overall stress will be greater for small cross-sectional areas and lesser for large cross-sectional areas. Computing the stress for c and d in Figure 8–2 gives a more complete description of what is happening to the real material.

Stress is expressed in units of newtons per square meter or pascals. Stress also can be applied to surfaces using the same formulation (equation 7). In fact, a stress vector can be defined incorporating the directional characteristics of the force. For example, hydrostatic pressure on a surface is a stress or force per area and is always directed perpendicularly to the surface.

Stress is actually independent of material characteristics. The material characteristics, however, determine what an object will do when subjected to stress. Any stress will produce some sign of strain in real materials. The type of strain varies with the type of stress and the material characteristics. Stress that is perpendicular to each tiny cross-sectional area is called normal stress and tends to produce compression or elongation. Stress that is parallel to each tiny cross-sectional area is called shear stress and tends to produce bending, twist, or similar distortion. Material characteristics also play a part. Some materials have good strength in compression but are terrible in shear. A stack of blocks and water are two examples. Other materials have good strength in tension but are lousy in compression. Rope is an example. Often, materials convert one kind of external stress into other kinds of internal stress because of their internal structures and the interaction of their internal forces during deformation or strain. Compression of a structural member may produce significant shear stresses internally. The various types of strain responses to stress are formalized in dimensionless units expressing either a ratio of the change in length or a trigonometric function of the distortion angle associated with bending or twist.

For many materials, the relationship between a particular stress and the resulting strain can be rather simply expressed, as long as the stress is held within a limited range, obviously below the breaking point. In this so-called linear range, certain materials may act like springs, for example, and have a strain that is proportional to the stress, like a spring's displacement is proportional to the applied force. A real spring, however, loaded with a given constant force for a long time, will have a displacement that slowly continues to creep along slightly, almost as if the spring were relaxing under the persistent load. This behavior of initial stretching with a further tendency to creep or relax can be modeled by a combination of strain displacement and strain velocity, each proportional to stress, which is called a viscoelastic model (*elastic* for spring and *visco* for the flow of viscous fluids). Interestingly enough, these two characteristics can be used to describe the behavior of most materials in their linear range. Some are more like springs, whereas other materials are more like very viscous fluids, such as glycerine, less viscous fluids, such as water, or even less viscous fluids, such as air. Fluids also may be compressible or incompressible, which determines their utility as springs.

A few simple viscoelastic models are shown in Figure 8–3. Such models can be used to describe the behavior of materials subjected to stress, including such phenomena as strain rate dependence or frequency response and hysteresis, which is the tendency of strain characteristics to vary from the loading phase to the unloading phase. They do not describe the behavior of materials in their nonlinear range, at or near the breaking or yield points.

In situations of interest in impact protection, normal and shear stresses on the human body are directly produced at points of force application, indirect internal stresses are induced at other locations within the body, and gross center of mass accelerations occur. The resulting strains are tolerable when the situations are controlled to assure that yield points are not reached for structures of significance. The

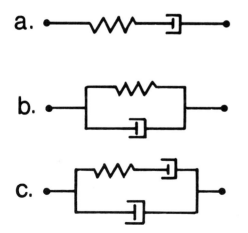

Fig. 8–3. Examples of viscoelastic models. ᴧᴧ spring: Force proportional to displacement. ⊣⊢ Damper: Force proportional to velocity.

techniques available to provide this control will be discussed in this chapter.

Rate Dependency and Frequency Response

The response of a mechanical system to an accelerating force depends not only on the magnitude, direction, and duration of the applied force but also on the rate at which the force builds up. If force is applied slowly, acceleration builds up slowly, can be accommodated, and is called sustained acceleration. If force is applied rapidly, acceleration builds up too rapidly for the mechanical system to track it and a transient or impact response occurs, which differs considerably from the steady-state response that would have resulted if the same force had been applied slowly. The interesting thing about all this is that slow application for one system is fast for another. In fact, slow application for an adequately restrained system may be too fast for the same system inadequately restrained. The ability of a system to track accelerating forces of varying application rates is described by its frequency response.

Frequency response is so named because the application of smoothly alternating or sinusoidal forces or vibration of varying frequencies allows the measurement of responses that reveal the system's tracking ability. Determination of frequency response under differing restraint conditions can serve as an evaluation of their relative effectiveness.

A significant characteristic of some mechanical systems is their natural tendency to respond to a nonsinusoidal, brief force application with a sinusoidal mechanical response at a fixed frequency. A familiar example is the tuning fork. A system's mechanical response is called its natural frequency, or its resonant frequency. If a system is subjected to sustained vibration at its natural frequency, it will respond at that frequency with increasing amplitude until restriction or mechanical failure is reached. The human body has natural frequencies not only for its gross structural elements, such as arms and legs, but also for various substructures such as internal organs. This fact may not seem particularly important since we are talking about impact and not vibration. Even the waveform of a limited duration impact pulse, however, can be described in mathematical terms involving a sum of various frequencies. It also has physical effects consistent with its frequency description and the frequency response of the system. For example, particular impact pulses can have more drastic effects on particular structures or substructures if there is a high power content in the impact pulse at the applicable natural frequency of the structure. This statement may sound somewhat odd, but you have probably subconsciously used this principle more than once. For example, why do you think some thumps on a tuning fork have more impressive effects than others? Have you noticed that a softer thumping surface works better for low-pitched forks? The softer surface slows the rate of force application and, therefore, lowers the frequency spectrum of the force pulse to better match the natural frequency of the fork.

Aerodynamics

Aerodynamics concerns itself with the flow of fluids around objects. This is of interest when situations such as high-speed ejection allow such flow to impose large forces, which result in transitory accelerations of the human body and its parts.

Aerodynamic forces are defined relative to the flight path. Forces perpendicular to the flight path, including side forces, are called lift. Forces along the flight path are called drag. Those forces tending to simply change the angle of the body as it moves along its flight path are called moments. On a wing, for example, the desired lift, or net upward force, derives both from an increase in pressure below the wing and from a decrease in pressure above the wing. One simplified way of thinking about the source of these forces begins with the observation that, with certain assumptions, energy of the flow in a steady state must be constant when no work is being done. That energy is determined by the sum of pressure energy, thermal energy, and speed energy. It follows, then, that when constant-temperature air moves faster over the top of a wing because of the wing's shape, the pressure must decrease for the energy to remain constant. The difference in pressure above and below the wing produces lift.

Two sources of drag force are similar to the lift situation. The most commonly quoted drag component is due to the pushing of the object from the front by the force of the moving wind. Aerodynamicists call this dynamic pressure, q, and point out that it is proportional to air density and the square of the velocity among other factors, such as air viscosity and elasticity. The drag force produced on a body by a given level of dynamic pressure is determined by its area, shape, and orientation. A less well-understood drag component is due to the sucking of the object from behind by the decreased pressure produced in its wake. This component can be quite significant. If a complete vacuum were to be produced in a wake at sea level, the available sucking drag would be over 0.98 kg/cm^2. That would be equivalent to the dynamic pressure, or pushing drag, imposed at an indicated airspeed of about 800 knots. Finally, a third drag component, not related to the lift analogy, is due to the surface friction of the air flowing around the object. This component also can be quite significant, depending on the roughness of the surface and the flow properties near the surface.

This area is complex, and aerodynamic descriptions frequently tend to be experimentally determined, even for smooth, simple, well-defined geometric structures in steady-state flow. Ejection seats and human arms are irregular, complex, and poorly defined, making them even less amenable to precise modeling for flow with rapidly changing speed. Some observations of relationships can nevertheless be made. Consider, for example, a coasting car with an initial speed of 100 km/hr. The car will be retarded by rolling friction and by aerodynamic drag and will decelerate at a rate determined by its mass and the retarding force (a = F/m). It the occupant extends an arm from the window, his arm will be forced back relative to the window unless he actively resists because the aerodynamic drag force relative to the arm's mass is greater than the aerodynamic drag and rolling friction force relative to the gross vehicle mass. The arm, therefore, decelerates at a greater rate.

The same situation exists for an unrestrained extremity protruding from a crewmember/ejection seat unit catapulted into a high-speed windstream. Limb flailing is produced by an inequality between the ratios of aerodynamic drag and mass for the flailing member, as compared to the overall occupant/seat unit. Injury can result simply from the differences in acceleration of the occupant and his flailing body parts. The flailing part also may strike a surface such as the seat edge, equalizing the velocities but producing injury in the process.

Application of Force

Penetrating Impact

Impact accelerations are produced by the sudden mechanical application of force requiring direct contact between an impacting object and the impacted structure. If the area over which the force is applied is small and/or if the impacted structure is fragile, the contact force may be sufficient to produce penetration into the impacted structure. Bullet wounds provide a typical example. If the impacting bullet passes completely through the impacted body part, the momentum transfer may be considerably less than would

have occurred if the impacting object lodged within the impacted structure. The amount of the difference depends on the penetrating object's residual velocity after passing through. Damage to the impacted structure from penetrating impact is typically determined more by the direct trauma associated with the penetration and less by the gross impact accelerations imposed on the involved body part. Therefore, the subject of penetrating impact will not be pursued further in this chapter.

Blunt Impact

The remaining impact force applications can be considered nonpenetrating impact, or blunt impact. This type of impact is the typical means of force application for restrained occupants of aerospace vehicles. The term, however, is most commonly applied to the more limited situation in which only a portion of the body is accelerated with respect to the rest of the body by localized, nonpenetrating force application. An example would be an aircraft birdstrike in which the bird shatters the windscreen and strikes the helmeted head of the pilot. Although penetration of the head may not occur, significant internal structural damage is still possible. These impacts are clearly of interest in aerospace medicine.

Whole-Body Acceleration

The primary concern of this chapter is with those nonpenetrating impact situations in which significant accelerations are imposed on the center of mass of a human being. The forces are typically applied bluntly by means of seat surfaces, restraints, distributed windblast force, or some combination of these factors. Typical localized blunt impact to inadequately restrained body parts also may ensue as a result of relative motions such as that of the head or extremities with respect to the torso. In these cases, the body part may strike a fixed surface such as the instrument panel or seat. Whole-body acceleration, then, involves generalized blunt impact and may secondarily include localized blunt impact.

IMPACT RESPONSE AND INJURY MECHANISMS

Subject Response

Mechanical Response

The human body responds to applied forces by a combination of acceleration and strain. Accelerations are force-dependent and are determined by the ratio of force to mass. Strains or deformations are stress-dependent and are determined by the ratio of force to area and by the viscoelastic characteristics of the material. The trick is to apply adequate accelerations over the appropriate times to produce the required velocity change while minimizing strain. Strain is associated with injury.

Descriptions of impact response usually concentrate on the displacements of the subject with respect to the vehicle and the accelerations of the subject with respect to an external fixed reference. Displacements with respect to the vehicle can be good or bad, depending on whether they increase or decrease the subject's accelerations with respect to an external fixed reference. They may increase accelerations in two ways. One way is by allowing the subject to strike a portion of the vehicle not designed for restraint. An instrument panel is a good example. This leads to increased accelerations during the collision. Elastic collisions not only stop the closing velocity but require more of the same acceleration to produce a separation velocity in the other direction. In other words, elastic collisions are bounces. They can involve nearly twice the momentum and energy transfer associated with inelastic collisions, which are nonbounce, or hit-and-stick collisions.

A second way in which displacements can increase accelerations can be seen by considering what occurs in a head-on vehicle crash into a fixed structure. The vehicle's initial velocity is rapidly decreased to zero relative to the structure if the collision is inelastic. If the vehicle and the structure were idealized rigid bodies, the velocity change would occur instantaneously and the acceleration would be infinite. In the real world, however, the vehicle and the fixed structure usually deform to some extent, allowing finite acceleration over some small time interval to produce the required velocity change. Clearly, for a given velocity change, shorter stopping distances require shorter stopping times and, therefore, higher accelerations.

In our vehicle crash, assume the occupant to be perfectly restrained to the vehicle from the bottom of the neck to the tips of the toes. Only the head and neck protrude from this otherwise perfect restraint system. Further, assume that vehicle acceleration in the crash is high but not infinite, of a duration that is short but not zero, such as a 25-m/sec velocity change in 1 m. In the crash, then, the occupant's body experiences acceleration identical to that of the vehicle. The head, however, does not. Some would say that the head is thrown forward. In point of fact, the head continues forward with the same velocity it had at the instant of impact, until some force acts to cause an acceleration. In this case, that force is provided by the neck, which is placed in tension as the head tries to keep going. In the upright position, the neck is initially well aligned to produce vertical forces on the head, but our crash requires horizontal force. From the neck, this force is initially off-axis with respect to the head's center of mass. Such off-axis forces are called torques and produce rotations. The head, therefore, is rotated to better align the center of mass with the required horizontal neck tension. This process takes time, during which the head continues forward with respect to the rest of the body. In fact, a velocity difference is built up between head and body because the body, in the early stages of the crash, does a much better job of stopping. In this case, the head will have to undergo much of the velocity change in less time than the body because the head starts late. Higher acceleration is required for the head simply as a result of the head displacement relative to the vehicle. Even worse, since necks have some springiness to them, the head not only moves forward and comes to a stop, but also pitches back again at the end. The result is similar to the case of an elastic collision, even without hitting anything, and implies a greater total velocity change for the head and, of course, more acceleration.

As mentioned earlier, however, some displacements of the subject with respect to the vehicle can be good. Such displacements may be produced to attenuate the effects of vibration or modest impacts. Consider our vehicle occupant perfectly restrained to the vehicle with metal seats and no springs or shock absorbers. A ride down a rough road would be most unpleasant. For this reason, some means of viscoelastic displacement of the occupant is built into most human restraint systems to allow much vibration and many sharp spike impacts to be minimized, particularly when little if any overall velocity change is required. Great care must be taken in the design of such systems to define the range of acceleration challenges that will be imposed. Otherwise, the displacement system can make things worse by bottoming out. The bone-jarring crunch at the bottom of a really deep pothole testifies to the limitations of automobile springs and shock absorbers. Similar limitations apply to any aerospace impact attenuation system.

The goal of restraint system design, then, is to match the characteristics of the restraint system to both the mechanical response of the human occupants and the potential accelerations that may be encountered. The matching criteria are maximum isolation from the vehicle during short-term events and minimum isolation from the vehicle during significant transitory accelerations that produce appreciable velocity changes. The contradictory nature of these criteria makes restraint system design a challenging task.

Biologic Response

When the human body or its parts are subjected to strain and acceleration, events may occur that are of structural and physiologic significance. These events may not be easily discernible through observation of the overt mechanical response. The most apparent effects are probably strains at points of stress appplication. These may include lacerations, contusions, joint injuries, and fractures. Acceleration of the body or its parts also may indirectly produce strains at points distant from direct stress applications. Examples are fractures of the spine during ejection acceleration and transection of the aorta during a forward-facing, head-on crash. Such strains result from internal structural loading or from differential acceleration of internal body parts that are attached to one another or are free to collide. Some of these effects may be subtle. For example, retinal or other hemorrhage may occur as a result of hydrodynamic blood surges or motion of a blood vessel with respect to the retina.

If each particle of the human body could be uniformly accelerated with respect to each adjacent particle, velocity changes could be accomplished without untoward physiologic response or injury. If there is no difference between the acceleration of each particle, there is no change in the respective positions of the particles. Thus, the deflections that cause mechanical failure of body tissues or stimulate adverse physiologic responses would not occur. This is a fundamental principle in understanding the mechanisms of injuries that result from transient acceleration and the approaches that are used to provide protection for the human body.

In their daily activities, people tend to minimize the deflections that might cause injury or discomfort by controlling the accelerations acting on their bodies. They accomplish this by the control of their body position, design of vehicles, and avoidance of collisions. When large velocity changes must be accomplished, the body is accelerated and decelerated gradually. A practical mechanical method to achieve simultaneous, uniform acceleration of each body particle has not been found when a relatively large velocity change must be accomplished in a short period of time. Such methods, unfortunately, remain in the domain of science fiction.

When a large acceleration is unavoidable, several methods are used to provide protection. The first is to minimize the applied acceleration as much as possible. For example, the magnitude of the acceleration may be reduced by distributing the velocity change over a longer period of time. The second method is to restrict the motion of the major body segments to reduce the relative displacements of the body segments and their internal organs. This method is most commonly accomplished by restraining the body segments to a supporting structure such as a vehicle seat.

The effectiveness of a transient acceleration protection system is evaluated in terms of how well it prevents injuries. The injuries may result from high-contact pressures under the restraints, impact of the body segments with vehicle structure, or whole-body acceleration, such as in spinal fractures incurred during the use of an ejection seat. In each case, the conditions of loading of the affected body element and the properties of the element, that is, its load-carrying viscoelastic characteristics and failure limits, determine the injury potential for any given set of acceleration conditions.

Injury Mechanisms

Human tolerance to transitory acceleration is defined in various ways. Under given conditions, it may be considered to be a maximum acceleration exposure level that generally does not result in significant injury or death. A given level, however, may result in no injury for one subject and death for another, so this definition is vague at best. Two observations explain its lack of precision. One observation is that resistance to injury varies from specimen to specimen, implying that a range of tolerance must be expected. The second observation, that the description of vehicle acceleration does not define the proximate cause of specific injuries, is more important. The end point of death or significant injury may be reached through various kinds of effects on different organs, structures, or systems. Therefore, before an assessment of the range of injury resistance or strength can be made, the way or ways must be defined in which the vehicle acceleration leads to imposition of the proximate cause of potential injuries. Defining the steps along the path from vehicle acceleration to localized stress is the process of defining the injury mechanism.

Injury mechanisms are usually difficult to work out in detail because force and stress measurements are increasingly difficult to make at the various steps beyond the vehicle acceleration stage. Many forces and stresses are internal to the subject. Compounding the force measurement problem are difficulties in defining or measuring the effective mass of body segments and the effective internal musculoskeletal and soft tissue forces. Experimental data are often in the form of kinematic descriptions that only define motions, without regard to force or mass. Kinetic descriptions would be far more useful from a protection viewpoint, because they would include the relation of the motion of masses to the forces acting on them to allow a more rational definition of protective interventions in the process, since the required protective forces and their own resulting stresses could be better assessed.

Precise injury mechanisms should meet the following criteria: (1) the load transmission path from seat structure and restraints to the point of injury should be clearly defined; (2) the defined load transmission path should be in accordance with physical principles by taking into account the origins of the loads, the motions of the transmitting structure under loading, and the capability of the transmitting structure to carry the presumed loads; and (3) the transmitted load should produce sufficient stress at the appropriate point to account for the injury. Even when these criteria are met, the proposed mechanism remains hypothetic. Verification often requires measurements that are inaccessible in conjunction with experiments that would be ethically inappropriate. Instead, proposed mechanisms generally achieve the status of working hypotheses on the basis of convincing argument, calculation with models, experimentation with human surrogates, and/or usefulness in devising successful protection schemes. The success of a protection concept, advanced on the basis of the presumed validity of a proposed mechanism, can still be misleading because alternate mechanisms also may be interrupted by a given protective intervention.

In the face of such difficulties, proposed mechanisms are often deficient. In the extreme, an alleged mechanism may simply identify a hyperflexion or similar injury mode and indicate that it is caused by vehicle acceleration. The result of such deficiencies in our knowledge of mechanisms is that adequate protection concepts become more difficult to define. To illustrate the problem, three injury types will be briefly examined with emphasis on the difficulties in defining precise mechanisms.

Concussion Resulting From Impact

The difficulty in defining the injury mechanism of concussion resulting from impact has historically been associated not so much with describing applied forces or load transmission paths. Instead, the trouble is encountered in defining the injury itself and its proximate cause. Concussion has been variously defined as usually requiring the traumatic loss of consciousness and/or post-traumatic disturbance of thought process or memory, usually without demonstrable gross anatomic damage to the brain. The last criterion is difficult to assure without postmortem examination and is often ignored or separately described when data allow. The cause of concussion is even less clear. Various hypotheses have been advanced, generally concentrating on the brain stem and the reticular activating system. The necessary and sufficient localized stress has been considered to be direct translational acceleration, pitch axis rotational velocity and displacement producing a pinching of the brain stem, or a variety of generalized traumatic effects at the cellular level produced by brain oscillations, fluid waves in the cerebrospinal fluid or brain stem tissue, resonance cavitation, vascular hemodynamic wave propagation, or other effects. One or more injury mechanisms may be proposed to produce each of the localized stresses as a result of a given impact event. In all likelihood, alterations in thought process can be produced by several of these stresses individually and in various combinations. The relative importance of the various causes in typical situations of interest in aerospace medicine is not clear. Current mechanisms are, therefore, deficient. From what we know, however, it appears prudent to minimize both head motions relative to the body and peak head accelerations.

Vertebral Fracture Resulting from Ejection

The difficulty in defining the injury mechanism of vertebral fracture resulting from ejection has not so much been in describing the injury and the required localized stress or even in defining the applied forces. Instead, the trouble is encountered in sorting out the stresses in the load transmission path, particularly with superimposed motions. The force imposed on a given vertebral body during upward ejection ultimately depends on the acceleration experienced by the vertebral body immediately below it and the time-varying effective mass above it, which must be supported or accelerated. Of course, the dynamic behavior of this force is further modified by the characteristics of the intervertebral disk and other associated connective and soft tissue. The importance of the effective supported mass may be appreciated by imagining an ejection of the lower portion of a man, the most superior point of which is the isolated, exposed first lumbar vertebra. The force imposed on the inferior face of this vertebral body could then be well approximated by the acceleration of the second lumbar vertebra multiplied by the mass of the first, neglecting gravity and the intervertebral disk. If more mass were to be attached to this preparation by stacking it on top of the vertebral body, the force would be increased accordingly.

In reality, the effective mass above a given vertebral body varies with the availability of alternate load paths. The arms, for example, may be supported and thus accelerated partially by contact with the anterior thighs or the seat structure. The time-varying remainder of the upper extremity's mass is accelerated by forces transmitted through the lower spine. Even these forces have alternate paths around portions of the upper spine. This derives from the fact that the bony articulation of the arm with the spine is not a determinate structure. Try working your way from arm to spine by following the bones. The humerus articulates with the scapula through a ball-and-socket joint held together by muscular attachments and a fibrous capsule. The scapula connects to the clavicle through a laterally placed fibrous attachment. The medial clavicle connects to the upper portion of the sternum in a similar fashion. Finally, most of the ribs connect to the sternum through fibrocartilaginous attachments of varying rigidity, and these ribs can be followed around to the spine. This connection is tenuous. Soft tissue-mediated load paths can be more significant than the strictly bony ones. They usually are variable and hard to trace.

In addition, the stress imposed by a given force varies dramatically with spinal orientation. Flexion or extension during the event can convert compression stress to tension or produce compression and tension stress on different portions of the same vertebral body. Measurement difficulties are profound. Surfaces are sufficiently complex so that simplifications necessary for modeling may obscure significant effects. Tissue behavior under stress is also poorly understood at high strain rates. Current understanding of injury mechanisms is, therefore, imprecise. From a protection point of view, however, minimizing relative motions certainly would make things more predictable, and the provision of alternate load paths around the spine would be reasonable under almost any set of assumptions.

Upper Extremity Injury Resulting from Windblast

The initial difficulty in defining the injury mechanism of upper extremity injury resulting from windblast has not been in describing the required localized stress or the load transmission path but in sorting out initial applied forces. Once the extremity is flailing around the side of the ejection seat, the forces of contact with the seat structure or forced motion beyond joint limitations are primarily of academic interest. The mechanism of injury begins with dislodgement of the extremity from a normal position. Therefore, research efforts have focused on the measurement of the forces and torques that cause dislodgement. Wind tunnel tests have been performed to measure these parameters using volunteer subjects at low airspeeds and rigid models of the human body at higher speeds.

The forces and torques acting to dislodge each body segment are a function of the flow field surrounding the segment and the aerodynamic characteristics of the segment. Unfortunately, the flow field around a segment is significantly influenced by the presence of nearby objects, and the aerodynamic characteristics are significantly influenced by individual variations, personal equipment, and body position. The aerodynamic forces and torques acting on a body segment of the seat occupant are, therefore, complex time functions. They are modified by the flow field changes caused by the aircraft fuselage, the ejection seat, and even the proximity of other body segments.[1] They vary from subject to subject and with orientation or voluntary muscle action. The difficulty of determining the direction and magnitude of these aerodynamic forces is further compounded by the typical lack of angular stability of the ejecting seat with respect to the incident wind and the presence of other forces, such as those generated by the ejection catapult and deployment of a drogue parachute to decelerate the seat more rapidly.

When these complexities are considered, the definition of a specific injury mechanism is usually no more than hypothetic. What does appear clear is that protective interventions should be applied as early in the event as possible and that seat angular stabilization techniques should be used to limit the direction and improve predictability of the aerodynamic and inertial forces.

IMPACT PROTECTION SYSTEMS

Range of Challenge

Transient accelerations that present an injury hazard occur inadvertently, as in vehicular crash, and by design, as in the case of spacecraft landings or aircraft emergency escape system performance. Whether inadvertent or deliberate, the acceleration magnitude, direction, and pulse shape are commonly quite variable. In most instances, if protective provisions are present, they are spartan. The reasons for this condition are clear. First, it is the nature of humans to believe that accidents will only happen to others. For this reason, it seems foolish to endure the additional inconvenience and cost of protection. The rationalizations cited are often elaborate and presented with considerable zeal and include references to the abridgement of individual freedoms. Second, when transient accelerations are an inherent feature of a system design, the system is usually a spacecraft or aircraft system where the weight of the protection system involves costs in the size of the launch system or range and performance of the aircraft. The challenge to the designer of protection equipment is immense.

The development of vehicular crash protection equipment is perhaps the most well-known challenge. The crash environment experienced in aviation accidents is quite difficult to predict. In commercial, military, and general aviation, primary emphasis is given to protection against acceleration vectors acting in the −x-axis, although y-axis and z-axis accelerations may be very high. Commercial airline passenger seats and restraints are usually designed to withstand −x-axis crash accelerations up to 9 G. Crew seats and rear-facing passenger seats in military transport aircraft are usually designed to 16-G crash conditions. The stiffer structures of military fighter aircraft provide less attenuation of crash loads, and, therefore, the seats are usually designed to withstand up to 40 G in the −x-axis.

The most comprehensive description of crash environments has been assembled to provide design criteria to improve the crashworthiness of military helicopters.[2]

These data describe the crash conditions in probabilistic terms for impact velocity, acceleration vector direction, and pulse shape.

The acceleration environment encountered during emergency escape from spacecraft or military aircraft is the most diverse and complex challenge to the designer. The escaping crewmember is first exposed to a high acceleration directed parallel to the spinal column to catapult the seat and occupant from the cockpit. The acceleration magnitude may be 10 to more than 20 G, depending on the type of ejection seat design, the mass of the occupant, the preignition temperature of the catapult propellant, and the normal variance in propellant performance. The catapult may produce a velocity ranging from 13 to 18 m/sec. As the seat separates from the aircraft, a rocket is ignited to develop additional velocity to assure clearance of the aircraft vertical stabilizer at high speed and to provide adequate trajectory height for parachute opening at low altitude. The rocket is aligned to apply its force vector through the expected center of gravity of the seat and occupant. When the rocket is mounted on the back of the seat, the rocket nozzle is aligned to produce an $+x$-axis acceleration component as well as a $+z$-axis acceleration.

At higher airspeeds, the effect of the $+x$-axis acceleration component of the rocket thrust becomes relatively small, as the effect of the aerodynamic pressure of the windstream becomes higher. The aerodynamic force increases as the square of the wind velocity. Therefore, at high airspeeds, the primary acceleration component acting on the seat occupant is the aerodynamic deceleration acting, at least initially, in the $-x$-axis. When the ejection airspeed is in the range of 500 to 600 knots, sea level equivalent, the aerodynamic deceleration level may be as high as 30 to 40 G for typical body and seat drag coefficients.

Once the velocity of the crewmember has been reduced to a safe parachute deployment speed of approximately 250 knots for conventional systems, the crewmember is exposed to another acceleration pulse known as parachute opening shock. This acceleration is created by the large drag force developed as the parachute canopy fills with air. The pulse is of relatively long duration, on the order of 1 to 2 seconds at 305 m, and may range in peak value from 10 to 20 G under ideal conditions. The acceleration magnitude is a function of the deployment velocity, air density, deployment orientation of the parachute canopy and lines, mass of the parachutist, and several other variables.

After completion of the parachute opening sequence and descent to the earth's surface, the ejectee is greeted by a final acceleration when he hits the ground. A military parachute will lower the parachutist to the earth at a velocity of approximately 6.4m/sec. The landing impact is equivalent to that experienced after a jump from a height of 2.1 m. The resulting impact forces are a function of the effectiveness of the parachutist's fall technique, that is, his ability to use his legs as impact attenuators, and the direction and velocity of his horizontal drift.

Range of Human Impact Tolerance

The primary factors that determine human tolerance to transient acceleration exposures are the direction, magnitude, and time history of the acceleration, the distribution of force to the human body, and the physical state of the human body. The variance and complexity of the acceleration environments encountered in aerospace design problems are generally well understood qualitatively, although too frequently not adequately quantified. Understanding the sources of variances associated with the human factors is also important.

The distribution of force to the human body is a function of the method of body support and restraint. The method that is used may have a very powerful effect on the tolerability of a specific set of acceleration conditions. For example, an individual restrained by a lap belt during a high-speed automobile crash has a much greater chance of survival than an individual without any restraint. Furthermore, an individual restrained by a lap belt and two shoulder straps can survive greater impacts than would be survivable with a lap belt alone. This relationship is illustrated by data collected with these two restraints, as shown in Figure 8–4.[3,4] The data, which were obtained in tests with baboons, show the very large difference between the mean lethal acceleration levels and the differences in the statistical variance for each restraint system.

The population to be protected is a key factor in the variance of acceleration tolerance. It is reasonable to expect that the variance will be greater in the general population than in a subset composed of military aviators. The factors that contribute to the variance in the tolerance of a given individual to a specific transient acceleration are primarily those that influence the physical state of the individual. These include age, size, body habitus or proportion, level of physical conditioning, and freedom from anatomic variations predisposing to injury. The extent to which each of the sources of variance contributes to the overall variation in an individual's capacity to withstand acceleration is currently not well defined. The general effects of factors such as age, however, are seen in laboratory tests of cadaver tissues, as well as experience with military aircraft escape systems.

Variation of the strength of materials under mechanical loading is not a problem that is unique to biologic materials. Large variability in the breaking strength of materials, components, and entire systems is recognized in most engineering design applications. For example, the mechanical properties of metal structural elements specified in engineering handbooks are usually based on minimum typical properties. In at least 99% of the samples of the element, the properties, such as tensile strength, are expected to exceed the minimum values. Other factors, such as material temperature, sensitivity to repeated loading, and service life, must be taken into consideration when these factors exceed the bounds of the original test conditions. In some cases, as in the case of human acceleration tolerance, it is not practical to quantify the effects of each of these factors in any detail. Therefore, a factor of safety is selected and added to the mechanical properties to assure a safe design. This same technical approach is appropriate for the specification of biologic material properties and the design of protection equipment.

Design Strategy

The design of protective equipment for aerospace applications must adhere to the same engineering principles that are applied to other components of vehicle design. The weight of the equipment must be minimized and, therefore, overdesign cannot be tolerated. On the other hand, underdesign could result in serious injuries that have major operational, humanitarian, and product liability implications.

The design process used to develop and evaluate protective equipment must include a comprehensive assessment of the severity of the acceleration environment,

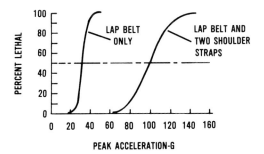

Fig. 8–4. Probability of lethal injury estimated from impact tests of baboons restrained by lap belt or lap belt and two shoulder straps.[3,4]

the characteristics of the personnel who are to be protected, and the normal mobility, performance, and comfort requirements for these personnel. This assessment is necessary to provide an objective basis for the selection of protection approaches and evaluation of the risks and benefits associated with these approaches.

Restraint Systems

The effectiveness of a restraint system depends on (1) how well the restraint configuration can transmit loads between the seat or vehicle structure and the occupant; (2) the ability of the restraint to control the motion of the restrained anatomic segments; (3) the restraint contact pressure; and (4) the load-carrying capability of the restrained anatomic segments. These factors are controlled by the choice of restraint material properties, restraint tie-down locations, belt area and flexibility, and anatomic-bearing areas. These choices are governed by the anticipated acceleration conditions, surrounding vehicle structure, space for body movement, encumbrance of occupant, and acceptance of risk, weight, and cost.

The first and most common restraint used in aerospace applications, the lap belt, provides a relatively low level of impact protection. The restraint loads are intended to be carried through the pelvis, and existing tolerance data are based on that presumption. Unfortunately, if the belt is improperly tightened or positioned or the acceleration vector is oriented to cause rotation of the pelvis, the belt will slip over the iliac crests and against the abdomen, causing the belt loads to be carried by the lumbar spine.

When the lap belt is the only restraint, the most common injuries are caused by the impact of body extremities with the vehicle. Figure 8–5 shows the strike envelopes of body extremities during forward-facing impact with lap belt and lap belt-double shoulder strap restraint configurations.[2] The reduction of the strike

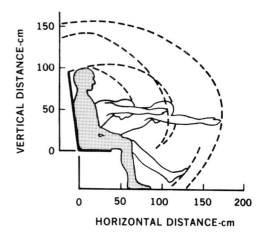

Fig. 8–5. Extremity strike envelopes with lap belt and lap belt-shoulder straps restraint configurations.[2]

envelope obtained through the use of two shoulder straps is demonstrated in this illustration. The use of shoulder straps also reduces the strike envelope for sideward and vertical impacts.[2] The use of shoulder straps also improves human tolerance to acceleration in any direction by increasing the restraint-bearing area, increasing the load paths into the torso mass, and reducing the relative motion between body parts. Where high upward acceleration components are anticipated, shoulder straps are mandatory to help maintain the alignment of the load-carrying spinal vertebrae.

Despite the aforementioned advantages of shoulder straps, the tension loads in these straps create a potentially serious problem if the straps are attached to the center of the lap belt, as they are in most military harness configurations. These strap loads, developed under forward-facing impact conditions, lift the lap belt over the iliac crests of the pelvis, allowing the belt to bear on the abdomen and the inferior costal margin. This problem has been observed in human tests at acceleration levels as low as 10 G with a velocity change of 5.5 m/sec. Stapp[5] reported that test subjects reached the threshold of voluntary tolerance with this restraint configuration at 17 G for impact velocities greater than 30 m/sec. All of the tests conducted by Stapp at higher acceleration were accomplished using a pair of crotch straps devised to carry the tension loads of the shoulder straps into the pelvis and seat structure. Each strap was attached to an adjacent rear corner of the seat and to the lap belt buckle, forming an inverted V. More contemporary restraint harnesses use a single strap that connects the lap belt buckle and the front central portion of the seat. The single crotch-strap installation is simpler and provides better restraint during vertical vibration, but its effectiveness has not been demonstrated at the high acceleration levels explored by Stapp.

In view of the large influence the restraint system has on the tolerability of impact, the restraint configuration must be considered when interpreting human test results and their operational implications. For example, Stapp successfully demonstrated that humans are capable of tolerating very severe transient acceleration exposures. Acceleration levels up to 45.4 G, with a rise time of 0.11 seconds and a velocity change of approximately 56 m/sec, were endured in a forward-facing body position.[5] The restraint system, however, was not a conventional military harness. The configuration was composed of 7.6-cm wide webbing and included a lap belt, two shoulder straps, inverted V crotch straps, and a strap that encircled the subject's chest at axillary height. The bearing area of the restraint was reported to be 553 cm². A conventional military harness, composed of two 4.5-cm wide shoulder straps and a 7.6-cm wide lap belt, has a bearing area of approximately 330 cm² and does not provide the effective coupling of the various parts of the torso that the Stapp configuration provided. Unfortunately, a harness configuration of the type Stapp used has not been practical in aerospace applications because of its multiple release points and the restriction of the occupant's mobility.

Efforts to develop a restraint system that will provide a high bearing area and better control of body segment motion during impact have been numerous, but the most innovative efforts have focused on the use of inflatable bags. This approach provides a restraint that does not encumber the vehicle occupant until the impact occurs. When predetermined acceleration levels are sensed on the vehicle structure, the bag restraint is inflated by compressed gas, pyrotechnic gas generators, or a combination of the two systems. In automotive applications, the inflatable bags are constructed of a porous material to control the forces transmitted to the occupant by allowing the gas to vent through the cloth during impact loading. Inflatable restraints considered for aircraft escape system applications have so far been designed only to provide additional body restraint and support to supplement existing harness configurations. Furthermore, because of the time available early in the escape sequences, they do not require the fast inflation capability of the automotive restraint.

Body Support Systems

Many aerospace designers have proposed that the ideal body support system is a rigid, individually contoured couch. This approach ensures that each external body segment will be simultaneously accelerated and that the support pressure exerted on the body surfaces will be minimized. Designs of this type have been found to be very effective in laboratory impact, vibration, and centrifuge tests. The rigid contour approach was used in the Project Mercury astronaut couch design and in the design of the seat and seatback used in Project Gemini. The disadvantages of the approach are the high cost of individual fitting and the discomfort of the rigid contour after a relatively short occupancy because only one body position matches the contour.

Attempts to circumvent the disadvantages of the rigid couch design have included the design of net couches. These designs provide relief from the comfort problems and high manufacturing costs of the rigid contour couches. Thus far, net body support systems have been found to be very effective in sustained acceleration but have not provided good protection in either vibration or impact. The problem has been related to the elasticity of the net material. In both vibration and impact tests, the net body suspension system tended to resonate at or near the major resonances of the body segments, and the motion of the body segments was not harmonious. The motion of each body segment was not in time phase with the motion of the other body segments.

The most successful body support systems that have aerospace vehicle applications have (1) slight contouring to control body position; (2) dimensions that accommodate large variations in body size; (3) relatively rigid, lightweight sheet metal structures; (4) padding to provide isolation from small-amplitude, high-frequency impacts and vibration; and (5) minimal cushioning of the seat to reduce flight fatigue without major degradation in impact protection. Armrests are often provided to increase comfort. If the armrests are properly positioned, they permit the mass of the arms to act through the armrest structure rather than through the spine during +z acceleration.

Impact Attenuation

The forces imposed on a vehicle occupant during a crash or other transient acceleration of the vehicle are influenced to a significant degree by the mechanical properties of the materials between the occupant and the source of the accelerating force. Unless these interposed materials in the vehicle structure or the body support and restraint system are nondeformable, they will alter the magnitude and time phase of the forces that the occupant will experience. At first glance, this character-istic appears to be intuitively desirable. One might expect that deformable materials and structures, like soft cushions, should always protect an individual during an impact. Unfortunately, this intuition may lead to a faulty if not injurious conclusion.

Materials positioned between the occupant and the acceleration source can amplify the acceleration to which the occupant will eventually be exposed in a number of ways. First, the materials may store energy during the impact and then release it in rebound. Thus, the occupant is exposed to a larger velocity change than the vehicle. This condition occurs when vehicle structure or body support and restraint system deformations are elastic. Second, these deformations may delay the acceleration of the occupant and create a large velocity difference between the occupant and the vehicle. Of course, the occupant acceleration must eventually exceed the vehicle acceleration to eliminate the velocity difference. An ejection seat cushion is a common component that can cause this second problem by virtue of the cushion material stiffness and the distance it creates between the seat structure and the seat occupant. During ejection, the seat will develop a higher velocity as it compresses the seat cushion, as shown in Figure 8–6. Once the seat cushion has been fully compressed, the occupant is then accelerated to the higher velocity of the seat and often beyond.

Impact attenuation is accomplished when the forces transmitted between the acceleration source and the occupant can be limited to less than the levels that would be experienced if the occupant were rigidly coupled to the source. The acceleration being transmitted to a vehicle occupant may be attenuated by vehicle structural deformation, impact attenuation devices mounted between the seat and the vehicle, body support and restraint materials, and impact-attenuating

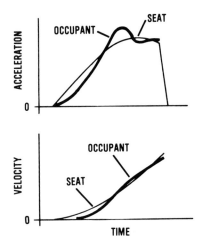

Fig. 8–6. Acceleration and velocity of ejection seat and occupant; the acceleration of the occupant is delayed by the soft-seat cushion.

materials mounted on the body such as in a flight helmet.

Attenuation of acceleration as it is transmitted through a vehicle structure, without failure of the structure, may occur because of the relatively low stiffness of the structure and its friction damping. Therefore, the high-frequency components of the acceleration cannot be transmitted through the low-frequency structure without being attenuated. This method is used in the design of automotive suspension systems. Automobile springs are selected so that the stiffness of the springs and the mass of the automobile body and occupants create a low-frequency mechanical system. Sharp impacts that occur along the roadway are attenuated into low-frequency, low-amplitude motion of the automobile body by the suspension system. Shock absorbers, which are viscous dampers, prevent the body from continued oscillation after the initial response.

In a vehicular crash, acceleration is attenuated by the collapse of structural members, but the occupied area of the vehicle must remain intact. The attenuation that is provided by structural collapse is a major factor in both aircraft and automotive crash protection because relatively

large attenuation distances are available. Unfortunately, the acceleration-limiting capability of an aircraft structure is not well controlled by design or adequately predictable by experimental results or numeric methods. For this reason, vehicles at high risk of crashing, such as some military helicopters, use seat-mounted impact attenuation devices to provide the final stage of acceleration limiting. These devices are intended to attenuate the imposed acceleration of the vehicle, as shown in Figure 8–7. This illustration shows how the attenuation device acts to limit the acceleration of the seat and occupant by providing additional stopping distance. Energy storage and rebound is usually avoided by using viscous or friction damping or permanently deforming materials such as metal tubes or bands. The performance of impact-attenuation devices, however, is limited by the

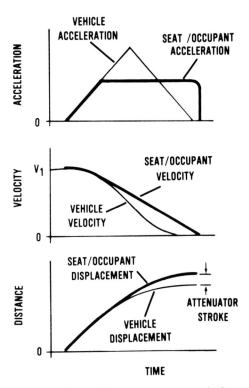

Fig. 8–7. Influence of impact attenuator on vehicle seat occupant acceleration, velocity, and displacement.

amount of stroke distance that is available. If the impact velocity exceeds the capability of the attenuation device, the stroke limit will be reached before the seat and occupant velocity are equal to the vehicle velocity. When this point is reached, the phenomenon referred to as bottoming occurs, and the acceleration of the seat and occupant will increase until the velocity of the vehicle is reached, as shown in Figure 8–8.

Commonly used impact-attenuation devices also may have other properties that limit their usefulness. These devices are

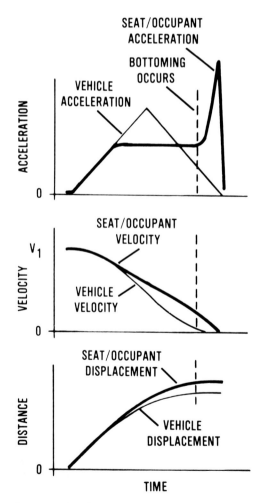

Fig. 8–8. The effects of bottoming of an impact attenuator on seat and occupant acceleration, velocity, and displacement.

often force-limiting mechanisms, and, therefore, their performance is predictable on the basis of occupant mass only if the seat and its occupant are rigid masses or if the vehicle acceleration rise time, t_r, is long enough to avoid causing significant transients in the occupant's acceleration response. If the rise time is too short and the mass of the seat is relatively low, the acceleration of the occupant may influence attenuator performance. Even if this condition is avoided, force-limiting attenuator performance will still vary as a function of variations in subject weight.

The degree of impact attenuation that can be provided by the body support and restraint system or padding that might be worn by an individual is limited by the small displacements that are available. The padding of body support structures is usually selected to provide some comfort and to attenuate structural vibrations and low-energy, high-frequency impacts. Restraint systems usually restrict the movement of the occupant to prevent the occupant's impact with surrounding structures. Attempts to provide impact-attenuating harnesses have so far been unsuccessful because designers have found it impractical to match the mechanical performance of the harness components' dynamic response characteristics to body segments for a large population. Therefore, the severity of impact injuries may be reduced in one anatomic area but increased in another.

MODELING IMPACT RESPONSE

Protection System Dynamics

A fundamental understanding of the impact-response characteristics of mechanical systems is a prerequisite for the meaningful analysis and interpretation of the impact responses of the human body and the influence of protection system designs. The dynamic responses of mechanical systems, whether these systems are steel beams, rubber tires, bones, or muscle, are governed by Newtonian mechanics and can be described in terms of mechanical analogies. These analogies are usually expressed in terms of abstract mathematical equations, but for most researchers, the use of more familiar physical models is necessary for the visualization of the analogy and understanding of its implications.

The physical models used to gain understanding of the principles of dynamic mechanical systems in this chapter are lumped parameter models. They are composed of elements such as springs, masses, and dampers, where each element represents only one mechanical property. In other words, the mass is a pure mass without elasticity or damping, whereas the spring and damper are massless. All of the elasticity of the modeled system is represented by the spring, and all the damping is represented by the damper. The lumped parameter model may be a single-degree-of-freedom system with one mass and one spring, where the position of the mass can be defined by a single coordinate, or a multidegree-of-freedom system composed of many masses, springs, and dampers.

The stiffness of the spring, k, is defined by the following equation:

$$k = \frac{F}{x} \qquad (8)$$

where F is the force required to deflect the spring a distance of x. The units of k are newtons per meter. The damper may represent several sources of friction in the mechanical system, but the damping that is most common to biologic systems is viscous damping, which is defined by the following equation:

$$c = \frac{F}{\dot{x}} \qquad (9)$$

where F is the force required to move the mass at a velocity of $\dot{x}$. The units of the

damping coefficient, c, are newton-seconds per meter. The velocity is designated in Newton's notation for a time derivative, as follows:

$$\text{velocity} = \dot{x} = \frac{dx}{dt} \text{ and}$$
$$\text{acceleration} = \ddot{x} = \frac{d^2x}{dt^2} \qquad (10)$$

The equation of motion for a simple system composed of a single mass and spring describes the forces that act on the system. These include a spring force, kx, an external force-time function, f(t), and the inertial reaction force m$\ddot{x}$, as follows:

$$F = -kx + f(t) + (-m\ddot{x}) = 0 \quad (11)$$

where the internal forces act in opposition to the external force and are, therefore, also functions of time.

The dynamic response characteristics of this physical model can be studied mathematically or empirically by observing the response of the model to various excitations. For the sake of simplicity, the mathematics have been minimized, and the response characteristics of the model will be demonstrated graphically. A more thorough treatment of this subject is available elsewhere.[6,7]

Because it is usual to specify human tolerance to transient acceleration in terms of acceleration measured at the input point to the human body, the response of the system to excitations at the base will be illustrated. The equation of motion in this case is as follows:

$$\ddot{y} = \ddot{x} + \frac{kx}{m} \qquad (12)$$

If an acceleration $\ddot{y}$ is instantaneously applied to the base of the spring-mass system to produce a constant continuing acceleration of the base, referred to as a step function, the system will respond as

shown in Figure 8–9. The peak acceleration of the mass, m, will be twice the acceleration of the base, and the spring force
(kx) will be twice as great as would be
experienced if the spring were a rigid
member.

By measuring the force in the spring of
the system as it is exposed to a series of
rectangular waveform accelerations applied at the base, the relationship between
the acceleration duration and the dynamic
response of the system can be seen, as
shown in Figure 8–10. The peak spring
force increases as the base acceleration
pulse duration increases, up to a peak
force. It then continues at that level for
longer pulse durations. This same experiment can be performed for other wave-

forms and similar results obtained. The
peak force is reached at a critical acceleration pulse duration, Δt_c. The value of
Δt_c depends on the natural frequency of
the system ω, as follows:

$$\Delta t_c = \frac{2}{\omega} \qquad (13)$$

where $\omega = \sqrt{\dfrac{k}{m}}$. If the acceleration pulse
duration is less the Δt_c, neither the duration nor the magnitude of the acceleration
are individually sufficient to determine
the response of the system. The critical
factor is their product, which is simply the
velocity change in a constant acceleration
pulse. If the acceleration pulse is longer
than Δt_c, the peak force in the system is
related to the peak input acceleration.
When the duration of the input pulse is
near Δt_c, the peak force is actually a complex function of the velocity change and
the acceleration magnitude.

At some force level, the spring of the
system that is represented by the mechanical model will reach a point of deflection
where it will fail. By knowing the relationship between the acceleration input
and the failure force level, the acceleration
tolerance of the system can be specified,
as shown in Figure 8–11. This graph
shows that for Δt less than Δt_c, the system
can be exposed to increasing acceleration
magnitudes as the duration of the acceleration pulse decreases.

When the acceleration pulse is longer
than Δt_c, the response of the dynamic system is also a function of the rise time, t_r,
of the acceleration. The acceleration waveform we have studied thus far has had a
rise time of zero. If the rise time of the
acceleration transmitted to the base of the
spring-mass system increases, the deflection of the spring will decrease and the
acceleration of the mass will decrease. The
theoretical relationship between the ac-

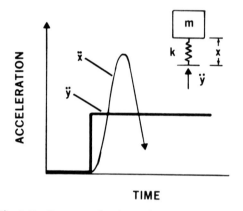

Fig. 8–9. Response of spring and mass system to step
function acceleration.

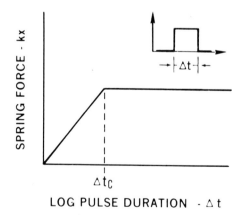

Fig. 8–10. Force response of a dynamic system to rectangular base accelerations of varying duration.

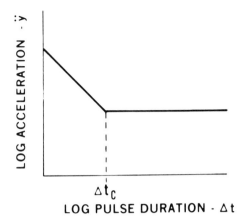

Fig. 8–11. Acceleration tolerance of a system with a known spring deflection tolerance.

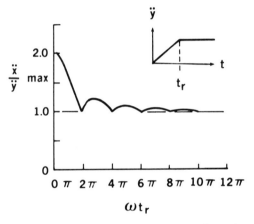

Fig. 8–12. Effect of rise time (t_r) on the peak acceleration of a mass ($\ddot{x}$).

celeration input rise time and the ratio of the acceleration of the mass to the acceleration input to the base of the system is shown in Figure 8–12.[7] For practical purposes, it may be assumed that the acceleration pulse has zero rise time if $t_r < 1/\omega$. The difference between the acceleration input magnitude and the resulting acceleration of the dynamic system can be ignored if $t_r > 10/\omega$.

Because damping exists to some degree in all real physical systems, its influence must be considered in the mechanical model. The equation of motion of the sin-

gle-degree-of-freedom model with damping is as follows:

$$F = -kx - c\dot{x} + f(t)$$
$$+ (-m\ddot{x}) = 0 \quad (14)$$

or

$$m\ddot{x} + c\dot{x} + kx = f(t)$$

The influence of viscous damping on a spring-mass-damper system subjected to a rectangular-shaped acceleration pulse applied at the base is illustrated in Figure 8–13. The degree of damping is expressed in terms of the damping coefficient ratio, ζ, expressed in terms of the actual damping coefficient, c, and the critical damping coefficient, c_c, as follows:

$$\zeta = \frac{c}{c_c} = \frac{c}{2m\omega} \quad (15)$$

The critical damping coefficient is the value of damping that is just adequate to allow the mass of the system to return from a displaced position to its initial position without oscillation. Figure 8–13 shows that as the damping coefficient ratio increases, the amplitude of the damped system's response decreases with each oscil-

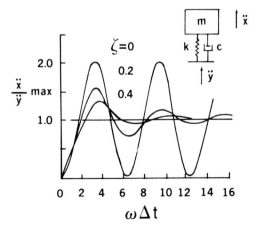

Fig. 8–13. Responses of a mechanical system with varying levels of viscous damping to step function base acceleration.

lation and the amplitude of the response also decreases. The deflection of the system or strain in the spring is no longer proportional to the total force as in the case of the undamped system because the damping force now contributes to the total force. A mechanical system with damping can tolerate higher impact acceleration levels before the deflection of the spring reaches the failure level. The relationship between the damping coefficient ratio and the amplification of an input acceleration pulse with rectangular waveform is shown in Figure 8–14.

Human Mechanical Response

Early investigators of human tolerance to transient acceleration recognized the importance of theoretical models in the analysis of experimental findings and in the guidance of further investigations. Kornhauser and Gold[8] proposed and then demonstrated by impact tests with mice that animals exhibit the same impact response characteristics as mechanical systems in terms of their sensitivity to injury. The data from impact tests of 329 mice conducted to determine lethal dose levels could be described in terms of critical velocity change or acceleration level. The relationship that was demonstrated between

the acceleration-time function and its lethality implied that the lethality rate corresponded to a critical maximum deflection or strain in a single-degree-of-freedom model. This important finding has been substantiated by other investigators for other animal species. It is important to recognize, however, that the implied model predicts a first-order effect only, that is, lethal dose. It does not predict the exact mode of lethal injury.

Lethal dose sensitivity curves may become more complex if the mode of injury is considered. The complexity occurs when more than one mode of injury exists, as shown in Figure 8–15.[9] This situation is likely because any complex biologic system will have a large number of potential injury modes. Most of the injury modes, however, will have no practical significance because the lethal dose will be determined by one or several that occur at lower stress levels due to their lower critical strain limits or their closer relationship to the stress input.

The potential for a complex, multimode injury curve can be conceptualized by considering a case in which a human would be accelerated by a force acting from back to chest. In this case, laboratory experience and observations of accident trauma suggest that the injury limit in the

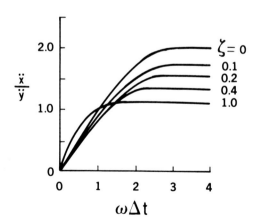

Fig. 8–14. Acceleration amplitude ratio as a function of base acceleration pulse duration for selected damping coefficient ratios.

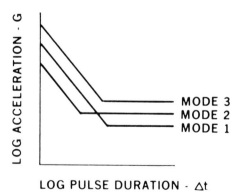

Fig. 8–15. Impact injury limit curves for three modes of injury. (Adapted from Stech, E.L., and Payne, P.R.: Dynamic Models of the Human Body. AMRL–TR–66–157, Aerospace Medical Research Laboratory, Wright-Patterson Air Force Base, Ohio, 1965.)

short-duration impulse region of the tolerance curve, where velocity change is the limiting factor, would be head injury. In the longer-duration impact region of the tolerance curve, injuries to the internal organs, such as the heart, liver, or spleen, would be more probable. In this case, it would be reasonable to describe the injury tolerance curve by two or more dynamic models in a parallel arrangement, that is, where there is no interaction between the motion of the models.

In many cases, however, a simple, single-degree-of freedom model may be adequate. This model is generally feasible if there is one injury mode, the direction of impact is controlled, and the exact location and severity of the injury are not important. In ejection seat design, such a model has been used to predict the probability of vertebral fractures in the lower spine.[10] This model is commonly used to evaluate the acceptability of ejection catapult designs and to analyze acceleration data collected during tests of escape systems. In these applications, the mathematical analog of this model is used to calculate the maximum deflection of the model in response to the total acceleration-time history. The maximum deflection value is then related to the probability of injury. The relationship that has been used is shown in Figure 8–16.[11] The out-

put of the model is expressed in terms of the Dynamic Response Index values, which have correlated well with United States Air Force operational ejection spinal injuries.[11]

The use of a dynamic model to evaluate the probability of spinal injury provides advantages over the method described earlier in the chapter. This method consists of a description of the acceleration-time history in terms of two or three limiting parameters. The usual limiting parameters were the rate of onset, that is, the slope of the rising portion of the acceleration-time history, and peak acceleration. In some applications, the duration of the acceleration pulse also was considered. This method was based on empiric evidence collected during the development and use of ejection catapults. The method was flawed in many respects. First, it was based on the false premise that there is an absolute limit beyond which injury will occur. Second, it assumed that there is a critical rate of onset that would cause injury. It did not recognize that there is a trade-off between the rate of onset and peak acceleration. Third, the method could not be used to evaluate complex acceleration waveforms. Therefore, it became obsolete when attempts were made to apply the method to problems such as space vehicle landing impact and more advanced aircraft escape system accelerations where complex waveforms are common. Fourth, the method did not provide a means of evaluating the influence of other factors such as the viscoelastic properties of ejection seat cushions.

A major advantage of dynamic models is that they are helpful in understanding the influences of the seat structure, cushion materials, restraint, or impact attenuation devices in modifying the acceleration transmitted to the human body.[7] Although the models of the protection system and the human body may be relatively complex, the fundamental principles of protection system dynamics can be illus-

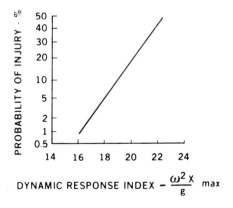

Fig. 8–16. Probability of spinal compression fracture as a function of the dynamic response index.

trated by the use of simple mechanical elements, as shown in Figure 8–17. The input to this model is the acceleration of the vehicle structure, which in most cases is the acceleration of the seat structure. The mass of the protection system or body support cushioning material is normally quite small in relation to the human occupant. For this analysis, it can be assumed that the body support and restraint material is sufficient to prevent injury due to non-uniform motion of the body segments and that the contact pressures will not cause injury.

If the restraint or body support material is very soft in contrast to the effective lumped stiffness of the human body model, the protection system will attenuate impulsive accelerations within the limits of its deflection capability, x_{max}. If the acceleration pulse duration is long enough to exceed x_{max}, however, the occupant will bottom out and will experience much higher acceleration than he would without the protection system. This general relationship is shown in Figure 8–17 for the human body model supported by a soft cushion and exposed to rectangular waveform acceleration inputs.

This simple analysis illustrates the importance of understanding the relationships among the spectrum of the acceleration pulses that might be encountered, the mechanics of the protection system, and the dynamic response properties of the human. It also serves as a warning that a protection system might appear acceptable under laboratory test conditions but prove unacceptable under more severe operational conditions. Restraint materials are commonly tested under static loads, where the influence of system dynamic response is ignored. They also are evaluated under very short-duration impulse loading, where the acceleration level may be the same as the operational condition but where the energy level is too low to produce the operational dynamic response (i.e., restraint strap tension). Tests using static or impulsive loads are acceptable only when these tests can be related to the operational loading conditions. If extrapolation is required, the dynamic response properties of the restraint occupant and the restraint system must be known. Therefore, test conditions should simulate the anticipated operational environment as closely as possible. Where feasible, the restraint system should be tested with volunteer subjects at subinjury levels and then evaluated with anthropomorphic dummies at the design limits.

EXPERIMENTAL IMPACT

Facilities

Impact tests to measure human responses and to evaluate protection equipment have been accomplished using a wide variety of methods. Pioneering work to establish performance limits for ejection seat catapults was conducted by ejecting prototype seats up extended ejection rails. The test subjects were often the engineers and scientists associated with the escape system development. Catapult acceleration limits were established when the subjects reached their voluntary tolerance levels or were injured. The escape

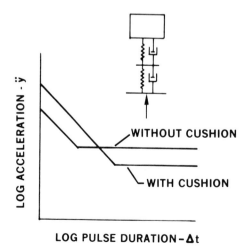

Fig. 8–17. Influence of cushion material dynamic response properties on acceleration tolerance of a system with a known spring deflection tolerance.

system was ultimately demonstrated by an in-flight ejection, first with anthropomorphic dummies as occupants and then with experimental test parachutists. This approach was used by the United States Air Force for nearly two decades.

The need to establish aeromedical design criteria for aircrew restraint systems for crash protection motivated a fundamental change in method. Experiments were begun at Muroc, California, using a sled propelled along a rail track by rockets. The seat and restraint system designs were evaluated, and the limits of human impact tolerance were explored by rapidly decelerating the sled with friction brakes.[5] These experiments were eventually extended to study the effects of transient deceleration and windblast associated with ejection from high-speed aircraft. These later tests were performed on rocket sled facilities at China Lake, California, and Holloman Air Force Base in New Mexico.[12] Deceleration was achieved by water brake scoops.

Facilities that can provide more precise control of the impact test conditions have been developed as the experimental efforts in this area matured beyond the initial field test approach. The facilities now used for impact experiments include (1) relatively simple towers that are used to drop test carriages onto decelerators such as metal-deforming devices or hydraulic cylinders; (2) horizontal tracks with various propulsion systems that are used to propel test carriages into decelerators; and (3) high-pressure gas actuators that are used to accelerate a test carriage along either vertical or horizontal rails. The gas-operated actuator facilities offer the greatest degree of impact control and reproducibility because initial conditions prior to the impact can be easily controlled.

Comparison of test data collected from different impact facilities is difficult and must be done cautiously. Factors such as body support and restraint system configuration, restraint pretension, subject brac-

ing, and similarity of the entire acceleration waveform must be considered. The conditions that exist prior to the impact are also critical. For example, the majority of the data gathered to explore human tolerance to $-x$-axis impact has been obtained using decelerator facilities. After accelerating the test sled to a desired velocity by use of a rocket or pyrotechnic catapult, the sled would then coast along the facility track until the deceleration mechanism was contacted. During the coasting phase, however, the test subject would be exposed to a deceleration due to sliding friction and aerodynamic drag. The level of deceleration generally exceeded 1.5 G, and the planned impact pulse sometimes was preceded by coasting deceleration as high as 15 G.

The deceleration level experienced during the sled-coast phase of contemporary horizontal deceleration facilities is about 0.3 G. Impact facilities that are designed to accelerate the sled and subject from a standing start impose no acceleration or velocity prior to the impact event. Recent experimental investigations with animal and human subjects have demonstrated that these preimpact conditions have significant measurable influence on the subject's responses and tolerance to the subsequent impact.[13]

These investigations have led to the concept of dynamic preload. Dynamic preload is defined as an imposed acceleration preceding, continuous with, and in the same direction as a subsequent impact. It should not be confused with static load conditions, such as pretension of the restraint, or subject bracing. The experimental investigations of dynamic preload have shown that volunteer subjects perceive their response to impact imposed by an accelerator to be more severe than their response to a comparable decelerator impact preceded by 0.25 G deceleration. Objective measures of the impact response, such as body segment accelerations and restraint loads, provided evidence that confirmed the subjective findings. Furthermore, tests conducted on a decelerator to compare measured forces and body segment accelerations in matched impacts preceded by 0.25 or 0.62 G preload showed that this increase in the dynamic preload will further decrease the measured subject responses.

The explanation for the response differences observed when the dynamic conditions preceding an impact are varied can be understood in part by recalling the properties of accelerated viscoelastic systems. In the case of the accelerated human body, in spite of restraint pretensioning and muscular bracing, many anatomic structures are poorly supported. The head, arms, legs, and various soft tissue masses and internal organs often must undergo some relative displacement before effective accelerating forces can be applied through joints, attachments, or direct contact with other supporting structures. The relative displacement of the lagging segment is a functional dead space. This phenomenon delays the acceleration of the lagging segments. Because of the developing velocity difference, however, the lagging segments will eventually experience a higher acceleration to catch up with the more efficiently accelerated portions of the body. The introduction of dynamic preload presumably acts to decrease the effective dead space and, therefore, the severity of the overall acceleration response.

Instrumentation

The results of the earliest impact tests with human subjects were assessed by simply asking, "How did that feel?" Subjective responses are still an important aspect of experimental findings. Objective measurements of mechanical responses and physiologic changes, however, are potentially more reliable experimental indicators of the stressfulness of an impact or the effectiveness of a protective technique. The basic problem is to determine what to measure, how to make the measurement, and how accurately the measurement must be made.

From the point of view of experimental impact mechanics, it would be desirable to measure the acceleration, velocity, and displacement of all the human body segments and internal organs as well as the test vehicle during each test. Furthermore, if possible, it would be useful to know what forces produced the observed body segment and organ motions and to determine how these forces may be controlled by various body support and restraint structures. From the point of view of the physician concerned about the injury potential, it also would be desirable to relate these motions and forces to tissue deformation or damage and to any changes that may occur in physiologic processes such as cardiac electrical activity. From a practical point of view, however, it is not feasible to measure all of these quantities during an impact test. Certainly, in tests with volunteer subjects, the measurement of internal organ movement is fraught with difficulties and hazards that make it impossible with current techniques.

The researcher must choose those measurements that are necessary and feasible and that will not cause untoward effects on the impact response or protective technique being studied. The physical measurements are usually made using electronic devices such as linear accelerometers, angular rate gyros, or force transducers. High-speed motion picture cameras also are used in conjunction with reference targets mounted on observable body segments.

The assessment of measurement accuracy involves more than a determination of the error from a true value. The investigator and those reviewing impact test results within the literature must understand the limitations of the measurements in terms such as resolution, linearity, dynamic range, repeatability, and frequency response. A systematic approach to the choice of accuracy is also vital. An inconsistent set of measurements, in which high accuracy in one measurement is wasted because of its use in a calculation with a low accuracy measurement, may result from the lack of error analysis during the experimental design. Because this factor may be neglected by some researchers, caution is advised in interpreting the results of tests in which the instrumentation and its accuracy are not adequately described.

The electronic devices used to measure impact responses are electromechanical transducers that convert a mechanical response within the instrument into an electric signal proportional to that response. Generally, the devices may be analyzed mathematically using spring-mass-damper models. Load cells are examples. They are basically rather stiff springs that deflect in proportion to the applied load. The small deflections are converted to an electrical potential by an element called a strain gauge that is attached to the spring. Although such a device may be quite accurate under single-axis loads, it may produce erroneous results if bending or off-axis loads are present. Therefore, it must be calibrated in a configuration representative of the experimental application.

The equipment used to process the outputs of the transducers also may be described in terms of a mathematical model of its response. It is critical to assess frequency response characteristics of these devices, particularly when the measurements are recorded as discrete samples over time. Frequencies of interest in measuring human impact responses range up to 20 to 30 Hz. A higher frequency response limit, however, allows measurement of the motion of the test fixture to include the highest frequencies that influence the lower frequency dynamic response of the human body. The limit commonly selected is 100 Hz.

Acceleration measurement is generally made with small, light, linear accelerometers. The simplest model of such a device is a mass, constrained to move in one direction, that is attached to its case by a spring. The electrical output of the accelerometer is proportional to the deflection of the spring and thus is actually a measure of force. For example, the accelerometer cannot distinguish between gravitational force at rest and the internal force produced during a 1-G acceleration. Furthermore, an accelerometer cannot distinguish between internal force produced by simple translational acceleration of the case and that produced by the rotational motion of the case. As a result, the output of the accelerometer cannot simply be integrated once to produce a measure of velocity and again to yield displacement, unless the acceleration is purely translational and the orientation with respect to the earth is known. Gyroscopic sensors provide more direct measurement of rotational accelerations than can be achieved even with arrays of linear accelerometers. Finally, acceleration data of any kind, when integrated, will produce velocity or position information with errors that increase with time.

To solve the problem of measuring displacement, most researchers have turned to photographic instrumentation. Displacement may be estimated from a series of photographs obtained from high-speed motion picture cameras. Here again, however, the same principles that apply to other forms of data collection and processing must be understood. Resolution and dynamic range are usually limited by the film grain size, frame coverage, and the relative size of the target. The frequency response is limited by the film frame rate and resolution.

Future applications should allow the use of optimal estimation theory to obtain the best estimates for the parameters of interest using the available data sources. Such techniques, exemplified by Kalman filtering, are extensively used in similar applications in inertial guidance. New transducers also may provide improved data for analysis.

Human Impact Test Results

Thousands of impact tests with human subjects are documented in the research literature. Direct comparisons among the results of these tests are usually difficult because of differences in acceleration conditions, restraints, instrumentation, subjects, and experimental procedures. An approximate understanding of tolerable conditions in a specific application, however, often can be gained by carefully choosing from among the previous test results. Summaries of substantial portions of the historical data base are available and can serve as useful guides to the literature.[14,15] Whenever possible, the original test documentation for the chosen cases should be reviewed to verify that the test conditions assure relevance of the data to the intended application.

Perhaps the most dramatic human impact test experience was gained by Stapp,[5] who conducted and often participated in rocket sled experiments. The highest acceleration exposure in this series, a 45.4-G deceleration with a velocity change of 56m/sec, was experienced by Stapp in a forward-facing seat (− x-axis). This test involved significant dynamic preload, specially designed restraints, and preimpact flexion of the neck. It resulted in retinal hemorrhage, but the post-test symptoms were less severe than in earlier tests in this series, in which the peak acceleration was above 38 G. The most severe effects were observed in a test at 38.6 G, in which the subject experienced definite symptoms of shock, several episodes of syncope, and was found to have albuminuria for 6 hours after the test. The greater severity of the 38-G exposures was attributed to the difference in the rate of onset of the acceleration waveforms. The rate of onset of the 45-G test ws 493 G/sec (t_r = 0.11 seconds), whereas the rate of onset for the 38-G tests was 1100 G/sec or greater (t_r = 0.035 sec-

onds). The limits of human tolerance in the − x-axis are much lower when the restraint system is less adequate, as previously discussed.

A restraining surface, such as a seatback in place of straps, and the structural arrangement of the human anatomy has allowed tolerance of very high onset rates when the acceleration vector was oriented in the + x-axis. Beeding and Mosley[16] exposed a subject to a peak acceleration of 40.4 G with a velocity change of 14.8 m/sec and rate of onset of 2139 G/sec (t_r = 0.022 seconds) on the Daisy decelerator at Holloman Air Force Base. Special restraints and a lower level of dynamic preload were involved. Symptoms of shock, including loss of consciousness after the test, also were experienced.

The limiting factor in + z-axis human impact is vertebral fracture. Early investigators observed vertebral fractures during laboratory ejection seat tests and estimated that acceleration levels of 18 to 20 G with a velocity change of up to 17.5 m/sec could be tolerated without injury. Operational experience with United States Air Force ejection seats has shown that these estimates were reasonable. For example, review of 175 ejections accomplished from four aircraft using catapults producing peak acceleration levels ranging from 17.5 to 18.4 G with velocities of 15.2 to 25.9 m/sec showe that vertebral compression fractures resulted from 7% of these ejections. The time to the peak acceleration produced by these catapults ranged from 0.1 to 0.18 seconds. The restraint system, which was identical for each of the seats, consisted of a lap belt and double shoulder straps. When the + z-axis accelerative forces are applied through a torso harness system, as in parachute opening shock, it appears that somewhat higher levels may be tolerable, although this has not been well defined.

Spinal fracture is also probably the limiting factor for acceleration applied in the − z-axis when the acceleration force is compressive, as in a head-first water impact. In a downward ejection seat, the $-z$-force is applied partly in traction, through the pelvis by the lap belt, and partly in compression, by the restraint harness shoulder straps. Under these conditions, volunteers have routinely tolerated acceleration peaks of 9 G with a velocity change of 12.7 m/sec. More elaborate restraint and body support have permitted even higher $-z$-axis acceleration levels to be endured. Subjects restrained to a rigid couch by double shoulder straps, cross-chest strap, lap belt, crotch strap, and leg straps were exposed to peak accelerations up to 18.5 G with a velocity change of 5.94 m/sec.[17]

Human responses to acceleration in the $-z$-axis provide a noteworthy example of the differences between the effects of sustained and impact acceleration. The acceleration limits for seated subjects, conventionally restrained, exposed to sustained acceleration in the $-z$-axis are less than half of the impact exposure levels. The sustained acceleration exposures are limited by head pain and red out, which are not observed in shorter duration impact exposures.

The severity of sideward impact is approximately equivalent in either direction given symmetric restraints and supports because the human body is fairly symmetric about the midsagittal plane. Volunteer subjects have been exposed to sideward impact up to 9.95 G with a velocity change of 4.6 m/sec when the subjects were restrained only by a lap belt.[18] These experiments were stopped because of the investigator's concern about lateral torso flexion of up to 30°. When a lap belt and double shoulder strap configuration was used, acceleration peaks up to 11.7 G with a velocity change of 4.5 m/sec were tolerated without irreversible injury.[19] The limiting factor was transient bradycardia and syncope, apparently related to impingement of the shoulder strap on the carotid body. Adding flat metal plates to support the head, torso, and legs has

permitted $\pm y$-axis impact exposures up to 23.1 G with an onset rate of 1210 G/sec (t_r = 0.04 seconds) and velocity change of 8.4 m/sec. The subject's complaints and physiologic responses to these test conditions suggested that subjective or objective tolerance had not been reached.

Experimental efforts to determine human exposure limits for impact directions involving more than one cardinal axis are limited to research conducted to evaluate a narrow range of impact conditions and a body support and restraint system proposed for a specific space vehicle. These experiments were conducted using a vertical deceleration tower, where the dynamic preload is the near-weightless condition of free fall, and a horizontal deceleration track with a dynamic preload of approximately 0.3 G. Seven impact vector directions were explored on the vertical decelerator using six acceleration profiles.[20] Peak accelerations measured on the rigid seat ranged from 23.0 to 26.6 G, with impact velocities of 8.0 to 8.6 m/sec and rates of onset of 980 to 1380 G/sec. These seven impact vectors were among 24 orientations explored on the horizontal decelerator in a series of 288 tests with volunteer subjects.[21] Maximum accelerations measured on the sled ranged from 11.1 G for the $-z$-axis to 30.7 G when the acceleration vector was acting from chest to back ($-x$-axis) and 45° left. Impact velocities were varied up to 13.7 m/sec. None of these tests exceeded voluntary tolerance, but transitory postimpact bradycardia was a consistent finding for those impact vectors in which a component of the acceleration vector acted in the $-z$-axis. Multiple potentiating interactions prevent simple superposition of the effects observed in the component cardinal axes. New limiting factors may be involved with acceleration directions that allow different injury mechanisms than are present along the cardinal axes.

Surrogate Tests

Tests with anthropomorphic dummies, cadavers, and animals afford the opportunities to test to impact levels that would be intolerable for human subjects and to make precise and sometimes invasive measurements that would be difficult or impossible with living humans. The difficulties in applying these data are formidable, however, because the errors that are introduced in making the transition from surrogate data to living human are frequently very large. Tests defining the physical properties of isolated tissue preparations may be particularly misleading because of such factors as donor characteristics, postmortem changes, absence of excised supporting tissue, loss of physiologic responsiveness, unrealistic force application, and inadequate strain rates.

The most reliable data always will be derived from tests of fully representative subjects under fully representative conditions. The usual problem is to draw the best conclusions from a combination of tests involving living human subjects under less than representative conditions and tests involving less than representative surrogates exposed to actual anticipated impacts.

DIRECTIONS IN IMPACT PROTECTION

Impact protection research promises continued improvements in our knowledge of how to accelerate people safely. Existing techniques will be refined. New techniques will be exploited. This chapter has presented a systematic overview of the fundamental physical and mathematical principles that form the basis for current practice in this important part of aerospace medicine. It also can be said with certainty that the same principles will be the basis for our future advancements.

Two tools of the trade deserve attention as we look to the future. The first of these is the mathematical model. Models have been used extensively in impact research and in this chapter. They will be more useful in the future. Models may be descriptive or predictive. Descriptive models are equivalent to fitting a deterministic curve

to empiric data. They are useful as a mathematical shorthand to describe findings and also may facilitate our understanding of the physical processes involved. Predictive models are descriptive models that may be used to extend our knowledge beyond what we have observed. Descriptive models are usually examples of the application of inductive reasoning in that they utilize specific findings to formulate general descriptions. The use of predictive models is an example of deductive reasoning in that general descriptions are applied to the prediction of specific untested results. Descriptive models can be, in a sense, validated by repeated observations with comparison to the hypothesized general description. They can even be used for interpolation between two tested conditions. A model used to predict or extrapolate cannot be validated by testing, however, for later use beyond tested regions. Each prediction in a new area must be verified by observation. It is imperative that models be used appropriately in the conduct of impact research. Descriptive models are necessary if we are to understand our data. Predictive models are helpful in devising new techniques and predicting their utility, but the predictions must be verified.

This brings us to the second tool of the trade, namely, human testing. If the fielding of untried techniques is to be avoided, human testing will continue to be a necessity. Particularly in impact research, it must be borne in mind that anthropomorphic dummies are simply mechanical manifestations of mathematical models. They are, therefore, subject to the limitations just described for such models. Animal surrogates and human cadavers are analogs with complex differences from the living human that are difficult to fully appreciate. These differences may, therefore, be the basis for erroneous conclusions from tests with surrogates. Particularly when the goal is to develop a protective system that does not injure the populations in which it is applied, it should be possible to responsibly and ethically design safe verification testing of proposed techniques with a carefully selected population of volunteers.

Impact protection techniques will improve as research provides the necessary basis for their refinement. Techniques of interest in aerospace medicine will continue to be divided into two basic approaches. One approach involves the protection of occupants of a vehicle subjected to impact. The second approach involves protection of an occupant who escapes from a vehicle, presumably prior to an anticipated impact.

Occupant impact protection places significant demands on the vehicle designer to provide an intrusion-free compartment for the occupant during vehicle impact. Survivable impact conditions are defined by the limiting factor in available occupant protection techniques. In many current applications, the vehicle compartment deficiencies are the limiting factors in survival. As vehicle design improves, however, new occupant protection approaches may be required to take full advantage of the improvements. In a vehicle crash, the basic tenet is to strike an optimum balance between two contradictory requirements on occupant displacement. In one sense, occupant displacement within the vehicle should be minimized to avoid secondary impacts with vehicle structures and to avoid the acceleration amplifications associated with dead space and bottoming. This is the rationale for restraints such as lap belts. In another sense, however, occupant displacement within the vehicle allows more time for the occupant to accomplish the required velocity change and, in turn, allows the controlled application of lower acceleration over a longer period than would have been the case without displacement. This is the rationale for stroking seats in some helicopters. Future applications may allow significant gains by exploiting dy-

namic preload in occupant protection. This technique would involve anticipatory acceleration of the occupant by a counterstroking seat, triggered by a reliable crash sensor, that would initiate the velocity change prior to the impact. Other novel techniques may become available in the areas of restraint, individual protection such as helmets, postcrash environmental protection against fire, and assisted postcrash egress. These developments should find broad application beyond the sphere of aerospace medicine in related endeavors such as automobile passenger protection.

The second impact protection approach involves escape systems. Current techniques employ ejection seats or separable crewstation escape modules, each with its own set of advantages and disadvantages. The open seat allows rapid parachute deployment but offers poor protection at high speed, even with current limb restraint techniques. The module provides extraordinary windblast protection at high speed but requires relatively long times for deceleration and parachute deployment. As a result, low-altitude escape attempts may be compromised, particularly with significant aircraft sink rates. Both systems may produce significant morbidity during escape, parachute opening, and at ground impact after parachute descent. Likely future directions in escape systems will involve the exploitation of the strong points of each system while addressing some of the other sources of injury as well. The resulting systems may involve some attributes of previous individual capsule systems. New techniques and materials should allow effective encapsulation of a seat occupant during the early stages of ejection. Other approaches that should see application involve decision-making functions to tailor the escape to the prevailing conditions by utilizing dynamic preload, variable thrust catapults, alternative escape path choices, and trajectory control. To ensure that expanded escape capabilities are utilized despite short decision times and severe aircraft accelerations that may be imposed, it is likely that assisted escape initiation techniques will be developed to provide alerting, warning, and, in extreme cases, automatic initiation. Systems will subserve multiple functions so that, for example, G-suits, windblast protection, parachute landing protection, flotation, and antiexposure suits may be integrated into one basic device. Escape systems will require such efficiency and innovation to meet the challenge of increasingly severe escape conditions, from high-speed, low-level ejection to orbital escape.

These and other protective techniques will be necessary to allow men to confidently venture forth in the flying machines of the future and accomplish the various tasks set before them. The required techniques will be as novel as the vehicles, missions, and conditions that demand them. The reassuring observation remains that an appreciation for the utilitarian framework of first principles still provides the best means to their achievement.

REFERENCES

1. Newhouse, H.L., Payne, P.R., and Brown, J.P.: Wind Tunnel Measurements of Total Force and Extremity Flail Potential Forces on a Crew Member in Close Proximity to a Cockpit. AMRL-TR-79-110, Aerospace Medical Research Laboratory, Wright-Patterson Air Force Base, Ohio, Dec., 1980.
2. Desjardins, S.P., Laananen, D.H., and Singley, G.T., III: Aircraft Crash Survival Design Guide. Vol. II. USARTL-TR-79-22B. Applied Technology Laboratory, United States Army Research and Technology Laboratories, Fort Eustis, Virginia, Dec., 1980.
3. Clarke, T.D., Sprouffske, J.F., Trout, E.M., Klopfenstein, H.S., et al.: Baboon tolerance to linear deceleration ($-G_x$): lap belt restraint. In Proceedings of the Fourteenth Stapp Car Crash Conference. New York, Society of Automotive Engineers, Inc., 1970, pp. 279–298.
4. Clarke, T.D., Sprouffske, J.F., Trout, E.M., Klopfenstein, H.S., et al.: Impact tolerance and resulting injury in the baboon: Air Force shoulder harness-lap belt restraint. In Proceedings of the Sixteenth Stapp Car Crash Conference. New York, Society of Automotive Engineers, Inc., 1972, pp. 365–411.
5. Stapp, J.P.: Human Exposures to Linear Deceleration. Part 2. The Forward-Facing Position and the Development of a Crash Harness. Air Force Technical Report 5915, Aero Medical Laboratory, Wright Air Development Center, Wright-Patterson Air Force Base, Ohio, 1951.
6. Harris, C.M., and Crede, C.E. (eds.): Shock and Vibration Handbook. 2nd Ed. New York, McGraw-Hill Book Co., 1976.
7. Payne, P.R.: The dynamics of human restraint systems. In Impact Acceleration Stress. Washington, D.C., National Academy of Sciences, National Research Council Publication 977, 1962.
8. Kornhauser, M., and Gold, A.: Application of the impact sensitivity method to animate structures. In Impact Acceleration Stress. Washington, D.C., National Academy of Sciences, National Research Council Publication 977, 1962.
9. Stech, E.L., and Payne, P.R.: Dynamic Models of the Human Body. AMRL-TR-66-157, Aerospace Medical Research Laboratory, Wright-Patterson Air Force Base, Ohio, 1965.
10. Payne, P.R.: Personnel Restraint and Support System Dynamics. AMRL-TR-65-127, Aerospace Medical Research Laboratory, Wright-Patterson Air Force Base, Ohio, 1965.
11. Brinkley, J.W., and Shaffer, J.T.: Dynamic simulation techniques for the design of escape systems: Current applications and future Air Force requirements. In Biodynamic Models and Their Applications. AMRL-TR-71-29-2, Aerospace Medical Research Laboratory, Wright-Patterson Air Force Base, Ohio, 1971.
12. Hanrahan, J.S., and Bushnell, D.: Space Biology: The Human Factors in Space Flight. New York, Basic Books, Inc., 1960.
13. Hearon, B.F., Raddin, J.H., Jr., and Brinkley, J.W.: Evidence For the Utilization of Dynamic Preload in Impact Injury Prevention. AMRL-TR-82-6, Aerospace Medical Research Laboratory, Wright-Patterson Air Force Base, Ohio, 1982.
14. Von Gierke, H.E., and Brinkley, J.W.: Impact accelerations. In Foundations of Space Biology and Medicine. Vol. II, Book I, Chapter 6. Edited by J. Calvin and O.G. Gazenko. Joint USA/USSR Publication. Washington, D.C., National Aeronautics and Space Administration, 1975.
15. Snyder, R.G. Impact. In Bioastronautics Data Book. Edited by J.F. Parker, Jr. and V.R. Weds. NASA SP-3006, Washington, D.C., National Aeronautics and Space Administration, 1973.
16. Beeding, E.L., Jr., and Mosley, J.D.: Human Tolerance to Ultra-High G Forces. AFMDC-TN-60-2, Aeromedical Field Laboratory, Air Force Missile Development Center, Holloman Air Force Base, New Mexico, Jan., 1960.
17. Highley, F.M., Jr., Critz, G.T., and Hendler, E.: Determination of Human Tolerance to Negative Impact Acceleration: Phase I. Naval Air Engineering Center, Pennsylvania. Presented at the 34th Annual Meeting of the Aerospace Medical Association, Los Angeles, California, 1963.
18. Zaborowski, A.V.: Human tolerance to lateral impact with lap belt only. In Proceedings of the Eighth Stapp Car Crash and Field Demonstration

Conference. Detroit, Wayne State University Press, 1966, pp. 34–71.

19. Zaborowski, A.V.: Lateral impact studies: Lap belt-shoulder harness investigation. *In* The Ninth Stapp Car Crash Proceedings. University of Minnesota, 1966, pp. 93–127.

20. Weis, E.B., Jr., Clarke, N.P., and Brinkley, J.W.: Human response to several impact acceleration orientations and patterns. Aerospace Med., *34(12):*1122–1129, 1963.

21. Brown, W.K., Rothstein, J.D., and Foster, P.: Human response to predicted Apollo landing impacts in selected body orientations. Aerospace Med. *37(4):*394–398, 1966.

Chapter 9

Biodynamics: Sustained Acceleration

Sidney D. Leverett, Jr. and James E. Whinnery

The time will come, when thou shalt lift thine eyes
To watch a long-drawn battle in the skies,
While aged peasants, too amazed for words,
Stare at the flying fleets of wondrous birds.

THOMAS GREY, 1737

The aeromedical consequences of excess acceleration acting on the human body did not become a concern until World War I, when fighter pilots began reporting visual changes occurring when pulling out of a dive or during aerial combat. Later, during the Schneider Cup Race in 1925, pilots complained of loss of vision while executing sharp turns around the pylons. In 1927, Captain Luke Christopher became the first person to be hospitalized because of overexposure to acceleration. During a test flight, he was reported to have experienced the effects of acceleration equal to over ten times that of gravity. In the mid 1920s, the French developed a centrifuge to investigate these disturbances; in 1934, Commander J.R. Poppen recorded blood pressure responses in dogs while maneuvering in a two-seater fighter aircraft. The Germans constructed a human centrifuge at their aeromedical laboratory in Berlin in 1935 and undertook a large number of experimental studies on human subjects to determine the cause of blackout (loss of vision) and subsequently to develop methods for protecting their aviators. In Canada, Wing Commander W.F. Franks, using the newly constructed human centrifuge in Toronto, developed the Franks Flying Suit, a water-filled, double-layered rubber suit. It used the principle of hydrostatic counterpressure as a means of protection. The suit was eventually combat-tested by the British Royal Air Force during the desert war in North Africa in World War II. At about this same time, the Mayo Clinic centrifuge group teamed up with the David Clark Company and Berger Brothers (both corset manufacturers) and scientists from Wright Field, Ohio, (Wright-Patterson AFB) to develop an inflatable G suit containing five interconnecting air bladders that covered the calves, thighs, and abdominal area. Air pressure replaced water as the counterpressure system. In a separate endeavor, Dr. F.S. Cotton of Sydney, Australia developed a pneumatic anti-G suit, using the Royal Australian Air Force centrifuge to conduct his tests. His inflatable G suit was successfully combat-tested in the South Pacific in 1942. In 1944, a five-bladder anti-G suit became a standard item of issue of United States Army Air Force fighter pilots. Because of pressing production problems, neither the Japanese nor the Germans ever furnished anti-G suits to their pilots. Some Japanese pilots did wrap their lower extremities and abdominal area with elastic material as a potential means of improving G tolerance, but this procedure was not operationally effective.

PHYSICAL PRINCIPLES

Speed and Velocity

Speed is a term used daily to describe a property of moving objects (e.g., "he's traveling 50 mph"). Therefore, speed signifies the rate at which an object is moving or changing position. It specifies a magnitude only, without direction; therefore, speed is a scalar quantity. The equation used to calculate speed is as follows:

$$\text{Speed} = \frac{\text{distance}}{\text{time}} \text{ or } \bar{v} = \frac{\Delta s}{\Delta t} \quad (1)$$

where $\bar{v}$ is the average linear speed in meters per second (m/sec), feet per second (ft/sec), miles per hour (mph), or nautical miles per hour (knots); Δs is the distance traveled in meters, feet, or miles; and Δt is the time elapsed in seconds or hours.

If the sampling time interval is approaching zero, one can refer to the term instantaneous speed (if magnitude only is expressed); thus, the equation becomes the first derivative of distance with respect to time, or:

$$\dot{s} = \frac{ds}{dt} \quad (2)$$

where ds is the infinitesimal distance cov-

ered in the fraction of time, dt, and $\dot{s}$ is the instantaneous linear velocity.

Velocity is sometimes incorrectly interchanged with speed because the units are the same. Velocity, however, is a vector quantity that describes both the rate of movement of a body and the direction in which it moves:

$$\text{velocity (v)} = \frac{\text{distance}}{\text{time}} = \frac{ds}{dt} \quad (3)$$

From this equation it can be seen that velocity is composed of both speed and direction. If velocity remains constant, speed and direction are not changed. If an aircraft alters its speed or direction or both, however, there is a change of velocity and this, in turn, produces an acceleration.

Acceleration

Acceleration is defined as the rate of change of velocity and is a vector quantity having both magnitude and direction. When the linear velocity of an object changes over time, the following formula applies:

$$a = \frac{v_2 - v_1}{\Delta t} \quad (4)$$

where v_1 is the initial velocity (m/sec, mph, ft/sec, or knots); v_2 is the final velocity; Δt is the elapsed time (seconds or hours); and a is the acceleration (m/sec² or ft/sec²). This provides the mean linear acceleration of the body. The instantaneous linear acceleration is expressed as follows:

$$\dot{v} = \frac{dv}{dt} \text{ or } \ddot{s} = \frac{d^2s}{dt^2} \quad (5)$$

where $\dot{v}$ and $\ddot{s}$ are the instantaneous linear acceleration, that is, the first derivative of velocity or the second derivative of distance with respect to time.

A special type of linear acceleration

called radial, or centripetal, acceleration results in curvilinear (usually circular) motion. Centripetal acceleration is that which occurs when the direction of motion of the body (or aircraft) is changed. The acceleration acts along the radius of the circle and is directed toward the center of rotation. This type of acceleration occurs when an aircraft pulls out of a dive, pushes over into a dive, or performs an inside or outside turn. The effects from this type of acceleration will be the main topic of discussion in this chapter.

The unit of linear and centripetal (radial) acceleration is the G, which is equal to G_o, the acceleration exhibited by a free-falling body near the surface of the earth. One G is 32.2 ft/sec² (or 9.81 m/sec²). In aviation medicine, the term G has been introduced as a measure of the strength of the gravitoinertial force environment. It is a dimensionless term arrived at by a relative comparison of weight:

$$a = \frac{w}{w_o} \qquad (6)$$

where w is the weight observed in the environment under consideration and w_o is the normal weight on the surface of the earth. This is true because the conventional physical definition of weight is w = ma and $w_o = mg_o$ where m is the mass; a is the acceleratory field (vector sum of actual linear acceleration plus an imaginary acceleration opposite the force of gravity); and g_o is the standard value of the acceleration of gravity (9.81 m/sec² or 32.2 ft/sec²). Hence:

$$G = \frac{w}{w_o} = \frac{ma}{mg_o} = \frac{a}{g_o} \qquad (7)$$

Therefore, the unit G represents either the ratio of weights or the ratio of accelerations. It is still a dimensionless number but allows a convenient method of expressing the magnitude of a force (or acceleration) acting on a body.

For example, a jet fighter was performing aerial combat maneuvers and subsequently failed to recover from one high G turn and impacted the ground. In the investigation of the mishap, it was determined that the pilot was flying at approximately 590 knots in a turn estimated to be 3000 ft. The question of excess G and subsequent loss of consciousness was raised. What was the $+G_z$ force during this turn? The answer is as follows:

$$a = \frac{v^2}{r} \qquad (8)$$

where a is the acceleration field in ft/sec²; v is the velocity of the turn in ft/sec; and r is the radius of the turn in feet.

$$a = \frac{590 \, \frac{\text{knots}}{\text{hr}} \times \frac{6080 \, \text{ft}}{\text{knots}} \times \frac{1 \, \text{hr}}{3600 \, \text{sec}}}{3000 \, \text{ft}}$$
$$a = 330.96 \, \text{ft/sec}^2 \qquad (9)$$
$$= G_z = \frac{a}{g_o} = \frac{330.96 \, \text{ft/sec}^2}{32.2 \, \text{ft/sec}^2} = +10.27 \, G_z$$

It is reasonable that there should be some question about the pilot's being conscious during this turn of $+10.27 \, G_z$.

Nomenclature

A system for describing the reaction forces in acceleration was proposed by Gell and adopted by the aerospace medical community in 1961. It is summarized in Table 9–1 along with other terminologies that have been used in the past. An example of the Gell terms would be, "An F-16 can pull 9 G during combat maneuvering," whereas an earlier system used for many years by the United States Navy would have stated, "the pilot in an F-16 pulls eyeballs-down G up to 9 G during combat maneuvering."

Gauer[1] defined prolonged acceleration as that force which acts on a body for a period longer than 60 seconds. Other researchers have suggested a spectrum of time intervals and G levels.[2] For the pur-

Table 9–1.   A Nomenclature System Describing the Reaction Forces in Acceleration

	Table A Direction of Acceleration	
Linear Motion	Aircraft Computer Standard	Acceleration Descriptive
Forward	$+a_x$	Forward acceleration
Backward	$-a_x$	Backward acceleration
Upward	$-a_z$	Headward acceleration
Downward	$+a_z$	Footward acceleration
To right	$+a_y$	Right lateral acceleration
To left	$-a_y$	Left lateral acceleration

	Table B Inertial Resultant of Body Acceleration		
Linear Motion	Physiologic Descriptive	Physiologic Standard	Vernacular Descriptive
Forward	Transverse, PA prone G; back to chest G	$-G_x$	Eyeballs-in
Backward	Transverse AP G; supine G; chest to back G	$+G_x$	Eyeballs-out
Upward	Positive G	$+G_z$	Eyeballs-down
Downward	Negative G	$-G_z$	Eyeballs-up
To right	Left lateral G	$+G_y$	Eyeballs-left
To left	Right lateral G	$-G_y$	Eyeballs-right

Gell, C.: Table of equivalents for acceleration terminology, recommended for general international use by the Aerospace Medical Panel, AGARD. Aerospace Med., 32:1109, 1961.

poses of this text, sustained acceleration is defined as a G vector manifesting itself for 1 second or longer.

CENTRIFUGES

During and following World War II, there was an upsurge of new human centrifuges at aeromedical facilities. The original use of the centrifuge was for research purposes, for example, to determine the cause of blackout and unconsciousness during simulated air combat maneuvering, to develop methods of increasing a pilot's tolerance to these increased G forces, or to develop training techniques that would, in a ground-based simulator, assist pilots in performing muscular straining maneuvers to improve G tolerance. In recent years, the workhorse centrifuge for this type of work has been the centrifuge at the United States Air Force School of Aerospace Medicine (USAFSAM) (Fig. 9–1). It has been used as a testing and training device for early astronaut candidates and United States Air Force space research pilots, as a stressing device to evaluate possible pathologic conditions in aircrew members who had been referred to USAFSAM for medical evaluation, and as an aeromedical research device.

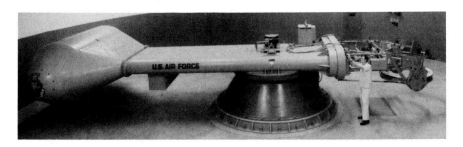

Fig. 9–1.   United States Air Force School of Aerospace Medicine, Brooks Air Force Base, TX Human Centrifuge, constructed in 1962.

The newest centrifuge is that at the Flug-medizinisches Institut der Luftwaffe, Für-stenfeldbruck, West Germany (Fig. 9–2). This centrifuge also will be used to train German Air Force fighter pilots to with-stand high G forces.

PHYSIOLOGIC RESPONSE TO ACCELERATION

Cardiovascular Function

The cardiovascular system is by far the most important system that determines the tolerance and response to $+G_z$ stress. It also is central to developing the best methods for combating the effects of $+G_z$ stress. Although much time and effort have been devoted to the cardiovascular system with excellent results, much re-mains to be thoroughly investigated.

Hydrostatic Column Effect

The most simplistic way to describe the effects of $+G_z$ stress on the circulatory sys-tem is to assume that a mechanical system is present that is nondistensible and with-out reflexes. This circulation model allows a simple estimation of the vascular pressures that develop as a result of $+G_z$ stress. The pressure at a particular point, then, becomes dependent on the hydro-static column and the magnitude of the $+G_z$ stress. The hydrostatic pressure at a specific point is the pressure exerted by the column of blood and is dependent on the height of the column of blood above the point and the weight per unit volume (density) of the blood. Assuming the weight per unit of blood does not change, the hydrostatic pressure is dependent only on the height of the column, that is, the point within the circulatory system at which one wishes to measure the pressure.

The model just described becomes most important with rapid-onset, short-dura-tion $+G_z$ stress. Figure 9–3 illustrates the hydrostatic column effect on systolic ar-terial pressure at $+1\ G_z$ and $+6\ G_z$. This diagram assumes a heart-to-brain (eye) distance of 30 cm that would exert a hy-drostatic column pressure of 22 mm Hg. The systolic arterial blood pressure is ap-proximately 120 mm Hg at heart level, of which 22 mm Hg is due to the hydrostatic

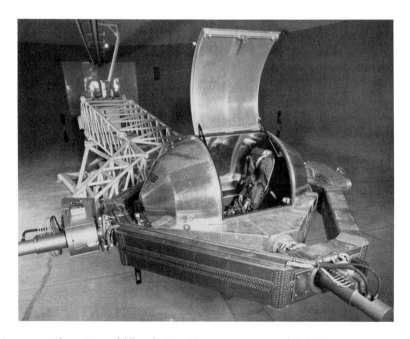

Fig. 9–2.   Human centrifuge, Fürstenfeldbruck, West Germany, constructed in 1982.

HYDROSTATIC COLUMN EQUIVALENTS (ARTERIAL SIDE)

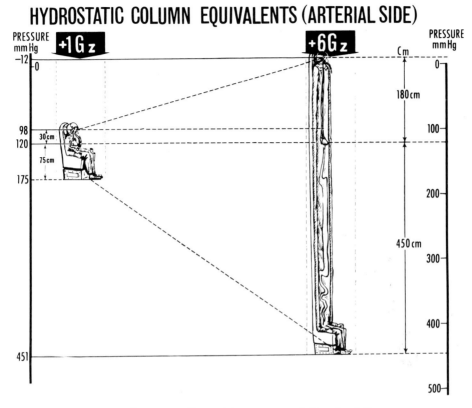

Fig. 9–3. Hydrostatic column effect on systolic arterial pressure at +1 G$_z$ and +6 G$_z$.

column effect. This leads to a predicted eye-level blood pressure of 98 mm Hg at +1 G$_z$. For each additional +1 G$_z$, the blood pressure at eye level will be reduced by another 22 mm Hg. This leads to a theoretical zero pressure at eye level at approximately +5.5 G$_z$ and a −12 mm Hg blood pressure at eye level at +6 G$_z$.

Any reduction in the heart-to-brain distance would reduce the hydrostatic column effect. This forms the basis of the protective effects of the tiltback seat. As shown in Figure 9–4, Burns has measured the heart (aortic valve)-to-eye distance at various seatback angles and configurations. One can easily predict the eye-level blood pressures at the various +G$_z$ levels using these heart-to-eye measurements and the simple hydrostatic column model.

The model does not accurately predict the pressure response to gradual-onset

+G$_z$ stress because continuous cardiovascular reflexes operate to compensate for the added +G$_z$ stress. In addition, even with rapid-onset +G$_z$ stress, the cardiovascular reflexes begin to make compensatory adjustments approximately 6 to 10 seconds after the onset of acceleration.

Reflex changes alter the pure hydrostatic column model and form the first line of defense against the effects of +G$_z$ stress. Due to the marked pooling of blood below heart level, the decrease in central blood pressure and apparent blood volume results in stimulation of both the high-and low-pressure systems within the vasculature. The major high-pressure stretch receptors are in the carotid sinus and the aortic arch. A fall in arterial pressure in these areas results in decrease in parasympathetic (vagal) inhibition and an increase in sympathetic stimulation. The heart rate

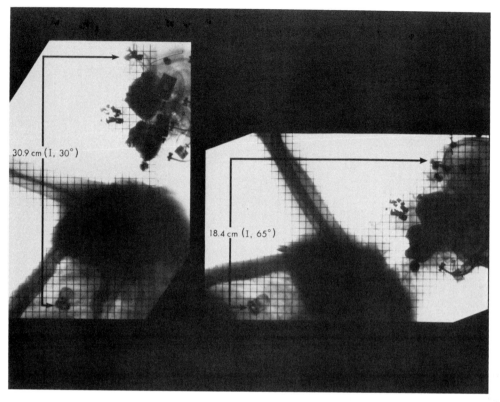

Fig. 9–4. Radiographic measurement of the human heart (aortic valve; as demonstrated by artificially replaced mechanical aortic valve)-to-eye (which is denoted by placement of a lead arrow at the lateral epicanthus of the eye) distance in a 30° and a 60° tiltback seat. $+G_z$ protection results from the decrease in heart-to-eye distance from 30.9 cm at 30° to 18.4 cm at 60° in relation to a vertical G vector.

increases, vasoconstriction and venocon-striction occur, and the cardiac contractile force increases, all in an attempt to restore homeostasis. Other more complex mechanisms, both mechanical and hormonal, also are present and form the basis of the integrated response to $+G_z$ stress.

Heart Rate Response to $+G_z$ Stress

The heart rate response to $+G_z$ acceleration both on a centrifuge and in flight actually begins before the onset of $+G_z$ stress. Generally, an increase in heart rate immediately preceding the $+G_z$ stress has been attributed to apprehension and anticipation of the upcoming stress. The magnitude of the prestress increase in heart rate in centrifuge studies was dependent on the anticipated level (and duration) of the stress. The higher the stress,

the higher the prestress heart rate. Table 9–2 shows the results of a specific study reported by Parkhurst and colleagues[3] that demonstrates the magnitude of this increase. As previously reviewed by Howard,[4] all reports agree that heart rates increased directly (but not linearly) with the maximum $+G_z$ level of exposure. The heart rate is known to vary, sometimes dramatically, not only from subject to subject but also in the same subject on different occasions. Burton and colleagues[5] suggested that the heart rate response during high, sustained $+G_z$ had three separate components: (1) physical work (straining); (2) acceleration; and (3) psychologic stress. This being the case, a wide individual variation in the heart rate response to $+G_z$ acceleration is to be expected because the amount of physical straining

Table 9–2. Heart Rates at Various Levels of +G$_z$ Acceleration*

G level	Number of Subjects	Preacceleration (beats/min)	Peak Acceleration (beats/min)
3	14	92 ± 3	109 ± 3
5	14	93 ± 3	125 ± 4
6	13	98 ± 3	142 ± 4
6.5	14	104 ± 3	153 ± 3
7.0	7	100 ± 9	159 ± 4
7.5	11	113 ± 3	162 ± 4
8.0	10	103 ± 4	156 ± 5
8.5	12	112 ± 4	162 ± 6
9.0	9	116 ± 6	167 ± 4

*The values shown are mean ± standard error.
From Parkhurst, M.S., Leverett, S.D., and Shubrooks, S.: Human tolerance to high, sustained +G$_z$ acceleration. Aerospace Med., 43:708, 1972.

performed by different individuals and the amount of psychologic stress perceived by each individual on each exposure could vary drastically. Only the reflex cardiovascular compensatory response to increased heart rate would be expected to be more uniform. Even this reflex response to +G$_z$ stress is subject to individual variation and has been shown to be dependent on a number of physiologic and anatomic factors such as height, age, sex, physical conditioning, and blood pressure.

In a rigidly controlled experiment to determine the reproducibility of +G$_z$ tolerance testing using trained centrifuge riders, it was found that the heart rate response to +G$_z$ was not as variable as previously considered. The gradual-onset (0.067 G/sec) and rapid-onset (1G/sec) runs with relaxed, highly trained centrifuge subjects were specifically designed to eliminate as much of the differential psychologic and muscular straining variation as possible to enhance the reflex response of heart rate to the +G$_z$ stress. The best reproducibility that could be achieved was 8 beats/min for the maximum heart rate response to gradual-onset and rapid-onset +G$_z$ stress in relaxed subjects. Even with the variation of straining performance using a gradual onset with straining +G$_z$ run, the same 8 beats/min variation was found. This amount of variation could be assumed to be close to the limit of

reproducibility of heart rate response to +G$_z$ stress. Heart rate response to +G$_z$ stress is illustrated in Figure 9–5.

The maximum heart rate response to +G$_z$ stress is directly related to the amount of +G$_z$ stress. Table 9–2 shows peak acceleration heart rates at various +G$_z$ levels from +3 G$_z$ through +9 G$_z$. The typical heart rate responses before, during, and after rapid-onset and gradual-onset exposures to +4.5 G$_z$ are shown in Figures 9–6 and 9–7, respectively. The rate at which the maximum heart rate is reached

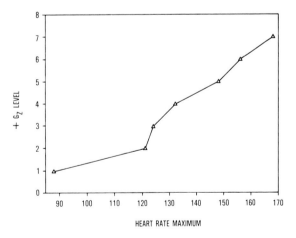

Fig. 9–5. The effect of increasing +G$_z$ on heart rate. The heart rate at +1 G$_z$ in the resting heart rate prior to acceleration exposure. The remainder of the heart rate data are taken from all runs on the United States Air Force School of Aerospace Medicine centrifuge over a 4-year period. Note the increase in heart rate as the +G$_z$ level increases.

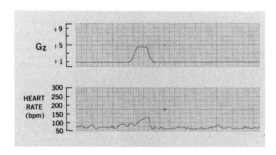

Fig. 9–6. Heart rate response before, during, and after exposure to a rapid-onset (+1 G$_z$/sec onset rate) run to +4.5 G$_z$. The duration at +4.5 G$_z$ was 15 seconds.

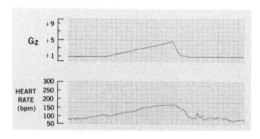

Fig. 9–7. Heart rate response before, during, and after exposure to a gradual-onset (0.067 G$_z$/sec onset rate) run to +4.5 G$_z$.

is dependent on the rate of onset of the G stress. In general, during rapid-onset runs with 1 G/sec onset, the time from onset of acceleration to the time for achieving maximum heart rate is 15 seconds. This coincides with the maximum heart rate being achieved within 5 to 10 seconds after reaching the maximum G level. After reaching a maximum level, the heart rate usually decreases slightly before it stabilizes, followed by a more gradual increase as maximal fatigue begins to occur. In certain individuals, a paradoxic decrease in heart rate may occur at the higher G levels. This phenomenon has been termed high-G bradycardia. Several reasonable explanations for this phenomenon are available, one of which is acute cardiac decompensation; therefore, an individual on a centrifuge with profound high +G$_z$ bradycardia during a run should be stopped to avoid possible complications.

The heart rate response has been con-

sidered to have little predictive value in determining +G$_z$ tolerance for the selection of personnel best suited to withstand +G$_z$ stress, although evidence indicates that heart rate does have a role in determining +G$_z$ tolerance. Anecdotal evidence consistent with this reveals that individuals able to withstand high, sustained +G$_z$ for very long durations frequently maintain a lower heart rate early in the run, even though the maximum heart rate at exhaustion is the same as for those individuals not able to sustain +G$_z$ for as long a period. This merely indicates that the individual with the lower heart rate is not stressed as much early in the run and, therefore, is more tolerant to that level of +G$_z$ stress for a longer period of time (less fatigue). Other evidence of the heart rate dependence of +G$_z$ tolerance is reflected in the specific group investigations of women and endurance-trained athletes. Women with high average +G$_z$ tolerance also had a higher than average maximal heart rate response during the gradual-onset (relaxed), rapid-onset (relaxed), and gradual-onset (with straining) +G$_z$ tolerance runs used to measure tolerance. The highly trained endurance athletes had lower than average +G$_z$ tolerance runs. Maximum heart rate response to +G$_z$ stress parallels the maximum heart rate response to other forms of stress, such as treadmill exercise testing, when factors such as age are coincidently considererd.

Cardiac Output

Cardiac output normally increases as a result of most forms of stress, including exercise. This increased cardiac output results from both an increase in stroke volume and an increase in heart rate (cardiac output equals stroke volume times heart rate). The stroke volume during exercise increases initially due to an increase in venous tone, which is mediated by the sympathetic nervous system, that results in increased venous return. The pumping action of exercising muscles, blood flow reflexly shunted from specific organ systems, and deep inspiration all result in enhancement of venous return. Although acceleration stress is a form of exercise and the above mechanisms are applicable, other perturbations are simultaneously occurring. Marked pooling of blood in the abdomen and lower extremities decreases venous return during $+G_z$ stress. The anti-G suit was designed to reduce this pooling and thereby enhance venous return. The most effective straining maneuvers used to combat $+G_z$ stress combine breathing techniques (M-1 or L-1 maneuvers) with muscular tensing of the abdominal and both upper and lower extremity muscles. The muscular tensing enhances venous return; however, a prolonged increase in intrathoracic pressure without short inspiratory efforts could inhibit venous return. Therefore, much importance should be placed on the correct performance of the M-1 or L-1 maneuver.

Measurement of cardiac output in the dynamic $+G_z$ environment has been and will continue to be difficult to perform. Decreases in heart volume have been demonstrated. Using radiographic size changes, Gauer[1] estimated that stroke volume was decreased 50 to 60% at $+4.6\,G_z$ and further concluded that with the concurrent increase in heart rate, cardiac output was only slightly below control levels. Howard[4] determined cardiac output using the direct Fick method at levels from $+2.0$ to $+2.4\,G_z$ and found a reduced stroke volume, as compared with the control levels, of 33 to 38%. Other techniques using dye-dilution at $+2$, $+3$, and $+4\,G_z$ found a progressive decrease in stroke index of 24%, 37%, and 49% compared with the control. A much easier measurement of the variation of cardiac output with G stress is the effect of changing from the horizontal ($0\,G_z$, $+1\,G_x$) to the vertical ($+1\,G_z$, $0\,G_x$) position, a change that can be observed in a routine clinical setting. Several investigators have shown that by this gravitational change alone cardiac output is decreased by an average of 25%.

As suggested by Glaister,[6] cardiac output is subject to abrupt and significant changes. A transient increase in cardiac output was noted as the initial response to $+G_z$ followed by a large decrease. Due to these variations, it was recommended that the subject spend at least 1 minute at G in an effort to achieve relative stability (steady state). This requirement becomes more and more difficult to adhere to at the higher $+G_z$ levels because tolerance to sustained G at $+7$ to $+9\,G_z$ may frequently be less than 1 minute. It, therefore, is apparent that cardiac output decreases as $+G_z$ increases. Because heart rate increases, a marked decrease in stroke volume must result in the decrement in output. Results to date have been obtained at relatively low $+G_z$ levels. Cardiac output measurements during high, sustained $+G_z$ stress have yet to be made. The most recent noninvasive measurement has included the echocardiographic determination of cardiac output, estimated by the product of the mitral valve area, the opening slope, and the diastolic interval of leaflet separation. These measurements again were made at low levels of $+G_z$ and revealed a decrease in cardiac output resulting from a 32% decrease in stroke volume at $+2\,G_z$ and a 46% decrease in stroke volume at $+3\,G_z$. The more promising noninvasive techniques for the future determination of cardiac output are echocardiographic and nuclear medicine techniques. The need for an accurate and reproducible beat-by-beat measurement of cardiac output will become more important in the future development of G-protective devices and techniques.

Coronary Blood Flow

Much of the recent aeromedical research in acceleration has centered on the assurance of adequate coronary artery blood flow during ever-increasing levels and durations of $+G_z$ stress. Because the

$+G_z$ environment is very complex and dynamic, the more routine methods of determination of coronary blood flow are unreliable and extremely difficult to use in a dynamic environment. Thus, much of the work has been related to indirect methods of assuring adequate coronary blood flow, such as the electrocardiographic response to $+G_z$. Several animal models have been used to determine coronary blood flow during $+G_z$ stress using more direct invasive techniques. Although not all studies agree, it appears that the majority of reports indicate that within the cardiovascular response stability limits of the animal (or human) coronary blood flow is adequate in the presence of completely normal coronary anatomy.

Under normal resting conditions, coronary blood flow is dictated by the existing myocardial oxygen consumption, which is determined by heart rate, myocardial wall tension, inotropic state, and myocardial fiber shortening. During $+G_z$ stress, the same determining factors are operable; however, there is a marked increase in myocardial oxygen consumption. The major determinants of adequate blood flow during $+G_z$ stress are heart rate, diastolic volume, aortic pressure (afterload), and arterial oxygen content. As previously described, heart rate increases with the $+G_z$ level, altered ventilation and perfusion occurs in the lungs during $+G_z$ and results in arterial hypoxemia, and ventricular pressures markedly increase. The combination of these factors should result in increased coronary blood flow. If the cardiac output is compromised by $+G_z$ decreased venous return, severe tachycardia, and a decreased arterial oxygen saturation, a compromise in adequate coronary blood flow could result.

Several investigators have shown that coronary blood flow was increased during $+G_z$ stress as long as their preparations were stable. These studies were carried out at relatively low $+G_z$ levels, very short durations of exposure, or in anesthetized animals. Laughlin and colleagues,[7] using unanesthetized miniature swine and radioactive microspheres, demonstrated increased blood flow even at $+7$ G_z in stable animals. Even the most susceptible layer, the endocardium, was found to have increased blood flow at $+7$ G_z. The results of Laughlin's study suggest that coronary blood flow is adequate during acceleration as long as aortic diastolic pressure is > 100 mm Hg. Aortic diastolic pressure may be the critical determinant in assuring adequate coronary blood flow.

From an aeromedical viewpoint, it is important to know that coronary blood flow is increased during moderate to high levels of sustained $+G_z$ stress. Defining man's upper limit of tolerance to $+G_z$ becomes important because the indications are that if cardiovascular tolerance is exceeded and aortic diastolic pressure drops precipitously, coronary blood flow will be compromised. In addition is the question of the effects of $+G_z$ stress on the coronary blood flow of an individual with subclinical coronary artery disease. Laughlin and colleagues[7] described one case of significant coronary artery disease in the left anterior descending coronary artery of a miniature swine. The animal developed fatal ventricular fibrillation after a 49-second exposure to $+7$ G_z and on autopsy was found to have areas of diffuse myocardial infarction. Because significant coronary artery disease can escape detection and remain subclinical, exposure of aircrewmen with this disease to the high $+G_z$ environment is likely. It, therefore, remains a double challenge to identify all individuals with significant coronary artery disease and to continue to define the upper limit of $+G_z$ tolerance that can be endured. Finally, it must be remembered that increased coronary blood flow alone does not necessarily compensate fully for the increased metabolic requirements of the heart.

Electrocardiographic Changes

The electrocardiogram (ECG) is an extremely useful tool for measuring the stress response to acceleration, for searching for pathologic changes in the heart resulting from higher and higher $+G_z$ levels, and as a noninvasive tool to further understand the physiologic response mechanisms to $+G_z$ stress. Although other forms of exercise stress, such as treadmill exercise testing, result in dynamic ECG changes, the additional volume shifts, cardiac displacement and distension, and reflex compensations make $+G_z$ stress uniquely complex.

Lead System

The major requirement for recording the electrocardiographic response to $+G_z$ stress is to obtain a noise-free tracing even during rapid-onset runs and offset of high $+G_z$ acceleration. The majority of high, sustained $+G_z$ runs also involve strenuous muscular and respiratory straining maneuvers, which add additional noise and artifacts to the tracing.

Satisfactory tracings have been obtained using a lead system consisting of two mutually perpendicular leads (sternal and biaxillary), which has allowed adequate monitoring of a diversity of individuals for rate and rhythm changes. Although other leads may be used for special purposes and perhaps different leads might be useful for pure diagnostic purposes, for routine monitoring this is a stable, rapidly attached system.

A large number of studies have documented the various electrocardiographic changes resulting from $+G_z$ stress. The majority of these reports have been most interested in documenting the presence or absence of ischemic changes in the ST segment and T-waves.

P-Wave

The changes observed in the P-wave reflect changes that affect atrial depolarization. Observations during exhaustive, high, sustained $+G_z$ simulated aerial combat maneuvers (SACM) verified an increased amplitude and duration of the P-wave. The time course of P-wave changes during a $+3$ G_z run followed by a $+4.5$ to $+7.0$ G_z SACM to exhaustion is shown in Figures 9–8 and 9–9. P-wave changes returned to control levels 3 minutes after the G stress. P-wave morphologic changes characteristic of ectopic atrial rhythm or chaotic atrial rhythm are covered in the section entitled "Rhythm Disturbances." During very stressful runs, the P-wave frequently merges into the T-wave. During the post-G-stress period, the P-wave frequently disappears completely, with excessive vagal inhibition of the sinoatrial pacemaker.

QRS Complex

Respiration, cardiac movement (displacement, distortion, and rotation), and altered ventricular function can alter QRS amplitude and configuration. The QRS response of normal individuals to $+G_z$ stress is such that the overall amplitude does not significantly change (Fig. 9–9). Depending on the lead, if the R-wave decreases in amplitude, a reciprocal deepening of the S-wave occurs. These changes probably signify a rotation of the electrical axis of the heart. Similar changes are, however, observed during other forms of stress (e.g., treadmill exercise). Other factors, therefore, may be additive, including decreased end systolic and diastolic volumes as compared with rest, increased end diastolic and end systolic pressure as compared with rest, increased catecholamines, and electrolyte disturbances. Which of these mechanisms (position, volume, catecholamines, electrolyte disturbance, or pressure) has the major influence on QRS amplitude and configuration is unknown.

T-Wave

ST segment and T-wave changes have received the most attention by acceleration cardiologists because of their possible association with myocardial ischemia or other disorders. Accurate assessment of ST segment changes has been hampered

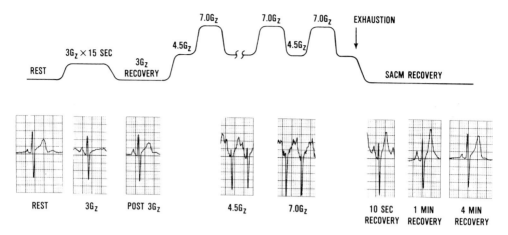

Fig. 9–8. Sample electrocardiographic P, QRS, and T-wave changes before, during, and after exposure to +3 G$_z$ followed by a +4.5 to +7.0 G$_z$ simulated aerial combat maneuver (SACM) profile.

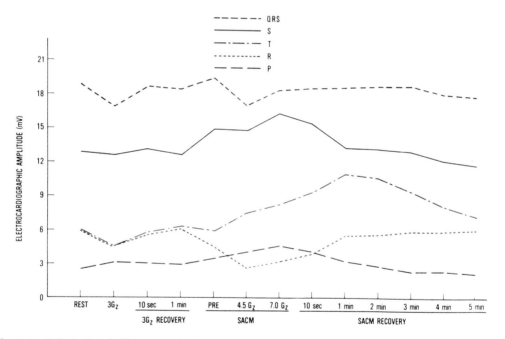

Fig. 9–9. P, R, S, T, and QRS amplitude alterations to the +G$_z$ exposures shown in Figure 9–8. Note that at 5 minutes postsimulated aerial combat maneuver (SACM), all wave changes have returned to baseline except for an increase in T-wave amplitude.

by frequent artifacts. Reported ST segment changes suggestive of myocardial ischemia are very infrequent. Individuals with a marked ST segment depression during or after +G$_z$ stress should be suspected of having ischemic heart disease until proven otherwise. T-wave changes, on the other hand, are very frequent. Early in the

course of +G$_z$ runs there is a decrease in T-wave amplitude, sometimes with flattening, diphasic or inverted T-wave, but these changes disappear later in the run. The characteristic response observed during SACM is shown in Figures 9–8 and 9–9.

Postacceleration T-wave changes following high, sustained $+G_z$ stress, especially strenuous SACM, consistently result in large, peaked T-waves. These changes are maximal between 1 and 2 minutes after the $+G_z$ stress and slowly return to normal thereafter. Even at 5 minutes after the $+G_z$ stress, the T-wave is not completely recovered. Similar changes occur during and after treadmill exercise. The exercise-induced changes in T-wave amplitude, especially in endurance-trained individuals and young adults post exercise, may be due to an increase in stroke volume that corresponds to an increased rate of decline in heart rate after exercise. The tall, peaked T-waves also are suggestive of the "tented T-waves" seen in association with hyperkalemia. Serum potassium is significantly elevated after the $+G_z$ stress; however, the magnitude of the change is small. The rate of change of electrolytes or other metabolites may be more important than the absolute magnitude of the change. Catecholamines also have been associated with the T-wave changes both during and after $+G_z$ stress. It has been suggested that a differential response to norepinephrine and epinephrine is responsible for the observed early and late T-wave changes.

Rhythm Disturbances

Lamb[8] nicely summarized the importance of cardiac rhythm disturbances in relation to the aeromedical environment:

> Cardiac arrhythmias are frequently the result of hypoxia and G forces and many of them may initiate syncopal episodes. Thus, they constitute a major segment of cardiac problems in flying populations. Cardiac arrhythmias are actually changes in the electrical mechanism of the heart and changes in cardiac rhythm which affect cardiac dynamics. They are not simply electrocardiographic findings. The electrocardiogram merely enables one to detect the changes in the dynamics which are occurring in the heart.

The electrocardiogram is a window into both pathologic and physiologic processes that affect the heart.

The in-flight aerial combat or aerobatic environment is a multistress environment with numerous factors occurring simultaneously. These factors, even when occurring alone, are known to be dysrhythmogenic. The major dysrhythmogenic stresses are listed in Table 9–3. They are not necessarily separate but are interrelated. It would be surprising if dysrhythmias were not observed during $+G_z$ acceleration stress. The aeromedical problem is the determination of which of the dysrhythmias are clinically significant, which are operationally significant, and which ones represent the normal response to the $+G_z$ stress environment.

A number of qualitative descriptions of the number and type of dysrhythmias that result from specific $+G_z$ exposures have been reported. Although it would seem that the occurrence of dysrhythmias during $+G_z$ is variable, it is evident that to accurately compare the frequency of occurrence, only similar populations being exposed to similar levels and durations of $+G_z$ stress under comparable environmental conditions are appropriate. The assurance of no pathologic changes resulting from $+G_z$ stress is costly and time-consuming. For this reason, electrocardiographically monitored high, sustained $+G_z$ runs will likely proceed before other techniques can be developed to monitor this dynamic environment.

Over a consecutive 3-year period at USAFSAM, the electrocardiographic responses to a multitude of $+G_z$ runs were tabulated to determine the spectrum of changes that would occur in a healthy asymptomatic male population during $+G_z$ exposure. All individuals (544 subjects) had successfully passed complete aeromedical evaluations prior to riding the centrifuge and were asymptomatic and considered healthy. The results are shown in Table 9–4. It is evident that a variety of rhythm disturbances and other electrocardiographic findings occur as a result of $+G_z$ stress.

These results unquestionably demon-

Table 9–3. Major Dysrhythmogenic Stresses*

Psychologic Stresses	Physiologic Stresses	Environmental Stresses
Anxiety	Exercise	Altitude
Fear	Respiratory alterations	Acceleration
Task overload	Mechanical distension or distortion	Temperature
Pain	Fatigue	Vibration
	Hormonal alterations	Noise
	Autonomic imbalance	
	Electrolyte alterations	
	Blood flow alterations	

*These stresses are listed arbitrarily. Many of these stresses are interrelated. This is not necessarily an all-inclusive list but represents many of the stresses that are documented to be dysrhythmogenic alone in a nonaviation environment. The aviation environment results in a combination of many or all of these stresses.

Table 9–4. Three-Year History of Acceleration-Related Dysrhythmias at the United States Air Force School of Aerospace Medicine*

Rank	Occurrences	Dysrhythmia Description
1	1566	Sinus arrhythmia (rate varying > 25 beats/min between successive beats)
2	1073	Premature ventricular contractions (PVCs)
3	768	Premature atrial contractions (PACs)
4	546	Sinus bradycardia (Rate < 60 beats/min)
5	372	Ectopic atrial rhythm
6	272	Premature junctional contractions (PJCs)
7	171	PVCs with bigeminy/trigeminy
8	126	Multiformed PVCs
9	104	AV dissociation
9	104	Paired PVCs

*Based on the exposure of 544 different subjects during 9831 $\pm G_z$ centrifuge runs.

Table 9–5. Time of Occurrence of the Most Frequent Dysrhythmias Associated With Centrifuge $+G_z$ Stress

Dysrhythmia	Time of Occurrence*			
	Pre-G	During G	Post-G	All of the Time
Premature ventricular contraction (PVC)	5	65	27	3
Premature atrial contraction (PAC)	5	61	31	3
Premature junctional contraction (PJC)	9	63	22	6
PVC with bigeminy	9	60	21	10
Multiformed PVCs	1	74	25	0
Paired PVCs	9	71	20	0
Sinus arrhythmia	2	4	94	0
Sinus bradycardia	5	8	87	0
Ectopic atrial rhythm	6	5	89	0
AV dissociation	2	7	91	0

*Given as a percentage of the total number of occurrences of each dysrhythmia.

strate the dysrhythmogenic nature of $+G_z$ stress. Previous investigators have questioned whether the various dysrhythmias most frequently encountered occurred during $+G_z$ stress or in the immediate recovery period. The time of occurrence of the various dysrhythmias reveals that certain dysrhythmias occur during $+G_z$ stress and others occur in the post G stress pe-

riod (Table 9–5). The cause of dysrhythmia distribution is probably the autonomic imbalance, with a sympathetic predominance before and during $+G_z$ stress and parasympathetic predominance in the post $+G_z$ stress period.

It is likely that the disparity in previous observations on the presence or absence of dysrhythmias, especially premature ventricular contractions (PVCs), is related to the comparison of different levels and types of G stress. The USAFSAM experience is heavily weighted to high, sustained $+G_z$, especially SACMs. These types of $+G_z$ runs are very stressful and should result in frequent ectopy if ectopy increases with the magnitude of the $+G_z$ stress. As shown in Figure 9–10, if the number of occurrences of PVCs is plotted for various $+G_z$ ranges, there is an increase with increasing $+G_z$ stress. If the number of occurrences is normalized to consider the number of runs within each $+G_z$ range, there is a steady increase in the ectopy as the $+G_z$ stress increases. Because heart rate increases with increasing $+G_z$ level, an increase in ectopy with increasing heart rate is to be expected. Indeed, as the stress increases, so does the ectopy. This is further verified by determining which type of $+G_z$ stress causes the most ectopy. As shown in Figure 9–11, a breakdown of the type of run associated with the incidence of PVCs reveals 54.2% of the PVCs that occurred during $+G_z$ happened during an SACM, whereas only 16.5% of the total runs were SACMs. Because SACMs most closely represent the in-flight $+G_z$ profile and require maxi-

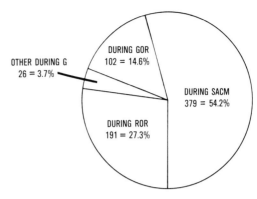

Fig. 9–11. Stage of occurrence of premature ventricular contractions (PVCs) during various types of $+G_z$ exposure (rapid-onset = ROR; gradual-onset = GOR). Note that 54.2% of the PVCs occurred during SACMs. Of all the runs, simulated aerial combat maneuvers (SACMs) were only 16.5% of the total number.

mum performance of protective straining maneuvers, they have the maximum summation of factors known to be dysrhythmogenic.

In asymptomatic healthy individuals with normal clinical evaluations, the entire spectrum of these dysrhythmias is probably benign. Even the more ominous ectopy, such as nonsustained ventricular tachycardia associated with $+G_z$ stress, is not necessarily considered an indication of pathologic change but rather a physiologic response to an extremely stressful environment. Specific dysrhythmias do have aeromedical significance. These are the ones that potentially could result in sudden incapacitation or an alteration in $+G_z$ tolerance. Included in this group are sinoatrial block (sinus arrest) with attendant asystole, atrioventricular dissociation during G, and ventricular tachycardia.

Sinoatrial Block (Sinus Arrest)

Prolonged sinoatrial block (sinus arrest) with failure of lower pacemakers to pick up the rhythm is very serious in the aerospace environment. The resultant loss of cardiac output can result in a loss of consciousness (as in a Stokes-Adams attack) or, if coincident with G-induced loss of consciousness, can lead to a resultant in-

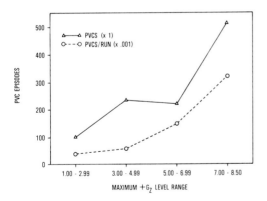

Fig. 9–10. Plot of the frequency of premature ventricular contractions (PVCs) and PVCs/run in various $+G_z$ ranges. Note that the frequency of PVC/run increases directly with increasing $+G_z$ level. Even without normalizing the PVC count for the frequency of exposure, there is an increase in PVC frequency.

creased time of incapacitation. An example of the latter instance is shown in Figure 9–12. In this example, the time of incapacitation was approximately 30 seconds, as compared with the average 15 seconds of incapacitation seen in pure $+G_z$ induced loss of consciousness. The most frequent cause of this disturbance in rhythm is very strong parasympathetic (vagal) tone. This can be due to a vigorous M-1 or L-1 straining maneuver or in the immediate $+G_z$ recovery period when the baroreceptors receive an unusually strong stimulation. There is some indication that certain individuals may be particularly sensitive to this problem. Such individuals may have developed a very high level of vagal tone such as that developed by extremely vigorous endurance training.

Atrioventricular Dissociation

A similar situation exists with the occurrence of atrioventricular (AV) dissociation. The loss of coordinated atrial function has been observed to result in a decrement in high, sustained $+G_z$ tolerance during SACM. An appropriately timed atrial systole is important for making a final contribution to ventricular filling and to assure crisp closure (without

regurgitation) of the AV valves. An example of AV dissociation is shown in Figure 9–13 during a $+4.5$ to $+7.0$ G_z SACM. The individual was able to tolerate $+4.5$ G_z and $+7.0$ G_z with appropriate atrial function but was unable to tolerate $+7.0$ G_z with AV dissociation. As previously suggested, the importance of atrial function may be apparent only during maximal stress or in an extremely ill individual when any decrement in cardiac output cannot be tolerated. The loss of atrial function could result in a blood pressure loss of as much as 30 mm Hg, a sufficient decrement to go from minimal grayout to blackout or loss of consciousness.

Ventricular Tachycardia

Any tachydysrhythmia, if at a sufficient rate to compromise cardiac output, may be considered as detrimental to $+G_z$ tolerance or performance. To compromise cardiac output, the tachydysrhythmia must be sustained. Short bursts of ventricular tachycardia are usually of no consequence. These short, three- to six-beat episodes may occur in completely healthy individuals in association with $+G_z$ stress. Although the possibility exists that this type of dysrhythmia has the capacity

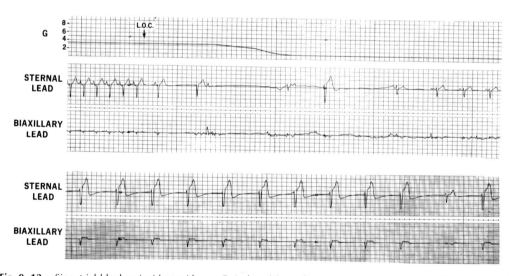

Fig. 9–12. Sinoatrial block coincident with a $+G_z$ induced loss of consciousness. The recovery illustrated in the lower tracing was by a slow idioventricular rhythm.

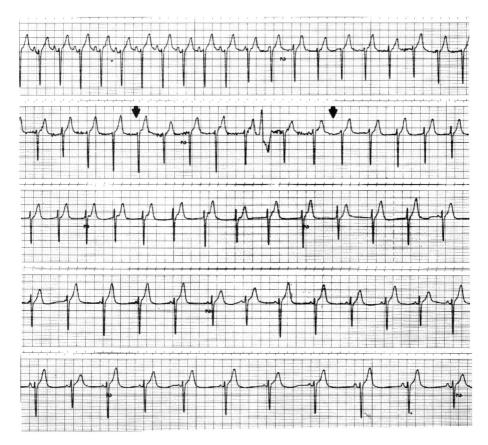

Fig. 9–13. $+G_z$ induced atrioventricular dissociation resulting in reduced $+G_z$ tolerance in an endurance-trained subject. The tracing is a continuous electrocardiogram starting with the subject at $+4.5$ G_z. The A-V dissociation occurs as the subject starts up to $+7.0$ G_z. The first arrow represents the attainment of $+7.0$ G_z. The subject had a complete blackout (second arrow) within 4 to 5 seconds at $+7.0$ G_z and returned to $+1.0$ G_z. AV dissociation with a variable P-wave persists into the recovery period. The subject was able to tolerate $+4.5$ G_z but not $+7.0$ G_z with AV dissociation.

to degenerate into the more severe ventricular fibrillation, it has not been documented in acceleration experiments. $+G_z$ induced ventricular tachycardia in flight has been documented in individuals with mitral valve prolapse.

Dysrhythmogenesis of $+G_z$ Acceleration

A comparison of the frequency and type of dysrhythmias induced by $+G_z$ stress, as compared with other types of stress, has not been thoroughly investigated. When the frequency of dysrhythmias before, during, and after treadmill exercise was compared with $+G_z$ stress, a significant increase in the frequency of $+G_z$ induced

dysrhythmias was found in a group of healthy males when maximum-stress $+G_z$ exposure was compared with maximal treadmill exercise and 24-hour Holter monitoring. In aircrewmen undergoing aeromedical evaluation, even with submaximal $+G_z$ stress, an equal frequency of rhythm disturbances was found, as compared with maximal treadmill exercise stress.

It is important that any comparisons of $+G_z$ induced dysrhythmias compare similar populations. It is the experience at USAFSAM that the frequency of $+G_z$ induced dysrhythmias is, among other things, age-dependent. Age is probably only one of many variables in the susceptibility to $+G_z$ induced dysrhythmias.

Pulmonary Function

The lungs are very important to acceleration physiology because tolerance, performance, and protection are all dependent on various aspects of pulmonary function. Isolated $+G_z$ acceleration stress profoundly affects pulmonary ventilation and perfusion, with marked changes apparent even between the supine (OG_z, $+1G_x$) and the upright ($+1G_z$, OG_x) positions. The additional stresses of using respiratory techniques to enhance $+G_z$ tolerance and anti-G suit inflation compressing abdominal contents upward further complicate pulmonary function. The major physiologic effects of $+G_z$ on the lungs fall into three areas: altered ventilation and perfusion resulting in hypoxemia, airway closure, and atelectasis. If man is exposed to sustained $+G_z$ levels above the currently investigated range ($+7$ to $+9$ G_z), pathophysiologic effects must be a consideration, including compromise of chest wall mechanics, pulmonary edema, and possible disruption of the anatomic integrity of the lung. Of maximum importance are the changes that occur in pulmonary function during dynamic fluctuations of G_z such as occur during high, sustained G_z maneuvering.

Respiration

The changes that result from progressively increasing $+G_z$ stress while wearing a standard United States Air Force anti-G suit and breathing room air are shown in Table 9–6. Measurements were made continuously for respiratory rate (f), heart rate (HR), tidal volume (V_T), and end tidal carbon dioxide tension (Pct_{CO_2}). Additional parameters measured during the final 20 seconds of the 45-second $+G_z$ exposure, with arterial blood being withdrawn from the radial artery, included arterial gas tensions (Pa_{O_2}, Pa_{CO_2}), arterial pH, and expiratory oxygen and carbon

dioxide (Pe_{O_2}, Pe_{CO_2}). The physiologic dead space (V_D) and V_D/V_T ratio were calculated from the data.

Respiratory rate increases as the $+G_z$ level increases. V_T also increases with the $+G_z$ level, but at $+7$ G_z, its increase is limited because of the mechanical limitations induced by the opposing downward $+G_z$ forces and the upward displacement of the diaphragm induced by the abdominal compression by the anti-G suit. The physiologic dead space increases, and in spite of increasing ventilation, Pa_{CO_2} changes very little as $+G_z$ increases. While breathing room air, the Pa_{CO_2} progressively drops toward 50 mm Hg at $+7$ G_z.

Regional Changes in Ventilation and Perfusion

When trying to understand the effects of acceleration on the lungs and to devise methods of increasing protection against $+G_z$, the regional changes in ventilation and perfusion must be defined. A large pressure gradient increasing from the apex to the base is markedly increased during exposure to $+G_z$ stress. This gradient results in regional changes in both ventilation and perfusion.

Ventilation is not evenly distributed during resting respiration in a normal individual. The distribution of ventilation is preferential to the dependent basilar area of the lung matching the increased blood flow in the dependent basilar area. The distribution pattern of ventilation is dependent on lung mechanics, specifically the lung volumes. It is profitable to discuss the ventilation distribution in view of conditions under which the lung volume is either greater or lesser than the functional residual capacity.

The apex of the lung is relatively more expanded than the basilar region because of the increase in the pleural pressure gradient from apex to base. The more distended units are at the top of the lung. With an incremental increase in pressure, less ventilation occurs at the top than at

Table 9–6. Mean Values ± Standard Deviation (in Parentheses) of Nine Men Breathing Air and Exposed to 45 Seconds of Various Levels of +G_z

| Parameter | Acceleration | | | |
	1 G	3 G	5 G	7 G
f	18.6	23.4	32.6	38.9
	(3.0)	(4.8)	(7.5)	(13.2)
HR	75.0	109.0	147.0	164.0
	(7.0)	(18.0)	(22.0)	(19.0)
V_T	0.68	0.93	1.20	1.13
	(0.11)	(0.21)	(0.31)	(0.44)
Pct_{CO_2}	33.6	27.3	20.2	15.8
	(3.5)	(4.6)	(3.6)	(3.3)
Pa_{O_2}	91.6	84.7	60.2	50.1
	(7.9)	(14.8)	(9.9)	(7.3)
Pa_{CO_2}	35.0	32.0	32.1	33.2
	(4.1)	(4.0)	(3.0)	(2.0)
pH	7.422	7.422	7.444	7.418
	(0.022)	(0.036)	(0.025)	(0.034)
Pe_{O_2}	119.2	127.2	132.2	136.0
	(2.8)	(3.8)	(4.5)	(2.3)
Pe_{CO_2}	22.7	20.0	15.5	12.8
	(1.9)	(1.9)	(3.5)	(2.8)
V_D	0.200	0.307	0.579	0.551
V_D/V_T	0.35	0.38	0.52	0.52

Abbreviations: f is respiratory rate; HR is heart rate; V_T is tidal volume; Pct_{CO_2} is end tidal carbon dioxide tension; Pa_{O_2} is arterial oxygen tension; Pa_{CO_2} is arterial carbon dioxide tension; pH is arterial pH; Pe_{O_2} is expiratory oxygen; Pe_{CO_2} is expiratory carbon dioxide; V_D is the physiologic dead space; and V_D/V_T is the dead space to tidal volume ratio.

the bottom of the lung. During increased +G_z acceleration, the pleural pressure gradient is markedly increased, accentuating the differences in expansion between the apex and base of the lung. As long as the lung volume is greater than the functional residual capacity, ventilation should remain preferentially to the basilar region even as the +G_z level increases. This regional distribution should continue until the excess mechanical forces resulting from the downward +G_z and upward displacement of the abdominal contents on the diaphragm by the anti-G suit causes closure of the distal airways in the basilar regions, thereby decreasing ventilation in those basilar regions. These theoretical considerations have been verified at relatively low +G_z levels, but accurate measurements have yet to be obtained to confirm the true regional differences in ventilation during high, sustained +G_z stress.

The distribution of pulmonary blood flow results from the balance of the hydrostatic forces and the driving pressure from the right ventricle through the pulmonary artery. Pulmonary blood flow within the normal unstressed lung has been described as consisting of four zones. These zones are described on the basis of the relative magnitude of the arterial, venous, and alveolar pressures. Figures 9–14 A and B show the effects of acceleration (−4 through +8 G_z) on pulmonary blood flow distribution using radioactive human albumin microspheres in the miniature swine. The changes in regional perfusion can be followed by noting the shift in high flow areas. In general, +G_z results in both a posterior and caudal shift in blood flow, and −G_z results in both an anterior and posterior redistribution pattern. Because the right lung is anatomically larger in the miniature swine, the final relative equalization actually represents a greater reduction in the perfused area of the right lung posteriorly. The high flow areas anteriorly and posteriorly shift more laterally with increasing +G_z up to +6 G_z;

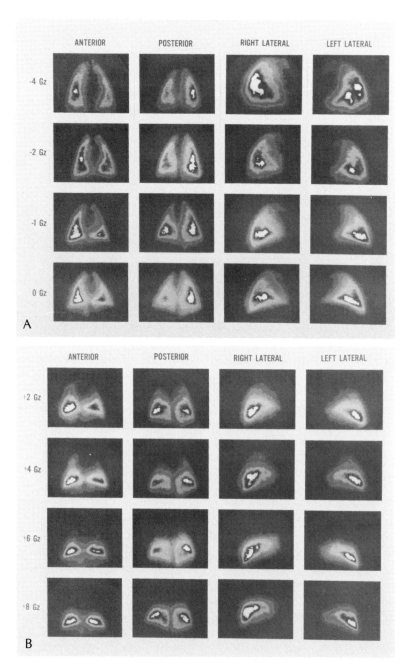

Fig. 9–14.   The effects of G_z on the distribution of pulmonary blood flow as demonstrated by perfusion scans using radioactive human albumin microspheres in the miniature swine.

however, at $+8$ G_z, the bilateral equalization results in a return of perfusion to the medial areas. The normal diaphragmatic curvature, evident in the lateral baseline scans, progressively disappears with increasing $+G_z$. The posterior caudal tips have progressively greater perfusion with a flattening of the diaphragmatic contour. The anterior scans reflect the cranial shift in flow induced by $-G_z$, with an overall thinning of the mediolateral thickness resulting in long, thin perfused areas at -4 G_z. The progressive disappearance of the posterior caudal tips is evident in the lateral scans at -2 G_z and -4 G_z. The progressive disappearance of the posterior caudal tips is evident in the lateral scans at -2 G_z and -4 G_z. In addition, the normal diaphragmatic curvature disappears, with a posterior rounding-off upward. The posterior scan initially shows a slight increase at -2 G_z, before having a decreased area of perfusion at -4 G_z, again reflecting the loss of posterocaudal perfusion and a simultaneous shift anteriorly.

It should be pointed out that in the baseline O G_z scan, the most dependent area is anterior due to the -1 G_z gravitational force from posterior to anterior. This -1 G_z gravitational force is constant and present in all scans except the -1 G_z scan, which was performed with the animal's head down. The loss of anterior perfusion in going from baseline to -1 G_z demonstrates the contribution of the -1 G_z present in the remainder of the scans.

The relative percentage changes for the serial G_z levels between $+8$ G_z and -4 G_z are shown in Figure 9–15. The maximum decrease in perfused areas due to $+G_z$ occurred at $+8$ G_z for all projections. The maximum increase in perfused area occurred at -4 G_z except for the posterior scan, which showed a maximum increase at -2 G_z.[9]

M-1 and Positive Pressure Breathing Effects on Lung Functions

Various straining maneuvers (M-1 and L-1) and positive pressure breathing have

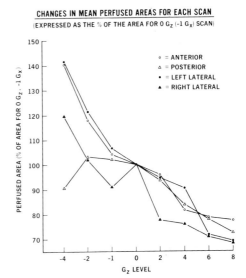

CHANGES IN MEAN PERFUSED AREAS FOR EACH SCAN
(EXPRESSED AS THE % OF THE AREA FOR 0 G_z (-1 G_x) SCAN)

o = ANTERIOR
△ = POSTERIOR
• = LEFT LATERAL
▲ = RIGHT LATERAL

Fig. 9–15. Quantitative description of the changes in pulmonary perfusion distribution with $+G_z$ and $-G_z$.

been shown to enhance $+G_z$ tolerance. The resultant arterial blood gas measurements on individuals performing the M-1 maneuver are given in Table 9–7 and on individuals using positive pressure breathing in Table 9–8. It has been suggested that the lower Pa_{O_2} values at $+3$ G_z and $+6$ G_z may be due to an increased oxygen requirement during performance of the M-1, indicating that positive pressure breathing might be the less strenuous protective procedure. Positive pressure breathing may, on the other hand, prevent dependent airway collapse and result in increased oxygenation at $+G_z$ levels below $+8$ G_z.

One Hundred Percent Oxygen Breathing

Breathing gas mixtures containing increased levels of oxygen, including 100% oxygen, have definite effects on the lungs when combined with $+G_z$ stress and the wearing of an anti-G suit. Vital capacity decreases are known to occur, and visible changes on post $+G_z$–stress chest radiographs are easily observable. The changes may be associated with no symptoms or with the symptoms characteristic of aero-

Table 9–7. Arterial Oxygen and Carbon Dioxide Tension and pH (Group Mean ± S.E.M. in Parentheses) Are Shown For Six Men Performing the M-1 Maneuver* and Exposed to Various Levels of +G$_z$ For 60 Seconds

	+1 G$_z$	+3 G$_z$	+6 G$_z$	+8 G$_z$†
Pa$_{O_2}$	101.3	73.1	56.3	48.3
	(3.7)	(5.5)	(6.0)	(0.33)
Pa$_{CO_2}$	27.4	31.1	32.0	29.7
	(2.1)	(1.1)	(1.1)	(2.0)
pH	7.43	7.44	7.44	7.44
	(0.02)	(0.01)	(0.01)	(0.02)

*Subjects were required to perform a maximum M-1 maneuver during 1 G exposure. The 3 G exposures did not require the M-1 maneuver.
†The 8 G means consist of only those subjects (three) who were capable of tolerating at least 50 seconds of 8 G.

Table 9–8. Arterial Oxygen and Carbon Dioxide Tensions and pH (Group Means ± S.E.M. in Parentheses) Are Shown For Six Men Using Positive Pressure Breathing and Exposed to Various Levels of +G$_z$ For 60 Seconds

	+1 G$_z$	+3 G$_z$	+6 G$_z$	+8 G$_z$
Pa$_{O_2}$	102.5	88.0	64.0	46.0
	(3.4)	(3.6)	(5.4)	(4.7)
Pa$_{CO_2}$	27.7	29.3	29.9	29.0
	(1.4)	(1.4)	(0.9)	(2.0)
pH	7.45	7.45	7.46	7.46
	(0.02)	(0.02)	(0.01)	(0.01)

*The +8 G$_z$ means consist of only those subjects (three) who were capable of tolerating at least 50 seconds of +8 G$_z$.

atelectasis. The magnitude of the vital capacity changes suggests that a greater decrease may occur in smokers than in nonsmokers. Kinetic studies have suggested that the airway closure may continue to occur even after the +G$_z$ stress is completed. Pulmonary function parameters at +1 G$_z$ and +5 G$_z$ while breathing 100% oxygen have been measured and are shown in Table 9–9.

Further work will be necessary to completely define the spectrum of optimum breathing mixtures for high-performance aircraft and the exact kinetics and mechanism of changes in pulmonary function of individuals exposed to high, sustained +G$_z$. There is no evidence to suspect irreversible pathologic changes to the lungs associated with current levels of +G$_z$ exposure.

Central Nervous System

The major acute limiting factors to high +G$_z$ stress in the central nervous system

Table 9–9. Respiratory Parameters During +G$_z$ Stress. Mean Values ± Standard Deviation (in Parentheses) of Four Men Breathing 100% Oxygen and Exposed to 45 Seconds of +1 G$_z$

	+1 G$_z$	+5 G$_z$
PA$_{O_2}$	663.0	660.0
Pa$_{O_2}$	616.0	570.0
	(21.0)	(48.0)
PA$_{CO_2}$	35.8	39.2
	(2.6)	(2.0)
pH	7.401	7.418
	(0.028)	(0.032)
Pa$_{CO_2}$	31.0	21.6
	(2.4)	(4.3)
f	17.7	24.1
	(2.2)	(13.2)
V$_T$	0.60	0.87
	(0.15)	(0.24)
HR	85.0	158.0
	(7.0)	(25.0)

Abbreviations: PA$_{O_2}$ is alveolar oxygen tension; Pa$_{O_2}$ is arterial oxygen tension; Pa$_{CO_2}$ is arterial carbon dioxide tension; f is respiratory rate; V$_T$ is vidal volume; HR is heart rate. PA$_{CO_2}$ is alveolar carbon dioxide tension.

are loss of vision and loss of consciousness. These symptoms result from decreased retinal and cerebral blood flow. A redistribution of blood flow has been found to occur near the $+G_z$ tolerance limit such that the cerebellum and brain stem blood flow is preserved even when blood flow to the cerebrum is diminished. Cerebral blood flow under normal conditions is controlled by autoregulation. During $+G_z$ stress, it has been proposed that flow is maintained by a combination of autoregulatory vasodilatation and the siphon effect. The siphon effect is thought to result from a pressure gradient established between the afferent carotid arterial system and the efferent jugular venous system; this pressure gradient is produced when very low cerebral perfusion pressures are present.

Maintainence of adequate retinal blood flow is necessary for a full field of vision. Loss of peripheral vision followed by loss of central vision leading to a complete blackout results from a decrement in retinal blood flow. These visual symptoms occur when the arterial perfusion pressure falls below the intraocular pressure (8 to 22 mm Hg). In a series of retinal photographs taken at intervals during a rapid-onset centrifuge run at $+3.1$ G_z on a human subject whose head-level arterial pressure was measured, blackout occurred at peak plus 1.6 seconds and lasted to peak plus 8.0 seconds. This coincided with a collapse of both the central retinal artery and vein and with a concurrent fall in head-level blood pressure. At 8.0 seconds, a recovery of pressure was observed, which coincided with a filling of the retinal artery (Fig. 9–16).

Electroencephalographic (EEG) studies have been performed in association with $+G_z$ stress both on the centrifuge and in flight. No cumulative or pathologic effects of $+G_z$ stress up to $+7$ G_z in man have been observed. The electrical activity of the brain is altered during and for a short time following $+G_z$ stress, even when blackout or loss of consciousness does not occur. The EEG measurements during $+G_z$ stress have not proven to be useful either for the selection of suitable aircrew or for use as a measure of the $+G_z$ tolerance end point. The following three basic processes influenced the EEG during $+G_z$ stress:

1. Absolute central nervous system blood flow (large-magnitude EEG changes).
2. Vestibular stimuli (transient changes in EEG intensity).
3. Metabolic processes in the central nervous system tissue and compensatory hemodynamic mechanisms (long-duration shifts in baseline intensities).

Renal System

Renal blood flow decreases when man assumes an upright posture. Exercise stress causes a decrease in renal blood flow in man. It would, therefore, be predicted that the $+G_z$ stress of aerial combat maneuvering requiring an anti-G suit would result in a marked decrease in renal blood flow because $+G_z$ and exercise are combined. Renal blood flow in man has not been measured; however, in dogs and miniature swine, renal blood flow has been found to be markedly decreased during $+G_z$ stress. Using a microsphere technique, Laughlin and colleagues[7] found zero blood flow throughout the cortex, juxtamedullary cortex, and medulla to be common at $+5$ G_z and $+7$ G_z. The decreased blood flow was observed to remain decreased for up to 10 minutes after the $+G_z$ stress, with no reactive hyperemia being observed. Inflation of the miniature swine anti-G suit to the appropriate pressures used during $+5$ G_z and $+7$ G_z in the absence of the $+G_z$ stress also caused marked reduction in renal blood flow (zero blood flow much of the time). Oliguria lasting 1 hour or more has been reported to occur following brief periods of

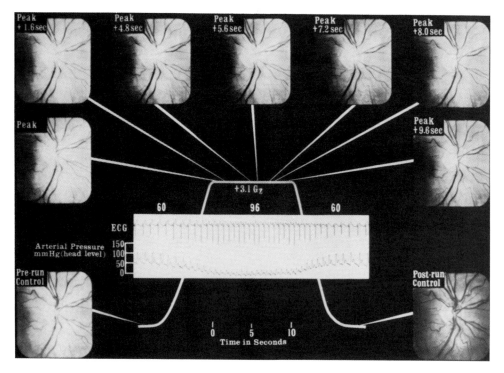

Fig. 9–16. Retinal photographs taken at intervals during a centrifuge run to $+3.1$ G$_z$.

$+$ G$_z$ stress, along with temporary sodium and potassium retention.

The mechanism for decreased renal blood flow appears to be related to a combination of factors, including direct mechanical impedance from wearing an anti-G suit, markedly increased alpha-adrenergic vascular constriction, and other humorally related mechanisms. A full investigation of the renin-angiotensin system has yet to be evaluated, although during low $+$ G$_z$ levels ($+2$ G$_z$ and $+2.5$ G$_z$), increased plasma renin levels have been measured. The renal system is important to consider when devising methods to enhance $+$ G$_z$ tolerance because even small deficits in sodium and water balance have been shown to decrease $+$ G$_z$ tolerance.

ACCELERATION-ASSOCIATED PATHOLOGIC CHANGES

Aerospace physicians and scientists have been particularly sensitive to the possibility of the stressful high $+$ G$_z$ environment resulting in pathologic changes in various body systems. The ultimate charge to the clinical aeromedical research community is to conduct research well ahead of exposure to environments in which possible pathologic changes might occur.

Although much effort has been put forth in trying to associate pathologic changes, especially cardiovascular changes, with G$_z$ stress, only one report documents a serious pathologic event in association with high $+$ G$_z$ stress. This was an isolated case of probable $+$ G$_z$ ($+9$ G$_z$) related temporary brain damage. The symptoms disappeared within 6 months. The remainder of reported possible pathologic changes have been observed in human analogs.

Cardiac Pathology

Because the most profound physiologic changes during $+$ G$_z$ stress are related to the cardiovascular system, the heart has received the most extensive investigation for possible $+$ G$_z$ related pathologic changes. Most of the early reports dealt with G_z levels (both $+G_z$ and $-G_z$) well in excess of the animal's tolerance. Although various animal studies have suggested possible myocardial injury from high $+G_z$ exposure, no pathologic changes have been detected in human centrifuge subjects. In addition, no pathologic cardiac findings suggestive of G-induced lesions have been found during autopsies carried out at the Armed Forces Institute of Pathology on high-performance fighter aircraft pilots killed in aircraft accidents. Electrocardiographic changes do not provide convincing evidence of suspected myocardial damage. It, therefore, is unlikely that myocardial damage due to $+G_z$ stress occurs within cardiovascular tolerance limits. This does not mean that experiments on the possible effects secondary to long-term chronic $+G_z$ exposure or of higher levels of sustained $+G_z$ stress should be discontinued.

Musculoskeletal Pathology

Back, neck, and limb injuries are most commonly associated with extremely high, rapid-onset acceleration forces. It remains a potential hazard that G_z forces, such as those experienced during aerial combat, aerobatics, or centrifuge exposure, could result in significant acute injury and that chronic exposure could result in degenerative disease in severely stressed areas. Further, there remains the question of deciding if certain skeletal abnormalities predispose an individual to problems related to $+G_z$ acceleration. Relatively few studies on this type of trauma have been reported. Two cases have been described of a ruptured intervertebral disk from in-flight $+G_z$ acceleration. The first case, which evidently occurred at $+9\ G_z$ involved the lumbar region between L-4 and L-5. The second case, occurring at $+5$ G_z affected the lumbosacral region. Both cases occurred during increased $+G_z$ with the back in a flexed and rotated position. It was suggested that this awkward flexed

position under $+G_z$ loading would result in severe strain on the posterior longitudinal ligament and its adjacent annulus fibrosis. The likelihood of posterior herniation of the nucleus pulposus was increased. The crouched position, used to enhance $+G_z$ tolerance, was considered detrimental from a spinal stability standpoint. The British previously reported similar problems and recommended that the crouch position be discontinued for these reasons. It has been estimated that spinal injury secondary to $+G_z$ stress while in an optimum position is unlikely until the $+20\ G_z$ range is reached, at which time the thoracic and lumbar vertebrae would be expected to fail.

Although no comprehensive study of $+G_z$ induced neck problems has been accomplished, flight surgeons at fighter aircraft bases are well aware of the frequency of neck-related problems. These problems are rarely of a long lasting, severe nature, but they do result in a decrement in performance and reduced $+G_z$ tolerance. Pilots of F-16 and F-15 aircraft regularly do neck-strengthening exercises and immediately prior to aerial combat sorties exercise the neck and shoulder muscles as a warm-up before pulling $+G_z$. Undoubtedly, the use of heavy helmets with an undesirable center of gravity exacerbates the problem, and future helmet designers must be aware of this increasing problem with high-G aircraft.

One documented case of $+G_z$ induced incapacitating paravertebral muscle sprain occurred at $+6.5\ G_z$ in an F-4 aircraft. The pilot was later found to have preexisting rotoscoliosis and a thoracic (T-11) healed vertebral compression fracture. Preexisting abnormalities such as excessive scoliosis, Scheuermann's disease, Schmorl's nodes, spondylolysis, spondylolisthesis, and degenerative disease of the vertebral column have been considered disqualifying for high $+G_z$ centrifuge experimentation. Spinal abnormalities must remain under constant scrutiny for aircrewmen who fly high-performance fighter aircraft.

Pulmonary Pathology

The lungs undoubtedly receive a major amount of stress during $+G_z$ with respect to ventilation and perfusion abnormalities and mechanical distortion and displacement. These physiologic changes are quickly reversible after the acceleration is stopped. The concern with respect to more serious structural damage to the pulmonary system is related to the major density differential between the lung and adjacent tissues. As acceleration is increased, the dense tissues are displaced more than the less dense tissues. No pathologic reports have appeared confirming structural lung damage during isolated in-flight or high $+G_z$ centrifuge stress in healthy individuals. The possible occurrence of a spontaneous pneumothorax would not be totally unexpected since an occasional pneumothorax occurs during other strenuous physical activities. At present, experience up to $+10 \ G_z$ has not demonstrated pulmonary pathologic changes. If higher and more sustained $+G_z$ stress is to be encountered, care must be taken to assure integrity of the pulmonary system.

Although $+G_z$ stress has not been associated with pathologic lung damage, higher $+G_z$ levels resulting from improved protective devices and procedures may pose threats to pulmonary integrity. Included in these protection-related procedures are positive pressure breathing and the aeroatelectasis syndrome related to breathing gas mixtures with high oxygen concentrations while wearing an anti-G suit. Positive pressure breathing has been investigated for enhancement of $+G_z$ tolerance. The potential hazards of positive pressure breathing include pneumothorax and air embolism. Although no problems have been encountered in the centrifuge experiments to date, if these methods do prove operationally useful, examination of the pulmonary system will

have added emphasis in high-performance aircraft aviator selection and retention.

Aeroatelectasis syndrome is associated with breathing oxygen-enriched gas mixtures, pulling high $+G_z$, and wearing an anti-G suit. Previous reports have documented the occurrence of aeroatelectasis in fighter pilots breathing 100% oxygen. The symptoms include retrosternal chest pain or discomfort, dyspnea, and paroxysmal coughing episodes. No residual effects are known to result from aeroatelectasis. This syndrome is related to the downward $+G_z$ forces and upward shift of the abdominal contents resulting from the inflation of the abdominal bladder of the anti-G suit, which compresses the lungs. If the distal alveoli are closed off and contain a large amount of oxygen, the gas is rapidly absorbed, causing the alveoli to collapse and resulting in atelectasis. The rate of gaseous absorption is dependent on the rate of the slowest absorbed gas in the alveolar mixture. This is normally nitrogen, which is very slowly absorbed. The problem can be reduced by avoiding breathing oxygen-rich mixtures. United States Air Force pilots currently do not breathe oxygen-rich mixtures over prolonged periods prior to aerial combat and, therefore, are not routinely affected. United States Navy pilots do routinely breathe 100% oxygen before, during, and after aerial combat, but, although they perhaps do have atelectasis, the symptoms are evidently of minimal consequence. No reports of significant problems to Navy operational aviation have been documented. For Air Force operations, the concern for aeroatelectasis has become more important with the development of newer methods of supplying aviator oxygen. Under current development is the onboard oxygen generating system, a molecular sieve system that concentrates oxygen while eliminating nitrogen. The maximum concentration capability results in approximately 95% oxygen and 5% argon, considered to be rich enough in oxygen to result in atelectasis, which has the potential for inducing symptoms. There is possibly a high degree of individual susceptibility to aeroatelectasis, and environmental factors, such as tobacco smoking, may be equally important in the development of the syndrome.

Peripheral Vascular Pathology

Symptoms related to the peripheral vascular system are the most frequent problems experienced by individuals exposed to $+G_z$ stress. Small, pinpoint, cutaneous petechiae occur in the dependent unsupported areas of the body during $+G_z$ stress. With pure $+G_z$ stress, this is predominantly in the feet and ankles, followed in decreasing frequency in the legs and arms. With an increasing $+G_x$ component, the buttocks and back are more frequently involved. It is probable that the petechiae result from rupture of the tiny peripheral capillaries secondary to the extremely high intravascular pressure. The petechiae, referred to by fighter pilots as "high-G measles," resolve in several days without particular problems. On occasion, they have a pruritic effect, probably due to the irritation of nerve endings by extravasated blood. It has been the experience at USAFSAM that frequent high $+G_z$ exposure results in the infrequent occurrence of petechiae, whereas on the initial reexposure after a long layoff, petechiae are more apt to occur over a larger area.

A less common but more painful problem results from the rupture of a larger blood vessel. One case of a $+G_z$ induced scrotal hematoma occurred at USAFSAM during a simulated aerial combat maneuver while the subject performed a vigorous straining maneuver. The hematoma resolved without sequelae, although initially it was very painful. The subject returned after complete resolution and continued to participate in high $+G_z$ acceleration research without further problems. At least one case of an in-flight incapacitation has been documented in an aviator with a varicocele who lost consciousness because of extreme pain during aerobatic training in a T-37 aircraft.

SELECTION CRITERIA AND STANDARDS FOR HIGH $+G_z$ ENVIRONMENTS

Increased $+G_z$ tolerance demands will continue to be placed on aviators flying high-performance fighter aircraft. Because of the high $+G_z$ stress, it has become increasingly important to accurately define human $+G_z$ tolerance limits. Future fighter aircraft promise even more stressful $+G_z$ environments. Future fighter pilot selection criteria may include G tolerance in the selection of individuals to fly high-performance aircraft. It is important to determine whether certain medical irregularities are associated with an altered $+G_z$ tolerance and if the condition is exacerbated during high $+G_z$ stress. Medical standards should utilize this information relative to $+G_z$ sensitivity that may compromise optimum performance or safety.

Centrifuge Research Standards

Some of the numerous reasons for exposing humans to increased $+G_z$ stress on a centrifuge include training, orientation, medical evaluation, and research. Although the basic concern for absolute well-being is the same, fundamental differences exist between human exposure to $+G_z$ stress for these various exposure reasons. Use of human volunteer subjects for research generally requires long-term intermittent exposure to $+G_z$ stress. Much of the time, the $+G_z$ levels are high and are sustained until the individual is completely exhausted. Training, orientation, and medical evaluation, on the other hand, generally require only one or two centrifuge exposures. For this reason, a rigorous medical evaluation is required for individuals who volunteer to be exposed to $+G_z$ stress as experimental subjects. The following is a list of the mandatory medical evaluation requirements for centrifuge volunteers, in the order of completion, as required at USAFSAM:

1. United States Air Force Flying Class II physical examination
   a. History and physical examination
   b. 12-lead electrocardiogram
   c. Clinical laboratory tests (blood and urine)
   d. Chest radiographs (PA and lateral)
2. Centrifuge orientation
   a. Medical evaluation protocol
   b. Minimum G-tolerance (ROR, +7 G_z × 15 seconds)*
3. Maximal treadmill exercise test
4. Echocardiogram
5. Complete spine radiograph series

The reasons for performing several of these tests are not the same as the reasons why they would be performed in a clinical diagnostic situation.

By using these stringent medical requirements, no disabling medical problems have been encountered at USAFSAM. The symptoms resulting from $+G_z$ stress were not significant, as evidenced by 3 years' experience (summarized in Table 9–10). These symptoms may be contrasted to the following list of potential problems that must be outlined, as re-

quired by the United States Air Force Advisory Committee on Human Experimentation, to any volunteer who is subjected to $+G_z$ stress:

1. Symptoms
   a. Blackout
   b. Loss of consciousness
   c. Seizures, convulsions, amnesia, confusion
   d. Vertigo
   e. Motion sickness, vomiting
   f. Dyspnea
   g. Pain, fatigue
2. Trauma
   a. Pneumothorax
   b. Muscle soreness
   c. Vertebral body compression fractures
   d. Herniated nucleus pulposus
   e. Petechial hemorrhages
   f. Swelling of the lower extremities
   g. Scrotal hematoma
   h. Hernia
3. Cardiac stress
   a. Dysrhythmias (tachycardia and bradycardia)
   b. Heart blocks
   c. Stress cardiomyopathy

Clinical Aeromedical Evaluation Using a Centrifuge

Since 1973, certain aircrew members undergoing conventional aeromedical evaluation at the USAFSAM Clinical Sciences Division have been referred for centrifuge testing in an effort to determine whether their medical condition was sensitive to $+G_z$ stress. This medical evaluation with $+G_z$ tolerance testing allows for both a determination of the suitability of the aircrew member for assignment to a high-performance aircraft and a determination of whether certain clinical parameters are consistently associated with either high or low $+G_z$ tolerance. Although it might be argued that only aviators with completely normal clinical evaluations should be selected for flying

Table 9–10. Type and Frequency of G_z Induced Symptoms Over a 3-Year Period on the USAFSAM Centrifuge

Frequency of Occurrence	Symptom Description
16	Abdominal pain
16	Arm pain
1	Clonic movements
5	Disorientation, vertigo
3	Hyperventilation
67	Loss of consciousness
2	Loss of consciousness with severe convulsion
15	Neck pain
16	Petechial hemorrhages
2	Scrotal hematoma/discomfort

*ROR is rapid-onset run at 1 G/sec.

high-performance fighter aircraft, there are two major drawbacks with this reasoning. The first drawback is the difficulty of defining accurately what a "normal" clinical evaluation really is, and the second drawback relates to the expertise and financial loss associated with disqualifying a fully qualified professional aviator.

Methods Used for G Testing

Clinical $+G_z$ tolerance measurement has been carried out using several techniques at different acceleration laboratories. Most investigators use at least two separate types of runs, including both rapid-onset and gradual-onset acceleration. The use of these two different types of runs allows an assessment of an individual's tolerance with (gradual-onset run) and without (rapid-onset run) cardiovascular reflex compensation. From the available G-time data, the rate of onset for a gradual-onset run should be slow enough to allow cardiovascular compensation to occur continually as the acceleration increases during the run. This type of gradual-onset run has an onset rate slower than approximately 0.25 G/sec. At USAFSAM, a gradual-onset run (GOR) has arbitrarily been established as 0.067 G/sec, an onset rate certainly below the required 0.25 G/sec upper limit. As shown in Figure 9–17, a rapid-onset run (ROR) is a run with an onset that is more rapid than cardiovascular reflexes can react to. A ROR would have a rate greater than 0.33 G/sec. At USAFSAM, a ROR has been set at 1.0 G/sec. The use of GORs and RORs, both relaxed and using a protective straining maneuver, allows the assessment of inherent tolerance to acceleration, the integrity of cardiovascular reflexes, and the proficiency in performance of the protective straining maneuver.

The aeromedical $+G_z$ stress protocol consists of a series of runs, including an initial relaxed GOR, GOR(1); a series of RORs; a second relaxed GOR, GOR(2); and a final GOR with performance of the pro-

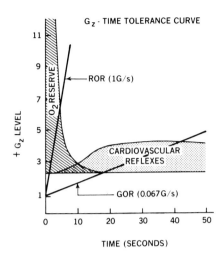

Fig. 9–17. $+G_z$ time-tolerance curve. Note the United States Air Force School of Aerospace Medicine rate of onset for a rapid-onset run (ROR) and a gradual-onset run (GOR). The GOR is slow enough to allow cardiovascular reflex compensation.

Table 9–11. G_z Tolerance Criteria For Centrifuge Profiles

	Profile Standard Values
Profile 1—GOR (1)	High—5.6 or greater
	Low—less than 4.0
	Average—4.0 thru 5.5
Profile 2—ROR (pass)	High—4.1 or greater
	Low—less than 3.1
	Average—3.1 thru 4.0
Profile 3—GOR (2)	High—5.3 or greater
	Low—less than 3.7
	Average—3.7 thru 5.2
Profile 4—GOR (S)	High—6.0 or greater
	Low—less than 4.6
	Average—4.6 thru 5.9

GOR = gradual-onset run (0.067 G/sec).
ROR = rapid-onset run (1.0 G/sec).

tective straining maneuver, GOR(S). The test results include the various $+G_z$ tolerance measurements, the electrocardiographic response, and any symptoms that occurred during the test period.

The G tolerance and heart rate response standards for this aeromedical evaluation protocol are given in Table 9–11. These standards were established using 425 healthy individuals on the USAFSAM centrifuge. The standards are given as a range of the mean, ± 2 standard deviations.

Additional G Tolerance Profiles

Although the above mentioned medical evaluation protocol serves a useful purpose in aeromedically evaluating individuals, it falls short of measuring the full spectrum of the in-flight aerial combat maneuvering environment. Although no centrifuge exposure can be an exact reproduction of the aircraft environment, certain centrifuge profiles have been developed to more closely simulate the in-flight $+G_z$ stress environment. These acceleration profiles have consisted of high $+G_z$ (greater than $+5$ G_z) RORs and SACMs. One specific high $+G_z$ ROR that has been of aeromedical use is $+7$ G_z for 15 seconds. This ROR has been considered as the minimum G-time profile that must be achieved for an individual to be fully recommended for flying high-performance fighter aircraft. Although successfully achieving $+7$ G_z for 15 seconds is an operational recommendation from clinicians, it is not an aeromedical standard that must be attained to remain on flying status. Perhaps with future higher $+G_z$ aircraft, mandatory minimum $+G_z$ tolerance standards will be adopted as part of the selection and retention criteria for fighter pilots. The currently recommended minimum tolerance of $+7$ G_z for 15 seconds was selected on the basis of experience in aeromedically evaluating aircrewmen referred for in-flight $+G_z$ induced loss of consciousness. None of these individuals referred for G tolerance evaluation and training who were able to achieve this minimum $+G_z$ standard subsequently have had operational in-flight difficulties with $+G_z$ stress upon their return to flying duty.

SACMs also have been utilized for the assessment of $+G_z$ tolerance. Typical examples of these profiles include an F-4 SACM and a $+4.5$ to $+7.0$ G_z SACM (onset rates of $+1$ G/sec). The F-4 SACM is a simulation of an actual in-flight F-4 aerial combat profile and lasts for 85 seconds

(Fig. 9–18). It is an extremely useful orientational profile for demonstrating the high $+G_z$ environment and probably is not atypical of most F-4, F-5, F-15, and F-16 flights. The $+4.5$ to $+7.0$ G_z SACM alternates for 15 seconds at each level (4.5 $+G_z$ and 7.0 $+G_z$) continuously until the subject terminates the run because of fatigue (Fig. 9–19). Tolerance using the exhaustive SACM is based on time of exposure, which represents reproducible fatigue levels. Although these SACMs more closely represent the in-flight aerial combat environment, they still are not completely satisfactory simulations. They do provide a useful method for testing the benefits of anti-G equipment. The SACMs do maximally stress the cardiovascular system and, therefore, provide a satisfactory $+G_z$ acceleration stress test profile.

Clinical Subgroup Trends

Efforts to correlate $+G_z$ tolerance with various anatomic and physiologic parameters have been made and include height and blood pressure. Because relative heart-to-eye distance in direct opposition to the G forces is a major factor in determining G tolerance, it would seem reasonable that individuals with a greater anatomic heart-to-eye distance would have a lower tolerance. Similarly, because a greater arterial driving pressure to the eyes and brain is necessary to maintain vision and consciousness, it would seem reasonable to postulate that individuals with a higher blood pressure might have enhanced tolerance.

A number of difficulties exist with respect to absolutely proving or disproving these predictions. The foremost problem is the sensitivity of the $+G_z$ tolerance testing methods. The differences in G tolerances due to isolated subtle anatomic and physiologic variations are frequently smaller than can be accurately measured. Individual differences in anxiety levels prior to $+G_z$ testing alone can more than mask the true tolerance changes.

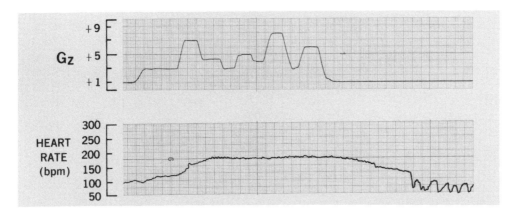

Fig. 9–18. The F-4 simulated aerial combat maneuver (SACM) with a typical heart rate response. The SACM lasts 85 seconds. Note the marked sinus arrhythmia in the recovery period.

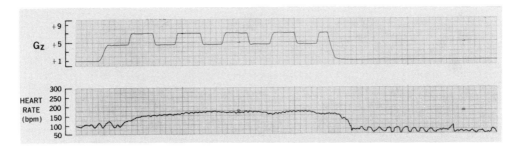

Fig. 9–19. The 4.5 to 7.0 $+G_z$ simulated aerial combat maneuver. The duration at 4.5 $+G_z$ and at 7.0 $+G_z$ is 15 seconds. The run is continued until the subject is exhausted. Note the marked sinus arrhythmia in the post $+G_z$ period.

For these reasons, many investigators have failed to find a relationship between stature (height, sitting height, or heart-to-eye distance), weight, blood pressure, various types of physical conditioning, or other parameters. Other researchers have found significant statistical correlation with weight, age, height, sitting height, blood pressure, muscle conditioning, and other parameters. Using the USAFSAM aeromedical evaluation protocol previously described, a series of clinical parameters were found to be associated with $+G_z$ tolerance. The high $+G_z$ prototype individual was found to have the parameters listed under the high-tolerance group (HTG) in Table 9–12. In addition, those individuals with clinically documented hypertension, as a group, were found to

have a higher $+G_z$ tolerance than other medical subgroups evaluated. Although the parameters are associated with increased $+G_z$ tolerance, they also are associated with increased risk for cardiovascular disease. The low $+G_z$ prototype individual characteristics are listed under the low-tolerance group (LTG). The definite existence of individuals with unusually low G_z tolerance is a real problem that frequently arises operationally. From documentation of in-flight physiologic incident reports and review of aircrewmen referred for aeromedical evaluation, it is evident that low-G tolerance individuals are frequently discovered among student pilots. These individuals are very likely predisposed to low G tolerance not only from a lack of experience but also from a

Table 9–12.   Clinical Parameters Associated With the High-G and Low-G Tolerance Subgroups*

Parameter	High-Tolerance Group (HTG)	Low-Tolerance Group (LTG)	Significance Level
Age (yr)	37 ± 5	32 ± 8	0.123
Height (in)	68.4 ± 1.6	71.3 ± 2.3	0.033†
Weight (lb)	172 ± 23	157 ± 19	0.243
Flying hours	3196 (high—5000; low—650)	1798 (high—3860; low—0)	0.165
Treadmill test			
Maximum heart rate (beats/min)	176 ± 7	186 ± 6	0.030†
Maximum time (min)	14.0 ± 3.1	14.1 ± 2.9	0.970
Maximum systolic blood pressure (mm Hg)	184 ± 11	171 ± 8	0.038†
Maximum diastolic blood pressure (mm Hg)	91 ± 13	72 ± 15	0.043†
Rest			
Heart rate (beats/min)	75 ± 17	69 ± 13	0.533
Systolic blood pressure (mm Hg)	135 ± 10	115 ± 13	0.014†
Diastolic blood pressure (mm Hg)	86 ± 19	68 ± 8	0.063
Lean body mass (lb)	132 ± 9	131 ± 19	0.941
Percent body fat	23 ± 8	18 ± 7	0.204
Hematocrit (%)	48.3 ± 0.8	45.2 ± 0.2	0.000†
Hemoglobin (g%)	15.8 ± 0.6	15.1 ± 0.6	0.068
Cholesterol (mg%)	222 ± 35	165 ± 10	0.003†
Triglyceride (mg%)	169 ± 77	92 ± 30	0.044†
Blood sugar (mg%)	112 ± 14	106 ± 11	0.463
Urine specific gravity	1.026 ± 0.004	1.021 ± 0.007	0.160

*Mean ± 1 standard deviation.
†Probability (p) > 0.05.

physiologic standpoint, because they usually have many of the low-G tolerance prototype attributes described in Table 9–12. The operational data available to the aeromedical community emphasizes that certain groups of individuals could be served very well by additional emphasis on methods for G protection and possibly specific G training.

Having an interest in continually trying to understand the factors that affect $+G_z$ tolerance, researchers have investigated special subgroups to determine if their specific characteristics are associated with altered tolerance.

Female $+G_z$ Tolerance

The entrance of more women into various aviation and aerospace disciplines has required some reinvestigation into certain physiologic responses and tolerances because much of the early work was accomplished exclusively on males. Although predictions could be made for female tolerance based on their previously documented differences in anatomic and physiologic parameters, the necessity to make $+G_z$ tolerance measurements to assure the absence of any decreased tolerance to this type of stress is essential from an aeromedical safety standpoint. Females collectively are smaller, less muscular, and have a higher percentage of body fat than their male counterparts. The effects of these and a multitude of other factors summate to determine their response to $+G_z$ stress. The preliminary results of a study to determine the response of healthy United States Air Force females to the standard aeromedical evaluation protocol previously described indicates that females do not have any impaired tolerance to $+G_z$ stress. Table 9–13 shows the heart rate and $+G_z$ tolerance response from the preliminary results of this study. Both heart rate response and tolerance were bet-

Table 9–13. $+G_z$ Tolerance and Heart Rate Response of Females to United States Air Force School of Aerospace Medicine Medical Evaluation Protocol*

G Profile	$+G_z$ Tolerance	Heart Rate Response (beats/min)
Rest	—	105.8 (15.5)
GOR (1)	4.77 (0.77)	160.5 (18.6)
ROR (pass)	3.40 (0.55)	137.4 (18.1)
GOR (2)	4.64 (0.83)	145.5 (20.3)
GOR (S)	5.55 (0.94)	169.4 (17.6)

*Mean ($\pm$15.0).

ter than previously determined data. No unusual symptoms or other problems were unique to these females with the exception of occasional urinary incontinence during high $+G_z$ while wearing an anti-G suit. There have been no documented unique problems from the Air Force operational community with respect to the female aviator exposed to in-flight $+G_z$ stress. Currently, a number of female flight surgeons have flown in fighter aircraft, including the F-15, and numerous female pilots and navigators have flown fighter-type aircraft, mostly T-37 and T-38 aircraft. The final determination of any unique problems, such as lack of upper body strength, during vigorous aerial combat maneuvering has yet to be determined.

Physical Fitness Extremes

Another special subgroup of interest are those individuals with high levels of aerobic conditioning. Although the benefits of a sound exercise program are well known and widely advocated, the unique environment of the high-performance fighter pilot may pose specific problems for the highly trained endurance individual. An overzealous endurance exerciser may develop grossly exaggerated vagal tone that predisposes him to a lowered syncopal threshold. Endurance training previously has been shown to reduce the effectiveness of blood pressure regulation. Both mean arterial pressure and heart rate fail to respond effectively to a decrease in ca-

rotid sinus pressure in endurance-trained athletes. It also has been shown that endurance-trained athletes have diminished lower-body negative pressure tolerance, an environment that simulates increased $+G_z$. In addition, vasoconstriction was less effective in these subjects than in untrained individuals. Moderate and not exclusively endurance-type exercise might well be more appropriate for those who are regularly exposed to high $+G_z$ environments. Endurance training not only causes an increase in parasympathetic activity but also a decrease in sympathetic tone. Previous work comparing the $+G_z$ tolerance of runners and weight lifters revealed that runners were less tolerant than weight lifters and further suggested that they might even be less tolerant than the control group. Other studies have failed to show any improvement in $+G_z$ tolerance with increased endurance capacity. A recent investigation of the strong vagal tone caused by heavy endurance training revealed that the vagal preponderance can suppress all automatic and conductive tissue of the heart. At times, this excess vagal tone was found to be so marked that sinoatrial or atrioventricular block developed and was associated with syncope. These observations on endurance training and $+G_z$ tolerance indicate that the type and magnitude of exercise used by fighter pilots deserve special consideration.

Using the aeromedical evaluation protocol, a group of military joggers and runners were evaluated for their response to $+G_z$ stress. The subject population (26 males) had to have been running for at least 2 years for a minimum of 20 miles per week. Although not a strict requirement, most of the subjects (23 of the 26) had previously and successfully completed a marathon. Preliminary investigation of the results in these individuals suggested that they had a low normal range of tolerance to $+G_z$ stress. The maximal heart rate response to all types of G_z stress was significantly lower than the average (Table 9–14). Interestingly, this group of individuals showed a predisposition to severe motion sickness, with 52% of the endurance-trained individuals becoming motion sick, as compared with 23% of other individuals exposed to $+G_z$ stress at USAFSAM. As previously predicted, some of these individuals did have episodes of marked cardiac slowing, with the longest sinus arrest being 4 seconds, which was associated with an episode of loss of consciousness.

ACCELERATION TOLERANCE END POINTS

$+G_z$ Stress

When the gravitoinertial forces act on the human body in a head-to-foot direction, many physiologic events take place simultaneously, any one of which could justifiably be used as an end point. For example, heart rate increases to levels approaching 200 beats/min in some individuals. The one event that is always impaired, however, is vision, varying from "fuzzy," "misting" or "veiling," "coning," "peripheral light loss" to total blackout (total loss of vision). In the early years of centrifuge research, many researchers used blackout as an end point. In some susceptible individuals, however, the difference between blackout and a loss of consciousness (LOC) can be as little as 0.1 G, thus creating a potentially and unnecessarily hazardous environment for the subject. Therefore, in recent years, con-

servative researchers use 100% peripheral light loss and 50% central light loss as the preferred end point. This is a very reproducible end point in experienced centrifuge subjects, but even using this end point, episodes of LOC do occur in the unwary. Fortunately for the subject, the LOC produces total amnesia of the event. A typical response is "What happened? Why did we stop?" Other visual end points include pupillary dilation at blackout, loss of ocular motility (blank stare), central retinal artery pulsation and then collapse at blackout, progressive and concentric narrowing of the visual fields, and a decline in visual acuity. In a typical $+G_z$ exposure approaching a subject's blackout tolerance, the individual will normally have clear vision for about 2 to 4 seconds after reaching peak G (onset rate = 1 G/sec), then peripheral vision will fail, with only a cone of central vision available for reading instruments. A second or so later, this will fail, and total blackout will occur. In about 2 more seconds, vision will suddenly return as compensatory reflexes are initiated to cause an increase in head-level blood pressure and a rise in heart rate. From that point to the end of the G exposure, vision will remain clear. The G level at which these events occur is defined as a person's blackout threshold.

Other body systems also respond to $+G_z$ and could be used as end points. For instance, respiratory frequency sometimes doubles, tidal volume decreases, there is a marked reduction in vital capacity, a

Table 9–14. $+G_z$ Tolerance and Heart Rate Response of Endurance-Trained Males to United States Air Force School of Aerospace Medicine Medical Evaluation Protocol*

G Profile	$+G_z$ Tolerance		Heart Rate (beats/min)	
	All Subjects	Upper 20%†	All Subjects	Upper 20%†
Rest	—	—	70 (14)	58 (11)
GOR (1)	4.8 (0.7)	4.5 (0.1)	125 (19)	126 (12)
ROR (pass)	3.4 (0.5)	2.9 (0.4)	104 (13)	103 (9)
GOR (2)	4.6 (0.8)	4.2 (0.7)	115 (22)	112 (15)
GOR (S)	5.6 (1.0)	5.3 (0.7)	141 (21)	143 (22)

*Mean (±15.0).
†G_z tolerance and heart rate response of the top 20% of the endurance-trained males to the USAFSAM medical evaluation protocol as determined by Vo_{2max} from treadmill exercise tolerance testing (5 subjects).

drop in total thoracic compliance, and a significant fall in arterial oxygen saturation (SaO_2). At high G levels, the subjects must continually be reminded to breathe, an action that decreases SaO_2 even more. From a cardiovascular standpoint, heart rate increases, systolic pressure at heart level falls about 30 mm Hg/G while diastolic pressure drops about 5 mm Hg/G, cardiac filling decreases, venous return falls, cardiac output falls, contractile force (dp/dt) of the ventricle increases, P-wave changes have been noted, there is some flattening of the ST segment, ectopic beats may occur, and a variety of cardiac arrhthymias can be seen, the most serious of which have been runs of ventricular tachycardia or short periods of complete asystole.

Subjectively, $+G_z$ exposure at high levels for extended periods or repeated exposures is very fatiguing. In testing an anti-G suit, a subject may endure eight to ten runs lasting 10 to 15 seconds each. Following the experiment, the subject is exhausted and ready for a rest. At extremely high levels ($+9\ G_z$ for 45 seconds in one experiment), most subjects had to be excused from work the remainder of the day and usually went immediately to bed. It is not unusual for a subject to stop a run simply due to exhaustion and fatigue. This end point was used in one study in which subjects were exposed to repetitive epochs of $+4.5$ to $7.0\ +G_z$ and back to $+4.5\ G_z$ (10 seconds at each level), never returning to 1 G until fatigue intervened and caused a halt in the run. Fighter pilots heavily engaged in aerial combat maneuvers also report great fatigue at the end of the day, sometimes missing supper and retiring for the night. Yet another event almost always seen in high-G centrifuge runs and described by all fighter pilots is the appearance of petechiae, usually in unsupported and distal dependent areas of the body. The ankles, legs, buttocks, and forearms are usually well covered with patches of petechiae. There is no pain associated with this event, and the petechiae disappear in several days. In high, repetitive $+G_z$ exposures, some ankle edema and ecchymosis are seen, and in one case, a painful scrotal hematoma occurred.

$-G_z$ Stress

The rapidly occurring and frequently debilitating symptoms seen in pilots exposed to $-G_z$ forces leave no doubt as to their severity, even at rather low levels of exposure (e.g., $-3\ G_z$ for 1 to 10 seconds). In $-1\ G_z$, the gravitoinertial forces are acting in a foot-to-head direction. One pilot exposed to $-4\ G_z$ for 30 seconds described his experience as a sense of expansion of the head together with a loss of hearing. He could not swallow, vision was disturbed, and severe pain in his head developed together with mental confusion. Pain in the eyes persisted for over an hour, and he had a severe headache for the rest of the day. Electrocardiographic recordings always reflect a severe bradycardia, and in at least one instance a 9-second asystole occurred. Arterial and venous blood pressures measured at head level indicate a decrease in the AV differential pressure, and this combined with the asystole can most certainly explain the mental confusion and subsequent loss of consciousness. Severe sinus pain, puffiness, and edema together with conjunctival vessel hemorrhage can all be explained by a sharp rise in head-level venous pressure, particularly as it approaches 100 mm Hg. For a time, it was feared that retinal hemorrhage could result from high $-G_z$ exposures, but experiments on goats, rhesus monkeys, large primates, and the accidental exposure of pilots have never shown this to be the case. The reported "red out" or "red veil" resulting from $-G_z$ can either be caused from the staining of lacrimal fluid with blood from ruptured conjunctival vessels or by the shining of bright light through the lower lid that is being forced upward over the pupil. The actual tolerance limit in humans is not known because extensive experiments have not been conducted. Experiments conducted in 1950, however, indicate tolerance to be -3 G_z for 15 to 30 seconds. On the other hand, experiments at the British Royal Air Force Institute of Aviation Medicine demonstrated a tolerance of -2 G_z for 5 minutes without undue discomfort. Finally, one United States Air Force pilot recovered from an aircraft accident that exposed him to an estimated -10 G_z for a period of 60 seconds as his aircraft was disintegrating and before he was able to initiate ejection procedures. Severe facial hemorrhage and edema resulted, but no irreversible injuries were sustained.

$+G_x$ Stress

The tolerance to $+G_x$ stress is usually related to circulatory, respiratory, and subjective end points and is heavily influenced by the angle of the spine with reference to the horizontal plane. Interest was high in exposures of this type when the Soviet Union and the United States entered the space program. Astronauts and cosmonauts both are launched from earth while recumbent in a couch, with the gravitoinertial vector acting in a chest-to-back direction. The couch $\dot{V}/\dot{Q}$ back angle varied from 8 to 12° and studies have been conducted on centrifuges with a back angle varying from 0 to 25°. Above $+8$ G_x, moderate to severe chest pain intervenes, heavy pressure develops in the chest, making respiration difficult, and there is a noticeable shift to abdominal breathing; some arrhythmias have been noted and have been related to $+G_x$ intensity and duration. Tidal volume decreases, vital capacity drops, a $\dot{V}a/\dot{Q}$ imbalance occurs, vision becomes blurred, and only hand and wrist movement is practical. With a 10° back angle, a significant $+G_z$ component develops above $+16$ G_x, leading to a loss of vision. Blackout occurs at $+10$ to $+12$ G_x when the subject is at a 25° back angle. To date, no irreversible injuries have resulted in studies carried out at a 10° back

angle to levels as high as $+26.5$ G_x for 8 seconds or at $+22$ G_x for 50 seconds. Beginning at $+8$ G_x, singly occurring ventricular extrasystoles and an occasional bigeminal pattern were evident, as was marked sinus arrhythmia. At a 0° back angle, intense pain in the retrosternal and epigastric areas, relative bradycardia with cardiac arrhythmias, and extensive changes in pulmonary function were reported, which were sufficient to reject this back angle in the experimental design. In another study with a 25° back angle, seated upright subjects lost vision at $+12$ G_x, whereas five of seven subjects blacked out below $+10$ G_x when placed in a semisupine position with the same 25° back angle in a free-swinging cab on a centrifuge. Therefore, it appears a back angle of 10° is probably optimum to increase tolerance in the $+G_x$ direction. In the $-G_x$ position (gravitoinertial force acting in a back-to-chest direction), there is no chest pain and no blackout, at least up to levels of -12 G_x. It is impossible to raise the body trunk, thighs, legs, or arms above 8 G_x, but forearm, hand, finger, and ankle movements are relatively unimpaired. When a counterbalance head restraint system is used, head movements and speech are possible at -12 G_x. In one study, tolerance at -12 G_x was stated to be longer than 30 seconds. Limiting factors were dyspnea, pooling of blood in dependent parts of the extremities, with petechial hemorrhage formation in the skin, postrun dizziness, edema of the periorbital tissues, and tachycardia.

PROTECTION AND ENHANCEMENT TECHNIQUES FOR $+G_z$

Physiologic Protection-Straining Maneuvers

In the research that led to the development of G suits, excellent physiologic studies addressed the cause of blackout and loss of consciousness.[10] It also was found that a pilot straining against stick pressure while pulling G improved his tolerance above that with the G suit alone. The rapid fall in head-level blood pressure that leads to decreased cerebral blood flow and eventually to a cessation in retinal blood flow can effectively be countered by performing a muscular straining maneuver while exhaling against a partially closed or fully closed glottis. Two straining maneuvers have been developed to assist pilots during strenuous aerial combat maneuvering: the M-1 and L-1 maneuvers.

M-1 Maneuver

Pilots commonly refer to the M-1 maneuver as the "grunt" maneuver because it approximates the physical effort required to lift a heavy weight. The M-1 maneuver consists of pulling the head down between the shoulders, slowly and forcefully exhaling through a partially closed glottis, and simultaneously tensing all skeletal muscles. Pulling the head downward gives some degree of postural protection by shortening the vertical head-to-heart distance; intrathoracic pressure is increased by strong muscular expiratory efforts against a partially closed glottis, and the contraction of abdominal and peripheral muscles raises the diaphragm and externally compresses capacitance vessels. For long-duration G exposures, the maneuver must be repeated every 4 to 5 seconds. When properly executed, the exhalation phase of the M-1 maneuver results in an intrathoracic pressure of 50 to 100 mm Hg, raising the arterial blood pressure at head level and thereby increasing $+G_z$ tolerance by at least 1.5 G. The inspiratory phase of the M-1 maneuver must be a fast "gasp," to be followed immediately by the slower exhalation phase, because mean blood pressure can fall to approximately zero during inspiration.

L-1 Maneuver

The L-1 maneuver is similar to the M-1 maneuver except that the aircrew member forcefully exhales against a completely closed glottis while tensing all skeletal

muscles. Using either maneuver, the pilot obtains equal protection, that is, 1.5 G greater than relaxed blackout level with or without the anti-G suit. In a 1972 study, subjects wearing anti-G suits and performing either the M-1 or L-1 straining maneuver were able to maintain adequate vision during a centrifuge exposure of $+9\,G_z$ for 45 seconds. Higher and longer runs have not been attempted. It is important to note, however, that forcefully exhaling against a closed glottis without vigorous skeletal muscular tensing (Valsalva maneuver) can reduce $+G_z$ tolerance and lead to an episode of unconsciousness at extremely low G levels. Therefore, instruction and training on the proper method of performing these straining maneuvers are essential.

In a number of cases when a fighter pilot is medically evaluated for low G tolerance, it is found that he is performing an improper or inadequate straining maneuver. Many cases of loss of consciousness in flight have been attributed to the performance of a Valsalva maneuver rather than an M-1 or L-1 maneuver. When these properly performed straining maneuvers are used in combination with G-suit inflation, the protection is additive.

Physical Condition

A recent study involved three separate groups of subjects: (1) ambulatory; (2) those in a running program; and (3) those in a weight-lifting program. Those individuals in a weight-lifting program had an improved tolerance to long-duration repetitive $+G_z$ stress. It was felt that these individuals could more effectively perform the required M-1 or L-1 straining maneuvers than subjects involved in only distance running or ambulatory subjects. A further study designed to specifically condition abdominal and thigh muscles demonstrated improved duration at G when compared with other subjects who conditioned only arm and back muscles. From a medical standpoint, it would be wise to encourage pilots of high-performance fighter aircraft to participate in physical conditioning programs that include both running and weight lifting. A definitive program to design a specific exercise regimen for fighter aircraft pilots awaits development.

Centrifuge Training

Training of selected fighter pilots on a centrifuge exposing them to G forces similar to those that occur in aerial combat has been successfully accomplished. Whether it improved their G tolerance or increased their ability to outmaneuver their adversary was not determined. Their comments, however, suggest that they were able to concentrate on learning a proper straining maneuver without the distraction of flying or maneuvering the aircraft while engaging other aircraft in aerial combat. A number of centrifuges throughout the world are currently training fighter pilots initially to high G environments. Other centrifuges being planned have G training as one of their missions.

Carbon Dioxide Breathing

It has been shown that breathing 5 to 7% carbon dioxide will increase tolerance by about 0.5 G in experienced subjects. The physiologic mechanism apparently is the action of carbon dioxide on the carotid-aortic chemoreceptors, leading to peripheral vasoconstriction, and by direct action on cerebral blood vessels, leading to vasodilatation. In addition, carbon dioxide shifts the oxygen dissociation curve to the right, increasing the unloading of oxygen to tissues and aiding oxygen uptake in areas with reduced blood flow due to the gravitoinertial effects. Whether carbon dioxide breathing would be operationally feasible remains to be seen.

Venous Constriction

Centrifuge studies in both canines and humans have shown that venous constriction occurs in response to a drop in the carotid-aortic arch pressure similar to arteriolar constriction during the imposition of $+G_z$ stress. Venous constriction, however, has the added benefit of potentially releasing large reservoirs of peripherally trapped blood, thus making it available for venous return and increasing cardiac output. The overall benefit of this venoconstriction in increasing $+G_z$ tolerance cannot be quantified, but it must be additive to the arterial pressor response, to the inflation of the G suit, and to the properly performed straining maneuver.

Mechanical Protection

The first anti-G device was an inflatable abdominal belt developed by Poppen,[11] who experimented with it in 1932. Further refinement by Armstrong and Heim inflated the belt with a carbon dioxide cartridge; however, this did not significantly improve the subject's tolerance to G forces. In Canada, Franks developed the first workable G suit with his water-filled device, but it was not acceptable because of its weight, production of a high heat load in pilots, and, most important, the impression by pilots that they were "free-floating" and could not get a feel for the aircraft's maneuvering. Finally, in 1944, the United States Army Air Force G-3A anti-G suit became a standard item of use for fighter pilots. The 1981 United States Air Force CSU 3-B/P anti-G suit is shown in Figure 9–20.

The anti-G valve used to inflate the anti-G suit was developed in January, 1944. It opened at about 2 G and delivered pressure to the suit at the rate of 1.5 psi/G to a maximum of 10.0 psi, at which point a pressure relief valve opened to avoid overinflation of the suit and severe, painful abdominal pressure on the pilot. The operational characteristics of anti-G valves throughout the world remained approximately the same until a high-flow ready-pressure anti-G valve was developed at the USAFSAM in 1979 for use in high-performance fighter aircraft. The function of

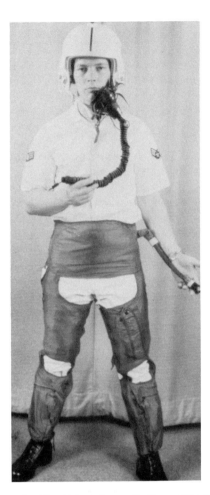

Fig. 9–20. The United States Air Force CSU 3-B/P anti-G suit.

the anti-G suit/valve combination is to provide counterpressure to the lower part of the body and the abdominal area during high-G maneuvering. It probably does very little to improve venous return because studies demonstrate that inflation of the leg bladders alone without inflation of the abdominal bladder increases tolerance by only 0.2 G. More likely, it improves tolerance in several ways. First, it increases peripheral resistance and thus aids in improving blood pressure. Second, it helps to prevent the rapid extravasation of plasma from the blood vessels into tissue during G stress by offering immediate counterpressure. Third, it may play some

role in increasing venous return, particularly with the simultaneous inflation of both the leg and abdominal bladders. Finally, it supports and raises the diaphragm, thus supporting the heart and decreasing the heart-to-eye distance.

Positive Pressure Breathing

Relatively few studies have been accomplished using positive pressure breathing as a means of improving G tolerance, but results indicate a significant increase in tolerance. The mechanism for improving $+G_z$ tolerance with positive pressure breathing is thought to be through a secondary stimulation of the baroreceptor apparatus, similar to that seen when arterial blood pressure falls in the carotid-aortic arch regions. When positive pressure breathing is used at 1 G, there is a rapid rise in systemic arterial pressure (Psa), and the elevated intrapleural pressure is applied directly to the heart and intrathoracic great vessels. This causes an initial rise in Psa equal to the increase in intrapleural pressure. Eventually, as a result of the rise in intrapleural pressure, venous return decreases, leading to a fall in Psa. This secondary fall in Psa then results in a baroreceptor response which leads to another rise in Psa that occurs 10 to 15 seconds after the beginning of positive pressure breathing at 1 G. In a 1973 study, Shubrooks showed a significant improvement in $+G_z$ tolerance in subjects who used positive pressure breathing at 30 to 40 mm Hg. He obtained direct Psa through a catheter system during positive pressure breathing. Positive pressure breathing at levels up to $+8 G_z$ was much less fatiguing than performing the M-1 straining maneuver, and this improvement in the ability to withstand high, sustained G increased with the addition of inflation of the anti-G suit. One of the difficulties of positive pressure breathing is the ability of a pilot to learn to breathe and communicate against pressures of up to 30 to 40 mm Hg. Brief training periods using positive pressure breathing have shown that it is easy to overcome the initial respiratory difficulty. In another study at the British Royal Air Force Institute of Aviation Medicine, in-flight studies were conducted with the pilot using positive pressure breathing through a valve regulated to increase or decrease the pressure breathing level depending on the G level imposed on the aircraft. Subjectively, it was found that the pilot could withstand high-G maneuvering for extended periods of time with less fatigue than with the anti-G suit. The pilots quickly learned to utilize positive pressure breathing while maneuvering the aircraft and felt they could adequately converse through the communications system. If chest counterpressure is added to positive pressure breathing and limb counterpressure, still-greater increases in systemic arterial blood pressure can be obtained, thus improving G tolerance. Frequently, the Psa reaches values greater than that of the applied breathing pressure. The optimum anti-G suit of the future may be one that employs the use of positive pressure breathing together with whole-chest counterpressure combined with limb counterpressure. Thus, the anti-G suit counterpressure system would extend from the limbs up to the chest region while the pilot was using positive pressure breathing. In this manner, both venous return and improved systemic arterial blood pressure would be achieved through physiologic and mechanical mechanisms that could potentially enhance $+G_z$ tolerance over that which exists today. Positive pressure breathing to levels of 30 to 40 mm Hg pressure for durations of up to 60 seconds does not appear to impede venous return and cardiac output to the extent that presyncopal symptoms result. It is well known, however, that performing positive pressure breathing at 1 G at levels above 80 to 100 mm Hg can lead to a rapidly occurring loss of consciousness. Therefore, there is an optimum balance between the effectiveness

of positive pressure breathing to improve systemic arterial blood pressure and the detrimental effect of positive pressure breathing, impeding venous return, which could lead to the catastrophic consequences of loss of consciousness in flight.

Water Immersion Protection

The use of water immersion as a method for protecting subjects from high gravitational forces has been investigated for many years. As early as the mid-1930s, the Germans proposed the use of hydrostatic counterpressure as a means of improving G tolerance. Theoretically, this could significantly improve G tolerance because hydrostatic pressure would serve as the perfect counterpressure to the gravitoinertial forces that cause blood to be pooled in the lower extremities. The Franks flying suit was a spinoff from this concept. The Mayo Clinic group actually built and tested a system in which subjects were immersed in water up to the third rib or to the sternum. It was found that an improvement in G tolerance could be achieved in those subjects immersed to the third rib but those who were immersed to the sternum had a decreased tolerance. This indicated that the gravitational forces acting through the water impeded cardiac output when the water level was above the heart; however, it tended to improve G tolerance when the water level was below the heart. The Wright Field group used an aluminum sarcophagus filled with water to evaluate the effectiveness of water immersion in improving $+G_x$ tolerance. The immersed, supine subject breathed through a scuba diver's valve and mask system and attempted to balance the breathing pressure across the chest to a comfortable level by regulating the level of the valve. Subjects were able to achieve $+12 G_x$ for approximately 4 minutes using this system but were unable to regulate the breathing pressure to a comfortable level. The final chapter in water immersion protection was conducted at the Naval Air Development

Center (NADC) centrifuge. Researchers constructed an "iron maiden" into which the seated, upright subject was placed. The iron maiden was installed on the arm of the centrifuge and was filled with water to the level of the subject's mouth. The subject then held his breath and the iron maiden was completely filled with water. The centrifuge was quickly accelerated up to the predetermined G level, in this instance $+16$ G_z for a short duration or as long as the subject could hold his breath. The researchers then modified the iron maiden with a standpipe that attempted to balance the hydrostatic pressure across the chest with increasing positive pressure breathing. With this modification, they were able to comfortably achieve $+31$ G_z for 5 seconds without difficulty. Finally, they exposed several primates to levels up to $+31$ G_z using the iron maiden and the standpipe. No further centrifuge studies have been conducted using this system due to some pathologic changes that occurred in the chimpanzees that were exposed to the extremely high levels of G. It should be stated, though, that the concept of water immersion for improving $+G_z$ tolerance has merit. It greatly improves the movement of arms and limbs under water during G. The difficulty at this time is achieving an adequate balanced breathing pressure across the chest wall and lung.

Body Positioning

Prone Position

Beginning in 1935, German investigators at their Aeromedical Research Institute in Berlin commenced investigations on the use of body positioning as a means of improving tolerance to G stress. Bührlen[12] exposed human subjects to ±17 G_x with the gravitoinertial vector acting in either the back-to-chest or chest-to-back direction. Subsequently, in-flight tests were conducted beginning in 1938 using a high-G research glider, the FS-17. This glider contained a prone bed with such

components as an adjustable chin and armrest and other supporting systems, as well as control devices and restraint systems. It had a maximum load factor of 14 G; the pilot had to initiate a dive to increase the glider's speed in order to produce G loads of long duration. Sustained G loads of up to $+8$ G_z and $+9$ G_z were routinely tested, and in at least one flight, the G load reached a peak of $+14$ G_z after a sharp pullout at low altitude. Subjectively, pilots reported that sustained G loads of $+8$ G_z and $+9$ G_z could easily be tolerated and did not interfere with their flight performance. There was no complaint about comfort, and the visibility forward and downward was judged to be superior to the conventional upright seated position. These studies later resulted in the development of the BV40, in which the pilot was in a prone-position couch with his head counterbalanced and resting on a chin rest; his controlling forearm was on an armrest for comfort. Seven prototypes of this glider fighter were constructed but were never placed in operational use due to higher priorities. In 1948, a prone bed was constructed at the Aerospace Medical Research Laboratory. This prone bed consisted of a nylon hammock net with an adjustable jaw rest, a counterweighted headrest support, and an adjustable footrest. In addition, special armrests were integral with the airplane controls. This prone bed was then inserted into an F-80E with an extended nose. Pilots flying the aircraft felt that it was satisfactory and that the aircraft was controllable. Forward and downward visibility was superb, and lateral visibility was adequate, but rearward and upward vision was very restricted. This was particularly noticeable in steep turns, where it was impossible to see more than an estimated 30° ahead of the aircraft. Vision is one of the limiting factors in the use of a prone-position seat in fighter aircraft. The improvement in G tolerance is well documented, and fighters potentially could be constructed that employed a prone-position seat. The emphasis now, however, appears to be on the use of a supinating seat.

Supine Position

The Germans again are given credit for early investigations into the improvement in G tolerance using the supine position. Bührlen[12] conducted many of these studies on the German centrifuge beginning in 1935. Also in 1935, a tailless glider, the Horten HoII, was developed as a pure flying wing to investigate the ability of a pilot to fly while in the supine position. In 1936, Wiesenhoefer developed a "flop-back seat" that automatically flopped back as the G load increased above $+3\,G_z$, allowing the seat back to be tilted backward and downward until a horizontal position was reached and allowing the seat to move forward. When the acceleration decayed, two spiral springs pulled the seat back again into the conventional upright position where it was automatically locked. This seat was installed in a biplane dive bomber, the Heinkle He50, and was flight-tested in the fall of 1938. Test subjects were exposed to $+G_x$ loads for 15 seconds up to peaks of $+7\,G_x$. At this point, the German Air Force high command deemphasized the efforts of protective aircrew positioning and all work on these systems was halted. In 1940, Stewart (of the British Royal Air Force) modified the observer seat of a light bomber, Fairey Battle, to support a wooden mockup that was inclined backward at the greatest angle possible. This was approximately 45° from the vertical due to structural limitations. The maximum G obtainable was 6 to 6.2 G, but most of the runs entailed accelerations of over 5 G for 10 to 20 seconds and a plateau of 6 G for 6 to 9 seconds.

Using this same concept, Stauffer, at the Naval Aviation Research Laboratory, developed another seat that would automatically reposition a conventionally seated pilot to a supinated position as G forces acted in the direction of head to hips and exceeded 3.9 G. The backrest of the seat rotated backward to place the subject in a modified supine position. This position was maintained until the G force had dropped below 2.7 G, when the backrest returned to its original position. Stauffer found that subjects could withstand stresses up to 12 G for 5 seconds in this position without further protection. An interesting aspect of the study was that if a subject lost his vision (blacked out) while sitting in the upright conventional position, his vision was restored when automatically tilted to the supine position. Gell reported on a supinating seat that was installed in the rear cockpit of a United States Navy F7F-2N airplane. The seat was controlled by the occupant, who could supinate himself to a point 87° backward from the upright position. The supinated pilot, when he desired, could take over control of the airplane through a PIK autopilot device. In the centrifuge portion of the study, Gell described a seat that could be tilted backward and fixed rigidly from the upright sitting position to angles of 15°, 25°, 35°, 45°, 55°, 65°, 77°, and 85°. Thus, the gravitoinertial vector at the higher angles would be in a progressively greater $+G_x$ direction. The 15° angle simulates the standard fighter seatback angle of today. Gell found that supination from 0 to 45° backward tilt offered no significant increase in G tolerance to blackout. Protection increased slowly until the 77° backward tilt position was reached, at which point the average increase in blackout level was no more than that afforded by an anti-G suit in its maximum inflation. G tolerance to blackout increases sharply beyond 77°, to 15 G or more at an 85° tilt. Apparently, the supine seat affords little protection against blackout until the subject is practically supine. Gell concluded that a healthy male subject could tolerate 15 G while supinated at 85° for 5 seconds with no indication of impending blackout. Later, Burns at USAFSAM conducted studies at varying seatback angles. Using vision as an end point, he found that there was no significant difference between relaxed tolerance at the control angle of 13° and 30°; however, at 45°, there was a significant increase in tolerance compared to control. Thereafter, tolerance continued to increase in an exponential manner to 8 G at 75°, an increase of 100% over control. He also found that as seatback angle increased from the vertical, the peak heart rate during acceleration decreased significantly. For subjects in which an esophageal balloon was used to measure intrathoracic pressure, it was found that the pressure decreased with increasing back angles, indicating that less work was required at the higher angles to perform the M-1 straining maneuver in order to maintain adequate vision at all back angles.[13]

Von Beckh[14] developed the PALE (pelvis and legs elevating) seat, which could automatically rotate a subject about his eye point and convert from a seatback angle of 13° to 75° in 1 second. This unique device was used in experiments at NADC. Some subjects were able to achieve 14 G at 75° for 45 seconds without a loss of peripheral vision. This same system was flight-tested in a helicopter to ensure that pilots could fly in a supine position. All three test pilots reported favorably on their ability to fly and preferred the 55° and 70° seatback angles.[14]

In G training experience, approximately 240 fighter pilots were exposed to levels of $+15$ G_x at USAFSAM. The duration above $+10$ G_x in this instance was 25 seconds. The back angle of the couch was 82° from the vertical. Only one subject in this group experienced an episode of loss of consciousness and this occurred as a result of breathholding while going over the top at $+15$ G_x; the loss of consciousness episode occurred at approximately $+13$ G_x on the way down. As the centrifuge came to an emergency stop, this pilot asked the typical question: "Why did you stop?" Other symptoms in these exposures included moderate to severe chest pain, cardiac arrhythmias, blurring of vision, difficulty in breathing, and an increase in heart rate. One pilot stated he felt "as if an elephant were sitting on my chest."

Operational Use of the Tiltback Seat

Today, the United States Air Force F-16 fighter and the Swedish Air Force Drachen have 30° seats. The pilots are very favorable in their opinion regarding the comfort of the seat. In addition, they feel they have a 2 G advantage over an adversary who is in a conventional 13° seat. One centrifuge study compared G tolerance in subjects at seatback angles of 23°, 28°, and 40° (seatback angle plus 10° angle of attack). This demonstrated improvement in relaxed tolerance in the 40° angle was significant only when compared with the 28° seat. The 40° seat, however, was more acceptable due to greater comfort, less fatigue, greater pilot acceptance, and a statistically significant reduction in the increased mean heart rate associated with G exposure.

The justification for use of a tiltback seat in high-performance fighter aircraft appears obvious if G protection is the only reason for placing the seat in the aircraft. Whether fighters will be required to maneuver at high G in air combat is an operational question. Air tactics may solely employ the use of air-to-air missiles that do not require high-G maneuvering to come into position for firing; however, a typical gun engagement is one requiring close-in firing from 450 m or less; thus, high-G maneuvering is essential. Air missile avoidance tactics will continue to require high-G maneuvers. If high-G maneuvering to 12 G or more is going to be a part of the tactical aircraft armamentarium of capabilities, it would appear that an automatic tiltback seat up to at least 55 to 65° supination will be required to achieve a tactical advantage over a similarly trained but upright adversary.

THE IN-FLIGHT ENVIRONMENT

The military in-flight environment is a unique multistress environment. The summation of altitude, mental, physical, emotional, thermal, and acceleration stress can be awesome. Continual monitoring of the in-flight environment is necessary to allow aerospace medicine physicians and scientists to assure safety and to continually improve the protective devices and procedures for assisting the aviator in higher stress situations.

Acceleration profiles are dependent not only on the type of aircraft but also on the type of mission flown. The most stressful environment is probably that of aerial combat. A complete description of the in-flight acceleration environment includes the following:

1. Duration of the flight and the length of the G maneuvering.
2. Rate of G onset/offset.
3. Peak G.
4. G-time integration.

Knowing these parameters allows a better approximation of the in-flight acceleration environment for use in aeromedical research and as an aid in clinical evaluation. In-flight G monitoring alone cannot result in a full appreciation of the total stress. Additional parameters, such as heart rate, respiratory rate, and body temperature, likewise can only approximate the true environment. Even with these limitations, there are all too few in-flight investigations of physiologic responses to the aerial combat environment. Burton's stress response investigation of high-performance fighter aircraft pilots (F-15 and F-106) during aerial combat maneuvers is one of these few critically needed studies.[15]

F-15 and F-16 Aircraft

The United States Air Force and Navy currently have the F-15, F-16, F-18, and F-14, which are air-superiority aircraft capable of high, sustained $+G_z$. These aircraft have high-onset acceleration rates of $+G_z$, above $+6$ G_z/sec. This capability makes them specifically liable for $+G_z$-induced symptoms that limit performance (grayout, tunnel vision, and blackout) or result in loss of consciousness. The seat-back angles in the F-15 and F-14 give no protection with regard to $+G_z$ stress. A wide field of vision is achieved with a bubble canopy. This allows the aviators to move about within the seat and cockpit to "check six," or look behind the aircraft. This movement during aerial combat can result in the head and neck being placed in extremely awkward positions during the highest levels of $+G_z$. This also puts a severe amount of strain on the musculoskeletal system of the neck, back, and shoulders. The amount of strain on the neck is not limited to being a sole function of $+G_z$ but is also dependent on the mass and center of gravity of the helmet and other attachments to the head and helmet. Thus, development of an extremely lightweight helmet with a low resultant center of gravity for high, sustained $+G_z$ maneuvering is needed.

Time tracings of simulated aerial combat for F-15 versus F-15 and F-15 versus F-5 recording the G levels experienced for the total flights have been recorded. The maximum $+G_z$ was $+7.5$ G_z. The maximum rate of onset was greater than $+6$ G_z/sec. The maneuvering time was approximately 300 seconds. The maximum $-G_z$ was -0.5 G_z. In-flight recordings of 1 hour aerial combat sorties (F-16 versus F-16, one on one) have also been obtained. The maximum $+G_z$ was $+9.0$ G_z. The maximum rate of onset was greater than $+6$ G/sec. The maximum $-G_z$ was -0.2 G_z. The F-16 has an aerodynamic G-limiter maximum of $+9.0$ G_z. As shown in Figure 9–21, the maximum angle of attack is related to the maximum $+G_z$ level.

The F-16 is a computer-controlled "fly-by-wire" system with a side stick controller. Both stick and rudder pedals are pressure-input controlled, thereby requiring

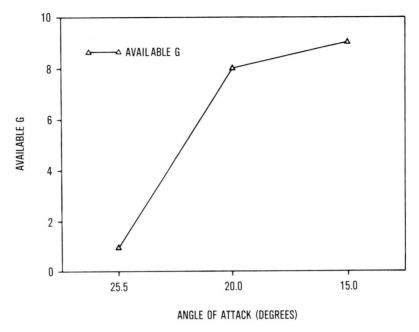

Fig. 9–21. Plot of the angle of attack versus the available $+G_z$ for the F-16 as controlled by the G-limiter.

only very slight actual movement. The seatback angle is 30°, with the heels elevated. The tiltback seat angle and seat configuration give added comfort not just during the short periods of high $+G_z$ but also during the longer cross-country trips. From an aeromedical/physiologic standpoint, one must agree with Colonel Ettinger's view on the benefits of the F-16's tiltback seat: "as more pilots fly the F-16s, I am personally convinced the United States Air Force will not produce another fighter without a slope back seat."[16]

Although first-line high-performance fighter aircraft should present the greatest challenge, other aircraft can produce severe stress to the aviators who fly them. Aircraft such as the A-10 and A-37 fall into this category. Gillingham has quantified the $+G_z$ stress for the A-10 aircraft. High $+G_z$ is not the only stress necessary for the induction of fatigue. The prolonged but lower $+G_z$ used in the "jinking" maneuvers of the low-flying A-10 carry a different set of stress parameters related to $+G_z$.

Indeed, high, sustained $+G_z$ is not even necessary to induce the most worrisome $+G_z$ symptom, which is loss of consciousness. Within a single 12-month period, over 30 episodes of $+G_z$ induced loss of consciousness were documented in United States Air Force T-37 aircraft. The mean $+G_z$ level for those episodes of loss of consciousness was only $+3.7$ G_z, with a range from $+2$ to $+6.5$ G_z. The individuals involved were mostly student pilots who theoretically fit a low G tolerance profile, not only because of a lack of experience but also from a physiologic standpoint. It is evident that many individuals are susceptible to $+G_z$ induced loss of consciousness at low $+G_z$ levels and that G-induced loss of consciousness incidents are probably more commonly documented in dual-seat aircraft.

Civilian In-Flight G_z Environment

Differences exist in the military and the civilian G_z environments. Although different, the civilian environment is by no means less stressful. Mohler's extremely fine treatise of the G effects on the pilot during aerobatics has served as a reference

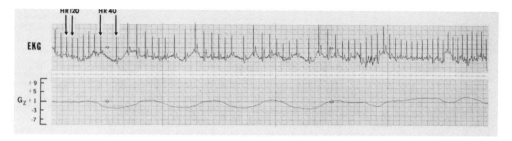

Fig. 9–22. Heart rate response to variable $+G_z$ and $-G_z$ during a typical civilian aerobatic profile. Note the abrupt slowing of heart rate during $-G_z$.

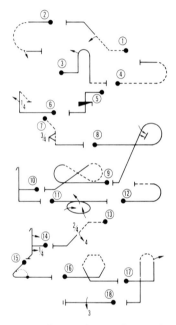

Fig. 9–23. Typical Aresti diagram for an advanced civilian aerobatic flight.

for those interested in this phase of aviation. Mohler's document was prompted by an overall lack of physiologic knowledge and coordinated aeromedical effort to assure aeromedical safety. Specific aerobatic maneuvers such as the vertical eight, if performed in the sequence of a negative G_z upper loop followed by a positive G_z lower loop, have been suggested to result in an unusually sensitive physiologic state that leaves the pilot prone to loss of consciousness. The reverse maneuver, with a positive G_z upper loop followed by a negative G_z lower loop, was found to reduce

susceptibility to loss of consciousness. Other researchers have indicated that certain competitive maneuvers may be unusually hazardous, such as when increased $+G_z$ rapidly follows increased $-G_z$. For these reasons, it is imperative that a continual vigil be maintained on the aerobatic community to help improve performance and maintain maximum safety. The question of safety should remain foremost for the aeromedical community as long as there are continued reports of aerobatic in-flight loss of consciousness and possible resulting accidents.

With the increased $-G_z$ levels, the question of the physiologic response to these maneuvers becomes important. Frazer described the effects of $-G_z$, with $-5 G_z$ for 5 seconds being the limit of tolerance. It is very likely that acclimatization to these maneuvers is attained with training and frequent exposures. Bloodwell made simultaneous heart rate and G_z recordings, and they do show marked heart rate variations: increased heart rate with $+G_z$ and decreased heart rate with $-G_z$ (Fig. 9–22). Advanced aerobatic sequences resulted in a minimum heart rate of 32 beats/min at $-3.8 G_z$. The heart rate in-flight prior to the onset of aerobatic maneuvering was 118 beats/min. The maximum heart rate was 188 beats/min at $+7.0 G_z$. The heart rate decreased from 175 to 40 beats/min within five beats during $+G_z$ to $-G_z$ maneuvering. The maximum rate of onset of $+G_z$ was $+6$ G/sec, with a maximum $-G_z$ rate of onset of -6 G/sec. Excursions from

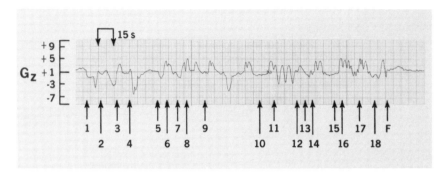

Fig. 9–24. The continuous electrocardiographic G_z profile for the Aresti diagram flight shown in Figure 9–23. The numbers refer to the start of the specific maneuvers. Note the rather high degree of $-G_z$ exposure.

$+5$ to -5 G_z over 3 seconds have occurred. The Aresti diagram for a typical "advanced known" aerobatic flight in a Pitts S-1 is given in Figure 9–23. The G_z profile for the aerobatic flight diagrammed in Figure 9–23 is shown in Figure 9–24. Such high-risk exposures should be documented and the information provided to the competitors and safety supervisors. It is important that the investigations serve not only to achieve safety but also strive to not unnecessarily limit vigorous aerobatic competition.

REFERENCES

1. Gauer, O.: The physiological effects of prolonged acceleration. In German Aviation Medicine, World War II, Vol. I. Washington, D.C., Government Printing Office, 1950.
2. Sharp, G.R., and Ernsting, J.: The effects of long duration acceleration. In Aviation Medicine: Physiology and Human Factors. Edited by G. Dhenin and J. Ernsting. London Tri-Med Books Ltd., 1978, pp. 208–241.
3. Parkhurst, M.S., Leverett, S.D., Jr., Shubrooks, S.: Human tolerance to high, sustained $+G_z$ acceleration. Aerospace Med., 43:708, 1972.
4. Howard, P.: The physiology of positive acceleration. In A Textbook of Aviation Physiology. Edited by J.A. Gillies. New York, Pergamon Press, 1965, pp. 551–687.
5. Burton, R.R., Leverett, S.D., Jr., Michaelson, E.D.: Man at high, sustained $+G_z$ acceleration: A review. Aerospace Med., 45(10):1115–1136, 1974.
6. Glaister, D.H.: The Effects of Gravity and Acceleration on the Lung. AGARDograph 133. England, Technivision Services, 1970.
7. Laughlin, M.H., Witt, W.M., Whittaker, R.N., and Jones, E.F.: Coronary blood flow in conscious miniature swine during $+G_z$ acceleration stress. J. Appl. Physiol., 49(3):462–470, 1980.
8. Lamb, L.E.: Cardiopulmonary aspects of aerospace medicine. In Aerospace Medicine. 2nd Ed. Edited by H.W. Randel. Baltimore, Williams & Wilkins Co., 1971.
9. Whinnery, J.E.: Acceleration effects of pulmonary blood flow distribution using perfusion scintigraphy. Aviat. Space Environ. Med., 51(5):485–491, 1980.
10. Wood, E.H., Lambert, E.H., Baldes, E.J., and Code, C.F.: Effects of acceleration in relation to aviation. Fed. Proc., 5(3):327–344, 1946.
11. Leverett, S.D., Jr., Whitney, R.U., and Zuidema, G.D.: Protective devices against acceleration. In Gravitational Stress in Aerospace Medicine. Edited by O.H. Gauer and G.D. Zuidema. Boston, Little, Brown and Co., 1961, pp. 211–220.
12. Bührlen, L.: Versuche uber die Bedeutung der Richtung beim Einwerken von Fliehkizaften auf den menschlichen Korper. Luftfahrtmed., 1:307–325, 1937.
13. Burns, J.W.: Re-evaluation of a tilt-back seat as a means of increasing acceleration tolerance. Aviat. Space Environ. Med., 46(1):55–63, 1975.
14. von Beckh, H.J.: The Development and Airborne Testing of the PALE Seat. NADC-81200-60, Naval Air Systems Command, Washington, D.C., Government Printing Office, June 20, 1981.
15. Burton, R.R., Storm, W.F., Johnson, L.W., and Leverett, S.D., Jr.: Stress responses of pilots flying high-performance aircraft during aerial combat manuevers. Aviat. Space Environ. Med., 48(4):301–307, 1977.
16. Ettinger, R.C.: The operational roles of the F-16. AGARD Conference Proceedings. 226, 1–1, 1980.

Chapter *10*

Vibration, Noise, and Communication

Henning E. von Gierke and Charles W. Nixon

Whoever, in the pursuit of science, seeks after immediate practical utility,
may generally rest assured that he will seek in vain.
HERMAN L.F. HELMHOLTZ, ACADEMIC DISCOURSE, 1862.

Aerospace systems produce perhaps the most severe noise and vibration environments experienced by man. These biomechanical force environments, singly and in combination, threaten the health, safety, and well-being of persons associated with or exposed to aerospace operations. Mechanical vibration transmitted to human operators can induce fatigue, degrade comfort, interfere with performance effectiveness, and, under severe conditions, influence operational safety and occupational health. Excessive exposure to airborne acoustic energy may interfere with routine living activities, induce annoyance, degrade voice communication, modify physiologic functions, reduce the effectiveness of performance, and cause noise-induced hearing loss. Both vibratory and acoustic effects may occur simultaneously with the onset of the stimulus or may be manifest only with the passage of time and repeated exposure, for example, noise-induced hearing loss and vibrational disease. The problems generated by the closely related phenomena of noise and vibration are addressed by the unifying field of biodynamics and dealt with on an individual or group basis by the field of aerospace medicine.

Human exposure to moderate vibratory and acoustic energy can be controlled to acceptable levels that do not jeopardize either the persons involved or the operational aerospace mission. Severe whole-body vibration and intense noise exposures of aerospace air and ground crews, however, may affect performance and even contribute to accidents. The results of noise and vibration research on physiologic and psychologic effects and on performance and comfort have provided an extensive technology pool that serve as the bases of exposure guidelines, criteria, and standards. Scientifically developed prediction schemes allow the nature and magnitude of biodynamic environments to be reliably estimated. Appropriate action may be initiated to minimize the impact of most exposures by treating the source, the propagation, and the exposed and by monitoring the influence of such exposures over time with hearing tests and medical observations. Certainly, research must continue to address the many gaps that exist in our knowledge of severe noise and vibration exposures, as well as less intense exposures to allow such environments to be controlled with even greater confidence. This chapter addresses the variety of effects on man of the vibratory and acoustic energy experienced in aerospace activities and the major operational control methods and procedures presently available and in use.

MEASUREMENT AND ANALYSIS OF SOUND AND VIBRATION ENVIRONMENTS

Definition and Measurement Units

Vibration Stimulus

Vibration is generally defined as the motion of objects relative to a reference position that is usually the object at rest. Specifically, vibration is a series of oscillations of velocity, an action that necessarily involves displacement and acceleration. Acceleration is typically used as the fundamental measure of vibration environments and is expressed as multiples of gravitational acceleration of the earth, G (G = 9.8 m/sec^2). Vibration is described relative to its effects on man in terms of frequency, intensity (amplitude), direction (with regard to anatomic axes of the human body), and duration of exposure.

FREQUENCY. The frequency of periodic motion (sound and vibrations) is the number of complete cycles of motion taking place in a unit of time, usually 1 second. The international standard unit of frequency is the hertz (Hz), which is 1 cycle/sec. Vibration in aerospace systems and activities is usually nonperiodic or random in nature. Random vibratory motion is adequately described in terms of frequency spectra using appropriate spectral analysis techniques. Vibrations with the energy concentrated in narrow regions or

at discrete frequencies may be analyzed by the measurement in frequency bands or by observation of the oscilloscope.

AMPLITUDE. The amplitude of vibration is defined as the maximum displacement about a position of rest. The displacement unit of choice in vibration work is the meter (m). The term amplitude is often used with a descriptor such as velocity-amplitude or acceleration-amplitude to describe the value of a vibration. Velocity and acceleration may be determined by the following formulas for sinusoidal vibrations for which the frequency and amplitude are known. Given the frequency, f, and the (displacement) amplitude, A:

$$\text{Velocity} - \text{amplitude} = 2\pi fA \quad (1)$$
$$\text{Acceleration} - \text{amplitude} = 4\pi^2 f^2 A$$

The same formulas may be used with narrow-band random vibration.

The intensity of nonperiodic or complex vibrations is a computed, time-averaged or root-mean-square (rms) value. In sinusoidal vibration, the rms value is $\frac{1}{\sqrt{2}}$ (0.707) times the maximum (peak) value. The relationships between sinusoidal vibration frequency, displacement, velocity, and acceleration may be determined from the nomograph in Figure 10–1.

DIRECTION OF VIBRATION. Vibration can have three linear and three rotational degrees of freedom. Man's response to linear vibration depends on the direction in which the force acts on the body. The directions of vibration entering the human body have been standardized relative to the anatomic axes illustrated in Figure 10–2. The description of the vibration should apply to the force or motion at the point of entry into the body when evaluating its effects on man. Care should be taken in the use of vibration data to ensure that its measurement relates to the coordinate system of anatomic axes and is not remote from the man. Rotational accelerations around a center of rotation are sep-

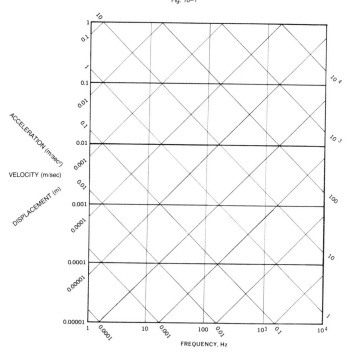

Fig. 10–1. Nomograph relating the principal parameters of sinusoidal vibration.

arated into pitch (rotation about the Y-axis), roll (rotation about the X-axis), and yaw (rotation about the Z-axis).

DURATION OF VIBRATION EXPOSURE. In general, human tolerance to continuous vibration declines with increasing duration of exposure.[1] Adaptation or habituation to vibration stress remains an open question because it has received little research attention. Long-term vibration sometimes denotes exposures exceeding 1 hour, whereas short-term (or short duration) vibration usually identifies exposures lasting 1 minute to 1 hour. Vibration lasting only a few seconds or a few cycles of motion can usually be treated as transient vibration, shock motion, or sometimes as impact.

Sound Stimulus

Sound waves are variations in air pressure above and below the ambient pressure. Sound is described in terms of its intensity, spectrum, and time history.[2]

INTENSITY. The intensity of a sound wave is the magnitude that the pressure varies above and below the ambient level. It is measured by a logarithmic scale that expresses the ratio of sound pressure to a reference pressure in decibels (dB). The decibel is a unit used to describe levels of acoustic pressure, power, and intensity.

Atmospheric or ambient pressure is measured in newtons/m² (N/m^2). The smallest ambient pressure change (sound wave), varying at a rate of about 1000 times per second, that can be detected by man is a pressure amplitude of about 0.00002 N/m^2. This just detectable pressure is the standard reference sound pressure for the decibel scale for sound measurement in gases in terms of sound pressure level (SPL). The intensity of a pressure (P), in terms of SPL, is defined as follows:

$$SPL = 20 \log_{10} \frac{P}{P_o} \qquad (2)$$

where $P_o = 0.00002 \ N/m^2$ and the SPL value is quoted in decibels referenced to

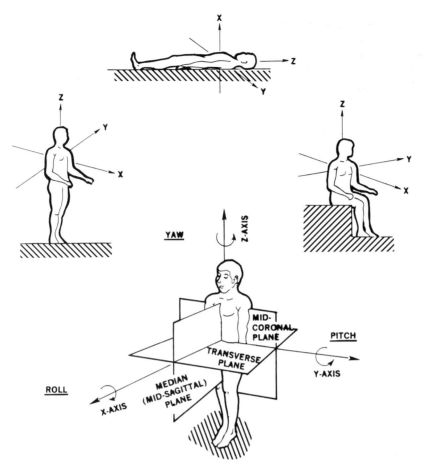

Fig. 10–2. Directions of coordinate system used in biodynamics for mechanical vibrations influencing humans.

0.00002 N/m². The relationship between sound pressure and SPL is shown in Table 10–1.

SPECTRUM. The spectrum of a sound represents the quantities present distributed across frequency (defined under vibration stimulus). It is commonly described in terms of levels of successive passbands of octave, half-octave, and third-octave bandwidths but can be any size successive bandwidth. Noises of concern to aerospace medicine are frequency-dependent in terms of their effects on man. The spectrum of acoustic energy important to

Table 10–1. Common Scales Used to Describe the Magnitude of Acoustic Energy

Sound Pressure Level (dB)	Sound Pressure (μbar)	Sound Pressure (N/m²)	Pressure (lb/in²)
174	100,000	10,000	1.47
134	1000	100	14.7×10^{-3}
94	10	1	147.0×10^{-6}
74	1	0.1	14.7×10^{-6}
54	0.1	0.01	1.47×10^{-6}
14	0.001	0.0001	14.7×10^{-9}
0	0.0002	0.00002	2.94×10^{-9}

man's perception ranges from less than 1 to over 20,000 Hz. The young, normal human ear is sensitive to acoustic energy of about 15 to 20,000 Hz, which is termed the audio frequency range. Infrasound, energy below about 15 Hz, can be perceived at high intensity levels. Ultrasound is classically defined as acoustic energy above 20,000 Hz; however, the term is applied to energy as low as 8000 to 10,000 Hz and above.

TIME HISTORY. Pressure-time histories describe variations in the sound pressure of a signal as a function of time. The frequency content is not quantified in pressure-time histories of signals. Analytic techniques must be applied to the signal to obtain frequency or spectrum characteristics. Steady-state sounds are those with a time course or duration greater than 1 second. Impulse sounds, individual pressure pulses of sudden onset and brief duration, are those with a duration of less than 1 second and a peak to rms ratio greater than 10 dB. Impulse sounds are typically described by their rise time, peak level, duration, and number of events or repetitions. The frequency content of impulsive sounds is determined by spectral-energy-density analysis.

Propagation

Theoretically, sound waves in open air spread spherically in all directions from an idealized point source. As a result of this spherical dispersion, the sound pressure is reduced to half of its original value as the distance is doubled, which is a 6-dB reduction in SPL. Sound propagation is further affected by such factors as atmospheric attenuation, air temperature, and topography, which generally result in propagation losses and distortion. The speed of sound in air is temperature-dependent and is about 344 m/sec at a temperature of 21° C.

Aerospace noises do not radiate uniformly in all directions, but follow forms or patterns characteristic of the source.

This directivity of sound propagation must be included in the evaluation of noise to ensure the appropriate placement of personnel and to avoid overexposure of communities in the vicinity of the noise sources.

Instrumentation

Vibration Measurement Instruments

The basic instrumentation components used for vibration measurement include a transducer, amplifier, and readout stage. The transducer is an acceleration (velocity or displacement) pickup that is available in models for measurement in one, two, or three (triaxial) mutually perpendicular directions and with different frequency and sensitivity ranges. Except for the transducer, the instrumentation is similar to that used for acoustic measurement, providing information on the level of the vibration and the frequency components present in the signal. The measurement of rotational vibration is infrequently accomplished because it is more sophisticated, requiring special pickups (rate gyros) and more complicated calibration.

A variety of vibration meters are available for general-purpose measurements, for monitoring, and for evaluating human response to vibration. Most devices operate in acceleration, velocity, and displacement modes. The amount of energy present at the various frequencies is obtained using conventional frequency analysis techniques and instrumentation. The frequency analysis component of the instrumentation is important for vibration measurement because the reduced comfort, fatigue-decreased proficiency, and safety criteria are presented in frequency or third-octave bands as a function of acceleration and exposure duration.[1] Care must be taken to ensure that all instrumentation components cover the whole frequency range of interest.

Sound Measurement Instruments

The basic instrumentation components used for sound measurement consist of a microphone, amplifier, and readout device. The basic sound level meter contains these components and responds to sound pressure levels referenced to 0.00002 N/m^2. It provides a single-number overall reading of the sound pressure level in the audible frequency range. Most sound level meters contain three standardized electrical weighting or filter networks, A, B, and C, which enable the instrument to measure the approximate loudness response of the human ear at the respective sound levels of 40, 70, and 100 dB. The sound level meter is an important instrument because most noise exposure standards and criteria are based on sound measurements made with the A-weighting scale of the device.

The sound level meter is used for general-purpose and survey work such as continuous monitoring of noise at a work station or the identification of noise-hazardous areas. When noise conditions exceed exposure criteria and noise control measures are indicated, an analysis of sound pressure level as a function of frequency is usually required. Instruments that perform this function are frequency analyzers, which commonly assess levels in frequency bandwidths of one octave or one-third octave and may be used independently or with sound level meters. Frequency analyzers are important because effective noise control measures deal with the problem areas in the frequency spectrum identified by octave or one-third octave descriptions of the sound.

Noise Dosimeters

Personal noise dosimeters are small, lightweight devices worn by individuals to indicate their noise exposure over a specified time period, typically for hearing-conservation purposes. A dosimeter consists of a microphone, a unit that integrates acoustic energy over time, and a readout that displays the exposure or dose at the time the unit is read. A dosimeter is designed with a specific built-in noise exposure standard like the Occupational Safety and Health Act standard of 90 dB(A) for 8 hours. Ideally, a 90-dB(A) exposure for 8 hours would read a dose of 100%, with greater and lesser exposures reading doses higher and lower than 100%, respectively. Various commercially available noise dosimeters differ somewhat in operation and readout, with some providing continuous 24-hour monitoring; however, the general principle of operation is essentially the same, with the final output indicating the percentage of the allowable daily noise dose actually experienced by the individual wearing the unit.

Aerospace Noise and Vibration Sources

Aerospace noises and vibrations that may impact man generally have common sources that are further influenced by the type of system, kind of operation, and environmental factors. A primary source, and usually the most intense, is the propulsion system required to power the aerospace vehicles.[5] These energy sources not only impact crew and support personnel but are radiated into surrounding areas and communities. Auxiliary ground equipment required for the maintenance and preflight support of both aircraft and space vehicles, as well as static engine firing, also produce a variety of noise and vibration environments. Onboard life-support systems generate different types and levels of acoustic energy that may be accompanied by vibration. Aerodynamic sources, wind gusts, and air turbulence also cause numerous combinations of biodynamic environments that gradually increase as vehicles fly closer and closer to the ground and subside at increasing altitude as the density of the atmosphere decreases, eventually to disappear for vehicles in space.

Substantial vibration is often present in

the operation of aviation and space vehicles. The primary sources during space operations are the propulsion systems, aerodynamic factors, and onboard powered systems and equipment. The intense combustion and powerful thrust required to propel the large space vehicle generate noise and movement that are transmitted throughout the structures and internally to the crew stations. Noise and vibration are worst during the maximum aerodynamic loads that occur immediately after launch as the vehicle is gathering speed and decrease as it moves through the more rarefied atmosphere into space. A similar but briefer effect occurs and subsides as the speed of the spacecraft is greatly reduced during the initial moments of reentry prior to deployment of the parachutes or landing of vehicles such as the space shuttle. Vibration from onboard equipment and apparatus may be present and even observable in some circumstances but is generally not a problem. Exceptions might be a low-level vibration that persists throughout the flight and is judged to be objectionable for a very delicate manual task whose performance is impacted by the vibration.

The maximum intensity of aerodynamically induced vibrations and noise occur when the aerospace vehicles are under the highest aerodynamic pressures. For space systems, this maximum intensity occurs during the first few minutes of acceleration after launch and during deceleration upon reentry into the atmosphere. Aerodynamically induced energy is maximum for aircraft during lift-off, climb-out, dives, supersonic dashes, and maneuvers. These categories of vibratory and acoustic energy are relatively high frequency and are more easily controlled than the low-frequency energy.

Crew and community noise exposure and the potential environmental impact from space operations are summarized in Table 10–2. Examples of aviation and space noise environments are compared with automobile and subway noises in Figure 10–3. Most aerospace noises shown are relatively intense; however, hearing protection and audio communications equipment provide adequate protection and information transfer in these hostile environments.

The crew is subjected to the highest maneuvering loads and vibration loads caused by air turbulence during the high-speed, low-altitude flight of military maneuvers. The transition in the force spectrum from low-frequency vibration to alternating G exposures to which the crew is exposed is continuous, and any dividing line between these areas is arbitrary and usually based on the difference in laboratory simulation equipment (centrifuge versus vibration table).

THE HUMAN BODY AS RECEIVER OF NOISE AND VIBRATION

Energy Absorption and Transmission

When the human body is exposed to airborne noise fields or comes in contact with vibrating structures such as aircraft floors or fuselage walls, there is a response to the physical force. Obviously, the alternating pressures or forces are transmitted to and propagated inside the body tissue. Basically, there is no longer any difference between sound and vibration once the energy is inside the tissue. There is a big difference, however, in the transmission of energy from air to body tissue compared with the transmission from a vibrating structure. Structures are solids and are similar to body tissue in their mechanical characteristics; consequently, vibrations are easily transmitted from the vibrating structure to tissue. At the body surface, the contact area, the tissue will be excited to the same vibration amplitude, that is, acceleration or velocity as the exciting structure. Most of the energy is transmitted from the structure to the body and propagates without much attenuation inside the tissue.[4] The situation is different, how-

Table 10–2. A Summary of Space Operations, Noise Exposure, and Potential Environmental Impact

Operation	Exposure	Spacecrew	Groundcrews	Community
Industrial support of space systems	Noise	Not applicable	Industrial noise exposure; 8 hr/day compliance with U.S. Dept. of Labor, 90 dB(A) criteria	Potential problems where noises intrude into neighboring communities
Launch	Noise	Brief exposures of 125–130 dB SPL in crew area; less than 120 dB at ear; hearing protection and voice communication adequate with current systems; no adverse effects due to protection and brief exposures	Very intense levels as high as 150 dB SPL at 600 ft from pad; adverse effects without protection provided by structures and/or hearing protectors	Intense levels perceived at great distances; low frequencies of 115 db 3 miles from pad; 105 dB at 10 miles; infrequent occurrence, brief duration contributes to acceptability
	Sonic boom	Not perceptible	Not perceptible	Not perceptible
Cruise	Noise	Onboard systems; ambient levels of 60–70 dB; noise levels higher during certain operations; levels tolerable for brief missions of several days; acceptable levels for missions of 6–18 mo not determined	Not applicable	Not applicable
Reentry	Noise	Noise similar to maximum aerodynamic noise at launch; greater duration; requires voice communication capability for space shuttle-type reentry	Brief, low-level exposures at landing	Negligible; infrequent
	Sonic boom	Not perceptible	Not perceptible; boom occurs some distance from landing site	Space shuttle-type reentry may expose large areas of Earth's surface; impact depends on number of people exposed.
Static firing	Noise	Not applicable	Very intense levels of 150 dB at 600 ft; must use protection; durations and frequency of occurrence much greater than launch	Noise propagates a far distance into communities; duration of runs; frequency of occurrence, time of day, will contribute to acceptability; this may be worst community exposure situation

ever, with respect to airborne sound waves. When they impinge on a solid surface, the wave is almost stopped, and the particle velocity at the interface is reduced to a small fraction of its free-field value. The sound wave is reflected at the body surface due to what is called the "mismatch" of the media, and only a small percentage of the sound energy enters the tissue.

The sound in our environment can carry important information to us about events,

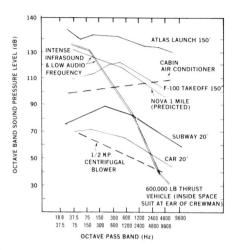

Fig. 10–3. Representative sources of acoustic energy depicting a variety of sound spectra and levels.

as well as messages from our fellow man; consequently, the ear has evolved as a special receiver of sound energy. By its intricate, dynamic design the mammalian outer and middle ear matches the receiver organ, the cochlea, to the acoustic characteristics of air. The tympanic membrane is the only part of the human body surface that absorbs almost 100% of the acoustic energy arriving through air in the frequency range of interest and transmits it to the cochlea to stimulate the receiver.

Mechanical Impedance

The amount of mechanical energy transmitted from one medium to another is best described by the match or mismatch of the mechanical impedance of the media. This mechanical impedance is the ratio of the force or pressure at the contact area to the velocity resulting from this force. For a simple sinusoidal motion, force and velocity can be out of phase. If the phase angle between force and velocity is $+90°$, one speaks of a mass reactance, that is, the medium acts at the interface like a pure inertial loading. If the phase angle is $-90°$, one speaks of an elastic reactance, that is, a pure spring. For phase angle $0°$, one speaks of a frictional resistance, that is, the energy transmitted through the boundary

is completely absorbed by the receiving medium.

Whole-Body Impedance

For an example of whole-body impedance, look at the mechanical impedance of a sitting human subject exposed to vibration (Fig. 10–4). At the low frequencies (below approximately 3 Hz), the body acts like a pure mass corresponding to the body weight (represented theoretically by the line mω). Depending on body dimensions, composition, muscle tension, and posture, there is a maximum of the impedance between 3 and 7 Hz, which is called a resonance. Above this frequency, the impedance decreases and more and more energy is absorbed by the elasticities of soft tissue and the damping inherent in the latter.

Such impedance curves are important and useful for the following reasons:

1. The impedance indicates in which frequency range maximum energy is transmitted to the subject, namely, in the resonance range. Where the maximum energy is transmitted, the maximum physiologic and potentially psychologic effects of the energy must be expected. It certainly explains why some frequencies are potentially more traumatic than others.

2. The impedance explains quantitatively why all vibration effects depend critically on body posture, restraint, and support. It indicates how to modify the energy transmission to the body.

3. The impedance is the first clue as to the mechanical structure of the human body and indicates how to describe this structure in mechanical/engineering terms. For example, for the standardized nominal impedance shown in Figure 10–4, a standardized engineering representation is shown in the insert. The network of masses, springs, and dampers of this mechanical system simulates at the

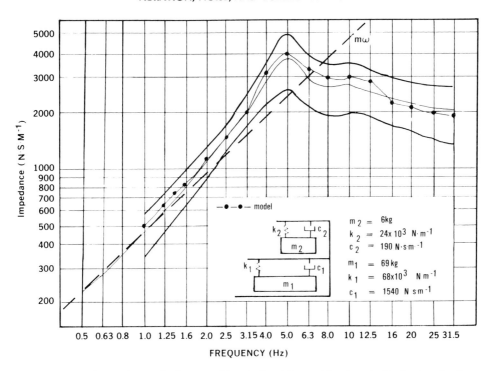

Fig. 10–4. Mechanical impedance of a human subject in the sitting position (standardized values for the mean, 20th percentile, and 80th percentile experimental data) on a rigid, flat seat; the subject's feet on a footrest move with the seat. Test accelerations are 1 to 2 m/sec². The subject's body weight is 51 to 94 kg. The impedance curve of a simple mechanical analog is also indicated. If the body would move as a rigid mass, the impedance would follow the $m\omega$ line.

input interface the complex mechanical impedance of the human body. The engineer considering vibration-attenuating seats or reduction of aircraft or automobile vibration can calculate numerically the effectiveness of vibration control measures by means of mechanical equivalents of the human body like the one shown in Figure 10–4. He also can design a physical analog of the human body, that is, a dynamic dummy that loads the seat or the vibration source dynamically the same way as a human subject. The impedance also indicates that anthropometric dummies, which simulate only dimensions and inertial properties of man without considering the elastic characteristics, cannot be expected to represent realistic loads above approximately 3 Hz and can lead to misleading re-

sults if used in tests containing higher frequencies.

The impedance of man is only linear as a first approximation, that is, the impedance value changes above certain displacements at constant frequency. For the same reason, the impedance changes with the static or inertial preload. For example, a person in an aircraft or space vehicle exposed to sustained acceleration maneuvers or to a zero-G environment reacts differently to vibration environments than in the normal environment on earth. These impedance changes are illustrated in Figure 10–5.[5] The curves explain why vibration and buffeting are perceived as less severe under acceleration preloads.

Because human susceptibility to transient acceleration and impact can be calculated for the simplified linear response condition from the steady-state response,

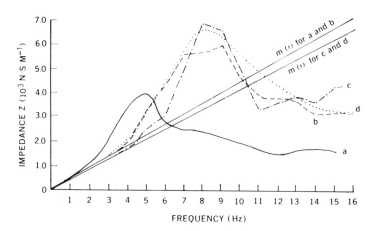

Fig. 10-5. The mechanical impedance of the sitting human body: (a) under normal gravity; (b) under $+2 G_z$; (c) under $+3 G_z$; and compared with (d) the mechanical impedance of a simple mass-spring-damper system with fo = 8 Hz, m = 65,000 dyne sec^2/cm, and $\delta = 0.575$.[5]

the vibration response discussed also is helpful in understanding human response to and protection against impact loads (see Chapter 8). The inertial preload effects illustrated in Figure 10–5 can alter and decrease human impact response. It is also the reason why vibration and impact response under zero G has been hypothesized to be more severe.

Acoustic Impedance

As another example of mechanical impedance, Figure 10–6 illustrates the acoustic impedance (mechanical impedance divided by the square of the area) of a small body area. The impedance of a 1-cm^2 surface area overlying soft tissue behaves at low frequencies like a mass reactance, whereas bony areas under the skin change the behavior to an elastic reactance. This figure also shows impedance values for the tympanic membrane and their proximity to the characteristic impedance of air. The transformer action of the middle ear is responsible for the high sensitivity of the ear to airborne sound compared with the rest of the body surface (curves a and b). Preloading of the tympanic membrane with static pressure, as, for example, due to atmospheric pres-

sure changes during ascent to or descent from altitude without pressure equalization through the eustachian tube shifts the elasticity of the transmission chain into the nonlinear range. As a result of this pressure differential, a decrease in auditory acuity or a temporary hearing loss can occur of as much as 8 to 10 dB for frequencies below 1500 and above 2300 Hz.

Transmission of Mechanical Energy

Impedance measurements at the body surface tell us how much energy enters the body; however, these measurements do not indicate how the energy is propagated and distributed inside the body. With respect to the human ear, the energy transmission from the tympanic membrane to the hair cells of the inner ear is well understood, and even the mechanical filtering and electrical filtering of the frequency components in the cochlea and peripheral nervous system are known in principle. The ear and auditory system as energy receivers hide no big secrets; however, the auditory system as information processor, analyzer, and pattern recognizer is still a serious challenge to science. Solving this puzzle will not only aid the medical therapy of speech and hearing disorders but

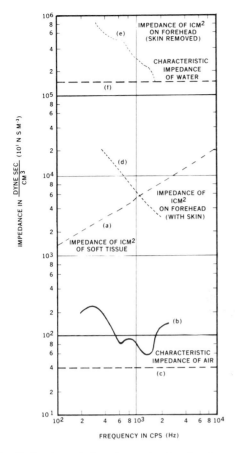

Fig. 10–6. Acoustic impedance at various locations on the body surface: (a) impedance of a 1-cm² area overlying soft tissue; (b) impedance measured at the tympanic membrane; (c) characteristic impedance of air; (d) impedance on the forehead; (e) impedance on the forehead without skin; and (f) characteristic impedance of water.[4]

ments of the transmission characteristics are available (Fig. 10–7); understandably, they vary greatly with the direction and the body support and restraint.

In explaining and describing energy transmission, mathematical models of the whole body and its subsystems have been of great assistance.[6] Although lumped parameter models (Fig. 10–8) with discrete masses, elasticities, and dampers can explain the basic behavior and have the advantage of illustrative insight, finite element models exercised on digital computers provide a geometric fidelity and detail of mechanical stress definition far beyond verification by available measurements. For example, the head-spine model, which is indicated in the computer graphics in Figure 10–8, not only incorporates details of the skeleton structure and the mechanical properties of the skeletal system but also the properties of the major tendons and muscles and of the internal organs. It allows calculation of rel-

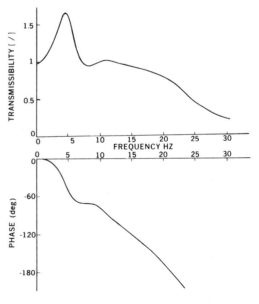

Fig. 10–7. Transmissibility (feet or buttocks to head) for the standing or sitting human subject. The transmissibility is essentially the same for both positions (based on ISO/DP7962 Mechanical Transmissibility of the Human Body. International Standards Organization, 1984).

also lead to further progress in the technology of automatic speech recognition, synthetic speech, and speech understanding.

Transmission of vibration and impact through the body structure is of primary interest with respect to explaining undesirable effects and trauma. Except for the case of direct energy transmission to the head, the effects are usually confined to the frequency range below 100 Hz and to the displacement of larger body parts such as the abdominal viscera, the arm and hand, or the head and eye. The measure-

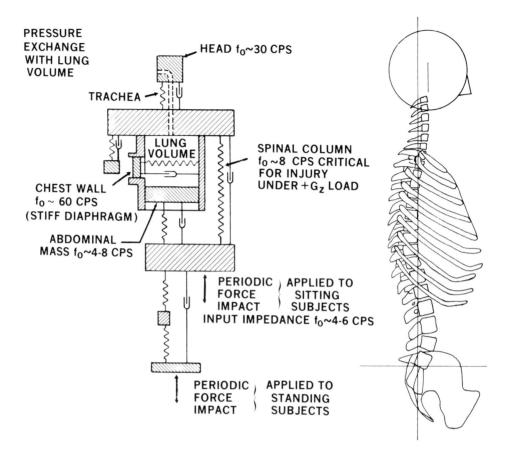

Fig. 10–8. Models for describing and predicting vibration response. The left side of the figure shows the lumped parameter model. The right side of the figure shows the finite element upper torso model.

ative displacement and deformation of major body parts, such as the head, spine, or abdominal viscera, and also compressive and bending stresses on vertebral bodies and disks. When excited at the buttocks with Z-axis vibrations, the head-spine model predicts the impedance of a sitting subject as measured. Today, the primary tool in predicting and assessing the mechanical response of human subjects to vibration, rotational oscillation, and impact are models such as the ones illustrated.

Sound and Vibration Reduction and Protection

Noise and vibration exposures exceeding established safety, health, or performance interference criteria must be reduced to desirable levels. Depending on the stimulus-response relationship considered, some criteria are defined by the effective exposure, that is, the product of stimulus intensity and exposure time, whereas other criteria give the desirable limits solely in terms of maximum or average sound pressure level or vibration.

Amplitude

To protect an operator from long-term health effects, exposure intensity and time are the factors requiring control. In the case of single events, such as impulse noise or shock, the intensity and number of events per day or week are the parameters to be controlled. Therefore, in most cases, it is desirable and economical to consider the whole system from the noise or vibration source over the transmission path to the human receiver and to analyze the feasibility of control at the source, in the intervening medium, or at the receiver. Engineering control and operational control through changes of the exposure time and exposure pattern are possibilities.

Noise Reduction

Noise control from the source to the receiver is a well-established engineering discipline that is amenable to quantitative analysis and design. Noise reduction of stationary sources on the ground can be accomplished through conventional engineering approaches, such as isolation, shock mounting, damping, or shielding, or enclosing the source to eliminate the radiation of airborne noise. Mufflers and hush houses for jet engines and aircraft are effective. Practical limits in noise control are dictated by operational and/or economical constraints. For example, the maintenance time of jet engines is increased because of the use of ground runup noise suppressors.

In closed facilities occupied by personnel, noise control is accomplished by sound treatment tailored to the specific noise situation. In aerospace vehicles, internal noise from air conditioning, blowers, and pneumatic pumps and external noise from the propulsion units and aerodynamic flow over the fuselage must be considered and controlled. Because weight and space are at a premium in flight vehicles, noise reduction is usually not designed to satisfy optimum comfort criteria but to guarantee allowable safe exposure conditions and communication capability for crew members. Whenever possible and practical, increasing the distance between the noise source and the receiver is a very effective noise control measure. The amount of attenuation to be expected can be grossly estimated by the inverse square law, which predicts a 6-dB change of sound pressure level for each halving or doubling of the distance between source and receiver.

PERSONAL PROTECTION. Whenever engineering control of the noise to desirable levels is not feasible, personal ear protection devices (i.e., earplugs, earmuffs, or helmets) must be worn. These devices attenuate the noise on its way from the surrounding air to the tympanic membrane. Because their effectiveness can vary considerably, depending on their basic performance and personal fit, it is important that a high-quality device be selected for use and that all personnel are well indoctrinated in size selection and use. The effectiveness of well-fitted personal protectors is demonstrated by Figure 10-9. The mean attenuation values presented are the so-called "real ear attenuation at threshold" determined by a standardized psychophysical method in the laboratory with human subjects. Under operational conditions, the acoustic fit of the protector can deteriorate due to various use factors, and an effectiveness of one or two standard deviations smaller than the average attenuation is frequently assumed. The maximum attenuation of 40 to 50 dB achievable with the best ear protectors is not attained due to leaks or sound passing through the protectors. Intense sound enters the head or upper torso through areas not covered by the ear protectors and reaches the inner ear through tissue and bone conduction, bypassing the physical barrier of the protectors. For the same reason, the protection provided by the combination of earplug plus earmuff, headset, or helmet is usually less than the sum of the individual attenuation values.

Active noise cancellation has made considerable progress in the recent past and might be practical and feasible in conjunction with future communication systems. This approach picks up the noise at the inside of the earmuff and feeds the noise with such phase and amplitude adjustments to an earphone under the muff as to cancel or minimize the noise in front

HEARING PROTECTION	FREQUENCY, Hz				
	1-20	20-100	100-800	800-8000	> 8000
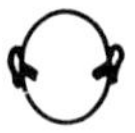 EARPLUGS	5-10	5-20	20-35	30-40	30-40
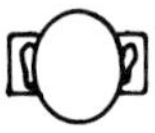 EARMUFFS	0-2	2-15	15-35	30-45	35-45
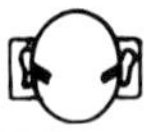 EARPLUGS AND EARMUFFS	10-15	15-25	25-45	30-60	40-60
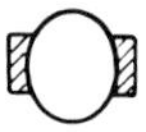 COMMUNICATION HEADSETS	0-2	2-10	10-30	25-40	30-40
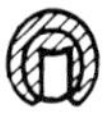 HELMETS	0-2	2-7	7-20	20-50	30-50
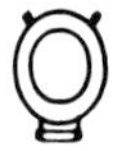 SPACE HELMET (TOTAL HEAD ENCLOSURE)	3-8	5-10	10-25	30-60	30-60

Fig. 10–9. The range of hearing protection expected for good protective devices shown represents the approximate minimum and maximum protection available.

of the tympanic membrane. This technology is particularly effective at the low frequencies (1000 Hz), where passive attenuation tends to decrease.

SPEECH COMMUNICATION WITH EAR PROTECTORS. Speech communication is not degraded for normal hearing listeners with ear protection in noises of 85 to 125 dB. Signal and noise are attenuated by the same amount, and the signal-to-noise ratio remains the same. As a matter of fact, experimental evidence suggests that with ear protection speech intelligibility is improved, probably through decreased distortion in the ear at the lower signal and noise levels.[7] The frequently expressed excuse for not wearing ear protection is that auditory warning signals such as bells and buzzers cannot be heard. This excuse is not valid for the same reason: better signal reception occurs in most practical situations when protection is worn. This does not necessarily apply when signal and noise are not in the same frequency band or are at very low signal-to-noise levels.

For operations with frequently interrupted high noise levels, where communication during the quiet periods is required and removal of the ear protectors is impractical, earmuffs that electronically transmit the speech signal from the outside to the inside of the muff are available. At high outside noise levels and impulse noise exposure, the electronic transmission is interrupted or limited and the passive muff attenuation is effective.

Vibration Reduction

Protection against undesirable vibration is accomplished by two means: (1) attenuation of the vibration delivered to the crew or isolation of the crew; and (2) restraining of the crewmember to the seatback and armrest to reduce relative displacement with respect to the seat, displays, and control handles and to minimize displacement of one body segment to another. Safety and performance criteria require vibration protection primarily in the frequency range below 12 Hz. Unfortunately, for many aerospace situations, the requirements for safety, comfort, and performance capability are not necessarily mutually compatible. In the low-frequency range, effective vibration isolation of a whole person requires large stroke distances, which are undesirable as long as displays and controls do not move with the person and are intolerable in space systems and military aircraft equipped with an ejection seat. Impact acceleration loads transmitted through an elastic seat or soft seat cushion usually lead to an amplification of the dynamic response of the human structure and an increased injury risk. The most common compromise is a seat cushion with a nonlinear stress-strain relationship. A soft elastic top layer provides comfort and isolation from annoying high-frequency vibration and the stiffer lower layers bottom out under high-amplitude impact accelerations.

Whole-body restraint in both commercial and military aircraft requires a compromise between acceleration, vibration, and impact protection and the mobility requirements for satisfying performance capability and comfort. Inertia reel-locking mechanisms employed for crash protection are actuated at higher forces and displacements than are usually involved in aircraft and spacecraft vibrations but can offer some protection against high-amplitude oscillations and displacement from the seat due to unexpected severe turbulence.

Another compromise to be considered in military aircraft and space systems is with respect to body positioning. Human tolerance to sustained G is maximum in the G_x (chest-to-back) direction, a fact which led to the use of the space couch for launch and reentry and the reclined seat proposals for high-performance military fighters. G_x vibrations transmitted to the crew through a couchlike body support expose the human head directly to the unattenuated input vibrations without the benefit of head isolation through the body structure in the seated position. Exposure criteria for this situation are available and must be considered.

Reducing direct vibration inputs to the hands, arms, or head usually presents no serious engineering problem once the necessity is predicted or recognized. Serious problems can exist with respect to occupational exposure to vibrations transmitted directly to the hand and arm from hand tools such as chipping hammers, pneumatic tools, and chain saws. Safety standards established for such exposures must be met for frequencies up to 1000 Hz by appropriate tool design, the wearing of protective gloves, and operational exposure time control.

EFFECTS OF AEROSPACE NOISES

The effects of aerospace noises on man have been divided into physiologic and psychologic responses. Physiologic responses, both auditory and nonauditory, involve changes in physiologic mechanisms or functions attributed to the noise. Auditory effects are confined to direct influences on the peripheral auditory system and the hearing function. Acoustic energy exposures can also impact the vestibular system, the autonomic nervous system, sleep, and startle and induce fatigue; however, with few exceptions, these nonauditory effects also are mediated through the auditory system. Psychologic response behavior to noise is influenced by man's perceptions, judgments, attitudes, and opinions, which may be either related or unrelated to the noise itself. Most noise exposures stimulate elements of both types of responses, which clearly affect and interact with one another.[8]

Human Hearing Function

The human auditory system is an extremely sensitive and highly specialized mechanism that is also quite resistant to the adverse effects of acoustic energy unless abused (Fig. 10–10). The audible frequency range in the normal, young human ear extends from about 16 to 20,000 Hz. The most sensitive region of hearing is from about 500 to 4000 Hz; this band is most important for understanding speech and is expressed in decibels relative to the normal threshold of hearing or standard hearing reference zero. In the infrasound region, below 20 Hz, signal detection by the human ear requires high sound-pressure levels, and tonal quality is lost below about 16 Hz. Airborne ultrasound, energy above 20,000 Hz, is not ordinarily perceived by the human ear. The harmonics of infrasound and subharmonics of ultrasound may be perceived outside their respective frequency regions. Although well below the upper boundary of hearing, in-

tense acoustic signals do produce tickle, discomfort, and even pain in the ear.

Hearing level is an individual's hearing sensitivity for standard test frequencies expressed in decibels relative to the normative hearing reference values. The range of normal hearing sensitivity is from −10 to 25 dB for a pure-tone air-conduction audiogram (Fig. 10–11). Hearing levels greater than 25 dB are considered below normal and constitute hearing loss. Conductive-type hearing losses, caused by impairment of outer and middle ear function, are relatively the same value for each test frequency and appear flat on the audiogram. Sensorineural or perceptive hearing loss, usually attributed to inner ear impairment, characteristically displays a growing loss of sensitivity with increasing frequency beginning around 1000 to 2000 Hz. Persons with hearing losses greater than 35 to 40 dB in the speech-frequency range (400 to 4000 Hz) are potential candidates for a hearing aid. Many conductive-type problems are amenable to medical treatment, whereas sensorineural problems usually consist of permanent intractable losses.

Excessive noise exposure is one of the situations that may produce either or both of these hearing loss syndromes, conductive hearing problems involving acoustic damage or mechanical stress to the tympanic membrane-middle ear system and sensorineural problems involving damage to the inner ear sensory system. The middle ear, mechanical-type acoustic trauma is the characteristic flat conductive hearing loss in which there is no sensorineural involvement. Noise-induced sensorineural hearing loss characteristically involves the higher audio frequencies and is a slow loss of sensitivity progressive with exposure time that is first observed between 2000 and 6000 Hz, with the greatest and most rapid decrease usually occurring at 4000 Hz. This loss increases in magnitude and spreads in frequency with continued exposure. The progression of noise-

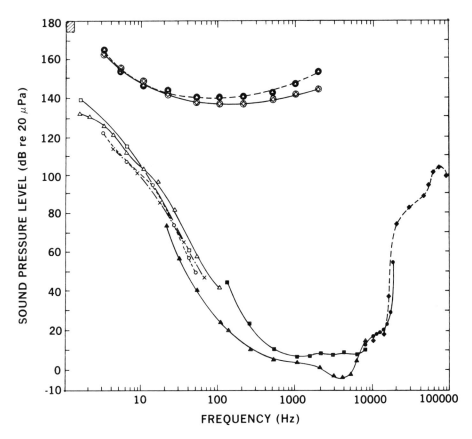

Fig. 10–10. Human auditory sensitivity and pain threshold levels. □ = von Békésy (1960) data-minimum audible pressure (MAP); ○ = Yeowart, Bryan, and Tempest (1969) data-MAP; △ = Whittle, Collins, and Robinson (1972) data-MAP; X = Yeowart, Bryan, and Tempest (1969) data-MAP for bands of noise; ■ = standard reference threshold values-MAP (American National Standard on Specifications for audiometers, 1969); ▲ = ISO R226-minimum audible field (1961); ● = Northern, et al. (1972) data; ◆ = Corso (1963) data-bone conduction minus 40 dB; ◎ = von Békésy (1960) data = tickle, pain; ⬡ = Benox; ▨ = static pressure-pain. (By permission of University Park Press, Measurement Procedures in Speech, Hearing and Language, 1975.)

induced sensorineural loss with the number of years of exposure has been widely documented.[9] Mixed hearing losses include both conductive and some sensorineural components.

A number of protective actions operate in the region of the middle ear to reduce the amount of acoustic energy transmitted to the inner ear. At high sound intensities, the motion of the stapes changes from a piston-like to a rocking action in the oval window due to temporary dislocation of the ossicular joints, thus reducing the efficiency of transmission. Also, the stapedic and tensor tympanic muscles

contract, increasing the stiffness and the damping of the ossicular chain. The response latency of this muscle reflex varies from 25 to over 100 milliseconds; consequently, it operates too slowly to provide protection against brief, impulsive sounds shorter than about 20 milliseconds.

Temporary Threshold Shift (TTS) and Permanent Threshold Shift (PTS)

Noise-induced hearing loss may be either temporary or permanent. Temporary threshold shift is a loss of sensitivity that returns to normal or preexposure hearing levels within a reasonable time

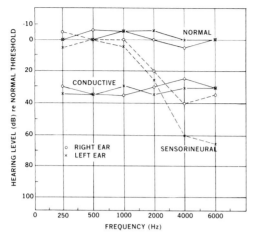

Fig. 10–11. Typical audiograms showing normal hearing, a conductive-type hearing loss that is relatively flat, and a sensorineural or perceptive hearing loss with the characteristic loss of sensitivity with increasing frequency.

following cessation of the noise exposure. Permanent threshold shift is a loss of hearing that persists, with no recovery of sensitivity, irrespective of the time away from the noise. Relationships have been established between recent noise exposure and TTS and between PTS and noise exposure experienced in daily activities performed over many years. Noise-induced TTS is considered to be an integral part of an essential precursor to noise-induced PTS. It is further assumed that noise exposures that do not produce TTS will not produce PTS, that PTS develops similarly to TTS but on a slower time scale, and, finally, that different noise exposures which produce equal amounts of TTS also are considered equally noxious with regard to PTS. These assumptions, based on TTS data from the laboratory and TTS/PTS data from actual field noise exposures, have provided a basis for formulating noise exposure standards and hearing risk criteria that relate noise exposure and hearing loss.[10,11]

Presbycusis

Noise-induced sensorineural hearing loss may be confounded by presbycusis,[9]

which is the gradual loss of high-frequency auditory sensitivity that accompanies advancing age. On the average, auditory sensitivity diminishes as a function of age at frequencies from 500 to 6000 Hz, beginning in the third decade of life. The higher the frequency, the greater the loss, with the maximum loss appearing at 4000 Hz. Aerospace medical evaluations of noise-induced hearing loss should discern that portion of the loss, if any, which is contributed by presbycusis. This may be accomplished statistically by subtracting the average presbycusis value for a non-noise–exposed population from the hearing loss values at each frequency. The remaining loss of hearing may be attributed to the noise exposure history of the individual, other factors considered.

Auditory Pain

Auditory pain due to intense noise is associated with excessive mechanical displacement of the middle ear system and is believed to occur in the threshold region where damage begins. Noise-induced auditory pain occurs almost independent of frequency at levels of 130 to 140 dB SPL and above. No pain is associated with overexposure of the inner ear; however, ringing or similar sounds in the ear produced by the noise do suggest that acceptable exposure limits have been exceeded and that the responsible exposure should not be repeated.

Static Air Pressure

Differential pressures may occur across the tympanic membrane with variations in pressure associated with changing atmospheric (flight) conditions and an eustachian tube that remains closed. Although a high pressure differential may cause noticeable discomfort or pain, lower pressure differences could cause an undetected decrease in hearing sensitivity of 8 to 10 dB for frequencies below 1500 and above 2300 Hz. These effects are usually transitory and may be relieved by the Valsalva maneuver or other means of equalizing ambient and middle ear pressures.

Individual Susceptibility

Individual ears vary greatly in their susceptibility to the adverse effects of noise. Although the ability to determine the noise susceptibility of an ear would be most valuable prior to a work assignment in noise, no satisfactory method for quantifying susceptibility has been developed. Exposure standards and criteria do not include a susceptibility factor because of this wide variance and the inability to predict TTS for a specific ear.

Nonauditory Effects of Continuous Noise

Generally, humans adapt quite well to stimuli such as noise; however, adaptation has not been demonstrated by the responses of a variety of nonauditory systems. Changes in physiologic responses to noise have been measured under laboratory conditions and in real-life situations; however, the magnitudes of these changes are frequently no greater than those experienced under typical daily living conditions. Although some physiologic reactions to certain noises occur at levels as low as 70 dB, the state of understanding is still unclear as to relationships between potential adverse physiologic effects and general noise exposure, as well as to the significance of the changes that do occur to general health and well-being.

General Physiologic Responses

Because most nonauditory effects are mediated through the auditory system, they may be avoided with the use of adequate hearing protection, which, unfortunately, is impractical in many situations (Fig. 10–9). Even with maximum hearing protection, exposure to sound pressure levels in excess of 150 dB should be prohibited because of mechanical stimulation of receptors other than the ear. Noise spectra containing intense low-frequency and infrasonic energy may excite body parts such as the chest, abdomen, eyes, and sinus cavities, causing concern, annoyance, and fatigue. The response of the vestibular system to extremely high levels of noise apparently mediated through the auditory system manifests itself by disorientation, motion sickness, and interference with postural equilibrium.

A number of investigators have reported general and specific physiologic responses to sound. The reported responses include effects on peripheral blood flow, respiration, galvanic skin response, skeletal muscle tension, gastrointestinal motility, cardiac response, pupillary dilation, and renal and glandular function. Recent emphasis has been directed toward hypertension, elevated blood pressure, and cardiovascular responses. Review of the European literature on the cardiovascular and related responses to noise primarily in industrial settings shows that the effects varied from study to study; however, the overall findings indicated adverse effects on the general health parameters investigated. Similar work in the United States has not demonstrated the same degree of adverse effects as shown in these European studies. Nevertheless, this area of concern is especially significant, and additional work is required to ensure that reasonable decisions that are safe for the exposed individuals are possible. In addition to these studies, subjective reports of fatigue, loss of appetite, irritability, nausea, disorientation, headache, and even loss of memory continue to be attributed to noise exposure. Caution should be exercised, however, in attributing such adverse effects solely to noise in various aerospace and industrial situations where numerous other factors may contribute to or create physiologic problems. The contribution of conditions such as temperature extremes, poor ventilation, threat of accidental injury or death, special task demands, and other non-noise elements that tend to grow as noise intensity grows cannot be ascertained without being controlled in test populations.

Subjective reports of disorientation, vertigo, nausea, and interference with postural equilibrium during high-intensity noise exposure suggest stimulation of the vestibular system. Empirical efforts to demonstrate the vestibular response to acoustic energy have been inconclusive; however, the evidence does suggest the vestibular system as the most probable site responding to the acoustic stimulation. Other than the vestibular system, mechanoreceptors and proprioreceptors may be the primary mediators of physiologic responses at SPLs above 140 dB.

SLEEP INTERFERENCE. Interference with sleep due to noise could be a serious effect because there is widespread agreement that adequate sleep is a physiologic necessity. Two general kinds of sleep interference are due to noise: actual arousal or wakening and changes within the sleeping individual who does not awaken. Sleep occurs in stages or levels, which are revealed by patterns of electrical activity in the brain. Individuals are more susceptible to awakening during some stages of sleep than during others. During sleep stage 2, subjects are more susceptible to behavioral wakening than during the other stages; they are more resistant to wakening during stage 4 and REM (rapid eye movements with dreaming) sleep. Sleeping individuals not awakened in response to noise stimuli still have shown changes in electroencephalographic recordings, as well as in peripheral vasoconstriction and heart rate. These responses confirm that measurable effects of noise on biologic responses occur in man during sleep, even though the sleeper is totally unaware of the acoustic exposure.

An interesting investigation of sleep was conducted by Myasnikov, who exposed subjects to broadband continuous noise at levels of 75 to 78 dB during simulated space flight. A dichotomy emerged: subjects who fell asleep rapidly slept well and awakened feeling well, and subjects who fell asleep with difficulty did not sleep well and did not feel well on awakening. Other effects were generally bimodal, corresponding to the two types of sleepers. Myasnikov concluded that the selection of candidates for astronauts should include screening of sleep characteristics to eliminate poor sleepers, especially for lengthy missions.

STARTLE. Startle may be evoked by a wide variety of stimuli but is particularly susceptible to sudden, unexpected noises. This response is more consistent among individuals than almost any other behavioral pattern. The physiologic aspects of the startle response are reasonably independent of the stimulus and include increased pulse rate, increased blood pressure, and diversion of blood flow to the peripheral limbs and gross musculature. Startle responses do not occur frequently or with any regularity in aerospace environments; consequently, they have not been an operational problem. The universality and uniformity of this reaction from one person to another suggests that startle is an inborn reaction that is modified little by learning and experience.

Several studies have been cited to point out that nonauditory physiologic responses to acoustic energy have been observed and measured among selected populations. At the same time, it should be emphasized that these findings are not sufficiently clear or consistent to demonstrate relationships reliable enough to generalize about any typical populations. The aerospace physician must evaluate potential adverse effects of aerospace noise environments on an individual basis, especially where they fall outside the conditions specified in existing standards and criteria for allowable noise exposures.

Psychologic Responses

Numerous psychologic factors in the lives of individuals, such as their perceptions, beliefs, attitudes, and opinions, contribute to the manner in which they respond to noise from aerospace activities. These responses are generally treated in terms of annoyance, performance, and speech communication, which is a special task addressed in a separate section of this chapter.

ANNOYANCE. Acoustic energy is undesirable when attention is called to it unnecessarily or when it interferes with routine activities in the home, office, shop, recreational area, or elsewhere. Individuals become annoyed when the amount of interference becomes significant. Numerous techniques based on measurement of the physical stimulus are used to assess noise exposure effects on people in work and living spaces and to estimate community reaction to noise. One concept maintains that the human reaction to a sound is determined by the annoyance or unwantedness of the sound instead of its loudness. This subjectively judged unwantedness of sounds is described as perceived noisiness (PN). Perceived noisiness may be adequately determined by using the physical measurements of the sound to calculate perceived noisiness in decibels, or PNdB.

Relationships between various PNdB levels and the nature of community reactions that correspond to them have been defined on the basis of data from airport noise experiences, as well as both laboratory and field research. These relationships are compiled for use in estimating reactions, and a step-by-step procedure is available for arriving at PNdB values from the measurement data of the noise. A comprehensive discussion of the concept of perceived noisiness is presented in detailed form in Kryter's discussion.[9]

A different concept of estimating annoyance incorporates both the duration and magnitude of all the acoustic energy occurring during a given time period. The measurement unit is the average sound level and is called the equivalent continuous sound level (Leq). The noise energy content of the continuous A-weighted level is equivalent to that of the actual fluctuating noise existing over the total observation period. Leq, which is the energy mean noise level, is defined as the level of the steady-state continuous noise having the same energy as the actual time-varying noise. The problem of quantifying environmental noise is greatly simplified using the statistical measures of the Leq. The Leq is one of the most important measures of environmental noise for assessing effects on humans because experimental evidence suggests that it accurately describes the development of noise-induced hearing loss and that it applies to human annoyance due to noise.

The equivalent continuous sound level (Leq) measured over a 24-hour period is the day-night average sound level (Ldn), which is weighted for night time exposures with a 10-dB penalty. Ldn is used to relate noise exposures in residential environments to interference with daily living activities and sleep, as well as to chronic annoyance. Most daily noise environments are repetitive in nature, with some variations occurring over weekends and with seasonal changes. It has been found useful to treat environmental noise as a long-term yearly average of the daily levels to account for these variations.

PERFORMANCE. The effects of noise on cognitive and sensorimotor performance remain unclear and somewhat of a puzzle. Degradation of performance has been found with different studies and, at times, even in the same study. The efficiency of vigilance tasks (requiring alertness) over long periods of time was degraded in noise environments of about 100 dB. Mental counting tasks were influenced in a complex manner, and time judgments were found to be distorted. High-frequency noise of sufficient intensity produces more harmful effects on performance than low-frequency noises. Sudden and unexpected changes in noise level, either up or down, may produce momentary disturbances. Noise ordinarily increases the number of errors but does not reduce the speed at which work is performed. High-level and moderate-level noises may act as stress factors and contribute to general fatigue and irritability. The general level of performance may be influenced by these responses.

SLEEP AND STARTLE. Both startle and sleep interference have substantial psychological components in addition to the clear-cut physiologic components discussed earlier. In fact, the major adverse reaction of annoyance is usually caused by being startled or awakened and not because of the changes in physiologic response that also occur. The personal feelings of the exposed individual regarding factors such as the reason for the disturbance, concern over those who are causing the disturbance, attempts to minimize and eliminate the disturbance, and other factors usually determine the degree of acceptance or annoyance to the acoustic energy.

Impulse Noise and Blast

Noise exposures generated by weapons fire, explosions, impact devices in industry, and sonic booms are impulsive or transient in nature and are not covered by continuous noise exposure data. Guidelines for the exposure to various kinds of impulses generated by these sources are contained in established standards and criteria. Some typical values of peak SPL for impulse noise are presented in Table 10–3.

Noise exposures with rapid rise times and durations of less than 1 second have been described as impulse noises. When impulsive noises occur repeatedly or at high levels, their potential for producing adverse effects on the auditory system is relatively high. Temporary threshold shift is systematically treated in the various exposure criteria cited above. The higher the peak pressure level of the impulse, the greater the risk of TTS. Other things being

Table 10–3. Some Typical Values of Peak Sound Pressure Levels (SPL) For Impulse Noise

SPL (in dB re 20 micropascals)	Example
190+	Within blast zone of exploding bomb
160–180	Within crew area of heavy artillery piece or naval gun when shooting
140–170	At shooter's ear when firing handgun
125–160	At child's ear when detonating toy cap or firecracker
120–140	Metal-to-metal impacts in many industrial processes (e.g., drop-forging, metal-beating)
110–130	On construction site during pile-driving

equal, longer impulse durations, higher repetition rates, and greater high-frequency energy in the spectrum of the impulse also pose greater risks to hearing. Although various impulsive sound exposures differ a great deal, TTS usually occurs in the 4000- to 6000-Hz region of hearing. Impulses repeated at a constant rate produce TTS that is generally predictable; however, TTS from single impulses and recovery both from single impulses and from serial impulses are more erratic and less predictable than from steady-state exposures.

The acoustic shock wave or blast noise generated by explosions is treated similarly to impulse noise by the ear even though the levels are much higher and the durations longer. The relationships between impulsive noise and the auditory system and function are generally the same for blast noise.

The eardrum may be ruptured by intense levels of blast noise or impulse noise. The high amplitude causes the operation of the middle ear system to exceed its mechanical limits, causing eardrum rupture and, in severe cases, disarticulation and damage to the ossicular chain. Acoustic signals of sufficient severity to rupture the eardrum membrane also often cause some sensorineural involvement. Eardrum rupture, however, which causes a flat 20 to 40 dB hearing loss, is usually repairable if it does not heal itself, and the conductive loss is restored. Eardrum rupture in response to these intense signals is considered to be a safety function that prevents the acoustic energy from reaching the inner ear. If the eardrum does not rupture, severe PTS at the high frequencies can be the result of the exposure. The threshold of eardrum rupture is 5 psi, with 50% of eardrums failing at 15 psi. The threshold for lung damage also is estimated to be in the region of 15 psi.

Sonic Boom

Research on the effects of sonic booms on people was concentrated in the late 1960s and early 1970s relative to potential overflights of land by commercial supersonic aircraft.[12] Decisions to stop the United States supersonic transport (SST) program and to prevent commercial overflights of land at supersonic speeds resulted in sharply reduced research on sonic boom effects. Today's knowledge of sonic booms is, with few exceptions, based on research conducted in those years (Table 10–4).

The sonic boom is again becoming an important issue for aerospace operations. The increasing numbers of high-performance aircraft being acquired by the United States Department of Defense have resulted in urgent requirements for new air space for supersonic training where some sonic booms will not be a problem. Present and future space programs will utilize vehicles that produce sonic booms during launch and reentry at more and more frequent intervals. Certain space-launch flight trajectories, as well as reentry from space at supersonic speeds, generate sonic booms that reach the ground. The impact on the population of these space vehicle-generated sonic booms, however, is expected to be small. The booms are generated at high altitudes with very long propagation distances and at infrequent intervals. The actual effects on communities of more frequent sonic booms anticipated for the future are yet to be determined.

Generally, sonic booms do not cause direct injury to humans, although both physiologic and psychologic changes may be stimulated by the sudden, unexpected loud sound. The potential effects of such acoustic exposures over many years, if any, have yet to be determined. The human auditory mechanism has shown no adverse effects of sonic booms in individuals exposed under special field and laboratory test conditions to numbers and intensities of booms greater than those that

Table 10–4. Sonic Boom and Blast Exposures: Measurements and Estimations

Peak Overpressure		Predicted and/or Measured Effects
lb/ft^2	dynes/cm^2	
0–1	0–478	No damage to ground structures; no significant public reaction day or night
1.0–1.5	478–717	Sonic booms from normal operational altitudes— Very rare minor damage to ground structures; probable public reaction
1.5–2.0	717–957	typical community exposures (seldom above 2 lb/ft^2) Rare minor damage to ground structures; significant public reaction, particularly at night
2.0–5.0	957–2393	Incipient damage to structures
20–144	9.57×10^3 6.8×10^4	Measured sonic booms from aircraft flying at supersonic speeds at minimum altitude; experienced by humans without injury
720	3.44×10^5	Estimated threshold for eardrum rupture (maximum overpressure)
2160	1.033×10^6	Estimated threshold for lung damage (maximum overpressure)

From von Gierke, H.E., and Nixon, C.W.: Human Response to sonic boom in the laboratory and the community. J. Acoust. Soc. Am. Part 2, *31*:5, May, 1966.

could occur under typical living conditions.[13]

Although alleged health effects of sonic booms have been reported, the major problems continue to be annoyance with the reaction caused by startle, fear associated with startle, interruption of activities, shaking and rattling of structures and buildings, sleep and rest interference, and attitudes toward those causing the sonic booms.

COMMUNICATION IN AEROSPACE ENVIRONMENTS

Voice communications effectiveness is influenced by environmental, personal, message, and equipment factors in aerospace operations. Noise, both acoustic and electrical, is the most predominant environmental factor; however, acceleration, whole-body vibration, artificial atmospheres, combinations of stressors, special task requirements, and environmental threats to personal safety also can alter communications. Audio communications may be further impacted by personal speech habits, dialects, word usage, hearing loss, the amount and type of communication experience, and even the emotional state of the individual. Speech reception also is affected by elements that include message set, type of material, vocabulary size, both familiar and unexpected terms, and infrequently used phrases. Communication equipment can be optimized for human speech using peak-clipping, spectrum-shaping, adequate passband, appropriate impedance, and the like to result in very little equipment degradation of speech.

Definition and Assessment of Speech Intelligibility

Various standardized methodologies measure the performance of the total voice communication system, with or without the man-in-the-loop, or of the various individual elements of the communication chain. These methodologies are based on the subjective measurement of intelligibility, which is the percentage of a given sample of speech presented to an observer that is correctly perceived, as well as the physical measurement of the communication system and environment. Everyday speech is difficult to quantify and measure, so that smaller collections of speech have been organized into groups of syllables, words, phrases, or sentences that can be more precisely specified relative to everyday communications. Most of these groups of materials, or tests of speech intelligibility, have been standardized with human operators in the loop to provide reliable measurements that can be generalized to other populations. Relating the physical measurements of the communications systems and environments to the speech intelligibility measurements allows the assessment of speech communications effectiveness.

The major operational threat to voice communications is noise that may mask or drown out the speech or produce a temporary hearing loss that interferes with the listener's ability to understand the message. Speech communication assessment techniques use physical measurements of the noise to assess the masking effect but do not account for temporary hearing loss that may be experienced by the communicators. Overall, the least sophisticated measurement method for estimating communications effectiveness is the sound level or the A-weighted sound level (dB(A)). Speech interference level (SIL) is the simplest method using octave-band descriptions of the noise. A more refined method developed for use in a wide range of applications is noise criteria (NC). The most comprehensive method for predicting speech communications in noise environments is the articulation index (AI). The most direct approach is to simulate the communication environmental and system variables and directly measure the intelligibility response of interest.

Communication vs. Sound Level

The A-weighting approximates sensitivity of the normal human ear to moderate-level sound. Measured values referenced in Figure 10–12 provide relationships between communication capability and noise (dB(A)). Speech communication as a function of type of communication and A-weighted sound level is provided in Table 10–5. This procedure is ideal for predicting intelligibility for survey and monitoring purposes; however, it is unsuited for noise control and engineering purposes because detailed spectral information is lacking in the descriptor. Additional accuracy with sound level data may be obtained using the correction factor for noise spectrum described in *Handbook of Noise Control*.[14]

Speech Interference Level

Speech interference level (SIL) procedures allow estimates of the maximum acceptable noise levels for satisfactory speech communication based on octave-band descriptions of the noise. The SIL is the arithmetic average of the sound pressure levels (dB) of the noise in the octave bands centered at 500, 1000, 2000, and 4000 Hz. SIL values for reliable communications at various distances and voice levels are shown in Figure 10–12.

Noise Criteria

Noise criteria (NC) are basically an expansion of SIL from a single number to sets of numbers representing octave-band values. The term NC is used interchangeably with preferred noise criterion (PNC). Noise criteria allow estimations of the quality of speech communication that may be expected with various indoor functional activities. Octave-band sound pressure levels for these functional activities are described in Table 10–6. To estimate the quality of communication for a given noise environment:

1. The noise in the octave bands must be described.
2. The octave-band spectrum must be

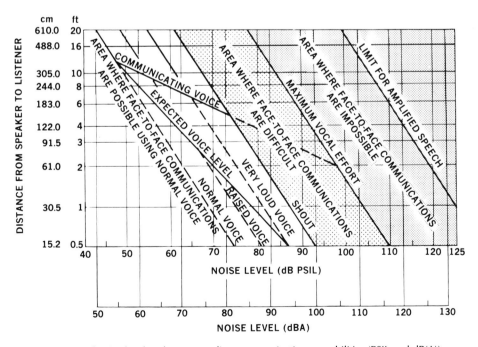

Fig. 10–12. Measures of noise level and corresponding communications capabilities (PSIL and dB(A)).

Table 10–5. Speech Communication Capabilities Versus A-Weighted Sound Level dB(A) of the Background Noise

Communication	Below 50 dBA	50 to 70 dBA	70 to 90 dBA	90 to 100 dBA	110 to 130 dBA
Face-to-face (unamplified speech)	Normal voice at distances up to 6 m	Raised voice level at distances up to 2 m	Very loud or shouted voice level at distances up to 50 cm	Maximum voice level at distances up to 25 cm	Very difficult to impossible, even at a distance of 1 cm
Telephone	Good	Satisfactory to slightly difficult	Difficult to unsatisfactory	Use press-to-talk switch and an acoustically treated booth	Use special equipment
Intercom system	Good	Satisfactory to difficult	Unsatisfactory using loudspeaker	Impossible using loudspeaker	Impossible using loudspeaker
Type of earphone to supplement loudspeaker	None	Any	Use any earphone	Use any in earmuff or helmet except bone conduction-type	Use insert-type or over-ear earphones in helmet or in earmuffs; good to 120 dBA on short-term basis
Public-address system	Good	Satisfactory	Satisfactory to difficult	Difficult	Very difficult
Type of microphone required	Any	Any	Any	Any noise-cancelling microphone	Good noise-cancelling microphone

Table 10–6. Octave-Band Sound Pressure Level (SPL) Values Associated With the Recommended 1971 Preferred Noise Criterion (PNC) Curves

Preferred Noise Criterion Curves	31.5 Hz	63 Hz	125 Hz	250 Hz	500 Hz	1000 Hz	2000 Hz	4000 Hz	8000 Hz
PNC-15	58	43	35	28	21	15	10	8	8
PNC-20	59	46	39	32	26	20	15	13	13
PNC-25	60	49	43	37	31	25	20	18	18
PNC-30	61	52	46	41	35	30	25	23	23
PNC-35	62	55	50	45	40	35	30	28	28
PNC-40	64	59	54	50	45	40	35	33	33
PNC-45	67	63	58	54	50	45	41	38	38
PNC-50	70	66	62	58	54	50	46	43	43
PNC-55	73	70	66	62	59	55	51	48	48
PNC-60	76	73	69	66	63	59	56	53	53
PNC-65	79	76	73	70	67	64	61	58	58

compared with the appropriate PNC curve in Table 10–6.

3. The criterion value just above the highest octave-band level must be used to describe the noise environment.

4. The quality of communication to be expected for that environment must be determined (Table 10–7).

Articulation Index

The articulation index (AI) is calculated from physical measurements made on a communication system that describes the intelligibility that might be expected for that system under actual conditions. The speech spectrum and effective masking spectrum at the ear of the listener are required for the computation. The method is applicable for communication situations that involve male talkers.

Procedures for calculating the AI are based on the spectrum level of the noise and of speech present in 20 contiguous bands of frequencies, octave bands, or one-third octave bands of frequencies. The greatest precision is obtained with the 20-band procedure, the least precision is obtained with the octave-band method. An appropriate worksheet must be used to calculate the AI. A sample worksheet is shown in Figure 10–13, and Figure 10–14 is a sample calculation of an AI by the octave-band method for a relatively flat noise spectrum of moderate intensity. This calculation procedure may be followed in the example in Figure 10–14, which provides an AI of 0.54. The procedure is as follows:

1. The octave-band levels of the steady-

Table 10–7. Recommended Noise Criteria Ranges For Steady Background Noise as Heard in Various Indoor Functional Areas

Type of Space (and Acoustic Requirements)	PNC Curve	Approximate Sound Level dB(A)
For sleeping, resting, relaxing, bedrooms, sleeping quarters, hospitals, residences, apartments	25 to 40	34 to 47
For fair-listening conditions; laboratory work spaces, drafting and engineering rooms, general secretarial areas	40 to 50	47 to 56
For moderately fair-listening conditions; light maintenance shops, office and computer equipment rooms	45 to 55	52 to 61
For just-acceptable speech and telephone communication; shops, garages, powerplant control rooms. Levels above PNC-60 are not recommended for any office or communication situation	50 to 60	56 to 66
For work spaces where speech or telephone communication is not required, but where there must be no risk of hearing damage	60 to 75	66 to 80

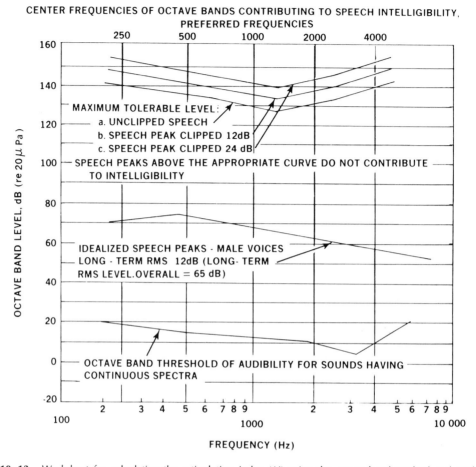

Fig. 10–13. Worksheet for calculating the articulation index (AI) using the octave-band method and preferred frequencies.

state noise reaching the listener's ears must be plotted.

2. The idealized speech peaks curve must be adjusted to reflect the speech curve in the system under test.

3. The difference in decibels at the band center frequencies between the speech and the noise spectra must be determined. (Assign 0 to differences less than 1 and 30 to differences greater than 30.)

4. The difference values in each band must be multiplied by the weighting factor for that band and the resulting numbers added to obtain the AI.

A number of factors that influence speech intelligibility scores, either individually or in combinations, may be quantitatively evaluated using the AI. Some of the factors are (1) masking by steady-state noise; (2) masking by nonsteady-state noise, including the interruption rate; (3) frequency distortion of the speech signal; (4) amplitude distortion of the speech signal; (5) reverberation time; (6) vocal effort; and (7) visual cues. The many factors not evaluated by AI include (1) the sex of the talker; (2) multiple transmission paths; (3) combinations of distortions; (4) monaural versus binaural presentation; and (5) asymmetric clipping, frequency shifting, and fading.

The relationship of AI to the various measures of speech intelligibility is shown

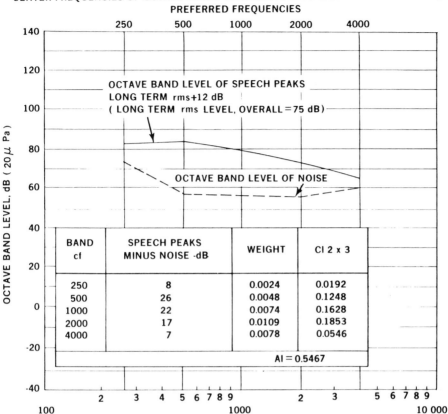

Fig. 10–14. Example of an articulation index (AI) calculation using the octave-band method.

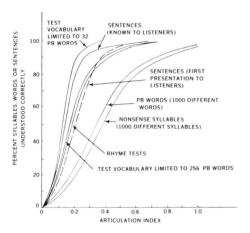

Fig. 10–15. Relation between the articulation index and the various measures of speech intelligibility. These relationships are approximate.

in Figure 10–15. The intelligibility score is dependent on the constraints placed on the message, that is, the greater the constraint, the higher the intelligibility score. No single-value AI can be established as a universally acceptable communications criterion because of variations in the proficiency of talkers and listeners and in the nature of the messages to be transmitted. The AI is a consistent, reliable procedure for predicting the relative performance of communications systems operating under given conditions. Modern communications systems usually have design goals of AIs in excess of 0.5. An AI of 0.7 appears appropriate as a goal for systems that will operate under a variety of stress conditions and with many different talkers and listeners of varying degrees of skill.

Measurement of Intelligibility

In some situations, the speech and/or noise characteristics may not satisfy the basic assumptions underlying the standard calculation procedures. Unusual noise environments, whole-body vibration in noise, audio communications jamming, artificial atmospheres, are examples. The communication efficiency with talkers and/or listeners in the environment of interest must then be measured. One sensitive test of speech intelligibility is the Phonetically Balanced (PB) Monosyllable Word Intelligibility Test. This test consists of trained talkers reading lists of phonetically balanced material to trained listeners using the communication system features being evaluated. A score of about 70% on the PB word lists corresponds to more than 90% intelligibility for sentences. Another standardized intelligibility measure is the Modified Rhyme Test (MRT), a test of choice for evaluating the performance of aerospace voice communications systems in the presence of environmental noise. Trained talkers read to trained listeners materials that consist of lists of 50 one-syllable words that are equivalent in intelligibility. Test words are presented imbedded within a carrier phrase that is the same for each item. The MRT is easy to administer, score, and evaluate, and it does not require extensive training of the listeners. The MRT word intelligibility has been sufficiently standardized to allow the relative intelligibility of such materials as closed message sets and sentences to be estimated on the basis of corresponding measured MRT scores. Scores of 80% and above are acceptable for aerospace and military systems; scores of 70% to 80% are generally marginal, and scores below 70% represent unacceptable voice communications for such applications.

Effects of Noise on Speech Reception

It has been established that the primary effect of noise on speech communication is interference with or masking of the speech signal. Intense noise levels at the ear also may cause aural overload and distortion that accompany the masking, producing additional interference with reception. The effectiveness of the acoustic masker varies with the frequency content of the noise and with the ratio of the signal level to the noise level (S/N ratio). The most effective noise for masking speech contains the same energy that is present in the long-term average speech spectrum of the signal to be masked. Long-term average speech spectra vary slightly from talker to talker and substantially for different levels of vocal effort. Although there is some upward spread of masking, intelligibility generally increases as the noise spectrum is maximum above or below the speech spectrum.

Generally, the speech signal level must be greater than the noise level at the ear for good intelligibility. Intelligibility as a function of the S/N ratio, however, does vary with the type of speech material. The intelligibility of sentences is approximately 0% correct at -12 dB S/N and greater than 95% correct at 0 dB S/N (range of 12 dB), whereas nonsense syllables that are also 0% corrrect at -12 dB S/N ratio require about $+15$ dB S/N to exceed 95% correct (range of 27 dB). Both the spectra and level of aerospace noises must be considered to avoid masking of the speech signal and ensure successful communication.

Direct Communication

The relationships between background noise, in terms of A-weighted sound level and SIL, and the distances between talker and listener, where face-to-face communication is satisfactory, are summarized in Figure 10–12. These data show that satisfactory communication, about 90 to 95% correct perception of sentences, is expected with a normal voice at a distance of about 3 m in a noise at a level of 55 dB(A) (48 dB SIL). At the same distance apart, direct communications are difficult at a noise level of about 74 dB(A), where talkers must shout to be understood. As the background noise reaches a level where the talker must increase his vocal output, the voice level is increased from 3 dB (lower noise levels) to 6 dB (higher noise levels) for every 10-dB increase in noise level.

The data in Figure 10–12 show the effect of noise on voice communication and demonstrate that conversation with a normal voice is not possible in most high-noise environments at distances greater than about 1 m. This means that aerospace work environment noises that require an above-normal voice effort place additional stress on both the talkers and listeners. The amount of stress on the communicator and strain on the vocal cords is dependent on the amount of vocal effort and frequency or amount of communication required. Infrequent or occasional raised voices and shouts may be tolerable; however, personnel should not be required to maintain frequent or continuous face-to-face communication under conditions requiring above-normal vocal effort. Electronically aided communications should be considered for these situations to protect the health and well-being of the personnel and to minimize errors due to inadequate communications.

Communication Equipment Effectiveness

State-of-the-art communications systems and accompanying terminal equipment are satisfactory for most modern speech communications tasks in noise. The equipment is designed to optimize the speech signal by techniques that include a passband similar to the long-term average speech spectrum, peak-clipping, low impedance, and automatic gain control. Microphones and earphones are housed in noise-excluding shields and earcups and designed with frequency responses ideal-

ized for human speech. Noise-cancelling microphones significantly reduce the sensitivity of the microphone to low-frequency noise without affecting their sensitivity to the speech signal. In some aerospace environments, such as helicopters, navy flight decks, jet engine test stands, and near field rocket firings, improved voice communications effectiveness is still needed. In these situations, the noise-excluding features of the terminal equipment are not always adequate for the high levels of noise in which the equipment is used; however, in most other situations, the equipment does not contribute to degradation of voice communications.

Communication in In-Flight Environments

The noise exposure at an in-flight crew station is composed of some combination of propulsion system, auxiliary equipment, and aerodynamic noise. The noise exposure for a particular flight sequence or profile can be analyzed in terms of frequency content, levels, and durations and appropriate equipment selected to operate under the worst-case conditions. All aircraft and space vehicles must contend with these propulsion system, auxiliary equipment, and aerodynamic noises. The duration of intense propulsion system noise and aerodynamic noise during space launches is so brief that communications equipment can be selected to operate in the presence of the lower noise levels of the equipment operating during cruise. These auxiliary and life-support system noises ordinarily pose no threat to voice communications, so that small, lightweight, headset-microphone systems are satisfactory. High-performance aircraft require voice communications equipment to be integrated with the flight helmet-oxygen mask system. Typically, this includes a high-performance, altitude-compensated earphone inside the helmet and a noise-cancelling microphone in the oxygen mask. Both the helmet and oxygen mask act as noise shields. Crewmembers of other types of military aircraft may use the flight helmet with a noise-cancelling microphone mounted on a boom or simply a headset with a noise-cancelling boom microphone. These terminal equipment items typically have been designed specifically for the kinds of noise environments in which they are used, and their performance is usually reliable.

The flight crew compartments of most commercial passenger aircraft have been sufficiently sound-treated to minimize or eliminate noise as a voice communications problem. The situation is different with general aviation aircraft where cabin noise can pose a threat to voice communications. Communications terminal equipment, that is, the headset-microphone system, should be selected specifically for the cabin noise environment in which it will be used because the performance in noise of such systems may vary widely. It is of interest that the preferred ambient noise levels for commercial airline passengers is about 67 dB(A), a level that generally masks conversations at a distance of about 1 m from the talker. Ambient noise levels below this value do not provide acoustic privacy for conversations of passengers seated close to one another and result in speech interference and dissatisfied passengers.

Helicopters generate environments in which present communications equipment, for special phases of flight, may become marginal or inadequate. This is particularly true for aircrew members required to work in large open vehicles or to be external to the vehicle fuselage. For example, medical rescue personnel immediately outside the helicopter in the direct downwash of the rotating blades may find both the transmitting and receiving of voice communication to be marginal to unacceptable. Part of the problem can be attributed to the helicopter noise spectrum, which is particularly high in the low-frequency regions where the noise-at-

tenuating properties of flight helmets are least effective. Although substantial progress has been made in the development of noise-excluding headwear, some helicopter situations need continued improvement in communications equipment. A concept now under development to provide low-frequency noise cancellation in communications helmets may provide significant help for helicopter crewmembers.

Communication in Ground Environments

Ground communication headset-microphones provide adequate to marginal communications in noise levels up to 130 to 135 dB SPL. Units consist of noise-cancelling microphones housed in noise shields and high-output earphones mounted in noise-excluding earcups. These units must be properly manufactured and in good working order to provide the maximum design performance. The Air Force standard ground communication headset-microphone (H-133) can be modified to provide satisfactory voice communications in some environments that exceed 140 dB. The modification involves the use of a custom-molded earplug (with long canal) equipped with a button microphone that is worn under the earcup. The standard earphone is removed and the leads reconnected to the button earphone. This modification has provided adequate voice communications in jet engine test cell noise, where communications were not satisfactory with the standard unit. Although demonstrated on the Air Force system, this modification concept should improve voice communications of most earcup-enclosed earphone terminal equipment.

Voice communications problems may occur in activities such as in-flight control centers, air traffic control facilities, C[3] (command, control, and communications), and surveillance operations due to noise generated by the equipment in use, as well as by external sources. Many of these problems can be alleviated by the identification and treatment of the noise source. Such treatment may range from the use of sound-absorbing materials and enclosures to rearrangement of the equipment to locate noise sources away from the crew positions. When the noise at crew positions is not adequately reduced by treatment of the source and propagation, it may be necessary to add noise-cancellation and noise-exclusion features to the headset-microphones in use.

Machine Speech Recognition and Production

Aerospace operations comprise a very fertile area for the successful application of developing new technologies of voice control and voice response. Voice control utilizing automatic speech recognition has been, for several decades, a technologic goal with virtually unlimited applications. The ultimate functional objective is a totally reliable, talker-independent device that requires virtually no training and will operate with an unlimited vocabulary. Human speech has proven to be a much more complex and sophisticated acoustic signal for this application than initially estimated; consequently, these objectives have necessarily been revised to realistically correspond to the present limited voice control technology. Voice response devices, those generating synthetic speech, have appeared only in the recent past but are already seen in numerous applications such as educational toys, games, status report systems, novelties, prompting, and the like. The voice response technology is growing much faster than voice control primarily because the problems associated with its generation and use are relatively less difficult and challenging than those associated with voice control technology.

Automatic Speech Recognition (Voice Control)

Automatic speech recognition systems are commercially available and in various stages of development for use in situations relatively free of interfering environmental factors. Although these systems operate using techniques such as template matching, linear predictive coding, or phoneme recognition, they are characterized in terms of vocabulary size, speaker dependency, word or phrase recognition, and reliability. Vocabulary size may vary from as few as 20 words to as many as a few hundred words. Speaker-dependent systems require training for each talker and retraining before use by another talker. Training consists of from one to numerous repetitions of the total vocabulary by the talker, depending on the system. Speaker-independent systems theoretically can be directly used by any talker without their participation in the training. Isolated word recognition systems ordinarily require a brief pause between words to allow each word to be recognized. Connected-word or connected-speech systems function more quickly and allow several words to be spoken as a phrase. The reliability of present systems is degraded by unfavorable operating conditions. Reliability or correct word recognition may vary from 95 to +99% under ideal conditions but may drop to essentially 0% under the most severe conditions such as high-level ambient noise environments.

Present automatic speech recognition systems are being evaluated and developed for adaptation to different applications, with varying degrees of success. Among these applications are human operator interfaces with data processing equipment, voice queries for information, the filing of information such as flight plans, voice instead of manual control of buttons, switches, and knobs, as well as of naval and aircraft avionics, flight controls, and weapons delivery. One of the areas of highest potential payoff is that of excessive human operator work load, which consists of too many visual and manual tasks, time-critical tasks, or highly specialized situations, such as high-speed, low-level flight, where looking down into the cockpit to perform a manual task is a threat to safety. Clearly, numerous situations exist that would profit from the use of a voice interactive system, having crewmembers speak appropriate key words, to control various aerospace vehicle operations typically activated with manual controls.

A major problem with current systems is their vulnerability to environmental stressors, which in aerospace operations means noise, vibration, and acceleration. Several programs are presently under way to produce robust versions of voice interactive systems that will operate in various aerospace vehicles, including helicopters, tactical aircraft, and space vehicles. The comparatively severe stressors present in helicopter and tactical aircraft environments require a much more robust system than demanded by the cruise portions of space flight. For example, voice control of cameras during most portions of a space mission may be within the state of the art. Generic systems are being developed and adapted to tasks instead of being designed for specific applications that require robust systems; perhaps this approach, along with the limitations in speech technology, is contributing to the difficulties experienced in achieving satisfactory systems for stress environments.

Advances in computer processing time, increased memory, coding techniques, and microprocessor development hold high promise for expanded application and increased reliability of voice interactive systems in spite of the absence of recent significant breakthroughs in speech recognition technology. Numerous companies are actively working in the voice recognition technology area, and specific applications in nonstressed environments will be implemented from time to time. The full application of voice control in the hostile environments of various aerospace systems, however, is not expected in the immediate future.

Machine Voice Response

Voice response systems are appearing on the commercial market in increasing numbers and at decreasing costs, resulting in a ready supply for applications activities. Microprocessors provide a wide variety of preprogrammed words and phrases in reasonably typical male or female voices. Speech synthesis systems can be custom-developed for a particular user and application, including specific vocabulary and male or female voice. Speech synthesis already has been successfully demonstrated in numerous contemporary situations where radios, automobiles, computers, clocks, games, educational toys, and various other devices provide information by "talking." The technology is well developed and will continue to be refined with virtually unlimited applications opportunities.

Machine voice response does not experience the same vulnerability to environmental stressors as voice control. It is susceptible to noise-masking, and favorable synthetic speech-to-noise ratios are required for effective operation. Voice response systems produce speech that varies to different degrees in quality or naturalness, and many systems sound cryptic, disconnected, poorly articulated, and lacking in inflection. In some applications, such as voice warning, the unnaturalness may be desirable as an "attention-getter," whereas during long-term space missions, natural-sounding synthetic speech would be preferred. Although preliminary, there are some indications that human responses to synthetic speech may differ slightly from responses to human speech; for example, the reaction time to synthetic speech was observed to be slightly longer than to human speech.

Among the aerospace applications of machine voice responses are advisory, validation, and warning functions. Appropriate rules for information management via the auditory, visual, and other sensory channels must be developed; however, many of the status conditions of aerospace vehicles could be provided by synthetic speech. These audio advisories would greatly relieve many of the visual requirements for monitoring dials, gauges, and annunciator panels. Validation functions could operate as feedback loops, actually telling the operator by voice the action that was performed, such as confirming "wheels down," talking avionics, repeating the newly tuned radiofrequency, and stating other changes in aircraft control as activated by the crewmember. In space, or missile control centers, and air traffic control-type environments, voice responses can accompany selected visual displays as a redundant means of increasing the effectiveness of audiovisual information transfer.

High interest has been shown in optimizing and integrating voice warning into the total warning networks of aerospace systems. The initial voice warning system in the United States Air Force B-58 Hustler aircraft consisted of tape recordings of words and phrases spoken by a female. Although novel at the time and of scientific interest, the technical approach eventually proved unacceptable. Present microprocessor-type systems are highly flexible and can be developed to be adaptive in terms of message management, including priorities. Additional investigative work is needed to develop a data base of the trade-offs and optimum usage of voice warnings. The application of this voice response data base involves the effective integration of voice warning with nonvoice-warning signals, visual displays, annunciator indicators, and the audio communications function.

Future Communication in Aerospace Environments

Aerospace requirements for secure, reliable communications have fostered the application of rapidly developing technologies to audio communications. The procedures involved in providing secure, jam-resistant communication utilize a variety of voice-processing techniques that may alter or even completely transform the signal. These techniques generally require a very wide bandpass, reduced sensitivity to noise, digitizing, and multiplexing, as well as other features that are not normally present in contemporary communications equipment. Future communications systems, including aerospace radios, must be designed to incorporate these new developments, as well as those of noise cancellation for communications systems, fiber optic technology, adaptive frequency response, and voice control. These highly advanced systems will display marked miniaturization of components, extremely high reliability, and robustness and will be completely wireless, resulting in essentially personal communication units, which together will comprise a communications system or net.

EFFECTS OF VIBRATION ON AVIATION PERSONNEL

Operational Vibration Exposures

Operators and passengers of all types of transportation vehicles, be it in air, space, on the ground, or underwater, are exposed to some kind of vibration during some phases of the operation. The oscillations of the vehicle motions around a reference stationary state, at rest, or during constant velocity and/or acceleration are transmitted to the occupants through the supporting seat and floor or through wall vibrations or vibrating handles. This transmission results in motions of the whole human body or body parts. In studying biomechanical interaction, it is somewhat artificial to separate body motions into sustained, transient, rotational, or impact acceleration and linear oscillations, although this is driven in part by our analytic, experimental, and laboratory simulation tools. In taking this conventional approach, it is important to keep its limitations in mind and not to forget that vibrations are only a small part of the total mechanical force or motion spectrum. The physical, physiologic, and performance effects to be discussed for the vibration spectrum of interest, from 0.5 Hz to a few hundred hertz, often occur simultaneous with and are modified by the effects of sustained and/or transient accelerations. Table 10–8 indicates the simultaneous occurrence of some of these mechanical environments during various phases of aerospace flight and denotes the degree of performance capability usually required or desired. Low-altitude, high-speed flight in military operations and storm and clear-air turbulence in commercial and general aviation cause the most severe vibration exposures of concern. Their severity depends on the input gust velocities and acceleration spectra, as well as on the aerodynamic properties and flexibility of the aircraft. In military aircraft with manual or automatic terrain-following control systems, maneuvering loads with maxima between 0.01 and 0.1 Hz are superimposed on the gust-response spectra of the aircraft and crew. Prediction of human effects and protective measures required for all phases indicated in Table 10–8 requires the forecasting or measurement of the environments in all six degrees of freedom and for the total mechanical spectrum.

Pathophysiologic and Physiologic Effects of Vibration

As elaborated in the earlier section entitled "The Human Body as a Receiver of Noise and Vibration," it depends on the frequency range and the exposure conditions which part of the human body is exposed to maximum vibration stress and responds most severely. Unlike sound exposure, in which most effects are mediated through the ear, there is no specific target area or organ for low-frequency, whole-body vibration, and the mechanical stresses imposed can potentially lead to interference with bodily functions and tissue damage in practically all parts of the body. Fortunately, operational stresses are almost never that high, and vibration exposures remain below injury and interference levels. Severe buffeting in one military aircraft led to a few oscillations best described as repetitive impacts that resulted in spinal fractures. Based on scanty human evidence and animal studies, damage to renal functions and pulmonary hemorrhages are suspected of being the first signs of injury from acute overexposure in the frequency range of maximum abdominal response (4 to 8 Hz). Whole-body vibration of intensities voluntarily tolerated by human subjects up to the limit of severe discomfort or pain has not resulted in demonstrable harm or injury.[15] Minor kidney injuries in truck and tractor drivers have been suspected to be due to vibration exposure of long duration at levels that produce no apparent acute effects, but epidemiologic studies have yet to prove any clear correlation. Similarly higher incidences of back pain in helicopter pilots and tractor operators have been assumed to be related to the vibration produced by the vehicles; in spite of several studies and plausible arguments, hard data are lacking and difficult to obtain. Modern exposure limits for health and safety reasons are, therefore, primarily based on voluntary tolerance limits, pain thresholds, and experiences with occupational exposures assumed to be safe. Most physiologic effects in the 2- to 12-Hz frequency range are associated with the resonance of the thoracoabdominal viscera. It has been shown to be responsible for pain occurring in the 1 to 2 g_z (peak) and 2 to 3 g_x ranges suspected to be caused by the stretching of the perichondrium and periosteum at the chondrosternal and interchondral joint capsules and ligaments. Movement of abdominal viscera in and out of the thoracic cage, in both X- and Z-axis excitation, is responsible for the interference of vibration with respiration. It causes the involuntary oscilla-

Table 10–8. Vibration, Acceleration, and Other Environments Associated With Aerospace Flight

Environment	Military		General Aviation		Space		
	Escape	Low-Altitude, High-Speed Flight	Storm and Clear-Air Turbulence	Helicopter and V/STOL Operations	Boost Phase of Spaceflight	Reentry Phase of Spaceflight	Weightlessness
Simple sustained acceleration	M	C	—	—	C	C	—
Complex sustained acceleration	M	C	C	—	C	C	—
Angular and linear vibration	E	C	C	C	C	C	C
Rotation	E	—	—	—	—	—	C
Transient acceleration	E	C	C	C	—	E	—
Complex transient acceleration	E	C	C	C	—	E	C
Overpressure	E	—	—	—	—	—	—
Windblast	E	—	—	—	—	—	—
Infrasonic noise	—	R	R	R	C	C	—
Acoustic noise	E	C	—	C	C	C	—
Thermal extremes, fire	E	—	—	—	—	R	R
Reduced atmospheric pressure	E	—	—	—	—	R	R
Ballistic impact	E	—	—	—	—	—	—

*The level of performance required is indicated by the letter code. The presence of a letter code indicates that the environment occurs during the indicated aerospace operation. Performance code: E = retain ability to escape and evade; M = retain monitor function; C = retain ability to control vehicle; and R = perform during repeated exposure.

tion of a significant volume of air in and out of the lungs, leading to an increase in minute volume, alveolar ventilation, and oxygen consumption. In some experimental exposures to g_z vibrations, PCO_2 decreased and clinical signs of hypocapnia were observed, suggesting hyperventilation. Dyspnea results from short exposures to high amplitudes.

Cardiovascular functions change similarly in response to X-axis, Y-axis, and Z-axis excitation.[16] The test results, indicating an increase in mean arterial blood pressure, cardiac index, and heart rate in humans, are illustrated in Figure 10–16. In general, the combined cardiopulmonary response to vibration in the 2- to 12-Hz range resembles the response to exercise. Although the increased muscular effort of bracing against the vibration and psychologic factors may account for some of the response, observance of the same general pattern in anesthetized animals speaks for the stimulation of various mechanoreceptors.

The resonance of the abdominal viscera, with its resulting distortions and stretching, is also responsible for the epigastric or periumbilical discomfort and testicular pain reported at high amplitudes. Headache is frequently associated with exposure to frequencies above 10 Hz. Particularly in $G_x \pm g_x$ and $G_x \pm g_y$ exposures (space couch positions), vibrations are transmitted to the head directly from the headrest, which can lead to extremely uncomfortable and disturbing impacts of the head against the headrest. Raising the head away from the headrest and attempts to counteract the forces leads to neck muscle strain, spasm, and soreness. Restraining the head to follow the motion can result in disorientation during the exposure.

Rubbing of body surfaces against the

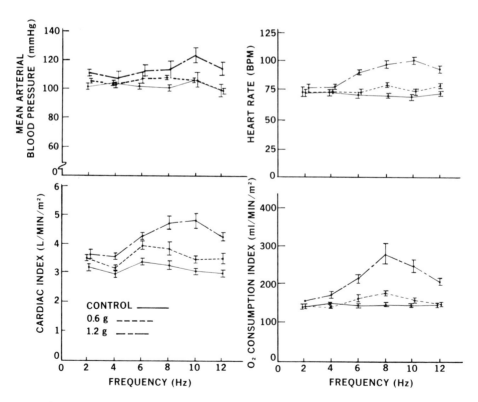

Fig. 10–16. Effect of amplitude and frequency of $G_z \pm g_x$ sinusoidal whole-body vibration on mean arterial blood pressure, cardiac index, heart rate, and oxygen consumption.[17]

seat, backrest, or restraint straps (e.g., "back scrub" in some tractor or vehicle arrangements) can lead to discomfort and skin injuries.

The severe vibration responses and injuries observed in animal experiments have not been reported in humans due to appropriate safety criteria.[17] In interpreting animal experiments, it is of utmost importance to consider appropriate scaling laws due to the changed body dimensions and resonances, and, therefore, maximum-effects frequencies are considerably higher in small animals.

The Vibration Syndrome

The only specific vibration-induced disease with well-supported etiologic data is the vibration disease, or "white finger syndrome,"caused by habitual occupational exposure over months and years to the vibration of machinery and certain hand tools such as chain saws, chipping hammers, and other pneumatic tools.[18] Although epidemiologic research over the last decade has documented various patterns and stages of the disease affecting the blood vessels, nerves, bones, joints, muscles, or connective tissues of the hand and forearm, the earliest and most clearly established manifestations are Raynaud's phenomenon, impairment of the blood circulation to the hands, or disorders of the peripheral nervous system. Individual susceptibility to the disease and the influence of other factors affecting peripheral circulation such as cold and smoking are not yet well understood. The physical impact of the handtool vibrations is clearly modified by working methods (tightness of handgrip, i.e., "let the tool do the work") and the intermittency of exposure. With respect to the effectiveness of various frequencies, constant input velocity appears to result in equal injury potential over most of the effective frequency range (8 to 1000 Hz). Consequently, curves of equal risk of developing disorders from exposure to hand-transmitted vibration are

assumed to have the shape shown in Figure 10–17, and filters with the inverse function have been standardized for measuring and weighting hand-arm vibrations. The overall weighted level so obtained in approximately 40 studies in various countries on workers exposed to hand-transmitted vibrations in their job for periods of up to 25 years has been related to the exposure time for the onset of vascular disorders in selected percentiles of the population (Fig. 10–18). This dose-effect relationship allows the estimation of the risk involved in various exposure conditions.[19] The particular curves in Figure 10–17 predict for a weighted acceleration of 2.9 m/sec² the onset of disorders in 50% of the population after 25 years. The lower curve A is for a broad-band spectrum that reaches the curve in each third-octave frequency band; the upper curve is for a weighted acceleration spectrum coinciding with the curve in a third-octave band

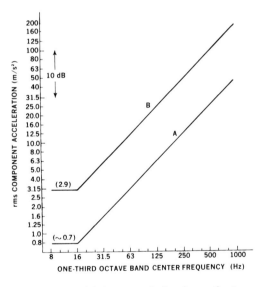

Fig. 10–17. Weighting curves for hand-arm vibrations. Both curves correspond to a weighted overall acceleration level of 2.9 m/sec²: curve A applies to broad band spectra, of which all one-third octave band levels coincide with the curve; curve B applies to spectra that are composed of a single band, which coincides with the criteria curve. Both curves represent curves of equal risk for the onset of disorders in 50% of a population after 25 years of using hand tools for approximately 4 hr/day.

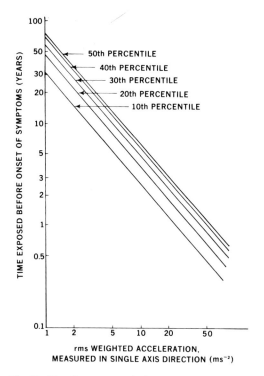

Fig. 10–18. Occurrence of vibration-induced vascular symptoms in various percentiles of a population using hand tools on a daily basis as a function of the weighted hand acceleration.

only while all other bands are 20 dB lower. All other possible spectra with the same weighted acceleration value will fall between these two curves.[20]

Effects on Task Performance

The vibration environment can interfere with the sensory and motor aspects of tasks. It has less effect on cognitive performance and central nervous system processing through its general stress component. The performance requirements under vibration conditions during various phases of aerospace flight are indicated in Table 10–8. They can vary from the gross monitoring of instrument panels and single gross motor tasks to detailed monitoring, reading of complex displays, and high work load motor functions required to control an aircraft in turbulent, low-level flight. In military missions, low-level navigation and weapon delivery and the ma-

neuvering loads associated with pull-ups and push-overs for terrain following increase task demands as well as environmental stress. With manual control, pull-ups are in the range of $+2.0\,G_x$, push-overs in the range of $+0.5\,G_x$. Aircraft and spacecraft design specifications with respect to vibration acceptability for satisfactory performance are based primarily on flight test data and subjective pilot evaluations. Realistic simulations of the vibration environment on moving-base simulators adds to this body of knowledge and gives confidence to specific designs or task requirements. Controlled laboratory experiments are designed to explore in detail interference effects as a function of frequency, amplitude, task design, and exposure time. These studies are the keys to improved designs of vibration-resistant controls and displays.

Motor Performance

The involuntary motions of the body and the extremities introduced by vibrations are superimposed as disturbances on the active control motions of a human operator. The greater the vibration amplitude of hand or foot in comparison with the required control motion (through strong original excitation or through resonance reinforcement), the larger the undesirable interference. The complexity of the overall control situation and of the various interference paths is shown in Figure 10–19. In laboratory tracking experiments, errors increase in the 2- to 12-Hz frequency range at seat accelerations above approximately $0.05\,g_z$ rms. The maximum decrement is usually in the range of 4 Hz, which is the main body resonance. For X-axis and Y-axis vibration, the largest decrements are at 1.5 to 2 Hz. In all cases, tracking errors tend to be largest in the direction of the disturbing vibration stimulus. The magnitudes of the decrements cannot be generalized because they depend too much on the specific details of the control task (e.g., position, velocity or force control, ampli-

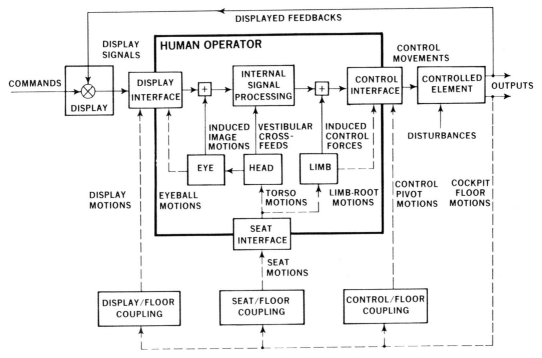

Fig. 10–19. The human operator performing a manual task in a biodynamic environment.

tude of required control motion) and the hand-arm or foot-leg support. Design guides for vibration-resistant controls are available, however. The ability to perform fine manipulative tasks such as writing or setting cursors should be verified by simulation before relying on them in operational situations.

The severity of the vibration interference can be influenced to some extent by the operator's control strategy. For example, under turbulent flight conditions, pilots often postpone motor activity during short bursts of high-amplitude vibrations and introduce corrective action as soon as the burst is over. Under sustained turbulence, very low frequencies can excite "pilot-induced oscillations," which are caused by inappropriate control inputs. The pilot apparently has time to correct for the disturbance inputs, but due to misinterpretations of kinesthetic cues or the response characteristics of the motor system, he does not do it in an appropriate

way at some frequencies and adds through his inputs to aircraft instabilities.

Effects on Vision

Difficulties in reading instruments and performing visual searches occur when vibrations introduce relative movement of the eye with respect to the target. Although persons and instruments might be excited by the same structural vibrations, their response is completely different, causing different displacements in different frequency ranges. A complex relationship exists between all of the relevant parameters, such as vibration frequency, amplitude and direction, viewing distance, illumination, contrast, and the shape of the viewed object. Large effects on the resolution of visual detail occur under Z-axis, whole-body vibration and for Y-axis and Z-axis vibration of viewed objects. The main difference between the object versus the subject vibration is the compensating ocular reflexes mediated by the vestibular system (vestibulo-ocular reflex) and by proprioceptors in the head (colliculo-ocular reflex), which enable the eye to compensate for body and head motions, thereby fixating the gaze on the target. Although effectiveness of the vestibulo-ocular reflex drops off above 1 Hz, it has been shown to affect results up to 8 Hz. Analysis and prediction of visual capability are further complicated by the fact that translational body motion results not only in translational but also in rotational head movements. The latter influence passive eye movement, as well as vestibular feedback. The same compensatory reflexes have been shown to degrade remarkably visibility on head-mounted or helmet-mounted displays under vibration when the display moves with the head.

Although mechanical eye resonances have been investigated in several studies up to 90 Hz, their influence on vision is apparently of secondary importance, and no sharp resonance phenomena as a function of frequency have been observed.

Unfortunately, the large number of test results cannot yet be presented in uniform curves allowing the prediction of visual decrement. The large number of variables, such as, for example, small changes in subject posture and restraint, affecting translational and rotational head responses and large intersubject intervariability and other variables prevent generalization of the results. The examples of Figure 10–20 should, therefore, be accepted as specific test results and not generally valid design guidance. The levels of vibration below which no interference with visual acuity normally is expected are indicated.

For $G_z \pm g_x$, g_y, and g_z vibrations and for $G_x \pm g_z$ vibrations, the largest effects were found in the 11- to 15-Hz range. Decoupling the head from the headrest improved capability in this frequency range, whereas head restraint generally reduced reading errors at 6 Hz and below. The type of helmet and restraint, however, is crucial for these experiments. All of these results underline the previously stated conclu-

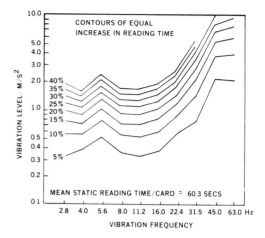

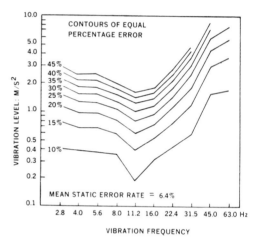

Fig. 10–20.   Mean vibration levels required to produce contours of equal percentage reading errors and equal percentage increases in reading time, ten subjects.

sion that because of the complexity and large number of variables, important vehicle performance requirements should be tested for each specific configuration in realistic simulations.

Effects on Speech Communication

Although hearing ability is practically not affected by vibration, the quality of speech can be impaired. Movements of the thoracoabdominal viscera induce modulations of the airflow in the respiratory system and, consequently, a tremolo-type modulation of the voice with the frequency of vibration. Vibrated speech is masked by noise to a greater extent than might be expected. Speech progressively deteriorates with increasing intensity of vibration. In addition, the pitch of the voice is increased, presumably due to the increased muscle tension. As a result of all these effects, speech intelligibility can be slightly impaired at some frequencies and amplitudes, as shown in Figure 10–21. In addition, the rate of talking can be slowed down.

Effects on Cognitive Functions

The central nervous system appears to be relatively unaffected by the vibration stress. Simple cognitive functions were unaffected in laboratory tests (pattern recognition and monitoring of dials and warning lights); more demanding tasks involving mental arithmetic and short-term memory during a 0.5 g_z (peak) vibration at frequencies below 15 Hz resulted in significantly slower performance. Other

studies, however, indicate that vibration can increase the level of arousal similar to observations in noise, depending on the exposure intensity, exposure time pattern, and the activity of the subject. This effect was particularly demonstrated in several studies on the combined effects of vibration and noise. In one such test, 100 dB(A) noise and 0.36 rms g_z vibration (5 sinusoids from 2.6 to 16 Hz combined) were used as stressors individually and in combination while the subjects performed a complex counting task. The task was sensitive to both the noise and vibration. Vibration and noise combined, however, resulted in less performance decrement than either of these stimuli alone.

The possibility of nonspecific central nervous system alterations due to continuing long-term exposure to vibrations in industrial situations and its contribution to general fatigue has been addressed in several studies, primarily in eastern European countries. The results are not uniform and not convincing. Habituation to monotonous vibration environments in aircraft or on ships is probably a central nervous system phenomenon, although some adaptation on the receptor level has been proposed.

Exposure and Design Guidance

General Basis for Guidelines

Discussion of the various vibration-induced physiologic and psychologic effects in the previous sections should have made it clear that no simple exposure limits and assessment procedures are applicable to all environmental, human posture and restraint, and task performance conditions. Too many factors can influence these conditions. A detailed interference analysis and simulation is desirable whenever expensive or irreversible decisions are at stake, particularly for the design of aircraft cockpits and spacecraft command modules when new environments or new visual or manipulatory tasks are involved.

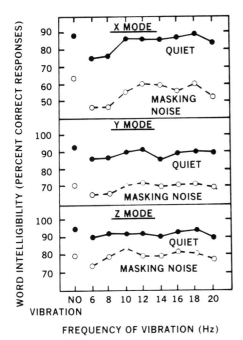

Fig. 10–21. Mean word intelligibility of talkers exposed to $G_x \pm g_x$, g_y, or g_z whole-body sinusoidal vibration (0.35 g (rms)). Quiet condition was with 70-dB speech and no masking noise; noise condition was with 70-dB speech and 70-dB masking noise.

For the evaluation of existing situations and the assessment of complaints and guidance with respect to good preventive medicine and ergonomic practices, however, the following guidelines should be helpful. These guidelines are a summary of present national and international standards and military specifications on this subject.

EXPOSURE CRITERIA. The guidelines give exposure criteria, considered on the basis of laboratory and field experiences, as protective with respect to the potential consequences stated.[21] They should not be exceeded without considered and compelling reasons. Criteria are proposed for the following conditions:

1. Preservation of health and safety exposure limits. These limits should not be exceeded without special justification and awareness of a potential health risk to a nonselected population. The limits are approximately doubled in amplitude in military specifications, where they are close to the pain threshold for healthy young subjects.
2. Preservation of working efficiency "fatigue or decreased proficiency boundary." As discussed, this limit cannot apply uniformly to all tasks and work loads. It is representative, however, of typical control situations in transportation vehicles and to a large extent based on aircraft pilot evaluations.
3. Preservation of comfort or reduced comfort boundary. The fatigue-decreased proficiency boundaries for Z-axis, X-axis, and Y-axis vibration are shown in Figure 10–22. To obtain the exposure limits, the curves should be raised by a factor of 2 (6 dB). The reduced comfort boundaries are obtained by dividing the curves in Figure 10–22 by 3.15 (10 dB). The dependence of the criteria on the vibration frequency is assumed to be

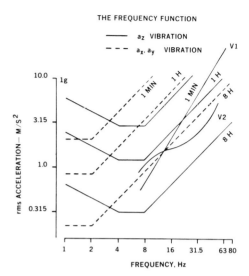

Fig. 10–22. Vibration exposure criteria for the g_z and g_x, g_y directions. The curves represent the "fatigue-decreased efficiency" boundary. For "exposure limit," curves should be raised by a factor of 2. For "reduced comfort," curves should be divided by 3.15. Object vibrations above curve V_1 and whole-body vibration above curve V_2 will lead to reductions in visual acuity.

the same for all three types of criteria: the Z-axis curve has maximum sensitivity in the resonance range of the thoracoabdominal system (4 to 8 Hz), whereas the X-axis and Y-axis curves have their maximum sensitivity below 2 Hz. The curves apply to the seated or standing subject without significant support by a backrest. A backrest will primarily affect the x-axis curve and make it increase less with frequency. In Figure 10–22, all criteria are a function of the average daily exposure time. This dependence, which might primarily apply to the exposure limits and the comfort boundary and is questionable with respect to task performance, is illustrated in Figure 10–23. The boundaries are defined in terms of rms value for single-frequency exposure or rms value in the third-octave band for broad-band vibration. The limits presented are valid at least for crest

THE EXPOSURE TIME FUNCTION

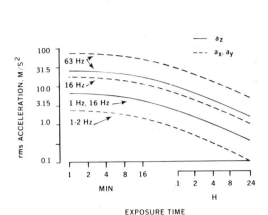

Fig. 10–23. "Fatigue-decreased efficiency" exposure criteria as a function of daily exposure time.

factors (maximum peak value to rms value over a 1-minute or longer period) of 3. Weighted accelerations with crest factors as great as 6 are still meaningfully interpreted by this approach.

WEIGHTED ACCELERATION. Frequently, it is desirable to characterize a vibration environment by a single quantity. Recent research on comfort and performance has shown that filtering the acceleration signal between 1 and 80 Hz with an electronic network having an insertion loss equivalent to the response curves of Figure 10–22 results in a single weighted acceleration value that correlates well with comfort and performance. The method weights each frequency according to its relative effectiveness with respect to human response. This weighting method is coming into wider and wider use, and the filtering networks for evaluating X-axis, Y-axis, and Z-axis whole-body vibrations and for evaluating hand-arm vibrations are incorporated into commercial human-response vibration meters. The overall weighted acceleration values are to be compared with the boundary values in the most sensitive frequency bands (4 to 8 Hz for Z-axis and 1 to 2 Hz for X-axis and Y-axis vibration).

Depending on the vibration spectrum, particularly if the spectrum rises outside the most sensitive frequency band, this weighting method can result in an overconservative assessment of the environment compared with the one-third octave-band analysis method. In this case, when the weighted values are close to the limits of acceptability, the one-third octave-band method should be used for numeric comparison with the criteria.

MULTIDIRECTIONAL AND ROTATIONAL VIBRATIONS. If vibrations are present in several directions simultaneously, the accelerations for each direction are to be assessed separately by the corresponding exposure criteria. When the g_x and g_y acceleration components multiplied by 1.4 have similar values to the g_z component, the combined motion can be more severe than the individual components would indicate. In this case, it is recommended that the weighted accelerations, g_w, be combined in the following way:

$$g_w = \sqrt{(1.4\ g_{xw})^2 + (1.4\ g_{yw})^2 + g_{zw}^2} \quad (3)$$

This amount of the vector sum can be compared for comfort and performance evaluations with the weighted acceleration values for Z-axis vibration.

Data on the acceptability of rotational or angular vibrations have been collected only recently, and generalized or standardized criteria are not available. Pure roll was perceived as producing more discomfort than the same amplitude and frequency of pure pitch oscillations. Examples of such data are shown in Figure 10–24. Yaw discomfort apparently varies considerably with a backrest support. If the operator is seated away from the axis of rotation, both the rotational vibration and the translational component must be considered. For many situations, prediction of response is adequate if only the most severe component is taken into consideration.

VIBRATIONS PRODUCING MOTION SICKNESS. Although the symptoms and causes

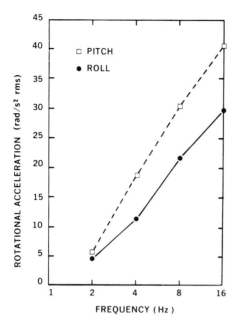

Fig. 10–24. Levels described as uncomfortable for pure rotational vibration.

of and therapeutic measures for motion sickness are discussed in Chapters 11 and 17, the frequency and amplitude range of vibrations producing the discomfort or acute distress associated with motion sickness shall be briefly mentioned in this chapter. The frequency range for vertical (Z-axis) vibration leading to this disability starts below 1 Hz, that is, right below the frequency range so far discussed. Motion sickness symptoms cause the curves shown in Figure 10–22 to drop sharply below 1 Hz. A continuous transition of the criteria curves shown in Figure 10–22 (e.g., of the reduced comfort boundary) is not desirable because the sensations, symptoms, and susceptibility of the population are quite different in the motion sickness range and are not comparable to those described for the higher vibrations. Because vibration-caused motion sickness can occur in most transportation systems and controlling vibrations in one frequency range can easily magnify the amplitudes in another frequency range, design guidance with respect to motion

sickness shall be briefly mentioned here. Curves of equal sensitivity in the 0.1- to 1-Hz range have the shape shown in Figure 10–25. The absolute levels for severe discomfort after 30-minute, 2-hour, and 8-hour exposures are very tentative and open to many variables. The boundaries as presented apply to infrequent, inexperienced travelers and are assumed to cover approximately 95% of such a population (5% probably never adapt to motion below 1 Hz). Civil and military vehicle operators and many travelers clearly have much higher discomfort and tolerance levels due to habituation and selection.

THE SUPINE POSITION. The criteria in Figure 10–22 apply to the normal standing or sitting position. Vibration transmission is changed in the supine or semisupine position, which is used in space operations and experimental military applications for its increased protection against sustained acceleration. In this position, X-axis vi-

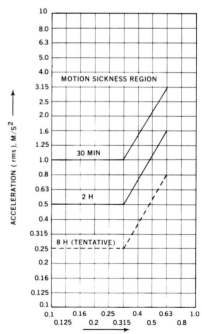

Fig. 10–25. Motion sickness weighting function for g_z oscillations. These are approximate boundaries for severe discomfort for a general population not accustomed to motion.

brations are most unpleasant and disturbing because of the direct transmission of the vibrations to the head (Fig. 10–26). Helmet properties are most significant, influencing tolerance as well as visual and speech capabilities.

SUSTAINED ACCELERATION COMBINED WITH VIBRATION. Limited experimental evidence suggests that accelerations and vibration are not synergistic. On the contrary, it appears as if vibration tolerance at 11 Hz 3 g_x was increased by the simultaneous application of 3.8 G_x. This finding can be theoretically explained by the inertial preload effect of the sustained acceleration, which at the same time has a static preload or restraining effect on the subject. On the other hand, it can be argued that the vibrations partially alleviate or counteract the circulatory and respiratory manifestations of sustained acceleration.

In this chapter, after reviewing the basic definitions and units of sound (decibel) and vibration (g [rms]) environments and their frequency ranges (in hertz), examples of their occurrence and intensity inside aerospace vehicles and radiating from the vehicles were discussed. The human body as receiver of mechanical energy was explained, including the absorption and reflection of sound at the body surface and the transmission of sound and vibration through the body structure. The special transformer design of the middle ear enables the high sensitivity and broad-bandwidth of the human auditory system so essential for speech communication. The requirements and technical possibilities for noise reduction and vibration control were elaborated. The effects of aerospace noise were reviewed in detail: the sensitivity (temporary and permanent threshold shift), the physiologic effects, potential health effects, startle, and annoyance. The measure of speech intelligibility, the masking of speech communication by noise, and the communication quality and reliability required operationally were described. Communication equipment effectiveness and the rapidly advancing areas of mechanical speech recognition and production were assessed.

Whole-body vibration exposure can result in various pathologic and physiologic effects located in different body regions, which are determined by the exposure frequency. For most operational exposures, however, effects on task performance and interference with activities were found to be of primary concern. The only well-documented vibration-induced disease is the "white finger syndrome" caused by habitual exposure to vibrating hand tools. The standards for safety, performance capability, and comfort for whole-body vibration (1 to 80 Hz) and for risk assessment of hand-tool vibration (8 to 1000 Hz) were recommended as practical guidelines for the assessment of operational vibration exposure. The guidance for the evaluation of vibration in air, spacecraft, and other transportation vehicles was supplemented by weighting curves (0.1 to 0.63 Hz) to estimate the incidence of motion sickness in vertical vibrating motions.

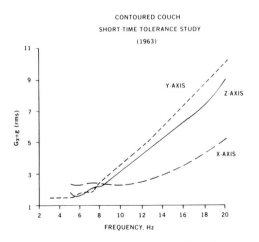

Fig. 10–26. Acceleration tolerance in three directions of vibration in a contoured couch.

REFERENCES

1. von Gierke, H.E., and Goldman, D.E.: Effects of shock and vibration on man. *In* Shock and Vi-

bration Handbook. 2nd Ed. Edited by C.M. Harris and C.E. Crede. New York, McGraw-Hill Book Co., 1979.

2. Harris, C.M., and Crede, C.E. (eds.): Handbook of Noise Control. 2nd Ed. New York, McGraw-Hill Book Co., 1979.

3. von Gierke, H.E. (ed.): Vibration and Combined Stress in Advanced Systems. NTIS, Springfield, Virginia, AGARD Conference Proceedings No. 145, 1975.

4. von Gierke, H.E.: Transmission of vibratory energy through body tissue. In Medical Physics III. Edited by O. Glasser. Chicago, YearBook Medical Publishers, Inc., 1960, pp. 651–669.

5. von Gierke, H.E., Nixon, C.W., and Guignard, J.: Noise and vibration. In Foundations of Space Biology and Medicine. Vol. II. Book 1. Joint USA/USSR Publication. Washington, D.C., National Aeronautics and Space Administration, 1975.

6. Symposium on Biodynamic Models and their Application. Aviat. Space Environ. Med., 49:109–348, 1978.

7. Nixon, C.W.: Exessive noise exposure. In Measurement Procedures in Speech, Hearing and Language. Edited by S. Singh. Baltimore, University Park Press, 1975.

8. Environmental Health Criteria 12: Noise. Geneva, Switzerland, World Health Organization, 1980.

9. Kryter, K.D.: The Effects of Noise on Man. New York, Academic Press, 1970.

10. Acoustics, Determination of Occupational Noise Exposure and Estimation of Noise-Induced Hearing Impairment. ISO/DIS 1999. International Standards Organization, 1982.

11. Hammernik, R.P., Henderson, D., and Salvi, R. (eds.): Noise-Induced Hearing Loss. New York, Raven Press, 1980.

12. Proceedings of the Sonic Boom Symposium. J. Acoust. Soc. Am. Part 2, 31:5, May, 1966.

13. von Gierke, H.E., and Nixon, C.W.: Human response to sonic boom in the laboratory and the community. J. Acoust. Soc. Am., 51:766–782, 1972.

14. Webster, J.: Effects of noise on speech communication. In Handbook of Noise Control. 2nd Ed. Edited by C.M. Harris and C.E. Crede. New York, McGraw-Hill Book Co., 1979.

15. Lippert, S. (ed.): Vibration Research. New York, Pergamon Press, 1963.

16. Hood, C.M., et al.: Cardiopulmonary effects of whole-body vibration in man. J. Appl. Physiol., 21:1725–1731, 1966.

17. Guide for the Evaluation of Human Exposure to Whole-Body Vibration. ANSI S3.18-1979, Standards Secretariat, New York, Acoustical Society of America, 1979.

18. Taylor, W., and Pelmear, P.L. (ed.): Vibration White Finger in Industry. New York, Academic Press, 1975.

19. Guide for the Measurement and the Assessment of Human Exposure to Vibration Transmitted to the Hand. Draft International Standard ISO/DIS 5349.2. International Standards Organization, 1984.

20. Proceedings of the International Occupational Hand-Arm Vibration Conference. Edited by D.E. Wasserman and W. Taylor. United States Department of Health, Education and Welfare. Publication No. 77–170. Washington, D.C., Government Printing Office, 1977.

21. Guide to the Evaluation of Human Exposure to Whole-Body Vibration. 2nd Ed. International Standard ISO 2631, 1978-01-15. Also, Amendment 1, ISO 2631/DAM, 1, Addendum 1, Acceptable Magnitudes of Vibration, and Addendum 2, Evaluation of Exposure to Whole-Body Z-Axis Vertical Vibration in the Frequency Range 0.1 to 0.63 Hz, International Standards Organization, 1980.

Chapter *11*

Spatial Orientation in Flight

Kent K. Gillingham and James W. Wolfe

Appearances often are deceiving.

AESOP

MECHANICS

Operators of today's and tomorrow's air and space vehicles must understand clearly the terminology and physical principles relating to the motions of their craft so they can fly with precision and effectiveness. These crewmembers also must have a working knowledge of the structure and function of the various mechanical and electrical systems of which their craft is comprised to help them understand the performance limits of their machines and to facilitate trouble-shooting and promote safe recovery when the machines fail in flight. So, too, must practitioners of aerospace medicine understand certain basic definitions and laws of mechanics so that they can analyze and describe the motional environment to which the flyer is exposed. In addition, the aeromedical professional must be familiar with the physiologic bases and operational limitations of the flyer's orientational mechanisms. This understanding is necessary to enable the physician or physiologist to speak intelligently and credibly with aircrew about spatial disorientation and to

enable him to contribute significantly to investigations of aircraft mishaps in which spatial disorientation may be implicated.

Motion

There are only two types of physical motion: *linear motion* or *motion of translation*, and *angular motion* or *motion of rotation*. Linear motion can be further categorized as rectilinear, meaning motion in a straight line, or curvilinear, meaning motion in a curved path. Both linear motion and angular motion are composed of an infinite variety of subtypes, or motion parameters, based on successive derivatives of linear or angular position with respect to time. The most basic of these motion parameters, and the most useful, are displacement, velocity, acceleration, and jerk. Table 11–1 classifies linear and angular motion parameters and their symbols and units and serves as an outline for the following discussions of linear and angular motion.

Linear Motion

The basic parameter of linear motion is linear displacement. The other parame-

Table 11–1. Linear and Angular Motion—Symbols and Units

Motion Parameter	Linear		Angular	
	Symbols	Units	Symbols	Units
Displacement	x	meter (m); nautical mile (=1852 m)	θ	degree; radian (rad) (=360/2π degree)
Velocity	v, $\dot{x}$	meter/second (m/sec); knot (≈0.514 m/sec)	ω, $\dot{\theta}$	degree/sec; rad/sec
Acceleration	a, $\dot{v}$, $\ddot{x}$	m/sec^2; g (≈9.81 m/sec^2)	α, $\dot{\omega}$, $\ddot{\theta}$	degree/sec^2; rad/sec^2
Jerk	j, $\dot{a}$, $\ddot{v}$, $\dddot{x}$	m/sec^3 g/sec	γ, $\dot{\alpha}$, $\ddot{\omega}$, $\dddot{\theta}$	degree/sec^3; rad/sec^3

ters—velocity, acceleration, jerk—are derived from the concept of displacement. Linear displacement, x, is the distance and direction of the object under consideration from some reference point; as such, it is a vector quantity, having both magnitude and direction. The position of an aircraft located at 25 nautical miles on the 150° radial of the San Antonio vortac, for example, describes completely the linear displacement of the aircraft from the navigational facility serving as the reference point. The meter (m), however, is the unit of linear displacement in the International System of Units (SI) and will eventually replace other units of linear displacement such as feet, nautical miles, and statute miles.

When linear displacement is changed during a period of time, another vector quantity, linear velocity, occurs. The formula for calculating the mean linear velocity, v, during time interval, Δt, is as follows:

$$v = \frac{x_2 - x_1}{\Delta t} \quad (1)$$

where x_1 is the initial linear displacement and x_2 is the final linear displacement. An aircraft that travels from San Antonio, Texas to New Orleans, Louisiana in 1 hour, for example, moves with a mean linear velocity of 434 knots (nautical miles per hour) on a true bearing of 086°. Statute miles per hour and feet per second are other commonly used units of linear speed, the magnitude of linear velocity;

meters per second (m/sec), however, is the SI unit and is preferred. Frequently, it is important to describe linear velocity at a particular instant in time, that is, as Δt approaches zero. In this situation, one speaks of instantaneous linear velocity, $\dot{x}$ (pronounced "x dot"), which is the first derivative of displacement with respect to time, $\frac{dx}{dt}$.

When the linear velocity of an object changes over time, the difference in velocity, divided by the time required for the moving object to make the change, gives its mean linear accelertion, a. The following formula:

$$a = \frac{v_2 - v_1}{\Delta t} \quad (2)$$

where v_1 is the initial velocity, v_2 is the final velocity, and Δt is the elapsed time, is used to calculate the mean linear acceleration, which, like displacement and velocity, is a vector quantity with magnitude and direction. Acceleration is thus the rate of change of velocity, just as velocity is the rate of change of displacement. The SI unit for the magnitude of linear acceleration is meters per second squared (m/sec^2). Consider, for example, an aircraft that accelerates from a dead stop to a velocity of 100 m/sec in 5 seconds; the mean linear acceleration is 100 m/sec − 0 m/sec ÷ 5 seconds, or 20 m/sec^2. The instantaneous linear acceleration, $\ddot{x}$ ("x double dot") or $\dot{v}$, is the second derivative of displacement or the first deriva-tive of velocity, $\dfrac{d^2x}{dt^2}$ or $\dfrac{dv}{dt}$, respectively.

A very useful unit of acceleration is g, which for our purposes is equal to the constant g_o, the amount of acceleration exhibited by a free-falling body near the surface of the earth—9.81 m/sec². To convert values of linear acceleration given in m/sec² into g units, simply divide by 9.81. In the above example in which an aircraft accelerates at a mean rate of 20 m/sec², one divides 20 m/sec² by 9.81 m/sec² per g to obtain 2.04 g.

A special type of linear acceleration, radial or centripetal acceleration, results in curvilinear, usually circular, motion. The acceleration acts along the line represented by the radius of the curve and is directed toward the center of the curvature. Its effect is a continuous redirection of the linear velocity, in this case called tangential velocity, of the object subjected to the acceleration. Examples of this type of linear acceleration are when an aircraft pulls out of a dive after firing on a ground target or flies a circular path during aerobatic maneuvering. The value of the centripetal acceleration, a_c, can be calculated if one knows the tangential velocity, v_t, and the radius, r, of the curved path followed:

$$a_c = \frac{v_t^2}{r} \qquad (3)$$

For example, the centripetal acceleration of an aircraft traveling at 300 m/sec (approximately 600 knots) and having a radius of turn of 1500 m can be calculated. Dividing (300 m/sec)² by 1500 m gives a value of 60 m/sec², which, when divided by 9.81 m/sec² per g, comes out to 6.12 g.

One can go another step in the derivation of linear motion parameters by obtaining the rate of change of acceleration.

This quantity, j, is known as linear jerk. Mean linear jerk is calculated as follows:

$$j = \frac{a_2 - a_1}{\Delta t} \qquad (4)$$

where a_1 is the initial acceleration, a_2 is the final acceleration, and Δt is the elapsed time.

Instantaneous linear jerk, $\dddot{x}$ or $\dot{a}$, is the third derivative of linear displacement or the first derivative of linear acceleration with respect to time, that is, $\dfrac{d^3x}{dt^3}$ or $\dfrac{da}{dt}$, respectively. Although the SI unit for jerk is m/sec³, it is generally more useful to speak in terms of g-onset rate, measured in g's per second (g/sec).

Angular Motion

The derivation of the parameters of angular motion follows in a parallel fashion the scheme used to derive the parameters of linear motion. The basic parameter of angular motion is angular displacement. For an object to be able to undergo angular displacement it must be polarized, that is, it must have a front and back, so that it can face or be pointed in a particular direction. A simple example of angular displacement is seen in a person facing east. In this case, the individual's angular displacement is 90° clockwise from the reference direction, which is north. Angular displacement, like linear displacement, is a vector quantity, having both magnitude (90°) and direction (clockwise). Angular displacement, symbolized by θ, is generally measured in degrees, revolutions (1 revolution = 360°), or radians (1 radian = 1 revolution ÷ 2π, approximately 57.3°). The radian is a particularly convenient unit to use when dealing with circular motion (e.g., motion of a centrifuge) because it is necessary only to multiply the angular displacement of the system, in radians, by the length of the radius to find the value of the linear displacement along the circular path. The radian is the angle subtended by a circular arc the same length as the radius of the circle.

Angular velocity, ω, is the rate of change of angular displacement. The mean angular velocity occurring in a time interval, Δt, is calculated as follows:

$$\omega = \frac{\theta_2 - \theta_1}{\Delta t} \qquad (5)$$

where θ_1 is the initial angular displacement and θ_2 is the final angular displacement.

Instantaneous angular velocity is $\dot{\theta}$, or $\frac{d\theta}{dt}$. As an example of angular velocity consider the standard-rate turn of instrument flying, in which a heading change of 180° is made in 1 minute. Then $\omega = (180° - 0°) \div 60$ seconds, or 3 degrees per second (degrees/sec). This angular velocity also can be described as 0.5 revolutions per minute (rpm) or as 0.052 radians per second (rad/sec) (3 degrees/sec divided by 57.3 degrees/rad). The fact that an object may be undergoing curvilinear motion during a turn in no way affects the calculation of its angular velocity: an aircraft being rotated on the ground on a turntable at a rate of half a turn per minute has the same angular velocity as one flying a standard-rate instrument turn (3 degrees/sec) in the air at 300 knots.

Because radial or centripetal linear acceleration results when rotation is associated with a radius from the axis of rotation, a formula for calculating the centripetal acceleration, a_c, from the angular velocity, ω, and the radius, r, is often useful:

$$a_c = \omega^2 r \qquad (6)$$

where ω is the angular velocity in radians per second. One can convert readily to the formula for centripetal acceleration in terms of tangential velocity if one remembers the following:

$$v_t = \omega r \qquad (7)$$

To calculate the centripetal acceleration generated by a centrifuge having a 10-m arm and turning at 30 rpm, equation 6 is used after first converting 30 rpm to π radians per second. Squaring the angular velocity and multiplying by the 10-m radius, a centripetal acceleration of 10 π^2 m/sec², or 10.1 g is obtained.

The rate of change of angular velocity is angular acceleration, α. The mean angular acceleration is calculated as follows:

$$\alpha = \frac{\omega_2 - \omega_1}{\Delta t} \qquad (8)$$

where ω_1 is the initial angular velocity, ω_2 is the final angular velocity, and Δt is the time interval over which angular velocity changes.

$\ddot{\theta}, \dot{\omega}, \frac{d^2\theta}{dt^2}$, and $\frac{d\omega}{dt}$ all can be used to symbolize instantaneous angular acceleration, the second derivative of angular displacement or the first derivative of angular velocity with respect to time. If a figure skater is spinning at 6 revolutions per second (2160 degrees/sec, or 37.7 rad/sec) and then comes to a complete stop in 2 seconds, the rate of change of angular velocity, or angular acceleration, is (0 rad/sec − 37.7 rad/sec) ÷ 2 seconds, or − 18.9 rad/sec². One cannot express angular acceleration in g units, which measure magnitude of linear acceleration only.

Although not commonly used in aerospace medicine, another parameter derived from angular displacement is angular jerk, the rate of change of angular acceleration. Its description is completely analogous to that for linear jerk, but angular rather than linear symbols and units are used.

Force, Inertia, and Momentum

Linear and angular motions by themselves are of little physiologic importance. It is the forces and torques which result in or appear to result from linear and angular velocity changes that stimulate or compromise the crewmember's physiologic mechanisms.

Force and Torque

Force is an influence that produces, or tends to produce, linear motion or changes in linear motion; it is a pushing or pulling action. Torque produces, or tends to produce, angular motion or changes in angular motion; it is a twisting or turning action. The SI unit of force is the newton (N). Torque has dimensions of force and length because torque is applied as a force at a certain distance from the center of rotation. The "newton meter (Nm)" is the SI unit of torque.

Mass and Rotational Inertia

Newton's Law of Acceleration states the following:

$$F = m\ a \qquad (9)$$

where F is the unbalanced force applied to an object, m is the mass of the object, and a is linear acceleration.

To describe the analogous situation pertaining to angular motion, the following equation is used:

$$M = j\ \alpha \qquad (10)$$

where M is unbalanced torque (or moment) applied to the rotating object, j is rotational inertia (moment of inertia) of the object, and α is angular acceleration.

The mass of an object is thus the ratio of the force acting on the object to the acceleration resulting from that force. Mass, therefore, is a measure of the inertia of an object—its resistance to being accelerated. Similarly, rotational inertia is the ratio of the torque acting on an object to the angular acceleration resulting from that torque—again, a measure of resistance to acceleration. The kilogram (kg) is the SI unit of mass and is equivalent to 1 N/(m/sec²). The SI unit of rotational inertia is merely the N m/(radian/sec²).

Because F = m a, the centripetal force, F_c, needed to produce a centripetal acceleration, a_c, of a mass, m, can be calculated as follows:

$$F_c = m\ a_c \qquad (11)$$

Thus, from equation 3:

$$F_c = \frac{m\ v_t^2}{r} \qquad (12)$$

or from equation 6:

$$F_c = m\ \omega^2\ r \qquad (13)$$

where v_t is tangential velocity and ω is angular velocity.

Newton's Law of Action and Reaction, which states that for every force applied to an object there is an equal and opposite reactive force exerted by that object, provides the basis for the concept of inertial force. Inertial force is an apparent force opposite in direction to an accelerating force and equal to the mass of the object times the acceleration. An aircraft exerting an accelerating forward thrust on its pilot causes an inertial force, the product of the pilot's mass and the acceleration, to be exerted on the back of the seat by the pilot's body. Similarly, an aircraft undergoing positive centripetal acceleration as a result of lift generated in a turn causes the pilot's body to exert inertial force on the bottom of the seat. More important, however, are the inertial forces exerted on the pilot's blood and organs of equilibrium because physiologic effects result directly from such forces.

At this point it is appropriate to introduce G, which is used to measure the strength of the gravitoinertial force environment. (Note: G should not be confused with G, the symbol for the universal gravitational constant, which is equal to 6.70 × 10⁻¹¹ N m²/kg².) Strictly speaking, G is a measure of relative weight:

$$G = \frac{w}{w_o} \qquad (14)$$

where w is the weight observed in the environment under consideration and w_o is the normal weight on the surface of the earth. In the physical definition of weight,

$$w = m\,a \qquad (15)$$

and

$$w_o = m\,g_o \qquad (16)$$

where m is mass, a is the acceleratory field (vector sum of actual linear acceleration plus an imaginary acceleration opposite the force of gravity), and g_o is the standard value of the acceleration of gravity (9.81 m/sec²). Thus, a man having a mass of 100 kg would weigh 100 kg times 9.81 m/sec² or 981 N on earth (although conventional spring scales would read "100 kg"). At some other location or under some other acceleratory condition, the same man could weigh twice as much—1962 N—and cause a scale to read "200 kg." He would then be in a 2-G environment, or, if he were in an aircraft, he would be "pulling" 2 G. Consider also that since

$$G = \frac{w}{w_o} = \frac{m\,a}{m\,g_o}$$

then

$$G = \frac{a}{g_o} \qquad (17)$$

Thus, the ratio between the ambient ac-

celeratory field (a) and the standard acceleration (g_o) also can be represented in terms of G.

Therefore, g is used as a unit of acceleration (e.g., a_c = 8 g), and the dimensionless ratio of weights, G, is reserved for describing the resulting gravitoinertial force environment (e.g., a force of 8 G, or an 8-G load). When in the vicinity of the surface of the earth, one feels a G force equal to 1 G in magnitude directed toward the center of the earth. If one also sustains a G force resulting from linear acceleration, the magnitude and direction of the resultant gravitoinertial G force can be calculated by adding vectorially the 1-G gravitational force and the inertial G force. An aircraft pulling out of a dive with a centripetal acceleration of 3 g, for example, would exert 3 G of centrifugal force. At the bottom of the dive, the pilot would experience the 3-G centrifugal force in line with the 1-G gravitational force, for a total of 4 G directed toward the floor of the aircraft. If the pilot could continue his circular flight path at a constant airspeed, the G force experienced at the top of the loop would be 2 G because the 1-G gravitational force would subtract from the 3-G inertial force. Another common example of the addition of gravitational G force and inertial G force occurs during the application of power on takeoff or on a missed approach. If the forward acceleration is 1 g, the inertial force is 1 G directed toward the tail of the aircraft. The inertial force adds vectorially to the 1-G force of gravity, directed downward, to provide a resultant gravitoinertial force of 1.414 G pointing 45° down from the aft direction.

Just as inertial forces oppose acceleratory forces, so do inertial torques oppose acceleratory torques. No convenient derived unit exists, however, for measuring inertial torque; specifically, there is no such thing as angular G.

Momentum

To complete this discussion of linear and angular motion, the concepts of momentum and impulse must be introduced. Linear momentum is the product of mass and linear velocity, m v. Angular momentum is the product of rotational inertia and angular velocity, j ω. Momentum is a quantity that a translating or rotating body conserves, that is, an object cannot gain or lose momentum unless it is acted on by a force or torque. A translational impulse is the product of force, F, and the time over which the force acts on an object, Δt, and is equal to the change in linear momentum imparted to the object. Thus:

$$F \Delta t = m\, v_2 - m\, v_1 \qquad (18)$$

where v_1 is the initial linear velocity and v_2 is the final linear velocity.

When dealing with angular motion, a rotational impulse is defined as the product of torque, M, and the time over which it acts, Δt. A rotational impulse is equal to the change in angular momentum. Thus:

$$M \Delta t = j\, \omega_2 - j\, \omega_1 \qquad (19)$$

where ω_1 is the initial angular velocity and ω_2 is the final angular velocity.

The above relations are derived from the Law of Acceleration, as follows:

$$F = m\, a$$
$$M = j\, \alpha$$

since
$$a = \frac{v_2 - v_1}{\Delta t}$$

and
$$\alpha = \frac{\omega_2 - \omega_1}{\Delta t}$$

Directions of Action and Reaction

A number of conventions have been used in aerospace medicine to describe the directions of linear and angular displacement, velocity, and acceleration and of linear and angular reactive forces and torques. The more commonly used of those conventions will be discussed in the following sections.

Vehicular Motions

Because space is three-dimensional, linear motions in space are described by reference to three linear axes and angular motions by three angular axes. In aviation, it is customary to speak of the longitudinal (fore-aft), lateral (right-left), and vertical (up-down) linear axes and the roll, pitch, and yaw angular axes, as shown in Figure 11–1.

Most linear accelerations in aircraft occur in the vertical plane defined by the longitudinal and vertical axes because thrust is usually developed along the former axis and lift is usually developed along the latter axis. Aircraft capable of vectored thrust are now operational, however, and vectored-lift aircraft are currently being flight-tested. This means that in the relatively near future, aircraft will operate in a complete, three-dimensional, linear acceleration environment. Spacecraft already have this capability, to a limited extent. Most angular accelerations in aircraft occur in the roll plane (perpendicular to the roll axis) and, to a lesser extent, in the pitch plane. Angular motion in the yaw plane is very limited in normal flying, although it does occur during spins and several other aerobatic maneuvers. Certainly, aircraft and space vehicles of the future can be expected to operate with considerably more freedom of angular motion than those of the present.

Physiologic Acceleration and Reaction Nomenclature

Figure 11–2 depicts a practical system for describing linear and angular accelerations acting on man.[1] This system is used extensively in aeromedical scientific writing. In this system, a linear acceleration of the type associated with a conventional takeoff roll is in the $+a_x$ direction, that is, it is a $+a_x$ acceleration. Braking to a stop during a landing roll results in $-a_x$ acceleration. Radial acceleration of the type usually developed during air combat maneuvering is $+a_z$ acceleration—foot-to-

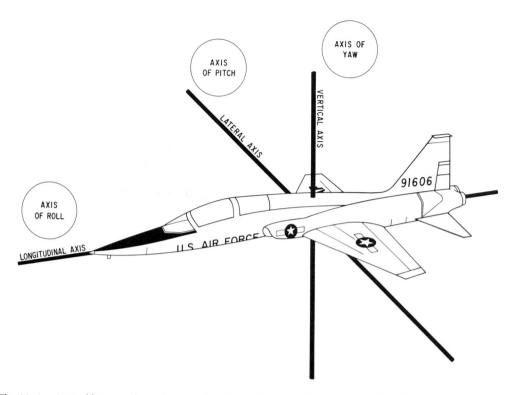

Fig. 11–1. Axes of linear and angular aircraft motions. Linear motions are longitudinal, lateral, and vertical, and angular motions are roll, pitch, and yaw.

head. The right-hand rule for describing the relationships between three orthogonal axes aids recall of the positive directions of a_x, a_y, and a_z accelerations in this particular system: if one lets the forward-pointing index finger of the right hand represent the positive x-axis, and the left-pointing middle finger of the right hand represent the positive y-axis, the positive z-axis is represented by the upward-pointing thumb of the right hand. A different right-hand rule, however, is used in another convention, one for describing vehicular coordinates. In that system, $+a_x$ is noseward acceleration, $+a_y$ is to the right, and $+a_z$ is floorward; an inverted right hand illustrates that set of axes.

The angular accelerations, α_x, α_y, and α_z, are roll, pitch, and yaw accelerations, respectively, in the system shown in Figure 11–2. Note that the relation between the positive x-axis, y-axis, and z-axis is identical to that for linear accelerations. The direction of positive angular displacement, velocity, or acceleration is described by another right-hand rule, wherein the flexed fingers of the right hand indicate the direction of angular motion corresponding to the vector represented by the extended, abducted right thumb. Thus, in this system, a right roll results from $+\alpha_x$ acceleration, a pitch down results from $+\alpha_y$ acceleration, and a left yaw results from $+\alpha_z$ acceleration. Again, it is important to be aware of the inverted right-hand coordinate system commonly used to describe angular motions of vehicles. In that convention, a positive roll acceleration is to the right, positive pitch is upward, and positive yaw is to the right.

The nomenclature for the directions of gravitoinertial (G) forces acting on humans is also illustrated in Figure 11–2. Note that

PHYSIOLOGIC ACCELERATION NOMENCLATURE

PHYSIOLOGIC REACTION NOMENCLATURE

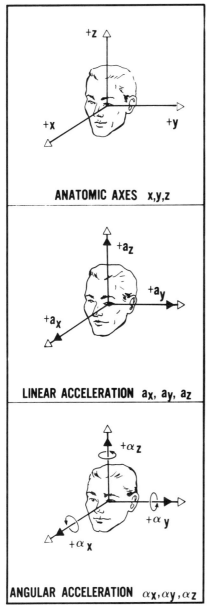

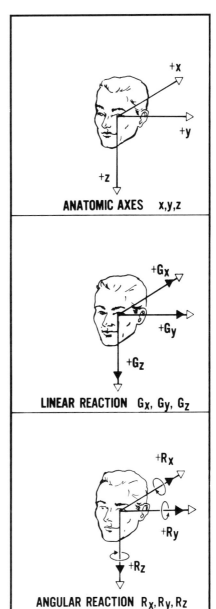

Fig. 11–2. System for describing accelerations and inertial reactions in humans. (Adapted from Hixson, W.C., Niven, J.I., and Correia, M.J.: Kinematics Nomenclature For Physiological Accelerations, With Special Reference to Vestibular Applications. Monograph 14. Naval Aerospace Medical Institute, Pensacola, Florida, 1966.)

the relation of these axes to each other follows a backward, inverted, right-hand rule. In the illustrated convention, $+a_x$ acceleration results in $+G_x$ inertial force, and $+a_z$ acceleration results in $+G_z$ force. This correspondence of polarity is not achieved on the Y-axis, however, because $+a_y$ acceleration results in $-G_y$ force. If the $+G_y$ direction were reversed, full polarity correspondence could be achieved between all linear accelerations and all reactive forces, and that convention has been used by some authors. An example of the usage of the symbolic reaction terminology would be: "An F-16 pilot must be able to sustain $+9.0$ G_z without losing vision or consciousness."

The "eyeballs" nomenclature is another useful set of terms for describing gravitoinertial forces. In this system, the direction of the inertial reaction of the eyeballs when the head is subjected to an acceleration is used to describe the direction of the inertial force. The equivalent expressions, "eyeballs-in acceleration" and "eyeballs-in G force," leave little room for confusion about either the direction of the applied acceleratory field or the resulting gravitoinertial force environment.

Inertial torques can be described conveniently by means of the system shown in Figure 11–2, in which the angular reaction axes are the same as the linear reaction axes. The inertial reactive torque resulting from $+\alpha_x$ (right roll) angular acceleration is $+R_x$ and $+\alpha_z$ (left yaw) results in $+R_z$; however, $+\alpha_y$ (downward pitch) results in $-R_y$. This incomplete correspondence between acceleration and reaction coordinate polarities again results from the mathematical tradition of using right-handed coordinate systems.

It should be apparent from all of this that the potential for confusing the audience when speaking or writing about accelerations and inertial reactions is great enough to make it a virtual necessity to describe the coordinate system being used. For most applications, the "eyeballs" convention is perfectly adequate.

VISUAL ORIENTATION

Vision is by far the most important sensory modality subserving spatial orientation, especially so in moving vehicles such as aircraft. Without it, flight as we know it would be impossible, whereas this would not necessarily be the case in the absence of the vestibular or other sensory systems that provide orientation information. For the most part, the function of vision in spartial orientation is obvious, so a discussion proportional in size to the importance of that function in orientation will not be presented here. Certain recent developments in our understanding of visual orientation deserve mention, however. First, there are actually two separate visual systems, and they have two distinct functions: object recognition and spatial orientation. A knowledge of these systems is extremely important, both to help in understanding visual illusions in flight and to appreciate the difficulties inherent in using flight instruments for spatial orientation. Second, the realization that visual and vestibular orientation information are integrated at very basic neural levels helps in understanding why spatial disorientation so frequently is not amenable to correction by higher-level neural processing.

Anatomy of the Visual System

General

The retina, an evaginated portion of the embryonic brain, consists of an outer layer of pigmented epithelium and an inner layer of neural tissue. Contained within the latter layer are the sensory rod and cone cells, the bipolar and horizontal cells that comprise the intraretinal afferent pathway from the rods and cones, and the multipolar ganglion cells, the axons of which are the fibers of the optic nerve. The cones, which number approximately 7 million in the human eye, have a relatively high threshold to light energy. They are responsible for sharp visual discrimination and color vision. The rods, of which there are over 100 million, are much more sensitive to light than the cones; they provide the ability to see in twilight and at night. In the retinal macula, near the posterior pole of the eye, the cone population achieves its greatest density; within the macula, the fovea centralis—a small pit totally comprised of tightly packed slender cones—provides the sharpest visual acuity and is the anatomic basis for foveal, or central, vision. The remainder of the eye is capable of far less visual acuity and subserves paracentral and peripheral vision.

Having dendritic connections with the rods and cones, the bipolar cells provide axons that synapse with the dendrites or cell bodies of the multipolar ganglion cells, whose axons in turn course parallel to the retinal surface and converge at the optic disk. Emerging from the eye as the optic nerve, they meet their counterparts from the opposite eye in the optic chiasm and then continue in one of the optic tracts, most likely to terminate in a lateral geniculate body, but possibly in a superior colliculus or the preoptic area. Second-order neurons from the lateral geniculate body comprise the geniculocalcarine tract, which becomes the optic radiation and terminates in the primary visual cortex, the striate area of the occipital cerebral cortex (Area 17). In the visual cortex, the retinal image is represented as a more or less point-to-point projection from the lateral geniculate body, which receives a similarly topographically structured projection from both retinas. The lateral geniculate body and the primary visual cortex are thus structurally and functionally suited for the recognition and analysis of visual images. The superior colliculi, on the other hand, project eventually to the motor nuclei of the extraocular muscles and muscles of the neck and thus appear to provide a pathway for certain gross ocu-

lar reflexes of visual origin. Fibers entering the pretectal area are involved in pupillary reflexes. In addition, most anatomic and physiologic evidence indicates that information from the parietal cerebral cortex, the frontal eye movement area (Area 8), and the occipital visual association areas (Areas 18 and 19) is relayed through the paramedian pontine reticular formation to the nuclei of the cranial nerves (III, IV, and VI) innervating the extraocular muscles. Via this pathway and perhaps others involving the superior colliculi, saccadic (fast) and pursuit (slow) eye movements are initiated and controlled. Interestingly, saccadic eye movements appear to originate in the contralateral hemisphere, whereas pursuit movements are under ipsilateral cortical control.[2]

Visual-Vestibular Convergence

It is now known that visually perceived motion information and probably other visual orientational data reach the vestibular nuclei in the brain stem.[3,4] The hypothesis that the superior colliculi project through the reticular formation to the vestibular nuclei is attractive because of the demonstrated responsiveness of most superior colliculus neurons to moving rather than stationary visual stimuli; however, this hypothesis is not yet supported by anatomic evidence. Most likely, the cerebellum is involved in visual-vestibular convergence via the recently discovered accessory optic system. Visual information from the retina reaches the inferior olive by way of the accessory optic tract and central tegmental tract. Fibers from the inferior olive provide inputs to the Purkinje cells of the cerebellar flocculus, which have inhibitory connections in ipsilateral vestibular nuclei. Because this area of the cerebellum receives mossy fibers directly from vestibular end-organs, visual-vestibular interactions also can occur within the cerebellum; and as the Purkinje cells project onto the vestibular end-organs themselves (at least in some species), such interactions can take place peripherally as well as centrally. There also are possible visual-vestibular interactions that occur as a result of cerebral cortical projections to the pontine nuclei and thence into the cerebellar vermis and cerebellar hemispheres. Of course, the confluence of visual and vestibular pathways in the paramedian pontine reticular formation makes possible the integration of visual and vestibular inputs to the final common pathway to the nuclei of cranial nerves III, IV, and VI. As might be expected, there also are afferent vestibular influences on visual system nuclei; these influences have been demonstrated in the lateral geniculate body and superior colliculus.

Visual Information Processing

Primary control of man's ability to move and orient himself in three-dimensional space is mediated by the visual system, as exemplifed by the fact that individuals without functioning vestibular systems ("labyrinthine defectives") have virtually no problems with spatial orientation unless they are deprived of vision. The underlying mechanisms of visual orientation-information processing are revealed by receptive field studies, which have been accomplished for the peripheral retina, nuclear relays, and primary visual cortex. Basically, these studies show that there are several types of movement-detecting neurons and that these neurons respond differently to the direction of movement, velocity of movement, size of the stimulus, its orientation in space, and the level of illumination. Functionally, however, vision must be considered as two separate systems, one involved with object recognition and the other involved with spatial orientation. These two systems, the focal and ambient visual systems, respectively, will be described in the following sections, as will certain functions of yet another visual system, the one responsible

for generating eye movements to facilitate the acquisition of orientation information.

Focal Vision

Liebowitz and Dichgans[4] have provided a very useful summary of the characteristics of focal vision:

[The focal visual mode] is concerned with object recognition and identification and in general answers the question of "what." Focal vision involves relatively fine detail (high spatial frequencies) and is correspondingly best represented in the central visual fields. Information processed by focal vision is ordinarily well represented in consciousness and is critically related to physical parameters such as stimulus energy and refractive error. The vast majority of studies in "vision" as well as most existing tests for evaluating performance or individual differences are concerned with focal function.

Focal vision is thus not primarily involved with orienting the individual in the environment but is used in some instances to acquire visual information about orientation. Certainly, focal vision is necessary for reading flight instruments; however, a complex cognitive process, that is, instrument flying skill, is required to convert such focally acquired orientation cues into usable orientation information.

In the visual as opposed to instrumental flight environment, focal visual cues provide the primary means by which judgments of distance and depth are made. Tredici[5] categorized these cues as being either monocular or binocular. The monocular cues are (1) size constancy, the size of the retinal image in relation to known and comparative sizes of objects; (2) shape constancy, the shape of the retinal image in relation to the known shape of the object (e.g., the foreshortening of the image of a known circle into an ellipsoid shape means one part of the circle is farther away than another); (3) motion parallax, the relative speed of movement of images across the retina—when an individual is moving linearly in his environment, the retinal images of nearer objects move faster than those of objects farther away; (4) interposition, the partial obstruction from view of more distant objects by nearer ones; (5) texture or gradient, the apparent loss of detail with greater distance; (6) linear perspective, the convergence of parallel lines at a distance; (7) illumination perspective, which results from the tendency to perceive the light source to be above an object and from the association of more deeply shaded parts of an object with being farther from the light source; and (8) aerial perspective, the perception of objects to be more distant when the image is relatively bluish or hazy. The binocular cues to depth and distance are (1) stereopsis, the visual appreciation of three-dimensional space that results from the fusion of slightly dissimilar retinal images of an object; (2) vergence, the medial rotation of the eyes and the resulting direction of their gaze along more or less converging lines, depending on whether the viewed object is closer or farther, respectively; and (3) accommodation, or focusing of the image by changing the curvature of the lens of the eye. Of all the cues listed, size and shape constancy and motion parallax appear to be most important for deriving distance information in flying because they are available at and well beyond the distances at which binocular cues are useful. Stereopsis can provide orientation information at distances up to only about 200 m; it is, however, more important in orientation than vergence and accommodation, which are useless beyond about 6 m.

Ambient Vision

Liebowitz and Dichgans[4] have provided a summary of ambient vision:

> The ambient visual mode subserves spatial localization and orientation and is in general concerned with the question of "where." Ambient vision is mediated by relatively large stimulus patterns so that it typically involves stimulation of the peripheral visual field and relatively coarse detail (low spatial frequencies). Unlike focal vision, ambient vision is not systematically related to either stimulus energy or optical image quality. Rather, provided the stimulus is visible, orientation responses appear to be elic-ited on an "all or none" basis. . . . The conscious concomitant of ambient stimulation is low or frequently completely absent. Interest in ambient visual function has a long history, but analysis of psychophysical properties, [etc.], . . . have been initiated primarily within the past ten to fifteen years.

Ambient vision, therefore, is primarily involved with orienting the individual in the environment. Furthermore, this function is completely independent of the function of focal vision. This becomes evident in view of the fact that one can fully occupy central vision with the task of reading while simultaneously obtaining sufficient orientation cues with peripheral vision to walk or ride a bicycle. It is also evidenced by the ability of certain patients with cerebral cortical lesions to maintain visual orientation responses even though their ability to discriminate objects is lost ("blindsight," which is presumably mediated through subcortical structures).

The function of ambient vision in orientation can be thought of as two processes, one providing motion cues and the other providing position cues. Large, coherently moving contrasts detected mainly with peripheral vision result in a percept of self-motion, or vection. If the moving contrasts revolve relative to the subject, he perceives rotational self-motion, or angular vection, which can be in the pitch, roll, yaw, or any intermediate plane. If the moving contrasts enlarge and diverge from a distant point, become smaller and converge in the distance, or otherwise indicate linear motion, the percept of self-motion that results is linear vection, which also can be in any direction. Vection can, of course, be veridical or illusory, depending on whether actual or merely apparent motion of the subject is occurring. One can appreciate the importance of ambient vision in orientation by recalling the powerful sensations of self-motion generated by certain scenes in wide-screen motion pictures (e.g., flying through the Grand Canyon).

Position cues provided by ambient vision are readily evidenced in the stabilization of posture that vision affords patients with defective vestibular or spinal proprioceptive systems. The essential visual parameter contributing to postural stability appears to be the motion of the retinal image that results from minor deviations from desired postural position. Visual effects on posture also can be seen in the phenomenon of height vertigo. As the distance from (height above) a stable visual environment increases, the amount of body sway necessary for the retinal image movement to be above threshold increases. Above a certain height, the ability of this visual mechanism to contribute to postural stability is exceeded, and vision indicates posture to be stable despite large body sways. The conflict between visual orientation information, indicating relative stability, and the vestibular and somatosensory data, indicating large body sways, results in the unsettling experience of vertigo.

One more distinction between focal and ambient visual function should be emphasized. In general, focal vision serves to orient the perceived object relative to the individual, whereas ambient vision serves to orient the individual relative to the perceived environment. When both focal and ambient vision are present, orienting a focally perceived object relative to the ambient visual environment is easy, whether the mechanism employed involves first orienting the object to oneself and then orienting oneself and the object to the environment or whether the object is oriented directly to the environment. When only focal vision is available, however, it can be difficult to orient oneself correctly to a focally perceived environmental orientation cue because the natural tendency is to perceive oneself as stable and upright and to perceive the focally viewed object as oriented otherwise with respect to the stable and upright egocentric reference frame. This phenomenon can cause a pilot to misjudge his approach to a night landing, for example, when only the runway lights and a few other focal visual cues are available for spatial orientation.

Eye Movements

The maintenance of visual orientation in a dynamic environment is greatly enhanced by the ability to move the eyes, primarily because the retinal image of a moving object or environment can be stabilized by appropriate eye movements. Very basic and powerful mechanisms involved in reflexive vestibular stabilization of the retinal image will be discussed in the section entitled "Vestibular Function." Visually controlled eye movements that provide image stabilization are the slow pursuit movements and the rapid saccadic movements. Pursuit movements adequately track targets moving at less than 60 degrees/sec; targets moving at higher velocities necessitate either saccadic eye movements or voluntary head movements for adequate tracking. Saccadic eye movements are used voluntarily or reflexively to acquire a target or to catch up to a target that cannot be maintained on the fovea by pursuit movements. Under some circumstances, pursuit and saccadic eye movements alternate in a pattern of reflexive slow tracking and fast backtracking called optokinetic nystagmus. This type of eye-movement response is typically elicited in the laboratory by surrounding the subject with a rotating striped drum; however, one can exhibit and experience optokinetic nystagmus quite readily in a more natural setting by watching railroad cars go by while waiting at a railroad crossing. Movement of the visual environment sufficient to elicit optokinetic nystagmus provides a stimulus that can either enhance or compete with the vestibular elicitation of eye movements, depending on whether the visually perceived motion is compatible or incompatible, respectively, with the motion sensed by the vestibular system. Vergence movements, which aid binocular distance and motion perception at very close range, also are visually controlled, but are of relatively minor importance in spatial orientation when compared with the image-stabilizing pursuit and saccadic eye movements.

Even though gross stabilization of the retinal image aids object recognition and spatial orientation by enhancing visual acuity, absolute stability of an image is associated with a marked decrease in visual acuity and form perception. This stability-induced decrement is avoided by continual voluntary and involuntary movements of the eyes, even during fixation of an object. We are unaware of these small eye movements, however, and the visual world appears stable.

Voluntary scanning and tracking movements of the eyes are associated with the appearance of a stable visual environment, but why this is so is not readily apparent. Early investigators postulated that proprioceptive information from the extraocular muscles provided not only feedback signals for the control of eye movement but also the afferent information needed to correlate eye movement with retinal image movement and arrive at a subjective determination of a stable visual environment. In 1960, Brindley and Merton[6] demonstrated that in man there is no subjective eye position sense, that is, no conscious extraocular muscle proprioception. An alternative mechanism for oculomotor control and the subjective appreciation of visual stability then became plausible: the "corollary discharge" or feed-forward mechanism first proposed by Sperry.[7] From his studies of the motor effects of surgical rotation of the eye in fish, Sperry concluded: "Thus, an excitation pattern that normally results in a movement that will cause a displacement of the visual image on the retina may have a corollary discharge into the visual centers to compensate for the retinal displacement. This implies an anticipatory adjustment in the visual centers specific for each movement

with regard to its direction and speed." The theoretical aspects of visual perception of movement and stability have been expanded over the years into various models based on "inflow" (afference), "outflow" (efference), and even hybrid sensory mechanisms.

VESTIBULAR FUNCTION

The role of vestibular function in spatial orientation is not so overt as that of vision but is extremely important for three major reasons. First, the vestibular system provides the structural and functional substrate for reflexes that serve to stabilize vision when motion of the head and body would otherwise result in blurring of the retinal image. Second, the vestibular system provides orientational information with reference to which both skilled and reflexive motor activities are automatically executed. Third, the vestibular system provides, in the absence of vision, a reasonably accurate percept of motion and position, as long as the pattern of stimulation remains within certain naturally occuring bounds. Because the details of vestibular anatomy and physiology are not usually well-known by medical professionals and because a working knowledge of them is essential to the understanding of spatial disorientation in flight, these details will be presented in the following sections.

Vestibular Anatomy

End-Organs

The vestibular end-organs are smaller than most people realize, measuring just 1.5 cm across; the whole vestibular sensory apparatus would fit inside the bowl of a typical smoker's pipe. They reside well-protected within some of the densest bone in the body, the petrous portion of the temporal bone. Each temporal bone contains a tortuous excavation known as the bony labyrinth which is filled with perilymph, a fluid much like cerebrospinal fluid in composition. The bony labyrinth consists of three main parts: the cochlea, the vestibule, and the semicircular canals (Fig. 11–3). Within each part of the bony labyrinth is a part of the delicate, tubular, membranous labyrinth, which contains endolymph, a fluid characterized by its relatively high concentration of potassium. In the cochlea, the membranous labyrinth is called the cochlear duct or scala media; this organ converts acoustic energy into neural information. In the vestibule lie the two otolith organs, the utricle and the saccule. They translate gravitational and inertial forces into spatial orientation information—specifically, information about position and linear motion of the head. The semicircular ducts, contained in the semicircular canals, convert inertial torques into information about angular motion of the head. The three semicircular canals and their included semicircular ducts are oriented in three mutually perpendicular planes, thus inspiring the names of the canals: anterior vertical (or superior), posterior vertical (or posterior), and horizontal (or lateral).

The semicircular ducts communicate at both ends with the utricle, and one end of each duct is dilated to form an ampulla. Inside each ampulla lies a crest of neuroepithelium, the crista ampullaris. Atop the crista, occluding the duct, is a gelatinous structure called the cupula (Fig. 11–4a). The hair cells of which the crista ampullaris is composed project their cilia into the base of the cupula, so that whenever the cupula moves, the cilia are bent.

Lining the bottom of the utricle in a more or less horizontal plane is another patch of neuroepithelium, the macula utriculi, and on the medial wall of the saccule in a vertical plane is still another, the macula sacculi (Fig. 11–4b). The cilia of the hair cells comprising these structures project into overlying otolithic membranes, one above each macula. The otolithic membranes are gelatinous structures containing many tiny calcium carbonate crystals, called otoconia, which are held together by a network of connective tissue. Having almost three times the density of the surrounding endolymph, the otolithic membranes displace endolymph and shift

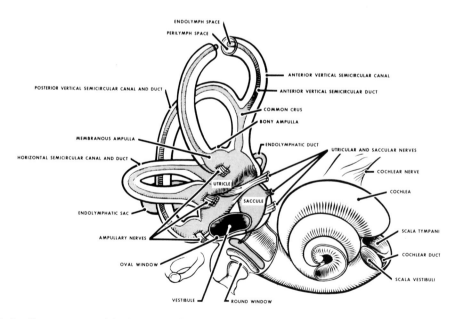

Fig. 11–3. Gross anatomy of the inner ear. The bony semicircular canals and vestibule contain the membranous semicircular ducts and otolith organs, respectively.

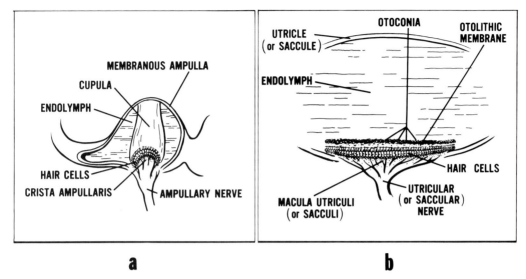

a   **b**

Fig. 11–4.   The vestibular end-organs. *a.* The ampulla of a semicircular duct, containing the crista ampullaris and cupula. *b.* A representative otolith organ, with its macula and otolithic membrane.

position relative to their respective maculae when subjected to changing gravito-inertial forces. This shifting of the otolithic membrane position results in bending of the cilia of the macular hair cells.

The hair cell is the functional unit of the vestibular sensory system. It converts spatial and temporal patterns of mechanical energy applied to the head into neural information. Each hair cell possesses one relatively large kinocilium on one side of the top of the cell and up to 100 smaller stereocilia on the same surface. Hair cells thus exhibit morphologic polarization, that is, they are oriented in a particular direction. The functional correlate of this polarization is that when the cilia of a hair cell are bent in the direction of its kinocilium, the cell undergoes an electrical depolarization, and the frequency of action potentials generated in the vestibular neuron attached to the hair cell increases above a certain resting frequency; the greater the deviation of the cilia, the higher the frequency. Similarly, when its cilia are bent away from the side with the kinocilium, the hair cell undergoes an electrical hyperpolarization, and the frequency

of action potentials in the corresponding neuron in the vestibular nerve decreases (Fig. 11–5).

The same basic process described above occurs in all the hair cells in the three cristae and both maculae; the important differences lie in the physical events that cause the deviation of cilia and in the directions in which the various groups of hair cells are oriented. The hair cells of a crista ampullaris respond to the inertial torque of the ring of endolymph contained in the attached semicircular duct as the reacting endolymph exerts pressure on the cupula and deviates it. The hair cells of a macula, on the other hand, respond to the gravitoinertial force acting to displace the overlying otolithic membrane. As indicated in Figure 11–6a, all of the hair cells in the crista of the horizontal semicircular duct are oriented so that their kinocilia are on the utricular side of the ampulla. Thus, utriculopetal endolymphatic pressure on the cupula deviates the cilia of these hair cells toward the kinocilia, and all the hair cells in the crista depolarize. The hair cells in the cristae of the vertical semicircular ducts are oriented in the opposite fashion, this is, their kinocilia are all on the side

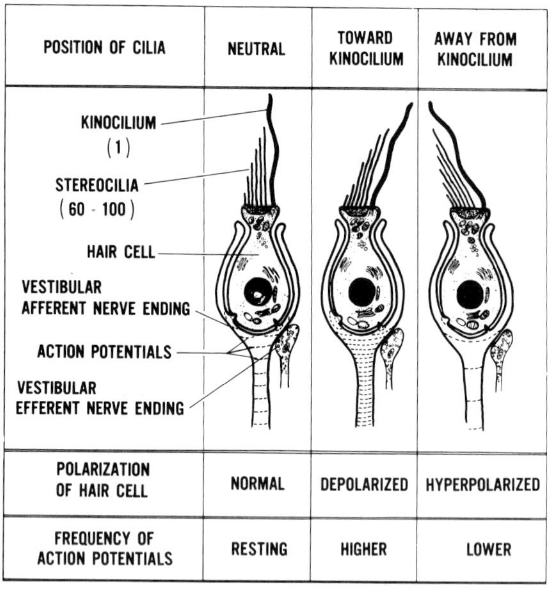

POSITION OF CILIA	NEUTRAL	TOWARD KINOCILIUM	AWAY FROM KINOCILIUM
KINOCILIUM (1) STEREOCILIA (60 - 100) HAIR CELL VESTIBULAR AFFERENT NERVE ENDING ACTION POTENTIALS VESTIBULAR EFFERENT NERVE ENDING			
POLARIZATION OF HAIR CELL	NORMAL	DEPOLARIZED	HYPERPOLARIZED
FREQUENCY OF ACTION POTENTIALS	RESTING	HIGHER	LOWER

Fig. 11–5. Function of a vestibular hair cell. When mechanical forces deviate the cilia toward the side of the cell with the kinocilium, the hair cell depolarizes and the frequency of action potentials in the associated afferent vestibular neuron increases. When the cilia are deviated in the opposite direction, the hair cell hyperpolarizes and the frequency of action potentials decreases.

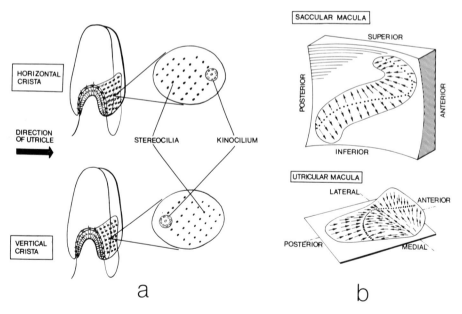

Fig. 11–6. Morphologic polarization in vestibular neuroepithelia. *a.* All the hair cells in the cristae of the horizontal semicircular ducts are oriented so that their kinocilia are in the direction of the utricle; those hair cells in the cristae of the vertical ducts have their kinocilia directed away from the utricle. *b.* The maculae of the saccule (above) and utricle (below) also exhibit polarization—the arrows indicate the direction of the kinocilia of the hair cells in the various regions of the maculae. (Adapted from Spoendlin, H.H.: Ultrastructural studies of the labyrinth in squirrel monkeys. *In* The Role of the Vestibular Organs in the Exploration of Space. NASA-SP-77, Washington, D.C., National Aeronautics and Space Administration, 1965.)

away from the utricle. In the ampullae of the vertical semicircular ducts, therefore, utriculopetal endolymphatic pressure deviates the cilia away from the kinocilia, causing all the hair cells in these cristae to hyperpolarize. In contrast, the hair cells of the maculae are not oriented unidirectionally across the neuroepithelium: the direction of their morphologic polarization depends on where they lie on the macula (Fig. 11–6b). In both maculae, there is a central line of reflection, on opposing sides of which the hair cells assume an opposite orientation. In the utricular macula, the kinocilia of the hair cells are all oriented toward this line of reflection, whereas in the saccular macula, they are oriented away from it. Because the line of reflection on each macula curves at least 90°, the hair cells, having morphologic polarization roughly perpendicular to this line, exhibit virtually all possible orientations on the plane of the macula. Thus, the orthogonality of the planes of the three semicircular ducts enables them to detect angular motion in any plane, and the perpendicularity of the planes of the maculae plus the omnidirectionality of the orientation of the hair cells in the maculae allow the detection of gravitoinertial forces acting in any direction.

Neural Pathways

To help the reader better organize the potentially confusing vestibular neuroanatomy, a somewhat simplified overview of the major neural connections of the vestibular system is presented in Figure 11–7. The utricular nerve, two saccular nerves, and the three ampullary nerves converge to form the vestibular nerve, a portion of the VIIIth cranial or statoacoustic nerve. Within the vestibular nerve lies the vestibular (or Scarpa's) ganglion, which is comprised of the cell bodies of the vestibular neurons. The dendrites of these bipolar neurons invest the hair cells of the cristae and maculae; most of their axons terminate in the four vestibular nuclei in

the brain stem—the superior, medial, lateral, and inferior nuclei—but some axons enter the phylogenetically ancient parts of the cerebellum to terminate in the fastigial nuclei and in the cortex of the flocculonodular lobe and other parts of the posterior vermis.

The vestibular nuclei project via secondary vestibular tracts to the motor nuclei of the cranial and spinal nerves and to the cerebellum. Because vestibulo-ocular reflexes are a major function of the vestibular system, it is not surprising to find ample projections from the vestibular nuclei to the nuclei of the oculomotor, trochlear, and abducens nerves (cranial nerves III, IV, and VI, respectively). The major pathway of these projections is the ascending medial longitudinal fasciculus (MLF). The basic vestibulo-ocular reflex is thus served by sensor and effector cells and an intercalated three-neuron reflex arc from the vestibular ganglion to the vestibular nuclei to the nuclei innervating the extraocular muscles. In addition, indirect multisynaptic pathways course from the vestibular nuclei through the paramedian pontine reticular formation to the oculomotor and other nuclei. The principle of ipsilateral facilitation and contralateral inhibition via an interneuron clearly operates in vestibulo-ocular reflexes, and numerous crossed internuclear connections provide evidence of this. The vestibulo-ocular reflexes that the various ascending and crossed pathways support serve to stabilize the retinal image by moving the eyes in the direction opposite that of the motion of the head. Via the descending MLF and medial vestibulospinal tract, crossed and uncrossed projections from the vestibular nuclei reach the nuclei of the spinal accessory nerve (cranial nerve XI) and motor nuclei in the cervical cord. These projections form the anatomic substrate for vestibulocollic reflexes, which serve to stabilize the head by appropriate action of the sternocleidomastoid and other neck muscles. A third projection is that from pri-

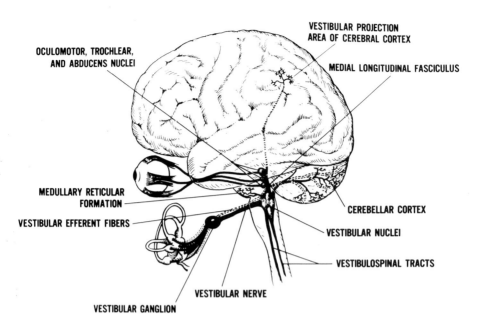

Fig. 11–7. Major connections and projections of the vestibular system.

marily the lateral vestibular nucleus into the ventral gray matter throughout the length of the spinal cord. This important pathway is the uncrossed lateral vestibulospinal tract, which enables the vestibulospinal (postural) reflexes to help stabilize the body with respect to an inertial frame of reference by means of sustained and transient vestibular influences on basic spinal reflexes. Secondary vestibulocerebellar fibers course from the vestibular nuclei into the ipsilateral and contralateral fastigial nuclei and to the cerebellar cortex of the flocculonodular lobe and elsewhere. Returning from the fastigial and other cerebellar nuclei, crossed and uncrossed fibers of the cerebellobulbar tract terminate in the vestibular nuclei and in the associated reticular formation. There are also efferent fibers from the cerebellum, probably arising in the cerebellar cortex, which terminate not in nuclear structures but on dendritic endings of primary vestibular afferent neurons in the vestibular neuroepithelia. Such fibers are those of the vestibular efferent system, which appears to modulate or control the

information arising from the vestibular end-organs. The primary and secondary vestibulocerebellar fibers and those returning from the cerebellum to the vestibular area of the brain stem comprise the juxtarestiform body of the inferior cerebellar peduncle. This structure, along with the vestibular end-organs, nuclei, and projection areas in the cerebellum, collectively constitute the so-called vestibulocerebellar axis, the neural complex responsible for processing primary spatial orientation information and initiating adaptive and protective behavior based on that information.

Several additional projections, more obvious functionally than anatomically, are those to certain autonomic nuclei of the brain stem and to the cerebral cortex. The dorsal motor nucleus of cranial nerve X (vagus) and other autonomic cell groups in the medulla and pons receive secondary vestibular fibers, largely from the medial vestibular nucleus; these fibers mediate vestibulovegetative reflexes, which are manifested as the pallor, perspiration, nausea, and vomiting—motion sickness—

that can result from excessive or otherwise abnormal vestibular stimulation. Via vestibulothalamic and thalamocortical pathways, vestibular information eventually reaches the primary vestibular projection area of the cerebral cortex, thought to be located in the parietal or parietoinsular cortex (not in the temporal lobe as previously suspected). This projection area is provided with vestibular, visual, and somatosensory proprioceptive representation and is evidently associated with conscious spatial orientation and with integration of sensory correlates of higher-order motor activity. In addition, vestibular information can be transmitted via long polysynaptic pathways through the brainstem reticular formation and medial thalamus to wide areas of the cerebral cortex; the nonspecific cortical responses to vestibular stimuli that are evoked via this pathway appear to be associated with an arousal or alerting mechanism.

Vestibular Information Processing

As the reader probably deduced while reading the discussion of the anatomy of the vestibular end-organs, angular accelerations are the adequate, that is, physiologic, stimuli for the semicircular ducts, and linear accelerations and gravity are the adequate stimuli for the otolith organs. This statement, illustrated in Figure 11–8, is the cardinal principle of vestibular mechanics. How the reactive torques and gravitoinertial forces stimulate the hair cells of the cristae and maculae, respectively, and produce changes in the frequency of action potentials in the associated vestibular neurons already has been discussed. The resulting frequency-coded messages are transmitted into the several central vestibular projection area as raw orientational data to be further processed as necessary for the various functions served by such data. These functions are the vestibular reflexes, voluntary movement, and the perception of orientation.

Vestibular Reflexes

As stated so adequately by Melvill Jones[9], "...for control of eye movement relative to space the motor outflow can operate on three fairly discrete anatomical platforms, namely: (1) the eye-in-skull platform, driven by the external eye muscles rotating the eyeball relative to the skull; (2) the skull-on-body platform driven by the neck muscles; and (3) the body platform, operated by the complex neuromuscular mechanisms responsible for postural control."

In humans, the retinal image is stabilized mainly by vestibulo-ocular reflexes, primarily those of semicircular-duct origin. A simple demonstration can help one appreciate the contribution of the vestibulo-ocular reflexes to retinal-image stabilization. Holding the extended fingers half a meter or so in front of the face, one can move the fingers slowly from side to side and still see them clearly because of visual (optokinetic) tracking reflexes. As the rate, or correspondingly, the frequency, of movement becomes greater, one eventually reaches a point where the fingers cannot be seen clearly—they are blurred by the movement. This point is at about 60 degrees/sec or 1 or 2 Hz for most people. Now, if the fingers are held still and the head is rotated back and forth at the frequency at which the fingers became blurred when they were moved, the fingers remain perfectly clear. Even at considerably higher frequencies of head movement, the vestibulo-ocular reflexes initiated by the resulting stimulation of the semicircular ducts function to keep the image of the fingers clear. Thus, at lower frequencies of movement of the external world relative to the body or vice versa, the visual system stabilizes the retinal image by means of optokinetic reflexes. As the frequencies of such relative movement become greater, however, the vestibular system, by means of vestibulo-ocular reflexes, assumes progressively more of this

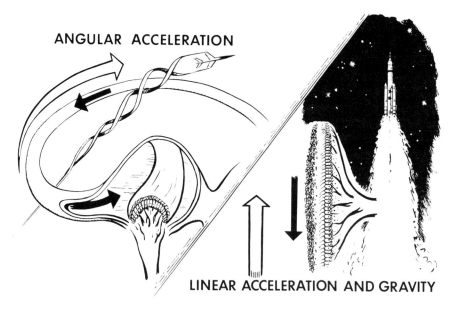

Fig. 11–8. The cardinal principle of vestibular mechanics: angular accelerations stimulate the semicircular ducts; linear accelerations and gravity stimulate the otolith organs.

function, and at the higher frequencies of relative motion characteristically generated only by motions of the head and body, the vestibular system is responsible for stabilizing the retinal image.

The mechanism by which stimulation of the semicircular ducts results in retinal image stabilization is simple, at least conceptually (Fig. 11–9). When the head is turned to the right in the horizontal (yaw) plane, the angular acceleration of the head creates a reactive torque in the ring of endolymph in (mainly) the horizontal semicircular duct. The reacting endolymph then exerts pressure on the cupula, deviating the cupula in the right ear in a utriculopetal direction, depolarizing the hair cells of the associated crista ampul-

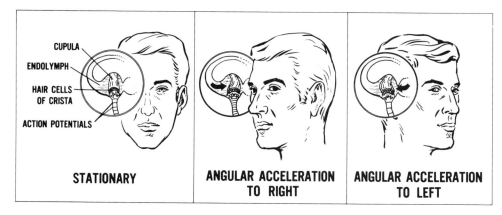

Fig. 11–9. Mechanism of action of a horizontal semicircular duct and the resulting reflex eye movement. Angular acceleration to the right increases the frequency of action potentials originating in the right ampullary nerve and decreases those in the left. This pattern of neural signals causes extraocular muscles to rotate the eyes in the direction opposite that of head rotation, thus stabilizing the retinal image with a compensatory eye movement. Angular acceleration to the left has the opposite effect.

laris and increasing the frequency of the action potentials in the corresponding ampullary nerve. In the left ear, the endolymph deviates the cupula in a utriculofugal direction, thereby hyperpolarizing the hair cells and decreasing the frequency of the action potentials generated. As excitatory neural signals are relayed to the contralateral lateral rectus and ipsilateral medial rectus muscles, and inhibitory signals are simultaneously relayed to the antagonists, a conjugate deviation of the eyes results from the described changes in ampullary neural activity. The direction of this conjugate eye deviation is thus the same as that of the angular reaction of the endolymph, and the angular velocity of the deviation is proportional to the pressure exerted by the endolymph on the cupula. The resulting eye movement is, therefore, compensatory; that is, it adjusts the angular position of the eye to compensate for changes in angular position of the head and thereby prevents slippage of the retinal image over the retina. Because the amount of angular deviation of the eye is physically limited, rapid movements of the eye in the direction opposite the compensatory motion are employed to return the eye to its initial position or to advance it to a position from which it can sustain a compensatory sweep for a suitable length of time. These rapid eye movements are anticompensatory, and because of their very high angular velocity, motion is not perceived during this phase of the vestibulo-ocular reflex.

With the usual rapid, high-frequency rotations of the head, the rotational inertia of the endolymph acts to deviate the cupula as the angular velocity of the head builds, and the angular momentum gained by the endolymph during the brief acceleration acts to drive the cupula back to its resting position when the head decelerates to a stop. The cupula-endolymph system thus functions as an integrating angular accelerometer, that is, it converts angular acceleration data into a neural signal pro-

portional to the angular velocity of the head. This is true for angular accelerations occurring at frequencies normally encountered in terrestrial activities; when angular accelerations outside the dynamic response range of the cupula-endolymph system are experienced, the system no longer provides accurate angular velocity information. When angular accelerations are relatively sustained or when a cupula is kept in a deviated position by other means, such as caloric testing, the compensatory and anticompensatory phases of the vestibulo-ocular reflex are repeated, resulting in beats of ocular nystagmus (Fig. 11–10). The compensatory phase of the vestibulo-ocular reflex is then called the slow phase of nystagmus, and the anticompensatory phase is called the fast or quick phase. The direction of the quick phase is used to label the direction of the nystagmus because the direction of the rapid motion of the eye is easier to determine clinically. The vertical semicircular ducts operate in an analogous manner, with the vestibulo-ocular reflexes elicited by their stimulation being appropriate to the plane of the angular acceleration resulting in that stimulation. Thus, a vestibulo-ocular reflex with downward compensatory and upward anticompensatory

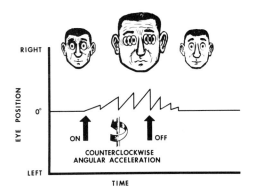

Fig. 11–10. Ocular nystagmus—repeating compensatory and anticompensatory eye movements—resulting from vestibular stimulation. In this case, the stimulation is a yawing angular acceleration to the left, and the anticompensatory, or quick-phase, nystagmic response is also to the left.

phases results from the stimulation of the vertical semicircular ducts by pitch-up $(-\alpha_y)$ angular acceleration, and with sufficient stimulation in this plane, up-beating vertical nystagmus results. Angular accelerations in the roll plane result in vestibulo-ocular reflexes with clockwise and counterclockwise compensatory and anticompensatory phases and in rotary nystagmus. Other planes of stimulation are associated with other directions of eye movement such as oblique or horizonto-rotary.

As should be expected, there also are vestibulo-ocular reflexes of otolith-organ origin. Initiating these reflexes are the shearing actions that bend the cilia of macular hair cells as inertial forces or gravity cause the otolithic membranes to slide to various positions over their maculae (Fig. 11–11). Each position that can be assumed by an otolithic membrane relative to its

macula evokes a particular spatial pattern of frequencies of action potentials in the corresponding utricular or saccular nerve, and that pattern is associated with a particular set of compatible stimulus conditions such as backward tilt of the head or forward linear acceleration. These patterns of action potentials from the various otolith organs are correlated and integrated in the vestibular nuclei and cerebellum with orientational information from the semicircular ducts and other sensory modalities; appropriate orientational percepts and motor activities eventually result. Lateral (a_y) linear accelerations can elicit horizontal reflexive eye movements, including nystagmus, presumably as a result of utricular stimulation. Similarly, vertical (a_z) linear accelerations can elicit vertical eye movements, most likely as a result of stimulation of the saccule; the term elevator reflex is sometimes used to

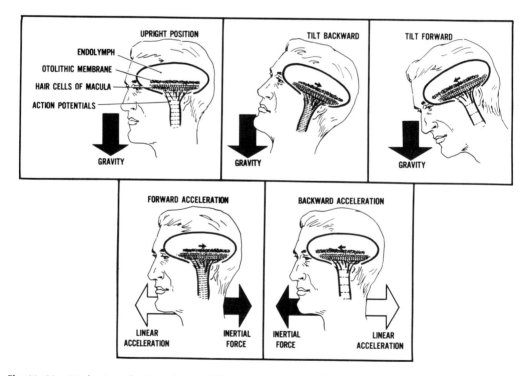

Fig. 11–11. Mechanism of action of an otolith organ. A change in direction of the force of gravity (above) or a linear acceleration (below) causes the otolithic membrane to shift its position with respect to its macula, thereby generating a new pattern of action potentials in the utricular or saccular nerve. Shifting of the otolithic membranes can elicit compensatory vestibulo-ocular reflexes and nystagmus, as weil as perceptual effects.

describe this response because it is readily provoked by the vertical linear accelerations associated with riding in an elevator. The utility of these horizontal and vertical vestibulo-ocular reflexes of otolith-organ origin is readily apparent: like the reflexes of semicircular-duct origin, they help stabilize the retinal image. Less obvious is the usefulness of the ocular countertorsion reflex (Fig. 11–12), which repositions the eyes about their visual (anteroposterior) axes in response to the otolith-organ stimulation resulting from tilting the head laterally in the opposite direction. Presumably, this reflex contributes to retinal image stabilization by providing a response to changing directions of the force of gravity.

Our understanding of the vestibulocollic reflexes has not developed to the same degree as our understanding of the vestibulo-ocular reflexes, although some clinical use has been made of measurements of rotation of the head on the neck in response to vestibular stimulation. Perhaps this situation reflects the fact that vestibulocollic reflexes are not as effective as the vestibulo-ocular reflexes in stabilizing the retinal image, at least not in humans. Such is not the case in other species, however; birds exhibit extremely effective reflex control of head position under con-

ditions of bodily motion—even nystagmic head movements are quite easy to elicit. The high level of development of the vestibulocollic reflexes in birds is certainly either a cause or a consequence of the relative immobility of birds' eyes in their heads. Nonetheless, the ability of a human (or any other vertebrate with a mobile head) to keep the head upright with respect to the direction of applied gravito-inertial force is maintained through tonic vestibular influences on the muscles of the neck.

Vestibulospinal reflexes operate to assure stability of the body. Transient linear and angular accelerations, such as those experienced in tripping and falling, provoke rapid activation of various groups of extensor and flexor muscles to return the body to the stable position or at least to minimize the ultimate effect of the instability. Everyone has experienced the reflex arm movements that serve to break a fall, and most have observed the more highly developed righting reflexes that cats exhibit when dropped from an upside-down position; these are examples of vestibulospinal reflexes. Less spectacular, but nevertheless extremely important, are the sustained vestibular influences on posture that are exerted through tonic activation of so-called "antigravity" muscles such as hip and knee extensors. These vestibular reflexes, of course, help keep the body upright with respect to the direction of the force of gravity.

Voluntary Movement

It has been shown how the various reflexes of vestibular origin serve to stabilize the body in general and the retinal image in particular. The vestibular system is also important in that it provides data for the proper execution of voluntary movement. To realize just how important such vestibular data are in this context, one must first recognize the fact that skilled voluntary movements are ballistic, that is, once in-

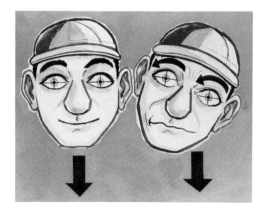

Fig. 11–12. Ocular countertorsion, a vestibulo-ocular reflex of otolith-organ origin. When the head is tilted to the left, the eyes rotate to the right to assume a new angular position about the visual axes, as shown.

itiated, they are executed according to a predetermined pattern and sequence, without the benefit of simultaneous sensory feedback to the higher neural levels from which they originate. The simple act of writing one's signature, for example, involves such rapid changes in speed and direction of movement that conscious sensory feedback and adjustment of motor activity are virtually precluded, at least until the act is nearly completed. Learning an element of a skill thus involves developing a computer-program-like schedule of neural activations that can be called up, so to speak, to effect a particular desired end product of motor activity. Of course, the raw program for a particular voluntary action is not sufficient to permit the execution of that action: information regarding such parameters as intended magnitude and direction of movement must be furnished from the conscious sphere, and data indicating the position and motion of the body platform relative to the surface of the earth—that is, spatial orientation information—must be furnished from the preconscious sphere. The necessity for the additional information can be seen in the signature-writing example cited above: one can write large or small, quickly or slowly, and on a horizontal or vertical surface. Obviously, different patterns of neuromuscular activation, even grossly different muscle groups, are needed to accomplish a basic act under varying spatial and temporal conditions; the necessary adjustments are made automatically, however, without conscious intervention. Vestibular and other sensory data providing spatial orientation information for use in either skilled voluntary or reflexive motor activity are processed into a preconscious orientational percept that provides the informational basis upon which such automatic adjustments are made. Thus, one can decide what the outcome of his action is to be and initiate the command to do it, without consciously having to discern the direction of the force of grav-

ity, analyze its potential effects on planned motor activity, select appropriate muscle groups and modes of activation to compensate for gravity, and then activate and deactivate each muscle in proper sequence and with proper timing to accomplish the desired motor activity. The body takes care of the details, using stored programs for elements of skilled motor activity, and the current preconscious orientational percept. This whole process is the major function and responsibility of the vestibulocerebellar axis.

Conscious Percepts

Usually as a result of the same information processing that provides the preconscious orientational percept, one also is provided a conscious orientational percept. This percept can be false, that is, illusory, in which case the individual is said to experience an orientational illusion. (The term pilot vertigo refers to an illusory conscious orientational percept experienced by a pilot. Although clinical use of the word vertigo usually, but by no means always, denotes a pronounced sensation of turning, in aeromedical usage no such sensation is implied—only a false conscious orientational percept.) One can be aware, moreover, that what his body is telling him is his spatial orientation is not what he has concluded from other information such as flight instrument data. Conscious orientational percepts thus can be either natural or derived, depending on the source of the orientation information and the perceptual process involved, and an individual can experience both natural and derived conscious orientational percepts at the same time. Because of this, pilots who have become disoriented in flight commonly exhibit vacillating control inputs, as they alternate indecisively between responding first to one percept and then to another.

Thresholds of Vestibular Perception

Often, an orientational illusion occurs because the physical event resulting in or from a change in bodily orientation is below the threshold of perception. For that reason, the student of disorientation should be aware of the approximate perceptual thresholds associated with the various modes of vestibular stimulation.

The lowest reported threshold for perception of rotation is 0.035 degrees/sec^2, but this degree of sensitivity is obtained only with virtually continuous angular acceleration and long response latencies (20 to 40 seconds). Other observations put the perceptual threshold between roughly 0.1 and 2.0 degrees/sec^2; reasonable values are 0.14, 0.5, and 0.5 degrees/sec^2 for yaw, roll, and pitch motions, respectively. It is common practice, however, to describe the thresholds of the semicircular ducts in terms of the angular acceleration-time product, or angular velocity, which results in just perceptible rotation. This product, known as Mulder's constant, remains fairly constant for stimulus times of about 5 seconds or less, although the observed values of this constant range between 0.2 and 8.0 degrees/sec, depending on the subjects and methods used to determine it. Using the reasonable value of 2 degrees/sec for Mulder's constant, an angular acceleration of 5 degrees/sec^2 applied for half a second would be perceived because the acceleration-time product is above the 2-degree/sec angular velocity threshold. But a 10-degree/sec^2 acceleration applied for a tenth of a second would not be perceived because it would be below the angular velocity threshold; nor would a 0.2-degree/sec^2 acceleration applied for 5 seconds be perceived.

The perceptual threshold related to otolith-organ function necessarily involves both an angle and a magnitude because the otolith organs respond to linear accelerations and gravitoinertial forces, both of which have direction and intensity. A 1.5° change in direction of applied G force is perceptible under ideal (experimental) conditions. The minimum perceptible intensity of linear acceleration has been reported by various authors to be between 0.001 and 0.03 g, depending on the direction of acceleration and the experimental method used. Values of 0.01 g for a_z and 0.006 g for a_x accelerations are appropriate representative thresholds, and a similar value for a_y acceleration is probably reasonable. Again, these absolute thresholds apply when the acceleration is either sustained or applied at relatively low frequencies. The threshold for linear accelerations applied for less than about 5 seconds is a more or less constant acceleration-time product, or linear velocity, of about 0.3 to 0.4 m/sec.

Unfortunately for those who would like to calculate exactly what orientational percept results from a particular set of linear and angular accelerations, such as might have occurred prior to an aircraft mishap, the actual vestibular perceptual thresholds are, as expressed by one philosopher, "constant except when they vary." Probably the most common reason for an orientational perceptual threshold to be raised is inattention to orientational cues because attention is directed to something else. Other reasons might be a low state of mental arousal, fatigue, drug effects, or innate individual variation. Whatever the reason, it appears that a given individual can monitor his orientation with considerable sensitivity under some circumstances and with relative insensitivity under others, which inconsistency can itself lead to perceptual errors that result in orientational illusions.

Of paramount importance in the generation of orientational illusions, however, is not the fact that absolute vestibular thresholds exist or that vestibular thresholds are time-varying. Rather, it is the fact that the components of the vestibular system, like any complex mechanical or electrical system, have characteristic frequency responses, and stimulation by patterns of acceleration outside the optimal, or "design," frequency-response ranges of the semicircular ducts and otolith organs causes the vestibular system to make errors. In flight, much of the stimulation resulting from the acceleratory environment is indeed outside the design frequency-response ranges of the vestibular end-organs; consequently, orientational illusions occur in flight. Elucidation of this important point is provided in the section entitled "Spatial Disorientation."

Vestibular Suppression and Enhancement

Like all sensory systems, the vestibular system exhibits a decreased response to stimuli that are persistent (adaptation) or repetitious (habituation). Even more important to the aviator is the fact that, with time and practice, one can develop the ability to suppress natural vestibular responses, both perceptual and motor. This ability is termed vestibular suppression. Closely related to the concept of vestibular suppression is that of visual dominance, the ability to obtain and use spatial orientation cues from the visual environment despite the presence of potentially strong vestibular cues. Vestibular suppression seems to be exerted, in fact, through visual dominance because it disappears in the absence of vision. The opposite effect, that of an increase in perceptual and motor responsiveness to vestibular stimulation, is termed vestibular enhancement. Such enhancement can occur when the stimulation is novel, as in an amusement park ride, threatening, as in an aircraft spinning out of control, or whenever spatial orientation is perceived to be especially important. It is tempting to attribute to the efferent vestibular neurons the function of controlling the gain of the vestibular system so as to effect suppression and enhancement, and some evidence exists to support that notion. The actual mechanisms involved appear to be much more complex than would be necessary to merely provide gross changes in gain of the vestibular end-organs. Precise control of vestibular responses to anticipated stimulation, based on sensory efferent copies of voluntary commands for movement, is probably exercised by the cerebellum via a feed-forward loop involving the vestibular efferent system. Thus, when discrepancies between anticipated and actual stimulation generate a neural error signal, a response is evoked, and vestibular reflexes and heightened perception occur. Vestibular suppression, then, involves the development of accurate estimates of vestibular responses to orientational stimuli repeatedly experienced, and the active countering of anticipated responses by spatially and temporally patterned sensory efferent activity. Vestibular enhancement, on the other hand, results from the lack of available estimates of vestibular responses because of the novelty of the stimulation, or perhaps from a revision in neural processing strategy obligated by the failure of normal negative feed-forward mechanisms to provide adequate orientation information. Such marvelous complexity of vestibular function assures adaptability to a wide variety of motional environments and thereby promotes survival in them.

OTHER SENSES OF MOTION AND POSITION

Although the visual and vestibular systems play dominant roles in spatial orientation, the contributions of other sensory systems to orientation cannot be overlooked. Especially important are the nonvestibular proprioceptors—the muscle, tendon, and joint receptors—and the cutaneous exteroceptors, because the orientational percepts derived from their functioning in flight generally support those derived from vestibular information processing, whether accurate or inaccurate. The utility of these other sensory modalities can be appreciated in view of the fact that, in the absence of vision, our vestibular, muscle, tendon, joint, and skin receptors allow us to maintain spatial orientation and postural equilibrium, at least on the earth's surface. Similarly, in the absence of vestibular function, vision and the remaining proprioceptors and cutaneous mechanoreceptors are sufficient for orientation and balance. When two components of this triad of orientational senses are absent or substantially compromised, however, it becomes impossible to maintain sufficient spatial orientation to permit postural stability and effective locomotion.

Nonvestibular Proprioceptors

Sherrington's "proprioceptive" or "self-sensing" sensory category includes the vestibular (or labyrinthine), muscle, tendon, and joint senses. Proprioception generally is spoken of as though it means only the nonvestibular components, however.

Muscle and Tendon Senses

All skeletal muscle contains within it complex sensory end-organs, called muscle spindles (Fig. 11–13a). These end-organs are comprised mainly of small intrafusal muscle fibers that lie parallel with the larger, ordinary, extrafusal muscle fibers and are enclosed over part of their length by a fluid-filled bag. The sensory innervation of these structures consists mainly of large, rapidly conducting afferent neurons that originate as primary (annulospiral) or secondary (flower-spray) endings on the intrafusal fibers and terminate in the spinal cord on anterior horn cells and interneurons. Stretching of the associated extrafusal muscle results in an increase in the frequency of action potentials in the afferent nerve from the intrafusal fibers; contraction of the muscle results in a decrease or absence of action potentials. The more interesting aspect of muscle spindle function, however, is that the intrafusal muscle fibers are innervated by motoneurons (gamma efferents and others) and can be stimulated to contract, thereby altering the afferent information arising from the spindle. Thus, the sensory input from the muscle spindles can be biased by descending influences from

higher neural centers such as the vestibulocerebellar axis.

Although the muscle spindles are structurally and functionally in parallel with associated muscle groups and respond to changes in their length, the Golgi tendon organs (Fig. 11–13b) are functionally in series with the muscles and respond to changes in tension. A tendon organ consists of a fusiform bundle of small tendon fascicles with intertwining neural elements, and is located at the musculotendinous junction or wholly within the tendon. Unlike that of the muscle spindle, its innervation is entirely afferent.

The major function of both the muscle spindles and the tendon organs is to provide the sensory basis for myotatic (or muscle stretch) reflexes. These elementary spinal reflexes operate to stabilize a joint by providing, in response to an increase in length of a muscle and concomitant stimulation of its included spindles, monosynaptic excitation and contraction of the stretched agonist (e.g., extensor) muscle and disynaptic inhibition and relaxation of its antagonist (e.g., flexor) muscle through the action of an inhibitory interneuron. In addition, tension developed on associated tendon organs results in disynaptic inhibition of the agonist muscle, thus regulating the amount of contraction generated. The myotatic reflex mechanism is, in fact, the foundation of posture and locomotion. Modification of this and other basic spinal reflexes by organized facilitatory or inhibitory intervention originating at higher neural levels, either through direct action on skeletomotor (alpha) neurons or through stimulation of fusimotor (primarily gamma) neurons to muscle spindles, results in sustained postural equilibrium and other purposive motor behavior. Some researchers have speculated, moreover, that in certain types of spatial disorientation in flight, this organized modification of spinal reflexes is interrupted as cerebral cortical control of motor activity is replaced by lower brain-

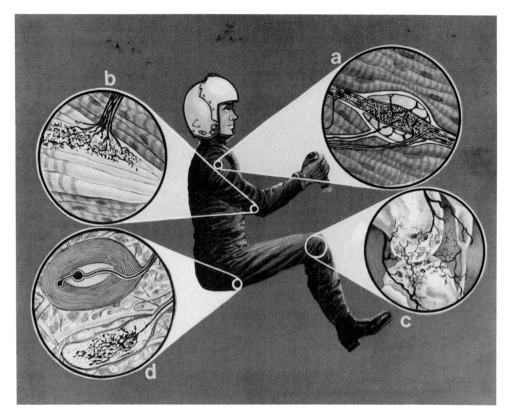

Fig. 11–13. Some of the nonvestibular proprioceptive and cutaneous exteroceptive receptors subserving spatial orientation. *a.* Muscle spindle, with central afferent (sensory) and more peripheral efferent (fusimotor) innervations is shown. *b.* Golgi tendon organ. *c.* Lamellated, spray-type, and free-nerve-ending joint receptors. *d.* Two of the many types of mechanoreceptors found in the skin : lamellated Pacinian corpuscles and spray-type Ruffini corpuscles.

stem and spinal control. Perhaps the "frozen-on-the-controls" type of disorientation-induced deterioration of flying ability is a reflection of primitive reflexes made manifest by disorganization of higher neural functions.

Despite the obvious importance of the muscle spindles and tendon organs in the control of motor activity, there is little evidence to indicate that their responding to orientational stimuli (such as occur when one stands vertically in a 1-G environment) results in any corresponding conscious proprioceptive percept. Nevertheless, it is known that the dorsal columns and other ascending spinal tracts carry muscle afferent information to medullary and thalamic relay nuclei and thence to the cerebral sensory cortex. Furthermore,

extensive projections into the cerebellum, via dorsal and ventral spinocerebellar tracts, ensure that proprioceptive information from the afferent terminations of the muscle spindles and tendon organs is integrated with other orientational information and is relayed to the vestibular nuclei, cerebral cortex, and elsewhere as needed.

Joint Sensation

In contrast to the situation with the so-called "muscle sense of position" just discussed, it has been well established that sensory information from the joints does reach consciousness. In fact, the threshold for perception of joint motion and position can be quite low: as low as 0.5 degree for the knee joint when moved at greater than

1.0 degree/sec. The receptors in the joints are of three types, as shown in Figure 11–13c: (1) lamellated or encapsulated Pacinian corpuscle-like end-organs; (2) spray-type structures, known as Ruffini-like endings when found in joint capsules and Golgi tendon organs when found in ligaments; and (3) free nerve endings. The Pacinian corpuscle-like terminals are rapidly adapting and are sensitive to quick movement of the joint, whereas both of the spray-type endings are slowly adapting and serve to signal slow joint movement and joint position. There is evidence that polysynaptic spinal reflexes can be elicited by stimulation of joint receptors, but their nature and extent are not well understood. Proprioceptive information from the joint receptors projects via the dorsal funiculi eventually to the cerebral sensory cortex and via the spinocerebellar tracts to the anterior lobe of the cerebellum.

One must not infer from this discussion that only muscles, tendons, and joints have proprioceptive sensory receptors. Both lamellated and spray-type receptors, as well as free nerve endings, are found in fascia, aponeuroses, and other connective tissues of the musculoskeletal system, and they presumably provide proprioceptive information to the central nervous system.

Cutaneous Exteroceptors

The exteroceptors of the skin include the mechanoreceptors, which respond to touch and pressure, thermoreceptors, which respond to heat and cold, and nociceptors, which respond to noxious mechanical and/or thermal events and give rise to sensations of pain. Of the cutaneous exteroceptors, only the mechanoreceptors contribute significantly to spatial orientation.

A variety of receptors are involved in cutaneous mechanoreception: spray-type Ruffini corpuscles, lamellated Pacinian and Meissner corpuscles, branched and straight lanceolate terminals, Merkel cells, and free nerve endings (Fig. 11–13d). The response patterns of mechanoreceptors also are numerous: eleven different types of response, varying from high-frequency transient detection through several modes of velocity detection to more or less static displacement detection, have been recognized. Pacinian corpuscles and certain receptors associated with hair follicles are very rapidly adapting and have the highest mechanical frequency responses, responding to sinusoidal skin displacements in the range of 50 to 400 Hz. They are thus well suited to monitor vibration and transient touch stimuli. Ruffini corpuscles are slowly adapting and, therefore, respond primarily to sustained touch and pressure stimuli. Merkel cells appear to have a moderately slowly adapting response, making them suitable for monitoring static skin displacement and velocity. Meissner corpuscles seem to detect primarily velocity of skin deformation. Other receptors provide other types of response, so as to complete the spectrum of mechanical stimuli that can be sensed through the skin. The mechanical threshold for the touch receptors is quite low— less than 0.03 dyne/cm^2 on the thumb. (In comparison with the labyrinthine receptors subserving audition, however, this threshold is not so impressive: a 0-dB sound pressure level represents 0.0002 dyne/cm^2, more than 100 times lower.) Afferent information from the described mechanoreceptors is conveyed to the cerebral cortex mainly by way of the dorsal funiculi and medullary relay nuclei into the medial lemnisci and thalamocortical projections. The dorsal spinocerebellar tract and other tracts to the cerebellum provide the pathways by which cutaneous exteroceptive information reaches the cerebellum and is integrated with proprioceptive information from muscles, tendons, joints, and vestibular end-organs.

Auditory Orientation

On the surface of the earth, the ability to determine the direction of a sound source can play an important role in spatial orientation. The major auditory cues providing this ability are differences between the ears in arrival times of congruent acoustic stimuli and interaural differences in the magnitude and phase of arriving stimuli. A revolving sound source can create a sense of self-rotation and even elicit reflex compensatory and anticompensatory eye movements called audiokinetic nystagmus. In aircraft, binaural sound localization is of little use in spatial orientation because of high ambient noise levels and the absence of audible external sound sources. Pilots do extract some orientation information, however, from the auditory cues provided by the rush of air past the airframe: the sound frequencies and intensities characteristic of various airspeeds and angles of attack are recognized by the experienced pilot, and he uses them in conjunction with other orientation information to create a percept of velocity and pitch attitude of his aircraft. As aircraft have become more capable, however, and the pilot has become more insulated from such acoustic stimuli, the importance of auditory orientation cues in flying has diminished.

SPATIAL DISORIENTATION

The evolution of man saw him develop over millions of years as an aquatic, terrestrial, and even arboreal creature, but never an aerial one. In this development, he subjected himself to and was subjected to many different varieties of transient motions, but not to the relatively sustained linear and angular accelerations commonly experienced in aviation. As a result, man acquired sensory systems well suited for maneuvering under his own power on the surface of the earth but poorly suited for flying. Even the birds, whose primary mode of locomotion is flying, are unable to maintain spatial orientation and fly safely when deprived of vision by fog or clouds. Only bats seem to have developed the ability to fly without

vision, and then only by replacing vision with auditory echolocation. Considering man's phylogenetic heritage, it should come as no surprise that his sudden entry into the aerial environment resulted in a mismatch between the orientational demands of the new environment and his innate ability to orient. The manifestation of this mismatch is spatial disorientation.

Illusions in Flight

An illusion is a false percept. An orientational illusion is a false percept of one's position, attitude, or motion, relative to the plane of the earth's surface. Thus, misperceptions of displacement, velocity, or acceleration—either linear or angular—result in orientational illusions. A great number of orientational illusions occur during flight: some named, others unnamed; some understood, others not understood. Those that are sufficiently impressive to cause pilots to report them, whether because of their repeatability or because of their emotional impact, have been described in the aeromedical literature and will be discussed here. The illusions in flight are categorized into those resulting primarily from visual misperceptions and those involving primarily vestibular errors.

Visual Illusions

The two different modes of visual processing are the focal (foveal) mode and the ambient (peripheral) mode. Generally speaking, focal vision is concerned with object recognition, and ambient vision is concerned with spatial orientation. Some visual orientation tasks in flying require a great deal of focal vision, however, and such tasks can be made extremely difficult by illusions resulting from the misinterpretation of focal visual cues. Runway illusions and approach illusions illustrate this fact.

Aerial Perspective

Figure 11–14a shows the pilot's view of the runway during an approach to landing

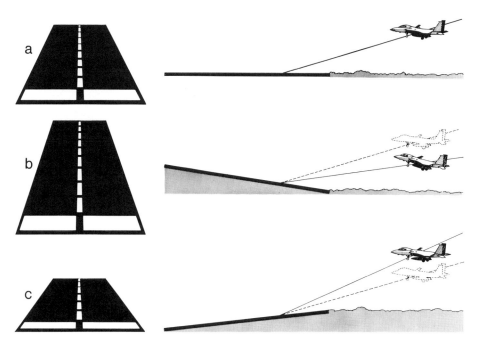

Fig. 11–14. Effect of runway slope on the pilot's image of runway during final approach (left) and potential effect on the approach slope angle flown (right). *a.* Flat runway—normal approach. *b.* An upsloping runway creates the illusion of being high on approach—pilot flies the approach too low. *c.* A downsloping runway has the opposite effect.

and demonstrates the linear perspective and foreshortening of the runway that the pilot associates with a 3° approach slope. If the runway slopes upward 1° (a rise of only 35 m in a 2-km runway), the foreshortening of the runway for a pilot on a 3° approach slope is substantially less (the height of the retinal image of the runway is greater) than it would be if the runway were level. This can give the pilot the illusion that he is too high on the approach. The pilot's natural response to such an illusion is to reshape his image of the runway by seeking a shallower approach slope (Fig. 11–14b). This response, of course, could be hazardous. The opposite situation results when the runway slopes downward. To perceive the accustomed runway shape under this condition, the pilot must fly a steeper approach slope than usual (Fig. 11–14c).

A runway that is narrower than that to which a pilot is accustomed also can create a hazardous illusion on the approach

to landing. Size constancy causes the pilot to perceive the narrow runway to be longer and farther away (i.e., that he is higher) than is actually the case, and he may flare too late and touch down sooner than he expects (Fig. 11–15b). Likewise, a runway that is wider than what a pilot is used to can lead him to believe he is closer to the runway (i.e., lower) than he really is, and he may flare too soon and drop in from too high above the runway (Fig. 11–15c). Both of these runway-width illusions are especially troublesome at night when peripheral visual orientation cues are largely absent. The common tendency for pilots to flare too high at night results at least partly from the fact that the runway lights, being displaced laterally from the actual edge of the runway, make the runway seem wider, and therefore closer, than it actually is.

The slope and composition of the terrain under the approach path also can influence the pilot's judgment of his height

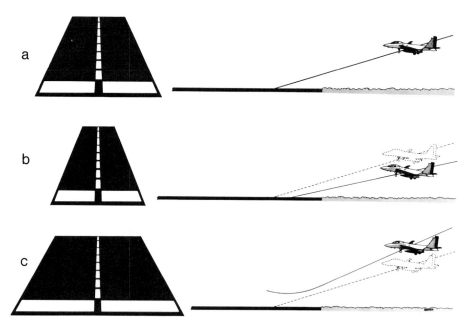

Fig. 11–15.   Effect of runway width on the pilot's image of runway (left) and the potential effect on approach flown (right). *a.* Accustomed width—normal approach. *b.* A narrow runway makes the pilot feel he is higher than he actually is, so he flies the approach too low and flares too late. *c.* A wide runway gives the illusion of being closer than it actually is—the pilot tends to approach too high and flares too soon.

above the touchdown point. If the terrain descends to the approach end of the runway, the pilot tends to fly a steeper approach than he would if the approach terrain were level (Fig. 11–16a). If the approach terrain slopes up to the runway, on the other hand, the pilot tends to fly a less steep approach than he would otherwise (Fig. 11–16b). Although the estimation of height above the approach terrain depends on both focal and ambient vision, the contribution of focal vision is particularly clear: consider the pilot who looks at a building below him and, seeing it to be closer than such buildings usually are, seeks a higher approach slope. By the same token, focal vision and size constancy are responsible for poor height and distance judgments pilots sometimes make when flying over terrain having an unfamiliar composition (Fig. 11–17). A reported example of this is the tendency to misjudge the approach height when landing in the Aleutians, where the evergreen trees are much smaller than those to which

most pilots are accustomed. Such height-estimation difficulties are by no means restricted to the approach and landing phases of flight. One fatal mishap occurred during air combat training over the Southwest desert when the pilot of a high-performance fighter presumably misjudged his height over the desert floor because of the small, sparse vegetation and was unable to arrest his deliberate descent to a ground-hugging altitude.

A well-known pair of approach-to-landing situations that create illusions because of the absence of adequate focal visual orientation cues are the smooth-water (or glassy-water) and snow-covered approaches. A seaplane pilot's perception of height is degraded substantially when the water below is still: for that reason, he routinely just sets up a safe descent rate and waits for the seaplane to touch down, rather than attempting to flare to a landing when the water is smooth. A blanket of fresh snow on the ground also deprives the pilot of visual cues with which to estimate

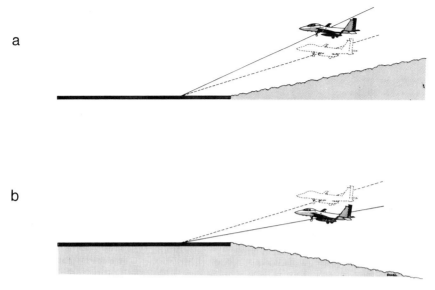

Fig. 11–16. Potential effect of the slope of the terrain under the approach on the approach slope flown. *a.* The terrain slopes down to runway; the pilot thinks he is too shallow on the approach and steepens it. *b.* Upsloping terrain makes the pilot think he is too high, so he corrects by making the approach too shallow.

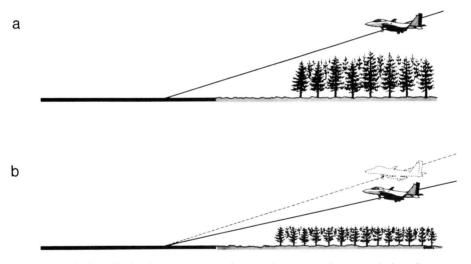

Fig. 11–17. Potential effect of unfamiliar composition of approach terrain on the approach slope flown. *a.* Normal approach over trees of familiar size. *b.* Unusually small trees under the approach path make the pilot think he is too high, so he makes his approach lower than usual.

his height, thus making his approach more difficult—extremely difficult if the runway is also covered with snow. Again, approaches are not the only regime in which smooth water and fresh snow cause problems. A number of aircraft have crashed as a result of pilots maneuvering over smooth water or snow-covered ground and misjudging their height above the surface.

Aerial perspective also can play a role in deceiving the pilot. In daytime, fog or haze can make a runway appear farther away as a result of the loss of visual discrimination. At night, runway and approach lights in fog or rain appear less bright than they do in clear weather and can create the illusion that they are farther away. It has even been reported that a pilot can have an illusion of banking to the right, for example, if the runway lights are brighter on the right side of the runway than they are on the left. Another hazardous illusion of this type can occur during approach to landing in a shallow fog or haze, especially during a night approach. The vertical visibility under such conditions is much better than the horizontal visibility, so that descent into the fog causes the more distant approach or runway lights to diminish in intensity at the same time that the peripheral visual cues are suddenly occluded by the fog. The result is an illusion that the aircraft has pitched up, with the concomitant danger of a nose-down corrective action by the pilot.

Peripheral Cues

Another condition in which a pilot is apt to make a serious misjudgment is in closing on another aircraft at high speed. When he has numerous peripheral visual cues by which to establish both his own position and velocity relative to the earth and the target's position and velocity relative to the earth, his tracking and closing problem is not much different from what it would be on the ground if he were giving chase to a moving quarry. When relative position and closure rate cues must come from foveal vision alone, however, as is generally the case at altitude, at night, or under other conditions of reduced visibility, the tracking and closing problem is much more difficult. An overshoot, or worse, a midair collision, can easily result from the perceptual difficulties inherent in such circumstances, especially when the pilot lacks experience in an environment devoid of peripheral visual cues.

Two runway approach conditions that create considerable difficulty for the pilot, and which (like the closure-rate problem just discussed) result from tasking focal vision to accomplish by itself what is normally accomplished with both focal and ambient vision, are the black-hole and whiteout approaches. A black-hole approach is one that is made on a dark night over water or unlighted terrain to a runway beyond which the horizon is indiscernible, the worst case being when only the runway lights are visible (Fig. 11–18). Without peripheral visual cues to help him orient himself relative to the earth, the pilot tends to feel he is stable and situated appropriately but that the runway itself moves about or remains malpositioned (is downsloping, for example). Such illusions make the black-hole approach difficult and dangerous and often result in a landing far short of the runway. A particularly hazardous type of black-hole approach is one made under conditions wherein the earth is totally dark except for the runway and the lights of a city on rising terrain beyond the runway. Under these conditions, the pilot may try to maintain a constant vertical visual angle for the distant city lights, thus causing his aircraft to arc far below the intended approach slope as he gets closer to the runway (Fig. 11–19). An alternative explanation is that the pilot falsely perceives through ambient vision that the rising terrain is flat and he lowers his approach slope accordingly.

An approach made under whiteout conditions can be as difficult as a black-hole approach, and for essentially the same reason—lack of sufficient ambient visual orientation cues. There are actually two types of whiteout, the *atmospheric whiteout* and the *blowing-snow whiteout*. In the atmospheric whiteout, a snow-covered ground merges with a white overcast, creating a condition in which ground textural cues are absent and the horizon is indistinguishable. Although visibility may be unrestricted in the atmospheric whiteout, there is essentially nothing to see except the runway or runway markers; an approach made in this condition must therefore be accomplished with a close eye on

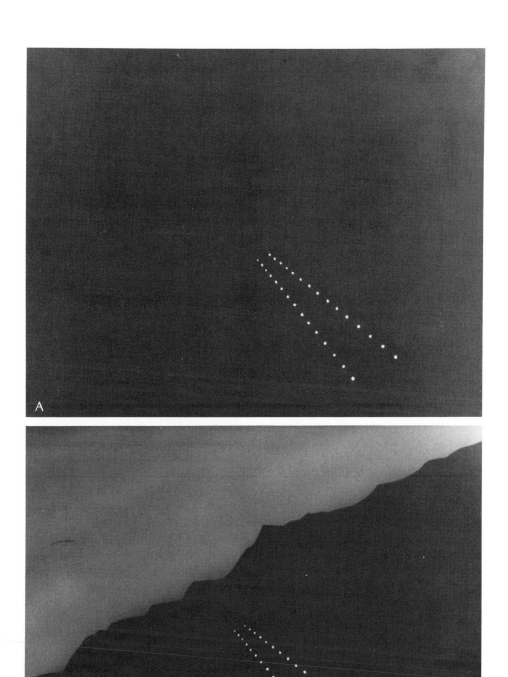

Fig. 11–18. Effect of loss of peripheral visual orientation cues on the perception of runway orientation during a black-hole approach. *A.* When peripheral visual orientation cues are absent, the pilot feels horizontal and (in this example) perceives the runway to be tilted left and upsloping. *B.* With the horizon visible, the pilot orients himself correctly with peripheral vision and the runway appears horizontal in central vision.

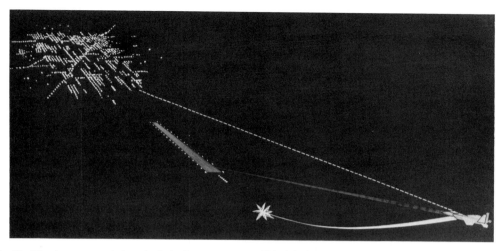

Fig. 11–19. A common and particularly dangerous type of black-hole approach, in which the pilot perceives the distant city to be flat and arcs below the desired approach slope.

the altitude and attitude instruments to prevent spatial disorientation and inadvertent ground contact. In the blowing-snow whiteout, visibility is restricted drastically by snowflakes, and often those snowflakes have been driven into the air by the propeller or rotor wash of the affected aircraft. Helicopter landings on snow-covered ground are particularly likely to create blowing-snow whiteouts. Typically, the helicopter pilot tries to maintain visual contact with the ground during the sudden rotor-induced whiteout, gets into an unrecognized drift to one side, and shortly thereafter contacts the ground with sufficient lateral motion to cause the craft to roll over. Pilots flying where whiteouts can occur must be made aware of the hazards of whiteout approaches, as the disorientation induced usually occurs unexpectedly under visual rather than instrument meterological conditions.

Autokinesis

One puzzling illusion that occurs when visual orientation cues are minimal is visual autokinesis (Fig. 11–20). A small, dim light seen against a dark background is an ideal stimulus for producing autokinesis. After 6 to 12 seconds of visually fixating

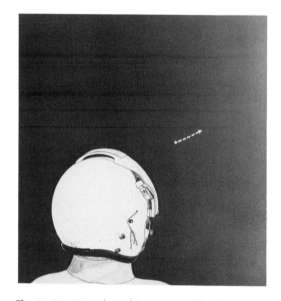

Fig. 11–20. Visual autokinesis. A small, solitary light or small group of lights seen in the dark can appear to move, when in fact they are stationary.

the light, the pilot can observe it to move at anywhere between 0.2 and 20 degrees/ sec in one particular direction or in several directions in succession. Peripheral visual autokinesis is associated with smooth apparent movements and large apparent displacements, whereas central visual autokinesis is often saccadic or jerky and results in little apparent displacement of the object fixated. In general, the larger and brighter the object, the less the autokinetic effect. The shape of the object seems to have little effect on the magnitude of the illusion, however. Nor does providing a larger number of objects necessarily reduce the illusory effect because multiple objects can appear to move, either as a unit or independently, as vigorously as a single object. The physiologic mechanism of visual autokinesis is not understood; in fact, it has not even been established with certainty whether actual eye movements are associated with autokinesis. One suggested explanation for the autokinetic phenomenon is that the eyes tend to drift involuntarily, perhaps because of inadequate or inappropriate vestibular stabilization, and that checking the drift requires efferent oculomotor activity having sensory correlates that create the illusion.

Whatever the mechanism, the effect of visual autokinesis on pilots is of some importance. Anecdotes abound of pilots who fixate a star or a stationary ground light at night, and seeing it move because of autokinesis, mistake it for another aircraft and try to intercept or join up with it. Another untoward effect of the illusion occurs when a pilot flying at night perceives a relatively stable aircraft, one that he must intercept or follow, to be moving erratically when in fact it is not; the unnecessary and undesirable control inputs the pilot makes to compensate for the illusory movement of the target aircraft represent increased work and wasted motion at best and an operational hazard at worst.

To help avoid or reduce the autokinetic illusion, the pilot should try to maintain a well-structured visual environment in which spatial orientation is unambiguous. Because this is rarely possible in night flying, it has been suggested that (1) the pilot's gaze should be shifted frequently to avoid prolonged fixation of a target light; (2) the target should be viewed beside or through and in reference to a rel-

atively stationary structure such as a canopy bow; (3) the pilot should make eye, head, and body movements to try to destroy the illusion; and (4) as always, the pilot should monitor the flight instruments to help prevent or resolve any perceptual conflict. Equipping aircraft with more than one light or with luminescent strips to enhance recognition at night probably has helped reduce problems with autokinesis. It has not abolished them, however.

Vection Illusion

So far, this chapter has dealt with visual illusions created by excessive orientation-processing demands being placed on focal vision when adequate orientation cues are not available through ambient vision or when strong but false orientation cues are received through focal vision. Ambient vision can itself be responsible for creating orientational illusions, however, whenever orientation cues received in the visual periphery are misleading or misinterpreted. Probably the most compelling of such illusions are the vection illusions. Vection is the visually induced perception of motion of the self in the spatial environment (self-motion) and can be a sensation of linear motion (linear vection) or angular motion (angular vection).

Nearly everyone who drives an automobile has experienced one very common linear vection illusion: when a driver is waiting in his car at a stoplight and a presumably stationary vehicle in the adjacent lane creeps forward, a compelling illusion that his own car is creeping backward can result (prompting a swift but surprisingly ineffectual stomp on the brakes). Similarly, if a passenger is sitting in a stationary train and the train on the adjacent track begins to move, he can experience the strong sensation that his own train is moving in the opposite direction (Fig. 11–21a). Linear vection is one of the factors that make close formation flying so difficult because the pilot can never be sure whether

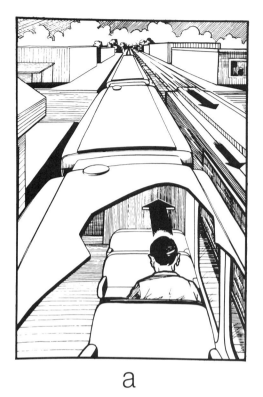 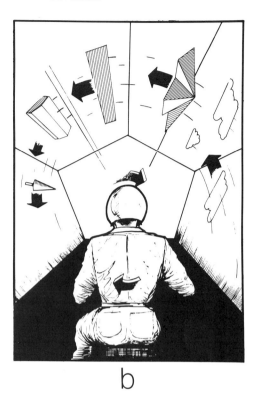

a   b

Fig. 11–21. Vection illusions. *a.* Linear vection. In this example, the adjacent vehicle seen moving aft in his peripheral vision causes the subject to feel as though he is moving forward. *b.* Angular vection. Objects seen revolving around him cause the subject in the flight simulator to sense self-rotation in the opposite direction—in this case, a rolling motion to the right.

his own aircraft or that of his lead or wingman is responsible for the relative motion of his aircraft.

Angular vection occurs when peripheral visual cues convey the information that one is rotating; the perceived rotation can be in pitch, roll, yaw, or any other plane. Although angular vection illusions are not common in everyday life, they can be generated readily in a laboratory by enclosing a stationary subject in a rotating striped drum. Usually within 10 seconds after the visual motion begins, the subject perceives that he rather than the striped drum is rotating. A pilot can experience angular vection if the rotating anticollision light on his aircraft is left on during flight through clouds or fog: the revolving reflection provides a strong ambient visual stimulus signaling rotation in the yaw plane.

Fortunately, vection illusions are not all bad. The most advanced flight simulators depend on linear and angular vection to create the illusion of flight (Fig. 11–21b). When the visual flight environment is dynamically portrayed in wide-field-of-view flight simulators, the illusion of actual flight is so complete and compelling that additional mechanical motion is rendered superfluous.

False Visual Cues

Another result of false ambient visual orientational cuing is the lean-on-the-sun illusion. On the ground, we are accustomed to seeing the brighter visual surround above and the darker below, regardless of the position of the sun. The direction of this gradient in light intensity thus helps us orient with respect to the surface of the earth. In clouds, however, such a gradient usually does not exist, and when it does, the lighter direction is generally toward the sun and the darker direction is away from it. But the sun is almost never directly overhead; as a consequence, a pilot flying in a thin cloud layer tends to perceive falsely the direction of the sun as directly overhead. This misperception causes him to bank in the direction of the sun, hence the name of the illusion. A variant of this phenomenon involves a somewhat different mechanism: occasionally, a pilot remembers the relative bearing of the sun when he first penetrated the weather, and he unconsciously tries to keep the sun in the same relative position whenever it peeks through the clouds. On a prolonged flight in intermittent weather, the changing position of the sun in the sky can cause the pilot to become mildly confused and fly his aircraft with less precision than he would in either continuously visual or continuously instrument meteorologic conditions.

Often the horizon perceived through ambient vision is not really horizontal. Quite naturally, this misperception of the horizontal creates hazards to flight. A sloping cloud deck, for example, is very difficult to perceive as anything but horizontal if it extends for any great distance in the pilot's peripheral vision (Fig.

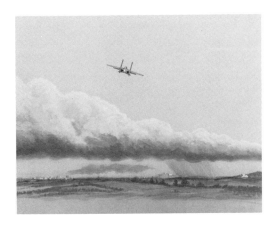

Fig. 11–22. A sloping cloud deck, which the pilot misperceives as a horizontal surface.

11–22). Uniformly sloping terrain, particularly upsloping terrain, can create an illusion of horizontality with disastrous consequences for the pilot thus deceived. Many aircraft have crashed as a result of the pilot's entering a canyon with an apparently level floor, only to find that the floor actually rose faster than his airplane could climb. A distant rain shower can obscure the real horizon and create the impression of a horizon at the proximal edge (base) of the rainfall. If the shower is seen just beyond the runway during an approach to landing, the pilot can misjudge the pitch attitude of his aircraft and make inappropriate pitch corrections on the approach.

Pilots are especially susceptible to misperception of the horizontal while flying at night (Fig. 11–23 A and B). Isolated ground lights can appear to the pilot as stars, and this causes him to think he is in a nose-high or one-wing-low attitude. Flying under such a false impression can, of course, be fatal. Frequently, no stars are visible because of overcast conditions. Unlighted areas of terrain can then blend with the dark overcast to create the illusion that the unlighted terrain is part of the sky. One extremely hazardous situation is that in which a takeoff is made over an ocean or other large body of water that cannot be distinguished visually from the night sky. Many pilots in this situation have perceived the shoreline receding beneath them to be the horizon, and some have responded to this false percept with disastrous consequences.

Pilots flying at high altitudes can sometimes experience difficulties with control of aircraft attitude, because at high altitudes the horizon is lower with respect to the plane of level flight than it is at the lower altitudes where most pilots are accustomed to flying. As a reasonable approximation, the angle of depression of the horizon in degrees equals the square root of the altitude in kilometers. A pilot flying at an altitude of 15 km thus sees the ho-

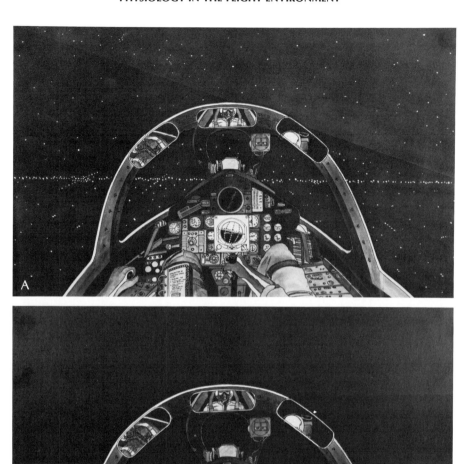

Fig. 11–23. Misperception of the horizontal at night. *A.* Ground lights appearing to be stars cause the earth and sky to blend and a false horizon to be perceived. *B.* Blending of overcast sky with unlighted terrain or water causes the horizon to appear lower than is actually the case.

rizon almost 4° below the extension of his horizontal plane. If he visually orients to the view from his left cockpit window, he might be inclined to fly with the left wing 4° down to level it with the horizon. If he does this and then looks out his right window, he would see the right wing 8° above the horizon, with half of that elevation due

to his own erroneous control input. He also might experience problems with pitch control because the depressed horizon can cause him to perceive falsely a 4° nose-high pitch attitude.

Finally, the disorienting effects of the northern lights and of aerial flares should be mentioned. Aerial refueling at night in high northern latitudes often is made quite difficult by the northern lights, which provide false cues of verticality to the pilot's peripheral vision. In addition, the movement of the auroral displays may make the pilot susceptible to vection illusions. Similarly, when aerial flares are dropped, they may descend vertically or they may drift with the wind, creating false cues of verticality. Their motion also may create vection illusions. Another important factor is that the aurora and aerial flares can be so bright as to reduce the apparent intensity of the aircraft instrument displays and thereby minimize their orientational cuing strength.

Vestibular Illusions

The vestibulocerebellar axis processes orientation information from the vestibular end-organs, the nonvestibular proprioceptors, and the peripheral visual fields. In the absence of adequate ambient visual orientation cues, the inadequacies of the vestibular and other orienting senses can, and generally do, result in orientational illusions. It is convenient and conventional to discuss the vestibular illusions in relation to the two functional components of the labyrinth that generate them—the semicircular ducts and the otolith organs.

Somatogyral Illusion

The somatogyral illusion results from the inability of the semicircular ducts to register accurately a prolonged rotation, that is, sustained angular velocity. When a person is subjected to an angular acceleration about the yaw axis, for example, the angular motion is at first perceived accurately because the dynamics of the cupula-endolymph system cause it to respond as an integrating angular accelerometer (i.e., as a rotation-rate sensor) at stimulus frequencies in the physiologic range (Fig. 11–24). If the acceleration is followed immediately by a deceleration, as usually happens in the terrestrial environment, the total sensation of turning

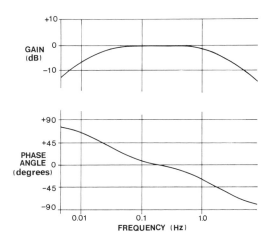

Fig. 11–24. Transfer characteristics of the semicircular duct system as a function of sinusoidal stimulus frequency. Gain is the ratio of the magnitude of the peak perceived angular velocity to the peak delivered angular velocity; phase angle is a measure of the amount of advance or delay between the peak perceived and peak delivered angular velocities. Note that in the physiologic frequency range (roughly 0.05 to 1 Hz), perception is accurate; that is, gain is close to unity (0 dB) and phase shift is minimal. At lower stimulus frequencies, however, the gain drops off rapidly, and the phase shift approaches 90°, which means that angular velocity becomes difficult to detect and that angular acceleration is perceived as velocity. (Adapted from Peters, R.A.: Dynamics of the vestibular system and their relation to motion perception, spatial disorientation, and illusions. NASA-CR-1309. Washington, D.C., National Aeronautics and Space Administration, 1969.)

one way and then stopping the turn is quite accurate (Fig. 11–25). If, however, the angular acceleration is not followed by a deceleration and a constant angular velocity results instead, the sensation of rotation becomes less and less and eventually disappears as the cupula gradually returns to its resting position in the absence of an angular acceleratory stimulus (Fig. 11–26). If the rotating subject is subsequently subjected to an angular deceleration after a period of prolonged constant angular velocity, say after 10 seconds or so of constant-rate turning, his cupula-endolymph system signals a turn in the direction opposite that of the prolonged constant angular velocity, even though he is really only turning less rapidly in the same direction. This is because the angular mo-

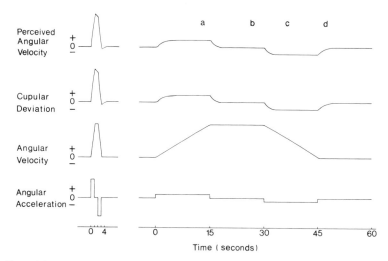

Fig. 11–25. Effect of the stimulus pattern on the perception of angular velocity. On the left, the high-frequency character of the applied angular acceleration results in a cupular deviation that is nearly proportional, and perceived angular velocity that is nearly identical, to the angular velocity developed. On the right, the peak angular velocity developed is the same as that on the left, but the low-frequency character of the applied acceleration results in cupular deviation and perceived angular velocity that appear more like the applied acceleration than the resulting velocity. This causes one to perceive: (a) less than the full amount of the angular velocity; (b) that he is not turning when he actually is; (c) a turn in the opposite direction from that of the actual turn; and (d) that turning persists after it has actually stopped. These false perceptions are somatogyral illusions.

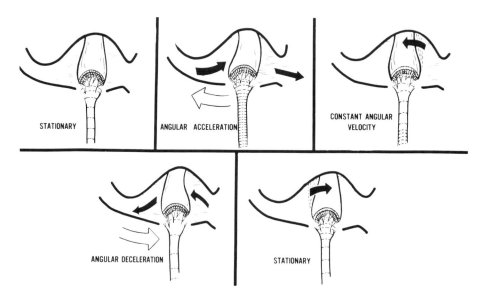

Fig. 11–26. Representation of the mechanical events occurring in a semicircular duct and resulting action potentials in the associated ampullary nerve during somatogyral illusions. The angular acceleration pattern applied is that shown in the right side of Figure 11–25.

mentum of the rotating endolymph causes it to press against the cupula, forcing the cupula to deviate in the direction of endolymph flow, which is the same direction the cupula would deviate if the subject were to accelerate in the direction opposite his initial acceleration. Even after rotation actually ceases, the sensation of rotation in the direction opposite that of the sustained angular velocity persists for several seconds—half a minute or longer with a large decelerating rotational impulse. Technically speaking, a somatogyral illusion is the sensation of turning in the opposite direction that occurs whenever one undergoes angular deceleration from a condition of persisting angular velocity. It is practical, however, to include in this category of illusions the sensation of turning more slowly and eventually ceasing to turn while angular velocity persists, because the two illusions have a common underlying mechanism and they inevitably occur in pairs. An even broader definition of somatogyral illusion is "any discrepancy between actual and perceived rate of self-rotation that results from an abnormal angular acceleratory stimulus pattern." The term "abnormal" in this case implies the application of low-frequency stimuli outside the useful portion of the transfer characteristics of the semicircular duct system.

In flight under conditions of reduced visibility, somatogyral illusions can be deadly. The graveyard spin is the classic example of how somatogyral illusions can disorient a pilot with fatal results. This situation begins with the pilot intentionally or unintentionally entering a spin, let's say to the left (Fig. 11–27). At first, he perceives the spin correctly because the angular acceleration associated with entering the spin deviates the appropriate cupulae the appropriate amount in the appropriate direction. The longer the spin persists, however, the more the sensation of spinning to the left diminishes as the cupulae return to their resting positions.

If the pilot tries to stop the spin to the left by applying the right rudder, the angular deceleration causes him to perceive a spin to the right, even though the only real result of his action is termination of the spin to the left. A pilot who is ignorant of the possibility of such an illusion is then likely to make counterproductive left-rudder inputs to negate the unwanted erroneous sensation of spinning to the right. These inputs keep the airplane spinning to the left, which gives the pilot the desired sensation of not spinning but does not bring the airplane under control. To extricate himself from this very hazardous situation, the pilot must read the aircraft flight instruments and apply control inputs to make the instruments give the desired readings (push right rudder to center the turn needle, in this example). Unfortunately, this may not be so easy to do. The angular accelerations created by both the multiple-turn spin and the pilot's spin-recovery attempts can elicit strong but inappropriate vestibulo-ocular reflexes, including nystagmus. In the usual terrestrial environment, these reflexes help stabilize the retinal image of the visual surround; in this situation, however, they only destabilize the retinal image because the visual surround (cockpit) is already fixed with respect to the pilot. Reading the flight instruments thus becomes difficult or impossible, and the pilot is left with only his false sensations of rotation to rely on for spatial orientation and aircraft control.[11]

Although the lore of early aviation provided the graveyard spin as an illustration of the hazardous nature of somatogyral illusions, a much more common example occurring all too often in modern aviation is the graveyard spiral (Fig. 11–28). In this situation, the pilot has intentionally or unintentionally gotten himself into a prolonged turn with a moderate amount of bank. After a number of seconds in the turn, the pilot loses the sensation of turning because his cupula-endolymph system cannot respond to constant angular veloc-

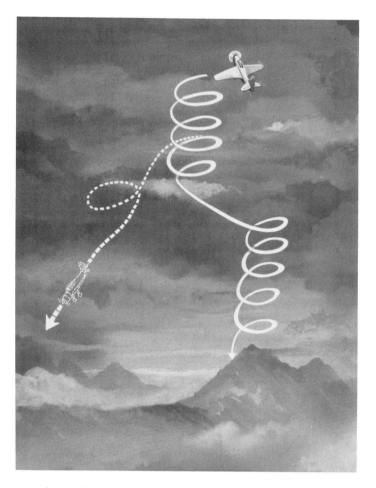

Fig. 11–27. The graveyard spin. After several turns of a spin the pilot begins to lose the sensation of spinning. Then, when he tries to stop the spin, the resulting somatogyral illusion of spinning in the opposite direction makes him reenter the original spin. (The solid line indicates actual motion; the dotted line indicates perceived motion.)

ity. The percept of being in a bank as a result of the initial roll into the banked attitude also decays with time because the net gravitoinertial force vector points toward the floor of the aircraft during coordinated flight (whether the aircraft is in a banked turn or flying straight and level), and the otolith organs and other graviceptors normally signal that down is in the direction of the net sustained gravitoinertial force. As a result, when the pilot tries to stop the turn by rolling back to a wings-level attitude, he not only feels he is turning in the direction opposite that of his original turn, but he also feels he is banked in the direction opposite that of his orig-

inal bank. Unwilling to accept this sensation of making the wrong control input, the hapless pilot rolls back into his original banked turn. Now his sensation is compatible with his desired mode of flight, but his instruments say he is losing altitude (because the banked turn is wasting lift) and still turning. So he pulls back on the stick and perhaps adds power to arrest the unwanted descent and regain the lost altitude. This action would be successful if the aircraft were flying wings-level, but with the aircraft in a banked attitude it tightens the turn, serving only to make matters worse. Unless the pilot eventually recognizes his error and rolls out of

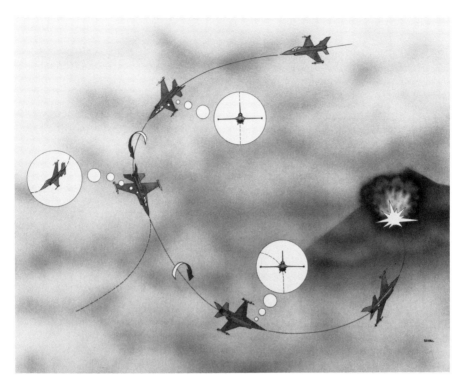

Fig. 11–28. The graveyard spiral. The pilot in a banked turn loses the sensation of being banked and turning. Upon trying to reestablish a wings-level attitude and stop the turn, he perceives that he is banked and turning in the opposite direction from his original banked turn, that is, he experiences a somatogyral illusion. Unable to tolerate the sensation that he is making an inappropriate control input, the pilot banks back into the original turn.

his unperceived banked turn, he will continue to descend in an ever-tightening spiral toward the ground, hence the name graveyard spiral.

Oculogyral Illusion

Whereas a somatogyral illusion is a false sensation, or lack of sensation, of self-rotation in a subject undergoing unusual angular motion, an oculogyral illusion is a false sensation of motion of an object viewed by such a subject. For example, if a vehicle with a subject inside is rotating about a vertical axis at a constant velocity and suddenly stops rotating, the subject experiences not only a somatogyral illusion of himself rotating in the opposite direction, but also an oculogyral illusion of an object in front of him moving in the opposite direction. Thus, a somewhat oversimplified definition of the oculogyral

illusion is that it is the visual correlate of the somatogyral illusion; however, its low threshold and lack of total correpondence with presumed cupular deviation suggest a more complex mechanism. The attempt to maintain visual fixation during a vestibulo-ocular reflex elicited by angular acceleration is probably at least partially responsible for the oculogyral illusion. (A similar mechanism underlies the illusory movement of the moon when one tries to fixate it visually while the relative movement of surrounding clouds is eliciting an optokinetic tracking reflex.) In an aircraft during flight at night or in weather, an oculogyral illusion generally confirms a somatogyral illusion: the pilot who falsely perceives that he is turning in a particular direction also observes his instrument panel to be moving in the same direction.

Coriolis Illusion

The vestibular Coriolis effect, also called the Coriolis cross-coupling effect, vestibular cross-coupling effect, or simply the Coriolis illusion, is another false percept that can result from unusual stimulation of the semicircular duct system. To illustrate this phenomenon, let us consider a subject who has been rotating in the plane of his horizontal semicircular ducts (roughly the yaw plane) long enough for the endolymph in those ducts to attain the same angular velocity as his head: the cupulae in the ampullae of his horizontal ducts have returned to their resting positions, and the sensation of rotation has ceased (Fig. 11–29a). If the subject then nods his head forward in the pitch plane, let's say a full 90° for the sake of simplicity, he is completely removing his horizontal semicircular ducts from the plane of rotation and inserting his two sets of vertical semicircular ducts into the plane of rotation (Fig. 11–29b). Although the angular momentum of the subject's rotating head is forcibly transferred at once out of the old plane of rotation relative to his head, the angular momentum of the endolymph in the horizontal duct is dissipated more gradually. The torque resulting from the

continuing rotation of the endolymph causes the cupulae in the horizontal ducts to be deviated, and a sensation of angular motion occurs in the new plane of the horizontal ducts—now the roll plane relative to the subject's body. Simultaneously, the endolymph in the two sets of vertical semicircular ducts must acquire angular momentum because these ducts have been brought into the plane of constant rotation. The torque required to impart this change in momentum causes deflection of the cupulae in the ampullae of these ducts, and a sensation of angular motion in this plane—the yaw plane relative to the subject's body—results. The combined effect of the cupular deflection in all three sets of semicircular ducts is that of a suddenly imposed angular velocity in a plane in which no actual angular acceleration relative to the subject has occurred. In the example given, if the original constant-velocity yaw is to the right and the subject pitches his head forward, the resulting Coriolis illusion experienced is that he and his immediate surroundings are suddenly rolling to the right and yawing to the right.

A particular perceptual phenomenon experienced occasionally by pilots of relatively high-performance aircraft during instrument flight has been attributed to the Coriolis illusion because it occurs in conjunction with large movements of the head under conditions of prolonged constant angular velocity. It consists of a convincing sensation of rolling and/or pitching that appears suddenly after the pilot diverts his attention from the instruments in front of him and moves his head to view some switches or displays elsewhere in the cockpit. This illusion is especially deadly because it is most likely to occur during an instrument approach, a phase of flight in which altitude is being lost rapidly and cockpit chores (e.g., radio frequency changes) repeatedly require the pilot to break up his instrument crosscheck. Whether the sustained angular ve-

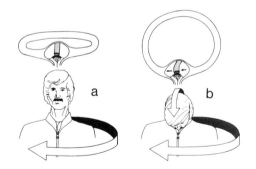

Fig. 11–29. Mechanism of the Coriolis illusion. A subject rotating in the yaw plane long enough for endolymph to stabilize in semicircular duct *(a)* pitches his head forward *(b)*. Angular momentum of endolymph deviates the cupula, causing the subject to perceive rotation in the new plane of the semicircular duct, even though no actual rotation occurred in that plane. The total Coriolis illusion is the combined effect of such stimulation on all six semicircular ducts.

locities associated with instrument flying are sufficient to create Coriolis illusions of any great magnitude is debatable, however, and another mechanism (the G-excess effect) has been proposed to explain the illusory rotations experienced with head movements in flight. Even if not responsible for spatial disorientation in flight, the Coriolis illusion is useful as a tool to demonstrate the fallibility of our nonvisual orientation senses. Nearly every military pilot living today has experienced the Coriolis illusion in the Barany chair or some other rotating device as part of his physiological training, and for most of these pilots it was then that they first realized their own orientation senses really cannot be trusted—the most important lesson of all for instrument flying.

The otolith organs are responsible for a set of illusions known as somatogravic illusions. The mechanism of illusions of this type involves the displacement of otolithic membranes on their maculae by inertial forces in such a way as to signal a false orientation when the resultant gravitoinertial force is perceived as gravitational (and therefore vertical). The most common example of the somatogravic illusions, the illusion of pitching up after taking off into conditions of reduced visibility, is perhaps the best illustration of this mechanism. Consider the pilot of a high-performance aircraft holding his position at the end of the runway waiting to take off. Here, the only force acting on his otolithic membranes is the force of gravity, and the positions of those membranes on their maculae signal accurately that down is toward the floor of the aircraft. Suppose the aircraft now accelerates down the runway, rotates, takes off, cleans up gear and flaps, and maintains a forward acceleration of 1 g until reaching the desired climb speed. The 1 G of inertial force resulting from the acceleration displaces the otolithic membranes toward the back of the pilot's head. In fact, the new positions of the otolithic membranes are nearly the same as they would be if the aircraft and pilot had pitched up 45°, because the new direction of the resultant gravitoinertial force vector, if one neglects the angle of attack and climb angle, is 45° aft relative to the gravitational vertical (Fig. 11–30). Naturally, the pilot's percept of pitch attitude based on the information from his otolith organs is one of having pitched up 45°; and the information from his nonvestibular proprioceptive and cutaneous mechanoreceptive senses supports this false percept, because the sense organs subserving those modalities also respond to the direction and intensity of the resultant gravitoinertial force. Given the very strong sensation of a nose-high pitch attitude, one that is not challenged effectively by the focal visual orientation cues provided by the attitude indicator, the pilot is tempted to push the nose of the aircraft down to cancel the unwanted sensation of flying nose-high. Pilots succumbing to this temptation characteristically crash in a nose-low attitude a few miles beyond the end of the runway. Sometimes, however, they are seen to descend out of the overcast nose-low and try belatedly to pull up, as though they suddenly regained the correct orientation upon seeing the ground again. Pilots of carrier-launched aircraft need to be especially wary of the somatogravic illusion. These pilots experience pulse accelerations lasting 2 to 4 seconds and generating peak inertial forces of +3 to +5 G_x. Although the major acceleration is over quickly, the resulting illusion of nose-high pitch can persist for half a minute or more afterward, resulting in a particularly hazardous situation for the pilot who is unaware of this phenomenon.[12]

Do not be misled by the above example into believing that only pilots of high-performance aircraft suffer the somatogravic illusion of pitching up after takeoff. More than a dozen air transport aircraft are believed to have crashed as a result of the somatogravic illusion occurring on takeoff.[13] A relatively slow aircraft, accelerat-

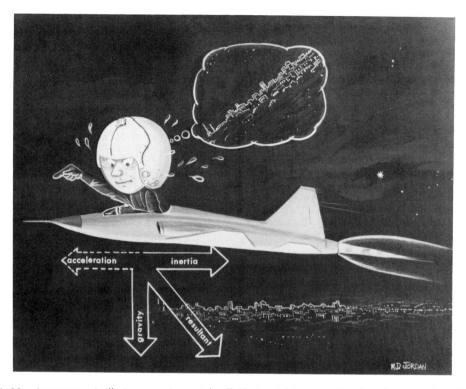

Fig. 11–30. A somatogravic illusion occurring on takeoff. The inertial force resulting from the forward acceleration combines with the force of gravity to create a resultant gravitoinertial force directed down and aft. The pilot, perceiving down to be in the direction of the resultant gravitoinertial force, feels he is in an excessively nose-high attitude and is tempted to push the stick forward to correct the illusory nose-high attitude.

ing from 100 to 130 knots over a 10-second period just after takeoff, generates $+0.16$ G_x on the pilot. Although the resultant gravitoinertial force is only 1.01 G, barely perceptibly more than the force of gravity, it is directed 9° aft, signifying to the unwary pilot a 9° nose-up pitch attitude. Because many slower aircraft climb out at 6° or less, a 9° downward pitch correction would put such an aircraft into a descent of 3° or more—the same as a normal final-approach slope. In the absence of a distinct external visual horizon or, even worse, in the presence of a false visual horizon (e.g., a shoreline) receding under the aircraft and reinforcing the vestibular illusion, the pilot's temptation to push the nose down can be overwhelming. This type of mishap has happened at one particular civil airport so often that a notice has been placed on navigational charts cautioning pilots

flying from this airport to be aware of the potential for loss of attitude reference.

Although the classic graveyard spiral was indicated earlier to be a consequence of the pilot's suffering a somatogyral illusion, it also can be said to result from a somatogravic illusion. A pilot who is flying "by the seat of his pants" applies the necessary control inputs to create a resultant G-force vector having the same magnitude and direction as that which his desired flight path would create. Unfortunately, any particular G vector is not unique to one particular condition of aircraft attitude and motion, and the likelihood that the G vector created by a pilot flying in this mode corresponds for more than a few seconds to the flight condition desired is remote indeed. Specifically, once an aircraft has departed a desired wings-level attitude because of an unperceived roll, and the pilot does not correct the resulting bank, the only way he can create a G vector that matches the G vector of the straight and level condition is with a descending spiral. In this condition, as is always the case in a coordinated turn, the centrifugal force resulting from the turn provides a G_y force that cancels the G_y component of the force of gravity that exists when the aircraft is banked. In addition, the tangential linear acceleration associated with the increasing airspeed resulting from the dive provides a $+G_x$ force that cancels the $-G_x$ component of the gravity vector that exists when the nose of the aircraft is pointed downward. Although the vector analysis of the forces involved in the graveyard spiral is somewhat complicated, a skillful pilot can easily manipulate the stick and rudder pedals to cancel all vestibular and other nonvisual sensory indications that his aircraft is turning and diving. In one mishap involving a dark-night takeoff of a commercial airliner, the recorded flight data indicate that the resultant G force which the pilot created by his control inputs allowed him to perceive his desired 10 to 12° climb angle and a net G force between 0.9 and 1.1 G for virtually the whole flight, even though he actually levelled off and then descended in an accelerating spiral until the aircraft crashed nearly inverted.

Inversion Illusion

The inversion illusion is a type of somatogravic illusion in which the resultant gravitoinertial force vector actually rotates backward so far as to be pointing away from rather than toward the earth's surface, thus giving the pilot the false sensation that he is upside down. Figure 11–31 shows how this can happen.[14] Typically, a steeply climbing high-performance aircraft levels off more or less abruptly at the desired altitude. This maneuver subjects the aircraft and pilot to a $-G_z$ centrifugal force resulting from the arc flown just prior to level-off. Simulta-

neously, as the aircraft changes to a more level attitude, airspeed picks up rapidly, adding a $+G_x$ tangential inertial force to the overall force environment. Adding the $-G_z$ centrifugal force and the $+G_x$ tangential force to the 1-G gravitational force results in a net gravitoinertial force vector that rotates backward and upward relative to the pilot. This stimulates the pilot's otolith organs in a manner similar to the way a pitch upward into an inverted position would. Even though the semicircular ducts should respond to the actual pitch downward, for some reason this conflict is resolved in favor of the otolith-organ information, perhaps because the semicircular-duct response is transient while the otolith-organ response persists, or perhaps because the information from the nonvestibular proprioceptors and other mechanoreceptors reinforces the information from the otolith organs. The pilot who responds to the inversion illusion by pushing forward on the stick to counter the perceived pitching up and over backward only prolongs the illusion by creating more $-G_z$ and $+G_x$ forces, thus aggravating his situation. Turbulent weather usually contributes to the development of the illusion; certainly, downdrafts are a source of $-G_z$ forces that can add to the net gravitoinertial force producing the inversion illusion. Again, do not assume one must be flying a jet fighter to experience this illusion. Several reports of the inversion illusion involve crews of large airliners who lost control of their aircraft because the pilot lowered the nose inappropriately after experiencing the illusion. Jet upset is the name, however, for the sequence of events that includes instrument weather, turbulence, the inability of the pilot to read his instruments, the inversion illusion, a pitch-down control input, and difficulty recovering the aircraft because of resulting aerodynamic or mechanical forces.[15]

The G-excess illusion also can be considered a form of somatogravic illusion, because it involves an abnormal magni-

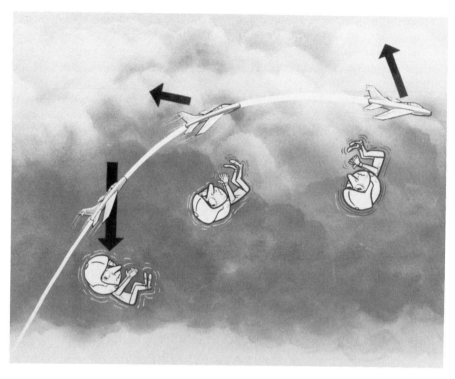

Fig. 11–31. The inversion illusion. Centrifugal and tangential inertial forces during a level-off combine with the force of gravity to produce a resultant gravitoinertial force that rotates backward and upward with respect to the pilot, causing him to perceive that he is suddenly upside down. Turbulent weather can produce additional inertial forces that contribute to the illusion. (Adapted from Martin, J.F., and Jones, G.M.: Theoretical man-machine interaction which might lead to loss of aircraft control. Aerospace Med., 36:713–716, 1965.)

tude and/or direction of applied gravito-inertial force that results in false perception of body position, and the perceptual response can be determined at least qualitatively by a simple mechanical analysis (Fig. 11–32). Let us assume that a subject is sitting upright in a $+1\ G_z$ environment and tips his head forward 30°. As a result of this change in head position, the subject's otolithic membranes slide forward the appropriate amount for a 30° tilt relative to vertical, say a distance of x μm. Now suppose that the same subject is sitting upright in a $+2\ G_z$ environment and again tips his head 30° forward. This time, the subject's otolithic membranes slide forward more than x μm because of the doubled gravitoinertial force acting on them. The displacement of the otolithic membranes, however, now corresponds not to a 30° forward tilt in the normal 1-

G environment but to a much greater tilt, theoretically as much as 90° (2 sin 30° = sin 90°). The subject had initiated only a 30° head tilt, however, and expects to perceive no more than that. The unexpected additional perceived tilt is thus referred to the immediate environment; that is, the subject perceives his vehicle, if he is in one, to have tilted by the amount equal to the difference between his actual and expected percepts of tilt. In a high-performance aircraft, the G-excess illusion can occur as a result of the moderate amount of G force pulled in a turn—a penetration turn or procedure turn, for example. If the pilot has to look down and to the side to select a new radio frequency or to pick up a dropped pencil while in a turn, he should experience an uncommanded tilt in both the pitch and roll planes due to the G-excess illusion. As noted previ-

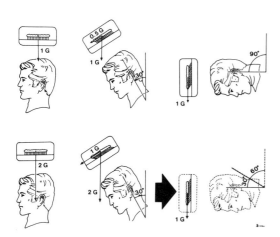

Fig. 11–32. Mechanism of the G-excess illusion. The subject in a 1-G environment (upper half of figure) experiences the result of a 0.5-G pull on his utricular otolithic membranes when he tilts his head 30° off the vertical, and the result of a 1-G pull when he tilts his head a full 90°. The subject in a 2-G environment (lower half of figure) experiences the result of a 1-G pull when he tilts his head only 30°. The illusory excess tilt perceived by the subject is attributed to external forces (lower right).

ously, the G-excess illusion may be responsible for the false sensation of pitch and/or roll generally attributed to the Coriolis illusion under such circumstances.

Oculogravic Illusion

Another illusion of otolith-organ origin, but not classified as a somatogravic illusion because it involves a visual perceptual effect, is the oculogravic illusion. The oculogravic illusion can be thought of as a visual correlate of the somatogravic illusion and occurs under the same stimulus conditions. A pilot who is subjected to the deceleration resulting from the application of speed brakes, for example, experiences a nose-down pitch because of the somatogravic illusion. Simultaneously, he observes the instrument panel in front of him to move downward, confirming his sensation of tilting forward. The oculogravic illusion is thus the visually apparent movement of an object that is actually in a fixed position relative to the subject during changing magnitude and/or direction of the net gravitoinertial force.

Like the oculogyral illusion, the oculogravic illusion probably results from the attempt to maintain visual fixation during a vestibulo-ocular reflex, elicited in this case by the change in magnitude or direction of the applied G vector rather than by angular acceleration.

The elevator illusion is a special type of oculogravic illusion that results from an increase or decrease in the magnitude of the $+G_z$ force acting on a subject. When an individual is accelerated upward, as in an elevator, the increase in $+G_z$ force elicits a vestibulo-ocular reflex of otolith-organ origin (the elevator reflex) that drives the eyes downward. Attempting to stabilize visually the objects in a fixed position relative to the observer causes those objects to appear to shift upward when the G force is increased. The opposite effect occurs when the individual is accelerated downward; the reduction in the magnitude of the net gravitoinertial force to less than $+1\ G_z$ causes a reflex upward shift of the direction of gaze, and the immediate surroundings appear to shift downward. (The latter effect also has been called the oculoagravic illusion because of its occurrence during transient weightlessness.) The importance of the elevator illusion in aviation is not well documented. In one tragic mishap, however, it was probably experienced by the pilot of a military transport aircraft who became disoriented shortly after leveling off abruptly from a prolonged steady descent on a dark night over desert terrain. The transient increase in $+G_z$ force that occurred as the pilot leveled off at pattern altitude most likely provoked the elevator illusion, and seeing his instrument panel rise, the pilot compensated by pitching downward during the subsequent fatal turn to final approach. It is also assumed that updrafts and downdrafts produce elevator illusions in pilots penetrating turbulent weather (Fig. 11–33).

The Leans

By far the most common vestibular illusion in flight is the leans. Virtually every

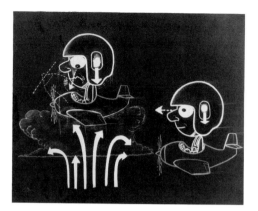

Fig. 11–33. Elevator illusion resulting from an updraft. In this type of oculogravic illusion, the increase in $+G_z$ force elicits a vestibulo-ocular reflex of otolith-organ origin which, when visual fixation is attempted, results in a falsely perceived upward motion of the object fixated—the instrument panel in the example shown.

instrument-rated pilot has had or will get the leans in one form or another at some time during his flying career. The leans consists of a false percept of angular displacement about the roll axis, that is, is an illusion of bank, and is frequently associated with an attempt by the pilot to compensate for the illusion by leaning in the direction of the falsely perceived vertical (Fig. 11–34). The usual explanations of the leans invoke the known deficiencies of both otolith-organ and semicircular-duct sensory mechanisms. As indicated previously, the otolith-organs are not reliable sources of information about the exact direction of the true vertical because they respond to the resultant gravitoinertial force, not to gravity alone. Furthermore, other sensory inputs can sometimes override otolith-organ cues and result in false perception of the vertical, even when the gravitoinertial force experienced is truly vertical. The semicircular ducts can provide such false inputs in flight by responding accurately to some roll stimuli but not responding at all to others because they are below threshold. If, for example, a pilot is subjected to an angular acceleration in roll so that the product of the acceleration and its time of application does

not reach some threshold value, say 3 degrees/sec, he does not perceive the roll. Suppose that this pilot, who is trying to fly straight and level, is subjected to an unrecognized and uncorrected 2-degree/sec roll for 10 seconds: a 20° bank results. If the pilot suddenly notices the unwanted bank and corrects it by rolling the aircraft back upright with a suprathreshold roll rate, say 15 degrees/sec, he experiences only half of the actual roll motion that took place, the half resulting from the correcting roll. As he started from a wings-level position, he is left with the illusion of having rolled into a 20° bank in the direction of the correcting roll, even though he is again wings-level. At this point, he has the leans; and even though he may be able to fly the aircraft properly by the deliberate and difficult process of forcing the attitude indicator to read correctly, his illusion can last for many minutes, seriously degrading his flying efficiency during that time.

Interestingly, pilots frequently get the leans after prolonged turning maneuvers and not because of alternating subthreshold and suprathreshold angular motion stimuli. In a holding pattern, for example, the pilot rolls into a 3-degree/sec standard-rate turn, holds the turn for 1 minute, rolls out and flies straight and level for 1 minute, turns again for 1 minute, and so on until traffic conditions permit him to proceed toward his destination. During the turning segments, the pilot initially feels the roll into the turn and accurately perceives the banked attitude. But as the turn continues, his percept of being in a banked turn dissipates and is replaced by a feeling of flying straight and level, both because the sensation of turning is lost when the endolymph comes up to speed in the semicircular ducts (somatogyral illusion) and because the net G force being directed toward the floor of the aircraft provides a false cue of verticality (somatogravic illusion). Then when the pilot rolls out of the turn, he feels he has rolled into a banked turn in the opposite direction.

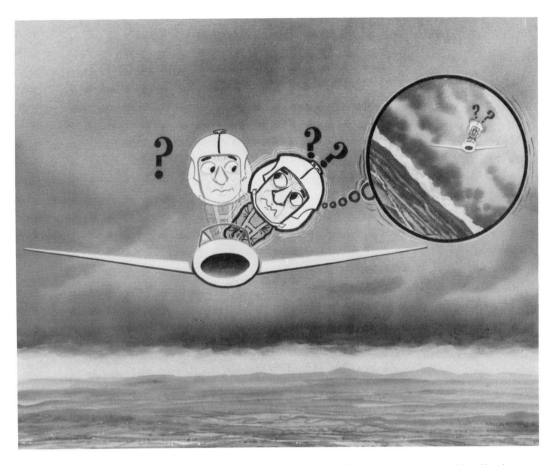

Fig. 11–34. The leans, the most common of all vestibular illusions in flight. Falsely perceiving himself to be in a right bank, but flying the aircraft straight and level by means of the flight instruments, this pilot is leaning to the left in an attempt to assume an upright posture compatible with his illusion of bank.

With experience, a pilot learns to suppress this false sensation quickly by paying strict attention to the attitude indicator. Sometimes, however, the pilot finds he cannot dispel the illusion of banking— usually when he is particularly busy, unfortunately. The leans also can be caused by misleading peripheral visual orientation cues, as mentioned in the section entitled "Visual Illusions." Roll angular vection is particularly effective in this regard, at least in the laboratory. One thing about the leans is apparent: there is no single explanation for this illusion. The deficiencies of several orientation-sensing systems in some cases reinforce each other to create an illusion; in other cases, the inac-

curate information from one sensory modality for some reason is selected over the accurate information from others to create the illusion. Stories have surfaced of pilots suddenly experiencing the leans for no apparent reason at all or even of experiencing it voluntarily by imagining the earth to be in a different direction from the aircraft. The point is that one must not think that the leans, or any other illusion for that matter, occurs as a totally predictable response to a physical stimulus: there is much more to perception than stimulation of the end-organs.

Disorientation in Flight

An orientational illusion has been defined as a false percept of position, attitude, or motion, relative to the plane of the earth's surface. Spatial disorientation and the equivalent term, pilot vertigo, are usually taken to mean the experiencing of an orientational illusion in flight. There is a major qualitative difference, however, between simply experiencing an orientational illusion and having to control an aircraft under conditions of misperceived or conflicting orientation cues. Furthermore, this difference becomes very important in the analysis of mechanisms involved in aircraft mishaps due to orientational illusions, and in the development of training aids for educating pilots about the potential for loss of aircraft control while under the influence of orientational illusions. For those reasons, it is necessary to restrict the use of the term spatial disorientation to the condition wherein one not only has an orientational illusion but also needs to have correct perception of orientation for controlling his position, attitude, or motion. When an individual has an orientational illusion but has no need for correct information about his orientation, he is said to have spatial unorientation. This distinction is exemplified by the contrast between the experience of a pilot, who must fly his vehicle on a desired path through space by responding to available orientation cues (and to whom such cues are, therefore, highly relevant), and the experience of an airborne communications monitor, who can perform his duty regardless of his spatial orientation (and to whom orientation cues, whether true or false, are essentially irrelevant). Obviously, it is spatial disorientation, not spatial unorientation, that causes aircraft mishaps and warrants investigative and educational efforts to prevent it.

It is also useful to make the distinction between unrecognized (type I) and recognized (type II) spatial disorientation. As the term implies, unrecognized spatial disorientation refers to the situation in which a pilot, oblivious to the fact that he is disoriented, controls his vehicle completely in accord with and in response to his false orientational percept. In recognized spatial disorientation, the pilot realizes something is wrong with his ability to fly the vehicle, but he may or may not actually realize that the source of his problem is spatial disorientation. Even further out in the spectrum of types of disorientation is the situation in which the pilot not only recognizes that he cannot control his vehicle effectively because of spatial disorientation, but he also cannot obtain correct orientation information because the violence of the motion imposed is blurring his vision with counterproductive vestibulo-ocular reflexes (nystagmus). For want of an adequately descriptive simple term, this type of disorientation is called vestibulo-ocular disorganization, or type III spatial disorientation.

Examples of Disorientation

The last of four F-15 Eagle fighter aircraft took off on a daytime sortie in bad weather, intending to follow the other three in a radar in-trail departure. Because of a navigational error committed by the pilot shortly after takeoff, he was unable to find the other aircraft on his radar. Frustrated, the pilot elected to intercept the other aircraft where he knew they would be in the arc of the standard instrument departure, so he made a beeline for that point, presumably scanning his radar diligently for the blips he knew should be appearing at any time. Meanwhile, after ascending to 1200 m above ground level, he entered a descent of approximately 700 m/min as a result of an unrecognized 3° nose-low attitude. After receiving requested position information from another member of the flight, the pilot either suddenly realized he was in danger of colliding with the other aircraft or he suddenly found them on radar because he then made a steeply banked turn, either to avoid a perceived threat of collision or to join up with the rest of the flight. Unfortunately, he had by this time descended far below the other aircraft and was going too fast to avoid the ground, which became visible under the overcast just before the aircraft crashed. This mishap resulted from an episode of unrecognized, or type I, disorientation. The specific illusion responsible appears to have been the somatogravic illusion, which was created by the forward acceleration of this high-performance aircraft during takeoff and climb-out. The pilot's preoccupation with the radar task compromised his instrument scan to the point where the false vestibular cues were able to penetrate his orientational information processing. Having unknowingly accepted an inaccurate orientational percept, he controlled the aircraft accordingly until it was too late to recover.

Examples of recognized, or type II, spatial disorientation are easier to obtain than are examples of type I because most experienced pilots have anecdotes to tell about how they "got vertigo" and fought it off. Some pilots were not so fortunate, however. One F-15 Eagle pilot, after climbing in his aircraft in formation with another F-15 at night, began to experience difficulty in maintaining spatial orientation and aircraft control upon leveling off in clouds at 8,200 m. "Talk about practice bleeding," he commented to the lead pilot. Having decided to go to another area because of the weather, the two pilots began a descending right turn. At this point, the pilot on the wing told the lead pilot, "I'm flying upside down." Shortly afterward, the wingman considered separating from the formation, saying, "I'm going lost wingman." Then he said, "No, I've got you," and finally, "No, I'm going lost wingman." The hapless aircraft then descended in a wide spiral, crashing into the desert less than a minute later, even though the lead pilot advised the wingman several times during the descent to level out. In this mishap, the pilot probably suffered an inversion illusion upon leveling off in the weather, and entered a graveyard

spiral after leaving the formation. Although he knew he was disoriented, or at least recognized the possibility, he still was unable to control the aircraft effectively. That a pilot can realize he is disoriented, see accurate orientation information displayed on the attitude indicator, and still fly into the ground always strains the credulity of nonaviators. Pilots who have had spatial disorientation, who have experienced fighting oneself for control of an aircraft, are less skeptical.

The pilot of an F-15 Eagle, engaged in vigorous air combat tactics training with two other F-15s on a clear day, initiated a hard left turn at 5200 m above ground level. For reasons that have not been established with certainty, his aircraft began to roll to the left at a rate estimated at 150 to 180 degrees/sec. He transmitted, "Out-of-control autoroll," as he descended through 5000 m. The pilot made at least one successful attempt to stop the roll, as evidenced by the momentary cessation of the roll at 2400 m; then the aircraft began to roll again to the left. Forty seconds elapsed between the time that the rolling began and the time that the pilot ejected—but too late. Regardless of whether the rolling was caused by a mechanical malfunction or was induced by the pilot himself, the certain result of this extreme motion was vestibulo-ocular disorganization, which not only prevented the pilot from reading his instruments but also kept him from orienting with the natural horizon. Thus, type III disorientation probably prevented him from taking appropriate corrective action to stop the roll and keep it stopped; if not that, it certainly compromised his ability to assess accurately the level to which his situation had deteriorated.

Statistics

Despite continuing efforts to educate pilots about spatial disorientation and the real hazard it represents, the fraction of aircraft mishaps caused by or contributed to by spatial disorientation has remained fairly constant over the three decades between 1950 and 1980. A number of statistical studies of spatial disorientation mishaps bear this out for the United States Air Force. In 1956, Nuttall and Sanford[16] reported that, in one major air command during the period of 1954 to 1956, spatial disorientation was responsible for 4% of all major aircraft mishaps and 14% of all fatal aircraft mishaps. In 1969, Moser[17] reported a study of aircraft mishaps in another major air command during the 4-year period from 1964 to 1967: he found that spatial disorientation was a significant factor in 9% of major mishaps and 26% of fatal mishaps. In 1971, Barnum and Bonner[18] reviewed the Air Force mishap data from 1958 through 1968 and found that in 281, or 6%, of the 4679 major mishaps, spatial disorientation was a causative factor; fatalities occurred in 211 of those 281 accidents, accounting for 15% of the 1462 fatal mishaps. A comment by Barnum and Bonner summarizes some interesting data about the "average pilot" involved in a spatial disorientation mishap: "He will be around 30 years of age, have 10 years in the cockpit, and have 1500 hours of first pilot/instructor-pilot time. He will be a fighter pilot and will have flown approximately 25 times in the three months prior to his accident." Barnum[19] next analyzed the mishap data for the 3-year period from 1969 to 1971 and concluded that spatial disorientation mishaps again accounted for 6% of major mishaps, but only for 10% of fatal mishaps during this period. In an independent 1973 study, Kellogg[20] found the relative incidence of spatial disorientation mishaps in the years 1968 through 1972 to range from 4.8 to 6.2% and confirmed the high proportion of fatalities in mishaps resulting from spatial disorientation. In 1980, Gillingham and Page (unpublished data) reviewed the Air Force aircraft mishaps of 1979 and determined that at least 9 of the 94 major mishaps (9.6%) and 9 of the 49 fatal mishaps (18.4%) occurring that year would not have occurred had the pilots not been spatially disoriented at some time during the mishap sequence. The cost of the Air Force aircraft destroyed each year in disorientation mishaps until recently has been on the order of $20 million per year. In 1979, it was $40 million, and the figure continues to rise, mainly as a result of the rapidly rising cost of new military aircraft. Statistics on the incidence of disorientation-related aircraft mishaps in the United States Army and Navy (7.11 and 6.75% of total mishaps, respectively) are remarkably similar to those of the Air Force, even though the flying missions of the several military services are somewhat different.

Although statistics indicating the relative frequency of spatial disorientation mishaps in air-carrier operations are not readily available, it would be a serious mistake to conclude that there have been no air-carrier mishaps caused by spatial disorientation. Fourteen such mishaps occurring between 1950 and 1969 were reportedly due to somatogravic and visual illusions that resulted in the so-called "dark-night takeoff accident."[13] In addition, 26 commercial airliners were involved in jet-upset incidents or accidents during the same period.[15] Spatial disorientation also is a problem in general (nonmilitary, nonair-carrier) aviation. Kirkham and colleagues[21] reported in 1978 that although spatial disorientation is a cause or factor in only 2.5% of all general aviation aircraft accidents in the United States, it is the third most common cause of fatal general aviation accidents. Of the 4012 fatal general aviation mishaps occurring in the years 1970 through 1975, 627 (15.6%) involved spatial disorientation as a cause or factor. Furthermore, the contribution of spatial disorientation to the second most common cause of fatal general aviation accidents—continued visual flight rules (VFR) flight into adverse weather—is undoubtedly highly significant. Notably,

90% of general aviation mishaps in which disorientation is a cause or factor are fatal.

Dynamics of Spatial Orientation and Disorientation

It is naive to assume that a certain pattern of physical stimuli always elicits a particular veridical or illusory perceptual response. Certainly, when a pilot has a wide, clear view of the horizon, ambient vision supplies virtually all of his orientation information, and potentially misleading linear or angular acceleratory motion cues do not result in spatial disorientation (unless, of course, they are so violent as to cause vestibulo-ocular disorganization). When a pilot's vision is compromised by bad weather conditions, the same acceleratory motion cues can cause him to develop spatial disorientation, but he usually avoids it by referring to his aircraft instruments for orientation information. If the pilot is unskilled at interpreting the instruments or if the instruments fail, those misleading motion cues inevitably cause disorientation. Such is the character of visual dominance, the phenomenon in which one incorporates visual orientation information into his percept of spatial orientation to the exclusion of vestibular and nonvestibular proprioceptive, tactile, and other sensory cues. Visual dominance falls into two categories: the congenital type, in which ambient vision provides dominant orientation cues through natural neural connections and functions, and the acquired type, in which orientation cues are gleaned through focal vision and are integrated as a result of training and experience into an orientational percept. The functioning of the proficient instrument pilot illustrates acquired visual dominance: he has learned to decode with foveal vision the information on the attitude indicator and other flight instruments and to reconstruct that information into a concept of where he is, what he is doing, and where he is going, and he refers to that

concept when controlling his aircraft. This complex skill must be developed through training and maintained through practice, and it is the fragility of this acquired visual dominance that makes spatial disorientation such a hazard.

Vestibular Suppression

The term vestibular suppression often is used to denote the active process of visually overriding undesirable vestibular sensations or vestibulo-ocular reflexes. An example of this aspect of visual dominance is seen in well-trained figure skaters who, with much practice, learn to abolish the postrotatory dizziness and nystagmus that normally result from the high angular decelerations associated with suddenly stopping rapid spins on the ice. But even these individuals, when deprived of vision by eye closure or darkness, have the very dizziness and nystagmus we would expect to result from the acceleratory stimuli produced. In flight, the ability to suppress unwanted vestibular sensations and reflexes is developed with repeated exposure to the linear and angular accelerations of flight. As is the case with the figure skaters, however, the pilot's ability to prevent vestibular sensations and vestibulo-ocular reflexes is compromised when he is deprived of visual orientation cues—when he must look away from his attitude indicator to manipulate a radio frequency-selector knob, for instance.

Vestibular Opportunism

At this point, the concept of vestibular opportunism should be introduced. Vestibular opportunism means the propensity of the vestibular system to fill an orientation-information void swiftly and surely with vestibular information. When a pilot flying in instrument weather looks away from his artificial horizon for a mere few seconds, this is usually long enough for erroneous vestibular information to break through the pilot's defenses and become incorporated into his orientational percept. In fact, conflicts between focal visual and vestibular sources of orientation information tend to resolve themselves very quickly in favor of the vestibular information, without providing the pilot an opportunity to evaluate the information. It would seem that any orientation information reaching the vestibular nuclei—whether vestibular, other proprioceptive, or ambient visual—should have an advantage in competing with focal visual cues for expression as the pilot's sole orientational percept because the vestibular nuclei are primary terminals in the pathways for reflex orientational responses and are the initial level of integration for any eventual conscious concomitant of perception of spatial orientation. In other words, although acquired visual dominance can be maintained by diligent attention to artificial orientation cues, the challenge to this dominance presented by the processing of natural orientation cues through primitive neural channels is very potent and ever present.

The lack of adequate orientation cues and conflicts between competing sensory modalities are only a part of the whole picture of a disorientation mishap. Why so many disoriented pilots, even those who know they are disoriented, are unable to recover their aircraft has mystified aircraft accident investigators for decades. There are two possible explanations for this phenomenon. The first suggests that the psychologic stress of disorientation results in a disintegration of higher-order learned behavior, including flying skills. The second describes a complex psychomotor effect of disorientation that causes the pilot to feel the aircraft itself is misbehaving.

Disintegration of Flying Skill

The disintegration of flying skill perhaps begins with the pilot's realization that his spatial orientation and control over the motion of his aircraft have been compromised. Under such circumstances,

he pays more heed to whatever orientation information is naturally available, monitoring it more and more vigorously. Whether the brain stem reticular activating system or the vestibular efferent system or both are responsible for the resulting heightened arousal and enhanced vestibular information flow can only be surmised; the net effect, however, is that more erroneous vestibular information is processed and incorporated into the pilot's orientational percept. This, of course, makes matters only worse. A positive-feedback situation is thus encountered, and the vicious circle can now be broken only with a precisely directed and very determined effort by the pilot. Unfortunately, complex cognitive and motor skills tend to be degraded under conditions of psychologic stress such as occurs during type II or type III spatial disorientation. First, there is a coning of attention. Pilots who have survived severe disorientation have reported that they were concentrating on one particular flight instrument instead of scanning and interpreting the whole group of them in the usual manner. Pilots also have reported that they were unaware of radio transmissions to them while they were trying to recover from disorientation. Second, there is the tendency to revert to more primitive behavior, even reflex action, under conditions of severe psychologic stress. The highly developed, relatively newly acquired skill of instrument flying can give way to primal protective responses during disorientation stress, making appropriate recovery action unlikely. Third, it is often suggested that disoriented pilots become totally immobilized—frozen to the aircraft controls by fear or panic—as the disintegration process reaches its final state.

The giant hand phenomenon described by Malcolm and Money[15] undoubtedly explains why many pilots have been rendered hopelessly confused and ineffectual by spatial disorientation, even though they knew they were disoriented and should have been able to avoid losing control of their aircraft. The pilot suffering from this effect of disorientation perceives falsely that his aircraft is not responding properly to his control inputs because every time he tries to bring the aircraft to the desired attitude, it seems actively to resist his effort and fly back to another, more stable attitude. A pilot experiencing disorientation about the roll axis (e.g., the leans or graveyard spiral) may feel a force—like a giant hand—trying to push one wing down and hold it there, whereas the pilot with pitch-axis disorientation (e.g., the classic somatogravic illusion) may feel the airplane subjected to a similar force trying to hold the nose down. Pilots who are unaware of the existence of this phenomenon and experience it for the first time can be very surprised and confused by it, and may not be able to discern the exact nature of their problem. A pilot's radio transmission that the aircraft controls are malfunctioning should not, therefore, be taken as conclusive evidence that a control malfunction caused a mishap: spatial disorientation could have been the real cause.

Giant Hand Phenomenon

What mechanism could possibly explain the giant hand? To try to understand this phenomenon, we must first recognize that an individual's perception of orientation results not only in the conscious awareness of his position and motion but also in a preconscious percept needed for the proper performance of voluntary motor activity and reflex actions. A conscious orientational percept can be considered rational, in that one can subject it to intellectual scrutiny, weigh the evidence for its veracity, conclude that it is inaccurate, and to some extent modify the percept to fit facts obtained from other than the primary orientation senses. In contrast, a preconscious orientational percept must be considered irrational, in that it consists only of an integration of data relayed to the brain stem and cerebellum by the primary orientation senses and is not amenable to modification by reason. So what happens when a pilot knows he has become disoriented and tries to control his aircraft by reference to a conscious, rational percept of orientation that is at variance with his preconscious, irrational one? Because only the data comprising one's preconscious orientational percept are available for the performance of primitive orientational reflexes (e.g., vestibulo-ocular and postural reflexes), higher-order reflexes (e.g., aversive responses), and skilled voluntary motor activity (e.g., walking, running, bicycling, driving, flying), it is to be expected that the actual outcome of these types of actions will deviate from the rationally intended outcome whenever the orientational data on which they depend are different from the rationally perceived orientation. The disoriented pilot who consciously commands a roll to recover aircraft control may experience a great deal of difficulty in executing the command, because the informational substrate in reference to which his body functions indicates that such a move is counterproductive or even dangerous. Or he may discover that the roll, once accomplished, must be reaccomplished repeatedly as his body responds automatically to the preconsciously perceived orientational threat resulting from his conscious efforts and actions to regain control. Thus, the preconscious orientational percept influences Sherrington's "final common pathway" for both reflex and voluntary motor activity, and the manifestation of this influence on the act of flying during an episode of spatial disorientation is the giant hand phenomenon. To prevail in this conflict between his will and his skill, the pilot must decouple his voluntary acts from his previously learned flying behavior by accomplishing those motions that produce directly the desired readings of the flight instruments, rather than by flying the airplane to an attitude corresponding to the desired readings of the flight instruments.

The salient features of the dynamics of spatial orientation and disorientation are diagrammed in Figure 11–35; the concepts of visual dominance, vestibular suppression, vestibular opportunism, disintegration of flying skill, conscious and preconscious orientational percepts, and the giant hand phenomenon are presented therein as they relate to the overall scheme of orientation-information processing.

Conditions Conducive to Disorientation

From his knowledge of the physical bases of the various illusions of flight, the reader can readily infer many of the specific environmental factors conducive to spatial disorientation. Certain visual phenomena produce characteristic visual illusions such as false horizons, linear and angular vection, and autokinesis. Prolonged turning at a constant rate, as in a holding pattern or procedure turn, can precipitate somatogyral illusions or the leans, and Coriolis illusions conceivably can occur with head movements under these conditions. Relatively sustained linear accelerations, such as occur on takeoff, can produce somatogravic illusions, and head movements during G-pulling turns can elicit G-excess illusions.

But what are the regimes of flight and activities of the pilot that seem most likely to allow these potential illusions to manifest themselves? Certainly, instrument

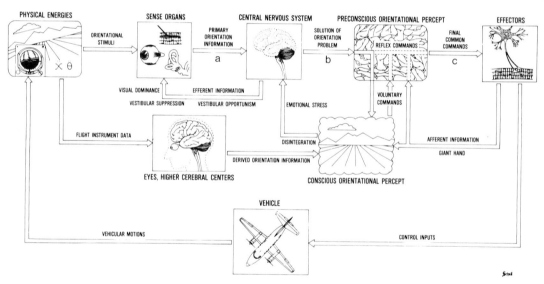

Fig. 11–35. Flow of orientation information in flight. The primary information flow loop involves stimulation of the visual, vestibular, and other orientation senses by visual scenes and linear and angular accelerations; processing of this primary orientation information by the brainstem, cerebellum, and lower cerebral centers; incorporating the solution into a data base for reflex and skilled voluntary motor activity (preconscious orientational percept); and effecting control inputs which produce aircraft motions that result in orientational stimuli. A secondary path of information flow involves the processing of largely numeric data from flight instruments into derived orientation information by higher cerebral centers. Subloop a provides for feedback between various components of the nervous system and includes efferent system influences on the sensory end-organs themselves. The phenomena of visual dominance, vestibular suppression, and vestibular opportunism occur in conjunction with the functioning of this loop. Subloop b generates the conscious perception of orientation, both from the body's naturally obtained solution of the orientation problem and from orientation information derived from flight instrument data. Voluntary control commands arise in response to conscious orientational percepts; and the psychic stress resulting from conflicting orientation information or from apparently aberrantly responding effectors can influence the manner in which orientation information is processed, leading ultimately to disintegration of flying skill. Subloop c incorporates feedback from the muscles, tendons, and joints involved in making control inputs and provides a basis for the giant hand phenomenon.

weather and night flying are primary factors. Especially likely to produce disorientation, however, is the practice of switching back and forth between the instrument flying mode and the visual, or contact, flying mode; a pilot is far less likely to become disoriented if he gets on the instruments as soon as out-of-cockpit vision is compromised and stays on the instruments until continuous contact flying is again assured. In fact, any event or practice requiring the pilot to break his instrument cross-check is conducive to disorientation. In this regard, avionics control switches and displays in some aircraft are located where the pilot must interrupt his instrument cross-check for more than just a few seconds to interact with them and are thus known (not so affectionately) as "vertigo traps." Some of these vertigo traps require substantial movements of the pilot's head during the time his cross-check is interrupted, thereby providing both a reason and an opportunity for spatial disorientation to strike.

Formation flying in adverse weather conditions is probably the most likely of all situations to produce disorientation; indeed, some experienced pilots get disoriented every time they fly wing or trail in weather. The fact that a pilot has little if any opportunity to scan his flight instruments while flying formation on his lead aircraft in weather means that he is essentially isolated from any source of accurate orientation information, and misleading vestibular and ambient visual cues arrive unchallenged into his sensorium.

Of utmost importance to a pilot in preventing spatial disorientation is competency and currency in instrument flying. A noninstrument-rated pilot who penetrates instrument weather is virtually assured of developing spatial disorientation within a matter of seconds, just as the most competent instrument pilot would develop it if he found himself flying in weather without functioning flight instruments. Regarding instrument flying skill,

one must "use it or lose it," as they say. For that reason, it is inadvisable and usually illegal for one to act as a pilot in command of an aircraft in instrument weather if he has not had a certain amount of recent instrument flying experience.

Finally, conditions affecting the pilot's physical or mental health must be considered capable of rendering the pilot more susceptible to spatial disorientation. The unhealthy effect of alcohol ingestion on neural information processing is one obvious example; however, the less well-known ability of alcohol to produce vestibular nystagmus (positional alcohol nystagmus) for many hours after its more overt effects have disappeared is probably of equal significance. Other drugs, such as barbiturates, amphetamines, and even the quinine in tonic water, are suspected of possibly having contributed to aircraft mishaps resulting from spatial disorientation. Likewise, physical and mental fatigue, as well as acute or chronic emotional stress, can rob the pilot of his ability to concentrate on his instrument cross-check and can, therefore, have deleterious effects on his resistance to spatial disorientation.

Prevention of Disorientation Mishaps

Spatial disorientation can be attacked in several ways. Theoretically, each link in the physiologic chain of events leading to a disorientation mishap can be broken by a specific countermeasure (Fig. 11–36). Many times, spatial disorientation can be prevented by modifying flying procedures to avoid those visual or vestibular motion and position stimuli that tend to create illusions in flight. Improving the capacity of flight instruments to translate aircraft position and motion information into readily assimilable orientation cues will help the pilot to avoid disorientation. Through repeated exposure to the environment of instrument flight, the pilot becomes proficient in instrument flying; this involves developing perceptual processes

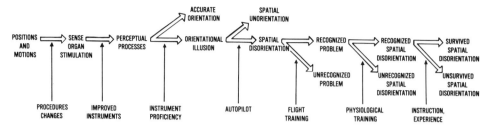

Fig. 11–36. The chain of events leading to a spatial disorientation mishap, and where the chain can be attacked and broken. From the left: Flight procedures can be altered to generate less confusing sensory inputs. Improved instrument presentations can aid in the assimilation of orientation cues. Proficiency in instrument flying helps to assure accurate orientational percepts. In the event the pilot suffers an orientational illusion, having the aircraft under autopilot control avoids disorientation by substituting unorientation. Proper flight training allows the disoriented pilot to recognize he is having a problem controlling his craft. Once he knows he is having a problem, the pilot's physiological training helps him realize that his problem is spatial disorientation. With appropriate instruction and/or firsthand experience, the pilot with recognized spatial disorientation can apply the correct control forces to recover the aircraft and survive the disorientation incident.

that result in accurate orientational percepts rather than orientational illusions. If a pilot who is experiencing an illusion can relinquish control of his aircraft to an autopilot, he can convert his situation from one of hazardous spatial disorientation to one of irrelevant spatial unorientation and reclaim control once the orientational illusion has subsided. Use of the autopilot, not only to help the pilot recover from disorientation, but also to help prevent the disorientation in the first place, has a considerable potential for saving lives, particularly in general aviation. If a pilot who has developed spatial disorientation can be made to recognize that he is disoriented, he is halfway along the road to recovery. Recognizing disorientation is not necessarily easy, however. First, the pilot must be aware that he is having a problem holding his altitude or heading; this he cannot do if he is concentrating on something other than the flight instruments—the radar scope, for instance. Only through proper flight training can the discipline of continuously performing the instrument cross-check be instilled. Second, the pilot must recognize that his difficulty in controlling the aircraft is a result of spatial disorientation. This ability is promoted through physiological training. It was just stated that the pilot who suspects he is disoriented is halfway down the road to

recovery: why not most of the way? Because a pilot's ability to cope with the effects of disorientation on his control inputs to the aircraft comes through effective flight instruction, proper physiological training, and experience in controlling his vehicle in an environment of conflicting orientation cues—his simply being aware that he is disoriented by no means ensures his survival.

Education and Training

Physiological training is the main weapon against spatial disorientation at the disposal of the flight surgeon and aerospace physiologist. This training ideally should consist of both didactic material and demonstrations. There is no paucity of didactic material on the subject of disorientation: at least eight films, two videocassette tapes, three slide sets, two handbooks, and numerous chapters in books and manuals have been prepared for the purpose of informing the pilot about the mechanisms and hazards of spatial disorientation. Although the efforts to generate information on spatial disorientation are commendable, there has been a tendency for the didactic material thus far produced to dwell too much on the mechanisms and effects of disorientation without giving much practical advice on how to deal with it. Money and Malcolm[22] noted that none of the available films on spatial disorientation gives sufficient emphasis on what the pilot should do when he suspects disorientation. Although several of the films recommend that the pilot believe his instruments, this message is too subdued and, by itself, is inadequate. Money and Malcolm argue that under some circumstances (e.g., panic) a pilot may in fact believe the instruments but continue to fly the aircraft according to his false orientational percept. If a pilot is told in addition, "Make the intruments read right, regardless of your sensation," he has simple, definite instructions on how to bring the aircraft under control when disorientation strikes. We strongly advise, therefore, that every presentation to pilots on the subject of spatial disorientation emphasize the need to make the instruments read right, as well as to believe them, when responding to disorientation stress.

The traditional demonstration accompanying lectures to pilots on spatial disorientation is a ride on a Barany chair or other smoothly rotating device. The subject, sitting in the device with his eyes closed, is accelerated to a constant angular velocity and asked to signal with his thumbs his perceived direction of turning. After a number of seconds (usually from 10 to 20) at constant angular velocity, the subject loses the sensation of rotation and signals this fact to the observers. The instructor then suddenly stops the rotation, whereupon the subject immediately indicates that he feels he is turning in the direction opposite to his original direction of rotation. The subject usually is asked to open his eyes during this part of the demonstation and is amazed to see that he is actually not turning, despite the strong vestibular sensation of rotation. After the described demonstration of somatogyral illusions, the subject is again rotated at a constant velocity with his eyes closed, this time with his head down (facing the floor). When the subject indicates his sensation of turning has ceased, he is asked to raise

his head abruptly so as to face the wall. The Coriolis illusion resulting from this maneuver is one of a very definite roll to one side: the startled subject may exhibit a protective postural reflex and may open his eyes to help him visually orient during his falsely perceived upset. The message delivered with these demonstrations is not that such illusions will be experienced in flight in the same manner, but that the vestibular sense can be fooled, that is, is unreliable, and that only the flight instruments provide accurate orientation information.

Over the years, at least a dozen different devices have been developed to augment or supplant the Barany chair for demonstrating various vestibular and visual illusions and the effects of disorientation in flight. These devices, collectively known as antivertigo trainers, fall into two basic categories: orientational illusion demonstrators and spatial disorientation demonstrators. The majority are illusion demonstrators, in which the subject rides passively and experiences one or more of the following: somatogyral, oculogyral, somatogravic, oculogravic, Coriolis, G-excess, vection, and autokinetic illusions. In an illusion demonstrator, the subject typically is asked to record or remember the magnitude and direction of the orientational illusion and then is told or otherwise allowed to experience his true orientation. A few antivertigo trainers are actually spatial disorientation demonstrators that allow the subject to experience the difficulty in controlling the attitude and motion of the trainer while being subjected to somatogravic, somatogyral, and/or Coriolis illusions. Figure 11-37 shows two antivertigo trainers presently in use. One must be aware that the name given to any particular antivertigo trainer does not necessarily describe its function: the United States Air Force School of Aerospace Medicine (USAFSAM) Spatial Disorientation Demonstrator, for example,

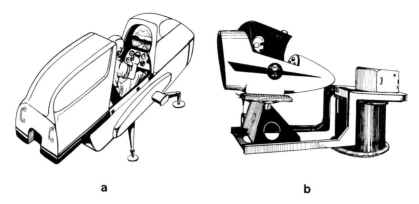

a   b

Fig. 11–37. Two types of antivertigo trainers currently in use. *a.* The Vertigon, an orientational illusion demonstrator, allows the subject to experience Coriolis and somatogyral illusions while performing tracking and dial-setting tasks. *b.* The Vertifuge, a spatial disorientation demonstrator, subjects the trainee to somatogravic, Coriolis, and somatogyral illusions that generate orientational conflicts as he tries to control the attitude and motion of the device by referring to true-reading flight instruments.

was actually an orientational illusion demonstrator.

Although the maximum use of antivertigo trainers in the physiological training of pilots is to be encouraged, it is important to recognize the great potential for misuse of such devices by personnel not thoroughly trained in their theory and function. Several antivertigo trainers have aircraft-instrument tracking tasks for the subject to perform while he is experiencing orientational illusions but is not actually controlling the motion of the trainer. The temptation is very strong for unsophisticated operating personnel to tell the subject he is "fighting disorientation" if he performs well on the tracking task while subjected to the illusion-generating motions. Because the subject's real orientation is irrelevant to the tracking task, any orientational illusion is also irrelevant, and he experiences no conflict between visual and vestibular information in acquiring cues on which to base his control responses. This situation, of course, does not capture the essence of disorientation in flight, and the trainee who is led to believe he is fighting disorientation in such a ground-based demonstration may develop a false sense of security about his ability to combat disorientation

in flight. The increasing use of spatial disorientation demonstrators in which the subject must control the actual motion of the trainer by referring to true-reading instruments while under the influence of orientational illusions will most likely reduce the potential for misuse and will improve the effectiveness of presentations to pilots on the subject of spatial disorientation.

Flight training provides a good opportunity to instruct pilots about the hazards of spatial disorientation. In-flight demonstrations of vestibular illusions are included in most formalized pilot training curricula, although the efficacy of such demonstrations is highly dependent on the motivation and skill of the individual flight instructor. Somatogyral and somatogravic illusions and illusions of roll attitude usually can be induced in a student pilot by a flight instructor who either understands how the vestibular system works or knows from experience which maneuvers consistently produce illusions. The vestibular-illusion demonstrations should not be confused with the unusual-attitude–recovery demonstrations in the typical pilot training syllabus: the objective of the former is for the student to experience orientational illusions and recognize them as such, whereas the objective of the latter is for the student to learn to regain control of an aircraft in a safe and expeditious manner. In both types of demonstration, however, control of the aircraft should be handed over to the student pilot with the instruction, "Make the instruments read right."

Part of flight training is continuing practice to maintain flying proficiency, and the importance of such practice in reducing the likelihood of having a disorientation mishap cannot be overemphasized. Whether flying on instruments, in formation, or engaged in aerobatic maneuvering, familiarity with the environment—based on recent exposure to it—and proficiency at the flying task—based on recent practice at it—result not only in a greater ability to avoid or dispel orientational illusions but also in a greater ability to cope with disorientation when it does occur.

In-Flight Procedures

If a particular in-flight procedure frequently results in spatial disorientation, it stands to reason that modifying or eliminating that procedure should help to reduce aircraft mishaps due to disorientation. Night formation takeoffs and rejoins are examples of in-flight procedures that are very frequently associated with spatial disorientation, and the United States Air Force wisely has officially discouraged these practices in most of its major commands.

Another area of concern is the "lost wingman" procedure, which is used when a pilot has lost sight of the aircraft on which he has been flying wing. Usually the loss of visual contact is due to poor visibility and occurs after a period of vacillation between formation flying and instrument flying; this, of course, invites disorientation. The lost wingman procedure must, therefore, be made as uncomplicated as possible while still allowing safe separation from the other elements of the flight. Maintaining a specified altitude

and heading away from the flight until further notice is an ideal lost wingman procedure in that it avoids frequent or prolonged disorientation-inducing turns and minimizes cognitive work load. Often, a pilot flying wing in bad weather does not lose sight of the lead aircraft but suffers so much disorientation stress as to make the option of going lost wingman seem safer than that of continuing in the formation. A common practice in this situation is for the wingman to take the lead position in the formation, at least until the disorientation disappears. This avoids the necessity of having the disoriented pilot make a turn away from the flight to go lost wingman, a turn that could be especially difficult and dangerous because of his disorientation. One should question the wisdom of having a disoriented pilot leading a flight, however, and some experts in the field of spatial disorientation are adamantly opposed to this practice, with good reason.

The manner in which others communicate with the pilot who is disoriented can mean the difference between life and death for that pilot and his passengers. Unfortunately, no clear-cut procedure exists for ensuring appropriate communications. Should the pilot be hounded mercilessly with verbal orders to get on the instruments or should he be left relatively undistracted to solve his orientation problem? The extremes of harassment and neglect are definitely not appropriate; a few forceful, specific, action-oriented commands probably represent the best approach. "Level the artificial horizon!" and "Roll right 90°!" are examples of such commands. One must remember that the pilot suffering from spatial disorientation may be either so busy or so functionally compromised that friendly chit-chat or complex instructions may fall on deaf ears. Simple, emphatic directions may be the only means of penetrating the disoriented pilot's consciousness.

To illustrate how official recommendations regarding in-flight procedures are disseminated to pilots in an effort to prevent spatial disorientation mishaps, a message from a major United States Air Force command headquarters to field units is excerpted here:

"... Review SD procedures in [various Air Force manuals] ... Discuss the potential for SD during flight briefings prior to flight involving night, weather, or conditions where visibility is significantly reduced ... Recognize the [SD] problem early and initiate corrective actions before aircraft control is compromised.

A. Single ship:
   (1) Keep the head in the cockpit. Concentrate on flying basic instruments with frequent reference to the attitude indicator. Defer nonessential cockpit chores.
   (2) If symptoms persist, bring aircraft to straight and level flight using the attitude indicator. Maintain straight and level flight until symptoms abate—usually 30 to 60 seconds. Use autopilot if necessary.
   (3) If necessary, declare an emergency and advise air traffic control. Note: It is possible for SD to proceed to the point where the pilot is unable to see, interpret, or process information from the flight instruments. Aircraft control in such a situation is impossible. A pilot must recognize when physiological/psychological limits have been exceeded and be prepared to abandon the aircraft.

B. Formation flights:
   (1) Separate aircraft from the formation under controlled conditions if the weather encountered is either too dense or turbulent to insure safe flight.
   (2) A flight lead with SD will advise his wingmen that he has SD and he will comply with procedures in Paragraph A. If possible, wingmen should confirm straight and level attitude and provide verbal feedback to lead. If symptoms do not abate in a reasonable time, terminate the mission and recover the flight by the simplest and safest means possible.
   (3) Two-ship formation. Wingman will advise lead when he experiences significant SD symptoms.
      (a) Lead will advise wingman of aircraft attitude, altitude, heading, and airspeed.
      (b) The wingman will advise lead if problems persist. If so, lead will establish straight and level flight for at least 30 to 60 seconds.
      (c) If the above procedures are not ef-

fective, lead should transfer the flight lead position to the wingman *while in straight and level flight*. Once assuming lead, maintain straight and level flight for 60 seconds. If necessary, terminate the mission and recover by the simplest and safest means possible.
   (4) More than two-ship formation. Lead should separate the flight into elements to more effectively handle a wingman with persistent SD symptoms. Establish straight and level flight. The element with the SD pilot will remain straight and level while other element separates from the flight."

Cockpit Layout and Flight Instruments

One of the most notorious vertigo traps is the communications-transceiver frequency selector or transponder code selector located in an obscure part of the cockpit. To manipulate this selector requires the pilot not only to look away from his flight instruments, which interrupts his instrument scan, but also to tilt his head to view the readout, which potentially subjects him to Coriolis or G-excess illusions. Aircraft designers are now aware that easy accessibility and viewing of such frequently used devices minimize the potential for spatial disorientation; accordingly, most modern aircraft have communications frequency and transponder code selectors and readouts located in front of the pilot near the flight instruments.

The location of the flight instruments themselves is also very important. They should be clustered directly in front of the pilot, and the attitude indicator, the primary provider of orientation cueing and the primary instrument by which the aircraft is controlled, should be in the center of the cluster (Fig. 11–38). When this principle is not respected, the potential for spatial disorientation is increased. One modern fighter aircraft, for example, was designed to have the pilot sitting high in the cockpit to enhance his field of view during air-to-air combat in conditions of good visibility. This design relegates the attitude indicator to a position more or less

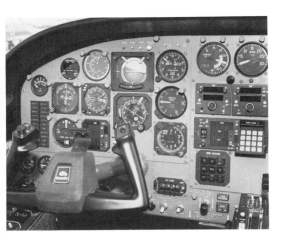

Fig. 11–38. A well-designed instrument panel, with the attitude indicator located directly in front of the pilot and the other flight instruments clustered around it. Radios and other equipment requiring frequent manipulation and viewing are placed close to the flight instruments to minimize interruption of the pilot's instrument scan and to obviate his having to make head movements that could precipitate spatial disorientation. (Photo courtesy of Gen-Aero Inc. of San Antonio, Texas.)

between the pilot's knees. As a result, at night and during instrument weather, the pilot is subjected to potentially disorienting peripheral visual motion and position cuing by virtue of his being surrounded by a vast expanse of canopy, while he tries to glean with central vision the correct orientation information from a relatively small, distant attitude indicator. The net effect is an unusually difficult orientation problem for the pilot, and a greater risk of developing spatial disorientation in this aircraft than in others with a more advantageously located attitude indicator.

A relatively new concept in flight instrumentation, the heads-up display (HUD), projects numeric and other symbolic information to the pilot from a combining glass near the windscreen, so that he can be looking forward out of the cockpit and simultaneously monitoring flight and weapons data. When the pilot selects the appropriate display mode, the pitch and roll attitude of the aircraft are observed on the "pitch ladder" (Fig. 11–39), and heading, altitude, airspeed, and other

parameters are numerically displayed elsewhere on the HUD. Its up-front location and its close-together arrangement of most of the required aircraft control and performance data make the HUD a possible improvement over the conventional cluster of instruments with regard to minimizing the likelihoood of spatial disorientation. Pilots' acceptance and use of the HUD for flying in instrument weather has not been universal, however. Many pilots prefer to use the HUD under conditions of good outside visibility and use the conventional instruments for flying at night and in weather. This preference may result from the fact that the horizon on the conventional instrument looks more like the natural horizon than does the zero-pitch indicator on the HUD pitch ladder.

The verisimilitude of the flight instruments is, in fact, a major factor in their ability to convey readily assimilable orientation information. The old "needle, ball, and airspeed" indicators (a needle pointer showing the direction and rate of turn, a ball showing whether the turn is being properly coordinated with the rudders, and an airspeed indicator showing whether the airplane is climbing or diving) required a lot of interpretation for the pilot to perceive his spatial orientation through them; nevertheless, this combination sufficed for nearly a generation of pilots. When the attitude indicator (also known as the gyro horizon, artificial horizon, or attitude gyro) was introduced, it greatly reduced the amount of work required to spatially orient during instrument flying because the pilot could readily imagine the artificial horizon line to be the real horizon. In addition to becoming more reliable and more versatile over the years, it became even easier to interpret: the face was divided into a gray or blue "sky" half and a black or brown "ground" half, with some models even having lines of perspective converging to a vanishing point in the lower half. Such a high degree of similarity to the real world has made the

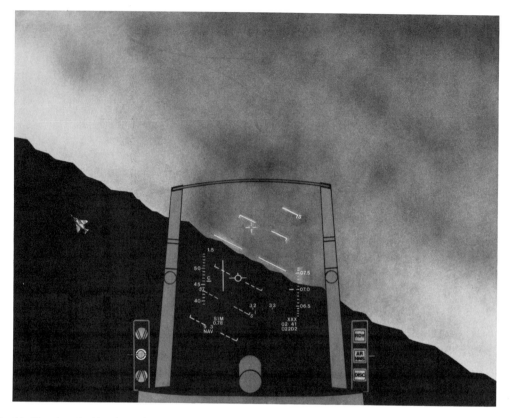

Fig. 11–39. A typical heads-up display (HUD). The pitch ladder in the center of the display provides pitch and roll attitude information.

attitude indicator the mainstay of instrument flying today.

As good as it may seem, the attitude indicator is not the perfect flight instrument for assuring spatial orientation. It suffers from the basic design deficiency of presenting visual spatial orientation information to the wrong sensory system—the focal visual system. Two untoward effects result. First, the pilot's focal vision not only must serve to discriminate numeric data from a number of instruments but also must take on the task of spatially orienting the pilot. Thus, the pilot has to employ his focal visual system in a somewhat inefficient manner during instrument flight, with about 70% of his time spent viewing the attitude indicator, while his ambient vision remains unutilized. Second, the fact that focal vision is not naturally

equipped to provide primary spatial orientation cues causes difficulty for pilots in interpreting the artificial horizon directly. There is a tendency, especially among novice pilots, to sense the displayed deviations in roll and pitch backward and to make initial roll and pitch corrections in the wrong direction. Several approaches have been taken to try to improve the efficiency of the pilot's acquisition of orientation information from the attitude indicator and associated flight instruments. One has been to make the artificial horizon stationary but to roll and pitch the small aircraft on the instrument to indicate the motion of the real aircraft. Theoretically, this configuration relieves the pilot of having to orient himself spatially before trying to fly his aircraft: he merely flies the small aircraft on his attitude instrument and the real aircraft follows. Another approach involves letting the artificial horizon provide pitch information but having the small aircraft on the attitude instrument provide roll information, and collocating heading, vertical velocity, airspeed, throttle setting, and navigation parameters with the aircraft attitude information on a 7-cm instrument face. Such an instrument is the Crane Alweather Flitegage (Fig. 11–40). Neither of these approaches, however, frees foveal vision from the unnatural task of processing spatial orientation information. Another concept, the peripheral visual horizon display (PVHD), also known as the Malcolm horizon, attempts to give at least pitch and roll cues to the pilot through his peripheral vision, thus sparing foveal vision for tasks requiring a high degree of visual discrimination. The several varieties of PVHD that have been developed as of this writing project across the instrument panel a long, thin line of light representing the true horizon; this line of light moves directly in accordance with the relative movement of the true horizon (Fig.

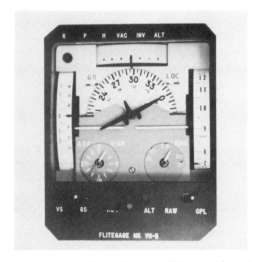

Fig. 11–40. The Crane Alweather Flitegage. The artificial horizon provides pitch information in the usual manner, but the small airplane on the instrument rolls in accordance with the rolling motion of the real aircraft. Other important flight data are displayed on the instrument face, thus minimizing the work involved in the cross-check.

11–41). The potential for further development and eventual pilot acceptance of PVHD-type aircraft attitude displays appears good because the PVHD is based on the physiologically sound concept of providing primary spatial orientation cuing through ambient vision, that is, in the natural fashion.

Other Sensory Phenomena

Flicker vertigo, fascination, and target hypnosis are traditionally described in conjunction with spatial disorientation, although, strictly speaking, these entities involve alterations of attention rather than aberrations of perception. Neither is the break-off phenomenon related directly to spatial disorientation, but the unusual sensory manifestations of this condition make a discussion of it here seem appropriate.

Flicker Vertigo

As most people are aware from personal experience, viewing a flickering light or scene can be distracting, annoying, or both. In aviation, flicker is sometimes created by helicopter rotors or idling airplane propellers interrupting direct sunlight or, less frequently, by such things as several anticollision lights flashing in nonunison. Pilots report that such conditions are indeed a source of irritation and distraction, but there is little evidence that flicker induces either spatial disorientation or clinical vertigo in normal aircrew. In fact, one authority insists there is no such thing as flicker vertigo and that the original reference to it was merely speculation.[23] Certainly, helicopter rotors or rotating beacons on aircraft can produce angular vection illusions because they create revolving shadows or revolving areas of illumination; vection does not result from flicker, however. Symptoms of motion sickness also can conceivably result from the sensory conflict associated with angular vection, but, again, these symptoms

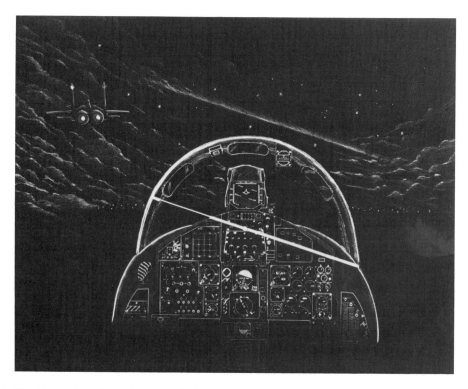

Fig. 11–41. The peripheral visual horizon display (PVHD), or Malcolm horizon. An artificial horizon projected across the instrument panel moves in accordance with the real horizon, and the pilot observes the projected horizon and its movement with his peripheral vision. Theoretically, this enables the pilot to process spatial orientation information in the natural fashion and spares his foveal vision for tasks requiring a high degree of visual discrimination.

would be produced by revolving lights and shadows and not by flicker.

Nevertheless, one should be aware that photic stimuli at frequencies in the 8- to 14-Hz range, that of the electroencephalographic alpha rhythm, can produce seizures in those rare individuals who are susceptible to flicker-induced epilepsy. Although the prevalence of this condition is very low (less than 1 in 20,000), and the number of pilots affected are very few, some helicopter crashes are thought to have been caused by pilots suffering from flicker-induced epilepsy.

Fascination

Coning of attention is something everyone experiences every day, but it is especially likely to occur when one is stressed by the learning of new skills or by the relearning of old ones. Pilots are apt to concentrate on one particular aspect of the flying task to the relative exclusion of others when that aspect is novel or unusually demanding. If this concentration is of sufficient degree to cause the pilot to disregard important information to which he should respond, it is termed fascination. An extreme example of fascination is when the pilot becomes so intent on delivering weapons to the target that he ignores the obvious cues of ground proximity and flies into the ground. Mishaps of this sort are said to result from target hypnosis; no actual hypnotic process is suspected or should be inferred, however. Other examples of fascination in aviation are the monitoring of one flight instrument rather than cross-checking during particularly stressful instrument flight; paying so much attention to flying precise formation that other duties are neglected; and the aviator's most ignominious act of negligence, landing an airplane with the landing gear up, despite the clearly perceived warning from the gear-up warning horn. These examples help us to appreciate the meaning of the original definition of fascination by Clark and colleagues: "a condition in which the pilot fails to respond adequately to a clearly defined stimulus situation in spite of the fact that all the necessary cues are present for a proper response and the correct procedure is well known to him."[24] From the definition and the examples given, it is clear that fascination can involve either a sensory deficiency or an inability to act, or perhaps both. It also is known that fascination, at least the type involving sensory deficiency, occurs not only under conditions of relatively high work load but also can occur when work load is greatly reduced and tedium prevails. Finally, the reader should understand that coning of attention, such as occurs with fascination, is not the same thing as tunneling of vision, which occurs with G stress: even if all pertinent sensory cues could be made accessible to foveal vision, the attentional lapses associated with fascination still could prevent those cues from being perceived or eliciting a response.

Break-off

In 1957, Clark and Graybiel[25] reported a condition that is perhaps best described by the title of their paper: "The break-off phenomenon—a feeling of separation from the earth experienced by pilots at high altitude." They found that 35% of 137 United States Navy and Marine Corps jet pilots interviewed by them had had feelings of being detached, isolated, or physically separated from the earth when flying at high altitudes. The three conditions most frequently associated with the experience were high altitude (5000 to 15,000 m, with a median of 10,000 m), being alone in the aircraft, and not being particularly busy with operating the air-

craft. The majority of the pilots interviewed found the break-off experience exhilarating, peaceful, or otherwise pleasant; over a third, however, felt anxious, lonely, or insecure. No operational importance could be ascribed to the break-off phenomenon; specifically, it was not considered to have a significant effect on a pilot's ability to operate his aircraft. The authors nevertheless suggested that the break-off experience might have significant effects on a pilot's performance when coupled with preexisting anxiety or fear, and for that reason, the phenomenon should be described to pilots before they go alone to high altitudes for the first time. Break-off may, on the other hand, have a profound, positive effect on the motivation to fly. Who could deny the importance of this experience to John Gillespie Magee, Jr., who gave us "High Flight," the most memorable poem in aviation?

> "Oh, I have slipped the surly bonds of earth . . .
> Put out my hand, and touched the face of God."

MOTION SICKNESS

Motion sickness is a perennial aeromedical problem. This important syndrome is discussed in this chapter to emphasize the critical importance of the spatial orientation senses in its pathogenesis; so closely entwined, in fact, are the mechanisms of spatial orientation and those of motion sickness that orientation sickness is sometimes (and legitimately) used as the general term for the category of related conditions that are commonly referred to as motion sickness.

Definition, Description, and Significance of Motion Sickness

Motion sickness is a state of diminished health characterized by specific symptoms that occur in conjunction with and in response to unaccustomed conditions existing in one's motional environment. These symptoms usually progress from lethargy, apathy, and stomach awareness to nausea, pallor, and cold eccrine perspiration, then to retching and vomiting, and finally to total prostration if measures are not taken to arrest the progression. The sequence of these major symptoms is sufficiently predictable that vestibular scientists have devised a commonly used scale, consisting of five steps from malaise I through frank sickness, to quantify the severity of motion sickness according to the level of symptoms manifested.[26] Other symptoms sometimes seen with motion sickness are headache, increased salivation and swallowing, decreased appetite, eructation, flatulence, and feeling warm. Although vomiting sometimes provides temporary relief from the symptoms of motion sickness, more commonly the motion-sick individual will continue to be sick if the offending motion or other condition to which he is not accustomed continues, and the vomiting will be replaced by nonproductive retching, or "dry heaves." A wide variety of motions and orientational conditions qualify as offensive, so there are many species of the generic term motion sickness. Among them are seasickness, airsickness, car sickness, train sickness, amusement-park-ride sickness, camel sickness, motion-picture sickness, flight-simulator sickness, and the most recent addition to the list, space sickness.

Military Experience

Armstrong[27] has provided us with some interesting statistics on airsickness associated with the World War II military effort:

> ...it was learned that 10 to 11 percent of all flying students became air sick during their first 10 flights, and that 1 to 2 percent of them were eliminated from flying training for that reason. Other aircrew members in training had even greater difficulty and the air sickness rate among them ran as high as 50 percent in some cases. It was also found that fully trained combat crews, other than pilots, sometimes became air sick which affected their combat efficiency. An even more serious situation was found to exist among air-borne troops. Under very unfavorable conditions as high as 70 percent of these individuals became air sick and upon landing were more or less temporarily disabled

at a time when their services were most urgently needed.

More recent studies of the incidence of airsickness in United States and British military flight training reveal that approximately 40% of aircrew trainees become airsick at some time during their training. In student pilots, there is a 15 to 18% incidence of motion sickness that is severe enough to interfere with control of the aircraft. Airsickness in student aviators occurs almost exclusively during the first several training flights, during spin training, and during the first dual aerobatic flights. The adaptation of which most people are capable is evidenced by the fact that only about 1% of military pilot trainees are eliminated from flight training because of intractable airsickness. The percentage of other aircrew trainees eliminated because of airsickness is considerably higher, however.

Although trained pilots almost never become airsick while flying the aircraft themselves, they surely can become sick while riding as a copilot or as a passenger. Other trained aircrew, such as navigators and weapon systems operators, are likewise susceptible to airsickness. Particularly provocative for these aircrew are flights in turbulent weather, low-level "terrain-following" flights, and flights in which high G forces are repeatedly experienced, as in air combat training and bombing practice. Both the lack of foreknowledge of aircraft motion, which results from not having primary control of the aircraft, and the lack of a constant view of the external world, which results from having duties involving the monitoring of in-cockpit displays, are significant factors in the development of airsickness in these aircrew.

Not surprisingly, seasickness is a hazard to aircrew who bail out over water. A life raft bobbing in the ocean is a notoriously provocative stimulus for seasickness; in one study, three fourths of the subjects became seasick and over half vomited during

1 hour of exposure to artificial wave motion while riding in a life raft. The debilitating and demoralizing effect of seasickness on the ability and will of downed aircrew to survive should be considered when planning sea rescue operations.

Flight-simulator sickness is getting increased attention now as aircrew spend more and more time in flight simulators capable of ever greater realism. Interestingly, simulator sickness is more likely to occur in pilots having considerable experience in the aircraft that the simulator is simulating than in pilots without such experience. The symptoms of simulator sickness are for the most part those of other forms of motion sickness, with nausea occurring in over 70% of pilots flying certain simulators. The progression of symptoms to the point of vomiting is uncommon in simulator sickness, however. Simulators providing wide-field-of-view visual presentations are reported to produce the additional symptoms of kinesthetic aftereffects, involuntary visual flashbacks, and disturbances of balance and locomotion for up to 10 hours after exposure. For that reason, it is recommended that pilots get a good night's sleep before flying real aircraft again after training intensively in wide-field-of-view flight simulators.

Civil Experience

The incidence of airsickness in the flight training of civilians can only be estimated but is probably somewhat less than that for their military counterparts because the training of civil pilots usually does not include spins or other aerobatics. Fewer than 1% of passengers in today's commercial air-transport aircraft become airsick, largely because the altitudes at which these aircraft generally fly are usually free of turbulence. This cannot be said, however, for passengers of most of the lighter, less capable, general aviation aircraft, who often must spend considerable portions of their flights at the lower, "bumpier" altitudes.

Space Sickness

The challenge of space flight includes coping with space sickness, a form of motion sickness experienced first by cosmonaut Titov and subsequently by approximately 29% of spacecrew (46 of 157 as of this writing). The incidence of sickness aboard the more recently launched, larger spacecraft is even greater (43%). The potential impact of space sickness on manned space operations must be acknowledged, and that impact must be minimized by appropriate mission planning. The sheer expense associated with each space launch, the high task loading of spacecrew, and the relative irrevocability of each space mission once committed make space sickness a hazard of primary importance.

If the duration of a space mission is long enough to allow crewmembers to adapt to the motional environment of space, they also risk disadapting to that of earth, and can consequently suffer earth sickness upon returning from the zero-G to the 1-G condition. Another type of space sickness will be encountered in the event that large space stations are rotated to generate G-loading for the purpose of alleviating the fluid shift, cardiovascular deconditioning, and skeletal demineralization that occur in the zero-G environment. Vestibular Coriolis effects created in occupants of such rotating systems are very potent producers of motion sickness and would be expected to plague the occupants for several days after arrival. Again, to the extent that the space station personnel were able to adapt to the rotating environment, they would risk disadapting to the nonrotating one and would suffer from motion sickness upon leaving the rotating space station.

Etiology of Motion Sickness

Man has speculated about the causes of and reasons for motion sickness for thousands of years. Largely because of the scientific interest in motion sickness that has been generated by naval and aerospace activities of the present century, we may now have a satisfactory explanation for this puzzling malady.

Correlating Factors

As already mentioned, motion sickness occurs in response to conditions to which one is not accustomed existing in his motional environment. Motional environment means all of the linear and angular positions, velocities, and accelerations that are directly sensed or secondarily perceived by an individual as determining his spatial orientation. The primary quantities of relevance here are mechanically (as opposed to visually) perceived linear and angular acceleration—those stimuli that act on the vestibular end-organs. Certainly, the pitching, rolling, heaving, and surging motions of ships in bad weather are clearly correlated with motion sickness, as are the pitching, rolling, yawing, and positive and negative G-pulling of aircraft during maneuvering. Abnormal stimulation of the semicircular ducts alone, as with a rotating chair, can result in motion sickness. So also can abnormal stimulation of the otolith organs alone, as occurs in an elevator or a four-pole swing. Whether the stimulation provided is complex, as is usually the case on ships and in aircraft, or simple, such as that generated in the laboratory, the important point is that abnormal labyrinthine stimulation is associated with the production of motion sickness. Not only is a modicum of abnormal vestibular stimulation sufficient to cause motion sickness, but some amount of vestibular stimulation is also necessary for motion sickness to occur. Labyrinthectomized experimental animals and humans without functioning vestibular end-organs (so-called "labyrinthine defectives") are completely immune to motion sickness.

The visual system can play two very important roles in the production of motion sickness. First, motion sensed solely through vision can make some people sick. Examples of this phenomenon are: motion-picture sickness, in which widescreen movies of rides on airplanes, rollercoasters, and ships in rough seas are provocative; microscope sickness, in which susceptible individuals cannot tolerate viewing moving microscope slides; and flight-simulator sickness, in which widefield-of-view visual motion systems create motion sickness in the absence of any mechanical motion. Abnormal stimulation of ambient (peripheral) vision rather than focal (foveal) vision appears to be the salient feature of visually induced motion sickness. The fact that orientation information processed through the ambient visual system converges on the vestibular nuclei makes visually induced motion sickness a less mysterious phenomenon, even if it is not totally explicable. The second role of vision in the etiology of motion sickness is illustrated by the well-known fact that the absence of an outside visual reference makes persons undergoing abnormal motion more likely to become sick than they would be if an outside visual reference were available. Good examples of this are the sailor who becomes sick below deck but prevents the progression of motion sickness by coming topside to view the horizon, and the aircrewman who becomes sick while attending to duties inside the aircraft (e.g., radarscope monitoring) but alleviates the symptoms by looking outside.

Other sensory systems capable of providing spatial orientational information also are capable of providing avenues for motion-sickness-producing stimuli. The auditory system, when stimulated by a revolving sound source, is responsible for audiogenic vertigo, audiokinetic nystagmus, and concomitant symptoms of motion sickness. Nonvestibular proprioceptors may contribute to the development of motion sickness when the pattern of stimulation of these senses by linear and angular accelerations is unfamiliar. Perhaps more important than the actual sensory channel employed or the actual pattern of stimulation delivered, however, is the degree to which the spatial orientational information received deviates from that anticipated. The experience with motion sickness in various flight simulators bears witness to the importance of unexpected patterns of motion and unfulfilled expectations of motion. Instructor pilots in the 2-FH-2 helicopter hover trainer, for example, were much more likely to become sick in the device than were student pilots. It is postulated that imperfections in flight simulation are perceived by pilots who, as a result of their experience in the real aircraft, expect certain orientational stimuli to occur in response to certain control inputs. Pilots without time in the real aircraft, on the other hand, have no such expectations, and therefore notice no deviations from them in the simulator. Another example of the role played by the expectation of motion in the generation of motion sickness is seen in the pilot who does not become sick as long as he has control of the airplane but does become sick when another pilot is flying the same maneuvers in the same airplane. In this case, the pilot's expectation of motion is always fulfilled whenever he is controlling the airplane but is not fulfilled when someone else is flying.

Several other variables not primarily related to spatial orientation seem to correlate well with motion sickness susceptibility. Age is one such variable: susceptibility increases with age until puberty and then decreases thereafter. Sex is another: women are more susceptible to motion sickness than men at any given age. The personality characteristics of emotional lability and excessive rigidity are also positively correlated with motion sickness susceptibility. Whether one is mentally occupied with a significant task during exposure to motion or is free to dwell on orientation cues and the state of

one's stomach seems to affect susceptibility—the latter, more introverted state is more conducive to motion sickness. Likewise, anxiety, fear, and insecurity, either about one's orientation relative to the ground or about one's likelihood of becoming motion sick, seem to enhance susceptibility. We must be careful, however, to distinguish between sickness caused by anxiety and sickness caused by motion: a paratrooper who vomits in an aircraft while waiting to jump into battle may be suffering either from extreme anxiety or from motion sickness, or both. Finally, it must be recognized that many things, such as mechanical stimulation of the viscera and malodorous aircraft compartments, even though they are commonly associated with conditions that result in motion sickness, do not in themselves cause motion sickness.

A mildly interesting but potentially devastating phenomenon is conditioned motion sickness. Just as Pavlov's canine subjects lerned to salivate at the sound of a bell, student pilots and other aircrew, with repeated exposure to the conditioning stimulus of sickness-producing aircraft motion, can eventually develop the autonomic response of motion sickness to the conditioned stimulus of being in or even just seeing an aircraft (Fig. 11–42). For this reason, it is advisable to initiate aircrew gradually to the abnormal motions of flight and to provide pharmacologic prophylaxis against motion sickness, if necessary, in the early instructional phases of flight.

Unifying Theory

Current thinking regarding the underlying mechanism of motion sickness has focused on the "sensory conflict," or "neural mismatch," hypothesis proposed originally by Claremont in 1931. In simple terms, the sensory conflict hypothesis states that motion sickness results when incongruous orientation information is generated by various sensory modalities, one of which must be the vestibular sys-

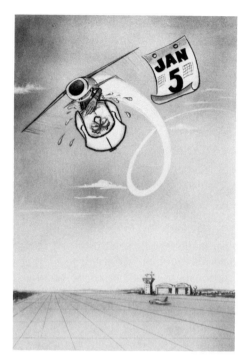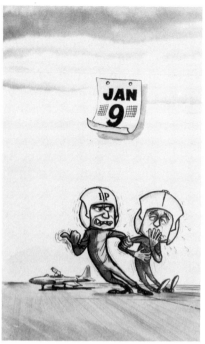

Fig. 11–42. Conditioned motion sickness. A student aviator who repeatedly gets airsick during flight can become conditioned to develop symptoms in response to the sight or smell of an aircraft even before flight. Use of antimotion-sickness medication until the student adapts to the novel motion can prevent conditioned motion sickness.

tem. In virtually all examples of motion sickness, one can, with sufficient scrutiny, identify the sensory conflict involved. Usually the conflict is between the vestibular and visual senses or between the different components of the vestibular system, but conflicts between vestibular and auditory or vestibular and nonvestibular proprioceptive systems are also possible. A clear example of sickness resulting from vestibular-visual conflict is that which occurs when an experimental subject wears reversing prisms over his eyes so that his visual perception of self-motion is exactly opposite in direction to his vestibular perception of it. Another example is motion-picture sickness, the conflict being between visually perceived motion and vestibularly perceived stationarity. Airsickness and seasickness are most often a result of vestibular-visual conflict: the vestibular signals of linear and angular motion are not in agreement with the visual

percept of being stationary inside the vehicle. Vestibular-visual conflict need not even be in relation to motion but can be in relation to static orientation: some people become sick in antigravity houses, which are built in such a way that the visually apparent vertical is quite different from the true gravitational vertical. Intravestibular conflict is an especially potent means of producing motion sickness. When vestibular Coriolis effects cause the semicircular ducts to signal falsely that angular velocity about a nonvertical axis is occurring, and the otolith organs do not confirm a resulting change in angular position, the likelihood of developing motion sickness is great. In a zero-gravity environment, when an individual moves his head away from the vertical, the semicircular ducts sense rotation, but the otolith organs cannot sense any resulting change of angular position relative to a gravity vector; the generation of this intravestibular conflict is believed to be the underlying mechanism of space sickness. It also can be argued, however, that the sensory conflict responsible for space sickness is between the otolith organs, which detect no gravitational vertical, and the eyes, to which structures within the space vehicle take on apparent verticality by virtue of some familiar aspect of their configuration.

What determines whether orientation information is conflicting or not? It is one's prior experience in the motional environment and the degree to which orientation information expected on the basis of that experience agrees with the actual orientation information received. The important sensory conflict is thus not so much an absolute discrepancy between information from the several sensory modalities as it is between anticipated and actual orientation information. Evidence of this can be seen in the gradual adaptation to sustained abnormal motional environments, such as the sea, space, slow rotation, and the wearing of reversing prisms, and in the readaptation to the normal environment that must take place upon returning to it. It can also be seen that being able to anticipate orientation cues confers immunity to motion sickness, as evidenced by the fact that pilots and automobile drivers almost never make themselves sick and by the fact that we actively subject ourselves to many motions (jumping, dancing, acrobatics) that would surely make us sick if we were subjected to them passively. It appears, then, that the body refers to an internal model of orientational dynamics, both sensory and motor, to effect voluntary and involuntary control over orientation. When transient discrepancies between predicted and actual orientation data occur, corrective reflex activity is initiated or the internal model is updated or both. But when sustained discrepancies occur, motion sickness is the result.

Teleology

Even if the mechanism of motion sickness could be described completely in terms of cellular and subcellular functions, the question would remain: "What purpose, if any, does motion sickness serve?" The idea that a chance mutation rendered countless generations of vertebrates potential victims of motion sickness, and that the relatively recent arrival of transportation systems gave expression to that otherwise innocuous genetic flaw, strains credulity. Steele[28] has suggested that the symptoms of motion sickness are "caused by cardiovascular inadequacy secondary to diversion of circulating blood to the muscles in response to a threatened need for vigorous muscular action on the basis of an inadequately perceived inertial and dynamic environment." A more recent hypothesis and, in our opinion, a more satisfying explanation of motion sickness is that of Treisman.[29] He proposed that the orientation senses, in particular the vestibular system, serve an important function in the emetic response to poisons. When an animal ingests a toxic substance and experiences its effects on the central nervous system, namely, deterioration of the finely tuned spatial orientation senses and consequent degraded predictability of sensory responses to motor activity, reflex vomiting occurs and the animal is relieved of the poison. The positive survival value of such a mechanism to eliminate ingested poisons is obvious. The essentiality of the vestibular end-organs and certain parts of the cerebellum, and the role of sensory conflict as manifested through the functioning of those structures, are provided a rational basis in Treisman's theory. Finally, experimental support for Treisman's theory recently has been provided: labyrinthectomized animals, in addition to being immune to motion sickness, exhibit marked impairment of the emetic response to certain naturally occurring poisons.

Prevention and Treatment of Motion Sickness

The variety of methods at our disposal for preventing and treating motion sickness is less an indication of how easy motion sickness is to control than it is of how incompletely effective each method can be. Nevertheless, logical medical principles are generally applicable; several specific treatments have survived the test of time and become traditionalized, and some newer approaches appear to have great potential. Additional information on the treatment of airsickness is contained in Chapter 17, "Neuropsychiatry in Aerospace Medicine."

Physiologic Prevention

An obvious way to prevent motion sickness is to avoid the environments that produce it. For most individuals in today's world, however, this is neither possible nor desirable. The most common and ultimately most successful way is to adapt to the novel motional environment through constant or repeated exposure to it. The rapidity with which adaptation occurs is highly variable, depending mainly on the strength of the challenge and on the adaptability of the individual involved. Usually, several days of sustained exposure to mild orientational challenges (like sea and space travel) or several sessions of repeated exposure to vigorous challenges (like aerobatics or centrifuge riding) will confer immunity. The use of antimotion-sickness medications to prevent symptoms during the period of adaptation does not appear to compromise the process of adaptation and is recommended where practicable.

The selection of individuals resistant to motion sickness, or screening out those unusually susceptible to it, has been considered as a method for reducing the likelihood of motion sickness in certain operations, such as military aviation training. The fact that susceptibility to motion sickness is so complex a characteristic makes selection less efficacious a means of prevention than might be supposed. At least three separate factors are involved in motion sickness susceptibility: (1) receptivity, the degree to which a given orientational information conflict is perceived and the intensity with which it is experienced and responded to; (2) adaptability, the rate at which one adjusts to a given abnormal orientational environment as evidenced by his becoming less and less symptomatic; and (3) retentivity, the ability to remain adpated to the novel environment after leaving it. These factors appear to be independent. This means that a particular prospective aviator with high receptivity also might adapt very rapidly and remain adapted for a long time, so that it would be unwise to eliminate him from flying training on the basis of a history of motion sickness or even a test of susceptibility. Nevertheless, although the great majority of aircrew trainees do adapt to the aerial environment, use of either vestibular stimulation or a motion sickness questionnaire reveals that sensitivity to motion sickness is inversely related to success in flight training. Furthermore, sound judgment dictates that an attempt to select against crewmembers with a high probability of becoming motion sick is appropriate for some of the more critical and expensive aerospace operations.

Some promising results have been obtained with biofeedback-mediated behavior modification for desensitizing fliers with chronic airsickness. This technique is discussed in Chapter 17.

Physiologic Treatment

Once symptoms of motion sickness have developed, the first step to take to bring about recovery is to escape from the environment that is producing the symptoms. If this is possible, relief usually follows rapidly; symptoms can still progress to vomiting, however, and nausea and drowsiness can sometimes persist for many hours, even after termination of the offending motion. If escape is not possible, assuming a supine position or just stabilizing the head seems to offer some relief. As mentioned previously, passengers subjected to motion in enclosed vehicles can help alleviate symptoms by obtaining a view of the natural horizon. One of the most effective physiologic remedies is turning over control of the vehicle to the symptomatic crewmember. Generations of flight instructors have used this technique to avert motion sickness in their students, even though they were probably unable to explain how it works in terms of reducing conflict between anticipated and actual orientation cues. Another procedure that has proved useful in practice is to cool the affected individual with a blast of air from the cabin air vent; such thoughtfulness on the part of their instructors has undoubtedly saved many student pilots from having to clean up the cockpit.

Pharmacologic Prevention

The most effective single medication for prophylaxis against motion sickness is scopolamine, 0.3 to 0.6 mg, taken orally 30 minutes to 1 hour before exposure to motion. Unfortunately, the side effects of scopolamine when taken in orally effective doses (i.e, drowsiness, dry mouth, pupillary dilation, and paralyzed visual accommodation) make the routine oral administration of this drug to aircrew highly inadvisable. When prophylaxis is needed for prolonged exposure to abnormal motion (e.g., an ocean voyage), oral scopolamine can be administered every 4 to 6 hours; again, the side effects are troublesome and may preclude repeated oral administration. A novel and promising approach to the problem of prolonged prophylactic administration of scopolamine is the Transderm-Scōp system, in which 0.5 mg of scopolamine is delivered transcutaneously over a 3-day period from a small patch worn on the skin behind the ear. The side effects associated with this system of administration are reportedly less than with oral scopolamine.

The antimotion-sickness preparation most commonly used in aircrew is probably the "scope-dex" combination, which is 0.3 to 0.6 mg of scopolamine and 5 to 10 mg of dextroamphetamine taken orally 1 hour prior to exposure to motion. Not only is this combination more effective than scopolamine alone, but the stimulant effect of the dextroamphetamine counteracts the drowsiness side effect of the scopolamine. Another very useful oral combination is 25 mg each of promethazine and ephedrine, taken approximately 1 hour before exposure. Because the individual response to the several effective antimotion-sickness preparations is highly variable, it may be worthwhile to perform individual assessments of different drug combinations and dosages to obtain the maximum benefit. The reader is referred to Graybiel and colleagues[30] and Johnson and associates[31] for additional information on the efficacy of antimotion-sickness preparations.

Pharmacologic Treatment

If motion sickness progresses to the point of nausea, and certainly if vomiting occurs, oral medication is useless. If the prospect of returning soon to the accustomed motional environment is remote, it is important to treat the condition to prevent the dehydration and electrolyte loss that result from protracted vomiting. The intramuscular injection of scopolamine, 0.3 mg, or promethazine, 25 mg, is recommended. Scopolamine administered intravenously or even by nasal spray or drops is also effective. Promethazine rectal suppositories are used to control vomiting in many clinical situations, and their use in the treatment of motion sickness also should be successful. If the parenteral administration of scopolamine or promethazine does not provide relief from vomiting, sedation with intravenous phenobarbital may be necessary to prevent progressive deterioration of the patient's condition. Of course fluid and electrolyte losses must be replaced in patients who have been vomiting for prolonged periods.

Aeromedical Use of Antimotion-Sickness Preparations

As mentioned previously, the routine use of antimotion-sickness drugs in aircrew is not appropriate because of the undesirable side effects of these drugs. Prophylactic medication can be very useful, however, in helping the student aviator cope with the novel motions that can cause sickness during flight training—thus promoting better conditions for learning, and preventing the development of conditioned motion sickness. Prophylaxis also can help reduce a student's anxiety over becoming motion sick, which can develop into a self-fulfilling vicious circle. After using medication, if necessary, for two or three dual training sorties (usually at the beginning of flight training and again during the introduction to aerobatics), student pilots should no longer need antimotion-sickness drugs. The use of drugs for solo flight should absolutely be forbidden. A more liberal approach can perhaps be taken with other aircrew trainees, such as navigators, because of their greater propensity to become motion sick and their less critical influence on flight safety. Trained aircrew, as a rule, should not use antimotion-sickness drugs. An exception to this rule is made for spacecrew, whose exposure to the zero-gravity condition of space flight is usually very infrequent and whose premission adaptation by other means cannot be assured. Spacecrew also should be expected to need prophylaxis for reentry into the normal gravitational environment of the earth after a prolonged stay at zero gravity. Airborne troops, who must arrive at the battle zone fully effective, are also candidates for antimotion-sickness prophylaxis under cer-

tain circumstances, such as prolonged low-level flight in choppy weather. In all such cases, the flight surgeon must weigh the risks associated with developing motion sickness against the risks associated with the side effects of the antimotion-sickness drugs and arrive at a judgment of whether to medicate. Decisions of this sort are the very essence of his profession.

Thus we see how man's recent transition into the motional environment of aerospace has introduced him not only to new sensations but also to new sensory demands. If he fails to appreciate the fallibility of his natural orientation senses in this novel environment, he succumbs to spatial disorientation. If he recognizes his innate limitations, however, he can meet the demands of the environment and function effectively in it. We see also how man's phylogenetic heritage, by means of orientational mechanisms, renders him susceptible to motion sickness. That same heritage, however, enables him to adapt to new motional environments. The profound and pervasive influence of our orientation senses in aerospace operations cannot be denied or ignored; through knowledge and understanding, however, it can be controlled.

REFERENCES

1. Hixson, W.C., Niven, J.I., and Correia, M.J.: Kinematics Nomenclature for Physiological Accelerations, With Special Reference to Vestibular Applications. Monograph 14. Pensacola, Florida, Naval Aerospace Medical Institute, 1966.
2. Henn, V., Young, L.R., and Finley, C.: Vestibular nucleus units in alert monkeys are also influenced by moving visual fields. Brain Res., 71:144–149, 1974.
3. Dichgans, J., and Brandt, T.: Visual-vestibular interaction: Effects on self-motion perception and postural control. In Handbook of Sensory Physiology. Volume VIII. Perception. Edited by R. Held, H.W. Liebowitz, and H.-L. Teuber. Berlin, Springer-Verlag, 1978.
4. Liebowitz, H.W., and Dichgans, J.: The ambient visual system and spatial orientation. In Spatial Disorientation in Flight: Current Problems. AGARD-CP-287. Neuilly-sur-Seine, France, North Atlantic Treaty Organization/1980.
5. Tredici, T.J.: Visual illusions as a probable cause of aircraft accidents. In Spatial Disorientation in

Flight: Current Problems. AGARD-CP-287. Neuilly-sur-Seine, France, North Atlantic Treaty Organization/1980.

6. Brindley, G.S., and Merton, P.A.: The absence of position sense in the human eye. J. Physiol., 153:127–130, 1960.
7. Sperry, R.W.: Neural basis of the spontaneous optokinetic response preceded by visual inversion. J. Comp. Physiol. Psych., 43:482–489, 1950.
8. Spoendlin, H.H.: Ultrastructural studies of the labyrinth in squirrel monkeys. In The Role of the Vestibular Organs in the Exploration of Space. NASA-SP-77. Washington, D.C.: National Aeronautics and Space Administration, 1965.
9. Jones, G.M: Disturbance of oculomotor control in flight. Aerospace Med., 36:461–465, 1965.
10. Peters, R.A.: Dynamics of the vestibular system and their relation to motion perception, spatial disorientation, and illusions. NASA-CR-1309. Washington, D.C., National Aeronautics and Space Administation, 1969.
11. Jones, G.M.: Vestibulo-ocular disorganization in the aerodynamic spin. Aerospace Med., 36:976–983, 1965.
12. Cohen, M.M., Crosbie, R.J., and Blackburn, L.H.: Disorienting effects of aircraft catapult launchings. Aerospace Med., 44:37–39, 1973.
13. Buley, L.E., and Spelina, J.: Physiological and psychological factors in "the dark-night takeoff accident." Aerospace Med., 41:553–556, 1970.
14. Martin, J.F., and Jones, G.M.: Theoretical man-machine interaction which might lead to loss of aircraft control. Aerospace Med., 36:713–716, 1965.
15. Malcolm, R., and Money, K.E.: Two specific kinds of disorientation incidents: Jet upset and giant hand. In The Disorientation Incident. AGARD-CP-95. Part 1. Edited by A.J. Benson. Neuilly-sur-Seine, France, North Atlantic Treaty Organization/1972.
16. Nuttall, J.B., and Sanford, W.G.: Spatial disorientation in operational flying. Publication M-27-56. United States Air Force Directorate of Flight Safety Research, Norton Air Force Base, California, Sept. 12, 1956.
17. Moser, R.: Spatial disorientation as a factor in accidents in an operational command. Aerospace Med., 40:174–176, 1969.
18. Barnum, F., and Bonner, R.H.: Epidemiology of USAF spatial disorientation aircraft accidents, 1 Jan. 1958–31 Dec. 1968. Aerospace Med., 42:896–898, 1971.
19. Barnum, F.: Spatial disorientation aircraft accidents, 1 Jan. 1969–31 Dec. 1971: A comparison. Presented at the Annual Scientific Meeting of the Aerospace Medical Association, Las Vegas, Nevada, May, 1973.
20. Kellogg, R.S.: Letter report on spatial disorientation incidence statistics. From The Aerospace Medical Research Laboratory, Wright-Patterson Air Force Base, Ohio to AMD/RDL; Mar. 30, 1973.
21. Kirkham, W.R., et al.: Spatial disorientation in general aviation accidents. Aviat. Space Environ. Med., 49:1080–1086, 1978.
22. Money, K.E., and Malcolm, R.E.: Assessment of films and slides for orientation training of military pilots. In Orientation/Disorientation Training of Flying Personnel: A Working Group Report. AGARD-R-625. Edited by A.J. Benson, Neuilly-sur-Seine, France, North Atlantic Treaty Organization/1974.
23. Wick, R.L.: No flicker vertigo. Letter to the editor. Business/Commercial Aviat., 51:16, July, 1982.
24. Clark, B., Nicholson, M., and Graybiel, A.: Fascination: A cause of pilot error. J. Aviat. Med., 24:429–440, 1953.
25. Clark, B., and Graybiel, A.: The Break-off phenomenon—a feeling of separation from the earth experienced by pilots at high altitude. J. Aviat. Med., 28:121–126, 1957.
26. Miller, E.F., II, and Graybiel, A.: Comparison of five levels of motion sickness severity as the basis for grading susceptibility. Aerospace Med., 45:602–609, 1974.
27. Armstrong, H.G.: Air sickness. In Aerospace Medicine. Edited by H. G. Armstrong. Baltimore, The Williams & Wilkins Co., 1961.
28. Steele, J.E.: Motion sickness and spatial perception—a theoretical study. In Symposium on Motion Sickness with Special Reference to Weightlessness. AMRL-TDR-63-25. Aerospace Medical Research Laboratory, Wright-Patterson Air Force Base, Ohio, 1963.
29. Treisman, M.: Motion sickness: An evolutionary hypothesis. Science, 197:493–495, 1977.
30. Graybiel, A., et al.: Human assay of antimotion sickness drugs. Aviat. Space Environ. Med., 46:1107–1118, 1975.
31. Johnson, W.H., Money, K.E., and Graybiel, A.: Airborne testing of three antimotion-sickness preparations. Aviat. Space Environ. Med., 47:1214–1216, 1976.

Chapter 12

Beyond the Biosphere

Arnauld E. Nicogossian and James F. Parker

That's one small step for a man, one giant leap for mankind.

NEIL ARMSTRONG

The historical view of space has been that of an empty and alien realm sharing none of the characteristics we associate with our comfortable terrestrial biosphere. Although from the standpoint of the unprotected human, space is indeed inhospitable, in a physical sense the distinction between the two environments is not as clear-cut as was once believed. We now know that the earth's atmosphere and space are in equilibrium. Rather than being two completely distinct zones, they form a continuum whose shape and constitution are acted on by forces that are both terrestrial and extraterrestrial in origin. Within our solar system other bodies, notably the sun and planets, are likewise in physical equilibrium with space and impact our own local environment and equilibrium with space in various ways.

THE ORBITAL ENVIRONMENT

The Transition to Space

The gaseous envelope that forms our atmosphere is acted on principally by two forces: the terrestrial gravitational force that binds it to earth and solar thermal radiation, which causes its gases to expand into the surrounding space. Because these two forces are in relatively constant balance, the atmosphere exhibits a fairly distinct vertical profile of density and pressure. As the distance from earth increases, the density of the gaseous medium decreases (Fig. 12–1). What we define as the border of the atmosphere occurs at the point where collisions between air molecules become immeasurably infrequent. This "collision limit" occurs at about 700 km above the earth's surface.

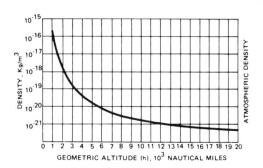

Fig. 12–1. Atmospheric density as a function of altitude. The rapid decrease in density is correlated with a decrease in both the pressure and partial pressure of oxygen. (Adapted from Air Force Surveys in Geophysics, No. 115, August, 1959.)

382

Above this level is the exosphere, a zone of free-moving air particles that gradually thins out into true space. Even in space, however, the density of gas particles is about one to ten gas particles per cubic centimeter.

What concerns us as humans—as organisms adapted to life at the planet's surface—is the capacity of the atmosphere at various altitudes to support life. Predominant among these considerations are the atmosphere's breathability, its barometric pressure, and its protective effect as a shield against harmful radiation emanating from space. Each of these life-support capabilities of the atmosphere is diminished with increasing altitude, and at a certain point, each ceases to function. These functional limits of atmospheric effects determine, for man, the true border between the terrestrial biosphere and space. Although the physical border of the atmosphere is considered to be at 700 km, its functional limits are reached at considerably lower altitudes.

Manned flight in near-earth orbit, at altitudes in the order of 240 km, requires a space vehicle well beyond the functional limits of the earth's biosphere. Designers of manned space vehicles must account for the new operating environment (weightlessness), the lack of a life-supporting atmosphere, radiation, and the danger of collision with small objects in space (micrometeoroids).

Zero Gravity

The various forces that act, or cease to act, on an astronaut in space are an important feature of his environment because these forces can affect his work efficiency, his health, and even his survival. The most significant aspect of the force environment in orbital flight is the loss of the normal gravitational force that acts on us at all times on earth. This loss of gravity, or "weightlessness," occurs when the gravitational force vector is exactly counterbalanced by the centrifugal force im-

parted to the spacecraft as its travels tangentially to the earth's surface (Fig. 12–2).

To live and work in a world in which there is no gravity is a totally new experience for first-time space travelers. It is an experience characterized mostly by its novelty, but one having a broad range of important medical and behavioral consequences as well.

The dynamics of human existence are continuously shaped by the all-pervading force of gravity within the earth's biosphere. Every conscious movement is made in a manner that accounts for gravity. Such a simple motor act as leaning forward brings into play a number of muscle systems that control the movement of the body as its center of gravity shifts. These are highly skilled acts, and yet they require no conscious thought. On initial entry into a gravity-free environment, however, each movement and act must be done differently, and a period of relearning is required. Fortunately, the problems of relearning have not proved to be as difficult as was predicted by some. Dr. Joseph Kerwin, in recounting his experiences as a crewmember in Skylab 2, noted that, "The primary theme was one of pleasant surprise at all the things that didn't change, at all the things that were pleasant and easy to do."[1] Berry, summarizing the early Apollo experiences, noted that the absence of gravity could represent a bonus for locomotion because locomotion in zero gravity requires much less work than on earth.[2] In addition, in-flight activities are frequently aided by the ease with which minimal velocities can be imparted to large objects that must be moved.

The zero-gravity environment also affects the physiologic functioning of major body systems; changes here are less obvious than the changes in locomotion but are of greater medical consequence. On entry into weightlessness, the body fluids are redistributed. The function of the vestibular system, which is uniquely sensitive to gravity, is disturbed. Other systems

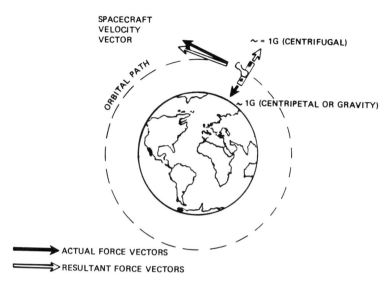

SPACECRAFT
VELOCITY
VECTOR

~ = 1G (CENTRIFUGAL)

ORBITAL PATH

~ 1G (CENTRIPETAL OR GRAVITY)

→ ACTUAL FORCE VECTORS
⇒ RESULTANT FORCE VECTORS

Fig. 12–2. Representation of the balance of forces that produces weightlessness (0 G) in earth orbit.

begin a slow process of adaptation to the altered environment. For example, the cardiovascular system adjusts to a new situation in which the demands placed on it are greatly decreased. The result is a "deconditioned" system that functions appropriately for life in zero gravity but may have real difficulty when called on to readjust suddenly to a 1-g environment.

Atmosphere

A major requirement for a manned spacecraft is the provision of a life-supporting atmosphere. The two key parameters of such an atmosphere are oxygen and pressure. Important additional requirements involve the control of carbon dioxide and maintaining comfortable temperature and humidity levels.

Humans function well when oxygen is supplied at a pressure between 160 mm Hg (3.1 psi—equivalent to sea level) and 110 mm Hg (2.1 psi—equivalent to an altitude of 3048 m). Provided that an appropriate pressure level is maintained, the atmosphere can be 100% oxygen, with no nitrogen or other diluent gas present. Early spacecraft, such as that used in project Gemini, provided a 100% oxygen atmosphere at a pressure of 5 psi. The obvious

fire hazard found with a pure oxygen atmosphere was controlled to some extent in project Apollo through the use of a 60% oxygen and 40% nitrogen mixture at the time of launch. Through time, gas leakage was made up through the provision of oxygen only until the spacecraft achieved a 100% oxygen level, again at 5 psi. The suits used for extravehicular activity during project Apollo were pressurized with 100% oxygen at 3.8 psi. No problems with hypoxia, dysbarism, or oxygen toxicity were experienced during any of the Apollo missions.

Another key parameter of the atmosphere is that of pressure. When the body is exposed to reduced pressure, nitrogen in the tissues tends to form bubbles that then enter the vascular system and can result in severe neurologic problems, which are termed "decompression sickness." Instances of this affliction occurring after exposure for an hour or longer at altitudes as low as 5486 m have been recorded. The pressure at 5486 m is 380 mm Hg (7.3 psi). Humans can function at lower pressures, such as the 5-psi pressure of the Apollo spacecraft, provided the tissue nitrogen is removed by breathing 100% oxygen for a period of several hours prior to exposure to the lower pressure.

The atmosphere in the space shuttle is essentially identical to that found at sea level on earth, with the oxygen supply, pressure, and humidity carefully controlled. The atmosphere consists of 22% oxygen and 78% nitrogen at a pressure of 760 mm Hg (14.7 psi) and provides complete comfort during normal shuttle activities. The only issue arises when astronauts must transfer into a pressurized suit for extravehicular work. For this type of shuttle work, generally conducted in the unpressurized cargo bay, the cabin is decompressed from 14.7 to 10.2 psi at least 12 hours prior to the work to allow some nitrogen removal from tissues. This procedure is followed by a 40-minute period in the pressure suit at 10.2 psi breathing 100% oxygen before final decompression to a suit pressure of 4.3 psi. These procedures remain under review and may change when new equipment becomes available or as mission requirements dictate.

Radiation

The vacuum of space, although a more perfect vacuum than can be achieved in any facility on earth, nevertheless contains a great deal of matter that interests the planners of space missions. Radiation, particularly the submicroscopic particles of ionizing radiation, is a topic of major concern for biomedical scientists.

The radiation encountered during orbital flight can be classed as primary cosmic radiations, geomagnetically trapped radiations (Van Allen belts), and radiation due to solar flares. The latter two classes determine the unique quality of radiation found in near-earth space. Indeed, these two classes of radiation are important factors in determining the scheduling and trajectories of orbital flights. Anticipated radiation levels always are taken into account prior to a given mission.

The atmosphere of earth serves as a protective blanket to shield organisms on the surface from virtually all potentially damaging radiation. Particle radiation is slowed by collision with air atoms, whereas the ionosphere reflects most portions of the electromagnetic spectrum back into space. Only two "windows" in the ionosphere allow radiation from the sun and from deep space to pass through to the earth. One window covers the visible light frequencies and part of the ultraviolet and infrared frequencies. Another window covers radio frequencies of approximately 10^9 Hz. The protection afforded earth's inhabitants also has insulated us from knowledge of the radiation's physical characteristics. Thus, most of what has been learned concerning space radiation has come from space missions and probes flown during the past 30 years.

COSMIC RADIATION. Galactic cosmic radiation consists of particles that originate outside the solar system, probably resulting from cataclysmic events such as the supernova explosion witnessed by Chinese astronomers in the year 1054. A.D. Data from space probes show that these particles consists of 87% protons (hydrogen nuclei), 12% alpha particles (helium nuclei), and 1% heavier nuclei, ranging from lithium to iron. The individual particle energies are extremely high—in some instances up to 10^{20} eV. It has been estimated that this amount of energy per particle, if converted to mechanical work, could lift a normal-sized book about 1 m off the ground.[3] The extreme particle energies mean that galactic cosmic particles, which fortunately are of very low flux density, are virtually unshieldable. At present, principal interest is in determining the extent to which periodic or continuous exposure to this radiation will affect career limits for space crewmen.

TRAPPED RADIATION. In 1958, a project team led by Dr. James Van Allen conducted experiments in the United States Explorer satellite series, in which they discovered the existence of bands of geomagnetically trapped particles encircling the earth. These radiation belts consist of electrons and protons of the solar wind, which encounter the earth's magnetic field and become entrapped and begin to oscillate back and forth along the lines of magnetic force. The trapped particles follow the magnetic field completely around the earth (Fig. 12–3).

The Van Allen belts have two main portions, with effects being evident at altitudes as high as 55,000 km. The inner Van Allen belt begins at an altitude of roughly 300 to 1200 km, depending on latitude. The outer belt begins at about 10,000 km,

with its upper boundary dependent on the activity of the sun.

In the low earth orbit to be followed in space shuttle missions, radiation from the Van Allen belts will be negligible. A discontinuity in the earth's geomagnetic field in the southern hemisphere, known as the South Atlantic anomaly, must be avoided to the extent possible in planning mission flight paths, however. At this location, which extends from about zero to 60° west longitude and 20 to 50° south latitude, the intensity of trapped protons having energies more than 30 MeV is, at 161 to 322 km altitude, equivalent to that found at 1287 km altitude elsewhere.

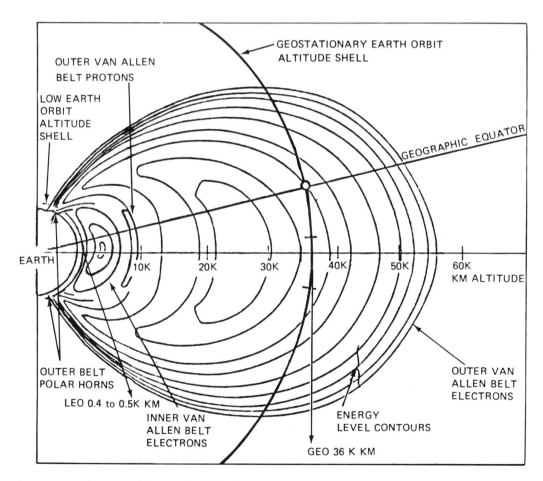

Fig. 12–3. Configuration of the Van Allen belts of particles trapped within the earth's magnetic field. (Adapted from Radiation issues. Extracted from Extravehicular Crewman Work System (ECWS) Study Program (SP 04J77). Presented at National Aeronautics and Space Administration, L.B.J. Space Center, Houston, Texas, October, 1977.)

SOLAR FLARES. Solar flares are a major source of radiation concern, possibly the most potent of the radiation hazards. The sun follows approximately an 11-year cycle of activity. When activity peaks, spectacular disturbances can occur on the surface of the sun. A solar flare is in fact a solar magnetic storm. These storms build up over several hours and last for several days. Although their occurrence cannot be forecast, the onset of buildup can be detected. As the flare builds, an increase in visible light first takes place, accompanied by disturbances in the earth's ionosphere, which are probably due to solar x-rays. The principal problem, though, is with the high-energy protons that are produced during the storm. The energy of these protons ranges from about 10 million to about 500 million eV. The flux also may be quite high. As a result, the radiation hazard for space crewmen could be quite serious, with a possibility of receiving a lethal dose.[4]

OTHER RADIATION EFFECTS. The Skylab missions provided an opportunity to evaluate yet another radiation hazard in space, the energetic neutron. Neutrons were recognized as one component of space radiation before Skylab, but the magnitude and, in particular, the source of this radiation were not well understood. Neutrons are of biomedical importance because, upon colliding with a hydrogen nucleus (a proton), there is a high probability of an energy exchange. Because humans contain an abundance of hydrogen-rich compounds, such as proteins, fat, and especially water, neutron exposure could cause considerable damage. Ambient neutron flux within a space vehicle, therefore, must be understood.

Free neutrons are not stable. With a half-life of 11 minutes, neutrons decay into a proton and an electron. Thus, neutrons detected in a space vehicle must be generated either within the spacecraft or within the earth's atmosphere and must represent products of the nuclear reactions caused by strikes of primary radiation. Skylab measurements showed that neutron flux within a spacecraft is higher than had been predicted—too high, in fact, to be attributed to solar neutrons, earth albedo neutrons, or even neutrons induced by cosmic rays in space-station materials. It was concluded that the neutrons were produced through bombardment of spacecraft material by trapped protons in the Van Allen belt. Fortunately, the flux level was not high enough to be considered a biologic hazard for crewmembers.

An interesting visual phenomenon that obviously was related to space radiation was first noted in the Apollo program. During the time of trans-earth coast, crewmembers of Apollo 11 reported seeing faint spots or flashes of light when the cabin was dark and they had become dark-adapted. From these reports and more systematic studies on later Apollo flights, it was concluded that the light flashes resulted from high-energy, heavy cosmic rays penetrating the spacecraft structure and the crewmembers' eyes. The fact that prior dark adaptation is necessary indicates that the phenomenon is connected with the retina rather than with a direct stimulation of the optic nerve.

Measures made during the Skylab program corroborated the light-flash finding of Apollo. Light-flash observations were made in two particular orbits to provide data on the effects of both latitude and the South Atlantic anomaly. During each session, the astronaut donned a blindfold, allowed 10 minutes for adaptation to darkness, and then recorded his observation of each flash. The results are shown in Figure 12–4. Two conclusions were drawn.[3] First, the occurrence of light flashes correlates with the flux of cosmic particles. Second, the greatly increased number of flashes in the South Atlantic anomaly probably results either from trapped protons in this region or from trapped heavier nuclei.

BIOMEDICAL SIGNIFICANCE. The biomed-

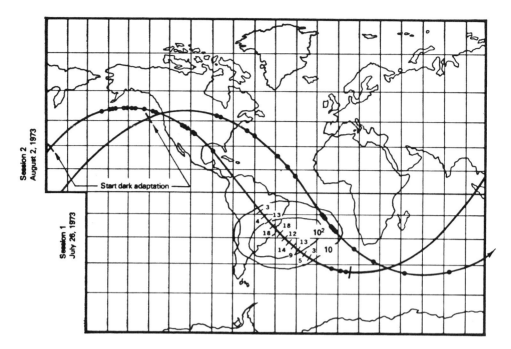

Fig. 12–4. Light flashes observed during two particular orbits selected to provide data on the effects of latitude and the South Atlantic anomaly.

ical significance of the radiation encountered in spaceflight can be assessed through a review of the radiation doses received by crewmen with varying times of exposure. Table 12–1 presents the measured radiation doses for three astronauts in the Apollo program and for three astronauts in the Skylab program.[5] These values are compared with the estimated total dose of radiation these individuals had received, based on their age, from diagnostic radiographs and other sources of radiation on earth. When the space radiation dose is compared with National Aeronautics and Space Administration (NASA) career limits, expressed in rem units for blood-forming organs, skin, and the lens of the eye, these exposures are of negligible consequence. The Skylab 4 crewmen, who showed the highest exposures, could fly a mission comparable to one 84-day Skylab 4 mission per year for 50 years before exceeding the career limits for radiation exposure.[6]

Table 12–1.   Representative Career Radiation Exposures For Astronauts

Astronaut	Career Time (years)	Exposure Time	Space Radiation Dose (in rem)	Diagnostic X-Ray and Other Radiation Doses (in rem)
X	15	9 days, 15 minutes	0.64	2.29
Y	10	12 days, 11 hours, 4 minutes	0.18	2.01
Z	18	22 days, 2 hours, 45 minutes (four flights)	1.83	2.76
A	15	28 days	1.66	2.82
B	15	59 days	3.71	2.36
C	2	84 days	8.01	2.65

From Radiation Protection in Manned Space Flight.[5] A presentation to the Occupational Safety and Health Administration, United States Department of Labor. National Aeronautics and Space Administration and the Lyndon B. Johnson Space Center, Houston, Texas, March 10, 1981.

Micrometeoroids

A number of solid objects regularly pass through the orbital environment of the earth. The largest of these are the meteors, or "shooting stars," that appear on occasion as long streaks in the sky. Composed of solid matter heated to incandescence by friction with the atmosphere, meteors are primarily of two types, with about 61% being stone, 35% iron, and 4% a mixture of the two. Remnants of meteors that reach the earth's surface are called meteorites.

The terms meteoroid and micrometeoroid describe the small solid objects found in interplanetary and orbital space. Micrometeoroids often are referred to as interplanetary dust. Most of the extraterrestrial matter reaching the earth's surface, estimated at 10,000 metric tons per day, is in the form of micrometeorites.

The presence of micrometeoroids in space has long been recognized. The extent to which such objects might represent a hazard for manned spaceflight, however, has not been known. Therefore, all missions have included some means of protection for crewmembers. In some instances, protection has been provided through the shielding afforded by the spacecraft itself. By contrast, during the Apollo program, astronauts who were scheduled for periods on the lunar surface were provided with an integrated thermal micrometeoroid garment.

The Skylab program presented an opportunity to obtain measures over an extended period of the incidence of micrometeoroids in orbital space. Because a number of these objects were expected to strike Skylab, an experiment was developed in which thin foils and polished metal plates were exposed on the exterior of the Skylab vehicle to record penetrations by micrometeoroids. On return to earth, the exposed materials were studied with optical microscopes and scanning electron microscopes at magnifications of 200X and at 500X. Table 12–2 shows the

Table 12–2. Micrometeoroid Impacts Recorded During Skylab Experiments (Exposed Area = 1200 cm²)

Sample Period (days)	Number of Impacts
1–34	23
2–46	17
3–34	21

Adapted from Lundquist, C.A. (ed.: Skylab's Astronomy and Space Sciences. NASA SP-404. Washington, D.C., Government Printing Office, 1979.

results of these analyses. Because the exposed plates were located at different positions on Skylab and at different orientations, these figures represent an approximation of the micrometeoroid flux in orbit.

The size of the craters measured in the Skylab experiment showed all of the impacting particles to be quite small, with only one believed to have been as large as 0.1 to 0.2 mm in diameter. The particles did have considerable power, as witnessed by their ability to produce craters in a stainless steel surface. Even though Skylab's micrometeoroid protective shield was lost during launch, however, the Orbital Workshop's wall, 3.8-mm thick, was not penetrated. There appears to be little, if any, micrometeoroid hazard to spacecraft in orbit with an exterior of such thickness.

Spacecraft Cabin Environment

In the absence of atmospheric protection, the space traveler is protected from these space factors by a pressurized space capsule containing various life-support systems. The hull itself provides the first line of protection against the near-vacuum of space, as well as against solar thermal radiation, particle radiation of various kinds, and micrometeoroids. Internal systems provide air and water regeneration while maintaining the necessary pressure, temperature, and humidity levels. The modern space vehicle is thus insulated against space and, in fact, constitutes a "shirt-sleeves environment" in which crewmembers can move, breathe, converse, and otherwise live in as normal a fashion as possible while they go about their daily routines.

The internal environment of the spacecraft, however, also includes factors that are significant in the overall health and well-being of the inhabitants. Although these environmental factors are generated by man and are thus not a "natural" aspect of the space environment, such as radiation and zero gravity, for instance, they are nonetheless space environmental issues in the context of manned missions.

The principal concern here is with contaminants present in the cabin atmosphere. Although materials used in the construction of manned spacecraft and onboard equipment are selected with great care, a certain amount of offgassing of organic and inorganic products inevitably occurs. Many of these gases have toxicologic significance. In addition, contaminants are produced by man himself as metabolic by-products. Some of these contaminants are listed in Table 12–3, along with acceptable concentration levels in the onboard atmosphere.

PLANETARY ENVIRONMENTS

The spectacular successes of the American Pioneer, Viking, and Voyager unmanned missions and the Soviet Venera missions have provided a wealth of scientific information concerning the nature of our nearest planetary neighbors. In recent years, the rate of acquisition of data concerning the solar system has been such that it may be a decade or more before all of it can be analyzed. Yet, even as we develop detailed descriptions of the solar planets, new questions are raised. For example, changes seen in the Martian polar regions have still not been explained; nor did the Viking missions provide insight as to the evolutionary processes that produced the puzzling differences between the Martian surface and soil and those of Earth. Voyager spacecraft sent back pho-

Table 12–3.   Space Cabin Contaminants— Provisional Limits For 90 and 1000 Days

Air Contaminant	Air Limit (ppm)	
	90 Days	1000 Days
N-butanol	10	10
2-butanone	20	20
Carbon monoxide	15	15
Chloroform	5	1
Dichloromethane	25	5
Dioxane	10	2
Ethyl acetate	40	40
Formaldehyde	0.1	0.1
2-methyl butanone	20	20
Trichloroethane		2
1,1,2-trichloro-1,2,2-trifluoroethane and related congeners	1000	200

Provisional Emergency Limits		
Air Contaminant	Air Limit for 60 Minutes	
	ppm	mg·m^{-3}
2-butanone	100	294
Carbonyl fluoride	25	68
Ethylene glycol	100	254
2-methyl butanone	100	352
1,1,2-trichloro-1,2,2-trifluoroethane and related congeners	30,000	2320

Data from the National Academy of Sciences, Space Science Board, 1968.

tographs of the moons of Jupiter and the rings of Saturn that are striking beyond belief. The nature of the processes occurring on some of Jupiter's moons remains unclear, as do the physics involved in the configuration of some of Saturn's rings. An understanding of our solar system and, indeed, of our universe requires that questions such as these be answered.

Because the essence of the human spirit is that partial descriptions and unresolved scientific issues provoke action, man will inevitably venture past the moon and on into interplanetary space. Interplanetary missions will require a new era of research and planning if man is to be sustained during these long ventures and if he is to carry out all assigned activities. The information we now have concerning interplanetary space, as well as the orbital and surface environments of the planets, suggests that such missions will not be simple. The following brief descriptions of the four planets that have been probed most extensively to date indicate the kinds of issues to be confronted by biomedical scientists participating in the planning of interplanetary missions.

Venus

Venus, together with Earth, Mercury, and Mars, is known as a terrestrial planet, being composed of rocky materials and iron and having a density quite similar to that of the earth. Passing 24 million miles from the earth at its point of closest approach, Venus is the earth's nearest planetary neighbor. It is a logical candidate for exploration missions within the solar system.

The first successful mission to Venus took place in 1962, when a United States Mariner 2 spacecraft flew to within 35,000 km of the planet and radioed back information concerning the near-environment of Venus. One of the more interesting of these discoveries was that Venus, for all practical purposes, has no surrounding magnetic field. From 1962 to 1982, the Soviet Union, with its Venera series, and the United States, with its Mariner and Pioneer programs, have sent 17 spacecraft to Venus.

Most of the information obtained in the American exploration of Venus has been through the Pioneer program. In December, 1978, the Pioneer-Venus spacecraft arrived in orbital flight around Venus. While the bus spacecraft remained in orbit, four entry probes were launched toward the Venusian surface. The gross topology of Venus was defined by a radar mapping system in the orbiting craft (Fig. 12–5). The probes provided much information on the structure of the atmosphere and more detailed surface effects. One probe transmitted for 67 minutes from the surface of Venus before heat rendered it ineffective.

The Soviet Venera spacecraft were the first to accomplish a landing on the planet's surface. The Venera-9 vehicle transmitted black-and-white photographs to

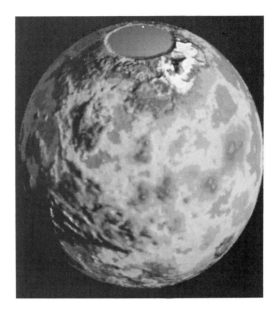

Fig. 12–5. This global view of Venus was taken by the radar altimeter of the Pioneer spacecraft, so that the planet's cloud cover is eliminated. The large feature at the top of the picture is Venus' northern "continent," Ishtar. (Photo courtesy of the National Aeronautics and Space Administration.)

earth on October 22, 1975, showing a Venusian landscape with considerably more light than had been expected under the heavy cloud cover and with sharply sided rocks indicating little of the expected erosion effects. More recently, in March, 1982, Venera 13 and 14 landed and transmitted photographs taken by imaging systems that permitted color reconstruction. Both landers also succeeded in analyzing samples of soil scooped up from their landing sites.

Although Venus has a number of features similar to earth, such as its size and density, there are some striking differences. The Venusian atmosphere is nearly 90 times more massive than that of the earth, and its predominant gaseous component is carbon dioxide. Sulfuric acid clouds encompass the entire planet, whereas the water clouds on earth only partially cover the planet. Water vapor and sulfur dioxide also have been detected in the lower atmosphere. Nitrogen is present,

PHYSIOLOGY IN THE FLIGHT ENVIRONMENT

on the order of 3% by mass. The large volume and density of the atmosphere, however, mean that the amount of atmospheric nitrogen on Venus is about three times greater than on earth. The planet's surface temperature is extremely high—more than 450° C. Material analyzed by Venera 13 and 14 was shown to be basalt, an igneous rock similar to material found on volcanically active midocean ridges on earth. This finding suggests recent or ongoing volcanic activity on Venus.

Three fourths of the solar energy that impinges on Venus is reflected back into space by the planet's atmosphere and clouds, with 60% of the remainder absorbed in the heavy cloud layer. This layer consists chiefly of 1- to -3-μm particles that are believed to be sulfuric acid.

One of the more interesting findings during the earlier probes of Venus was evidence of lightning activity in the lower atmosphere. Both the American and Soviet data indicate that lightning discharges may occur as often as 25 times per second in relatively small areas above the Venusian surface. Terrestrial lightning, on the other hand, occurs only on the order of 100 times per second over the entire earth. The electrical characteristics of Venusian storms, therefore, may be both different and more severe than those to which we are accustomed.

It was also learned that Venus has no planetary magnetic field to shield it from the solar wind. As a result, the Venusian ionosphere reacts strongly with the stream of particles from the sun. Both ion density and the height of the top of the ionosphere are affected by solar wind speed and pressure.

The picture of Venus pieced together from the various probes demonstrates that, although orbital observations certainly would be possible, the surface characteristics are not conducive to manned exploration of this planet. The great heat and barometric pressure at the surface and the composition and turbulence of the atmos-

phere make the planet quite inhospitable to human life. In addition to these physicochemical barriers, the rotation of Venus is much different from that to which we are accustomed, resulting in a day of 243 earth-days and a year of 224 earth-days. Thus, a day on Venus is longer than a Venusian year. Venus is not a planet that beckons visitors.

Mars

Mars is the closest neighbor of earth as one proceeds away from the sun. It also is a planet about which we have an unparalleled fund of scientific information, due mainly to data provided through Project Viking. By the beginning of the 1980s, the United States and the Soviet Union had sent 16 probes to Mars. The three most successful as planetary exploration missions were Mariner 9 and Viking 1 and 2.

The Viking program was a masterful blend of science and technology, for the first time carrying an automated scientific laboratory to a soft landing on the surface of another planet. The Viking 1 spacecraft landed on Mars on July 20, 1976 and was followed by Viking 2 on September 3. These spacecraft were each comprised of an orbiter-lander combination, which traveled through space as a single unit, separating only after orbit had been achieved around Mars and the appropriate landing site selected. The orbiter served as a relay station to transmit to earth information received from the lander. In addition, each orbiter took many thousands of high-resolution photographs of Mars as its orbit carried it over different areas of the planet. In combination, these four spacecraft have provided information concerning the Martian surface and its atmospheric environment that may be analyzed and studied fruitfully for many years.

The Martian atmosphere is totally unlike that found on Venus. For one thing, it is extremely thin. Pressures measured at various times by the Viking spacecraft were in the range from 6.5 to 7.7 mb, a value less than 1% of the earth's atmospheric pressure at sea level. Nevertheless, it is an active atmosphere. The Mariner 9 spacecraft, which orbited Mars in late 1971, photographed huge dust storms that obscured the surface for a 2-month period until they quieted enough for photographs to be made of the surface. The primary constituent of the Martian atmosphere is carbon dioxide, just as on Venus, with nominal amounts of neon, argon, and oxygen.

Thanks to the remarkable photographs transmitted by Viking, the surface features of Mars now are familiar (Fig. 12–6). Mars has a very heterogeneous surface, with extensive cratering and evidence of volcanos over vast areas of the planet. Much of the northern hemisphere is covered by volcanic fields. Widespread evidence of catastrophic flooding is apparent, but no collection basins such as lakes or oceans have been found, and the source and sink of the water are still conjectural. The only water found on Mars to date occurs in the polar ice caps. These caps contain substantial amounts of water ice, are covered seasonally by carbon dioxide frost, and vary in size seasonally.

A major objective of the Viking project

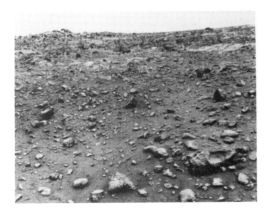

Fig. 12–6. This view of the Martian surface and sky was taken by Viking 1. Color reconstruction showed that orange-red surface materials (possibly limonite) overlie darker bedrock and that the sky is pinkish-red. (Photo courtesy of the National Aeronautics and Space Administration.)

was to search for any indication of life on Mars. A number of photographs of the surface were taken, some at close range, to determine if any organism—large or small—could be seen. The results were entirely negative. Beautiful pictures of the soil and rocks were obtained, but nothing lifelike was noted.

A more scientific approach to the detection of life was made through the use of the automated laboratory carried in the Viking landers. Samples of Martian soil were used for three experiments in the Biology Instrument Package, as follows:

1. *Gas exchange experiment.* This experiment was conducted in two parts. The first part tested whether the presence of moisture and appropriate environmental conditions would produce metabolic activity in simple, prebiologic organic complexes that might be present in the soil in a dormant state. Although gas-chromatographic analysis indicated a chemical generation of oxygen, as well as physical desorption of some gases, nothing suggested the presence of metabolic activity. The second part of the experiment tested for the presence of heterotrophic organisms using organic compounds to satisfy their metabolic requirements. Extended incubation in the presence of organic nutrients and moisture resulted in a steady production of carbon dioxide, although no gases attributable to living systems were found.

2. *Pyrolytic release experiment.* It was assumed that both carbon dioxide and carbon monoxide are found in the atmosphere of Mars; thus, organisms might have developed the capacity to assimilate one or both of these gases and convert them to organic matter. This experiment was conducted under conditions that approximated the Martian environment

to the extent feasible. Incubations were carried out either in light or in dark for 5-day periods. Although weak responses were noted, the results appear to rule out any biologic explanation.

3. *Labeled-release experiment.* This experiment tested the assumption that Martian organisms would be capable of decomposing the simple organic compounds reported to be produced in the so-called "primitive reducing atmospheres" in laboratory simulations. The soil was moistened with nutrients tagged with carbon-14. Upon incubation, the sample immediately started to emit labeled gas. The radioactive gas release leveled off over the next several days until additional nutrients were added. Samples that had been heat-sterilized did not show this release of the gas. Young notes that, although the release of tagged carbon dioxide in a nominally terrestrial soil would have been indicative of an extremely active biota, under Martian conditions this might only suggest the presence of highly reactive soil-oxidizing agents.[7] In short, the fact that the sterilized control samples did not show the reaction may mean either that the active run was biologic in nature or that the earlier heating of the sterilized samples had exhausted the reaction.

The general conclusion is that the Martian surface is very different from earth in terms of its chemistry and that this difference seriously affects the interpretation of the biology experiments. The bulk of the evidence, however, favors a nonbiologic explanation of the observed phenomenon.

Mars remains an attractive candidate for further exploration. It has a thin atmosphere mostly comprised of carbon dioxide and a surface that could be traversed readily by exploration vehicles. The soil resembles that on earth but apparently has an intriguing increase in oxidative qualities. Of particular importance is the water supply contained in the large polar ice caps. This resource would be invaluable to an exploration team.

Jupiter

As one travels somewhat more than 240 million miles past Mars and on toward the outer solar system, the next planet to be encountered is Jupiter, the first of the giant planets. Jupiter is the largest planet, with a mass 318 times larger than the mass of earth. Its density (1.33 g/cm^3), however, is ony one-fourth that of earth and just slightly greater than the density of water.

The United States has launched four successful fly-by missions to Jupiter. The first of these, Pioneer 11, reached its closest point to the planet (130,000 km) on December 3, 1973. The most recent, Voyager 2, passed within 650,000 km of the planet on July 9, 1979. The two Pioneer and the two Voyager spacecraft returned a wealth of scientific information plus thousands of photographs of Jupiter. Although much of the interior of the planet remains a mystery, the outer surface of Jupiter, its satellites, and the conditions in the space surrounding it are now well documented. This information is contributing much to an understanding of the processes whereby the solar system was formed.

Jupiter is a gas planet, more massive than all of the other planets combined. It has no surface, in the usual sense, and many scientists believe that Jupiter is an entirely fluid planet with no solid core. Recent studies, however, postulate that the planet may have a small core of rocks and ice that constitutes about 4% of its mass.

In many respects, Jupiter resembles a star; in fact, had it been 70 times more massive, it would have contracted during the time of its early formation into a star. Had this occurred, the sun would have been a double star and the solar system would be much different. Since 1969, it has been known that Jupiter radiates more heat than it receives from the sun. Thus, Jupiter must have an internal heat source. The internal heat is believed to represent the conversion of gravitational potential energy from the contraction of a giant cloud of gas beginning some 4.6 billion years ago. The surface heat, about 10^{17} W of power, flows from the dynamic processes within its luminous interior, which is believed to be about 30,000°K. Jupiter is composed of the same elements as the sun and stars, primarily hydrogen and helium. Most of its interior is metallic hydrogen held under enormous pressure, with normal molecular hydrogen appearing nearer the surface. In the upper regions, the hydrogen is a gas.

The great mass of Jupiter and its powerful gravity mean that all gases and solids available during its early stages of condensation should remain today. Jupiter, therefore, has the same basic composition as the sun, with hydrogen and helium being the two principal constituents. There is an abundance of additional elements and compounds, however.

The atmosphere of Jupiter is a mass of complex motion. Some of the atmospheric changes are quite fleeting; others, such as the Great Red Spot, remain relatively unchanged for centuries. The dominant features in the atmosphere of Jupiter are banded belts and zones, the Great Red Spot, and three white ovals (Fig. 12–7). The Great Red Spot is larger than the earth, and the ovals are about the size of our moon. All show anticlonic, counterclockwise motion. Materials within the Great Red Spot can be seen to rotate about once every 6 days.

Within the Jovian atmosphere, clusters of lightning bolts have been seen on the night side of the planet. One Voyager photograph showed the electrical discharges of 19 "superbolts" of lightning. This evidence of extensive electrical activity con-

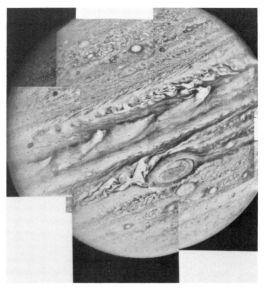

Fig. 12–7. This mosaic of Jupiter was assembled from nine individual photographs taken by Voyager 1 when it was 7.8 million km from the planet. Shown are the Great Red Spot, the banded cloud features, and several white ovals. (Photo courtesy of the National Aeronautics and Space Administration.)

firms the disturbed condition of the atmosphere of Jupiter.

The similarities between the weather systems of Jupiter and Earth are matched by likenesses in the surrounding magnetic fields. The interior pressures of Jupiter are so great that hydrogen becomes an electrical conductor. The rotation of the planet thus causes a current to flow through the metallic core and to produce a surrounding magnetic field. The strength of the Jupiter field, however, is about 4000 times that found around the earth. A key effect of this field is to trap atomic particles arriving as part of the solar wind. The boundaries of the magnetosphere, in the direction toward the sun, lie between 4 and 8 million km from the planet. Within the magnetosphere, charged particles can be accelerated to high energies, with some subsequently escaping and being encountered far from Jupiter. On Voyager 1, one stream of hot plasma was encountered almost 50 million km from the planet. Certain "hot spots" are inside the magnetosphere. Voyager 1 also detected such a plasma about 5 million km from Jupiter and measured its temperture at 300 to 400 million degrees. This is the highest temperature encountered anywhere within the solar system. (It should be noted that the low particle densities found in such a stream make the concept of temperature almost meaningless from a physiologic standpoint.)

One of the most spectacular features of the Voyager missions was the photographs taken of the principal satellites of Jupiter. Jupiter now is known to have 14 satellites, with the four largest being termed the Galilean moons, in consideration of their discovery by Galileo in 1610. These moons (Io, Europa, Ganymede, and Callisto) are considered "terrestrial" space bodies. They are similar to the planets of the inner solar system, including earth, in both size and composition. Io, the innermost Galilean satellite, gained a measure of fame when it was found, by chance observation, to have an active volcano. A more careful search then revealed that there were no fewer than eight active volcanos on Io throwing up plumes from 70 to 300 km high. The next satellite, Europa, was found to be crisscrossed by stripes and bands that may represent filled fractures in the satellite's icy crust. It is believed that water, in solid and liquid form, constitutes about 20% of Europa's mass. The next satellite, Ganymede, is the largest of Jupiter's moons. A most noticeable feature of this moon is an immense dark area, the remnant of an ancient crust showing the impact of many meteorites. Finally, there is Callisto, at a distance of 1.8 million km from the planet. Callisto is about the size of the planet Mercury and shows the effects of billions of years of cratering. It also shows a number of concentric rings that encircle the satellite. These rings are believed to have been formed dynamically by the impact of a large body early in the developmental cycle of the satellite.

Future explorations of Jupiter, particularly if there is any requirement for close observation, will almost certainly be through unmanned space probes. The planet itself is most interesting because it retains many features from the early developmental period of the solar system. It also possesses a system of satellites that are quite different from one another and should offer unique insights into the dynamics of early planetary development. The region itself, however, is not hospitable. An immense band of trapped radiation surrounds Jupiter. The planet itself is extremely hot toward the interior and offers no reasonable landing site. Any conceivable manned mission would have to be to one of the satellites.

Saturn

The rings of Saturn are without doubt one of the most spectacular features in the solar system. These rings, which were first observed by Galileo in July, 1610, are the distinguishing characteristics of Saturn. Observations from earth could easily distinguish three of the rings but provided little insight into the ultimate number and complexity of these rings until close observations were made by American spacecraft.

The Pioneer 11 spacecraft accomplished a successful fly-by mission to Saturn on September 1, 1979. Considerable scientific information was returned, including a number of images from a photopolarimeter, which achieved up to 20 times the resolution provided in earth-based photographs. A major accomplishment of Pioneer was its demonstration that a spacecraft can safely cross the ring plane of Saturn. Although Pioneer was struck at least five times during the encounter by particles at least 10 μm in diameter, there was no real threat to its survival. Pioneer paved the way for the much more ambitious Voyager flights that followed immediately.

The missions of the Voyager 1 and 2 spacecraft provided thousands of startling photographs of the features of Saturn (Fig. 12–8). Voyager 1 made its closest approach to the cloud tops of Saturn on November 12, 1980. Thirty-eight months after launch and nearly 1.6 billion km from Earth, Voyager 1 passed the giant planet at a distance of 200,000 km. The Voyager 2 encounter with Saturn occurred on August 25, 1981 at a distance of less than 100,000 km. Each spacecraft photographed the planet, its rings, and its satellites. The passage of each spacecraft carried it through an area of the ring structure.

The surface of Saturn is covered by dense clouds, preventing any direct observation. Much is known of the structure of the planet, however. Saturn is a gas planet, like Jupiter. Its mass is 95 times that of earth. Recent estimates indicate that Saturn may have at the bottom of its gaseous and molten levels a solid core which could constitute about 25% of its mass. The outermost layer of the planet has a liquid mixture of hydrogen and helium, with the hydrogen in molecular form. Beneath this is a metallic liquid layer of hydrogen. The core is presumed to be made of rock and ice. It also is known that Saturn has a source of internal heat, presumably from the conversion of gravitational potential energy.

The atmosphere of Saturn is similar to that of Jupiter, although muted by a thick haze layer. It contains dark belts, white-banded zones, and circulating storm regions. Maximum wind speeds are at the equator and can reach speeds of about 1600 km/hr. Temperatures near the cloud tops range from −152°C to −146°C. Although auroral emissions have been seen near the poles, lightning has not yet been observed. Saturn also has been found to have a red spot, approximately 11,263 km in length, which resembles Jupiter's red spot. This relatively stable spot is believed to be the upper surface of a convective cell.

The rings of Saturn are most fascinating. The particles that make up these rings are believed to be primarily rock and ice. They have been described as having the size and appearance of "dirty snowballs." Voyager measurements indicate that the particle size in the ring structure ranges from micrometers to meters, with all sizes in between. The well-known A, B, and C rings were found to consist of hundreds of rings or ringlets, a few of which are elliptic in shape. The F ring is more complex and may consist of three interwoven rings that seem to be bounded by two "shepherding" satellites. It is believed that the "spokes" observed in the B ring may be due to fine, electrically charged particles above the ring, perhaps resulting from lightning occurring within the ring.

The flight of Voyager 1 resulted in the discovery of three new satellites of Saturn, bringing the total of known satellites to 15 at that time. Analyses of data from the Voyager 2 encounter, combined with new information from the Voyager 1 flight, now brings the number of known Saturnian satellites to between 21 and 23. The two "possible" satellites were seen in only one observation each, so their orbits could not be confirmed. Scientists at the Jet Propulsion Laboratory in California are continuing their extensive review of Voyager 2 data, and it is possible that additional satellites may yet be confirmed.

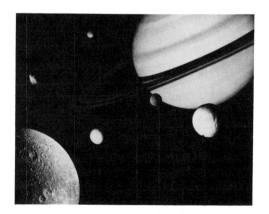

Fig. 12–8. This montage of Saturn, its rings, and six of its moons was taken by Voyager 1. Shown clockwise from the right are Tethys, Mimas (with large crater), Enceladus, Dione (at lower left), Rhea, and Titan.

With the exception of one—the satellite

Titan—all of the moons of Saturn are covered with water, ice, and, in some instances, are composed mainly of water ice. For the most part, these satellites show evidence of heavy cratering through the years.

The most interesting of the moons is Titan. Voyager 1 passed within 7000 km of Titan, the closest encounter between either of the Voyager spacecraft and any planet or moon. This was done to obtain as much information as possible. Titan is the second largest moon observed in the solar system, with a radius of 2575 km. It is the only moon in the solar system with a measurable atmosphere, found to be largely nitrogen with lesser amounts of methane, ethane, acetylene, ethylene, and hydrogen cyanide. The atmosphere of Titan is three times as dense and ten times as deep as that on earth. It also is quite cold, with a temperature near the surface of −146°C. The surface pressure is 1.6 bars, or 60% more than that found at the earth's surface. Titan's surface, which is not visible through the atmosphere, may be liquid methane or liquid nitrogen.

The real value of observations of Titan is that this moon, which in many ways resembles a primitive earth maintained in a deep-freeze condition, might provide considerable information concerning the manner in which earth has developed. Titan might serve as a natural laboratory within which to realistically study the interaction of environmental forces and chemical factors.

The Voyager missions have shown Saturn and its environment to be a most complex and dynamic scene. As many as 1000 identifiable bands may be within its complicated ring structure. The known moons of Saturn now number at least 21. The planet has a strong magnetic field and an extensive magnetosphere containing energetic charged particles. It also has the only satellite in the solar system, Titan, known to have a measurable atmosphere.

In all, future missions to Saturn would be a highly recommended step as we attempt to understand better the nature and origin of our solar system. Indeed, planning is being done now for possible insertion of an instrumented probe into the atmosphere of Titan at some future date. It is entirely feasible for such a probe to be launched from a manned laboratory orbiting within the near-space of Saturn. A manned mission, allowing direct control over the data collection plan and the operation of onboard instrumentation, would provide a wealth of scientific information and would represent a tremendous stride in the exploration of the solar system.

INTERSTELLAR SPACE

Today, manned spaceflight beyond the solar system remains a topic for science fiction. Probably within the next 100 years, however, serious planning will begin for manned missions beyond the most remote planets. Definitive data showing that the nearest stars have planetary systems similar to that of our sun certainly serves to spur such planning.

Missions into interstellar space will require new technologies. The challenges in engine development will be tremendous. Lightweight engines capable of imparting a continuous accelerative force over a period of days or months will be necessary. For the life sciences, a completely regenerative life-support system will be needed. Obviously, no opportunity will be available for resupply of any kind.

The interstellar environment within which a manned spacecraft will operate is sparse but by no means empty. Considerable gaseous matter is in the interstellar medium, although at densities substantially lower than the best vacuum achievable on earth. Approximately 90% of this gas is neutral hydrogen, radiating at a characteristic wavelength of 21 cm and thus readily detectable. Nearly all of the remaining 10% of gas is made up of atoms of helium. Most of the hydrogen is believed to have been formed during the explosive events that occurred in the creation of the universe approximately 13 to 15 billion years ago. Some of the helium perhaps was formed from primordial hydrogen at the same time, with the rest being manufactured in stars and distributed through supernova explosions. The remaining 1% or less of interstellar gases consists principally of carbon, nitrogen, oxygen, aluminum, and iron. All of these, including still scarcer elements such as aluminum, were formed in nuclear reactions within stars.

In recent years, complex molecules such as cyanogen and formaldehyde also have been detected in interstellar space. These molecules are of considerable interest as possible precursors of living matter. They also demonstrate that, although much is being learned about the interstellar environment, a number of mysteries remain. For example, certain small, dense clouds of gas within the Milky Way appear to have substantial concentrations of formaldehyde molecules. Radio observations of these clouds show that the formaldehyde absorbs energy from its microwave background, rather than radiating energy. The formaldehyde appears to be about 1.7°K colder than the background. Because one would expect that over time the formaldehyde normally would be warmed to match the temperature of the microwave background radiation, some unspecified action is working within the gas clouds to keep the formaldehyde chilled. Whether this interstellar refrigerator, as well as other features yet to be observed, is of any consequence for manned missions remains to be determined. The finding of such effects does underscore the work remaining before such missions can be attempted. When man looks up toward the heavens, he is looking toward his future.

REFERENCES

1. Kerwin, J.P.: Skylab 2 crew observations and summary. In Biomedical Results from Skylab. Edited by R.S.Johnston and L.F. Dietlein. NASA SP-377. Washington, D.C., Government Printing Office, 1977.
2. Berry, C.A.: Biomedical findings on American astronauts participating in space missions: Man's adaptation to weightlessness. Paper presented at The Fourth International Symposium on Basic Environmental Problems of Man in Space. Yerevan, Armenia, U.S.S.R., October 1–5, 1971.
3. Lundquist, C.A. (ed.): Skylab's Astronomy and Space Sciences. NASA SP-404. Washington, D.C., Government Printing Office, 1979.
4. Radiation issues. Extracted from Extravehicular Crewman Work System (ECWS) Study Program (SP 04J77). Prepared by Hamilton Standard under Contract NAS 9-15290. Presented at the National Aeronautics and Space Administration, and the Lyndon B. Johnson Space Center, Houston, Texas, October, 1977.
5. Radiation Protection in Manned Space Flight. A presentation to the Occupational Safety and Health Administration, United States Department of Labor. National Aeronautics and Space Administration and the Lyndon B. Johnson Space Center, Houston, Texas, March 10, 1981.
6. Bailey, J.V., Hoffman, R.A., and English, R.A.: Radiological protection and medical dosimetry for the Skylab crewmen. In Biomedical Results from Skylab. Edited by R.S. Johnston and L.F. Dietlein. NASA SP-377. Washington, D.C., Government Printing Office, 1977.
7. Young, R.S. Viking on Mars: A preliminary survey. Am. Sci., 64(6):620–627, 1976.

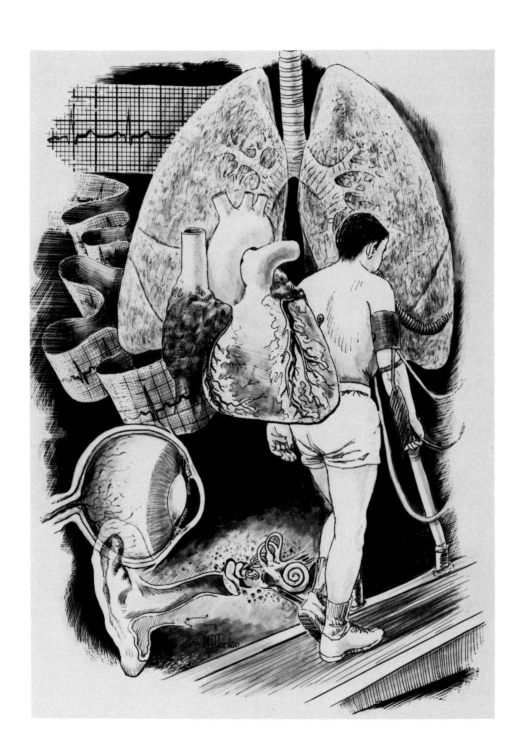

Section *III*

Clinical Practice of Aerospace Medicine

Because the aerospace environment can be demanding on an aviator or astronaut, it is recognized that those controlling flight need to meet a standard of medical fitness. Thus, it is usual for the candidate aircrew person to undergo a medical examination. The standards for the examination are dependent on the nature of the crew duty anticipated. Each body system may be examined, and standards have been developed over time that are responsive to the sophistication of the examination techniques available and the dynamics of experience.

Once performing aircrew duties, the airman receives periodic health assessments. Again, the frequency and level of examination is dependent on the nature of the crew duties performed. The flight surgeon can have a major impact during this periodic examination by taking advantage of the opportunity to advise on wellness and to institute a program of perspective

health. Should the examination reveal the early signs of preclinical disease, active steps can be initiated to ameliorate the process.

In assessing the balance between the public safety and the desires of the crewmember when disease becomes evident, it is frequently necessary to turn to the appropriate clinical specialist. A broad body of knowledge exists regarding the diseases of various body systems and their impact on continued activities in flying. This data is reviewed in the chapters that follow.

SUGGESTED READING LIST

1. Ad Hoc Committee on S-Hemoglobinopathies. The S-Hemoglobinopathies: An Evaluation of Their Status in the Armed Forces. National Academy of Sciences, National Research Council, Washington, DC, 1973.
2. Adler, H.F.: Dysbarism. Aeromedical Review 1-64. United States Air Force School of Aerospace Medicine, Brooks Air Force Base, Texas, 1964.
3. Air Force Occupational Safety and Health

401

(AFOSH) Standard 161-10. Health Hazards Control for Laser Radiation. Washington, D.C., Department of the Air Force, May 30, 1980.

4. Aircraft Instrument and Cockpit Lighting by Red or White Light. Conference Proceedings No. 26, Advisory Group for Aerospace Research and Development (AGARD)/North Atlantic Treaty Organization (NATO), Washington, DC, Oct., 1967.

5. American College of Cardiology: Cardiovascular problems associated with aviation safety. Am. J. Cardiol., 36:573–628, 1975.

6. American Medical Association: Neurological and neurosurgical conditions associated with aviation safety. Arch. Neurol. 36:729–812, 1979.

7. American National Standards for the Safe Use of Lasers. ANSI-Z136.1, 1976. New York, American National Standards Institute, 1976.

8. Armstrong, H.G., and Heim, J.W.: The effect of flight on the middle ear. JAMA, 109:416, 1937.

9. Brown, F.M.: Vertigo due to increased middle ear pressure: Six-year experience of the Aeromedical Consultation Service. Aerospace Med., 42:999, 1971.

10. Carr, J.E.: Behavior therapy and the treatment of flight phobia. Aviat. Space Environ. Med., 49:1115–1119, 1978.

11. Dalessio, D.J.: Wolff's Headache and Other Head Pain. 3d Ed. New York, Oxford University Press, 1972.

12. Devine, J.M.: Navy flight surgery: From biplanes to Skylab. U.S. Navy Med., 69:21–25, March, 1978.

13. Dhenin, G. (ed.): Aviation Medicine. London, Tri-Med Books Ltd., 1978.

14. Fregly, A.R.: Handbook of Sensory Physiology. Berlin, Springer-Verlag, 1974.

15. Gangarosa, E.J., Kendrick, M.A., Lowenstein, M.D., Merson, M.H., et al.: Global travel and travelers' health. Aviat. Space Environ. Med., 51(7):265–270, 1980.

16. Gastaut, H., and Broughton, F.: Epileptic Seizures: Clinical and Electrographic Features, Diagnosis and Treatment. Springfield, Illinois, Charles C Thomas, 1972.

17. Jones, D.R.: Suicide by aircraft. Aviat. Space Environ. Med., 48:454–455, 1977.

18. Kazarian, L.E., and Belk, W.F.: Flight Physical Standards of the 1980s: Spinal Column Considerations. Aeromedical Research Laboratory Technical Report 79–74. AMRL Wright-Patterson AFB, OH, 1979

19. Mohler, S.R.: Medication and Flying: A Pilot's Guide. Boston, Boston Publishing Co., 1982.

20. Moses, R.A.: Adler's Physiology of the Eye, Clinical Applications. St. Louis, C.V. Mosby Co., 1981.

21. McFarland, R.A.: Human Factors in Air Transportation. New York, McGraw-Hill Book Co., 1953.

22. Orford, R.R., and Carter, E.T.: Preemployment and periodic physical examination of airline pilots at the Mayo Clinic, 1939–1974. Aviat. Space Environ. Med., 47:180–184, 1976.

23. Perry, C.J.G. (ed.): Psychiatry in Aerospace Medicine. International Psychiatry Clinics 4. Boston, Little, Brown and Co., 1967.

24. Pitts, D.G.: Visual Illusions and Aircraft Accidents. SAM-TR-67-28, United States Air Force School of Aerospace Medicine, Brooks Air Force Base, Texas, April, 1967.

25. Plum, F., and Posner, J.B.: Diagnosis of Stupor and Coma. Philadelphia, F.A. Davis Co., 1972.

26. Procedures for Testing Color Vision. Report of Working Group #41, Committee on Vision, National Academy of Sciences, National Research Council. Washington, D.C., National Academy Press, 1981.

27. Rayman, R.B.: Clinical Aviation Medicine. New York, Vantage Press, Inc., 1982.

28. Sarnoff, C.A.: Medical Aspects of Flying Motivation. United States Air Force School of Aviation Medicine, Brooks Air Force Base, Texas, 1957.

29. Sours, J.E., Ehrlich, R.E., and Phillips, P.B.: The fear of flying syndrome: A reappraisal. Aerospace Med., 35:156–166, 1964.

30. Tredici, T.J.: Screening and management of glaucoma in flying personnel. Milit. Med., 145:1, 1980.

31. United States Naval Flight Surgeons Manual. GPO, Washington, D.C., 1978.

32. Ursano, R.J., and Jones, D.R.: The individual's vs. the organization's doctor: Value conflicts in psychiatric aeromedical evaluation. Aviat. Space Environ. Med., 52:704–706, 1981.

33. Wulfeck, J.W., et al: Vision in Military Aviation. WADC Technical Report 58–399, Wright Air Development Center, Wright-Patterson Air Force Base, Ohio, Nov. 1958.

34. Youngling, E.W., et al: Feasibility Study to Predict Combat Effectiveness for Selected Military Roles: Fighter Pilot Effectiveness. Report No. MDC E1634. St. Louis, Missouri, McDonnell-Douglas Corporation, April 29, 1977.

Chapter *13*

Aircrew Health Care Maintenance

Russell B. Rayman

And it is well to superintend the sick to make them well, to care for the healthy to keep them well, also to care for one's own self, so as to observe what is seemly.

HIPPOCRATES

What Hippocrates said centuries ago has as much relevance to today's practitioners of aerospace medicine as it did to the healers of ancient days. The aeromedical specialist is charged not only with the care of the aviator, but also with the prevention of illness and injury. To fulfill this obligation, the flight surgeon must fully understand the aviation environment and the physiologic stresses it imposes on aircrew members. Forearmed with this knowledge, that which was prescribed by Hippocrates can be fulfilled: to care for the aviator when he is not well and to keep him healthy when he is well.

MEDICAL ASPECTS OF AIRCREW SELECTION

Historical Background

In the skies over Flanders Fields, Verdun, and other World War I battlegrounds, most Allied losses were due not to enemy fire but rather to poor techniques in the selection of airmen and practically nonexistent physical standards. This stark re-

alization prompted the founding of aeromedical laboratories such as the one at Mineola, Long Island, New York in 1917 to investigate human factors as a cause of aircraft losses and to establish physical standards for aviators. These early flight surgeons working in primitive laboratories revolutionized aircrew selection by establishing the first aircrew physical standards. Almost immediately, the number of losses over the battlefields of France, Germany, and the Low Countries was significantly reduced.

These early physical standards were only the beginning. Through the years, with the astounding worldwide proliferation of the airlines, general aviation, and military aviation and with the increasing experience of practitioners of aviation medicine, selection techniques and physical standards have continued to evolve.

One of the original selection tests that has survived to this day, introduced by Major Raymond F. Longacre in 1930, is the Adaptability Rating for Military Aeronautics (ARMA). The ARMA is a psychologic/personality inventory interview required of all United States Air Force aircrew candidates and is conducted by a flight surgeon. During this interview, the flight surgeon tries to determine the candidate's suitability for aviation by evaluating background, mental status, emotional stability, and motivation. Although the validity of this technique has not been proved, it is still an integral part of all Air Force aircrew candidate physical examinations and has been for over a half a century.

As World War II approached and it became clear to many that airpower would play a decisive role in the conflict, there was renewed interest in aircrew selection in overseas countries, as well as in the United States. By this time, a large number of test batteries had been designed and adopted by flying organizations according to their own needs and their faith in the validity of these tests. In general, aircrew selection was governed not only by physical examination, but also by composite scores of psychologic and personality testing, general intelligence, emotional stability, and mechanical aptitude. In the United States Army, composite scores of the test battery were calculated and graded 1 through 9; the higher the score, the better. This system was known as the Standard 9, or Stanine. There appeared to be a direct correlation between Stanine score and the successful completion of pilot training.

Curiously, no giant steps have been taken since World War II in the area of aircrew selection. For example, the United States Air Force still depends very much on a paper-pencil general intelligence test, the Air Force Officer Qualification Test (AFOQT), which was adopted in 1955. Certainly, most flying organizations now have minimum educational requirements and have adopted newer aptitude testing techniques and test batteries. These tests, however, have basic similarities to their predecessors and, like their predecessors,

purport to select those candidates with the greatest potential for success in flight training. Unfortunately, we continue to be frustrated in our quest for an aircrew selection test battery that is convincingly valid.

Conversely, aviation medicine has taken great strides in the development of the aircrew physical examination. Our diagnostic armamentarium is now much more sophisticated, and we have a much clearer understanding of what causes in-flight pilot incapacitation, the adverse effects of illness and medication on pilot performance and flying safety, and the stresses of flight on the human organism. Consequently, we are now better able to detect and eliminate those individuals who, for medical reasons, are unsuitable for a career in aviation.

Cogent reasons clearly exist for an effective aircrew selection process: to preserve flying safety, to select those whose promise of a successful career is highest, to eliminate those unsuitable for aviation, and to minimize economic loss because of student pilot wastage. It has been estimated that of every 1000 applicants for flight training, 750 will be rejected for medical or psychologic reasons and 100 will be rejected due to flying deficiencies, leaving 150 candidates who will be able to complete the course successfully.[1]

Aircrew Selection by Job Analysis and Testing

Although aircrew selection has long been of concern to flight surgeons and has been the subject of countless professional inquiries through the years, one needs only to consult Dr. Ross McFarland's classic textbook, *Human Factors in Air Transportation*, written 30 years ago, to understand the basic tenets as well as the inherent complexities of this subject. It was this pioneer of aviation medicine who recognized that the first step in the selection process of pilots is job or task analysis. That is, aircrew duties must be subjected to close scrutiny to identify their requirements in respect to reactions and responses, stresses, and component task skills. Next, those aptitudes must be identified that would be most desirable in accomplishing each task in question. The final step is to devise tests that could then be used to identify flight training applicants who are best endowed with these aptitudes because they presumably would be the most likely to succeed.

Although this sequitur, at first glance, appears to be ingenuously logical, it is fraught with pitfalls that, to this day, remain unresolved. For example, one can never be certain that the job analysis is entirely accurate because the analysis itself is based on subjectivity, which, in turn, invites differences. For example, if two pilots, current in the same aircraft, were asked to analyze their cockpit responsibilities, there undoubtedly would be differences of opinion in substance as well as degree. Likewise, there would probably be inconsistencies if the pilots also were asked what they considered to be desirable traits or aptitudes to accomplish successfully their tasks. Finally, even if pilots unanimously agreed on job analysis and desirable aptitudes, how does one validate those tests or procedures used to select aircrew applicants? The validation of selection tests is very difficult regardless of whether the criterion is the successful completion of flight training or the "success" of a flying career, perhaps over a 5- to 10-year period. Thus, the complexities of aircrew selection become painfully clear.

Over the past 65 years, various types of selection tests have been designed, adopted, and administered by flying organizations. These have included general intelligence, mechanical, psychologic, and personality tests.

Mechanical/apparatus testing was given a great deal of attention in previous decades. Pilot candidates were evaluated with a multitude of contraptions—some inge-

nious, others primitive—for reaction time, stick and rudder control, instrument interpretation, and two-hand coordination tests, to mention only a few. A lot of time and effort was devoted to this science in the belief that there was a positive correlation of apparatus scores and training outcome. In recent years, however, there appears to have been a decline in interest in these tests, due, in part, to the cost of purchasing large numbers of expensive devices, as well as the administrative costs of bringing student applicants to their locations.

A more realistic method of flying aptitude testing may be the use of simulators or Link trainers, which the British Royal Air Force first utilized in 1941. Another useful program was adopted by the United States Air force in recent years in which pilot applicants are required to complete an introductory flying course in a single-engine propeller aircraft. In this way, candidates with a flying deficiency can be identified early and eliminated before entering undergraduate pilot training.

Flight surgeons generally agree that certain personality types are better adapted than others for cockpit duties. For this reason, aircraft selection usually includes some type of personality inventory or evaluation. Those personality traits that are desirable for pilots were first described by McFarland almost four decades ago and are probably still relevant today. Among those desirable traits McFarland identified were mental ability, mechanical comprehension, judgment, alertness, observational ability, motor skill, emotional control, character, and leadership. Other investigators have found high correlations with intelligence, emotional stability, conscientiousness, and self-control.

Another method utilized by some flying organizations, the RAF in particular, is the group interaction technique, in which aircrew candidates are placed into groups and given problems to solve that require joint cooperation and coordination. By observing the group, skilled observers can identify those with leadership qualities, those who can function under stress, and those who effectively participate in problem solving. It is believed that these individuals would be eminently qualified for flight training, although not all flying organizations subscribe to this selection approach.

As an aside, a large American aircraft company recently published a comprehensive and detailed report outlining a program for the selection of fighter pilots who would be most effective in air-to-air combat.[2] The report identifies 45 attributes that are essential to the most combat-effective air-to-air fighter pilot. The report further describes what testing is available to identify those applicants with these attributes. This study, although new and innovative, really is based on the original principles of job analysis that McFarland described many years ago.

Although much controversy remains regarding the efficacy and validity of the various test batteries, most of them, to some degree, have predictive value in the identification of pilot candidates who will be successful. Clearly, more research needs to be done in this area. In the meantime, flying organizations must incorporate those testing procedures into their aircrew selection process that are cost-effective and would most efficiently identify aircrewmen who will best accomplish the mission requirements of that flying organization.

PERIODIC MEDICAL ASSESSMENT

Purpose

Although flying organizations may employ different aircrew selection techniques and physical standards, individuals must be in a good state of health to pass any aviation medical department physical examination. With time, however, even healthy aviators will develop illnesses, whether acute or chronic, seri-

ous or benign, as would be expected in any adult population regardless of age or occupation. Because of the requirements of cockpit duties, as well as the obligation of aviation for safety in the air, airmen, to ensure continued good health, are required to have a periodic medical assessment. The purpose of the periodic physical examination is really threefold: flying safety, health of the airman, and mission completion.

Scope

Aviation medical departments worldwide have, to some extent, different aeromedical programs and policies: what constitutes medical grounds for temporary or permanent removal from flying status, how often a periodic examination is required, and what physicians are qualified to administer the examination. This becomes apparent when one studies the policies of the International Civil Aviation Organization (ICAO), the Federal Aviation Administration (FAA), and the military services in the United States and abroad. To explore in detail these differences would not be particularly instructive because what may be policy one day may not be the next as flying organizations must readapt their standards to ever-changing conditions and requirements. Let it suffice to say that medical departments are obligated to establish physical standards tailored to their flying mission, with flying safety an uppermost consideration.

The periodic flight physical examination can be divided into five parts: history and physical examination, dental examination, laboratory procedures, subprofessional consultations, and specialty consultations. The history and physical examination is accomplished by the practitioner, and because of its universality, little need be said other than to repeat that old adage—the physician should do a complete history and physical examination.

Although dental disease is an unlikely cause of in-flight incapacitation (the rare occurrence of aerodontalgia is perhaps the one exception), it is advisable that airmen maintain a healthy dental status. A toothache can cause both considerable discomfort and performance decrement should it occur in flight or in an isolated location where immediate dental care might not be available. There are also military implications in that many aviators who were prisoners of war during the Vietnam War suffered because of preexisting dental disease and practically nonexistent treatment during captivity. Long-term captivity for an airman with dental disease means not only pain, but possibly poor nutrition because of an inability to chew.

Laboratory tests may include a variety of determinations such as a complete blood count and urinalysis, with some medical departments adding to these a fasting blood glucose, serologic evaluation, and lipid profile. Procedures that are often part of the periodic flight physical include chest radiographs, spirometry, electrocardiogram, and electroencephalogram. As is true for so many screening laboratory tests and procedures, there is considerable debate regarding their cost-effectiveness. The chest radiograph is an example. Although the vast majority of chest radiographs taken in conjunction with the flight physical are normal, silent lesions occasionally are found such as a benign or malignant tumor, small pneumothorax, or sarcoid. The expense of the procedure weighed against the number of pathologic conditions detected often causes questions regarding its necessity.

Spirometry is felt to be worthwhile, at least in the United States Air Force, to detect obstructive pulmonary disease, particularly that caused by excessive cigarette smoking. Besides the known pulmonary association of cigarettes with lung cancer and emphysema, there is the aeromedical consideration of increased carbon monoxide levels reducing the oxygen-trans-

port capability of hemoglobin. Hence, an explanation of this factor to the airman should reinforce the usual admonitions against smoking.

Because of the increased awareness of coronary artery disease during the past 10 to 20 years and its possible role in causing sudden in-flight incapacitation, all aviation medical departments require resting and/or stress electrocardiograms. Differences occur not only in the frequency of testing but also the method of stressing and the interpretation of results. Clearly, the main reason for a periodic electrocardiogram is to detect latent coronary artery disease.

Several medical departments require an electroencephalogram only on entry into flight training to identify those applicants with epileptogenic activity. Another reason is to have on record a baseline tracing that can be used for comparison should the individual sustain head trauma at some time in the future.

The paraprofessional portion of the examination is that which can be done by a technician. The physician's time need be spent only in the interpretation of abnormal findings. Measurements may include blood pressure and pulse determinations, audiometry, and several tests of vision. Because of the singular importance of vision in flight, the eye examination should include testing for near and far visual acuity, phoria-tropia-diplopia, accommodation, depth perception, visual fields, and color and night vision. Tonometry to rule out glaucoma is also advisable for older airmen.

Specialty consultations must be available in the event that illness is suspected, the diagnosis and treatment of which is beyond the expertise of the flight surgeon. Such consultation is particularly useful if the specialists are also aeromedical examiners or, at least, have had some training in the principles of aerospace medicine.

Effectiveness

The periodic flight physical examination can be considered a form of secondary preventive medicine, as defined by Lilienfeld:

> Secondary preventive measures are designed to detect the disease at a sufficiently early stage to permit intervention in order to decelerate the rate of progression of the disease, and to prevent complications, sequelae, disability, and premature mortality.[3]

To this definition the flight surgeon might add, "to remove from flying status, either temporarily or permanently, those aviators with illness which poses an added risk to flying safety."

Because the periodic physical examination really consists of a test battery (i.e., professional and paraprofessional examination and a number of laboratory procedures), it can be considered a form of multiphasic screening. Multiphasic screening has been a favorite, although controversial, subject of preventive medicine specialists in recent years. All of the arguments, pro and con, basically center on cost-effectiveness, that is, one questions whether, with limited health care delivery funds and finite physician time available, sufficient pathologic conditions are detected and effectively treated to make screening programs worthwhile.

For example, a study was done 11 years ago in the United States Air Force's Strategic Air Command to study the efficacy of the periodic flight physical examination. It was found that in a 1-year period, 28,000 physical examinations were administered, with each examination consuming 30 minutes of a physician's time and a total of 200 minutes of time if laboratory procedures, dental examinations, and administration were included. The authors found that very little disease was detected by the physician; rather, the majority of the pathologic disorders were discovered by those measurable portions of the examination, such as blood pressure, radiography, electrocardiography, blood

and urine tests, and visual and auditory testing, which can be done by a technician. Hence, it was concluded that too much time and money are given to the flight physical examination as we know it and that it would be far more economical to include only those measurable screening tests that can be performed by a technician.

Even if one accepts this, however, the flight surgeon reaps other benefits from the physical examination, which are unquantifiable in terms of cost-effectiveness yet clearly important. First, it affords the physician the opportunity to spend a little time in the quiet and privacy of the office. This time can be well spent reviewing the aviator's medical history, particularly the interval history since the last examination and just talking with the aviator. During these minutes, the flight surgeon can get to know the airman a little better and possibly gain better insight into his personal situation. If given the opportunity, airmen will often confide in the flight surgeon various problems, either relating to health, family, or some other difficulties affecting job performance. The flight surgeon has a chance not only to intercede if it is appropriate, but also to enhance rapport with the airman, something that is very important to any aviation medicine program. Furthermore, in this day of emphasis on healthy life-styles and health education, the flight surgeon has the opportunity to help the aviator identify poor health habits and to suggest ways of correcting such habits. For these reasons, the periodic flight physical examination is important and should continue to be an integral part of any aerospace medicine program.

THE FEMALE CREWMEMBER

Historical Background

The exigencies of World War II led to the creation of the famous Women's Army Service Pilots (WASPS) as a part of United States Army Aviation. Because every male

crewmember was needed for combat assignments, this first group of female pilots
was tasked with ferrying military aircraft
within the United States and to overseas
theaters. The saga of the WASPS and their
success is now history. By ferrying
hundreds of aircraft and logging thousands of hours, they clearly demonstrated
that women could accomplish cockpit responsibilities. In spite of their illustrious
record, however, women have been admitted to the ranks of primary crewmember, in commercial as well as military aircraft, only in recent years. Even then, their
admission was greeted with some degree
of reluctance and skepticism. Although
some of this skepticism may be emotional,
questions must be addressed before unrestricted admission to the cockpit will be
the modus operandi for aviation. The controversial issues of women in the cockpit
include anthropometric conformity to
standard cockpit design, ability to withstand the stresses of flight, and pregnancy
and menses.

At this time, the aerospace medicine literature has devoted few pages to these subjects. It is to be expected, however, that
more investigation will be accomplished
as more experience is accrued in the coming years and as the military and the commercial airlines gain confidence in their
selection procedures of women crewmembers. The employment of the full-fledged
female aviator is still new, and the search
continues for acceptable selection procedures and physical standards for women.
We will probably continue to grapple with
this problem in the coming years until
there is full confidence in and unqualified
acceptance of the military and commercial
aviatrix.

Man-Machine Interface

The science of aviation anthropometrics
was born in the early aeromedical research
laboratories just prior to World War II. It
was apparent that as cockpits were becoming more complicated and in-flight tasks

more demanding, aeronautic engineers
would have to take into consideration
man's physical limitations. Consequently,
cockpits, as well as flight clothing and life-
support equipment, were designed to accommodate the physical size and strength
characteristics of men between the 5th and
95th percentiles. All of these activities
came under the rubric, man-machine interface, which gives a subtle clue that
those physical characteristics of women,
size and strength in particular, were probably given little or no attention.

The average man is taller, heavier, and
stronger than the average woman. A number of studies have clearly demonstrated
that women have about 60% of the physical strength of men.[4] Another study indicated that the maximum force of a significant percentage of women would fall
below the design criteria of certain aircraft
controls (see Table 13-1). Although this
disparity may not be true for all types of
airplanes, the implication is that under
certain extreme conditions, some women
would not have sufficient strength to control the aircraft.

Over the years, cockpits have been designed to accommodate men anthropo-
metrically, that is, sitting height, reach,
and buttocks-to-knee distance, in the 5th
to 95th percentiles. Surveys of anthropometrics of women reveal that a significant

Table 13-1. Percent of Subjects Whose Maximum Force Was Below MIL-F-8782B Design Criteria

Control	Criteria kg	Criteria lb	Percent Below Criteria Males	Percent Below Criteria Females
Stick forward	34	75	0	28
Stick back	23	50	0	40
Stick left	16	35	5	95
Stick right	16	35	50	100
Left rudder	82	180	7	11
Right rudder	82	180	0	5

From McDaniel, J.W.: Male and female strength ca-
pabilities for operating aircraft controls. Preprints of the
Scientific Program of the Aerospace Medical Association
Meeting, May 4-7, 1981, p. 12.

proportion of them, fall below the 5th percentile of men in all measured parameters. For example, 77% of women fall below the 5th percentile for men in sitting height and 27% fall below the 5th percentile in buttocks-to-knee length.[5] Hence, a significant percentage of women cannot be accommodated in today's cockpits. This is not due to any feminine deficiency, however, as much as to the engineering design and configuration of aircraft cockpits, which heretofore took into account only male physical characteristics. The solution, therefore, can be found in aeronautic engineering textbooks. Simply stated, if the military services and the airline companies see that it is in their interests to employ larger numbers of female crewmembers, engineers will consider the physical attributes of women and design cockpits accordingly.

The Stresses of Flight

The physiologic stresses of flight have been well defined through several decades of intense research. For the most part, however, the effects of these stresses and the limitations of human beings have focused on male crewmembers. We are only now starting to examine how well women can tolerate these stresses and how the two sexes compare. Undoubtedly, a great body of literature will come to light in the near future on the female crewmember's tolerance of acceleration, hypoxia, decompression sickness, circadian rhythm, and noise and vibration, as well as a host of other physiologic stresses associated with aviation.

As an example of such research, the United States Air Force School of Aerospace Medicine (USAFSAM) has conducted studies on women and their tolerance to acceleration. These studies have revealed no evidence indicating that women are in any way inferior to men in G tolerance.[6]

These studies and others like it are now in progress in various research facilities around the world. More information will be forthcoming as an increasing number of female pilots are admitted to the cockpit and as their performance is observed. Even at this early stage, many experienced flight surgeons believe that a normal, healthy woman can tolerate the physiologic stresses of flight just as well as a normal, healthy man and that in good time this will be clearly demonstrated.

Menses and Pregnancy

Menses and pregnancy are the two physiologic processes that clearly separate women from men. Because of their usual indispositions, women's fitness for cockpit duties has been questioned. There are those who argue that dysmenorrhea is very common and can cause excessive absenteeism. Furthermore, there is the possibility that pain relief can be obtained only by medication, which might be disqualifying for flying duties. In support of this position, a study of 200 stewardesses indicated that 48% of them reported a change in menses—increased or decreased flow and/or pelvic pain and congestion—which was attributed to stress and internal desynchronization due to disruption of circadian rhythm.[7] At this time, however, there is no solid evidence that menses causes performance decrement or increased absenteeism among female pilots.

Many questions regarding the pregnant pilot remain unanswered. What undesirable effects will the stresses of flight cause for the pregnant woman and the fetus and when should a pregnant crewmember stop flying? Most authorities agree that the physiologic stresses of flight in normal airline operations are so slight that they cannot really threaten a fetus. Even the mild hypoxia caused by cabin altitudes of 1524 to 2134 m will cause no adverse effects. Hence, physiologically, a pregnant woman with a normal pregnancy should be able to fly safely from the time of conception to the eve of delivery. In aviation, however, there are other considerations, especially performance decrement, which demand disqualification from the cockpit at some time during the course of the pregnancy. For example, most pregnant women will normally experience nausea and vomiting, increased fatigue, and emotional lability, not to mention an increase in size and weight. Although the time for removal is somewhat arbitrary and at the discretion of the many airline companies, flight attendants are usually disqualified between 20 and 27 weeks of gestation; primary crewmembers are removed at the time of conception or shortly thereafter.

Regarding military aircraft that subject crews to special physiologic stresses such as low barometric pressures, in-flight decompressions, and accelerative forces, it would be prudent to disqualify the pregnant crewmember at the time of conception because we have no knowledge at this time of the ill effects these would have on the conceptus.

MEDICAL DISABILITY

Temporary and Permanent Disability

Regardless of the stringent selection procedures for flight training and of the number of applicants that are disqualified because of preexisting disease, it can be expected that most aviators over the years will develop illness necessitating either temporary or permanent disqualification from flying duty or a medical waiver. Because aviators cannot be expected to maintain perfect health throughout their careers, flying organizations must employ some system that permits these deviations while compromising neither flying safety nor the health of the aviator. Financial factors also cannot be ignored in that permanent disqualification and pilot wastage will create enormous dollar losses in both commercial and military aviation. Disqualification and waiver policies necessarily differ among flying organizations because of both the differences of the aircraft flown and air operations. Although

every flying organization has evolved its own rules and regulations governing these matters, in general, all of them have stringent entry physical examination requirements, with some degree of relaxation once the student crewmember or new employee is trained and operational.

In most cases, temporary disqualifications are for minor, self-limiting illness, illness requiring the temporary use of medication considered hazardous to the aviation environment (e.g., antihistamines, sedatives or analgesics), and treatable illness wherein cure is expected. In any event, once the condition is in remission and there are no sequelae that pose a threat to flying safety, it would be in order for the aeromedical specialist to recommend a return to flying status.

On the other hand, if the disease is of a more serious nature, permanent disqualification must be considered. Examples might include coronary artery disease, uncorrectable loss of visual acuity, or untreatable carcinoma. Again, all flying organizations determine those policies that govern permanent disqualification based on the type of aircraft flown and the flying mission.

Medical Waiver System

In some cases, crewmembers may develop illnesses that can be effectively treated, albeit with a potential for progression. Glaucoma, glomerulonephritis, and hypertension are classic examples. Clearly, airmen with illnesses such as these can be granted medical waivers for flying duty as long as the defect is static and the disease itself or the treatment pose no threat to flying safety and there is assurance of periodic follow-up. On the other hand, if the disease process progresses, permanent disqualification from the cockpit would have to be considered. A sensible waiver policy and administrative mechanism tailored to the needs of every flying organization is necessary, without which there is the risk of eliminating airmen unnecessarily and unfairly.

The military services and the FAA have their own medical and administrative procedures, policies, and regulations for processing temporary and permanent disqualification and medical waiver requests. Let it suffice to say that in the military services, no formal appeal process exists should the airman not agree with the recommendation of the flight surgeon; that is, the aeromedical services makes its recommendation to operational commanders regarding disqualification, and in practically all cases, these recommendations are not countermanded. In the case of the FAA, however, a system of appeals exists whereby individuals denied medical certification can petition the FAA or the National Transportation Safety Board for an exemption. These procedures are described in greater detail in Chapter 26.

Consultation Services

Occasionally, airmen develop complex or obscure medical conditions for which continued flying status is questionable. To make a diagnosis and/or recommend aeromedical disposition, the United States Army, Navy, and Air Force have established their respective aeromedical consultation services. These consultation services are staffed by physicians with specialty training, as well as considerable training and experience in aerospace medicine. Crewmembers who are disqualified for flying duties because of complex or obscure medical conditions are referred from bases worldwide to these centers for diagnostic evaluation and recommendations for flying status. Over the years, the staffs of these consultation services have examined thousands of airmen with a legion of diseases involving all body systems. They have, because of their expertise in aviation medicine, saved the government a considerable sum of money by recommending a return to flying status for many

airmen who otherwise would have been permanently disqualified.

OPERATIONAL STRESS

Since the infancy of aviation medicine, the physiologic stresses of flight have been the subject of intensive research in laboratories around the world. This great interest has been prompted by the realization that acceleration, hypoxia, vibration, and decreased barometric pressure, alone or in combination, pose a threat to flying safety, as well as to the personal safety of airmen. Through years of diligent research efforts, aerospace medicine scientists have developed excellent life-support equipment and systems to minimize this threat. Yet, even with these countermeasures, accidents and incidents continue to occur because of man's inability to fully accommodate himself to the extraterrestrial environment. It is for this reason that aviation organizations seek healthy, fit aircrew members whose constitutions are most resistant to the physiologic stresses of flight.

Acceleration

Although any type of aircraft can subject its crew to accelerative forces, we think more of aerobatics, crop-dusting, or high-performance military operations when discussing significant $+G_z$ or $-G_z$ stress. $+G_z$ affects primarily the cardiovascular system and can cause blackout or loss of consciousness—both clearly undesirable in flight—by decreasing blood flow to the brain. Countermeasures include the use of an anti-G suit and the proper performance of the M-1 maneuver, the latter giving an additional 1 to 2 G's of protection. With $-G_z$, blood is accelerated headward, causing stimulation of the carotid sinus and possible incapacitation by inducing various degrees of heart block. Unfortunately, there are no effective countermeasures for this type of acceleration other than the avoidance of $-G_z$ maneuvers such as outside loops.

Accelerative forces are potentially incapacitating, although countermeasures are protective to some degree. Because $+G_z$ and $-G_z$ acceleration primarily affect the cardiovascular system, it is extremely important that individuals who fly G-inducing aircraft be free of cardiovascular disease. This is one reason why the cardiovascular system is given such intense scrutiny during initial and periodic physical examinations.

Hypoxia

Because most aircraft cockpits do not pressurize to sea level pressures during normal operations, crewmembers are frequently hypoxic to some degree. Healthy individuals, however, should still be able to perform their cockpit tasks without difficulty as long as they are not exposed to altitudes above 3048 m. At higher altitudes, everyone will develop hypoxic symptoms that can cause some degree of performance decrement. Crewmembers are well protected from hypoxia by sophisticated life-support systems, the foremost being the pressurized cabin. Furthermore, oxygen masks with continuous-flow or pressure-demand systems are commonplace in commercial and military aviation.

There is little question that a normal, healthy crewman can tolerate mildly hypoxic environments without experiencing a significant performance decrement and without jeopardizing health. The same cannot be said, however, for individuals with cardiopulmonary disease. For example, in an hypoxic state, the coronary vessels must dilate to allow more blood to reach the oxygen-starved myocardium. The coronary vessels of individuals with coronary artery disease, however, do not dilate well, and this imposes an added burden on the heart muscle, which can have serious implications. Likewise, individuals with diseased lungs, such as those with emphysema, cannot absorb a normal complement of oxygen even under sea level conditions, and at altitude, oxygen absorption would be even more compromised.

Noise and Vibration

The noise emanating from any aircraft engine, jet or propeller, will eventually cause acoustic trauma if an unprotected individual is exposed for a sufficiently long time. This places not only aircrews at risk but also the large work force normally employed in the various shops and activities in the vicinity of the flight line. Because of the potential for developing partial or complete deafness due to acoustic trauma, aviation medical departments conduct hearing conservation programs, the objective of which is to prevent hearing loss. Although these programs may vary somewhat in design, they are basically alike, with protocols that require the identification of flight-line and in-flight hazardous noise areas, the issuing of earplugs and/or muffs to those individuals at risk, and the administration of baseline and follow-up audiograms. Generally, audiologists agree that some form of ear protection is advisable if noise intensity levels exceed 85 db.

It has been well established that vibration between 1 and 12 Hz will cause performance decrement in the cockpit. For example, low-frequency vibration can induce motion sickness, fatigue, shortness of breath, and abdominal and chest pain. Furthermore, considerable blurring of the instrument panel can make accurate reading of the dials extremely difficult. For these reasons, aeronautic engineers have gone to great lengths in designing aircraft to eliminate or at least minimize potentially hazardous vibration.

Decreased Barometric Pressure

As one gains altitude from the Earth's surface, the barometric pressure decreases accordingly from a sea level value of 760 mm Hg to the vacuum of space. Because of this natural phenomenon, man is at risk, if without adequate protection, of becoming hypoxic or of developing decompression sickness and barotrauma. Decompression sickness manifests itself in various forms, causing symptoms by bubble formation in the body fluids. Because significant bubble formation is unusual below altitudes of 5486 m, decompression sickness is rarely encountered in those aircraft normally pressurized to 1524 to 2438 m. The risk is far greater in military aircraft, which fly with higher cabin altitudes. The symptoms of evolved gas decompression sickness are many and include joint pain (bends), chokes, central nervous system disturbances, and neurocirculatory collapse. Hence, this syndrome is of great aeromedical significance not only because it can cause in-flight incapacitation, but also because it can be lethal.

Besides the ill effects of evolved gas, crewmembers can suffer serious discomfort if a pressure differential exists between the bony cavities, for example, the sinuses or middle ear, and the ambience. These forms of barotrauma can occur with any change in altitude, although they are most commonly associated with descent. The inability for gas to freely exchange can incapacitate the crewmember by causing excruciating pain.

Circadian Rhythm

With the advent of long-range aircraft capable of crossing oceans and continents without refueling, the term circadian rhythm has become part of the aerospace medicine vocabulary. Today, it is not at all unusual for international flights to cross as many as five to ten time zones. Hence, an aircrew may depart on a flight en route to a destination with an 8-hour time difference. As a result, the sleep/wake/meal time cycle at the destination will not be synchronized with that of the crew. This desynchrony can result in some degree of personal discomfort and inefficiency at the destination because of fatigue during the day and wakefulness at night, commonly referred to as jet lag. As a rule of thumb, it takes approximately 1 day per time zone crossed to fully recover from jet lag.

It is well known that the above phenomenon is not just a psychologic idiosyncrasy but rather is due to diurnal biochemical reactions that occur at set times during the day and night. Therefore, when suddenly going to another part of the world with a significant time difference, the diurnal reactions are not in harmony with the time of day or night at the destination.

The physical and psychologic problems of circadian desynchrony are matters of special concern for those crossing numerous time zones for purposes other than recreation. Politicians, statesmen, athletes, business persons, and military personnel can all be affected by desynchronization, resulting in lower efficiency, poor decision making, and compromised negotiation ability. For most people, studies have established that fewer problems occur with movement across the time zones from east to west. More time zones can be crossed with the same degree of physiologic disruption as going from west to east. For a few people, it would appear that the circadian cycle cannot be reversed when a set number of time zones have been crossed from west to east. For those individuals, recovery from desynchronization can be significantly prolonged. It is as if the body clock can only be reset in one direction, as in a clock that can only be turned clockwise for resetting.

Temperature and Humidity

With the development of modern environmental systems, cockpit temperature and humidity are reasonably well controlled in commercial aircraft; however, the same cannot be said for many types of military aircraft. Cockpits with poor environmental control are frequently hot and dry, causing some degree of dehydration due to fluid loss, which can result in subjective discomfort and performance decrement. The stresses of cockpit heat are particularly threatening to military crews operating in tropical or desert climates. It is not at all unusual for pilots to spend 15 to 20 minutes in preflight readiness of their aircraft in a hot revetment area and then to sit in the cockpit wearing cumbersome flying equipment and without the benefit of air conditioning for another 30 minutes while completing checklists, taxiing, and arming prior to takeoff. Pilots frequently report that they are wringing wet from perspiration under such circumstances. Then, temperature control in flight is notoriously poor in many fighter aircraft, causing further heat buildup during low-level or gunnery-range operations. The solution to the problem is improved engineering of environmental systems, which must come with future technologic advances.

Life-Support Equipment

Great technologic advances have occurred in life-support equipment over the years, without which flying operations as we know it would not be possible. Nevertheless, the benefits reaped are partially offset by the penalties, which, in the present state of the art, cannot be obviated. Some of the equipment is bulky and cumbersome, causing restriction of movement as well as heat retention and excessive perspiration—a significant imposition, particularly in hot, humid weather. These are special burdens in military aviation because a shirt-sleeves environment is the rule in commercial aircraft.

The fighter pilot's life-support equipment includes a helmet, visor, oxygen mask, anti-G suit, and survival vest, which are worn over the standard Nomex flight suit. It is easy to understand, therefore, how a buildup of body heat can occur, particularly when it takes as long as 30 minutes to do the preflight tasks, start the engines, taxi, arm, and take off. Another penalty pilots pay is restriction of visibility and limitation of movement of the head and neck due to the helmet/mask combi-

nation. This can be most critical in aerial combat maneuvers because scanning the skies and recognizing enemy aircraft early is a sine qua non of success in such operations. Furthermore, because the neck muscles must bear the entire weight of the helmet/oxygen mask combination, they tend to fatigue with repetitive G maneuvers.

For high-flying aircraft that normally operate at altitudes above 15,240 m, full- or partial-pressure suits must be worn. Although these suits can be lifesaving in the event of rapid decompression or ejection at high altitudes, they can cause considerable difficulties for pilots who must wear them—heat buildup, restriction of vision, and impaired movement of the head and limbs, to cite only a few problems.

A relatively new addition to life-support systems is the chemical defense ensemble, the purpose of which is to protect airmen on the ground, as well as in flight should an enemy utilize chemical weapons. These suits provide excellent protection, but, like the pressure suit, they restrict vision and movement, although their greatest liability is heat retention. Today, scientists are avidly continuing the quest for an improved suit that will protect the wearer while imposing minimum penalties.

Fatigue

In view of the many operational stresses of flight, it is clear that all of them induce fatigue to some degree. It can be said perhaps that fatigue is an inherent stress of aviation duties. Erratic schedules, hypoxic environments, noise and vibration, and imperfect environmental systems will eventually take their toll. Therefore, in aviation, fatigue is always a potential threat to flying safety. Although fatigue can be neatly defined as acute, chronic, or cumulative and correlated to some extent with biochemical aberrations, we are yet unable to determine objectively at what point an airman is fatigued enough to cause performance decrement. Therefore, until we can do so, the risk of fatigue must be reduced by preventive measures such as ensuring that reasonable flying schedules and hours logged are maintained and that good food, quarters, and accommodations are provided.

SELF-IMPOSED STRESS

The physiologic stresses of flight, which have been briefly described, in themselves are potentially threatening to flying safety. Even under the most benign conditions, aviation will impose some degree of stress on airmen. Clearly, a healthy individual with a strong constitution will be more resistant to these physiologic stresses and, therefore, will function more efficiently and more safely. Unfortunately, many airmen degrade this resistance by self-imposed, unhealthy behavior patterns and life-styles.

Self-Medication

The side effects of commonly prescribed medications are well known to practicing aeromedical specialists. Because of the potential threat to flying safety, physicians in aerospace medicine are particularly sensitive to the actions of any medication prescribed for airmen. Consider, for example, the many medicines that, in addition to their primary pharmacologic effects, also cause degradation of visual acuity, impaired coordination, increased reaction time, drowsiness, or hypotension. Those that come immediately to mind are the antihistamines, anticholinergics, tranquilizers, sedatives, antihypertensives, and analgesics. It is likely that the vast majority of prescribed drugs would fall into one of these categories.

To discuss the hundreds of various drugs and their side effects routinely prescribed is beyond the scope of this chapter. Suffice it to say that practically every drug in the physician's pharmacopoeia has the potential for some untoward effects that could be detrimental in the cockpit. Because of this potential, it is advisable to temporarily remove airmen from flying duties for the duration of treatment. Although this is a universal principle in aerospace medicine, exceptions can and have been made for those medications that have been judged to be of minimal risk. Medical waivers for these exceptions can be safely granted with the proviso that there is a reasonably close following by the flight surgeon. Examples might include certain antibiotics. thiazides, thyroid medications, and probenecid.

Organizational policies concerning medication and the aviator are somewhat difficult to enforce for several reasons. First, aviators may seek medical care from physicians who are unauthorized by the flying organization or who are not versed in aerospace medicine. Consequently, a physician may prescribe what he considers to be a benign medication, not fully appreciating the in-flight implications. Perhaps a far greater problem is the availability of over-the-counter medicines that have enjoyed a remarkable proliferation over the past two decades. Many of these medicines, which purport to cure colds, headaches, myalgias, as well as a host of other ailments suffered by mankind, are no different than prescription drugs in that they can cause side effects that are undesirable in the cockpit. Crewmembers often purchase over-the-counter drugs for a minor illness without realizing the potential danger of this practice. For this reason, self-medication can be considered one form of self-imposed stress.

It is the physician's obligation to discourage aircrewmen from this practice and to encourage them to report all illnesses to the appropriate medical authority. Only in this way can the proper medication be prescribed and proper follow-up be ensured. The flight surgeon can do this only by aircrew education in the form of talks and bulletins, as well as by establishing good rapport with the aviators of his organization.

Alcohol and Illicit Drug Abuse

The use of illicit drugs has become a global social phenomenon in recent decades, reaching into all socioeconomic strata. Their availability, therefore, extends not only to the underprivileged, but also to the middle and affluent classes, to which most members of the aviation community belong. Hence, with the ubiquity of illicit drugs, as well as their social acceptability, airmen may be tempted to become experimenters or abusers. Today's newspapers and periodicals devote many pages to the subject of drugs and to the "expert" opinions of those who advocate their free and legal usage. Although controversy does exist concerning the short-term and long-term effects of many drugs, as well as the social implications of their use, they are clearly unacceptable in any cockpit. Most illicit drugs cause side effects (drowsiness, euphoria, impaired mentation, hallucinations, and flashbacks) that categorically threaten flying safety. For this reason, legal and moral considerations aside, these substances must be condemned. The aviation medicine practitioner is obligated to have some knowledge of illicit drugs and hallucinogens and to discourage their use among the crewmen in his practice.

Of the various types of self-imposed stress, the misuse of alcohol is unquestionably the leader as the cause of aircraft accidents and loss of life. Although there has been improvement in recent years in the incidence of accidents attributed to alcohol, alcohol-associated fatal accidents in general aviation remain steady at about 16%.[8] It has been well established that even small amounts of alcohol, 20 to 77 mg/dL, can cause significant performance decrement.[9] This study is representative of many others, leading one to the inescapable conclusion that alcohol, even in modest amounts, has no place in the cockpit if flying safety is to be preserved.

Because alcohol is metabolized at an approximate rate of one-third ounce per hour, it may take considerable time for its elimination from the body, particularly if larger amounts are ingested. This is well illustrated in Figure 13–1. Hence, flying organizations have instituted minimum bottle-to-throttle times. Besides the undesirable effects of a high blood alcohol level, there is also the problem of hangover to consider. Even if an individual's blood alcohol level approaches zero, the symptoms of hangover (e.g., headache, impaired mentation, and fatigue) can compromise flying safety.

Smoking

Today's practitioners of medicine are nearing unanimity in their condemnation of cigarette smoking as a leading health hazard. Coronary artery disease, cancer, and chronic lung disease have been convincingly linked to this habit, which has been part of our culture for several hundred years. This should be reason enough for flight surgeons, as practitioners of preventive medicine, to discourage patients from smoking cigarettes. Even if

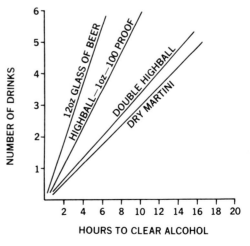

Fig. 13–1. Time required for the body to eliminate alcohol.

public health considerations can be momentarily set aside, can we as aviation medicine specialists answer the question: Is cigarette smoking a threat to flying safety?

Theoretically, it would seem reasonable to assume that under certain circumstances of flight, cigarette smoking is indeed a threat to safety. Carbon monoxide, a by-product of cigarette smoke, has an affinity for hemoglobin approximately 210 times that of oxygen. Hence, carbon monoxide will displace available oxygen from the hemoglobin molecule, reducing the oxygen-carrying capacity of the blood. Even at sea level, therefore, an individual who smokes will have a degree of hypoxia, albeit not necessarily to the point where symptoms will occur. Therefore, airmen who are slightly hypoxic at sea level because of cigarette smoke will be that much less resistant to the hypoxic environment of altitude, and this could be considered a threat to flying safety.

Investigators of the Civil Aeromedical Institute recently reviewed the literature on the subject of the hazards of smoking in aviation, reviewing 2660 fatal general aviation aircraft accidents occurring between 1973 and 1976 to see if they could find any evidence linking cigarette carbon monoxide to accidents.[10] In this study, smoking was not identified as a causal factor but may have contributed to five of the accidents. These investigators, however, concluded that smoking cessation programs should still be pursued to improve health and maintain levels of performance and safety. Therefore, in spite of the negative findings of the above study, the positive recommendations of the authors should be endorsed by all flight surgeons, and aggressive campaigns against cigarette smoking should be pursued.

Improper Nutrition

Only in recent years have the medical community and the public at large become so aware of nutrition and weight control.

As a result, the subject receives an unprecedented amount of space in lay periodicals and in the medical literature. Although there is some controversy about what exactly constitutes a healthy diet—cholesterol-containing foods and heart disease provides a classic example—recommendations can be made that are reasonably tenable scientifically, although precise evidence may still be lacking.

Unfortunately, common sense and the basic principles of proper nutrition are too often forgotten by the public. Many people are frequently attracted to self-acclaimed nutritionists who advocate various crash programs, weight-reducing diets, and food fads that are often unphysiologic. Aeromedical specialists, in their role as preventive medicine specialists, should be strong advocates of acceptable nutritional principles and weight-reduction programs and educate airmen accordingly.

Regarding proper eating habits and cockpit duties, common sense again is the best guide to flying safety. Flight-line eating facilities and in-flight kitchens should be available to airmen day and night, depending on the flying operations. These facilities should be periodically inspected by aeromedical personnel to ensure not only the adequacy of food selection but also sanitation. Airmen should be encouraged to utilize these facilities and to take their usual nourishment before flying, as well as in flight. The practice of having aircrew eat different meals at different times that is required by some flying organizations is to be commended. There continues to be the occasional incident of in-flight "food poisoning" among aircrew.

For those airmen flying aircraft with cabin altitudes well in excess of 1524 to 2438 m, special admonition is warranted. It is advisable for these crews to avoid preflight foods that are highly seasoned, greasy, or gas-forming (for example, cabbage, beans, and soft drinks). These foods can be extremely irritating to the gastrointestinal tract at altitude—recall that a given volume of gas in the gastrointestinal tract will be doubled at 5486 m. These dietary principles are well known to flight surgeons but need to be reviewed occasionally with aircrews.

Health Maintenance

The aviation environment, although not necessarily a hostile one, can be unfriendly to the aviator who is ill-prepared to accomplish his required duties. For this reason, a great amount of time and scientific effort have been directed toward studying the stresses of flight and developing appropriate life-support equipment to offer the airman maximum protection, and in this endeavor we have been eminently successful. The pressurized cabin is undoubtedly the single greatest development in life-support systems achieved during this century. Oxygen systems, flying clothing, temperature and humidity control, anti-G suits, and pressure suits are other contributions to aviation safety. For these advances, the aerospace medicine scientific community must be applauded because they have not only made flying safer, but have extended man's operational capabilities to the outer limits of his physiologic tolerances.

Perhaps we have reached a point wherein self-imposed stress is now more threatening than operational stress. Smoking, alcohol, drugs, obesity, and unhealthy life-styles have become commonplace in our culture. It is to these undesirable habits that physicians must direct their attention to ensure health maintenance of the aviation population. Today, the lay literature abounds with a multitude of recipes for a healthful life. Sometimes the advice is sensible, but too frequently it is not. After one has digested all of this material, it can probably be best summarized in these words: moderation and common sense.

If these rules, long ago given to us by the Greek philosophers, were applied to our daily lives, many of our health-related problems could probably be avoided. Moderation and common sense dictate proper rest prior to flight, proper nutrition, the discreet use of alcohol and tobacco, and regular exercise. As a preventive medicine specialist, the health maintenance of aviators should be an area of high interest for flight surgeons and aviation medical examiners. Besides accomplishing periodic physical examinations as a preventive medicine function, the practitioner must actively participate in health education programs aimed at the flying population. Speaking at flying squadron meetings and consulting and advising commanders or organizational executives, are excellent forums. Some flying organizations have embarked on even more ambitious programs that not only educate, but also intervene in life-style, the most popular example being the coronary artery disease risk factor intervention programs.

It is far too early to tell if these programs will be successful. In any event, they appear to be well founded and commensurate with the basic principles of preventive medicine. It is very much hoped that such intervention programs will reduce the incidence of coronary artery disease, which, in turn. would not only lessen the risk of an in-flight incapacitating event, but would also allow a longer and more productive career for the aviator.

REFERENCES

1. Hartman, B.O.: In Aerospace Medicine. 2nd Ed. Edited by H. W. Randel. Baltimore, Williams & Wilkins Co., 1971, p. 566.
2. Youngling, E.W., et al: Feasibility Study to Predict Combat Effectiveness for Selected Military Roles: Fighter-Pilot Effectiveness. St. Louis, Missouri, McDonnell-Douglas Corp. April, 1977.
3. Lilienfeld, A.: Chronic Diseases. In Preventive Medicine and Public Health. 10th Ed. Edited by P.E. Sartwell. New York, Appleton-Century-Crofts, 1973, p. 498.
4. Baetjer, A.M.: Industrial Health. In Preventive Medicine and Public Health. 10th Ed. Edited by P.E. Sartwell. New York, Appleton-Century-Crofts, 1973, p. 964.
5. McDaniel, J.W.: Male and female strength capabilities for operating aircraft controls. Preprints of the Scientific Program of the Aerospace Med-

ical Association Meeting, AsMA, Washington, DC, May 4–7, 1981, p. 12.

6. Gillingham, K.: Crew Technology Division, United States Air Force School of Aerospace Medicine, Brooks Air Force Base, Texas, June, 1981, personal communication.

7. Iglesias, R., and Terres A.: Disorders of the menstrual cycle in airline stewardesses. Aviat. Space Environ. Med., 51:518–520, 1980.

8. Ryan, L.C., and Mohler, S.R.: Current role of alcohol as a factor in civil aircraft accidents. Aviat. Space Environ. Med., 50:275–279, 1979.

9. Aksnes, E.G.: Effects of small dosages of alcohol upon performance in Link trainer. J. Aviat. Med., 25:680–683, 1954.

10. Dille, J.R., and Linden, M.K.: Effects of tobacco on aviation safety. Aviat. Space Environ. Med., 52:112–115, 1981.

Chapter 14

Clinical Aerospace Cardiology

James R. Hickman, Jr. and George M. McGranahan, Jr.

Consequently, we must select a man who has a responsive, elastic system, capable of compensating for the strain which it will encounter.

LOUIS H. BAUER, M.D.

The cardiovascular system represents a frequent crossing point for aerospace medicine, physiology, and clinical medicine. Cardiovascular disease is of great concern in several areas of aerospace medicine, including civil aviation certification, aerobatics, military high-performance flying, and zero-G flight. Military aviation cardiology especially has been challenged by the new generation of high-performance fighter aircraft. These aircraft have introduced degrees of rapid-G onset and sustained G that have placed unprecedented stress on the cardiovascular system. A number of subclinical conditions may be unmasked or exacerbated by high $+G_z$ loading, especially asymptomatic coronary artery disease. Although military aviation medical standards have been influenced by the advent of this advanced fighter technology, civilian aviation medicine standards essentially have been unaffected by these developments. Thus, the Federal Aviation Administration (FAA) has been able to apply less rigid decision rules than the United States Air Force for

a given cardiovascular diagnosis. These differences are easily understood in view of the rather different missions of these agencies. Whereas the Air Force has placed great emphasis on cardiovascular testing for the identification of subclinical disease states, the FAA has tended to apply specialized cardiovascular tests to assess the significance of a given condition and the likelihood of sudden impairment. In this regard, most conditions can be considered for exemption by the Federal Air Surgeon based on test results. The decision rules discussed in this chapter are derived from experience and data from United States Air Force aviators. It is more difficult to apply discrete decision rules in civil aviation cases, where exemptions for cardiovascular disease are oriented toward functional testing.

One of the unique aspects of aviation cardiology is its close relationship to epidemiology. In many instances, abnormal cardiovascular findings, such as left bundle branch block, represent abnormal tests rather than a discrete disease entity. Or,

421

alternatively, these abnormal findings do not represent a disease entity that can be defined in the subclinical state by available technology. Only through the elucidation of the natural history of these incidental findings in asymptomatic subjects will their significance become clear. In this regard, aeromedical policy is heavily dependent on epidemiologic studies of disease subsets. Aeromedical policy in the area of cardiovascular abnormalities has, of necessity, been quite conservative. This conservatism largely has been due to the following three factors:

1. The diagnostic criteria for virtually all cardiovascular entities have been derived from "sick patient" populations.
2. The natural history of most asymptomatic cardiovascular findings is unknown, and prognosis can only be estimated from clinical populations.
3. The common use of invasive tools, such as coronary angiography and electrophysiologic studies, and noninvasive tools, such as two-dimensional echocardiography, thallium scintigraphy, and radionuclide angiography, are relatively recent innovations. The anatomic definition of the cardiovascular system has provided a previously unavailable baseline for natural-history studies of asymptomatic disease.

Aeromedical standards are necessarily arbitrary when they are initially derived. Certification standards should be liberalized when the retrospective data for a given cardiovascular finding represent a favorable trend. These groups of subjects should then be prospectively followed closely over time. Subsequent standards should be relaxed or made more stringent based on these long-term observations.

This chapter will attempt to describe the data base currently available regarding some specific cardiovascular findings in apparently healthy men, especially in the areas of treadmill testing and scalar electrocardiographic findings.

CORONARY ARTERY DISEASE
Gwynne K. Neufeld
James R. Hickman

Incapacitation in flight from coronary artery disease (CAD) is a direct threat to flying safety and mission completion. Sudden cardiac death has resulted in documented loss of aircraft and passengers in civil and military aviation. Sudden death occurs without warning and is frequently the first symptom of CAD. No other medical condition results in as much disability and loss of life in adult men as CAD. Approximately 650,000 Americans die annually and an additional 2 million develop symptoms or signs of the disease. CAD is the leading cause of nonaccidental mortality among flyers in the United States Air Force.

Young adults are prime victims of CAD. Autopsy studies performed on battle casualties of the Korean and Vietnam wars, with a mean age in the early twenties, demonstrated that 31 to 42% of these soldiers studied had some degree of obstructive coronary atherosclerosis. In addition, approximately 10% of these soldiers had total or near-total occlusions of the lumen of at least one major artery.[1,2]

Pathophysiologic Factors

Coronary artery disease results from atherosclerosis of the blood vessels, leading to partial or total occlusion of the lumen. Atherosclerosis involves a thickening and hardening of the coronary arteries, with clinical events resulting from obstruction to blood flow or superimposed thrombosis at the site of a plaque. It is important to understand that critical obstruction of the coronary arteries is not always necessary for a catastrophe to occur. Frequently, an obstructing thrombus develops at the site of an ulcerated plaque of moderate severity, resulting in myocardial infarction or sudden death from arrhythmia.

Epidemiologic Factors

Knowledge of the epidemiology of CAD has been advanced significantly by several long-term prospective studies, of which the Framingham Heart Study is the best known.[3] These studies have followed several thousand men and fewer women who were free of cardiovascular disease at the inception of the study and were observed for the development of CAD. These studies have been complemented by numerous other investigations of specific variables, leading to the concept of "risk factors" for CAD. Naturally occurring traits that are associated more frequently with the development of CAD have been labeled risk factors. Modification of risk factors probably reduces the incidence of CAD, although this hypothesis for the most part remains unproven despite strong inferential data.

Demographic Variables

Mortality from CAD increases strikingly with increasing age. Male mortality rates are higher than female rates in all age groups, with a lag of 7 to 10 years between the two groups. Race, an independent variable, has not had a consistent effect on mortality. As much as a tenfold variation in mortality is seen among the different nations. Although genetic variation may play a role, studies of similar ethnic populations in different countries suggest that environmental factors are the basis for the observed differences in mortality rates. Mortality rates also vary over time, with the United States showing an increase over the first half of the twentieth century and a steady decline since 1968. The reasons for this encouraging decline are unknown, although changes in life-style and dietary habits have been postulated to play a role.

Lipids

Epidemiologic studies comparing cultures with different levels of dietary saturated fats and cholesterol have shown dramatic differences in the incidence of CAD. The relationship between blood lipids and CAD is the best-documented association among the postulated risk factors. The risk of CAD varies in proportion to the total serum cholesterol level. When evaluated independently from the other risk factors, triglycerides have not been shown to have a consistent relationship to the risk of CAD.

Recent investigations have evaluated not only the relationship of total cholesterol to the risk of CAD but also to the various forms in which cholesterol appears in the blood. High-density lipoprotein (HDL) cholesterol normally accounts for 20 to 25% of the total plasma cholesterol. The HDL level has shown a strong inverse relationship to CAD. The relationship between total serum cholesterol and HDL cholesterol is frequently expressed as a ratio of the two, and this ratio seems to be more sensitive in predicting CAD risk than either absolute value alone. Retrospective analysis of this ratio in aircrew members with abnormal treadmill tests undergoing cardiac catheterization at the United States Air Force School of Aerospace Medicine (USAFSAM) revealed that a total cholesterol/HDL cholesterol ratio of greater than 6 occurred in 88% of individuals with CAD, whereas a ratio of over 6 was seen in only 4% of those with no disease. Conversely, patients with a ratio of less than 4.3 had a low incidence of CAD (Fig. 14–1).[4]

HDL cholesterol can be influenced by many factors. It is independent of age during adult life. The dietary intake of cholesterol and saturated fats consistently reduces HDL cholesterol levels. Strict dietary control of fat should be recommended to all patients with abnormal cholesterol profiles. Moderate alcohol intake has an apparent beneficial effect on HDL levels. The ethical considerations and possible harmful effects of regular alcohol ingestion, however, preclude the recom-

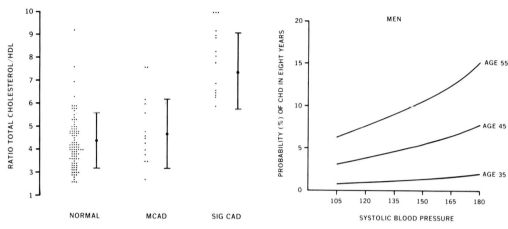

Fig. 14–1. Values for cholesterol/HDL cholesterol ratio plotted according to angiographic classification (normal, minimal coronary artery disease [MCAD] and significant coronary artery disease [Sig CAD]). A ratio greater than 6.0 predicted Sig CAD. (From Am. J. Cardiol. 48:903–910, 1981, published by permission.)

Fig. 14–2. Probability of developing CAD within 8 years according to systolic blood pressure levels in men with cholesterol levels measuring 235 mg/dl who are nonsmokers and have normal glucose tolerances. (From the Framingham Heart Study.)

mendation of this agent as a general therapeutic measure.

Physical activity elevates HDL cholesterol. This effect has been postulated as an explanation for the reported reduction in CAD among regular exercisers. This positive influence on HDL cholesterol is seen at moderate levels of exercise and seems to increase with more vigorous physical fitness programs. For example, marathon runners have higher levels of HDL cholesterol on the average than joggers.

Smoking decreases HDL cholesterol levels, suggesting that part of the increased rate of CAD in smokers may be through this mechanism.

Other Risk Factors

Elevated blood pressure is associated with an increased risk of developing CAD. This risk increases with increasing levels of either systolic or diastolic blood pressure (Fig. 14–2), even within the normal range of blood pressures.[5,6] The physician who counsels the aviator with a "high-normal" blood pressure measurement must be aware that this high-normal level carries a definitely increased risk of CAD as compared with the risk of a "low-normal" blood pressure.

Cigarette smoking is a potent risk factor for CAD, with the risk increasing as more cigarettes are smoked each day. In the Framingham study, men who smoked more than 20 cigarettes/day had a 2.15 relative risk of developing CAD as compared with nonsmokers. Pipe and cigar smoking also has been shown to have a small but consistent effect vis-a-vis increasing the risk of CAD.

Several prospective studies have shown that discontinuation of smoking decreases the risk of CAD. The excess risk of CAD declines within a few years of the discontinuation of smoking. Smoking is the most widely documented case in which modification of the risk factor has revealed a positive influence on subsequent cardiovascular morbidity. All aviators should be encouraged to abstain from smoking; this is mandatory in those who have any degree of CAD or in those with other significant risk factors. Major educational and behavioral modification programs should be instituted as early as possible in the young aviator who smokes.

Diabetes mellitus is a significant risk factor for CAD. In one large prospective study, an elevated fasting blood glucose was shown to be a significant predictor of subsequent CAD, even when other risk factors were controlled.[7] No evidence exists to show that control of hyperglycemia by any method reduces the elevated risk for cardiovascular disease. Despite this, prudence dictates the institution of dietary control and weight loss (if indicated) in all individuals who have persistently abnormal fasting glucose levels.

Stress is viewed as a major precursor of CAD by the general public and most physicians. Scientific investigation of this association has been hampered by difficulty in measuring and defining stress. The definition of Type A behavior by Rosenman and colleagues[8] has assisted in defining this relationship. Type A individuals are more aggressive, ambitious, and competitive than their Type B peers. Type A individuals tend to be successful and make excellent pilots and military officers. Many prospective studies have shown a definite association between Type A behavior and CAD. The mechanism for this is unclear, although chronic elevation in catecholamines and other stress hormones have been postulated to play a role.

A family history of documented cardiovascular events before age 65 is significantly associated with an increased risk of CAD, although this association is less impressive when adjusted for other traits that have a familial occurrence such as hyperlipidemia, hypertension, and glucose intolerance.

The evidence that a reduction in the incidence of CAD is possible with physical activity is controversial, and emotions have clouded the issue. A review of the currently available evidence reveals a trend in favor of a reduction in cardiovascular mortality in exercisers as compared with nonexercisers. This positive effect may be modulated through the documented positive influence of physical activity on HDL cholesterol. The risk of precipitating an ischemic event must be weighed against the apparent benefits of exercise in a patient with known CAD.

Other factors that have been reported to increase the risk of developing CAD include gout, obesity, carbohydrate consumption, and blood type A. In general, the influences of such factors diminish or disappear when the data are corrected for the other risk factors previously discussed.

Clinical Presentation of Coronary Artery Disease

Only a minority of patients with CAD are identified by screening tests while still asymptomatic. The vast majority present with symptoms of advanced disease, such as angina pectoris, myocardial infarction, or sudden cardiac death. An infrequent patient will present with symptoms resulting from arrhythmias such as syncope or palpitations. Clinical congestive heart failure is rarely the presenting symptom of the disease.

Classic angina pectoris is reported by the minority of patients as the presenting symptom of CAD. Such discomfort is predictable, occurs with exertion or emotion, is brief but usually lasts at least 1 minute, and is usually described as a "squeezing" or "heavy" sensation. The pain occurs retrosternally and radiates variably into the jaw or arms. It may be accompanied by dyspnea, diaphoresis, or nausea. Classic angina pectoris implies a high probability of CAD, although confirmatory tests are required for diganosis. Angina pectoris usually occurs in patients with stenosis of at least two coronary arteries.

"Atypical angina" describes unusual pain precipitated by classic factors or classic pain in an unusual clinical setting.

Myocardial infarction is the most common initial presentation of CAD in the general population. Unfortunately, many patients with myocardial infarction have had unreported or misinterpreted premonitory symptoms. Mortality following hospitalization depends on the location and size of the necrotic myocardium. Approximately 15% of patients with acute myocardial infarction die before hospital discharge, and an additional 10% die during the following 1-year period. Most of these subsequent deaths occur suddenly. Malignant arrhythmias are frequent in the healing phase of the infarction but can occur at any later time. For this reason, among others, it is not recommended that aircrew members with a history of myocardial infarction be allowed to return to the cockpit under any circumstances. Civil pilots with uncomplicated myocardial infarction, however, have been granted exemptions by the FAA following normal noninvasive examinations.

Silent myocardial infarction occurs occasionally. At USAFSAM, silent myocardial infarction was found on the routine electrocardiogram in 72 of 48,633 aviators screened over a 10-year period.[9] Of those aviators who were interviewed, most recalled no symptoms at all and the remainder had atypical symptoms.

Sudden cardiac death is the presenting symptom of CAD in an estimated 15 to 20% of all patients and is the mode of demise in approximately 60% of all patients who succumb to the disease. The mechanism of sudden death is primarily arrhythmic. Many patients do not have myocardial necrosis at the time of autopsy, although advanced atherosclerosis involving all three coronary arteries is usually present.

Screening Tests

The detection of asymptomatic CAD in aircrew members is the primary goal of aerospace cardiology. Although angiographic disease in asymptomatic aviators is usually single-vessel or low-grade multivessel disease, severe disease is still found with regularity. Even mild degrees of CAD can potentially lead to sudden incapacitation during $+G_z$ stress. Currently available screening methods include history, physical examination, resting electrocardiogram (ECG), exercise electrocardiography, exercise scintigraphy, and risk estimation. The dismal failure of history and physical examination in detecting subclinical disease is universally recognized. The resting ECG is often nondiagnostic unless silent myocardial infarction has occurred. Nonspecific ST and T-wave changes, especially T-wave flattening or inversion and ST depression, are occasional indications of the presence of CAD. Such abnormalities are only useful if comparison with previous ECGs can be performed. Over a 1-year period at USAFSAM, 32,000 referral ECGs were reviewed. Treadmill tests were performed for various nondiagnostic serial electroradiographic changes, resulting in 923 exercise ECGs, of which 779 were normal. Of the 144 patients with abnormal exercise ECGs, 90 were evaluated by cardiac catheterization, yielding 19 cases with any degree of CAD. Although the predictive value of an abnormal treadmill test in this population is low (21%), it is actually doubled, from 10% to 21%, by screening for serial nonspecific resting electrocardiographic changes.[10] A study by Piepgrass and colleagues[11] described the rather marked limitations of the exercise test in a population of United States Air Force aviators who were exercised without regard to scalar electrocardiographic changes or risk factors. The absence of some pretest stratification, which enhances predictive value, was shown to severely limit the usefulness of the exercise test as a first-order screening test in apparently healthy men.

As the above studies demonstrate, a major limitation of treadmill testing in asymptomatic populations has been the occurrence of false-positive results. A rational approach to stress testing involves the application of Bayes' theorem.[12] This theorem applies conditional probability analysis to any diagnostic test that is not perfect. The reliability of any less than perfect test is strongly influenced by the prevalence of the disease being sought in the study population. Understanding a few common epidemiologic terms is required. Predictive value is defined as the proportion of positive results that are truly positive and is dependent on the prevalence of the disease in the study population. Sensitivity is the percentage of positive results in patients with disease. Specificity is the percentage of negative results among those subjects without disease. For purposes of illustration, assume that a treadmill test with 75% sensitivity and 60% specificity is applied to a population of 10,000 subjects with a disease prevalence of 50%. Table 14–1 illustrates the predictive value of an abnormal test under these conditions. Therefore, this treadmill test applied to a population with a disease prevalence of 50% would correctly identify 3750 of the 5000 diseased patients and correctly classify 3000 of the 5000 nondiseased individuals. A population with a disease prevalence of 5%, similar to the prevalence in healthy male aviators, would reveal a marked decrease in the predictive power of the identical test (Table 14–2).

False-positive exercise tests have numerous causes, including mitral valve prolapse, electrolyte abnormalities, cardiomyopathies, pericardial disease, anemia, left ventricular hypertrophy, preexcitation, nonfasting state, vasoregulatory ab-

Table 14–1. Performance of a Test With 75% Sensitivity and 60% Specificity in a Population With 50% Prevalence of Disease

Subjects	Number of Abnormal Tests	Number of Normal Tests
5000 diseased	3750 (TP)	1250 (TN)
5000 nondiseased	2000 (FP)	3000 (TN)
Total	5750	4250

Predictive value of an abnormal test: $\dfrac{TP}{TP + FP}$ = $\dfrac{3750}{5750}$ = 65.2%. Note: TP = true-positives; FN = false-negatives; FP = false-positives; and TN = true-negatives.

Table 14–2. Performance of a Test With 75% Sensitivity and 60% Specificity in a Population With 5% Prevalence of Disease

Subjects	Number of Abnormal Tests	Number of Normal Tests
500 diseased	375 (TP)	125 (FN)
9500 nondiseased	3800 (FP)	5700 (TN)
Total	4175	5825

Predictive value of an abnormal test: $\dfrac{TP}{TP + FP}$ = $\dfrac{375}{4175}$ = 8.9. Note: TP = true-positives; FN = false-negatives; FP = false-positives; and TN = true-negatives.

normalities, and coronary spasm. The bulk of false-positive exercise tests with normal coronary arteriograms are of unknown etiology, however.

Another problem with exercise electrocardiography is the occurrence of false-negative ST segment responses. The frequency of false-negative ST segment responses is not accurately known in asymptomatic populations because such patients rarely undergo cardiac catheterization.

A number of variables may be evaluated during exercise ECGs. Exercise electrocardiography is abnormal when ST depression of a degree greater than a predetermined normal level develops with exercise or during recovery. All investigators accept horizontal or downsloping ST segment depressions of greater than 0.1 mV, when compared with baseline, as abnormal. Most investigators also accept upsloping ST segment depression as abnormal if the ST segment remains greater than 0.1 mV depressed 80 milliseconds after the termination of the QRS complex (the J point). We consider ST segment depression between 0.05 and 0.09 mV as "borderline," a category not universally recognized, but which we feel requires further testing for CAD. Additional variables evaluated during exercise electrocardiography include the occurrence of stress arrhythmias, maximum heart rate reached, maximum systolic blood pressure, and total QRS and R-wave amplitude. Decreased peak heart rate or falling systolic blood pressure with progressive exercise are possible indicators of CAD. Additional information, such as the inadequate rise of systemic blood pressure, early appearance of ST segment depression, and prolonged duration of ST segment depression after exercise, also have diagnostic importance. The most extensive angiographic correlation of these multiple treadmill variables in totally asymptomatic men has been performed by Hopkirk and colleagues,[13,14,15] who conducted an exhaustive minute-by-minute analysis of 255 exercise tests of asymptomatic United States Air Force aviators prior to angiography. This study attempted to identify a combination of electrocardiographic, hemodynamic, and risk factor data that would be of diagnostic value in asymptomatic subjects. The predictive value of more than 0.1 mV of ST segment depression was 24%. ST segment depression alone did not increase predictive value until a greater than 0.3-mV depression was reached, increasing the predictive value to 60%. The onset of a greater than 0.1-mV depression in early exercise proved to be a poor predictor of angiographic disease in asymptomatic men. Exercise-induced R-wave amplitude increases (or no change in amplitude) increased the predictive value to 40% but were markedly insensitive (18%). Further, a decreased percentage of maximal predicted heart rate achieved and exercise double product failed to enhance significantly the predictive value of the exercise test in asymptomatic men. The exercise test variables that performed best were a total treadmill time of less than 10 minutes on the USAFSAM protocol[16] (predictive value, 67%) and greater than 0.1 mV of ST segment depression persisting for at least 6 minutes after exercise (predictive value, 43%). Univariate analysis of cardinal risk factors did not increase the predictive value of the exercise test in asymptomatic

men, but the value of the ST segment response was enhanced modestly by the presence of three risk factors. The combination of one or more risk factors with the three most predictive exercise variables (greater than 0.3-mV depression early in exercise, greater than 0.1-mV depression persisting 6 minutes after exercise, or less than 10 minutes total performance) yielded a predictive value of greater than 80% for the detection of multivessel disease. Unfortunately, sensitivity was too poor to rely on this combination to rule out significant disease. Hopkirk and colleagues' work has underscored the limitations of exercise testing in apparently healthy men and has graphically demonstrated the diagnostic trade-offs between sensitivity and specificity as various criteria are examined. Of special concern in aerospace medicine is the usual loss in sensitivity when criteria of higher specificity are applied.

Exercise electrocardiography remains the most widely used screening procedure for asymptomatic CAD. A United States Air Force study by Froelicher and colleagues[17] analyzed the epidemiologic value of screening asymptomatic males with exercise electrocardiography. An abnormal ST segment response proved to be a potent predictor of subsequent symptomatic CAD. At USAFSAM, 640 aircrew members who underwent exercise electrocardiography over a 4-year period were reevaluated after a mean interval of 6.6 years. Marked differences were noted between those who originally had abnormal ST segment responses and those with normal responses. A fourteenfold increase in the risk for subsequent coronary events was found in those with an abnormal result, as compared with the group who had normal tests.[17] Although the treadmill test is an imperfect predictor of anatomic CAD, the potent epidemiologic risk of an abnormal result cannot be ignored.

Exercise Scintigraphy

Thallium-201(^{201}Tl) is a radioisotope that is rapidly cleared from the bloodstream and concentrated in the myocardium. This property makes ^{201}Tl ideal for assessing areas of relative underperfusion of the myocardium. Such areas of underperfusion are generally supplied by partially occluded coronary arteries. Complete absence of ^{201}Tl in a region of the myocardium indicates scar tissue and is highly specific for myocardial infarction. [201]Tl is generally injected at peak exercise, with images obtained within 5 minutes of the cessation of exercise. These images are then compared with either a resting scan performed on a separate day or with images obtained 3 to 6 hours following the exercise study, analogous to a resting scan.

Various sensitivities and specificities have been reported for ^{201}Tl scintigrams. The sensitivity of ^{201}Tl scanning is improved by utilizing tomographic analysis of computer-enhanced images. In a preliminary USAFSAM study involving 191 patients who underwent cardiac catheterization, the predictive value of a positive test was 74%, and the predictive value of a negative test was 92% in an asymptomatic population with abnormal treadmill tests.[18]

Using ^{201}Tl scintigraphy as an adjunct to exercise electrocardiography provides an improved sensitivity for the detection of CAD. A negative scan in a young individual with an abnormal exercise ECG indicates that the exercise test is most likely a false-positive result. We do not recommend cardiac catheterization in asymptomatic individuals under the age of 35 who have the combination of an abnormal exercise ECG and a normal ^{201}Tl scintigram unless significant risk factors for CAD are present. It is hoped that further refinement of nuclear imaging techniques will allow the same recommendation to be made regardless of age.

Various techniques are also available to label the circulating blood with Technetium-99m. The blood can then be imaged as it passes through the heart. "First pass" or "gated blood pool" studies are then performed, which are termed radionuclide angiograms. These studies allow the assessment of global and regional left ventricular contraction with exercise. Abnormalities of myocardial contraction that develop with exercise are highly specific for CAD. These procedures, however, appear to be less sensitive than thallium scintigrams in the overall detection of asymptomatic CAD.

Coronary Angiography

Coronary angiography remains the definitive procedure for the detection of CAD. The test, in the appropriate hands, can be performed with little discomfort and minimal risk. In general, it should be performed on all aircrew members in whom a significant possibility of CAD exists following appropriately administered noninvasive testing.

A new technique, termed digital subtraction radiography, may allow the acquisition of coronary images of diagnostic quality from the peripheral intravenous injection of x-ray contrast media. This technique, however, is still several years from clinical application.

Prevention

An aviator who is identified as having an increased risk for CAD is a candidate for modification of any adverse factor. A strong theoretical case can be made that modification of these risk factors will reduce the probability of subsequent CAD. The evidence is strongest that curtailment of cigarette smoking reduces the risk of subsequent ischemic cardiovascular complications. There is some evidence that reductions of moderate and severe levels of hypertension reduce subsequent cardiovascular mortality; however, much of this reduction is seen because of reduced incidence of stroke and congestive heart failure.[6] Modification of other risk factors has not been shown to reduce the risk of CAD, although this is the subject of an intense research effort.

Despite widespread awareness in the United States since the 1964 Surgeon General's report that cigarette smoking adversely affects health, many individuals continue to smoke. The American Heart Association Ad Hoc Committee on Cigarette Smoking in Cardiovascular Diseases has made the following recommendations for actively encouraging the elimination of cigarette smoking:

1. Do not allow medical staff in physician's offices to smoke.
2. Always raise the question of smoking in conection with the finding of cardiac or pulmonary disease and in general routine examinations (e.g., aviation medical examinations).
3. Support and refer patients to smoking cessation clinics when necessary.
4. Obtain help from the patient's family in the endeavor to cease smoking.
5. Check the patient's compliance with periodic advice.

The substitution of cigar or pipe smoking for cigarette smoking will not reduce the risk of CAD because the patient most likely will continue to inhale.

Dietary management of an elevated cholesterol or an abnormal ratio of total cholesterol to HDL cholesterol warrants detailed instructions to the patient and his family concerning reducing the intake of cholesterol and saturated fats. Individuals who have complex hyperlipoproteinemias should be referred to clinical dietitians for dietary recommendations. Follow-up should be aimed at assessing the degree of dietary compliance, as well as any improvement in the major blood lipids. If an adequate hypolipidemic effect is not seen with diet and weight loss, drug therapy should be instituted. Cholestyramine is a bile acid sequestrant that is frequently used as initial therapy for hyperlipidemias in aviators because it is not significantly absorbed through the gastrointestinal tract. The most frequent side effect is gastrointestinal intolerance, limiting the total dosage that can be taken in most cases. If adequate reduction in serum cholesterol is not seen with cholestyramine, other agents should be considered, although none have been evaluated from a flying safety standpoint.

Modification of Type A behavior requires a major life-style change, and major changes probably occur infrequently. Formal, supervised behavioral modification techniques to alter Type A behavior patterns are being evaluated at different medical centers, and preliminary results suggest that serum cholesterol levels may be reduced by such programs. No investigation has shown a reduction in the risk for CAD through modification of Type A behavior. A growing number of physicians advocate vigorous exercise programs in an effort to reduce the risk of CAD. Before exercise is recommended in patients over age 35, some commonsense precautions should be taken. Individuals who have risk factors for CAD should be screened with exercise electrocardiography. In those individuals who have previously been sedentary, a gradual increase in the level of physical activity over a period of weeks to months is desirable.

Hypertension should be aggressively sought and treated whenever present. Obesity is best managed as part of a total life-style modification that includes diet, exercise, and possibly psychotherapy.

Therapy of Coronary Artery Disease

In general, CAD is incompatible with flying safety, and the patient should be referred for appropriate long-term management. A preliminary study group has been instituted in the United States Air Force in which patients with minimal CAD have been allowed to return to the cockpit in non-high–performance dual-pilot aircraft.[19] Minimal CAD has been defined in this study as no single coronary lesion greater than 30% of the diameter of the lumen and no aggregate of lesions greater than 50%. Preliminary results suggest that such patients can be returned safely to the cockpit, although they occasionally reveal evidence of progression with serial follow-up. Repeat angiography is performed at 3-year intervals or less, depending on the risk-factor profile and the results of annual noninvasive testing, including thallium scintigraphy. The Eighth Bethesda Conference of the American College of Cardiology contains a series of recommmendations for civil pilots with CAD.[20] The recommendations include guidelines for the recertification of aviators with angina pectoris, myocardial infarction, or bypass surgery, based primarily on the results of coronary angiography. These recommendations, made by a task force comprised of military, governmental, and civilian specialists, have no regulatory stature but represent a consensus of opinion in this controversial area. These guidelines are considerably more liberal than aircrew standards for the United States armed forces.

Coronary artery angioplasty is a technique that involves the placement of an inflatable balloon at the site of coronary artery obstruction. The balloon is then inflated under pressure in an attempt to dilate the obstruction. Preliminary results from major medical centers suggest that this technique will reduce the severity of stenosis significantly in carefully selected candidates. The outcome of such procedures is currently being investigated. Conceivably, such patients should be considered for a return to flying status if successful dilatation of the arterial lesions is achieved and careful follow-up for restenosis is maintained.

Coronary artery bypass grafting precludes a return to flying in the military environment, regardless of the clinical or anatomic results. The FAA, however, was directed by the National Transportation Safety Board to medically certify civilian pilots after bypass surgery in a number of instances between 1978 and 1982. These certifications included aircraft commanders of commercial jet aircraft. In May, 1982, the FAA achieved amendments to Part 67 of the Federal Aviation Regulations, which required that applicants for certification have no medical history or clinical diagnosis of coronary disease that has required treatment or, if untreated, that has been symptomatic or clinically significant.[21] This amendment places more direct control over the CAD issues in the hands of the Federal Air Surgeon, and policy regarding untreated and asymptomatic CAD, as well as bypass surgery, is still evolving as of this writing. Many specialists in aerospace medicine consider bypass surgery to be a palliative procedure that does not diminish the potential for progression of the underlying disease. The disease substrate remains unchanged, and the disease may progress to involve vessels distal to the graft insertion or the graft itself. The 3% yearly graft occlusion rate (9% per year in a subject with three grafts) is an unacceptable risk in the view of many aviation specialists. The unpredictable and capricious nature of atherosclerotic lesions does not currently allow one to formulate a rational policy for the regular surveillance and return to the cockpit of aviators who have had bypass surgery. These same constraints also apply to the disposition of aviators with angiographically significant asymptomatic CAD. Preliminary data from the United States Air Force's study of the natural history of asymptomatic CAD by Hickman and colleagues[22] reveals a 6% per annum event rate (angina, infarction, or sudden death), with 75% of initial events occurring as angina. In the view of these authors, CAD of more than minimal degree remains incompatible with aviation safety.

HYPERTENSION
Paul V. Celio

As in clinical practice, one of the commonly encountered problems in the aviator population is hypertension, with a prevalence which parallels that of the general population, 10 to 20% of the adult population in the United States. Hypertension demands our utmost concern, not only because of documented increases in mortality and morbidity associated with hypertension, but because of complications resulting in sudden incapacitation. Although heart and renal failure are major presenting complications, stroke and myocardial ischemic events dominate the aeromedical risk.

Actuarial data clearly reveal that the mortality and morbidity of hypertension increases steadily with increasing levels of systolic, diastolic, or mean blood pressure. Because there is no level that clearly delineates increased risk, any definition of hypertension must be somewhat arbitrary, but most definitions identify a point that is associated with a 50% increase in mortality. In the United States, the most common prevailing definition of hypertension is a systolic pressure of 140 mm Hg and/or a diastolic pressure of 90 mm Hg.

Methodology

Blood pressure values should be measured with the patient seated and resting comfortably, with the arm hanging at the side. Blood pressure should be measured in both arms and one leg to exclude the possibility of aortic coarctation. Appropriate cuff size is essential because a cuff that is too small will yield a falsely high value. Although multiple blood pressure values are generally obtained, some studies have revealed an increased risk of future complications with even casual blood pressure elevations. Several ambulatory blood pressure devices are under evaluation, and a 24-hour blood pressure record eventually will be obtained with acceptable accuracy, thus improving the confidence with which preponderant blood pressures are derived.

Aeromedical Implications of Hypertension

Aerospace medicine is closely allied with preventive medicine. Nowhere has this relationship been more closely demonstrated than in hypertensive disease. Hypertension is one of the chronic diseases for which therapy has been of demonstrated effectiveness in the reduction of mortality and morbidity. Thus, a great premium is placed on the early identification and treatment of hypertension. Unlike many diagnostic procedures that require additional time-consuming testing in the pursuit of false-positive and false-negative findings, blood pressure determinations carry few such penalties. The diagnostic test for hypertension is almost ideal: inexpensive, safe, quick, painless, and easily repeated. In borderline or minimal elevations, one simply repeats the determinations under a wide variety of conditions until the presence or absence of a given diagnostic threshold is documented with confidence. Although unanimity of opinion is lacking regarding a blood pressure level that is abnormal, most aviation certification agencies leave the examiner little choice in this regard. Whereas the United States Air Force chooses a pressure of 140/90 mm Hg, irrespective of age, the United States Army allows a systolic level of 140 mm Hg at age 35 or less and a systolic level of 150 mm Hg over age 35 but allows only a diastolic level of 90 mm Hg at any age. Multiple variations of blood pressure standards are found among the civil and military authorities around the world. The most uniform requirement among all agencies, however, is the determination of preponderant blood pressures, implying multiple serial determinations. A minimum of six blood pressure readings over 3 days represents a reasonable consensus. Hull and colleagues[23] have documented the utility of the response to orthostatic stress in separating borderline hypertensive patients from normotensive individuals.

It is unfortunate that the detection and treatment of hypertension continues to represent one of the least successful areas in clinical and preventive medicine. Lamentably, the diagnosis of hypertension is frequently not documented or documented only belatedly in aviators. The underdiagnosis of hypertension in aviators is partially due to the potentially adverse effect of this diagnosis on airman certification. This reluctance to aggressively pursue the diagnosis of hypertension in aviators derives historically from the availability of a very limited number of drugs considered safe for aviation. The United States Air Force has extensively evaluated the thiazide diuretics for all classes of airmen.[24] The thiazides, with and without triamterene, remain the sole drugs available in both United States Air Force and Army aviation. The Canadian forces have evaluated propanalol and so far have found this beta blocker acceptable in non-high–performance flying. Likewise, the FAA has sanctioned the use of limited dose ranges of beta blockers for aviators with hypertension. Drugs for use in aviators must be exhaustively evaluated in terms of their effect on orthostatic stress response, $+G_z$ acceleration tolerance, aerobic exercise capacity, responses to hypoxia and lowered barometric pressure, cardiac rhythm stability, blood volume changes, metabolic homeostasis, and psychomotor function. Currently, several of the newer beta blockers are under evaluation at aeromedical centers. There is a broad general consensus that virtually all second-line drugs, after the thiazides, have severe practical and theoretical limitations for high-performance flying, and many of these agents are unacceptable for general aviation. Aviation medicine specialists are concerned about the masking effects of the beta blockers in aviators with asymptomatic coronary disease and the distinct possibility of obviating an ischemic response to exercise testing. The continuing evolution of the beta-blocker family of agents may reveal selectivity characteristics that are more acceptable for use in aviators. New agents should undergo rigorous evaluation before they are used in the aeromedical community.

Treatment of Hypertension in Aviators

Because the pharmacologic alternatives are quite limited in aviators, a great premium must be placed on dietary efforts to achieve ideal body weight and to restrict sodium intake in the treatment of hypertension. Although the population of hypertensive individuals can now be subdivided more accurately into high and low renin, as well as volume-dependent and sodium "sensitive" subsets, the flight surgeon is unable to exploit the currently available "tailored" drug therapy for these entities. Still, 50% of all aviators with a new diagnosis of hypertension can be adequately controlled with a combination of thiazide diuretics and dietary measures. Aviators should be restricted from flying duties for 30 days following the institution of drug therapy to assess treatment efficacy, metabolic derangements, and idiosyncratic reactions.

The diagnosis of hypertension remains the most pressing issue of the hypertensive problem in aviation. Although the therapeutic latitude is usually closely circumscribed by the certifying authority, the diagnosis is the province of the flight surgeon. The diagnosis of hypertension must not be avoided when the preponderant blood pressures are consistently elevated. The endless repetition of recumbent blood pressures in the near-somnolent aviator (after 2 hours of bed rest in a darkened room) must not be employed to derive a few acceptable blood pressures. Likewise, an aviator whose hypertension has begun to accelerate while on therapy will be poorly served by withholding a second drug, even though the consequences will be loss of certification for flying. Few occupations are more closely linked to good health than aviation. The flight surgeon who has established a close personal rapport with his aviators will serve them best by pursuing a timely diagnosis of this common disease.

DISPOSITION OF ELECTROCARDIOGRAPHIC ABNORMALITIES IN AVIATORS
William C. Wood
James R. Hickman

In this section, electrocardiographic abnormalities will be discussed in the context of their aeromedical significance. The prognostic implications of specific findings in electrocardiography traditionally have been based on clinical populations. The present criteria for the disposition of electrocardiographic abnormalities in aviators are based on findings within a flying population and on observation of the natural history of specific electrocardiographic characteristics. These recommendations are derived from the experience gained from the United States Air Force Central Electrocardiographic Library, which was established in 1957. Almost 1 million ECGs are on file in this facility.

Electrocardiography is not an exact science. It must be correlated with the history and physical examination. Extensive cardiac evaluation may be required to clarify a given finding. The significance of a specific finding and its aeromedical implication depend heavily on the presence or absence of underlying cardiovascular disease.

This section will be devoted primarily to a discussion of serial ST segment and T-wave changes, common arrhythmias, the Wolff-Parkinson-White electrocardiographic pattern, and conduction disturbances. The current aeromedical dispositions for these abnormalities will be discussed. The disposition of individuals with certain of these electrocardiographic findings will remain flexible. Aeromedical recommendations continue to evolve as more experience is accumulated with the natural history of these cardiovascular findings.

Electrocardiographic diagnostic criteria will not be addressed in this section, and the reader is referred to any one of the currently available excellent textbooks on electrocardiography.

The following is a list of the electrocardiographic findings that are considered normal variants:

1. Sinus pause—less than 2 seconds in duration
2. Atrial premature beats—rare
3. Junctional premature beats—rare
4. Ventricular premature beats, uniform—rare
5. Supraventricular rhythm, if slow*
6. Supraventricular escape beats, occurring after a pause of less than 2 seconds
7. Wandering atrial pacemaker
8. Terminal conduction delay of the QRS complex
9. Right axis deviation on an initial tracing in an individual less than 30 years old (QRS axis greater than +120 degrees)
10. Left axis deviation in an initial tracing (QRS axis less than −30 degrees)
11. $S_1S_2S_3$ pattern
12. Short PR interval (PR of 0.10 seconds duration or less)
13. Indeterminate QRS axis
14. Early repolarization pattern
15. Incomplete right bundle branch block pattern

These variants, however, may require further evaluation to ensure that the aircrew member is free of cardiac disease. The rhythm disturbances listed above will, in many cases, require treadmill exercise testing and ambulatory electrocardiography for further evaluation. A normal variant electrocardiographic finding by definition must occur in an individual who is free of underlying heart disease. The recommended evaluation procedures listed

---

*Refers to a nonsinus supraventricular rhythm such as atrial or junctional rhythm.

in Table 14–3 should exclude the more commonly associated abnormalities.

Prevalence of Electrocardiographic Abnormalities

In the United States Air Force, all aviators receive an initial ECG on entry into flying duties and annually after age 34. An analysis of all initial ECGs performed in the Air Force flying population reveals that 82.5% are normal and 17.4% are abnormal. Of the normal ECGs, 10% are labeled as normal variants. A normal variant is a finding that is common in normal individuals but not usually associated with underlying organic heart disease, incapacitating events, or a shortened life span. A normal variant ECG, however, may require an extensive evaluation to exclude organic heart disease. A normal variant may be defined in two ways. The first definition is based on the prevalence of the finding in the population. The second definition is based on the presence or absence of organic heart disease. The prevalence definition of an abnormal ECG means that the ECG is unlike the usually observed electrocardiographic patterns. To judge an ECG as normal or abnormal from the state of health of an individual requires more information than is usually available to the electrocardiographic technician. Diagnostic criteria based on prevalence are preferable in an asymptomatic population

to those based on the state of health. In an asymptomatic population, especially a population of healthy aviators, an abnormal tracing must be considered the tracing of an individual at an increased risk of a cardiovascular event. Many electrocardiographic abnormalities, when viewed alone, are nonspecific, but when compared with previous ECGs may represent a significant serial change. The serial follow-up of resting ECGs has been a key feature of the United States Air Force Central Electrocardiographic Library. The detection of a serial change of the ECG represents a valuable indicator of possible underlying disease. The scalar ECG remains the fundamental tool in the early detection of CAD, cardiomyopathy, and arrhythmias. Figures 14–3 through 14–9 are constructed from the United States Air Force Central Electrocardiographic Library data of Lancaster and Ord.[25]

Specific Electrocardiographic Findings by Age

Approximately 30% of aviators aged 50 years or older in the United States Air Force have an abnormal initial ECG (Fig. 14–3). The most common abnormality is that of repolarization changes, especially ST segment and T-wave abnormalities (Fig. 14–4). The prevalence of repolarization changes on the initial ECG is lowest in the 20- to 34-year-old age group, an age

Table 14–3. Cardiovascular Evaluation of Electrocardiographic Findings That May Represent Normal Variant Patterns

Pattern	Evaluation Indicated
Sinus tachycardia (sinus rate greater than 110 beats/min)	Metabolic determinations to exclude hyperadrenergic state and hyperthyroidism
Voltage criteria for left ventricular hypertrophy (SV_1 plus RV_5 or SV_2 plus RV_6 of >55 mm in individuals below age 35 and >45 mm in individuals age 35 and older)	Echocardiographic study
First-degree AV block (PR interval of >0.21 seconds)	Treadmill test for PR interval >0.22 seconds
Possible right ventricular hypertrophy (tall R in V_1 with or without secondary ST-T changes)	Echocardiographic study
Evidence of left or right atrial abnormality	Echocardiographic study
Left axis deviation (serial change)	Treadmill exercise test
Q-waves suggestive of myocardial abnormality	Vectorcardiography, echocardiographic study, and, when indicated, nuclear cardiologic studies

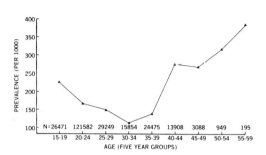

Fig. 14–3. Prevalence of total electrocardiographic abnormalities on the initial electrocardiogram in 5-year age groups of United States Air Force aviators.

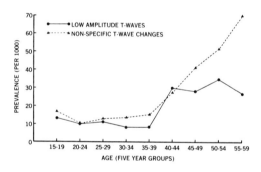

Fig. 14–4. Prevalence of repolarization abnormalities on the initial electrocardiogram in 5-year age groups of United States Air Force aviators.

range in which CAD, hypertension, and cardiomyopathy are infrequent. Further, most conduction disturbances and congenital heart diseases have been detected prior to this age. After an initial normal ECG, the prevalence of low-amplitude T-waves remains essentially unchanged, whereas the prevalence of nonspecific T-wave changes continues to increase to a maximum of 320 cases per 1000 aviators (Fig. 14–5). By age 50 to 54 years, other repolarization abnormalities, consisting of ST segment changes, have a strong correlation with age and are present in 28% of aviators by age 40.

Serial repolarization changes on a resting ECG increase the predictive value of the treadmill exercise test twofold. Serial repolarization changes require a repeat fasting 12-lead ECG, exercise electrocardiography, and a risk-factor analysis. An asymptomatic aviator with an abnormal ST segment response to exercise should be further evaluated by exercise thallium myocardial scintigraphy and in selected cases by angiography. The predictive value of exercise thallium scintigraphy in asymptomatic men is still under investigation and has not yet replaced coronary angiography for definitive aeromedical purposes.

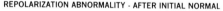
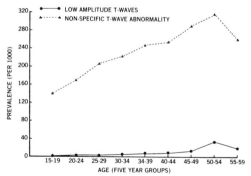

Fig. 14–5. Prevalence of serial repolarization abnormalities after a normal initial electrocardiogram in 5-year age groups of United States Air Force aviators.

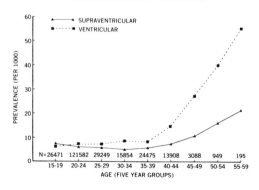

Fig. 14–6. Prevalence of premature beats on the initial electrocardiogram in 5-year age groups of United States Air Force aviators.

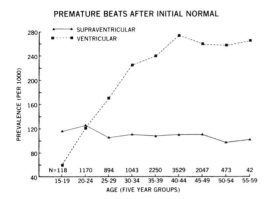

Fig. 14–7. Prevalence of premature beats after a normal initial electrocardiogram in 5-year age groups of United States Air Force aviators.

Premature Beats

A study of premature beats on the initial ECG reveals that ventricular premature beats are more common in the older age group (Fig. 14–6). Although the majority of individuals with premature atrial or ventricular beats have no clinical heart disease, the steady rise in the prevalence of ventricular ectopic beats with age parallels the increased prevalence of hypertension, CAD, and cardiomyopathy. After an initial normal ECG, the prevalence of supraventricular premature beats remains constant, whereas the prevalence of ventricular premature beats continues to rise, reaching a maximum prevalence of 260 aviators per 1000 at age 40 (Fig. 14–7).

Atrial Premature Beats

Atrial premature beats (APBs) or junctional premature beats (JPBs) are a common finding in ECGs. In one reported series, 56% of healthy subjects had APBs on ambulatory electrocardiographic monitoring.[26] APBs have special significance as precursors of supraventricular arrhythmias, including atrial tachycardia, atrial fibrillation, and atrial flutter. APBs may, in some cases, be related to excess caffeine ingestion or other stimulants. The presence of APBs warrants clinical evaluation, including history, physical examination,

and an ambulatory electrocardiographic study. Exercise electrocardiography, echocardiography, and thyroid function studies also may be needed.

Ventricular Premature Beats

Ventricular premature beats (VPBs) are a common finding in individuals, both with and without underlying heart disease. In Brodsky and colleagues' study of ambulatory electrocardiographic recordings, 50% of the apparently healthy individuals had VPBs.[26] VPBs may be associated with organic heart disease such as cardiomyopathy, hypertension, or CAD. Evaluation of a patient with VPBs should include a careful history, physical examination, risk-factor analysis, and ambulatory electrocardiographic recording. Cardiac echocardiography, exercise electrocardiography, and radioisotope studies also may be indicated. The ambulatory electrocardiographic study is particularly important in detecting complex VPBs and supplements the information acquired by treadmill exercise testing. Considerable debate has surrounded the relationship of VPBs to sudden death. Ventricular arrhythmias are particularly dangerous in individuals with prolonged QT syndromes. Individuals with QT intervals that are prolonged for heart rate should be investigated carefully for underlying heart disease or associated arrhythmias.

Ventricular Ectopy During Stress

VPBs and complex ventricular arrhythmias that are absent in the resting state may be produced by increasing sympathetic tone in the normal individual during exercise. An unfavorable oxygen supply-demand imbalance may produce similar arrhythmias in individuals with subclinical ischemic heart disease. In addition, both mechanisms may be operating simultaneously. Further, the increasing parasympathetic tone seen in individuals immediately post $+G_z$ acceleration may lead to "breakthrough" ectopy as the heart slows. All aviators undergoing an evaluation for ventricular arrhythmias should undergo centrifuge testing with electrocardiographic monitoring if high-performance flying is contemplated.

VPBs are commonly seen during exercise stress. Their presence alone is poorly predictive of the existence of underlying CAD. In a United States Air Force School of Aerospace Medicine (USAFSAM) study population, the prevalence, complexity, configuration, or time of occurrence of VPBs were not strong indicators of the presence of CAD among asymptomatic individuals.[27] The absence of a statistical relationship between exercise-induced VPBs and angiographic coronary disease is reassuring, but the true aeromedical significance of ventricular ectopy must await long-term follow-up studies of men with asymptomatic ectopy.

Exercise-Induced Ventricular Tachycardia

Exercise-induced ventricular tachycardia (EIVT), defined as three or more consecutive ventricular beats at a rate of 100 beats/min or greater, is seen in some apparently healthy aviators during exercise testing. At USAFSAM, EIVT has been noted in 0.5% of treadmill tests.[28] In a 6-year retrospective follow-up study of 43 aviators with EIVT, nine individuals (21%) had cardiac events (angina, myocardial infarction, or sudden death). Among these nine individuals with cardiac events, there were three deaths. The deaths occurred in patients with amyloidosis, myocardial infarction, and mitral valve prolapse at 9 months, 3 years, and 6 years, respectively. Six nonfatal events occurred, with four individuals developing angina pectoris and two sustaining nonfatal myocardial infarctions.

In aviators with EIVT, neither the length of the ventricular tachycardia, number of ventricular tachycardia episodes, rate of the ventricular tachycardia, ventricular

tachycardia configuration, heart rate at onset of ventricular tachycardia, ST segment response to exercise, ambulatory electrocardiographic data, nor echocardiographic data discriminated between those with and those without cardiac events. Further, the presence of warning arrhythmias (greater than 10 VPBs per minute, pairing of VPBs, multiformity, or ventricular bigeminy) did not separate those with and without events. All subjects were asymptomatic during EIVT. EIVT was usually unsustained, usually occurred in late exercise or early recovery at heart rates of less than 150 beats/min, and was usually an isolated event. Antecedent complex arrhythmias were usually absent. Almost one third of the EIVT subjects were initially referred for noncardiac reasons.

Seventeen of the EIVT subjects underwent cardiac catheterization with coronary angiography. Of these 17 individuals, 13 had normal coronary arteriograms, whereas four persons had CAD. Although men with EIVT as a group were at increased risk for cardiac events, none of the aviators with normal arteriograms in this group had subsequent cardiac events during follow-up.

Disposition of Ventricular Tachycardia in Aircrew

Adequate periods of ambulatory electrocardiographic monitoring are necessary in EIVT subjects to detect non-exercise–induced ventricular tachycardia, a condition for which the data base is currently insufficient for aeromedical decision making. Thus, non-exercise–induced ventricular tachycardia remains a disqualifying and nonwaiverable finding. Although not all subjects in the EIVT group received cardiac catheterization, the available angiographic and epidemiologic data supported a policy of return to flying duty of selected aviators. Aviators with EIVT and otherwise normal cardiac evaluations with normal coronary arteriograms may be returned to flying duty. These aviators should be restricted to non-high–performance aircraft with dual-pilot crews and should undergo annual cardiovascular reevaluations. These individuals constitute a long-term, ongoing natural history study at USAFSAM. Future aeromedical recommendations will be made on the basis of the follow-up of these aviators.

Supraventricular Tachycardia

Supraventricular tachycardia (SVT) may cause sudden incapacitation. Even in the healthy individual, rapid, sustained tachycardias with very short diastolic filling periods may lead to inadequate cardiac output or near or frank syncope. Further, individuals with subclinical CAD may develop symptoms of angina pectoris, heart failure, or cardiovascular collapse due to sustained tachyarrhythmia. Prior to 1974, all episodes of SVT were considered disqualifying for flying duties in the United States Air Force. Subsequently, aviators with isolated asymptomatic episodes of SVT have been returned to flying status following stringent evaluations.[27] The most favorable cases of SVT for return to flying status were those associated with classic precipitating factors for SVT in younger persons. The episodes of SVT often were related to a combination of fatigue, anxiety, hunger, alcohol, and stimulants such as caffeine. SVT occurring in such circumstances is frequently referred to as the "holiday heart syndrome" and accounts for most cases of SVT seen in healthy aviators. Such episodes of SVT are usually self-limited events that seldom recur if the precipitating factors are avoided.

The aeromedical disposition of SVT begins with a precise arrhythmia diagnosis. Whereas reentrant SVT and atrial fibrillation are potentially waiverable arrhythmias, atrial flutter is not waiverable because of the possibility of excessive ventricular rates. SVT with aberrancy must be distinguished from ventricular tachycardia. At present, non-exercise–induced ventricular tachycardia is a nonwaiverable arrhythmia because aeromedically acceptable subsets have not been identified.

Aeromedical Disposition of
Supraventricular Tachycardia

An aviator with a history of SVT must meet certain criteria before being considered for a return to flying duty. The criteria in the United States Air Force are as follows:

1. No syncope or vascular collapse
2. No recurrence of the arrhythmia
3. Six-month waiting period without SVT recurrence
4. No maintenance medication required

If these criteria are met, the aviator should undergo further cardiovascular evaluation. Coronary angiography and left ventriculography are performed in aviators over age 35 to exclude latent CAD. Even minimal CAD may become manifest during a rapid SVT, especially with the superimposed stress of high $+G_z$ acceleration. If the aviator has any degree of coronary stenosis, aeromedical disqualification follows. If the coronary arteriograms are completely normal and the left ventriculogram reveals no evidence of mitral valve prolapse, an electrophysiologic study must be performed to rule out concealed bypass tracts, detect abnormal refractory periods, and document unstable hemodynamics if the arrhythmia is induced in the cardiac catheterization laboratory. In aviators 35 years of age or younger, electrophysiologic studies alone are performed if the exercise ECG and thallium scintigram are normal.

Ninety-four cases of SVT have met the criteria for referral to USAFSAM. Of these individuals, 68 (72%) were returned to flying status, 15 (16%) were disqualified due to some degree of CAD, and 11 (12%) were aeromedically disqualified due to other causes. Rapid progress in electro-physiologic techniques, combined with increased observation of the natural history of asymptomatic arrhythmias, will likely lead to further identification of subsets with favorable prognoses.

Wolff-Parkinson-White Electrocardiographic Finding

The Wolff-Parkinson-White (WPW) electrocardiographic finding consists of a short PR interval (<0.10 seconds), a delta wave at the onset of the QRS complex, and a widened QRS complex. By definition, individuals with the WPW electrocardiographic finding who also have tachyarrhythmias have the WPW syndrome. The electrocardiographic finding of the WPW pattern indicates the presence of a bypass tract. The WPW electrocardiographic finding is disqualifying for entry into flight training in the United States Air Force. This electrocardiographic finding may be waiverable for continued flying duties if discovered in trained aviators in the absence of a history of tachyarrhythmia. Because the electrocardiographic finding of preexcitation may be intermittent, some cases of WPW are not discovered on entry into aircrew training and only appear on a subsequent ECG. Electrophysiologic studies for aeromedical assessment are not indicated in individuals with either the WPW electrocardiographic finding or in those with the WPW syndrome. An electrophysiologic study would not change the aeromedical disposition because the basic WPW pattern indicates the presence of a bypass tract, and the occurrence of tachyarrhythmias is a priori disqualifying in the WPW syndrome. The presence of the WPW pattern on the ECG requires thorough cardiovascular evaluation, including ambulatory electrocardiographic monitoring, treadmill exercise testing, and baseline thallium scintigraphy. Centrifuge stress testing is indicated for aircrew flying in high-performance aircraft.

In the experience of USAFSAM, the WPW electrocardiographic pattern is not a marker for CAD. The occurrence of CAD in aviators with the WPW syndrome, however, is of special concern because coronary artery stenosis is the condition that individuals with rapid tachyarrhythmias are least able to tolerate. Although a young aviator without coronary disease may remain asymptomatic during a paroxysmal tachycardia, the ability to tolerate the arrhythmia later in life may be compromised by the development of coronary disease. Coronary disease is the most frequently acquired heart disease in aviators. This fact, in our opinion, prohibits the training of individuals with the anatomic substrate for paroxysmal tachyarrhythmias. Further, the ST segment becomes uninterpretable during exercise in the majority of individuals with the WPW pattern. The loss of the exercise test as a noninvasive cardiovascular surveillance tool is most unfortunate. The flight surgeon is thus deprived of a means to screen serially for the one condition that individuals with the WPW syndrome can least tolerate in the face of tachyarrhythmias: coronary artery disease. The presence of a large number of aviators with the WPW pattern and an uninterpretable electrocardiographic ST segment response to exercise would present a formidable medical follow-up problem and would seriously complicate surveillance for CAD in this group. The increased risk of sustained tachycardia and the logistic difficulty of cardiovascular surveillance in these patients continue to make this disorder disqualifying for entry into flight training in the United States Air Force. Trained aviators without tachyarrhythmias may remain on flying status with periodic surveillance.

Individuals with shortened PR intervals (<0.10 seconds) who have a history of SVT without other features of the WPW syndrome are said to have the Lown-Ganong-Levine syndrome. Individuals with this syndrome are disqualified from flying duties in the United States Air Force. Those individuals with a shortened PR interval and no history of tachyarrhythmia may be entered into or continued on flying status.

Right and Left Bundle Branch Block

Both right and left bundle branch block are rare conduction disturbances in the United States aviation population (Fig. 14–8). Left bundle branch block (LBBB) occurs on the initial ECG in fewer than 2 of 1000 aviators under the age of 50. Right bundle branch block (RBBB) occurs on the initial ECG in fewer than 6 of 1000 aviators below age 50. Bifascicular and trifascicular blocks account for 90% of cases that ultimately develop complete heart block, whereas monofascicular blocks account for only 10% of cases that develop complete heart block.

Right Bundle Branch Block

Studies at USAFSAM have located the site of conduction delay in asymptomatic aviators with acquired RBBB.[29] Using endocardial mapping techniques, investigators found that aviators with acquired RBBB had normal His bundle to RBB conduction times and prolonged His bundle to right ventricular outflow times. Normal control data were obtained from subjects undergoing electrophysiologic studies for reasons other than acquired RBBB. Although the cause of the conduction delay is unknown, the distal location of the block suggests that a progressive conduction delay is unlikely. Indeed, complete heart block developed in only 1 of 372 aviators with RBBB followed for an average of 10 years.[30] Based on electrophysiologic and epidemiologic information, aviators with RBBB may be retained on flying status if a full noninvasive evaluation, including exercise electrocardiography and thallium scintigraphy, is normal. Electrophysiologic studies are still needed for aviators with RBBB if left axis deviation, marked right axis deviation, first-degree atrioventricular (AV) block, or second-degree AV block are present. Among the 164 aviators with RBBB previously evaluated at USAFSAM, 83% have been returned to flying duty. CAD was found in 13% of these aviators, and an abnormal His bundle electrogram was found in 1%.[27] Most cases of asymptomatic acquired bundle branch blocks were not due to coronary disease in early studies by Lancaster and colleagues.[31]

Left Bundle Branch Block

Coronary arteriography and electrophysiologic study are required by the United States Air Force for all aviators with acquired LBBB. Aviators with LBBB have tended to be slightly older in the USAFSAM series, and the prevalence of CAD and hypertension were slightly greater than in a control population.[30,31] Although the ST segment response to exercise is interpretable with RBBB,[32] the ST segment response during exericse is uninterpretable with LBBB. R-wave amplitude changes with exercise in LBBB subjects, however, may have diagnostic value.[33] The USAFSAM experience indicates that some aviators with LBBB and normal coronary arteriograms have an abnormal exercise thallium myocardial scintigram. The presence of abnormal thallium scintigrams in individuals with LBBB and normal coronary arteriograms suggests

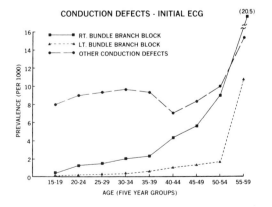

Fig. 14–8. Prevalence of conduction defects on the initial electrocardiogram in 5-year age groups of United States Air Force aviators.

that the basic defect in asymptomatic LBBB may be due to a process that is not confined to the conduction system but may stem from a common process affecting both myocardium and specialized conduction tissue. Aviators with acquired asymptomatic LBBB will continue to be the focus of a natural history study.

In a group of 63 aviators with LBBB evaluated at USAFSAM, all of whom underwent left heart catheterization and electrophysiologic study, 46 (73%) were returned to flying status, 14 (22%) had CAD and were medically disqualified, and three (5%) were disqualified due to other causes, including one aviator with a prolonged H-Q interval.[27]

Aviators with LBBB should have a complete cardiovascular evaluation with exercise electrocardiography, thallium myocardial scintigraphy, coronary angiography, and electrophysiologic studies. A waiver may be considered for those aviators in whom no underlying cardiovascular disease is demonstrated.

Atrioventricular Block

Atrioventricular (AV) block is classified as first-degree, second-degree, and third-degree block. Second-degree AV block is further divided into Mobitz Type I (Wenckebach) and Mobitz Type II blocks. For United States Air Force aviators, first-degree AV Block is defined as a PR interval on the resting ECG greater than 0.21 seconds in duration, irrespective of age and heart rate. The definition of first-degree AV block requires that, without exception, every sinus P-wave must be followed by a ventricular complex. First-degree AV block may occur anywhere in the AV conduction system proximal to the Purkinje fibers. The site of the conduction delay in first-degree AV block is nearly always in the AV node. First-degree AV block is usually a normal variant secondary to increased vagal tone in healthy aviators. Associated sinus bradycardia is common. Aviators with first-degree AV block should

undergo exercise electrocardiography to document that the PR interval shortens appropriately with increasing heart rate. In an asymptomatic aviator with a normal physical examination and a normal PR interval response to exercise, continuation of flying status is recommended. Follow-up examinations should include annual ECGs and repeat treadmill testing, if indicated.

In typical Mobitz Type I block, the PR interval of successive beats lengthens progressively until a P-wave appears, but no QRS complex follows as expected. The next beat after the pause that follows the nonconducted P-wave has a shorter PR interval than any subsequent PR interval in the Wenckebach cycle. Electrophysiologic studies have revealed that block occurs within the AV node in most cases of Mobitz Type I block. Rarely is Mobitz Type I block caused by a conduction delay below the level of the AV node. Aviators with Mobitz Type I AV block should undergo a complete cardiovascular examination, including exercise electrocardiography and an ambulatory electrocardiographic study. Centrifuge testing may be needed in some cases.

In Mobitz Type II AV block, some of the P-waves are not followed by QRS complexes. There is no progressive increase in the PR interval prior to the nonconducted P-wave, nor is there shortening of the PR interval following the nonconducted P-wave. Mobitz Type II block and third-degree AV block (complete heart block) will not be further discussed here because both of these conduction disorders are incompatible with flying safety.

Axis Deviation

Right axis deviation (RAD) is defined as a mean QRS axis of +120 degrees or more in the frontal plane. Left axis deviation (LAD) is defined as a mean QRS axis equal to or more negative than −30 degrees in the frontal plane. The prevalence of LAD on the initial ECG increases with age in the United States Air Force aviator, occurring in 5/1000 aviators below age 30 and 50/1000 aviators by age 60 (Fig. 14–9). LAD may be related to conduction disturbances or myocardial disease. In older aviators, pulmonary disease is the most common cause of RAD. RAD in young aviators is usually due to a persistent juvenile pattern, previously undetected congenital heart disease, or right ventricular hypertrophy unrelated to congenital heart abnormalities. In the absence of findings suggestive of organic heart disease, aviators with acquired left and right axis deviations may, in most cases, be adequately evaluated noninvasively.

LAD may be a part of the left anterior fascicular block pattern (LAFB). LAFB also includes a small q-wave in leads I and aVl, small r-waves in leads II, III, and aVf, and s-waves in leads V_5 and V_6. Similarly, RAD may be a part of left posterior fascicular block (LPFB). LPFB is associated with small q-waves in leads II, III, and aVf and with small r-waves in leads I and aVl. The diagnosis of LAFB or LPFB is contingent on the exclusion of other causes of axis deviation. Acquired LAFB or LPFB requires full noninvasive evaluation. In most cases, coronary arteriography and an electrophysiologic study will be needed prior to a consideration of return to flying.

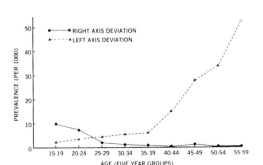

Fig. 14–9. Prevalence of axis deviation on the initial electrocardiogram in 5-year age groups of United States Air Force aviators.

Sinus Bradycardia

As a functional definition, the United States Air Force chooses 50 beats/min or less rather than 60 beats/min to define sinus bradycardia. Sinus bradycardia often is seen in healthy, athletic individuals and frequently is found in military aviators. Sinus bradycardia, however, cannot always be presumed to be due to physical conditioning. In particular, sinus bradycardia, as a serial change in an unconditioned individual, may be a pathologic finding. In a 10-month study conducted at USAFSAM, 64 subjects over age 30 were noted to have heart rates equal to or less than 50 beats/min as a serial change. Of those subjects under age 30, 24 had heart rates of less than 43 beats/min as a serial change. Surprisingly, 20% of the subjects who had newly diagnosed sinus bradycardia rarely engaged in exercise, and 40% failed to show an appropriate heart rate increase following intravenous atropine.[27] Sinus bradycardia as a serial change should suggest the possibility of sinus node disease. Sinus node dysfunction also must be suspected in cases of sinus arrest, sinus node exit block, unexplained syncope, and in episodes of SVT in which a bradycardia-tachycardia syndrome may be the underlying disorder. Evaluation of the aviator with sinus bradycardia should begin with a precise exercise history. If further evaluation is required, exercise electrocardiography is the next step. Failure of appropriate heart rate increase with exercise[34] should be further evaluated with atropine administration. Failure to respond after atropine necessitates an electrophysiologic study. Ambulatory electrocardiographic monitoring may be helpful in detecting associated arrhythmias and advanced degrees of AV block. Table 14–4 outlines the aeromedical evaluation of sinus bradycardia.

Sinus arrest must always be considered in the differential diagnosis of syncope or presyncope. Sinus pauses of greater than

Table 14–4. Evaluation of Sinus Bradycardia in Aircrew

Clinical Finding	Recommended Evaluation
Sinus bradycardia as an initial finding or serial change	Correlation with exercise history. If exercise history fails to account for bradycardia, treadmill exercise testing should be performed
Inadequate heart rate response to treadmill exercise	Administer atropine, 0.02 mg/kg intravenously, under physician's supervision. Failure of heart rate to increase to 100 beats/min or to double requires electrophysiologic testing of sinus node function
Appropriate heart rate increase with exercise or appropriate response to atropine indicates sinus bradycardia due to vagotonia	No further evaluation required

2 seconds should be considered abnormal until normal sinus node function is demonstrated by further testing. The most common causes of sinus arrest are increased vagal tone, as seen in well-trained athletes, digitalis use, and sinus node disease.

Follow-up of Aviators with Electrocardiographic Abnormalities

Aviators with electrocardiographic abnormalities who are returned to flying duties should receive adequate follow-up to ensure that the abnormal finding does not represent disease. Repetitive evaluations are mandatory because the natural history of many asymptomatic electrocardiographic abnormalities remains undefined. Only through detailed natural history follow-up studies will it be possible to determine the significance of certain electrocardiographic findings. Surveillance of aviators after an initial ECG should resume with annual ECGs at age 35. ECGs in asymptomatic aviators are most useful when viewed in a serial fashion. The collection of natural history data on electrocardiographic abnormalities and variant patterns remains an important challenge in aviation cardiology.

MITRAL VALVE PROLAPSE
George M. McGranahan

Mitral valve prolapse (MVP) is the most common valvular abnormality seen in the general population, occurring in approximately 5% of males and in from 10 to 12% of females. Prevalence figures for females vary widely, depending on selection factors. MVP may occur in a familial autosomal dominant pattern with variable penetrance. MVP also occurs secondary to abnormalities such as rheumatic heart disease, CAD, cardiomyopathy, and congenital heart disease.

Pathophysiologic Factors

In the common form of MVP, the spongiosa component of the valve proliferates, with acid mucopolysaccharide found in abnormal quantities. The pathologic changes in MVP are similar to those seen in Marfan's syndrome and related connective tissue disorders. Although increased spongiosa in the mitral leaflet occurs in apparently normal individuals of all ages, the changes are minor when compared with those of MVP. The term myxomatous degeneration has been applied to this process, but there is little evidence to support a degenerative process. Secondary epithelial changes may initiate platelet-fibrin complexes, which may lead to embolization. Qualitative platelet abnormalities also have been found in MVP. It is unclear whether these coagulation phenomena are related to the abnormal valve or whether both are related to a common cause.

The leaflets in MVP are known to be thinned and voluminous. One or both leaflets bulge back into the left atrium during ventricular systole. It is felt that this prolapse places abnormal stress on the attached chordae tendinae and papillary muscles. Presumably, abnormal tension also is placed on the myocardium surrounding the papillary muscle. This "ischemic theory" of MVP may partially explain the electrocardiographic abnormalities, chest pain, thallium scintigraphic abnormalities, and arrhythmias.

Clinical Presentation

The majority of individuals with MVP are asymptomatic and never come under any medical surveillance. Chest pain, palpitations, fatigue, dyspnea, syncope, near-syncope, or symptoms of transient cerebral ischemia, however, may occur as an initial manifestation. Unfortunately, albeit rarely, MVP subjects may experience catastrophic complications, including sudden death, myocardial infarction, rupture of chordae tendinae, infective endocarditis, incapacitating chest pain, significant arrhythmias, or stroke. MVP is now recognized as a leading cause of strokes in subjects under age 40. Disconcertingly, the subsets of patients with MVP at risk for catastrophic events have not been identified.

Physical Examination

The auscultatory hallmark of MVP is a midsystolic click, which may be associated with a late systolic murmur. The auscultatory findings vary with positional changes and pharamacologic interventions. A helpful way to view the dynamics in MVP is to observe that the mitral apparatus is functionally too large for the left ventricular cavity, and any maneuver or intervention that decreases cavity size will cause the valve to prolapse earlier in systole. Thus, the click and murmur will move toward the first heart sound. Any positional change or challenge that increases left ventricular cavity size will move the click and murmur later in systole, shortening the murmur. The intensity of the click and murmur depend on alterations in peripheral resistance. Figure

14–10 describes the effects of these interventions in MVP.

Other Findings

The resting ECG may reveal nonspecific ST-T wave changes in the inferior and lateral leads. Special attention must be paid to the QT interval because the prolonged QT syndrome is a recognized risk for sudden death in MVP, due to paroxysmal ventricular arrhythmias. The routine chest radiograph usually demonstrates a normal cardiac silhouette and pulmonary vascularity in the absence of significant mitral insufficiency. Thoracic skeletal anomalies, such as scoliosis, kyphosis, pectus abnormalities, and the straight back syndrome, also may be seen. A narrow anteroposterior chest diameter may compress the heart and increase the size of the cardiac silhouette in the posteroanterior view, mimicking cardiomegaly. MVP is a recognized cause of abnormal exercise tests in the absence of CAD. In one study, 25% of asymptomatic aviators with MVP had abnormal exercise ECGs.[35] The suspicion of an ischemic mechanism in MVP has been strengthened by the observation

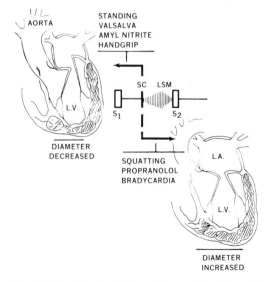

Fig. 14–10. Effects of intervention on the click and murmur of mitral valve prolapse. (Reproduced with permission of Dr. Robert O'Rourke and the American Heart Association.)

of perfusion defects with thallium scintigraphy and normal coronary arteriograms. Abnormal responses to cardiovascular stress are especially remarkable, consistent with the observed autonomic liability found in this condition.[36] Noncardiac presentations, such as neuropsychiatric symptoms, may be the initial manifestation in some patients with MVP.

Echocardiography

Two-dimensional echocardiography and M-mode echocardiography usually will confirm the clinical diagnosis of MVP. An apparently normal echocardiogram, however, should not deter one from the diagnosis when the auscultatory findings are typical. A normal M-mode echocardiogram may occur in 15% of individuals with MVP. Although two-dimensional studies are apparently more sensitive than M-mode echocardiograms, the sensitivity and specificity of two-dimensional echocardiography are not fully defined in MVP.

Aeromedical Considerations of Mitral Valve Prolapse

Most aviators with MVP are discovered incidentally during physical examinations. We believe that the healthy male aviator in whom MVP is discovered in the absence of chest pain, arrhythmias, or other symptoms represents the most benign end of the clinical spectrum of this disorder. Undoubtedly, some aviators with MVP are true normal variants with an excellent prognosis. Unfortunately, clinically identical subsets may experience sudden cardiac events. The current practitioner of aerospace medicine must recognize that the MVP subsets at risk for sudden events are not currently identifiable. USAFSAM is currently following over 200 cases of MVP in male aviators with serial clinical and noninvasive evaluations in an attempt to elucidate the natural history of this disorder. Of 253 documented cases, 75 aviators (30%) have been disqualified

from flying duties in the United States Air Force. Thirty-one (47%) of these 75 disqualifications were due to arrhythmias. Two thirds of the disqualifying arrhythmias were due to complex ventricular ectopy, including six cases of ventricular tachycardia, whereas one third of the disqualifying arrhythmias were due to supraventricular tachycardia. Eighteen (24%) of the 75 disqualifications were due to associated cardiac disease, including five aviators with CAD, six with conduction defects, and seven with associated disorders such as significant mitral regurgitation, aortic root disease (with and without aortic insufficiency), Marfan's syndrome, rheumatic heart disease, and aortic insufficiency due to myxomatous changes. It must be recognized that many of the flying disqualifications occurred early in the past decade, when a reservoir of more blatant MVP cases existed. In recent years, as the incidental diagnosis of MVP has increased, disqualifying MVP cases are less frequent. The latter group may well reveal a natural history more akin to a normal variant population.

Aeromedical Disposition of Mitral Valve Prolapse

Individuals with documented MVP are not enrolled in aviation training in the United States Air Force. Because MVP has only been diagnosed with regularity in recent years, the disposition of active aviators has required reasonable, albeit somewhat arbitrary, standards for retention for flying duties. In the absence of significant mitral regurgitation or underlying heart disease, aviators with asymptomatic MVP should be waivered for flying if no significant stress arrhythmias are present. The following is a list of the disqualifying rhythm disturbances in MVP:

1. Ventricular premature beats greater than 10 beats/min, or 20% of the exercise heart rate

2. Atrial premature beats occurring as above
3. Paired ventricular ectopic beats
4. Technical ventricular tachycardia (three consecutive premature beats)
5. Supraventricular tachycardia

Mitral valve prolapse with aortic valve prolapse or aortic root disease, suggesting a common myxomatous disorder, is not considered waiverable for aviation duties. MVP with more than minor mitral regurgitation should be followed with serial ejection fraction responses during progressive upright exercise in gated blood pool studies. When the ejection fraction response falls or fails to increase normally with exercise, the reduction in forward flow is excessive from an aeromedical standpoint. We recommend that aviators with MVP who fly high-performance aircraft should undergo centrifuge testing to screen for significant arrhythmias under $+G_z$ acceleration.

It must be recognized that commonly found conditions, such as complex ventricular ectopy and MVP, may occur coincidentally and be totally unrelated. For aeromedical purposes, however, one must consider these conditions to be related. A more intellectually satisfying aeromedical disposition of MVP must await recommendations based on natural history studies. Another problem in the aeromedical disposition of MVP involves the individual with borderline criteria for the diagnosis of MVP. Obviously, the elucidation of arrhythmias and other findings necessitates the pursuit of a definitive diagnosis. Because there are no standardized or quantitative diagnostic criteria for MVP, Engel and Hickman[37] have proposed cineangiographic, echocardiographic, and phonocardiographic (or auscultatory) criteria for MVP in an aeromedical setting. Invasive procedures may be needed when the aeromedical disposition hinges on the unequivocal diagnosis, as in an aviator with rhythm disturbances and possible

MVP. Lastly, we recommend that all aviators with MVP, including those with the midsystolic click only, receive bacterial endocarditis prophylaxis.

VALVULAR HEART DISEASE
George M. McGranahan

Valvular lesions, both congenital and acquired, are found often enough in an apparently healthy population to warrant a discussion of the aeromedical disposition of these abnormalities. Valvular lesions, when discovered incidentally in asymptomatic aviators, usually represent subtle subclinical disease that is compatible with continued aviation duties. The aeromedical disposition of each valvular lesion should include a consideration of all factors that could predispose to sudden incapacitation or an aggravation of coincidental disease processes such as unsuspected CAD. These aeromedical considerations are as follows:

1. Risk of tachyarrhythmias
2. Risk of thromboembolic phenomena
3. Adverse effect of some valvular lesions on coronary perfusion
4. Risk of abrupt heart failure
5. Abnormal hemodynamics under $+G_z$ acceleration
6. Risk of bacterial endocarditis

The Problem of the Innocent Murmur

Aviation examiners should be intimately familiar with the innocent murmur because it will be the most commonly encountered murmur in a healthy young population. It must be emphasized that an innocent murmur is produced by a normal cardiovascular system. An innocent murmur does not mean a slight murmur produced by a bicuspid aortic valve or hemodynamically insignificant mitral regurgitation; such lesions frequently progress, and the risk of endocarditis is always present. Although the prevalence of innocent murmurs decreases steadily in the fourth decade of life, they are by no means rare. Failure to recognize an innocent murmur has serious personal consequences for the patient in whom it is mistaken for an organic lesion. Such individuals are often needlessly restricted in life-style and occupational pursuits, rated for insurance purposes, or saddled with neurotic concerns about their hearts. On the other hand, failure to diagnose minimal organic valvular disease in an aviator leaves the risks of sudden incapacitation and endocarditis unaddressed.

Evaluation of Valvular Lesions

The examination of all cases of suspected valvular disease begins with a thorough history and physical examination. Occasionally, the history may direct one toward the central nervous system, as in mitral valve prolapse, or the musculoskeletal system, as in ankylosing spondylitis with aortic valvulitis. The physical examination should include prolonged auscultation with the patient's chest completely bare. Auscultation should be performed in a quiet room that is free of air-conditioner noise or other distractions. Applicable postural, mechanical, and pharmacologic interventions should be applied to differentiate the origin of the murmur. For aeromedical purposes, valvular lesions generally should be evaluated with a full noninvasive battery, as follows:

1. Resting electrocardiogram
2. Chest radiograph
3. Exercise electrocardiography
4. M-mode and two-dimensional echocardiography
5. Ambulatory electrocardiography
6. Isotope ventriculography (in some cases)
7. Thallium scintigraphy (in some cases)

Thallium scintigraphy should be employed in those cases with remarkable risk factors for concomitant coronary disease or other noninvasive evidence of ischemia. Abnormal scintigrams may, of course, be due to noncoronary factors, as in mitral prolapse, or due to oxygen supply-demand imbalance in aortic valve disease. Gated blood pool studies with progressive exercise are invaluable in the assessment of the hemodynamic significance of regurgitant lesions. Cardiac catheterization should be performed for aeromedical indications if any uncertainty regarding the presence or degree of valvular disease exists or if associated coronary disease is suspected. A high index of suspicion for coronary disease must be maintained because of the confounding effects of valvular and coronary disease. When a decision has been made to waiver the aviator with mild valvular disease for flying duties, serial noninvasive surveillance must then be instituted, preferably on an annual basis. The ejection fraction response to exercise, measured by gated blood pool studies, is an ideal way to follow aviators with valvular heart disease. Repeat cardiac catheterization is occasionally necessary to assess any deterioration in noninvasive test results, which suggests progression of the valvular abnormality. Left heart catheterizations done during an initial evaluation of a valvular lesion in an aviator should routinely include coronary angiography in those over age 35. This recommendation is necessary because of the implications of annual noninvasive studies for waivered personnel with valvular lesions. Abnormal noninvasive tests for ischemia arising during follow-up in this asymptomatic population are most probably falsely abnormal tests, a circumstance which can usually only be aeromedically clarified by angiography. In our experience, this situation has arisen often enough to warrant coronary angiography if an initial left heart catheterization is needed. This rule seems preferable to the performance of repeat catheterizations in a significant number of aviators. In United States Air Force aviators, the probability of the development of significant coronary disease within 10 years of completely normal coronary arteriograms is remote.

Aortic Valve Stenosis

The most common cause of isolated aortic valve stenosis is a congenitally bicuspid aortic valve, with 20 to 30% of isolated bicuspid valves eventually developing stenosis. It is extremely unusual to find isolated aortic valve diseases as a single valvular lesion in rheumatic heart disease. Degenerative changes produce aortic valve stenosis, but this is uncommon in a young flying population.

Pathophysiologic Factors

The aortic valve area is usually 2.5 to 3.5 cm^2. A valve area of 1.0 cm^2 or less leads to increased left ventricular work, whereas a valve area of less than 0.75 cm^2 usually produces symptoms. The left ventricle responds to such stenosis with concentric hypertrophy, thereby maintaining normal wall stress despite elevated tension. This compensatory mechanism in the absence of other cardiac abnormalities maintains a normal cardiac output, even with significant aortic valve stenosis. The systolic gradient across the aortic valve is dependent on the rate of blood flow and the valve area. The hypertrophied ventricle has decreased diastolic compliance, thus producing an elevated left ventricular end-diastolic pressure. Left atrial contraction then becomes necessary for adequate filling of the stiff ventricle. Any cardiac rhythm disturbance that abolishes the atrial contribution to left ventricular filling can lead to pulmonary edema. In time, progressive stenosis results in congestive heart failure. Cerebral complaints, such as syncope, are common. Syncope usually occurs during or immediately following exercise. The failure of cardiac output to increase normally with exertion, coupled with systemic vasodilatation related to effort, results in decreased cerebral perfusion and loss of consciousness. Syncope may be dysrhythmic in origin. Coronary

blood flow is decreased in aortic valve stenosis due to left ventricular hypertrophy, a shortened diastolic filling time, systolic compression of the coronary blood vessels, a reduced gradient across the coronary vascular bed due to elevation of left ventricular end-diastolic pressure, and, in some individuals, by associated aortic insufficiency. Increased myocardial oxygen demand and decreased coronary artery blood flow may produce angina pectoris, with or without associated coronary atherosclerosis.

Physical Examination

The carotid pulse is normal with minimal aortic valve stenosis, but with increased severity, a slowly rising carotid pulse is characteristic. Palpation of the cardiac apex in the left lateral decubitus position reveals the sustained, forceful lift of left ventricular hypertrophy. The apical impulse may be bifid, the initial impulse corresponding to the S$_4$ gallop heard on auscultation. The systolic ejection murmur, which is usually loudest over the primary aortic area, transmits well to the carotid arteries and to the cardiac apex. In a young population, an aortic ejection click is frequently audible. The ejection click frequently disappears when the valve becomes relatively fibrotic, calcified, and immobile. The first heart sound is usually normal in aortic valve stenosis, and inspiratory splitting of the second heart sound usually is maintained until a delay in left ventricular ejection causes the second heart sound to be either single in inspiration or paradoxically split in expiration. Commonly, there is an associated diastolic murmur of aortic insufficiency. An S$_4$ gallop is frequently audible due to the decrease in left ventricular diastolic compliance. The presence of an audible S$_4$ gallop usually correlates with at least moderate aortic valve stenosis in individuals under age 40. The recognition of an S$_3$ gallop in the younger population is not very meaningful. In individuals over age

40, however, the presence of an S_3 gallop may be one of the earliest signs of left ventricular decompensation.

Aeromedical Evaluation and Disposition

A complete cardiac noninvasive evaluation must be accomplished (see the list in the earlier section entitled "Evaluation of Valvular Lesions"). The ECG may reveal changes consistent with left ventricular hypertrophy. The chest radiograph or cardiac fluoroscopy may reveal calcification in the aortic valve. Echocardiographic studies may reveal findings consistent with a bicuspid aortic valve, thickened aortic leaflets, and left ventricular hypertrophy. Centrifuge testing should be strongly considered to assess $+G_z$ tolerance in aviators with high-performance flying duties. Provocative acceleration testing should not be performed if the noninvasive examination suggests anything more than mild stenosis. During high $+G_z$ loading in normal subjects, cardiac output and coronary blood flow may be reduced by as much as 60%. Any preexisting aortic valve gradient may become significant under $+G_z$ stress. Aortic valve stenosis is potentially waiverable for flying duties if hemodynamically insignificant and asymptomatic. Aortic valve stenosis is waiverable for continued flying if the mean systolic gradient is 20 mm Hg or less, and exercise capacity, exercise ejection fraction response, and other noninvasive studies are normal. No left ventricular hypertrophy should be found by any diagnostic mode. The Eighth Bethesda Conference authors[20] suggested that aortic valve stenosis should be waivered if asymptomatic, with systolic murmurs of grade III/VI or less, no S_4 gallop, no left ventricular hypertrophy, and a normal submaximal exercise test. The Bethesda consultants pointed out the occasional subject with a high valvular gradient but a normal ECG and a physical examination suggesting only mild stenosis. Although the Bethesda authors felt that cardiac catheterization is necessary in the aforementioned case, we strongly recommend catheterization in all aviators with aortic vlave stenosis who are deemed suitable for flying duties because estimation of hemodynamic significance (gradient and cross-sectional area) is difficult, even with a complete noninvasive data base. The disqualification of aviators with more marked aortic valve stenosis can be accomplished with considerable clinical confidence, often as a prelude to cardiac catheterization and/or surgery. The aeromedical disposition of mild to moderate cases demands a degree of discrimination unobtainable without invasive data. The frequency with which mild to moderate aortic valve stenosis is misjudged in clinical practice demands hemodynamic studies for hemodynamic criteria (20 mm Hg mean gradient). Any degree of coronary atherosclerosis other than intimal roughening should also be disqualifying for flying duties. Although the Bethesda authors would certify only those cases with a mean gradient of 20 mm Hg or less and a normal left ventricular end-diastolic pressure (12 mm Hg), we feel that the latter criterion is perhaps too restrictive because many normal subjects with no valvular, coronary, or myocardial disease exceed this 12-mm Hg limit. Mandatory annual noninvasive examinations are necessary for aviators who are returned to active flying with aortic valve stenosis because the rate of progression of this lesion is unknown but is clearly capricious. Entry into flight training for individuals with valvular heart disease is prohibited by the United States armed forces, and exceptions made for mild lesions are reserved for those already trained to fly.

Aortic Valve Insufficiency

The most common cause of isolated aortic valve insufficiency is a congenital abnormality. It is extremely unusual to find isolated aortic insufficiency secondary to rheumatic heart disease. Other causes of aortic insufficiency are infections, trauma, and diseases that cause aortic root dilation.

Pathophysiologic Factors

Aortic valve insufficiency results in an increased volume load on the left ventricle. The resultant left ventricular dilatation produces increased myocardial wall stress, which stimulates an increase in left ventricular muscle mass. This increase in diastolic compliance accommodates a large volume of blood without an increase in the diastolic filling pressure. Aortic insufficiency is associated with a wide pulse pressure. Ventricular ejection is quite rapid, decreasing wall tension during systole while maintaining a normal ejection fraction. The left ventricular stroke volume increases so as to maintain a normal net forward cardiac output, which is required to compensate for the regurgitant flow in aortic valve insufficiency. The amount of aortic regurgitation is dependent on the pressures in the aorta and left ventricle, peripheral resistance, and the duration of diastole. As compensatory mechanisms fail, ventricular failure results from elevation of left ventricular end-diastolic pressure and an increase in the time spent in systole by the left ventricle. Because the major portion of the coronary arterial blood flow occurs during diastole, the reduced time in diastole results in a discrepancy between left ventricular mass and myocardial oxygen demand. Angina pectoris is infrequent in pure aortic valve insufficiency, in contrast to cases with attendant aortic valve stenosis.

Physical Examination

With more than minimal aortic valve regurgitation, the peripheral pulses are hyperdynamic and the carotid artery pulsation may have a bisferious quality. On palpation, the apical impulse is hyperdynamic, consistent with diastolic overload of the left ventricle. The typical diastolic murmur is best heard in the third left intercostal space at the left sternal border, with the patient leaning forward during forced expiration. The murmur also may be heard in the primary aortic area, and it is not unusual for the murmur to transmit to the cardiac apex. Because the majority of cases of isolated aortic valve insufficiency are congenital in origin, an aortic valve ejection click is frequently audible. Because of the large stroke volume, an aortic ejection murmur most often is present, raising the possibility of associated aortic valve stenosis. The first heart sound may be decreased in intensity because of partial, premature closure of the mitral valve by the regurgitant flow into the left ventricle. The second heart sound maintains physiologic splitting until left ventricular failure ensues; paradoxic splitting may then occur. Aortic insufficiency commonly produces S_3 and S_4 gallops. An apical diastolic rumble in apparently pure aortic regurgitation is far more apt to represent an Austin Flint murmur (relative mitral valve stenosis) than anatomic mitral valve stenosis. Inhalation of amyl nitrite usually distinguishes the cause of this diastolic rumble. Following amyl nitrite inhalation, increases in cardiac output, tachycardia, and a fall in total peripheral resistance will increase the murmur of mitral valve stenosis, whereas the rumble associated with aortic valve insufficiency will decrease or disappear. Great care must be observed to avoid the administration of amyl nitrite to any patient with aortic valve stenosis.

Aeromedical Evaluation and Disposition

A complete noninvasive cardiac evaluation must be accomplished. The chest radiograph may demonstrate enlargement of the left ventricle and left atrium. The pulmonary vascular pattern is usually normal. The ECG often demonstrates prominent QRS voltage due to the increased volume load placed on the left ventricle. Echocardiography is the noninvasive procedure of choice to detect chamber enlargement. Cardiac catheterization should be performed if there is any question as to the cause or degree of aortic regurgitation. Pulsed Doppler echocardiography may suffice for the latter determination. Aortic valve insufficiency is the lesion most vulnerable to the effects of $+G_z$ acceleration because the "eyeballs-down" forces would adversely affect the perfusion column between the aortic valve and the cerebral circulation, lowering the threshold for visual grayout or frank syncope. Further, the Venturi effect, or the "sucking action" of the regurgitant aortic jet, may adversely affect coronary blood flow. As ventricular muscle mass increases to handle the regurgitant load, coronary blood flow may be inadequate to prevent subclinical ischemia, even in the absence of obstructive coronary lesions. Thus, abnormal thallium scintigrams in aortic regurgitation may not necessarily imply CAD.

Aortic insufficiency is acceptable for flying duties in hemodynamically insignificant and asymptomatic cases. Aortic insufficiency is well tolerated in a mild form for many years. In fact, the subclinical phase of this lesion extends throughout the active flying career of most military aviators.[38,39] For flying recertification, there should be no left ventricular hypertrophy, and the angiographic grading of aortic valve insufficiency should be 2+ or less, with a regurgitant fraction of 25% or less. The insufficiency should be due to a primary valvular abnormality. Aortic valve insufficiency secondary to aortic root disease is not waiverable for flying duties. Exercise capacity should be normal, with no significant exercise-induced arrhythmias. The lesion of aortic insufficiency is not usually a source of sudden incapacitation, and decrements in function are generally gradual and detectable. The United States Air Force follows aviators with aortic insufficiency at 1- to 2-year intervals. Echocardiography and ejection fraction response to exercise with gated blood pool studies are the primary noninvasive procedures used for surveillance of this population. Progressive left ventricular dilatation and/or a failure of the ejection fraction to rise appropriately with exercise (6% or greater increase) is grounds for disqualification, even if the aviator is asymptomatic. Although serial centrifuge evaluations are necessary in high-performance aircraft pilots, there is a growing concern that aortic valve insufficiency is one of several cardiovascular conditions which are potentially aggravated by repeated $+G_z$ exposure, and waivers for high performance flying are in a state of transition.[40] Certainly, aviators with aortic valve insufficiency should not be retrained into high-performance aircraft. We do not recommend the selection of individuals with aortic insufficiency for initial aviation training.

Mitral Valve Insufficiency

Pathophysiologic Factors

Mitral regurgitation increases the volume load and dilates both the left atrium and left ventricle. Contractility is maintained by early rapid decompression of the left ventricle. Forward cardiac output depends on the degree of mitral valve insufficiency and the total peripheral resistance. Effective forward cardiac output eventually will decrease due to an increasing portion of the regurgitant stroke volume entering the left atrium. As the left atrium enlarges, mitral regurgitation begets more mitral regurgitation. Eventually, left ventricular failure occurs, further decreasing forward cardiac output.

It must be remembered that mitral valve insufficiency is a multifaceted disorder, which is best understood by considering all structures comprising the mitral valve apparatus. The mitral valve apparatus is a complex mechanism consisting of valve leaflets, chordae tendinae, papillary muscles, mitral annulus, contiguous left ventricular wall, left atrial tissues, and the left ventricular outflow tract. Disease processes involving any of these structures may produce mitral valve insufficiency. Thus, one must make a decision as to whether the lesion is a primary leaflet abnormality or a more complex abnormality of the mitral valve apparatus.

Physical Examination

The left ventricular apical impulse is diffuse and hyperdynamic, consistent with a volume overload of the left ventricle. The typical murmur of chronic mitral valve insufficiency is a pansystolic, blowing murmur heard best at the cardiac apex in the left lateral decubitus position, transmitting well to the left axilla. The first heart sound may be decreased in intensity, whereas the second heart sound usually reveals exaggerated physiologic splitting due to rapid left ventricular decompression. The degree of mitral valve insufficiency may be assessed by listening carefully to early diastole in the left lateral decubitus position. The presence of an S_3 gallop in individuals over age 40 usually denotes moderate mitral regurgitation, whereas an S_3 gallop followed by a rumble usually indicates significant regurgitation. This should not be confused with an opening snap and rumble of true anatomic mitral valve stenosis. If diastole is quiet, the degree of regurgitation is usually mild.

Aeromedical Evaluation and Disposition

A complete noninvasive evaluation is required. A baseline ejection fraction response and wall motion study by gated blood pool technique should be performed on all aviators with mitral regurgitation who are being considered for a return to flying. As in aortic regurgitation, there are certain practical and theoretical objections to the exposure of aviators with mitral regurgitation to high $+G_z$ loads. The effect of repeated marked increases in afterload during straining maneuvers could reasonably be expected to acutely and transiently increase mild preexisting mitral regurgitation. The effect of high-performance

flying on the natural history of mild mitral regurgitation is unknown, but we feel that trained aviators with mitral regurgitation should not be placed into high-performance aircraft. Any aviator considered for return to a high-performance aircraft should receive a centrifuge evaluation. Cardiac catheterization should be performed if there is any question regarding the cause or degree of mitral regurgitation or to exclude coronary disease if suspected by noninvasive testing.

Aviators with mild valvular mitral regurgitation may be acceptable for flying duties if asymptomatic and if the regurgitation is not due to ruptured chordae tendinae, papillary muscle dysfunction, or left ventricular wall dysfunction. Further, there can be no associated mitral valve stenosis, other valvular disease, left ventricular or left atrial enlargement, or arrhythmia. Exercise capacity must be normal. If cardiac catheterization is performed, the radiographic estimate of regurgitation must be +2 or less, with a regurgitant fraction of 25% or less. Left ventricular end-diastolic pressure should be within the range of normal. Waivered aviators with mitral regurgitation must be evaluated annually, including serial gated blood pool studies. Individuals with mitral regurgitation should not be enrolled in initial aviation training.

Mitral Valve Stenosis

Mitral valve stenosis is the most capricious of the valvular lesions and seldom occurs as an isolated finding. Because of the risk of sudden incapcitation from atrial tachyarrhythmias, thromboembolic events, and abrupt pulmonary venous hypertension, no degree of mitral valve stenosis is waiverable for aviation duties. For the same reasons, tricuspid stenosis is a nonwaiverable disorder.

Pulmonary Valve Stenosis

Pathophysiologic Factors

Congenital obstruction to right ventricular outflow can be valvular, subvalvular, or supravalvular. Valvular pulmonary stenosis produces poststenotic dilatation of the main pulmonary artery and is often accompanied by dilatation of the left, but not the right, pulmonary artery. Valvular pulmonary stenosis commonly occurs as an isolated congenital anomaly. Subvalvular and supravalvular pulmonary stenosis are uncommon as isolated anomalies and will not be discussed here. In pulmonic stenosis, the systolic gradient across the pulmonary valve produces increased right ventricular pressure. The pulmonary artery pressure may be normal or decreased, and concentric right ventricular hypertrophy may develop.

Physical Examination

The jugular venous pulse is normal in mild pulmonary stenosis, but with moderate to severe obstruction, a prominent a-wave will be noted if the atrial septum is intact. A prominent v-wave and rapid descending y-wave will occur if there is associated tricuspid insufficiency. Precordial palpation may reveal a sustained and forceful left parasternal lift consistent with pressure overload of the right ventricle. Auscultation reveals a normal first heart sound. With mild pulmonary stenosis, the second heart sound reveals physiologic splitting and well-preserved pulmonic closure. A high-pitched, sharp ejection click is usually present and is heard best at the second through fourth left parasternal interspaces, loudest during expiration and decreasing during inspiration. This click is the only right-sided event that increases in intensity during expiration. A systolic ejection murmur, usually grade II to III/VI, is best heard at the second left intercostal space. The murmur usually increases in intensity during inspiration, is well transmitted to the left

infraclavicular area, and may be heard in the left scapular region. A right ventricular S_4 gallop is not unusual. An S_3 gallop and a murmur of tricuspid regurgitation may be present when right ventricular failure develops.

Aeromedical Evaluation and Disposition

The chest radiograph may demonstrate an enlarged right ventricle, prominent pulmonary artery trunk, or dilated left pulmonary artery. The pulmonary vascular pattern is usually normal. The ECG usually demonstrates a pattern consistent with right ventricular hypertrophy. Echocardiography may demonstrate right ventricular hypertrophy and an abnormal pulmonic valve.

A complete noninvasive cardiac evaluation must be accomplished. If the gradient across the pulmonary valve at cardiac catheterization is 20 mm Hg or less, the individual should be considered qualified for flying duties in the absence of other cardiac abnormalities. Complete noninvasive cardiac testing must reveal normal cardiac function on exercise and no evidence of conduction abnormalities. The individual must be asymptomatic. Cardiovascular reevaluation at 1- to 2-year intervals is mandatory. Any evidence of increasing pulmonic stenosis, right ventricular dilatation and failure, or deterioration in any other noninvasive cardiac tests would render the aviator unfit for flying duties.

Other Congenital Lesions

In military aviation, congenital heart disease, even if corrected by surgery, is grounds for rejection upon application for flight training. Certain congenital lesions, however, when discovered in a trained aviator, may be waiverable for continued flying. Decisions regarding waiverability of specific lesions depend on the individual anatomy, method of repair, residual hemodynamic findings after repair, and the history of the postsurgical results (when available for a significant cohort of individuals followed closely for sequelae). In a trained aviator, successful closure of a secundum atrial septal defect without hemodynamic abnormalities is sufficient for a return to flying status following a waiting period of 6 months. Completely normal cardiac function and a successful repair should be documented by cardiac catheterization before a return to the cockpit is contemplated. One United States Air Force aviator was returned to flying status following successful excision of a left atrial myxoma that presented as supraventricular tachycardia and syncope. A waiting period of 36 months with repeated noninvasive evaluations was observed to rule out the possibility of undetected recurrence of the tumor.

Although individuals with congenital heart disease, even if corrected by surgery, are unacceptable for military aviation training, increasing numbers of surgically treated adults with congenital heart disease are achieving such life spans that their cases are no longer oddities in civilian aviation medicine practice. The Eighth Bethesda Conference recommends that surgically treated atrial septal defect (secundum or sinus venosus), aortic coarctation, patent ductus arteriosus, tetralogy of Fallot, transposition of the great vessels, and ventricular septal defect are all potentially certifiable abnormalities following a minimum of 1 year's postoperative observation of the patient's clinical and hemodynamic state.[20]

Bacterial Endocarditis Prophylaxis

All acquired and congenital lesions require bacterial endocarditis prophylaxis, irrespective of hemodynamic significance. The majority of the lesions discussed in the previous sections are mild and compatible with extended subclinical courses, during which the greatest risk is endocarditis. The risks begin to alter later in the course of the lesions as hemodynamic consequences occur, but the flight surgeon must ensure that the aviator is aware of the small but definite risk of endocarditis in asymptomatic valvular lesions. A program of prevention should include wallet cards and specific earmarking of dental and medical records, with special attention to allergic and idiosyncratic drug histories. Guidelines published by the American Heart Association should be followed with regard to prophylaxis.

MISCELLANEOUS CARDIAC DISORDERS
Samuel B. Parker

A number of other cardiac abnormalities, although less frequent than those previously discussed in this chapter, may present special problems in the aircrew member. Although a host of miscellaneous cardiovascular disorders are disqualifying for flying, it will be most useful to focus on those conditions that may allow continued performance of aircrew tasks.

Pericardial Abnormalities

Congenital defects of the pericardium are uncommon, the most frequent being a deficient left parietal pericardium. Due to potential fatal herniation of the left atrial appendage as a result of the defect, this condition should preclude flying.[41] Likewise, total absence of the pericardium is a disqualifying defect for flight training or the continuation of aviation duties.

Undoubtedly, acute pericarditis, with or without associated tamponade, is the most common pericardial condition seen in the generally young aircrew population. The classic presentation is pleuritic retrosternal pain, radiating to the left trapezial ridge, and increasing on reclining in association with a pericardial friction rub, cardiac silhouette enlargement on chest radiography, and diffuse ST segment elevation of the ECG. Pericarditis may present as an influenza-like condition, associated with an enlarged cardiac silhouette on chest radiography. There are many causes of pericarditis, including idiopathic, infectious, metabolic, autoimmune, traumatic, iatrogenic (drugs and radiation), and neoplastic conditions. Echocardiography is presently the best noninvasive tool for the evaluation of the presence and amount of any associated effusion. Pericardiocentesis should be reserved for the emergency treatment of tamponade with circulatory compromise. After resolution of the acute pericarditis, an aviator should be observed for 6 months. This will allow for the detection of recurrence or the appearance of an underlying disease not apparent during the initial episode. If the 6-month waiting period is uneventful, meticulous reevaluation is recommended and should include exercise electrocardiography, ambulatory electrocardiographic monitoring, and echocardiography. Centrifuge stress testing is necessary in a high-performance aircraft crewmember. If such testing reveals normal cardiac function and reserve with no evidence of persistent effusion, pericardial constriction, or significant arrhythmias, a return to flying is appropriate. Any recurrence of pericarditis is grounds for disqualification.

Pericardial constriction may result from a variety of insults that produce inflammation of the pericardial tissues and associated exudation of fluid into the pericardial sac. Constriction is usually a chronic, insidious problem, although subacute effusoconstrictive conditions occur. Functionally, constriction produces a significant impairment of cardiac filling, a reduction in cardiac reserve, and a characteristic increase in systemic venous pressure. Pericardial constriction should be disqualifying for aircrew duties due to a propensity for arrhythmias, primarily atrial fibrillation.[42] The quite variable results of pericardial stripping for constriction generally necessitate permanent disqualification for aviators who are surgically stripped, but rare individuals could conceivably be returned to flying after lengthy observation.

Multiple benign tumors, primary malig-nancies, metastatic neoplasms, and lymphoreticular neoplasms can involve the pericardium. Included in this category are pericardial cysts, which may be asymptomatic lesions commonly located at the right heart border.[43] The potential for arrhythmias and symptoms precludes further flying duties in all patients with pericardial tumors and cysts.

Myocardial Abnormalities

Primary muscle diseases of the heart include a variety of unrelated conditions that may result eventually in similar symptoms and hemodynamic syndromes. Primary cardiomyopathies are customarily divided into congestive, restrictive, and hypertrophic categories. These cardiomyopathies are chronic, progressive diseases with a propensity for arrhythmias, thromboembolism, and sudden death. The arbitrary separation of hypertrophic cardiomyopathies into obstructive and nonobstructive categories is not justified aeromedically because of the similar risk of sudden death in both categories. All cardiomyopathies should preclude further flying.

Acute viral myocarditis, although relatively uncommon clinically, may occur more frequently than has been recognized. Viral myocarditis is usually recognized because of congestive heart failure during or following a viral illness. The viral etiology should be confirmed by serial viral titers. Following a 6-month waiting period, a return to flying may be considered if a complete noninvasive cardiac evaluation is normal. This evaluation should include a detailed study of left ventricular function by two-dimensional echocardiography and/or radionuclide angiography. Right and left heart catheterizations may be required to exclude residual myocardial dysfunction. An apparent potential for progression to a chronic cardiomyopathy exists, however, and may occur even years later.[44] Thus, cases of apparently resolved myocarditis require reevaluation on at least a yearly basis. Other potential causes of an acute myocarditis include connective tissue diseases, toxic damage from drugs or chemicals, and metabolic disorders.

A variety of tumors may involve the myocardium. Metastic tumors are the most common neoplasms that involve the heart. Sarcomas are collectively the most common primary malignancies of the heart that are associated with significant myocardial involvement. Because even the benign tumors may seriously alter cardiac function and predispose to significant arrhythmias, their presence should preclude further aircrew duties.

Athlete's Heart

In any discussion of heart disease in aviators, it is appropriate to discuss athlete's heart, a condition that superficially may be confused with a primary or secondary myocardial abnormality. In fact, the athletic heart is a variant of normal, representing a compensatory response to the enhanced requirements of strenuous and/or prolonged muscular exercise. The athletic heart is usually first recognized by a significant resting bradycardia, an enlarged heart, auscultation of diastolic gallops or an ejection murmur, or evidence of chamber hypertrophy. First-degree AV block, Mobitz Type I (Wenckebach) second-degree block, and junctional escape rhythms are common due to the high resting vagal tone in these individuals. Significant arrhythmias are uncommon in these trained athletes.[45] Echocardiography characteristically confirms enlarged chamber cavity sizes, particularly the right ventricle, and mild hypertrophy of the left ventricular walls, with excellent contractility. Exercise electrocardiography and radionuclide angiography reveal superior performance. In some difficult diagnostic circumstances, cardiac catheterization may be required to exclude cardiac disease. The long-term prognosis of athlete's heart is excellent, and continuation of flying duties is justified.

Endocardial Abnormalites

The primary endocardial disease of aeromedical significance is bacterial endocarditis. Endocarditis may occur even in a previously normal heart and is recognized as one of the great masqueraders, with diverse presentations.[44] It may present as an acute, subacute, or chronic condition. Although cures with antibiotics are generally the rule, complications are common, usually with at least residual minor degrees of damage to the infected tissue. Therefore, even an isolated bout of bacterial endocarditis with excellent therapeutic response is unacceptable for flying duties. The same disposition pertains to nonbacterial, infectious endocarditis and to all other proliferative endocardial diseases.

Myxomas are the most common primary cardiac tumors. Although myxomas occur in all chambers, they are slightly more common on the left side of the heart and may exist in more than one cavity simultaneously.[43] Myxomas may mimic valvular heart disease or systemic illness in their presentation. Systemic or pulmonic embolization may be an initial symptom. Surgical resection remains the treatment of choice and may be curative. Following a minimum of 6 months' observation after successful resection of a myxoma, an aviator may be returned to flying status if there are no arrhythmias and a meticulous two-dimensional echocardiographic study reveals no evidence of recurrence. A two-dimensional echocardiogram should be accomplished at 6-month intervals to detect recurrence or a multifocal tumor. Similar action is appropriate following resection of other benign intracavity tumors.

Intracavity thrombi, with their ever-present risk of embolization and their virtually universal association with significant underlying cardiac disease, preclude further aircrew duties.

Cardiac Trauma

Trauma to the heart, its main vessels, and the coronary arteries can be divided into penetrating and nonpenetrating injuries. Penetrating injuries to the heart involve at least a portion of the myocardium. Required reparative surgery and healing may increase the risk of future arrhythmias; therefore, such injuries are felt to exclude future flying duties. Blunt trauma to the heart may result in abnormalities ranging from subclinical chamber injury to vessel rupture and death. Pericardial responses to this form of injury may present and progress much like acute pericarditis and should be handled aeromedically in a similar fashion. Myocardial damage, including contusion, intradural hematoma, myocardial infarction, and rupture, should exclude the aviator from further flying. Traumatic damage to cardiac valves, valve apparatus, or to thoracic or coronary vessels is likewise disqualifying.

PULMONARY DISEASE
Paul V. Celio

Pulmonary function tests are required annually by the United States Air Force on all aviators over age 39. These tests screen for pulmonary disease and broadly categorize the nature of any pulmonary dysfunction into obstructive or restrictive forms. Such testing also quantitates the degree of impairment, assists in the prediction of subsequent functional impairment, and allows one to gauge therapeutic responses if pulmonary disease is identified. Physicians should be aware of two significant problems in the use of pulmonary function tests as screening tools. The first is that abnormal pulmonary function tests do not indicate the cause of the defect because many different respiratory diseases may have the same effect on pulmonary functioning; therefore, only the general class of disease is identified. The second problem is that pulmonary function tests are only gross indicators of function and become abnormal only after significant

disease exists. The most frequently used test for pulmonary screening is spirometry, which evaluates the mechanical properties of the lung to determine if restrictive or obstructive defects exist. Such defects are caused by abnormally high elastic forces in the lung or chest wall (restrictive disease) or by an increase in the flow-resistance properties of the airways (obstructive disease). Restrictive diseases are commonly evaluated by determining the vital capacity (VC), the maximum volume of air that can be expelled following a maximal inspiration. The VC obtained in a patient is compared with a predicted normal value according to age, sex, and height, and the result is expressed as some percentage of this predicted normal. A normal VC essentially excludes restrictive disease. A low VC value may represent restrictive disease (or an artifact due to a poor inspiratory effort) or obstructive disease. All lung volumes are decreased in patients with true restrictive disease, including the total lung capacity and the residual volume. Spirometry is also used to evaluate obstructive disease, which produces a decreased expiratory flow rate that indicates an increased airway resistance. Resistance is evaluated by measuring the volume of air expelled in 1 second during a forced exhalation (FEV_1). This value is generally reduced in a patient with obstructive disease but may also be reduced in restrictive disease when the VC is reduced. A more accurate value for determining obstructive disease is the ratio of the FEV_1 to the VC. In patients with obstructive disease, the FEV_1 is less than 75% of the VC. In restrictive disease, the FEV_1 also may equal the VC. Another useful value in assessing the possibility of obstructive disease is the mid-maximal expiratory flow rate (MMEF). This value can be calculated from the spirometry tracing and is useful because it is not dependent on expiratory effort. If significant obstructive or restrictive disease is identified in an aviator, a complete medical evaluation is necessary to determine the degree of functional impairment and the cause of the defect. Abnormal pulmonary function tests alone do not warrant disqualification from flying. If no functional limitation exists, such abnormalities should be followed closely to detect any further deterioration.

Spontaneous Pneumothorax

Spontaneous pneumothorax is usually associated with mild symptoms of pleuritic chest pain and dyspnea, although it may be incapacitating and life-threatening. Pneumothorax occurs when air is introduced into the pleural space, either via the chest wall or the lung parenchyma. Although occasionally associated with underlying pulmonary disease, such as sarcoidosis, infection, or neoplasm, pneumothorax frequently occurs in otherwise healthy young patients. In older patients, bullous lung disease is the usual cause of pneumothorax. The degree of symptoms is generally proportional to the amount of air introduced and the size of the resulting pneumothorax. A small pneumothorax may be asymptomatic or produce mild pleuritic pain. When a large quantity of air enters the pleural space, the lung collapse produces a shift of the heart, mediastinum, and trachea to the opposite side, causing severe dyspnea, cyanosis, or even death. The diagnosis of spontaneous pneumothorax should be suspected in the patient with a sudden onset of pleuritic pain and dyspnea, expecially if the patient is young. On physical examination, hyperresonance and a decrease in breath sounds are noted on the involved side. The chest radiograph confirms the diagnosis. A chest radiograph taken after full exhalation is useful in revealing a small pneumothorax that would otherwise be overlooked on an inspiratory chest radiograph. A small pneumothorax (10 to 15%) usually requires close observation but no active treatment. If the original leak seals spontaneously, the small amount of air will resorb over 1

to 2 weeks. Tube thoracostomy with suction drainage is usually necessary in patients with large pneumothoraces or in patients with significant symptoms. If a bronchopleural fistula is present and persists, surgical intervention may be necessary.

From an aeromedical standpoint, spontaneous pneumothorax occurring in flight is a distinct hazard, especially under conditions of decreased barometric pressure. The most distressing characteristic of spontaneous pneumothorax is its propensity to recur. In some series, nearly 50% of patients with a spontaneous pneumothorax will experience a recurrence. Spontaneous pneumothorax has been treated in the United States Air Force with tube thoracostomy for the first episode, followed by a return to flying if convalescence is complete, no secondary cause is identified, pulmonary function studies are normal, and an altitude chamber evaluation is unremarkable. A second episode of pneumothorax requires a definitive procedure, such as chemical pleurodesis or surgical pleurectomy. Hopkirk and colleagues[46] have reported the most compelling data on this problem. In a study of 152 subjects with pneumothoraces, 32 aircrewmen had four in-flight pneumothoraces, none of which was incapacitating. All 152 subjects underwent pleurodesis with 10% silver nitrate following pleuroscopy. Seven percent of subjects had recurrences on the same side, and 14% of individuals had recurrences on the opposite side. Eighteen percent of the subjects developed a pneumothorax on one side or the other. Hopkirk and colleagues also reported on the use of the Maxwell box to attempt the induction of an artificial pneumothorax. Absolute pleurodesis failure was 28% in aircrewmen when failure of this test was included. Clearly, a more vigorous approach in aircrewmen with pneumothorax seems indicated. Although pleurectomy is a major procedure, the mortality rate is quite low, and the procedure is essentially curative for same-side recurrences. Nevertheless, 12.5% of crew recurrences were contralateral and would be unaffected by unilateral surgery initially. No firm policy can be stated regarding pneumothorax and flying safety because a reduction of the recurrent risk would entail bilateral pleurectomy. Evaluation of other sclerosing agents, however, may reveal additional future alternatives.

Sarcoidosis

Sarcoidosis is generally considered a benign and self-limiting disorder of young adults, although it requires special attention in aviators. Sarcoidosis is a systemic disease of undetermined cause, which is characterized by the formation of noncaseating granulomas in the lymph nodes, lungs, skin, eyes, liver, spleen, bone, and heart. Its prevalence is approximately 10 cases per 100,000 people, and it is more common in black females. Stage one sarcoidosis represents a chest radiography pattern revealing only hilar or peritracheal adenopathy. Stage two sarcoidosis represents both hilar adenopathy and pulmonary parenchymal infiltrates, and stage three sarcoidosis represents only parenchymal infiltrates without hilar adenopathy. Stage zero disease is generally used to describe a patient with a normal chest radiograph after all signs of sarcoidosis have resolved. Most patients are entirely asymptomatic or develop mild symptoms of cough, fever, shortness of breath, easy fatigability, weight loss, or erythema nodosum. During the initial phase of the disease, many patients have mild and transient abnormalities in pulmonary function tests, anergy to tuberculin and other skin tests, elevated urinary calcium levels, increased serum globulins, and a positive Kveim test. The symptoms usually resolve rapidly, with the radiographic findings returning to normal within 6 to 24 months. A small percentage of patients (5 to 10%) progress to severe functional disturbances, including chronic pulmonary insuffi-

ciency and cor pulmonale secondary to pulmonary fibrosis.

A more insidious clinical complication of sarcoidosis results from myocardial involvement.[47] Autopsy studies have revealed a prevalence of myocardial sarcoidosis that is between 8 and 27% of all patients with sarcoidosis. The diagnosis of myocardial sarcoidosis is difficult and rarely made during life, even in cases of extreme involvement. A major difficulty in the diagnosis of myocardial sarcoidosis is the poor correlation of cardiac lesions with overt pulmonary involvement. In fact, some authors claim that patients with symptomatic involvement of other organs are less likely to have significant myocardial involvement.[48] It is clear that patients with myocardial sarcoidosis generally have little or no clinical evidence of the disease in organs other than the heart. Because such patients are usually diagnosed only at autopsy, the time course between the intial onset and resolution of pulmonary findings and the appearance of myocardial granulomas is impossible to determine. Although some patients have died with massive myocardial involvement within months of the appearance of hilar adenopathy, this complication may develop years after the initial onset of disease.

A serious hazard to flying safety is caused by the sudden, catastrophic presentation of patients with myocardial sarcoidosis. A review of 113 necropsy patients with myocardial sarcoidosis revealed that 89 patients (79%) had cardiac dysfuntion secondary to sarcoid involvement.[49] Of these 89 patients, 60 patients (67%) died suddenly, presumably from arrhythmias. Of these 60 patients, sudden death was the initial manifestation of sarcoidosis in 10 individuals (17%). Several other reports have confirmed the malignant nature of myocardial involvement. Cardiac symptoms are caused not only by active granulomas but also by areas of fibrosis from healed granulomas.

These fibrotic areas may be extensive and lead to the formation of ventricular aneurysms. These aneurysms may occur more frequently in patients treated with corticosteroids although the number of such patients studied is small. Granulomas may occur at any myocardial site but seem to have a predilection for the left ventricular wall, including the septum. Pericardial disease with pericardial effusion and tamponade is also well described. In addition, granuloma formation may affect any portion of the conduction system. Ventricular arrhythmias, including ventricular tachycardia and complete AV block are among the most frequent arrhythmias reported, but bundle branch block and atrial arrhythmias also are often noted.

Sarcoidosis in aviators is almost universally discovered on a routine chest radiograph. The initial evaluation must establish a clinical picture consistent with sarcoidosis while eliminating any condition that may mimic sarcoidosis. The diagnosis of sarcoidosis depends on the following:

1. A compatible clinical history and radiographic findings
2. Histologic evidence of noncaseating granulomas
3. Negative bacteriologic and fungal studies from sputum, biopsied material, or other sources, as appropriate

A number of fungal and bacterial diseases, such as tuberculosis and histoplasmosis, must be ruled out. Biopsy material is usually obtained by mediastinoscopy, transbronchial biopsy, or scalene node biopsy. Serum levels of angiotensin-converting enzyme (ACE) may be elevated in patients with active disease. Although elevated ACE levels are seen in other systemic diseases, differentiation usually can be made on a clinical basis. Once the diagnosis is confirmed, aviators with sarcoidosis should be removed from flying. During a period of observation, a complete clinical evaluation, including echocardiography, stress testing, ambulatory electrocardiography, complete pulmonary function studies with diffusion capacity, and thallium scintigraphy should be accomplished. Because myocardial sarcoidosis involves either active granulomas or fibrosis after healing of a granuloma, the defect is a space-occupying lesion. Although small asymptomatic lesions are probably undetectable by present techniques, most lesions are probably detectable by thallium scintigraphy.[49] Although one cannot exclude the possibility of a small lesion interrupting the conduction system or producing a significant arrhythmia, the majority of patients with cardiac symptoms have large, grossly visible lesions. Gallium is also concentrated in areas of active granuloma formation and may prove to be a complementary technique in locating myocardial sarcoidosis. Although arrhythmias are common in healthy populations, a significant arrhythmia in an asymptomatic aviator with documented sarcoidosis should alert the physician to the possibility of myocardial involvement.

No information is currently available to determine whether the prevalence of myocardial sarcoidosis in autopsy series bears any similarity to the situation in apparently healthy men with incidentally discovered sarcoidosis. The United States Air Force is following all aviators with resolved pulmonary sarcoidosis in a long-term natural history study. Air Force aviators remain grounded for 2 years from the date of the first radiographic diagnosis of sarcoidosis and are returned to flying if the parenchymal and lymph node abnormalities have resolved radiographically. There must be no evidence of myocardial involvement or significant residual pulmonary abnormalities. If steroids have been used to treat pulmonary sarcoidosis, 1 year should elapse following the cessation of steroids. Aviators with even a remote history of resolved sarcoidosis should be evaluated, and every aviator with sarcoidosis should be followed periodically. Low-grade residual gallium activity may persist in the lungs or nodes for years after radiographic clearing and should not constitute a disqualifying finding in the absence of other abnormalities. The above timetable and recommendations are based on the unknown time course between initial presentation and the development of myocardial disease. Further, the actual onset of sarcoidosis is defined quite imprecisely because an annual radiograph is the diagnostic source in most aviators. It is hoped that the observation period can be shortened on the basis of natural history studies. Aviators who are permanently disqualified from flying because of myocardial sarcoidosis should be considered for corticosteroid therapy because healing of granulomas may occur with these agents. There is some evidence, however, that steroids may lead to an increased likelihood of ventricular aneurysm. In view of the malignant nature of myocardial sarcoidosis, the benefits of therapy appear to outweigh the possible risks.

SUMMARY

Present aeromedical certification standards regarding cardiovascular disease, both military and civilian, reflect changes that are largely the result of natural history observations and rapid advancements in cardiovascular diagnosis. Nevertheless, the poor specificity of most diagnostic tests in a healthy population will continue to be a difficult problem. Efforts to correct poor specificity usually have resulted in a loss of sensitivity. Poor specificity imposes additional expense, inconvenience, and occasional diagnostic risk on those who are screened for subclinical disease. Poor sensitivity, however, poses an even greater potential threat in aerospace medicine because aviators with significant disease entities may be returned to the cockpit. The major challenge in aerospace cardiology is to accurately define the nat-

ural history of a host of abnormal tests and cardiovascular findings in the apparently healthy aviator. Such long-term studies should allow one to structure certification standards tailored to a variety of aviation categories. Epidemiologic studies should reveal disease subsets at the greatest risk of incapacitation, the poorest candidates for expensive aviation training, and define the serial cardiovascular tests that would be most useful. Careful natural history studies should benefit all certifying agencies because each agency can then clearly address selection and recertification criteria based on the demands of particular aerospace systems. Some asymptomatic cardiovascular findings may prove to be as unacceptable for high-performance jet flying as they are for recreational light-aircraft flying. If the aerospace medicine community is to serve the aviator best, we must pursue a data base that allows the widest latitude in aeromedical decision making.

REFERENCES

1. Enos, W.F., Holmes, R.H., and Beger, J.: Coronary disease among United States soldiers killed in action in Korea. JAMA, 152:1090, 1953.
2. McNammara, J.J., Molot, M.A., Stremple, J.F., and Cutting, R.T.: Coronary artery disease in combat casualties in Vietnam. JAMA, 216:1185, 1971.
3. Kannel, W.B., McGee, D., and Gordon, T.: A general cardiovascular risk profile: The Framingham study. Am. J. Cardiol., 58:46, 1976.
4. Uhl, G.S., Troxler, R.G., Hickman, J.R., and Clark, J.D.: Relation between high density lipoprotein cholesterol and coronary artery disease in asymptomatic men. Am. J. Cardiol., 48:903–910, 1981.
5. Kannel, W.B.: Role of blood pressure in cardiovascular disease: The Framingham study. Angiography, 26:1, 1975.
6. Veterans Administration Cooperative Study Group on Antihypertensive Agents. II. Results in patients with diastolic blood pressure averaging 90 through 114 mm Hg. JAMA, 213:1143, 1970.
7. Ostrander, L.D., Jr., Block, W.D., Lamphier, D.E., and Epstein, F.H.: Altered carbohydrate and lipid metabolism and coronary heart disease among men in Tecumseh, Michigan. In Vascular and Neurological Changes in Early Diabetes. Edited by R.A. Camercini-Davales and H.D. Lok. New York, Academic Press, 1973, p. 73.
8. Rosenman, R.H., Brand, R.J., Sholtz, R.I., and

Friedman, M.: Multivariate prediction of coronary heart disease during 8.5-year follow-up in the Western Collaborative Group Study. Am. J. Cardiol., 37:903, 1976.

9. Caris, T.N.: Silent myocardial infarction in USAF flyers detected solely by annual required electrocardiograms. Aerospace Med., 41(6):669–671, 1970.

10. Hickman, J.R., Jr.: Treadmill Testing For the Detection of Asymptomatic Coronary Disease in the Healthy Male. Advisory Group for Aerospace Research and Development (NATO) Report No. 681. National Technical Information Service (NTIS), Springfield, VA, 1980.

11. Piepgrass, S.R., et al.: The limitations of the exercise stress test in the detection of coronary artery disease in apparently healthy men. Aviat. Space and Environ. Med., 53:379–382, 1982.

12. Epstein, S.E.: Implications of probability analysis on the strategy used for noninvasive detection of coronary artery disease. Am. J. Cardiol., 46:491, 1980.

13. Hopkirk, J.A.C., Uhl, G.S., Hickman, J.R., Jr., and Fischer, J.: Predictive value of positive exercise electrocardiogram in asymptomatic men: Relation of level of exercise causing ischemia. Circulation, 62(4):268, 1980.

14. Hopkirk, J.A.C., Uhl, G.S., Hickman, J.R., Jr., and Fischer, J.: The magnitude of ST segment depression and predictive accuracy of exericse testing in asymptomatic men. Circulation, 62(4):268, 1980.

15. Hopkirk, J.A.C., et al.: Discriminant value of clinical and exercise variables in detecting significant coronary artery disease in asymptomatic men. J. Am. Coll. Cardiol., 3:887–94, 1984.

16. Wolthuis, R.A., et al.: New practical treadmill protocol for clinical use. Am. J. Cardiol., 39:697–700, 1977.

17. Froelicher, V.F., Thomas, M.M., Pillow, C., and Lancaster, M.C.: Epidemiologic study of asymptomatic men screened by maximal treatment testing for latent coronary artery disease. Am. J. Cardiol., 34:770, 1974.

18. Uhl, G.S., Kay, T.N., and Hickman, J.R., Jr.: Computer-enhanced thallium scintigrams in asymptomatic men with abnormal exercise tests. Am. J. Cardiol., 48:1037-1041, 1981.

19. McGranahan, G.M., Jr., et al.: Minimal coronary artery disease and continuation of flying status. Aviat. Space Environ. Med., 54:548, 1983.

20. Cardiovascular Problems Associated with Aviation Safety. Eighth Bethesda conference of the American College of Cardiology. Am. J. Cardiol., 36:573–628, 1975.

21. Federal Aviations Regulations, Part 67, Section 67.17(e)(1) (iii), USGPO, Washington, DC, May 1982.

22. Hickman, J.R., Jr., et al.: A natural history study of asymptomatic coronary disease. Am. J. Cardiol., 45(2):422, 1980.

23. Hull, D.H., et al.: Borderline hypertension versus normotension: differential response to orthostatic stress. Am. Heart J., 94:414–420, 1977.

24. King, W.H., Lancaster, M.C., and Lloyd, D.E.: Antihypertensive drug therapy in USAF flying personnel. Aviat. Space Environ. Med., 46:436–444, 1975.

25. Lancaster, M.C., and Ord, J.W.: The USAF Central Electrocardiographic Library. U.S. Air Force Med. Service Dig., 23(7):8–10, 1972.

26. Brodsky, M., Wu, D., Denes, P., and Rosen, K.M.: Arrhythmias documented by 24-hour continuous electrocardiographic monitoring in 50 medical students without apparent heart disease. Am. J. Cardiol., 39:390, 1977.

27. Hickman, J.R., Jr.: Disposition of Electrocardiographic Abnormalities in Aviators. Advisory Group for Aerospace Research and Development (NATO), Report No. 681:11–1 to 11–13, NTIS, Springfield, VA, 1980.

28. Alpert, B.L., Cook, R.L., Engel, P.J., and Hickman, J.R., Jr.: The prognosis of exercise-induced ventricular tachycardia in asymptomatic patients. Circulation, 58(4)II:238, 1978.

29. Alpert, B.L., Schnitzler, R.N., and Triebwasser, J.H.: Right ventricular conduction times in asymptomatic isolated right bundle branch block. Am. J. Cardiol., 41:385, 1978.

30. Rotman, M., and Triebwasser, J.H.: A clinical and follow-up study of right and left bundle branch block. Circulation, 51:477, 1975.

31. Lancaster, M.C., Schechter, E., and Massing, G.K.: Acquired complete right bundle branch block without overt cardiac disease: Clinical and hemodynamic study of 37 patients. Am. J. Cardiol., 30:32, 1972.

32. Whinnery, J.E., et al.: The electrocardiographic response to maximal treadmill exercise of asymptomatic men with right bundle branch block. Chest, 71:335, 1977.

33. Uhl, G.S., and Hopkirk, J.A.C.: Analysis of exercise-induced R-wave amplitude changes in detection of coronary artery disease in asymptomatic men with left bundle branch block. Am. J. Cardiol., 44:1247, 1979.

34. Wolthuis, R.A., Froelicher, V.F., Fischer, J., and Triebwasser, J.H.: The response of healthy men to treadmill exercise. Circulation, 55:153, 1977.

35. Engel, P.J., Alpert, B.L., and Hickman, J.R., Jr.: The nature and prevalence of the abnormal exercise electrocardiogram in mitral valve prolapse. Am. Heart J., 98(6):716–724, 1979.

36. Coghlan, H.E., et al.: Dysautonomia in mitral valve prolapse. Am. J. Med., 67:236–244, 1979.

37. Engel, P.J., and Hickman, J.R., Jr.: Mitral valve prolapse—review. Aviat. Space Environ. Med., 51:273–286, 1980.

38. Enders, L.J., and Caris, T.N.: Aeromedical consultation service report: Aortic insufficiency. Aerospace Med., 41:1076–1077, 1970.

39. Enders, L.J.: Aortic insufficiency in flying personnel. Aerospace Med., 38:623–628, 1967.

40. Hickman, J.R., Jr., Triebwasswer, J.H., and Lancaster, M.C.: Physical standards for high-performance fighter aircraft pilots. Aviat. Space Environ. Med., 51:1052, 1980.

41. Fowler, N.O.: Diseases of the pericardium. Curr. Prob. Cardiol., 2(10):6–38, 1979.

42. Hirshmann, J.V.: Pericardial constriction. Am. Heart. J., 96:110, 1978.
43. McAllister, H.A.: Primary tumors and cysts of the heart and pericardium. Curr. Prob. Cardiol., 4(2):7, 1979.
44. Braunwald, E.: Heart Disease: A Textbook of Cardiovascular Medicine. Philadelphia, W.B. Saunders Co., 1980.
45. Crawford, M.H., and O'Rourke, R.A.: The athlete's heart. In Advances in Internal Medicine. Vol. 26. Chicago, Yearbook Medical Publishers, Inc., 1979. pp. 311–327.
46. Hopkirk, J.A.C., Pullen, M.J., and Frazier, J.R.: Pleurodesis: The results of treatment for spontaneous pneumothorax in the Royal Air Force. Aviat. Space Environ. Med., 54:158–160, 1983.
47. Virmani, R., Bures, J.C., and Roberts, W.C.: Cardiac sarcoidosis. Chest, 77:423, 1980.
48. Roberts, C.W., McAllister, H.A., and Ferrans, V.J.: Sarcoidosis of the heart: A clinicopathologic study of 35 necropsy patients (Group I) and review of 78 previously described necropsy patients (Group II). Ann. J. Med., 63:86, 1977.
49. Bulkley, B.H., et al.: The use of thallium-201 for myocardial perfusion imaging in sarcoid heart disease. Chest, 72:27, 1977.

Chapter *15*

Ophthalmology in Aerospace Medicine

Thomas J. Tredici

And God said, "Let there be light."

Genesis 1:3

Vision has always held a dominant place in the attributes necessary for flying. This was recognized by early pioneers such as Drs. William Wilmer and Conrad Berens, who established the first laboratory to study the visual problems of the flyer in 1918 at the Air Service Medical Research Laboratory at Mineola, Long Island, New York.[1] This almost total dependence on vision is evident today as astronauts have reported the necessity of vision for orientation in space.

Vision occurs peripherally at the eye and centrally in the brain. In the eye, the retina receives electromagnetic energy (photons) and, through a photochemical reaction, converts it into electrical signals. These nervous impulses are relayed to the occipital area of the brain, where the signals are processed and interpreted as vision.

APPLIED ANATOMY AND PHYSIOLOGY

Embryology

The eye develops from neural and surface ectoderm and mesoderm. The neural ectoderm eventually develops into the ret-

ina, ciliary epithelium, the sphincter and dilator muscles, and the pigment layer of the iris. The surface ectoderm becomes the epithelial lining of the cornea, conjunctiva, and lids and their glands and also forms the lens. The mesoderm gives rise to all the permanent and transitory blood vessels, the sclera, sheath of the optic nerve, ciliary muscle stroma and endothelium of the cornea, stroma of the iris, and the extrinsic muscles of the eye.

Orbit

The bony orbits develop so as to afford both protection and support of the globe while allowing it maximum exposure for seeing. The bony orbit is shaped like a quadrilateral pyramid, which allows the cornea and conjunctiva to be exposed anteriorly and tapers down to the openings located at the apex. In an adult, the medial walls of the orbit are parallel and the lateral walls make an angle of 90° with each other. The posterior openings allow the cranial nerves and blood vessels from the brain to communicate with the eye, which is acting as an external sensor, gathering information and relaying it along neural paths for final processing in the central nervous system. All of the extraocular muscles except for the inferior oblique muscle originate from a fibrous ring, the annulus of Zinn, which is located at the orbital apex and in close approximation to the optic nerve. Thus, inflammation of the optic nerve (retrobulbar neuritis) may at times manifest as pain on motion of the eye. Fractures of the floor of the orbit, the so-called blowout fractures, may cause double vision, especially in upward gaze. The thinnest bones are in the medial wall, and orbital cellulitis may ensue secondary to a fracture of these delicate bones, creating a communication with the ethmoid sinuses or nasal cavity. A hemorrhage into the orbit following an injury may displace the globe, causing proptosis, immobility, and ensuing diplopia. The orbit also contains Tenon's capsule, which acts as an articular socket. The remainder of the orbit is completely filled with fat pads so that an accumulation of fluid in the body (edema) shows around the eyes as puffy lids, whereas the opposite (dehydration and/or starvation) causes the eyes to sink deeply into the orbit.

Globe

The globe measures approximately 25 mm in diameter. It has three coats. The two outer layers, the sclera and uveal coats, are involved with support, protection, and nutrition. The inner coat, the retina, contains the light-sensitive elements. The eye can be considered an external sensor, converting and then relaying signals to an internally located computer. The eye is beautifully developed to concentrate electromagnetic energy, or photons, onto the light-, or photon-, sensitive retina. Here, electromagnetic energy from 400 to 760 nm, a very narrow band within the electromagnetic spectrum, is absorbed by pigments in the retina; a photochemical reaction occurs, and this chemical activity is converted into electrical energy, which is transmitted through the retina and the

optic nerve onto the occipital area of the central nervous system, where these signals are interpreted as vision.

The sclera is the tough outer fibrous coat, which is composed of collagen bundles laced in an irregular fashion. The extraocular muscle tendons are continuous with the sclera and merge into it. The sclera has a radius of approximately 12 mm. The sclera has an anterior bulge, the cornea, which measures approximately 12 mm in diameter. The cornea has a shorter radius, measuring only 7.5 mm. The transition zone between the opaque sclera and the clear cornea is known as the limbus. Most surgical procedures for entering the anterior segment of the eye are done at the limbus. The sclera is thinnest (0.3 mm) under the insertion of the muscle tendons and is thickest (1.0 mm) at the posterior pole (Fig. 15–1).

The cornea is composed of collagen fibers similar to those found in the sclera. The cornea is transparent to visible radiation. Absorption by the cornea becomes apparent and increases steeply in the long ultraviolet range at about 370 nm. At 300 nm, only 25% of the incident radiation is transmitted through the cornea, and at 290 nm, a mere 2% of the radiation is transmitted into the inner eye. Corneal transparency is enhanced by its structural composition, that is, by the collagen fibers, which are laid down in regular layers of parallel fibers; by action of the endothelial cell pump mechanism, which keeps the cornea continuously dehydrated; and by the fact that there are no blood vessels or pigmented cells present in the corneal stroma. The cornea is thinnest in the center (0.6 mm) and thickens toward the edge (0.8 mm). The oxygen that is supplied to and metabolized in the cornea is derived from three sources: the aqueous humor, the perilimbal vascular supply, and the tear film bathing the epithelial cells. The oxygen supply to the epithelium is primarily derived directly from the atmosphere as it is absorbed by the tear layer

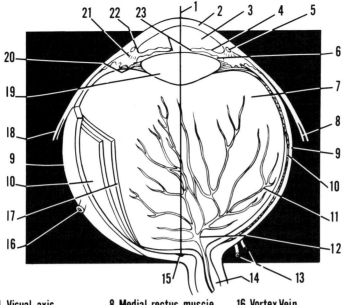

1. Visual axis
2. Cornea
3. Anterior Chamber
4. Iris
5. Schlemm's canal
6. Posterior chamber
7. Vitreous

8. Medial rectus muscie
9. Sclera
10. Choroid
11. Retinal vessels
12. Central retinal vessels
13. Ciliary artery & nerve
14. Optic nerve
15. Fovea centralis

16. Vortex Vein
17. Retina
18. Lateral rectus muscle
19. Lens
20. Ciliary zonule
21. Ciliary muscle
22. Angle of anterior chamber
23. Pupil

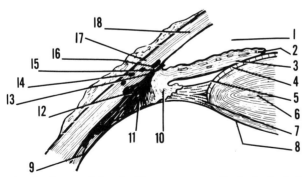

1. Anterior chamber
2. Iris sphincter muscle
3. Iris dilator muscle
4. Lens epithelium
5. Anterior lens capsule
6. Lens nucleus

7. Zonular fibers
8. Posterior lens capsule
9. Ciliary epithelium
10. Ciliary muscle (Circular)
11. Ciliary muscle (Radial)
12. Ciliary muscle (Meridional)

13. Angle of anterior chamber
14. Aqueous vein
15. Trabecular meshwork
16. Canal of Schlemm
17. Sclera
18. Corneal stroma

Fig. 15–1. Anatomy of the eye.

and passed directly into the epithelial cells. Capping this oxygen source, such as by placing some types of contact lens over the cornea, will reduce the oxygen tension at the corneal epithelium. The oxygen tension is reduced as an aviator goes to altitude; this is one of the reasons why contact lenses should be thoroughly evaluated before being fitted on aviation personnel.

As shown in Figure 15–2, the eye is approximately a 60-diopter (D) refracting system. Because the cornea separates elements of the greatest difference in indices of refraction (air/cornea), it is the most powerful component in the ocular refracting system. Approximately 45 D of the total refraction is due to the cornea, and 15 D is due to the unaccommodated lens. Because small changes in the cornea's radius can cause substantial changes in refraction, attempts are often made at altering the corneal curvature to change the refraction, such as by the use of contact lenses (orthokeratology) or the newer surgical procedures (e.g., radial keratotomy).

The uvea lies inside of the scleral coat. The uvea is the pigmented vascular portion of the eye and consists of the choroid posteriorly and the iris and ciliary body

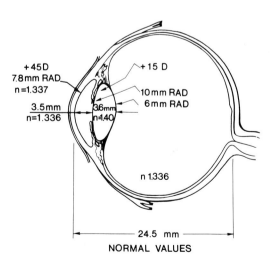

Fig. 15–2. The normal values for the optical properties of the eye (RAD = radius; D = diopter; n = index of refraction.)

anteriorly. The uveal tract contains melanin pigment. Anteriorly, the iris color is a function of the degree of pigmentation. For instance, brown eyes are heavily pigmented, whereas blue or green eyes have a rather sparsely pigmented iris. The outer half of the retina is nourished by the choroid's abundant vascular supply. Anteriorly, the choroid, along with the anterior extensions of the retina, becomes the ciliary body. The ciliary body is composed of smooth muscle running in circular, longitudinal, and radial directions. Also, over 70 ciliary processes are formed that extend centrally toward the lens. The ciliary muscle, innervated by the parasympathetic nervous system, supplies the contractile forces that are necessary for accommodation, which allows one to see clearly close up. Aqueous humor is produced by diffusion and secretion in the epithelium of the ciliary processes. This aqueous humor is derived from blood plasma. There is only one-one thousandth as much protein in the aqueous as there is in the blood. The iris is a thin circular disk that controls the amount of light entering the eye and affects the depth of field of the eye's optical system. The iris divides the anterior segment into an anterior and posterior chamber. The aqueous, formed in the ciliary processes, enters the posterior chamber, bathes the lens, flows through the pupillary opening into the anterior chamber, continues through the trabecular meshwork, where it meets sufficient resistance to keep the intraocular pressure between 10 and 22 mm Hg, continues into Schlemm's canal, and then flows into the aqueous veins and returns to the general circulation. The pupil is controlled by a delicate balance of the sympathetic and parasympathetic tone of the autonomic nervous system. The sympathetic system innervates the dilator of the iris while the parasympathetic system innervates the sphincter. This mechanism regulates the amount of light entering the eye, which is proportional to the square of the pupillary diameter. In the brightest daytime illumination, the pupil can constrict down to 1.5 mm and open to 8 mm in diameter in darkness. In the aviator's environment at altitude, even a 1.5-mm wide pupil will allow excess light to enter the eye for comfort; therefore, filters in the form of sunglasses can reduce the ambient illumination to a comfortable level. In darkness, even with an 8-mm wide pupil, there may not be sufficient light to stimulate the retinal receptors. Waiting 30 minutes in darkness, however, will allow another mechanism, adaptation, to come into play. Adaptation is a retinal mechanism that increases the light sensitivity many thousand times and will be discussed in more detail in the section entitled "Night (Scotopic) Vision" later in this chapter.

Lens

The lens is approximately 9 mm in diameter and 4 mm in thickness in its unaccommodated state. Its anterior radius is approximately 10 mm, whereas the posterior radius is shorter (6 mm). The lens is held in place by zonular fibers. These zonular fibers are inserted into the lens capsule and into the valleys between the ciliary processes on the ciliary body. In young individuals, the lens is quite malleable. Its elastic capsule deforms the lens to view near objects clearly. When accommodation takes place, there is an increase in the refractive power on the lens as the lens becomes more spherical. This is accomplished by constriction of the circular muscle of the ciliary body through parasympathetic innervation. The zonular fibers slacken, and the inherent elasticity of the lens capsule allows it to become more spherical and thus increase its diopteric power. In the young individual, this can be as much as 15 D over the amount of refractive power in the lens' resting state. At age 40, approximately 5 D of accommodative power remain, and when this amount drops to 4 D, the individual is considered to be presbyopic. Actually, most reading is done at 0.33 m, where it is necessary to exert 3 D to see clearly. One must maintain a 20 to 25% reserve of accommodation, however; otherwise, presbyopic symptoms will ensue. By age 65, only 1 D of accommodative power remains. The stimulus for accommodation is probably the blurred retinal image; however, chromatic aberration may play a substantial role in man's ability to focus rapidly. Monochromatic light systems, such as red cockpit lighting, work against this aspect of accommodative adjustment, and, perhaps much more important, monochromatic red light is focused 1 to 1.25 D behind the retina, in essence making the individual hypermetropic or more presbyopic. This extra accommodative requirement increases the difficulty for individuals who are farsighted or are early presbyopes. Therefore, from the visual system standpoint, it is a good thing that red cockpit lighting has almost disappeared. Low-level white light is much more effective for seeing in the cockpit, and, provided its intensity is kept low, the degradation of night vision is minimal. The reason that red light is focused behind the retina and monochromatic blue is focused in front of the retina is because of chromatic aberration in the optical system of the eye. The eye is in focus for monochromatic yellow only, being hypermetropic for red and myopic for blue.[2]

Retina

The retina is the innermost photosensitive layer and is protected and nourished by the sclera and choroid (Fig. 15–3). The outer half of the retina, from the inner nuclear layer out, is nourished by the choroid. From the internuclear layer to the inner limiting membrane, the retina is nourished by the retinal vasculature. Nutrients leave the choriocapillaris in the choroid, pass through Bruch's membrane, which separates the choroid from the retina, and into the single layer of the pigment epithelium. The tips of the receptors,

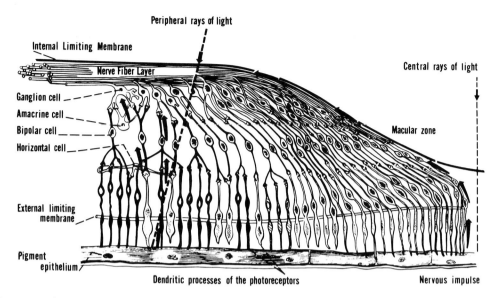

Fig. 15–3. The retina.

the rods and cones, are nestled in between these cells, and all metabolites of the outer retina pass through the retinal pigment epithelium. There are ten layers to the neurosensory retina. The light-sensitive elements are the rods and cones. The rods serve vision at low levels of illumination (scotopic vision), whereas the cones are effective both for medium and high levels of illumination (mesopic and photopic vision) and for color vision. The cones are mainly concentrated in the fovea centralis, where the density has been measured at 47,000 cones/mm^2. Fifteen degrees temporal to the optic disk lies the center of an avascular area known as the macula, as shown in Figure 15–4. The macular area is 1.5 mm in diameter and subtends 5° at the nodal point. The fovea centralis, where form vision is most acute, measures approximately 0.3 mm in diameter and subtends an arc of 54 minutes, or approximately 1°. In the center of this 1°, visual acuity can be as high as 20/10, whereas at the edge of the macula, or 2.5° from the center of the fovea, the visual acuity already has dropped to 20/50 (Fig. 15–4). This is why central serous retinopathy or a foveal macular burn is such a devastating

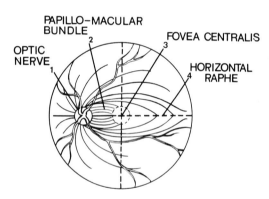

Fig. 15–4. Fundus of the eye.

condition for the aviator. The other retinal system, the rod receptors, are mainly useful in low illuminations because they are more sensitive than the cones and are better at motion detection. The rods reach a maximum density in the retina at 15 to 20° from the fovea centralis, and, therefore, looking 15° off-center maximizes one's scotopic vision. Rod receptors contain the photo pigment rhodopsin, which has its maximum sensitivity at 510 nm. The maximum sensitivity of a light-adapted human eye is at 555 nm. This change in luminosity function of the human eye is called the Purkinje shift (see Fig. 15–8).

To facilitate color vision, the cones have three different photosensitive pigments, one absorbing primarily in the blue wavelength at 440 nm, one in the green wavelength at 535 nm, and one in the red wavelength at 570 nm. Absorption at these wavelengths in varying amounts gives the human eye its color vision capabilities.[3] All the retinal nerve fibers combine into the optic nerve and leave the globe at the disk.There are no receptors here; thus, a functional "blind spot" is formed. The optic disk, or blind spot, is located 15° nasal from the fovea and covers an area 7° in height and 5° in width. Because one blind spot is covered by the functioning retina of the other eye, we are unaware of its existence unless the visual field is being mapped. The optic nerves extend through the optic foramina, decussate at the chiasma, and continue as optic tracts to the lateral geniculate body. From the lateral geniculate body, the optic radiations fan out over the temporal and parietal lobes, eventually reaching the occipital lobe and concentrating in the posterior calcarine fissure of Brodmann's area 17. Decussation of the nerve fibers allows us to have corresponding points in each retina, which facilitates stereoscopic vision, the highest order of the perception of depth obtainable.

The vitreous, a clear, colorless, gel-like structure, fills the posterior four fifths of the globe. The vitreous is firmly attached to the ciliary epithelium in the area of the ora serrata and surrounding the optic disk. The vitreous is composed of 99.6% water, with proteins and salt comprising the remainder. The proteins are important because they make up a scaffolding. These fine fibrils are composed of collagen. The spaces between the fibrils are filled with hyaluronic acid and form the molecular network in the vitreous. The complaint of vitreous floaters is universal and usually is innocuous. Floaters are probably due to collapse of the protein/collagen scaffolding, which causes thickening and casts a shadow on the retina. More ominous floaters, which must be investigated at once, are often referred to as a "shower" of floaters; these floaters are probably red blood cells following a hemorrhage into the vitreous. The complaint of a dark floating membrane that may obscure vision should be investigated for the possibility of a retinal detachment.

Adnexa

The adnexa of the eye are the extraocular muscles, the eyelids, and the lacrimal apparatus (Fig. 15–5). Six extraocular muscles are attached to each globe, and because of the strong desire for fusion and the maintenance of single binocular vision, both foveas are maintained on the object of regard by both reflex and voluntary action. This is done by the yoke muscles of each eye, which are driven by Hering's law of equal and simultaneous innervation to each yoke muscle. If there is a breakdown in either the nervous arc organization or in the actual muscles themselves, binocularity will break down and strabismus and diplopia will ensue. The elevators of the globe are the superior recti and inferior oblique muscles. The depressors are the inferior recti and superior oblique muscles, and the horizontal rotators are the medial and lateral recti muscles. The actions of the muscles are described with the eye in the primary position of gaze (see Fig. 15–24). The actions of these muscles change, however, depending on the position of the globe. In the eye examination for flying, the flight surgeon should be able to discern the difference between a tropia or strabismus (manifest deviation of the eyes) and a phoria or heterophoria, which is a latent deviation that becomes manifest only when fusion is interrupted by an opaque occluder, a Maddox rod, or a prism.

The corneal epithelium is covered by a thin, three-layer, precorneal tear film. The thin, outer, oily layer is derived from the meibomian glands of the tarsal plate. The

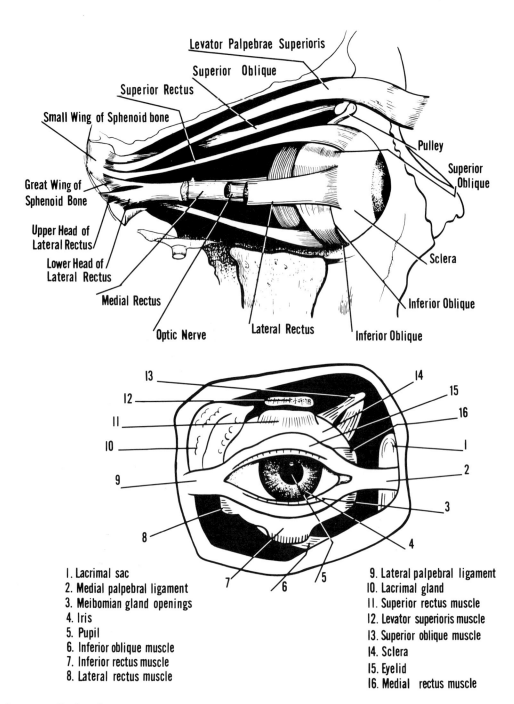

Fig. 15–5. Ocular adnexa.

1. Lacrimal sac
2. Medial palpebral ligament
3. Meibomian gland openings
4. Iris
5. Pupil
6. Inferior oblique muscle
7. Inferior rectus muscle
8. Lateral rectus muscle
9. Lateral palpebral ligament
10. Lacrimal gland
11. Superior rectus muscle
12. Levator superioris muscle
13. Superior oblique muscle
14. Sclera
15. Eyelid
16. Medial rectus muscle

middle aqueous layer is derived from the lacrimal glands, and the inner mucoid layer arises from the goblet cells of the conjunctiva. The external oily layer helps to retard evaporation of the tears and produces a smooth and regular anterior optical surface to the cornea. Ordinarily, a large part of the tear film evaporates each minute, with only the remainder passing through the lacrimal passages. This evaporation causes the tears to become slightly hypertonic, producing an osmotic flow of water from the anterior chamber through the cornea to the tear film. The lacrimal gland is situated in a bony fossa of the frontal bone just posterior to the superior and temporal rim of the orbit. It secretes the aqueous portion of the precorneal tear film layer. Accessory lacrimal glands, located in the conjunctiva, also can secrete tears. The drainage system for the tears consists of a small punctum, or opening, in the innermost edge of the upper and lower lids. These openings lead into a common canaliculus, then into the lacrimal sac, and finally into the nasolacrimal canals exiting under the inferior turbinate in the nose. Obstruction in any part of this system prevents normal drainage from the conjunctival sac, and a chronic conjunctivitis and dacryocystitis can result. Excess tearing will interfere with an aviator's visual capabilities; a dry eye due to lack of tears also will interfere with his visual efficiency.

The eyelids provide protection for the cornea and the remainder of the eye by reflexive, involuntary closing. The lids blink involuntarily six to eight times per minute, thus evenly distributing and smoothing the precorneal tear film to enhance the optical qualities of the cornea. The eyelids are closed by action of the orbicularis oculi muscle, which is innervated by the seventh cranial nerve, and are opened by the levator palpebrae superioris muscles, which are innervated by the oculomotor nerve (III cranial nerve), assisted by Müller's muscle, which is innervated by the sympathetic nervous system. Thus, pilots on long and exhausting missions may begin to have a droopy, sleepy look because of a lack or reduction in sympathetic flow to Müller's muscle. The lids are composed of four layers: the thin outer skin, which is the thinnest on the body and contains no subcutaneous fat; the muscle layer, which is formed by the orbicularis oculi muscle; the tarsal plate, which is a fibrous plate lending shape to the lids and inside of which lie the meibomian glands that secrete the oily portion of the precorneal tear film; and the conjunctiva, which is inside the lid and proximal to the cornea. The oily secretion of the tarsal glands is also spread over the lid edges, and when the lids are tightly closed, a watertight seal is formed. The lids have a very abundant vascular supply such that they heal quite rapidly even when severely injured. The ducts of the meibomian gland are located at the inner edge of the ducts from the glands of Moll, and the hair follicles are on the outer, or skin, edge of the lid. When the duct of the meibomian gland becomes occluded, the oily secretion remains in the tarsal plate, forming a small granuloma or chalazion. This "lump" in the lid usually will have to be removed surgically. It also should be differentiated from the hordeolum, or stye, which is an infection of the hair follicle and usually can be differentiated from the chalazion because the stye is red and painful and responds to heat and antibiotics. These are relatively minor afflictions, but in the aviator, it is important to determine whether the chalazion is applying pressure to the cornea, thus causing astigmatism and distortion of his vision or whether the stye is interfering with his optical appliances and headgear.

VISUAL PRINCIPLES

Vision is essential in all phases of flying and is most important in the identification of distant objects and in perceiving details of shape and color. The visual sense also allows the judgment of distances and gauging of movements in the visual field. In flying modern aircraft and spacecraft, near vision is also exceedingly important because it is absolutely necessary to be able to read the instrument panel, radio dials, charts, visual displays, and maps. At night, even though man's vision is reduced, he still must rely on his vision to safely fly the aircraft.

Physical Stimuli

The electromagnetic spectrum extends from the extremely short cosmic rays with wavelengths on the order of 10^{-16} m to the long radiowaves several kilometers in length (Fig. 15–6). The part of the spectrum that stimulates the retina is known as visible light and extends from 380 nm (violet) to about 760 nm (red). A nanometer is a millionth of a millimeter, or 1×10^{-9}m. Adjacent portions of the spectrum, although not visible, affect the eye and are, therefore, of interest. Wavelengths of 380 nm and shorter, down to 180 nm, are known as ultraviolet or abiotic rays. Exposure of the eyes to this portion of the electromagnetic spectrum produces ocular tissue damage; the severity of the damage depends on the intensity and duration of exposure. Wavelengths longer than 760 nm, up to the microwaves, are known as infrared or heat rays. These rays, too, may cause ocular tissue damage, depending on the intensity and exposure time. The light intensity in extraterrestrial space above 30,000 m is approximately 13,600 foot-candle (ft-c). At 3000 m on a clear day, the light intensity is about 12,000 ft-c and approximately 10,000 ft-c at sea level. The water vapor, dust particles, and air in the atmosphere absorb some of the sun's light; in addition, selective absorption occurs. Ultraviolet light shorter than 200 nm is absorbed by dissociated oxygen. The ultraviolet light between 200 and 300 nm is absorbed by the ozone layers in the atmosphere; this is fortunate because wavelengths from 200 to 300 nm are the most damaging to the eye. These wavelengths produce the actinic keratoconjunctivitis that welders suffer when they fail to wear protective lenses. These wavelengths from 200 to 300 nm are no problem until an altitude of approximately 40,000 m is reached. This is about the height of the second ozone layer. Above this altitude, these ultraviolet wavelengths must be considered. Recent work done in the space program shows that the most abiotic rays have a wavelength of 270 nm.[4] They must be filtered by protective visors, or they will severely limit the time that can be spent in extravehicular space activities. The rays

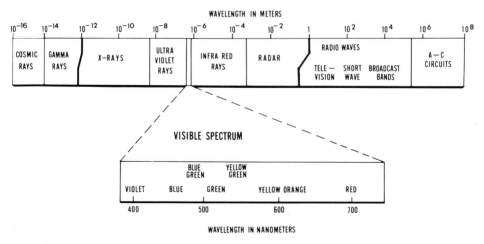

Fig. 15–6. The electromagnetic spectrum.

that concern us on earth, therefore, are from 300 to 2100 nm in wavelength, with an intensity varying between 10,000 ft-c at ground level to about 13,000 ft-c at presently attainable altitudes.

Visual Functions

The visual apparatus, stimulated by light, primarily must perform three basic functions. It must be able to perceive an object by the detection of light emitted or reflected from it; this is known as light discrimination. Second, it must be able to perceive the details of an object; this is known as visual acuity. Third, it must allow one to judge distances from objects and to perceive movement in the field of vision. These latter two functions combined are known as spatial discrimination. Obviously, all of these functions are perceived simultaneously; however, in this chapter, they will be discussed separately. Light discrimination consists of brightness sensitivity, which is the ability to detect a very dim light; brightness discrimination, which is the ability to detect a change or difference in the brightness of light sources; and color discrimination, which is the ability to detect colors. As noted in Figure 15–7, when the illumination is below a certain intensity , approximately 10^{-6} log ml, the eye will not respond and only total darkness will be seen. As the level of illumination increases, one begins to see shapes and objects; this is rod or scotopic vision. At best, this vision is on the order of 20/200 to 20/400 in scope. As illumination increases, such as with snow in full moonlight of 10^{-2} log ml, the threshold for the cones is reached, and this is known as mesopic vision; here, both rods and cones are functioning. A further increase in illumination (such as with white paper under 100 ft-c, equivalent to approximately 10^2 log ml, causes the cones alone to be functional; this is known as photopic vision. The cones are now sensitive to color, and minute details can be appreciated. Increasing the illumination

beyond 10^2 log ml enhances the visual efficiency very little. The upper limit of tolerance for normal vision is between 10^4 and 10^5 log ml of luminance. This would be equivalent to staring at the sun or at the detonation of a nuclear weapon. The eye can adapt to this tremendous range of illumination because of the dual system of rods and cones in the retina. The rods contain the photosensitive pigment rodopsin and are sensitive to minute quantities of light energy. They are also sensitive to motion but not to color. The cones contain photosensitive pigments with maximum absorption at 445 nm (blue), 535 nm (green), and 570 nm (red). The cones must have much more light energy than the rods to be stimulated; however, the cones can perceive fine detail in discriminate colors.

The three psychologic components to color are hue, saturation, and brightness. Hue is the component denoted by naming a color such as red, yellow, or orange. This is closely related to the wavelength of the light. Saturation refers to adding white light to the pure color so as to decrease the saturation of this color. For instance, a spectral red becomes pink when it is mixed with white light. The hue is still red, but its saturation has now been decreased. Finally, brightness relates to the amount of luminous flux reaching the eye. In essence, a source of high intensity or luminance will seem bright-colored, for example, bright red or bright yellow, whereas a source of low intensity or luminance will appear dark or dull-colored.[3]

At night or under low levels of illumination, the fovea, containing all the cones, becomes a relative blind spot. Therefore, best vision is attained at night by looking 10 to 15° off-center to utilize the part of the retina containing both cones and rods. As is noted in the dark adaptation curve (see Fig. 15–11), the cones adapt rather quickly, taking 6 to 8 minutes; however, the rods are much slower in adapting, requiring another 20 to 30 minutes in the dark. Another factor of interest is that the

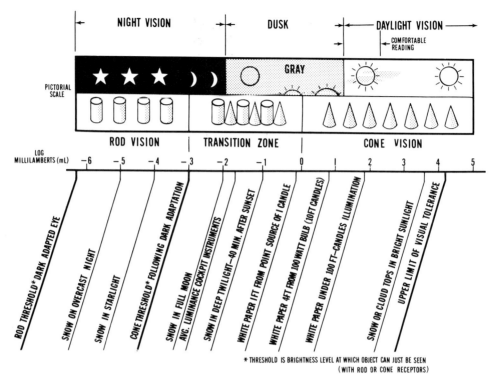

Fig. 15–7. Luminance under varying conditions of illumination.

rods and cones have different peak sensitivities. The relative luminosity curves of photopic and scotopic vision show that scotopic vision (rod function) peaks at 510 nm, whereas photopic vision (cone function) peaks at 555 nm, as shown in Figure 15–8. The difference in these peak sensitivities is the basis of the Purkinje shift. The luminosity curves also show why red filter goggles with a cutoff at 610 nm allow the cones to receive enough light for the individual to function while greatly reducing the light to the rods and allowing dark adapatation to take place.

The second of the basic functions, visual acuity, is the ability to see very small objects, to distinguish separate details, or to detect changing contours. This is usually measured in terms of the reciprocal of the visual angle subtended by the detail. The central (foveal) visual acuity is high, whereas the peripheral visual acuity is quite poor, less than 20/200. The retinal distribution pattern of rods and cones causes this difference in visual acuity, as shown in Figure 15–9. The cones are dense in the foveal and macular areas and even have a 1:1 nerve fiber-to-brain relationship in the fovea, whereas images outside of the macular area lose detail, becoming worse in the peripheral retina. In certain areas of the peripheral retina, many hundreds of rods may be connected to a single nerve fiber. This is an excellent system for picking up a minimum of light energy or detecting motion but quite poor for perceiving detail. Visual acuity is influenced by the refractive state of the eye. Visual acuity can be separated into four basic types: minimum visible, which is the ability to see a point source of light, with intensity determining whether it can be seen or not; minimum perceptible, which is the ability to see small objects against a plain background, where size (the angle subtended) and contrast become the determining factors; minimum separable, which is the ability to see objects as sep-

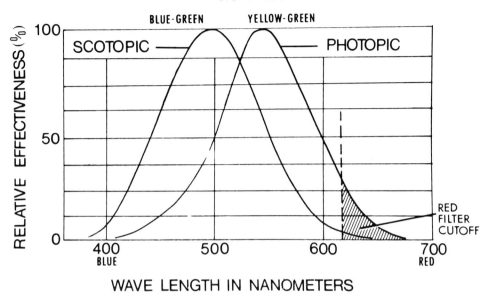

Fig. 15–8.   Luminosity curves for scotopic (rod) and photopic (cone) vision.

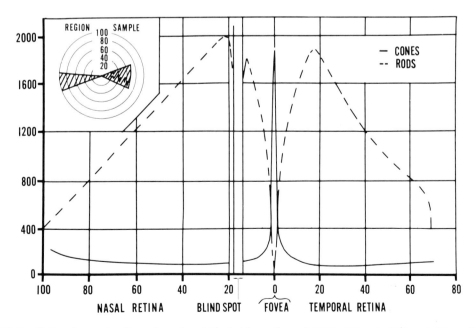

Fig. 15–9.   Rod and cone density in the retina. (Adapted from Chapanis,R.N.: Vision in Military Aviation. Wright Aeronautical Development Center, Wright Field, Ohio, Technical Report 58–399, November, 1958.)

arate when close together (also known as two-point discrimination); and minimum distinguishable, which is the form sense, usually measured on the Landolt C or Snellen charts and resolving a 1 minute of arc break in the C or thickness in letters at 20/20 visual acuity.

A new form of testing visual resolving power is by the use of contrast sensitivity and gratings (Fig. 15–10). The most useful form for visual testing is the sine form. The use of this sinusoidal form allows the ready application of a powerful mathematical tool, the Fourier transform. A sine grating of 30 cycles/degree visual angle may be compared with 1 minute of visual

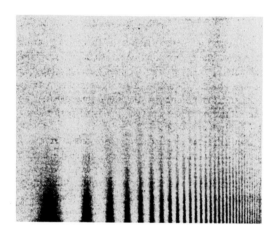

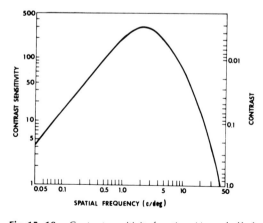

Fig. 15–10. Contrast sensitivity function. Upper half of figure: viewing, the sine gratings shows the effect of contrast and spatial frequency on visual resolution. Lower half of figure: normal contrast sensitivity curve.

angle or 20/20 Snellen equivalent. A contrast sensitivity plot shows that the human visual system is most sensitive in the area of 2 to 4 cycles/degree. This method of testing is presently a laboratory tool, but it is helping to clarify how the complex visual system works.[5]

The third important visual function necessary for aerospace flight is depth perception. This is the judging of distance and the perception of motion in the visual field. Distance judgment, or depth perception, is the ability to judge absolute distance or, more commonly, the relative distance of two or more objects. It is aided by conscious and subconscious cues learned from experience such as aerial perspective, relative motion, relative size, distribution of light and shadow, overlapping contours, and, perhaps the most important of these monocular factors, motion parallax.

The binocular factors of convergence and stereopsis also are involved in this process. Stereopsis, caused by the disparity of images on the retina of the two eyes, is the most important factor in judging the distance of near objects. In flying aircraft, however, it is felt that the maximum practical limit of stereopsis is only 200 m.

Thus, vision is a complex physiologic and psychologic process that necessitates a decoding or interpretation of the signals coming from the sensor (the eye) to the brain. Environmental stresses may disrupt the delicate physiologic balance necessary for maintaining clear vision and will be discussed in the ensuing sections.

VISION IN THE AEROSPACE ENVIRONMENT

The aviator and astronaut function in a hostile environment. In this section the effects of this environment on the eye and vision will be discussed. Some of the factors affecting vision are hypoxia, decompression, glare, high-speed acceleration, and, if one proceeds into space, excessive electromagnetic energy, zero gravity, and other factors. All of these factors can degrade vision and, therefore, the airman's ability to perform his duties at the most effective level possible.

Environment and the Eye

Hypoxia

Vision is the first of the special senses to be altered by a lack of oxygen, as evidenced by diminished night vision. The extraocular muscles become weakened and incoordinated and the range of accommodation is decreased, causing blurring of near vision and difficulty in carrying out near visual tasks. From sea level to 3000 m is known as the indifferent zone because ordinary daytime vision is unaffected up to this altitude. There is, however, a slight impairment of night vision such that all combat crews flying at night should use their oxygen equipment from the ground up. From 3000 to 5000 m is the zone of adaptation. Here, some impairment of visual function occurs; however, this impairment can be overcome sufficiently for duties to be performed. At this altitude, retinal vessels become darker and cyanotic, arterioles show a compensatory increase of from 10 to 20% in diameter, retinal blood volume increases up to four times, retinal arteriolar pressure, along with systemic blood pressure, increases slightly, the pupil constricts, and, at 5000 m, there is a loss of approximately 40% in night vision. Accommodation and convergence decrease, and one's ability to overcome heterophorias decreases. All of these changes can return to normal if the flyer returns to ground level or uses oxygen. Physiologic compensatory reactions will enable the flyer to carry out his tasks unless he remains at this altitude for a long period of time without oxygen. Between 5000 and 8000 m is the zone of inadequate compensation, so-called because the physiologic processes can no longer compensate for the lack of oxygen. The visual disturbances described above become

more severe, with reaction time and response to visual stimuli becoming sluggish. Heterophorias can no longer be compensated for and become heterotropias with double vision. Accommodation and convergence are so weakened as to cause blurred vision and diplopia. Night vision is most seriously impaired. Once again, if not subjected to too long a stay at this altitude, all changes will be reversed by the use of oxygen or a return to sea level. Above 8000 m is the zone of decompensation, or lethal altitude. Circulatory collapse occurs, with loss of vision and consciousness, and permanent damage to the retina and/or brain may result from the lack of circulation and hypoxia. Commercial aircraft and other aircraft with pressurized cabins maintain cabin equivalent pressures of 2500 m. None of the aforementioned visual effects are felt at this altitude except for an almost immeasurable effect on night vision. For smokers, the altitude zones can be considerably lower due to the effects of carbon monoxide.[6]

Reduced Barometric Pressure

Decompression sickness is a disturbance that affects the flyer as a result of reduced barometric pressure. Infrequently with decompression sickness, a transitory visual defect consisting of homonymous scotoma or even hemianopia may occur, followed by headache that closely resembles migraine. Even more rarely, the aviator may be afflicted by transitory hemiplegia, monoplegia, aphasia, and disorientation. In rare cases, permanent visual impairment will occur.

The Visual Environment

The aviator's visual environment is constantly changing. He goes from night to day, from sunlight to shadow, from well-structured scenes to empty visual fields. Fortunately, the eye is quite adaptable, functioning in light levels from 1×10^{-6} log ml to 1×10^{5} log ml. For example, the brightness of the full sun on a cloud is approximately 6×10^3 log ml, snow in full moonlight is 1×10^{-2} log ml, and snow in starlight is 1×10^{-4} log ml. As higher altitudes are attained, the sky darkens, being lighter at the horizon and darker at the zenith. This reverses what is considered normal light distribution, creating a bright view below and darkness above. At high altitudes, there is less haze and the sun's rays are much more intense, so that at 30,000 m, there is 13,600 ft-c of illumination. A higher proportion of ultraviolet rays are also found at this altitude. Glass sunglasses will decrease the intensity of the light and protect against the ultraviolet radiation as well. Plastic spectacle lenses must have attenuators in the plastic to filter out the ultraviolet radiation. New materials, however, such as polycarbonate, being used in the windscreens of modern aircraft substantially reduce the amount of ultraviolet radiation that enters the cockpit. This material cuts off most of the ultraviolet light below 380 nm. The aviator's vision is also affected by the lack of detail in the sky at altitude. This empty field, or space myopia, causes a decrement in his visual capabilities. Finally, changes occur in the appearance of the sunlight and areas of shadow. Areas in shadow are illuminated by scattered light, but there is less light scatter at altitude and brighter sunlight, so that the contrast between the sunlit and shadowed areas increases.

Visibility

Much of modern flying is done in the cockpit. This necessitates good near vision and is dependent on having an adequate amount of visual accommodation. In spite of instruments and radar scopes, one must still see outside the cockpit to land and take off, fly formation, navigate, and, especially, look out for other aircraft. Multiple related factors allow the aviator to see objects in his environment: (1) the size of the target, which is relative to its distance; (2) the luminance or overall brightness; (3) the degree of retinal adaptation; (4) the brightness and color contrast between the target and background; (5) the position of the target in the visual field; (6) the focus of the eye; (7) the length of time the object is seen; and (8) atmospheric attenuation.

The visibility of an object depends mostly on its size and its contrast with the background. In daylight, with the best of contrast (a black object on a white background), an object would be seen at near the threshold of visual acuity, subtending 0.5 minute of arc, or the equivalent of 20/10 vision. A speck of light against a black background, such as a star, can be seen even when it is much smaller and obviously at enormous distances; however, this example is not a function of visual acuity but of light perception only. A star appears bigger because it is brighter not because it subtends a larger visual angle. The visibility of objects is lost as the contrast is reduced between the object and its background. In such a case, the object, now with lower contrast, must be much larger or nearer before it can be seen. In conditions of haze or mist, there is such a marked loss of contrast that even a large object may not be seen at all. Newly emerging testing techniques (contrast sensitivity function tests) hold promise for the possible identification of individuals whose systems function more effectively at lower contrast thresholds. The visibility factors outlined above are, to a certain extent, interrelated, so that a reduction in one may be compensated for by an increase in one of the others. For instance, an object may be so small or so far away that it is just below the threshold of visibility. It may be made visible by an increased illumination or by improving the contrast between it and its background or both. In other instances, the object may be better perceived if more time is spent viewing it.

Targets in the periphery of the visual field must be proportionally larger to be seen. To get maximum visibility, the target will have to be seen within 1° of fixation (fovea). If the object in the peripheral field is moving, it will be easier to detect.

One final factor capable of degrading target acquisition is empty field or space myopia. Older theories explained that the resting state of the eye was one of zero accommodation. Recently, more sophisticated testing techniques (laser optometry) show that in some individuals, the resting state of the eye is actually one in which a small amount of accommodation is being exerted, thus defocusing the eye for distance vision. In the so-called resting states, these individuals show 0.75 to 1.00 D of myopia, thus degrading their distance visual acuity because their resting focus is at 1 or 1.5 m distant from the eye. This is said to occur in both emmetropic and myopic individuals. Moderately farsighted individuals (hypermetropes), however, may find that this accommodative tonus is actually advantageous and that their distance vision perhaps may be enhanced. In bright daylight, the small pupil produced will compensate somewhat for the space myopia by increasing the depth of focus; however, a better method of overcoming this induced myopia is to fix on a distant object. Actually, anything more distant than 15 to 18 m will help to relax the accommodation sufficiently to improve the distance visual acuity. Night myopia, which is similar to empty field and space myopia, only worse at times, is discussed in the following section on night vision.

Night (Scotopic) Vision

Night vision is extremely important in aviation. It is quite different from day or photopic vision. The eyes must be used differently at night if the aviator is to gain the maximum usefulness of vision. The aviator must understand the principles of night vision and must practice using his eyes at night to gain efficient night vision.

All parts of the retina are not alike in their reaction to light. A very small central area containing only cones is responsible for maximum visual acuity and for color discrimination, but it fails to operate under low intensities of illumination. This is the fovea, the area with which one reads and where one focuses objects in the direct line of vision. It gives us central vision, which is useful in high and moderate illumination (photopic and mesopic conditions).

In the remaining peripheral area, both the rod-type and cone-type receptors are present. The peripheral retina is capable of less acute visual perception and of only poor color determination, but it functions under very low illumination or scotopic conditions. According to the widely accepted duplicity theory of vision, the human eye is an eye within an eye. Central vision requires light of about 1×10^{-3} log ml intensity or greater. Bright moonlight gives about 1×10^{-2} log ml. Hence, in light that is less intense than moonlight, there is little central vision. Peripheral vision requires only one-thousandth as great an intensity 1×10^{-6} log ml or more. On a dark, starlit night, the individual sees only with the peripheral area of his retina. This explains why pilots often complain that they are able to see an aircraft at night only to have it disappear when they look directly at it. To keep an object in sight at night, one must learn to look off to the side at about a 10 to 15° angle. When the light intensity is between 1×10^{-3} and 10° log ml, both the rods and cones are functioning, and mesopic vision occurs (see Fig. 15-7).

An individual can determine which type of vision he is using by noting whether he has color sense. The cones perceive all colors. Rods pick up colors only as shades of gray. Most of the cones are in the central area of the retina, so that if color can be recognized at night, one has central vision; however, if everything appears in shades of gray, one has only peripheral or rod vision.

Dark adaptation is the process by which the eye adjusts for maximum efficiency in low illumination. It is commonly experienced when one first enters a theater or goes out into the dark from a brightly lit room. The central area of the retina dark-adapts in about 6 to 8 minutes, but this part of the retina is useless for night vision. The peripheral area dark-adapts in about 20 to 30 minutes, although further slight adaptation continues over a period of 2 days (see Fig. 15–11). It also happens that this peripheral area is not sensitive to dark red light (630 nm or longer in wavelength). Such light is not perceived even as gray, so dark adaptation goes on in the periphery in dark red light as though there were no light at all. This characteristic is fortunate because, by wearing red, light-tight goggles before a flight, pilots can read or rest in a brightly lit room while the peripheral areas of their retinas are dark-adapting.

Dark adaptation is an independent process in each eye. It is slow to develop in the dark and is quickly lost in the light. The aircrew must be so familiar with the location of their equipment and controls that lights are unnecessary for making adjustments in flight. The aviator should avoid gazing at exhaust stacks or any other bright light sources. When using light at night in the plane, such as in reading instruments, maps, or charts, as little light as possible should be employed and for as brief a time as possible, and red light should be used (although red lighting does create problems such as accommodative fatigue and reduction of color perception;

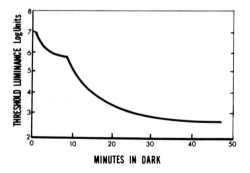

Fig. 15–11.   Dark adaptation curve.

thus, red light is no longer favored for cockpit visual activities). If the individual who is exposed to a very bright light closes one eye, the closed eye will remain dark-adapted, even though the exposed retina has been bleached.

Dark adaptation also depends on an adequate supply of vitamin A in the diet. Vitamin A is found in vegetables that are green or were green at some stage of development such as lettuce, carrots, cabbage, peaches, tomatoes, green peas, and bananas. Other sources of vitamin A are milk, eggs, butter, cheese, and liver. A deficient diet or an illness that decreases the vitamin A supply will impair night vision, and a return to normal, even when large doses of vitamin A are ingested, may take several months. Excessive vitamin A ingestion, such as in taking large doses of vitamin capsules, is worthless to a normal person. Various drugs also have been studied and have not been found to improve a normal person's dark adaptation.

Under conditions of low-intensity illumination, the peripheral area of the eye is most sensitive to green light and is least sensitive to red light; both colors are perceived as shades of gray, of course, but green light is picked up readily, whereas red light is spotted with difficulty. If a red light with a wavelength of 630 nm or longer is used at an intensity that makes it just visible to the central area of the eye, the individual can dark-adapt in 20 to 30 minutes and have the acute vision of his cones available. An observer cannot see this light with his peripheral vision at all, and can spot it with his central vision only if he is fortunate enough to look directly at it. Lest the aviator be concerned about it, the red warning light on the airplane wing has so much yellow and shortwave red that it easily can be seen at night.

Because of the central blind spot under low illumination, one should not look directly at the objects one needs to see but rather to one side of the object. This seems unnatural, and some practice is required to perfect this technique. The eyes also should not be held in a fixed position at night. The use of a scanning technique with intermittent stops at points of fixation is best for night observation. Objects are seen only by contrast at night, that is, they are either lighter or darker than their surroundings. Ordinarily, aircraft can be seen better if they are above and silhouetted against the sky. Contrast is reduced by fog, haze, and dirty or scratched windshields or goggles. For this reason, goggles, spectacles, and windshields should be scrupulously clean for night operation. Reflection of light from instruments on the surfaces also reduces the ability to sight planes at night.

An emmetropic or myopic observer will have a shift toward myopia under conditions of reduced illumination. This shift is thought to be due to the spherical aberration of the eye and to the involuntary accommodation exerted. This myopia is no different from the previously discussed space myopia. Individuals vary but may show from 0.75 to 1.25 D of increased myopia, which, in turn, means a decrease in functional visual ability.

Without supplemental oxygen, the average percent decrease in night vision capability is 5% at 1100 m altitude, 18% at 2800 m, 35% at 4000 m, and a 50% decrease in night vision capability at 5000 m altitude without supplemental oxygen. Oxygen lack, fatigue, and excessive smoking all reduce the ability to see well at night. Oxygen should be used from the time of takeoff if maximum visual acuity is desired. Fatigue should be prevented, insofar as possible, by obtaining adequate sleep prior to flying. Hypoxia resulting from carbon monoxide poisoning affects brightness discrimination and dark adaptation in the same way as altitude-induced hypoxia. As an example, 5% saturation with carbon monoxide has the same effect as flying at 3000 m without oxygen. Smoking three cigarettes before a flight may cause a carbon monoxide saturation of 4%,

with an effect on visual sensitivity equal to an altitude of 2800 m or a 15 to 18% decrease in night vision.

The rules for pilots' most effective use of night vision are as follows:

1. Eat a diet with adequate vitamin A
2. Become dark-adapted before takeoff
3. Avoid bright exterior or cockpit light. Make any exposure to light as brief as possible and use light of as low intensity as possible. Close one eye if exposed to a bright light source.
4. Look 10 to 15° off to one side of objects viewed
5. Develop a scanning technique to search the sky
6. In wartime situations, make use of contrast. Fly below an enemy when over dark ground and fly above when over snow, sand, or white clouds
7. Keep goggles, spectacles, and windshield clean
8. Use oxygen from the ground up because hypoxia reduces night vision (Fig. 15–12)

During World War II, much work was done on the use of red cockpit illumination. The use of a red light having a wavelength greater than 630 nm illuminating the cockpit is desirable from the viewpoint of dark adaptation. The intent was to retain the greatest rod sensitivity possible while permitting an effective illumination for foveal vision; however, with the increasing use of electronic devices for navigation as well as for enemy aircraft and target detection, the importance of the pilot's visual efficiency inside the cockpit has increased markedly. Therefore, low-intensity white cockpit lighting is presently advocated because it affords a more natural visual environment within the aircraft without degrading the color of objects that are not self-luminous. The disadvantages of the previously used red light is that red markings on aerial maps are invisible when viewed in the red light. Also, red light tends to create or worsen near-

THE EYE IN NIGHT VISION

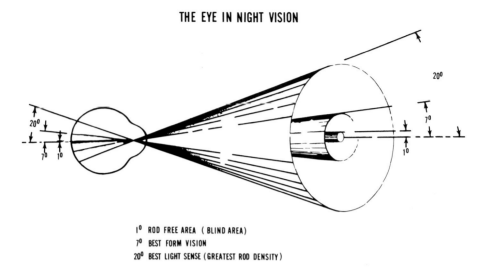

1⁰ ROD FREE AREA (BLIND AREA)
7⁰ BEST FORM VISION
20⁰ BEST LIGHT SENSE (GREATEST ROD DENSITY)

Fig. 15–12. Zones of sensitivity for night vision.

point blur in prepresbyopic, presbyopic, and, at times, hypermetropic pilots. Because of the chromatic aberration of the eye, man is hypermetropic for red.[7]

Ultraviolet light has been used for cockpit illumination and has a disconcerting side effect if it becomes reflected directly into the eye. These radiations produce a fluorescence of the crystalline lens in the eye, giving the pilot a sensation that he is flying in a fog. Properly adjusting the ultraviolet lamps and reducing their intensity can overcome this fluorescence problem to some degree. One might also add that the radiations from these lamps are not injurious to the eyes because, even at the highest intensity, they are still far below the threshold for affecting the corneal epithelium.

During World War II, the problem of night vision was studied intensively by numerous scientists, but no single satisfactory test of night vision was developed. The United States Air Force did develop the radium plaque night vision tester, which is a self-illuminating Landolt C target; however, because it contains radium, it is rarely used today.[8]

At present, the best test of night vision is the Goldmann-Weekers Dark Adapto-

meter. This instrument is capable of determining the dark-adaptation curve of an individual with great detail and accuracy. It obviously is not something that should be done on everyone because it is quite time-consuming, the apparatus is expensive, and only research institutions and larger clinics have it available. With this instrument, one can establish the threshold of night vision in an individual. The testing results in the very familiar dark-adaptation curve (see Fig. 15–11).

The most direct way of protecting and enhancing night vision is by adapting in the dark or wearing red goggles for at least 30 minutes and maintaining an adequate intake of vitamin A. Modern technology has also brought us night vision goggles, which enhance vision at night over and above that possible by the naked eye. Presently available night vision goggles can intensify ambient light about 1000 times. They are passive binocular image intensifiers and are sensitive to light from approximately 400 to 900 nm.

Spatial Discrimination, Stereopsis, and Depth Perception

In aviation, it is important to accurately localize oneself in three-dimensional space. If this cannot be done, one becomes spatially disoriented, a marked hazard to the flyer. Under + 1 G$_z$ acceleration, man orients himself on the earth by proprioceptive impulses from various parts of the body, from receptors in the semicircular canals and vestibular apparatus, and with the strongest cue to orientation, the visual system. Linear and angular accelerations are capable of producing spatial disorientation, especially when outside visual reference is excluded; however, when adequate external visual references are available, spatial disorientation usually does not occur. The pilot's ability to resist spatial disorientation, then, is greatly enhanced by adequate visual references and is diminished by mental stress. The visual cues to the perception of depth are both monocular and binocular. The monocular cues are learned, and some investigators feel that they can be improved by study and training. These cues, however, are the ones that can be the most easily tricked by illusions. On the other hand, stereopsis, which is the most important binocular cue, is innate and inescapable. If the flyer has this capability, it will remain with him, even when the learned cues are sparse such as at night, under conditions of low visibility, and in unfamiliar surroundings. Unfortunately for the flyer, however, the maximum range at which his stereoscopic vision is useful is only up to 200 m. This is not to imply that stereopsis is an absolute must in flying an aircraft because numerous individuals who lack stereopsis still make good aviators; however, if the pilot does have stereopsis, so much the better, and, therefore, stereoscopic testing procedures should be retained in the flight examination. The stereoscopic test for flying is probably the single most revealing component of the visual examination. The individual who truly passes the stereoscopic test down to 15 to 20 seconds of arc must, of necessity, have a well-functioning visual system. He must have two eyes; they must be equally balanced; the visual acuities must be excellent to attain this kind of arc disparity; he must have normal retinal correspondence; and his motility status must be functioning normally in at least the straight-ahead position. In essence, even if stereopsis had nothing at all to do with flying, retaining the stereopsis portion of the ophthalmologic examination is wise.

Depth Perception (Spatial Localization)

Depth perception is the mental projection onto visual space of a perceived object in real space. Correlation of the real object in real space with that projected in visual space results in accurate depth perception. There are both monocular and binocular cues to depth perception.

The monocular cues are as follows:

1. Size of the retinal image (size constancy)—being able to judge the known and comparative size of objects is an important cue
2. Motion parallax—the relative speed of motion of images across the retina. Objects nearer than fixation move against the observer's motion, distant objects move in the same direction as the observer's motion
3. Interposition—one object obscured from vision by another
4. Texture or gradient—detail loss at increasing distances
5. Linear perspective—parallel lines converging at distance
6. Apparent foreshortening—a circle appears as an ellipse at an angle, and so forth
7. Illumination perspective—light sources usually are assumed to be from above
8. Aerial perspective—distant objects appear more bluish and hazy than near objects

The binocular cues are as follows:

1. Convergence—the value of this cue

is questionable and is generally used only for very near distances

2. Accommodation—also useful only for near distances

3. Stereopsis—this is the visual appreciation of three dimensions during binocular vision, occurring during fusion of signals from slightly disparate retinal points, which are disparate enough to stimulate stereopsis but not so disparate as to cause diplopia

The two most important monocular factors for flying are considered to be motion parallax and size of the retinal images. All monocular cues are derived from experience and are subject to interpretation. Stereopsis is felt to be the most important binocular cue and is based on a physiologic process that is innate and inescapable. Like visual acuity, stereopsis can be graded and is known as stereo acuity, which is measured in seconds of arc of disparity. In administering the various tests of stereopsis, the finer the stereoscopic angle, the smaller the number of seconds of arc disparity appreciated (see Fig. 15–13).

The limiting distance for stereopsis is shown in the following equation as b_l. The interpupillary distance is 2a and the threshold disparity is n_t.

$$b_l = \frac{2a}{n_t} \quad (1)$$

The limiting distance varies directly as the interpupillary distance and inversely as the stereopsis threshold (stereo acuity). Theoretically, the limiting distance of stereopsis is about 1300 m; however, for all practical purposes, stereopsis is not reliable beyond 200 m.[9]

Stereopsis occasionally is called depth perception and is measured by several different instruments. One can measure stereopsis for near, on the Verhoeff depth-perception apparatus, where the stereo

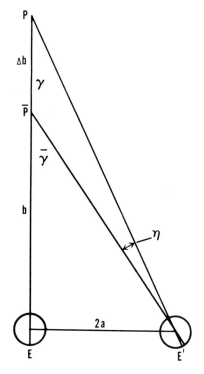

Fig. 15–13. Linear stereoscopic depth interval. The eyes fixate point $\bar{P}$; Δb is the linear stereoscopic interval; 2a is the interpupillary distance; b is the fixation distance; $\bar{\gamma}$ is the binocular parallax angle for point $\bar{P}$; γ is the binocular parallax angle for point P; and E and E' are the right and left eye, respectively.

acuity is measured at 1 m without any special optical devices. Stereopsis for near also can be measured by the Wirt (Titmus) circles. In this case, the eyes are dissociated with polarizing lenses. Stereoscopic vision for distance is measured in testing devices such as the Bausch and Lomb Ortho-Rater, Titmus, or Keystone instruments. Using these instruments, separate images are presented to each eye, and lenses in the instruments project the images to 6.1 m or infinity. In essence, these are tests of stereoscopic vision for distance, and many examiners are not aware that in some motility disturbances, such as microstrabismus, the candidate may have normal stereoscopic vision (depth perception) for near but not for distance or vice versa.

Color Vision

In 1920, Drs. William Wilmer and Conrad Berens noted in their article, "The Eye in Aviation,"[1] that the proper recognition of colors plays an important part in the success of all types of flyers. Can this still be said today, however? One would have to answer yes because a quick glance at what is required in the form of color discrimination by pilots and aircrew, both military and civilian, indicates that this is so. For instance, aviators and aircrew must be able to identify colored light signals, such as navigation lights, airport beacons, approach lights, runway lights, taxi strips, biscuit gun, Aldis lamp, and the various colors on the instrument panel, as well as the colors of various reflecting surfaces such as flags, panels, smoke, and flares. It is important to be able to identify colors used in the coding of electronic equipment, as well a for map reading, and, especially in the military, for ascertaining the subtle color differences in terrain. Therefore, even though the flyer uses largely form vision in the performance of his task, color vision is a bonus that increases his efficiency without demanding much further conscious effort.

Individuals with normal color vision can be identified with almost absolute certainty by using pseudoisochromatic plates, which screens normal and abnormal color vision. Another point to be considered, however, is that flying is done predominantly by males, and, unfortunately, the luck of the draw has dealt them a bad color-vision hand. Nearly 8.5% of all males are color-defective. Only 0.5% of females are color-defective. Congenital color vision defects are inherited as a sex-linked recessive trait. Approximately 3% of males with defective color vision fall into a category that is classified as mild, and these individuals have been shown to be safe for aviation duties. The problem is to separate this 3% of men from the 5.5 or 6% of individuals with moderate to severe

color vision deficiencies who are considered unsafe in the aviation environment. At present, this separation can best be done by lantern tests such as the United States Air Force School of Aerospace Medicine's Color Threshold Tester (CTT), which was devised by Dr. Louise Sloan at Randolph Field in Texas during World War II. Another lantern that can accomplish this test is the United States Navy Farnsworth lantern. Other more definitive tests of color vision are the 15-hue and 100-hue Farnsworth tests, the Nagel Anomalascope, and more recently devised tests. The flight surgeon and aeromedical examiner, however, need not go beyond the pseudoisochromatic plate test and perhaps one lantern test. One must point out here, however, that the pseudoisochromatic plate test, whether it be Ishihara, American Optical, or Dvorine, must be illuminated with light of proper Kelvin temperature. The most commonly used light is the MacBeth light, which has a temperature of about 6000°K.[10]

According to the Young-Helmholtz theory of color vision, three classes of cones are present in the macula. These cones absorb light with peak sensitivities of 445 nm (blue), 535 nm (green), and 570 nm (red), as shown in Figure 15–14. Any color of the spectrum may be constituted with varying combinations of these three primary colors, and when all three colors are stimulated, the color perceived is white. Individuals with defective color vision inherit their conditions. The most severe deficiency is known as monochromatism, a complete absence of color sensation. There are, perhaps, only 1:100,000 such individuals in the general population, with central visual acuities in the 20/200 range, and it is doubtful that they will enter aviation. Individuals with dichromatism constitute 2 to 3% of the males, and they recognize only two distinct hues. These individuals require only two primary colors to match all hues. The types are protanopia (1% of males, whose only

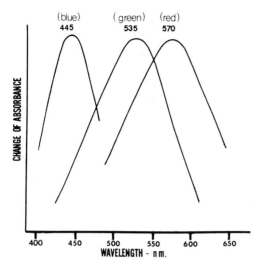

Fig. 15–14. Cone photosensitive pigments. Maximum absorption wavelengths.

Table 15–1.   Incidence of Color-Vision Deficiency

Males	Percent	Females	Percent
Protanopia	1.0	Protanopia	—
Deuteranopia	1.4	Deuteranopia ⎫	
Protanomaly	0.78	Protanomaly ⎭	0.4
Deuteranomaly	4.6	Deuteranomaly	—
Total*	8.0	Total*	0.4

*Monochromatism occurs in 1/100,000 individuals.

color sensations are blue and yellow and who confuse reds with greens and blue-greens), deuteranopia (also 1% of males, whose only color sensations are blue and yellow and who confuse purple with green), and tritanopia (exceedingly rare, only red and green are perceived).

The vast majority of individuals with defective color vision are anomalous trichromats. They recognize three distinct hues but have a weakness in one of the hues. Protanomaly, constituting 1% of the males, means red-weak, and these individuals require more red stimulation than normal people to acquire a color match. Deuteranomaly, affecting 5% of the males, means green-weak, and these individuals need more green stimulation than normal people to acquire a color match. Tritanomaly, a condition in which more blue stimulation is required to obtain a color match, is exceedingly rare. The pseudoisochromatic plates will screen out all of these anomalous types. The 3% of individuals with mild defective color vision will be anomalous trichromats and can be identified by the various color lantern testing procedures (Table 15–1).

There are also acquired color vision defects. They are, at least early in the disease,

not bilateral as are the congenital defects. These acquired color vision defects can be brought on by diseases and conditions of the cones in the retina, the optic nerve, and, occasionally, by brain injury. Some of the causes are central serous retinopathy; drug and toxic poisoning, such as by lead, tobacco, or alcohol; diseases of the central nervous system, such as multiple sclerosis; and brain injuries. One simple test that all examiners can use to separate the acquired color deficiency from the congenital deficiency (besides a good history) is to examine each eye separately when screening with the pseudoisochromatic color vision plates.

For a long time, designers have thought about engineering the necessity for color vision out of flying. Shape, size, numbers, configurations, and lights would be used rather than color itself. At first, this sounds like a good idea, but it appears to be exceedingly expensive, and tests have proven that it is actually much less efficient than the use of color in a coding system.

A new filter technique has been developed to "cure" color vision defects. It is the "X-chrome lens," a red, 15 to 20% transmitting-filter contact lens that is worn on only one eye. The lens has been touted as the device to put individuals with defective color vision into the cockpit; however, recent scientific evaluations have shown that disadvantages to this approach may be more significant than the fact that some individuals wearing this lens can actually pass the pseudoisochromatic plate test. This device has not made the individual's color vision normal; he still may not be able to identify colors in the real world in which the aviator performs and usually will fail the lantern tests.[11]

AIRCRAFT/ENGINEERING FACTORS

G Force (Gravity)

The visual system is profoundly affected in high-speed flight by acceleration (G forces), vibration, and a normal lag in human visual perception. On earth, the human body is constantly affected by gravity, and this force is termed 1 G. In flight, the speed, acceleration, and changes in direction can increase the amount and direction of this G force. These G effects are discussed in much more detail in Chapter 9; however, G forces have significant effects on the aviator's vision, and these effects will be discussed here. In flight, the aviator will encounter linear acceleration such as in catapult takeoff, aircraft carrier landings, ditching, and high-speed bailout. Radial acceleration is encountered in banks, turns, and pullouts from dives, loops, and rolls. Angular acceleration occurs in spins, in storms, and in tumbling following bailout from aircraft. It is the $+G_z$ acceleration that mainly concerns pilots, especially those of high-speed aircraft. When $+G_z$ are being pulled, the quantity of blood returning to the heart is diminished. The heart continues to beat, but diminution of the volume of systolic blood reduces the cardiac output, lowers the arterial tension, and causes a drop in pressure. Figure 15–15 shows that with increasing G forces, a point will be reached when the arterial pressure in the ophthalmic artery no longer exceeds the intraocular pressure. It is at this point that visual function is definitely impaired and blackout ensues. There is, however, sufficient perfusion pressure in the remainder of the central nervous system so that unconsciousness does not occur until the increasing G force further decreases the

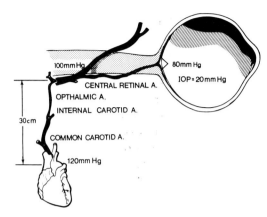

Fig. 15–15. Normal arterial blood pressures from the heart to the eye.

arterial pressure and the resulting pressure in the central nervous system is zero. On the average, the pilot will begin to lose his peripheral vision at $+3.5$ to $+4.5$ G_z. Blackout, or a complete loss of vision, occurs at $+4$ to $+5.5$ G_z. Hearing, however, will persist and orientation remains. From $+4.5$ to $+6$ G_z the pilot will lose consciousness. These are only average values, and they vary depending on the rapidity of onset of the G forces and the physical condition of the aviator. In the recent past, training, certain maneuvers, and protective clothing have enabled the aviator to reach higher G forces and maintain his efficiency for longer periods of time. These factors entail improving his physical condition, tensing of muscles, performing maneuvers such as the M-1, and wearing improved anti-G suits. G-force protection could be further enhanced if reclining, tilting seats were available.

Negative G forces are not often encountered. If these forces are prolonged, however, they will result in congestion of the blood vessels of the upper part of the body, leading to a violent headache. Visually, a so-called "red out" may occur. The actual cause of this phenomenon is still unknown; it may be due to looking through a congested lower lid, which then acts as a filter. At high speeds, in order to maintain functional vision, one must maintain a radius of turn large enough so as not to cause excessive G loading. Table 15–2 shows the radii of high-speed aircraft turns that produce +6 G forces.

For example, at a speed of 3200 kph, the pilot could not make a turn in a circle smaller than 29 km in diameter or he would black out unless he was performing the aforementioned protective maneuvers and was wearing a good anti-G suit. Figure 15–16 shows the effects of acceleration and time on vision.

Table 15–2. Radii of High-Speed Aircraft Turns Producing +6 G Forces

Kilometers Per Hour	Number of Meters
400	209
1200	1,882
1600	3,395
3200	13,597

Vibration

Vibration causes blurred vision and thus reduces the visual efficiency of the aviator. Studies have shown that during vertical sinusoidal vibrations at frequencies above 15 Hz, visual acuity is degraded. Particularly degrading to vision have been the frequency bands in the ranges of 25 to 40 and 60 to 90 Hz. When vibration cannot be avoided, its effect on visual performance can be reduced somewhat by the proper design of the visual instruments, displays, and printed materials, and an increase in their illumination and contrast.

Lag in Visual Perception

The length of time between an event and when the person sees the event depends on two factors: the length of time required for light to reach the eye and the conduc-

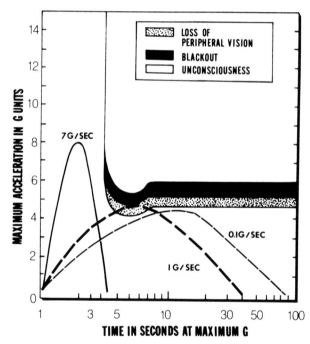

ACCELERATION AND TIME AT MAXIMUM G REQUIRED TO PRODUCE VISUAL SYMPTOMS AND UNCONSCIOUSNESS. CURVES SHOWING DIFFERENT RATES OF G DEVELOPMENT ARE GIVEN TO SHOW THE IMPORTANCE OF THIS PARAMETER FOR THE OCCURRENCE OF PERIPHERAL VISION AND BLACKOUT.

Fig. 15–16. Visual effects produced by various $+G_z$ environments.

tion time in the visual pathways and brain tracts. Because of the speed of light, the interval between the event and the eye is an unimportant factor, but the lag in the visual mechanism is appreciable and, at supersonic speeds, turns out to be an important factor. This is demonstrated in Figure 15–17. A pilot flying at 1000 kph sees an aircraft in his peripheral vision; he has traveled 28 m before the image is transmitted from the retina to the brain. He travels 300 m before he recognizes it. He travels more than 1 km before he has decided whether to climb, descend, or bank. He travels nearly 1.5 km before he can actually change his flight path. At 3000 kph, speeds that can be attained in advanced fighter aircraft, all of these distances are tripled. The times noted here are probably absolute minimums and are not reducible

by any mechanical or electronic ingenuity solely because they are unchanging characteristics of the human eye, mind, muscle, and nervous system. On the other hand, the distance traveled at each interval will undoubtedly increase as the speed of new-generation aircraft increases. Further, one must also be aware that anything that would interfere with the pilot's vision, whether a structural component of the aircraft, the windscreen, his clothing, his spectacles, haze, or grayout induced by G forces, could greatly stretch out the time required to perceive and recognize an event. The pilot has not only to identify the object as an aircraft, but he must decide whether it is a friend or foe. The recognition time will then probably stretch out to perhaps 1.5 seconds, and decision time would probably be in the 4- to 5-sec-

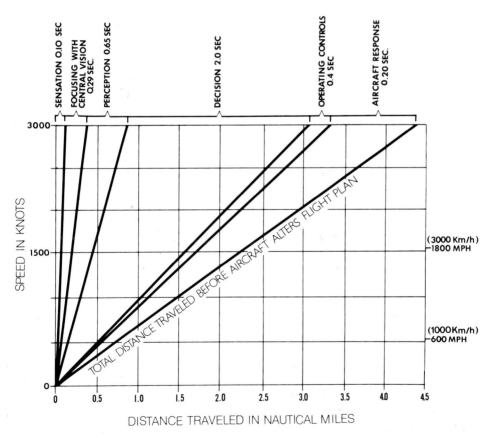

Fig. 15–17. Distance traveled as a function of aircraft speed and visual processing.

ond range rather than the 2 seconds indicated in the chart. A pilot may fly blind for thousands of feet while performing such simple operations as glancing at an instrument. At 1000 kph, his vision outside the aircraft is interrupted for nearly 1 km. At 3000 kph, his vision would be interrupted for 2 km. In shifting sight from outside the aircraft to the instrument panel and back, the accommodation time (the time required for the eyes to focus on the instrument), becomes important. Accommodation and relaxation take up a total of 1 second, or 1 km at 3000 kph.[12] This is an important factor for the aging pilot who is losing his ability to accommodate. Recognition of his instruments will consume a good deal more than 0.8 second if they are poorly designed or poorly lit. Likewise, if the sky is bright and the panel dim, the pilot will first have to adapt to the dim light in the cockpit, then readapt to the brightness outside. He can do little to speed up these times. All of this shows that the modern pilot, especially in fighter aircraft, must be given the best design possible in illuminated cockpit instruments. Skimping in this area will be penny-wise and pound-foolish, as the saying goes, because a drop in the pilot's visual efficiency will not allow him to take advantage of an otherwise superbly designed and powered aircraft.

Aircraft Windscreens

The pilot must, of necessity, look through several layers of transparent materials. He must look through the windscreen. He also may be using a visor, and, if he is ametropic, he will also have to wear a pair of spectacles. Vision through these multiple transparencies may be distorted; therefore, it is imperative that the transparencies have a minimum amount of distortion and that the pilot should use as few as possible. Aircraft windscreens are shaped for aerodynamic reasons, and at times these designs are not compatible with the requirements of good visibility.

When only flat panels of glass were used in aircraft windscreens, the problems of distortion and multiple images were minimal. Newer aircraft demand compound shapes that can only be fabricated in plastic, and flying high-speed aircraft at low altitudes has introduced another peril: bird strikes. The combination of the aircraft and bird speeds can easily fracture any glass windscreen, necessitating multiple layers of new-generation plastic, such as polycarbonate, to withstand the impact created by bird strikes. This, however, has introduced another problem. Because the plastic windscreens are made of multiple layers of the material, there is a reflection of the image at each layer, and these multiple images can become very annoying and contribute to confusing visual effects for the pilot. Light rays striking the windscreen can be displaced, deviated, or distorted, or can give rise to multiple images, as shown in Figure 15–18. Refracted light is displaced but remains parallel to the incident light. Deviations occur when the refracted light travels at an angle to the incident light, and distortion is relative deviation among numerous refracted rays. The false projection in displacement is so small that it can be ignored. In deviation, however, there is a larger false projection, whereas distortion gives rise to a misshapen appearance of the objects viewed. Displacement alone occurs only in plain parallel panels and is greater with an increased angle of incidence and an increased thickness of the panel. Deviation occurs when the panel is wedged (in other words, is shaped like a prism) and increases with the angle of incidence and thickness of the transparency and with a decrease in the radius of the curvature. Distortion occurs in irregular, wedged, and curved panels, and it increases with the irregularity of the panel and the angle of incidence, thickness of the glass or plastic, decrease in its radius of curvature, and increase in the distance of the observer from the transparency. Optically, a flat,

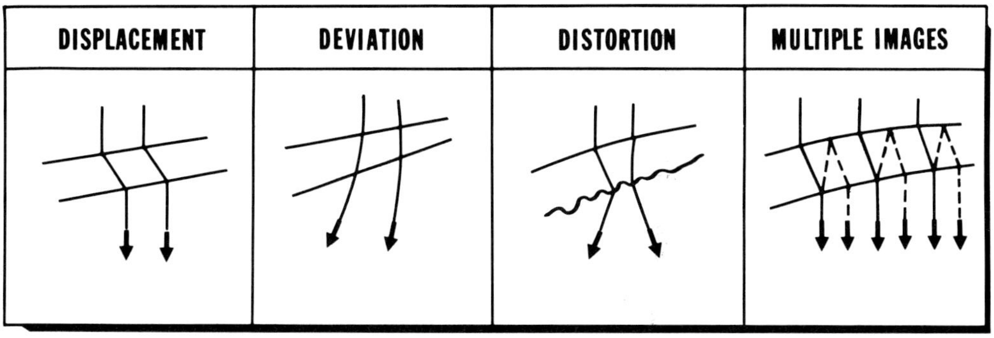

DISPLACEMENT	DEVIATION	DISTORTION	MULTIPLE IMAGES

Fig. 15–18. Windscreen optical effects.

thin glass or plastic would be the most desirable from the visual standpoint. For the reasons mentioned previously, however, curved, thick, and laminated transparencies are a necessity in today's aircraft. In the final design, a compromise has to be made between the aerodynamic, optical, and stress considerations.[13]

AVIATOR SELECTION—VISUAL STANDARDS

The visual selection of individuals for flying careers, the steps that need to be taken to maintain vision at peak efficiency, and the protection of the eyes from hazards that might affect the peak efficiency of the aviator's vision will be discussed in this section. It cannot be denied that vision is the most important sense needed to fly an aircraft or spacecraft. In the early days of scarf, helmet, goggles, and open cockpit, good distance vision was by far most important. With the advent of closed cockpits and cluttered instrument panels, both distance and near vision became absolutely necessary. In modern closed aircraft, flying with spectacles is now acceptable if the refractive error is not too extreme. In military flying, especially in the new advanced fighters, however, spectacles are still a nuisance and, at times, are a definite disadvantage, because of the following:

1. They are uncomfortable on long missions

2. High G forces may dislodge them
3. There is a reduction of light transmission through any transparency
4. There is one more transparency to look through
5. There is a limitation of the visual field
6. Spectacles have a tendency to fog
7. They give annoying light reflections at night
8. They are particularly difficult to integrate with other personal equipment
9. High refractive powers may cause aberrations and distortions of the image
10. High myopic corrections reduce the image size on the retina

Selection of Candidates for Flying

The techniques used for the visual selection of candidates for flying should not be so absolutely restrictive as to eliminate major segments of the population. There are different visual demands on the aviator, depending on his mission and aircraft. All missions do not require maximum visual capabilities. The examination techniques should be able to select those who have the ability to do the following:

1. Discriminate very small distant objects, as detected by
   Visual acuity tests for distance
   Stereoscopic/depth perception tests (confirmatory)
2. Appreciate the relationships be-

tween self/aircraft/other objects and the earth, as detected partially by
　Stereoscopic/depth perception tests
　Motility-red lens tests
3. Distinguish small objects at near, as detected by
　Near visual acuity tests
　Accommodation tests
4. Distinguish colors, as detected by
　Pseudoisochromatic plate tests
　Color threshold lantern, United States Air Force School of Aerospace Medicine's Color Threshold Tester
　Farnsworth lantern, United States Navy
　Other color testing lanterns
5. Distinguish objects in the peripheral field, as detected by
　Confrontation test
　Perimeter and tangent screen tests
6. See under reduced illumination, as detected by
　History
　Night vision test (radium plaque)
　Goldmann adaptometer
　Contrast sensitivity function test
7. Use both eyes simultaneously and fuse the images, as detected by
　Stereoscopic/depth perception tests
　Cover test
　Red lens test
　Heterophoria tests
8. Carry out previous function with eyes rotated in various directions, as detected by
　Cover test
　Heterophoria test
　Red lens test
　Near point of convergence
9. Maintain all of these functions throughout a flying career, as detected by
　Passing all previous testing procedures
　Ophthalmologic/fundus examination that reveals a disease-degeneration–free ocular status

Newer techniques just emerging will examine visual function in even greater depth, including contrast sensitivity function measurements, the dark focus examination, dynamic visual acuity tests, analysis of visual processing, electro-retinography, electro-oculography, and visual-evoked responses. At present, these are largely laboratory studies. Should these tests be more widely used in the visual examination, they would create even more new data to be considered. At this time, one would be hard put to decide how all this information would correlate with the performance of such a complex task as flying.

Examination Techniques

History

One should attempt to elicit a complete ocular history from the subject. This would include any ocular disease, injury, medication, operations, loss of vision, double vision, and/or use of glasses or contact lenses. It also would be useful to get a family history of any ocular disorders, especially a history of glaucoma, night blindness, crossed eyes, cataracts, or color blindness.

Equipment For the Ocular Examination

The following equipment will save time and make it easier to carry out the ocular exam:

1. A flashlight and a second flashlight with a bare bulb that can be used as a point source of light
2. A distance target, which can be the flashlight with the point source of light
3. A near target such as a tongue depressor with a small letter printed on it
4. Ophthalmoscope
5. Prisms to measure phorias and tropias if one is not using a vision screener

6. An occluder
7. A millimeter scale or a Prince rule
8. A loupe that magnifies approximately 2×.

General Eye Examination

External Examination

The orbits are examined for any abnormality or asymmetry; exophthalmus or enophthalmus are noted. The eyes are then observed for any gross motility disorders or nystagmus. The presence of any tearing or discharge is noted. The lids are examined for symmetry and the presence of any ptosis. Lashes are observed and any inversion or eversion of the lids noted. Inflammation, cysts, or tumors of the lids and margins can quickly be discerned. The palpebral and bulbar conjunctivas can then be examined by everting the upper lid and depressing the lower lid. Here, one looks for hyperemia, injection, discharge, tumors, or pigmentation. With the use of a flashlight, the pupils are examined. At this time, it should be noted whether any contact lenses are being worn. Soft contact lenses are more difficult to detect, and it may be necessary to use the magnification of the loupe to see them. The pupils are examined for size, symmetry, position, and reaction (i.e., reaction to the light—direct, consensual, and accommodative). The Marcus Gunn pupillary sign is an extremely valuable indication of an optic nerve or retinal lesion. It is present when pupillary response to light is greater consensually than on direct stimulation, and it is elicited by the swinging light test. For instance, with the light shining in the right eye, the right pupil reacts directly and the left pupil consensually; when the light is swung to the left eye, the left pupil reacts directly and the right pupil consensually. If an incomplete lesion is present in the right optic nerve, the right pupil will dilate somewhat when the light is switched back to the right from the left eye, that is, the consensual light response is greater than

the direct light response. This indicates a positive Marcus Gunn pupillary sign. The ocular examination is completed by observing the corneas, anterior chambers, irides, and as much of the lenses as possible with the flashlight and loupe. The corneas should be free of opacities and vascularization. With experience, the depth of the anterior chambers can be estimated, the irides observed for any cysts, tumors, or unusual pigmentation, and the lenses observed for opacities.

VISUAL ACUITY/REFRACTIVE ERRORS. At 6 m, the entire letter on the 20/20 line subtends the visual angle of 5 minutes of arc. As shown in Figure 15–19, each component of the letter subtends 1 minute of arc, so that 20/20 indicates that at 6 m this individual can identify the component parts of the test letters. Vision should be tested in each eye separately, first without spectacles and then with spectacle correction. If the subject has below-normal visual acuity without any correction and has no spectacles, he may be tested with a pinhole of 1.5 to 2 mm in diameter. An improvement in the visual acuity signifies that the subnormal vision is most likely due to a refractive error. If his visual acuity does not improve, there is most likely an opacity in the cornea or lens or a defect in the retina or optic nerve. If spectacles are used but do not improve the subject's visual acuity to 20/20, the pinhole test also can be used over the spectacles. An improvement in vision signifies that a change in the subject's prescription is indicated.

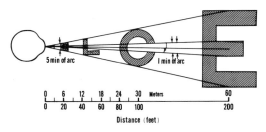

Fig. 15–19. Geometry of visual acuity. (Adapted from Adler, F.H., Physiology of the Eye: Clinical Application. St Louis, C.V. Mosby Co., 1970.)

Figure 15–20 shows the approximate visual acuity for spherical refractive errors up to +4 (hypermetropia) or −4 D (myopia).

Refractive errors are only rarely due to disease processes. They are mainly a mismatch between the diopteric power of the refractive system of the eye and the length of the globe. With a close match of these components, the individual is emmetropic, or nearly so. A mismatch can lead to hypermetropia (farsightedness) when the globe is too short for the refractive power, or the individual can be myopic (nearsighted) when the diopteric power of the refractive surfaces is too strong and the eye, therefore, is relatively too long. The third and most common aberration is astigmatism. This is most often due to an asphericity of the cornea; that is, one meridian of the cornea has a higher diopteric power or is more curved than a second meridian located at 90° from it. The rays of light passing through an astigmatic eye form a path known as Sturm's conoid. This form of astigmatism is known as regular astigmatism and can be corrected by cylindric and spherocylinder lenses. Occasionally, an eye is encountered that has irregular astigmatism; in this case, the as-

tigmatism's maximum and minimum powers are not at 90°, and this form of astigmatism can only be corrected by contact lenses. The hard contact lens can uniquely correct this deficiency because the tear film layer beneath the contact lens fills in the irregularities of the astigmatic cornea. If the candidate's vision is worse than 20/20, he should have a refraction. A cycloplegic refraction is preferable because it totally relaxes the accommodation and thus yields the true and total refractive error. This will especially help delineate the refractive errors in hypermetropic people because these young, farsighted individuals obscure the total amount of their error by exerting an accommodative effort, which corrects some part of the spherical error. Accommodation does not help to correct a myopic error, however. In fact, accommodation will increase the myopia and make the refractive error even worse. Astigmatic individuals may not be able to see clearly at either near or far. Only a cylinder or spherocylinder or contact lens correction can clear their vision. Accommodation may be of some help in mildly astigmatic individuals by shifting Sturm's conoid on the retina to the circle of least

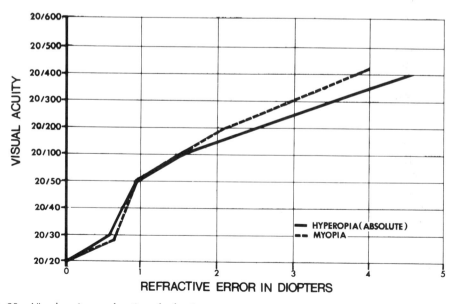

Fig. 15–20. Visual acuity as a function of refractive error.

confusion. As is the case with the hyper-metropic individual, however, this takes ciliary muscle effort, and symptoms of fatigue and blurred vision will ensue if the refractive error is not corrected.

To see clearly at near, the diopteric power of the crystalline lens must be increased an appropriate amount for the distance of the object seen. After the age of 45, most individuals will not retain sufficient accommodation to see clearly at reading distances of 33 to 35 cm. This condition is known as presbyopia and must be corrected by plus lenses if one wishes to be able to read at near.

Distant visual acuity can be examined in a 6-m lane with an eye chart or a projector chart. A smaller room, such as a 3- to 4-m room, can be used with reverse charts and mirrors. Perhaps the best way for a flight surgeon or aeromedical examiner to check the visual acuity and other visual functions as well is by using a vision screener such as the one shown in Figure 15–21. These instruments conveniently check a subject's distance and near visual acuities, phorias, and stereopsis. Without a screener, near vision also can be examined with a near vision test card held at 33 or 35 cm as per the instructions on the card. Each eye is tested separately.

Accommodation is tested in each eye separately using a Prince rule or its equivalent. One must be aware that if the subject has a refractive error, accommodation is tested through his spectacles. Should the subject be presbyopic and wearing bifocals or trifocals, he must be tested only through the upper, or distance, part of his spectacles and not through the bifocal or trifocal. Allowing the subject to look through the bifocal portion alters the test and adds accommodative amplitude equal to the value of the strength of the bifocal. Figure 15–22 shows that accommodation normally decreases with age at an almost constant rate. It becomes manifest at about age 45 because most reading materials subtend a visual angle that is too small to see if held much beyond 0.3 m from the eye.

MOTILITY. Normal ocular motility is expected in individuals who will be controlling aircraft. Diplopia or loss of stereopsis at a critical phase in flight could be devastating. The physician looks for straight eyes in the primary position of gaze and ensures that they remain so when taken into the six cardinal positions of gaze, as shown in Figure 15–23. As discussed earlier in this chapter, the six extraocular muscles rotate the eyes into infinite positions of gaze by the use of the yoke muscles operating under Hering's law of equal and simultaneous innervation to each yoke muscle. The yoke muscles and their actions are shown in Figure

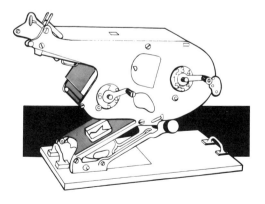

Fig. 15–21. Vision screener used to assess visual function.

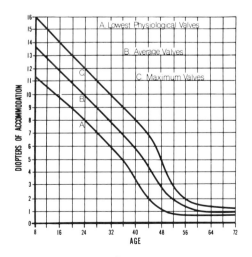

Fig. 15–22. Accommodation-age curve.

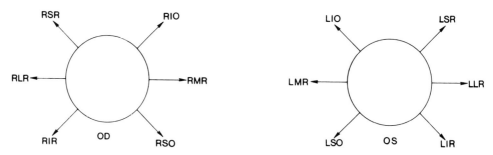

Fig. 15–23. Muscle actions in the cardinal positions of gaze.

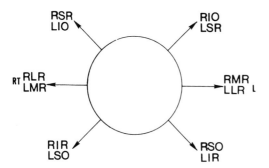

Fig. 15–24. Yoke muscles.

15–24. A manifest deviation of the eyes is known as a tropia and usually can be observed by inspection and quantitated by the Hirschberg test, that is, observing the position of the corneal light reflex in the deviating versus the fixing eye, as shown in Figure 15–25. A phoria, on the other hand, is a latent deviation. It is only present when fusion (binocular viewing) is interrupted such as by an occluder, a Maddox rod, or a red lens placed over one eye. Tropias are present in approximately 3% of the population, whereas phorias are present in nearly 100% of the population, meaning that, in essence, a phoria is normal unless it is extreme. It measures the resting state of the eyes. The eyes can be deviated in, which is an esotropia or esophoria; deviated out, which is an exotropia or exophoria; or up or down, signifying hyper- or hypo- tropia or phoria. An individual with a tropia (strabismus) may be seeing double, suppressing the vision in the deviated eye, or the eye may be amblyopic, with ensuing poor vision in that eye. Because almost all individuals have

a phoria, it is not of too great a concern unless it is excessive. If the phoria were excessive, a large neuromuscular effort would be required to maintain fusion and, therefore, single binocular vision. Any added stress might cause a breakdown of fusion, thus leading to diplopia and loss of stereopsis. Hypoxia and fatigue are common stresses to the aviator that can alter phorias; this is the principal reason for taking phoria measurements as part of the visual examination for flying. The easiest way for an aeromedical examiner to accurately measure phorias is by use of a vision screener. Ophthalmologists and optometrists mainly use a Maddox rod, occluder, and prisms in the eye lane to detect and measure phorias. As has already been mentioned, the Hirschberg (inspection) test will delineate a large-angle tropia. Small-angle tropias can only be detected by the cover test.

In doing the cover test, one uses an opaque occluder and has the patient fixate on a target at distance or one held at near while the examiner observes the position of the eyes. The right eye is covered and the left eye observed; if the left eye moves, it must not have been fixing, and the subject has a left tropia. This can be esotropia, exotropia, or hypertropia. Should the examiner cover the right eye and, while observing the uncovered left eye, note that the left eye does not move, he would then cover the left eye and observe the uncovered right eye. If the right eye moves, it signifies a tropia; if the right eye does not move, there is no tropia because both right

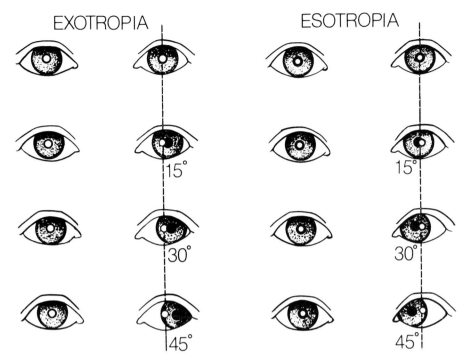

Fig. 15–25. Hirschberg reflex test used to detect tropias.

and left eyes were fixing on the target. If no tropia is noted on the cover test, the examiner can proceed to the alternate cover test in which the right eye is covered and then the left eye, and then back to the right eye, and back to the left eye, and so on. The examiner observes the uncovered eye. If there is movement to take up fixation on the target because the eye was deviated (phoric) under cover, this constitutes a phoria. Movement outward means the eye was in, or esophoric; movement inward means the eye was out, or exophoric. Should there be no movement of the uncovered observed eye, the examiner has noted a rare case of no phoria, or orthophoria.

The near point of convergence is also important in this examination because it, too, is influenced by hypoxia and fatigue. The near point has a tendency to recede under these conditions. Normally, the near point of convergence is 100 to 120 mm from the eye, but in military aviators, the near point of convergence is expected to be 70 mm or less. The Prince rule can be used to do this test. A small dim light or a small test target is brought forward along the rule until the subject breaks fusion and sees double. Simultaneously, the examiner will note one of the eyes deviates out. A measurement at that point will be the near point of convergence and should be within acceptable limits.

If the examiner notes nystagmus, whether it be pendular or rotary, when occluding an eye, he should refer the patient to an ophthalmologist for a complete evaluation.

COLOR VISION. The pseudoisochromatic plate test differentiates between individuals with normal color vision and those with defective color vision. Approximately 8.5% of the male population will fail this test. Approximately one third of these individuals can be classified as having only mild color deficiencies and are considered safe for flying. The other two-thirds, those with moderate and severe color deficiencies, are considered hazardous in the flying environment. The plates most commonly used are Ishihara, Dvorine, and American Optical. All of these must be administered with the proper illumination of approximately 6000° K temperature. These tests are best administered under the MacBeth lamp. Ordinary tungsten lighting will increase the pass rate for some people with defective color vision, especially those with deuteranomaly (green-weak). The Dvorine and American Optical tests consist of 14 plates and one demonstration plate. Ten or more correct responses are necessary for the subject to be considered as having normal color vision. The United States Armed Forces and the Federal Aviation Administration (FAA) utilize various color lanterns to test those who fail the pseudoisochromatic plate test. The United States Air Force uses the School of Aerospace Medicine Color Threshold Tester, in which eight different colors with eight different intensities are presented to the subject. A passing score of 50 or better of the 64 available colors identifies the individual with mildly defective color vision who would be eligible for aviation duties. The test is given in a darkened room at a 3-m distance. The United States Navy Farnsworth color lantern consists of nine presentations of two colored lights each, for a total of 18 colors. This test can be administered under room illumination or in a darkened room, also at a 3-m distance. If any errors are made on the first test, the subject is retested once or twice. An average of more than one error per series of nine color pairs is a failing score.

STEREOPSIS/DEPTH PERCEPTION. Tests of binocular vision given to aviators are usually referred to as depth perception tests. In reality, they are tests of stereopsis, one component in the perception of depth. Visual screeners, such as the Bausch and Lomb, Titmus, or Keystone, with excellent test slides quantify stereopsis down to as fine as 15 seconds of arc. Military flyers are expected to have stereopsis of at least

25 seconds of arc disparity. These tests, done in visual screeners, are at optical infinity; therefore, they are distance tests. Near tests of stereopsis are also available, such as the Verhoeff, with its three bars of varying width. This test is administered at 1 m without any special optical devices. The subject should be wearing his spectacles if he needs correction for distance, and he must have no failures in the eight presentations to pass the Verhoeff depth perception test. This equals approximately 32 seconds of arc disparity. Another commonly used near-stereoscopic test is the Wirt. This test necessitates using polarizing glasses but has the disadvantage of only going to 40 seconds of arc disparity. Normal room illumination is used for all three stereo tests.

FIELD OF VISION. Aeromedical examiners need only do confrontation fields, which compare the monocular field of the examiner and the subject. Any aberration in this field examination or history of neurologic disease or increase in intraocular pressure necessitates that a more exact perimetric study be done on a tangent screen or perimeter. The extent of normal visual fields is shown in Figure 15–26.

NIGHT VISION. Night vision is not routinely tested unless indicated by history.

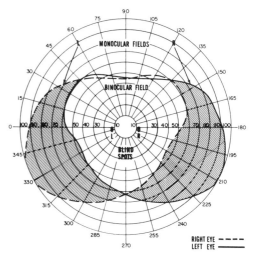

Fig. 15–26. Normal visual fields.

If a history of difficulty in seeing at night is elicited, dark adaptometry is indicated. This test will have to be accomplished by referring the subject to a center that has an adaptometer.

INTRAOCULAR PRESSURES. Glaucoma is a disease of maturity. Most of the glaucoma seen in aircrew members is of the open-angle variety, which is rarely found in individuals below the age of 40. The intraocular pressure measurements need only be done in individuals 35 years of age or older. If, however, there is a family history of glaucoma, intraocular pressure measurements should be done at any age. Schiøtz (indentation) tonometry is most readily available for the aeromedical examiner. Applanation tonometry is an excellent technique; however, this takes more practice and requires the availability of an expensive slit lamp. In any case, the results will be comparable regardless of which instrument is used. Space-age technology has brought us the air or puff tonometer. It, too, gives reliable results in experienced hands. Any intraocular pressures consistently over 22 mm Hg should be referred for a full glaucoma workup. Most of these individuals will be found to have only intraocular hypertension; that is, they will show an increase in intraocular pressure without any field loss or disk cupping. This condition generally requires no treatment; however, these individuals must be followed carefully at regular intervals, such as every 3 or 6 months, with intraocular pressure measurements, ophthalmoscopy, and visual field examinations. If their condition deteriorates, indicated by scotomas in the visual field or an abnormal cup-to-disk ratio, treatment is indicated and consultation should be sought from an ophthalmologist immediately.

Internal Examination

The final part of the examination for flying is an examination of the clear media and fundus of the eye. To get a good look at the fundus, the pupils should be dilated. In light-colored irides, two drops of 2.5% phenylephrine will suffice to dilate the pupil without altering the accommodation. With a darker-colored iris, a short-acting cycloplegic agent will probably have to be added to dilate the pupil sufficiently to view the fundus. One drop of 1% cyclopentolate or 1% tropicamide along with one drop of 2.5% phenylephrine will dilate the pupil for several hours. The examiner views the patient's right fundus with his right eye, then switches the direct ophthalmoscope to his left eye to view the patient's left fundus. A +6- or +8-D lens is rotated in the ophthalmoscope, and the red reflex is visualized at about 15 cm from the eye and examined for opacities, streaks, or any other alterations. If any of these conditions are noted, the patient probably deserves to be referred for a consultation. Moving closer to the pupil and simultaneously reducing the power of the plus lens, at some point near the zero power (if the subject and examiner have only minimal refractive errors), the optic disk and vessels of the fundus will come into view (Fig. 15–27). If they are not seen until high-powered minus lenses are rotated into the ophthalmoscope, the subject's refraction can be estimated. In this case, the subject would be myopic. If it takes plus lenses to view the subject's fundus, he is hypermetropic. The examiner now views the optic disk and cup and estimates the cup-to-disk ratio. Then he looks at the arter-

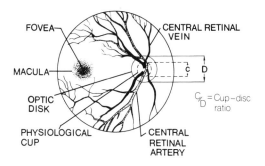

Fig. 15–27.   Normal fundus details.

ioles and veins as they leave the optic nerve in all four quadrants. Finally, the examiner looks at the macula and fovea. Normal fundus details are shown in Figure 15–27. If the examiner has trouble locating the fovea, he should simply ask the subject to look at the ophthalmoscope light, and this area will be brought into view by the patient as he fixates on the light. Individuals with fundus abnormalities should be referred to an ophthalmologist for diagnosis and possible treatment.

MAINTENANCE OF VISION

Individuals preparing for a lifelong career in aviation should have a thorough ophthalmologic examination. For a military flying career, long-term prediction of the health of the visual system is extremely important because it is expected that the aviator will serve for at least 20 years. Examiners should strive to select individuals with excellent visual capabilities that are up to the visual demands of the duties to be performed. The selection of individuals with disease-free visual systems will go a long way toward assuring a 20 + year flying career. Periodic reexaminations will aid in maintaining a disease-free ocular system. Proper nutrition is vital to the maintenance of the visual system. Vitamin A is necessary for night vision and to aid in the production of visual pigments, whereas the water-soluble B vitamins protect against nutritional amblyopia. Protection from physical forces in daily activites, sports, and in the aircraft is important. Protection from excess electromagnetic energy is also a necessity. This energy can be an occupational hazard encountered in aviation. If ocular disease or injury is found, proper, timely, and correct treatment will speed recovery. This treatment should be followed by a reevaluation to consider the degree of impairment, if any, and its possible effects on the aviator's flying efficiency. Finally, the aeromedical examiner or flight surgeon should educate all aircrew in the proper use and care of their eyes and vision.

Many drugs are used to diagnose and treat ocular conditions. Most of these drugs should be left to the use of the ophthalmologist; however, the aeromedical examiner should have a basic knowledge of the action of certain commonly used drugs on the eye. The eye is an excellent field to observe the pharmacodynamics of the autonomic nervous system. Both the sympathetic and parasympathetic parts of the autonomic nervous system innervate the pupil and ciliary body. The dilator muscle of the pupil is innervated by the sympathetic nervous system, and the sphincter is innervated by the parasympathetic nervous system. The ciliary muscle involved in accommodation is innervated by the parasympathetic nervous system. Some common ophthalmic drugs and their actions are summarized in Table 15–3.

The aeromedical examiner should consult an ophthalmologist if atropine or steroid preparations are to be prescribed. Finally, he should never prescribe ocular anesthetic agents for use by the patient.

Conditions Affecting the Aviator's Vision

Once selected with a disease-free visual system, the aviator will usually remain so for several decades except for minor refractive changes and the universal onset of presbyopia in the fifth decade of life. Young flyers, especially those who do not use spectacles, may become victims of ocular trauma. Ocular trauma can be devastating to a flying career. Aeromedical examiners should warn their patients to use protective goggles or impact-resistant spectacles for all sports in which a high-speed missile may be involved such as handball, tennis, squash, hockey, and so on. Injuries to the eye should be referred at once for definitive diagnosis and treatment. In the older aviators, glaucoma or intraocular hypertension (preglaucoma) is often encountered. With the latest medical

Table 15–3. Common Ophthalmic Drugs

Dilate Pupil	
Adrenergic (Sympathomimetic; Dilating, Direct-Acting)	Anticholinergic (Parasympatholytic; Competitive Antagonists to Acetylcholine)
Epinephrine (alpha and beta)	Atropine
Norepinephrine (alpha)	Scopolamine
Phenylephrine (alpha)	Homatropine
Isoproterenol (beta)	Cyclopentolate
Timolol (beta-blocking)	Tropicamide

Constrict Pupil—Cholinergic (Parasympathomimetic)	
Direct-Acting	Indirect-Acting (Anticholinesterase)
Pilocarpine	Edrophonium
Carbachol	Isofluorophosphate (DFP)
Methacholine	Echothiophate

Drug	Concentration	Begin Effect	Duration
Pilocarpine	0.5 to 6%	15 minutes	4–6 hours
Tetracaine (Pontocaine)	0.25 to 0.5%	1 minute	15 minutes
Proparacaine (Ophthaine)	0.5%	30 seconds	10 minutes
Lidocaine (Xylocaine)	1%, 2%	5 minutes	3–4 hours
Phenylephrine (Neo-Synephrine)	2.5%, 10%	10 minutes	2 hours
Atropine	0.5 to 2%	2 hours	7–14 days
Homatropine	2 to 5%	30 minutes	6 hours
Cyclopentolate (Cyclogyl)	0.5%, 1%, 2%	15–30 minutes	24 hours
Tropicamide (Mydriacyl)	0.5%, 1%	15–20 minutes	2–3 hours

philosophy on when treatment for glaucoma should be instituted and with new medications that do not secondarily affect vision, one need not fear the effects of glaucoma on a flyer's career. Observation and the treatment regimen pioneered at the United States Air Force School of Aerospace Medicine (USAFSAM) have kept 95% of these Air Force patients on flying status for a full career.[14] Those individuals with intraocular hypertension (intraocular pressure greater than 22 mm Hg but less than 30 mm Hg, without field defects) are observed at regular intervals without treatment. Those individuals with glaucoma (over 30 mm Hg or with visual field or optic disk changes at any pressure) are treated with either levo-epinephrine or timolol eye drops with remarkable success without creating secondary visual aberrations.

Retinal disorders also will be seen in the younger patients. Central serous retinopathy, an edema of the macula of unknown origin, plays havoc with a pilot's stereopsis/depth perception. Fortunately, about 80% of these afflicted individuals will recover and can be returned to full flight status.[15] Older flyers may develop macular degeneration that may eventually end their flying careers because there is presently no effective treatment.

A small number of flyers may develop keratoconus or irregular astigmatism, but almost all of these individuals can be returned to full flight status by the proper fitting of hard contact lenses.

A fair number of individuals suffer from migraine, but only a few flyers will complain of it to the aeromedical examiner. The most significant aspect of this condition for flying personnel is developing a central scotoma during an attack or becoming incapacitated by the headache that may follow.

Cataracts commonly will be seen in the older flying population or as a result of ocular trauma. If the opacity is dense enough, it will affect vision and, therefore, a flyer's career. Modern surgical procedures and operative or postoperative optical correction by either an intraocular lens placed into the eye at surgery or by a contact lens fitted after surgery should allow most individuals to pass the visual examination and return to flying.

Correction of Refractive Errors

Standard Techniques

Refraction is a procedure used to determine the lens power needed to correct a patient to emmetropia. The refractive error can be estimated by retinoscopy, which is usually done following the use of cycloplegic eye drops. A manifest or subjective refraction is done with lenses, crossed cylinders, or astigmatic dials, and a third and common way of calculating the refractive error is with a lensometer, which measures the patient's present spectacle correction. If his spectacles correct the patient's vision to 20/20, nothing further need be done concerning the refraction. The aviator's distance refraction will change very little during his 20s and 30s. After the age of 40, even though the error for distance may remain static, a correction for his early presbyopia will be necessary. Spherical plus lenses will correct the deficient accommodation. Once presbyopia has commenced, the subject will need to be reexamined every 2 years to maintain clear, comfortable near vision. A half-eye spectacle will suffice for the patient with no error in his distance vision, but bifocals will be needed to correct the error in those who also require a correction for distance. Figure 15–28 depicts all the refractive errors except presbyopia. Lenses used to correct each type of error also are shown.

The use of contact lenses to correct refractive errors began about 30 years ago. They have found moderate acceptance in civilian aviation, but today, even in their relatively refined state, contact lenses are only rarely used in military flying. There are hard lenses made of polymethylmethacrylate (PMMA) and soft contact lenses made of hydroxyethylmethacrylate (HEMA) and silicone plastics. The hard lenses are used in a limited manner by the military to correct visual defects such as irregular astigmatism, keratoconus, and aphakia. The soft contact lens is more comfortable to wear, less time is needed for adaptation, and the soft lens rarely alters the corneal curvature. Soft lenses, however, do have a significant drawback for aviators in that they cannot correct astigmatism of over 1 D. In certain individuals, hard lenses may temporarily or permanently mold the cornea to a different refractive status or curvature. This could fortuitously improve the vision or it could lead to corneal warpage and degrade visual acuity. Several nations' military forces are presently evaluating soft contact lenses for use in the military environment, but to date no definitive results are available.

New Techniques for Refractive Error Correction

In the preceding discussion, it was stated that hard contact lenses could mold the cornea and alter the refractive error. About a decade ago, some practitioners attempted purposefully to alter the corneal contour with contact lenses in the hope that it would improve the vision to where no contact lenses or spectacles would be necessary. This procedure is called orthokeratology (to straighten the cornea). Evaluation of the technique has shown that in some instances, corneas will change contours, usually flattening, reducing the myopia while one is wearing the lenses. On removal of the lenses, however, most corneas will revert to their original curvatures and refractive errors in several weeks' time. Occasionally, this procedure will result in a permanent increase in "with the rule" astigmatism, and in rare cases the cornea may warp so that

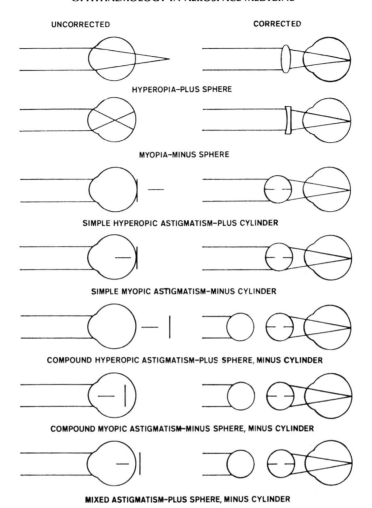

UNCORRECTED   CORRECTED

HYPEROPIA–PLUS SPHERE

MYOPIA–MINUS SPHERE

SIMPLE HYPEROPIC ASTIGMATISM–PLUS CYLINDER

SIMPLE MYOPIC ASTIGMATISM–MINUS CYLINDER

COMPOUND HYPEROPIC ASTIGMATISM–PLUS SPHERE, MINUS CYLINDER

COMPOUND MYOPIC ASTIGMATISM–MINUS SPHERE, MINUS CYLINDER

MIXED ASTIGMATISM–PLUS SPHERE, MINUS CYLINDER

Fig. 15–28.   Refractive errors and corrective lenses.

the condition cannot be distinguished from keratoconus. Orthokeratology indeed can alter the corneal curvature, but the procedure is highly unpredictable and is not permanent.[16] In the past several years, another new technique to alter the refractive status of myopic individuals has come forth. It is a surgical procedure called radial keratotomy. Radial K, as it is known, involves making 8 or 16 radial incisions in the corneal stroma down to the depth of Descemet's membrane, reaching radially to the limbus, and sparing a central 3- or 4-mm pupil. On healing, the cornea flattens in the center, thus altering the radius of curvature in that area and hopefully de-

creasing the myopia sufficiently to render the subject emmetropic. Just as in orthokeratology, this procedure is unpredictable; however, radial K is much more permanent.[17] Pilot aspirants willingly undergo this procedure in an attempt to pass entrance examinations. Presently, the United States Armed Forces are not accepting individuals who have had this surgery because of the unpredictability of results, frequently noted fluctuations in visual acuity, an increased susceptibility to glare, and, primarily, because the long-term (10 to 15 years) status of the corneal integrity is not known at this time.

In summary, it appears that even today

the most cost-effective and reliable way to correct refractive errors in aircrew is still by the use of spectacles.

PROTECTION OF VISION

Ocular Protective Materials

Since June, 1972, all spectacle lenses used in the United States have had to be impact-resistant by a Federal Drug Administration (FDA) ruling. Impact-resistant does not mean that they are unbreakable, just that a glass lens must withstand a ⅝-in diameter steel ball dropped on it from a 50-in height. Glass lenses are hardened to withstand the drop-ball test by heat or chemical tempering.

A plastic, allyldiglycol carbonate (CR-39) lens also may be used in place of glass. A new, space-age, transparent plastic polycarbonate (Lexan) is being used in helmet-mounted visors and as a cockpit transparency that is strong enough to withstand bird strikes. Bird strikes are a real hazard to low-flying, high-speed aircraft. The combination of a multilayered polycarbonate windshield and a visor of similar material for the aviator's helmet has markedly improved the protection against this lethal hazard. A dual-visor system, one clear and one tinted, allows for maximum protection under all flight conditions. experiments are ongoing to develop a polycarbonate lens for use in ordinary spectacles. This material would offer significant ocular protection in lenses that could correct refractive errors as well.

Filters and Sunglasses

The extent and effects of electromagnetic energy (light) on the eye have been previously discussed. As noted, light intensities in the aviation environment can be up to 30% higher than on earth. Abiotic ultraviolet radiation (200 to 295 nm) is filtered by the atmosphere but does begin to become significant at high altitudes. Ultraviolet radiation from 300 to 400 nm, which is abundant on earth, is now re-

puted to have some damaging effect on the human lens following long-term, chronic exposure. Infrared radiation above 760 nm is a contributor to solar and nuclear retinal burns. Sunlight falling on the earth is comprised of 58% infrared energy (760 to 2100 nm), 40% visible light (400 to 760 nm), and only 2% ultraviolet radiation (295 to 400 nm). At high altitude, ultraviolet radiation may be as high as 4 to 6% and makes up 8 to 10% of the solar energy spectrum in space. Sunglasses can protect the aviator from excessive and harmful electromagnetic energy.

The ideal sunglass for the aviator should do the following:
1. Correct refractive errors and presbyopia
2. Protect against physical energy (wind or foreign objects)
3. Reduce the overall light intensity
4. Transmit all visible energy but attenuate ultraviolet and infrared radiation
5. Not distort colors
6. Not interfere with stereopsis (depth perception)
7. Be compatible with headgear and flying equipment
8. Be rugged, inexpensive, and need minimal care

Five types of sunglasses are now in common use: colored filters, neutral filters, reflecting filters, polarizing filters, and photochromic filters. They all allow only a certain percentage of the total amount of incident light to get through to the eye but produce this effect in different manners. The colored, neutral, polarizing, and photochromic filters achieve this effect by absorbing some of the light and allowing the rest to pass. Spectral filtering is achieved in glass lenses by adding specific chemicals to the melt, producing a through-and-through tint. Also, the anterior surface of the glass lens may only be tinted, but this method is subject to scratching. Plastic lenses are usually dipped into dyes to produce their filtering effect.

Colored filters have the disadvantage of altering the color of viewed objects and might possibly reduce color discrimination of color-vision deficient persons.

Neutral filters adequately reduce the amount of light. Mainly, they do not distort colors and most will adequately eliminate the excessive infrared and ultraviolet radiation.

Reflecting filters can be coated uniformly. They eliminate the ultraviolet and infrared energy; however, this type of coating scratches and peels easily and gives a greenish tint to objects.

Polarizing filters reduce glare off water or highways. For the aviator, they can cause a problem, such as blind spots in windshields and canopies, due to stress polarization of the canopy matching that in the spectacles. Plastic polarized filters will scratch easily and, if laminated in glass, will be quite expensive and heavy.

Photochromic filters (variable light transmission) are photodynamic lenses that vary in intensity in response to the ultraviolet content of the incident light. Some flyers may find their darkest density sufficient; however, for military use it was found that the range of transmission variation is not adequate. The darker lenses remain too dark in the "open" state, and the lighter lenses are not dark enough at their maximum density.[18] Their cycling time was found to be slow, and the density is less in hot and low-ultraviolet environments, such as inside automobiles or cockpits, where the light must traverse another transparency. This is shown in Figure 15–29, which also compares these lenses with other filters.

Selection of Sunglasses for the Aviator

The lens material should be CR-39 or polycarbonate plastic or impact-resistant glass. After much experimentation, it was finally decided that a 15% transmitting lens was probably the best all-around com-

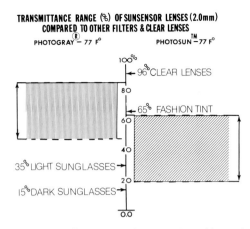

TRANSMITTANCE RANGE (%) OF SUNSENSOR LENSES (2.0mm) COMPARED TO OTHER FILTERS & CLEAR LENSES
PHOTOGRAY® – 77 F°   PHOTOSUN™ –77 F°

Fig. 15–29. Effectiveness of various tints of lenses in reducing light transmission.

promise for use by the aviator. Some individuals prefer a 25% transmitting lens for daily use (e.g., driving or sports) but switch to the 15% transmitting lens for aviation use. The lens should have a fairly flat curve in the visible energy range but attenuate the ultraviolet and infrared radiation. An ideal transmission curve is shown in Figure 15–30.

This type of lens allows a fairly equal amount of all spectral colors to pass through, and it will not distort the color of the overall scene. The difference in overall transmission between the two spectacle lenses should not be greater than 10%; otherwise, this difference in density will induce the Pulfrich effect, which, in turn, may affect stereoscopic vision and depth perception. When there is sufficient overall light intensity, such as in daylight, visual acuity through neutral density, 15% transmitting lenses will be as good as in the eye lane without filters.

Under extraordinary conditions, electromagnetic energy may reach such a magnitude that ordinary protective devices will not be adequate. Such tremendous amounts of energy can be released during a nuclear detonation or packaged in a laser beam that protection of the eye against these energy sources is a must; otherwise, permanent injury to the eye will ensue.[19]

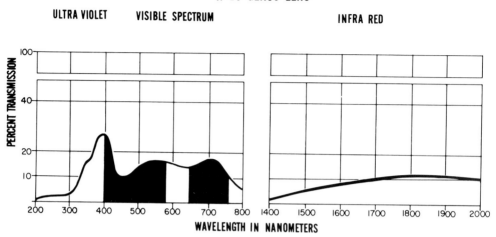

Fig. 15–30.   Ideal transmission curve for a sunglass for the aviator.

Nuclear Flash Protection

The eye is more susceptible to injury from nuclear explosions at far greater distances than any other organ or tissue of the body. When a pupil of a given size is exposed to a nuclear detonation at a given distance, it will result in a certain amount of energy being distributed over the image on the retina. If one doubles the distance from the detonation, the amount of energy passing through the same size pupil will be only one-fourth as great. The image area on the retina, however, will be only one-fourth as large; therefore, the energy per unit area will remain constant irrespective of the distance from the detonation except for the attenuation due to the atmosphere and the ocular media. The potential danger of flashblindness and chorioretinal burns resulting from viewing nuclear fireballs has now become a concern to aircrew members and thus has created new problems for the flight surgeon.

During daylight, with a high ambient illumination and through a small pupillary diameter, the retinal burn and flashblindness problem is greatly diminished. At night, with a large pupil, protection is a must. Many different ideas for eye protection have been advocated. Fixed-density filters, either on the pilot or the windscreen, electromechanical and electro-optical goggles, explosive lens filters, and phototropic devices have been developed. The sum total of all this work is that a 2% transmission-fixed filter, gold-plated visor gives adequate protection against retinal burns and reduces flashblindness to manageable proportions during daylight. This filter cannot be used at night, however. Another aid, a readily available countermeasure to flashblindness, day or night, is the ability to raise instrument panel illumination by auxiliary panel lighting to 125 ft-c. This increased illumination will significantly reduce the visual recovery time. The ideal "omni" protector against nuclear flash is still being sought. The most recently developed material for protecting against nuclear flash is a transparent ferro-electro-ceramic material (lead lanthanum zirconate titanate, PLZT) placed between crossed polarizers, as shown in Figure 15–31. It reacts to the light energy of detonation within 50 to 100 milliseconds, reaching an optical density of 3. Its biggest drawback is that in its open state, it transmits only 20% of the light.

Laser Eye Protection

Lasers (light amplification by stimulated emission of radiation) produce mon-

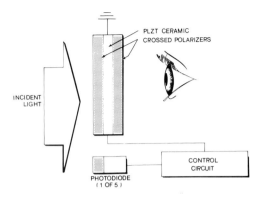

Fig. 15–31. Flashblindness protective goggles.

ochromatic, coherent, collimated light. The laser beam diverges very little, so that the energy of the beam decreases only minimally with increasing distance from the source. Laser energy is capable of severely injuring tissue in the eye that absorbs the beam energy. If a sufficiently powerful carbon dioxide laser (10.6 mm) strikes the eye, it could severely injure the cornea. Argon (480 nm), ruby (693 nm), and neodymium (1060 nm) lasers can injure the retina and choroid because they absorb these wavelengths. Lasers have now been classified by the American National Standards Institute standard Z-136.1 as follows:

> Class I—nonhazardous
> Class II—safe lasers but may produce retinal injury if looked at for long periods of time
> Class III—medium-power, medium-risk lasers
> Class IV—high-risk lasers, potentially hazardous by both direct and specular reflected beams.[20]

The military applications of lasers are increasing in the areas of target ranging and illumination. Pilots themselves are not usually at hazard from their own laser beams, but technicians and others working with such instruments should wear protective goggles or visors with an optical density that is considered safe at the laser wavelength being employed. Other safety factors also should be considered such as educating the worker in laser safety—not looking at the laser beam, examining for reflective materials in the laboratory or shop, posting warning signs, and operating a laser in well-lit rooms when possible (small pupils). Laser-safe working distances, the selection of protective materials, and safety programs are becoming quite complicated and involved for the flight surgeon to manage alone. He should have help from a bioenvironmental engineer or health physicist if at all possible.

The flight surgeon or aeromedical examiner is, however, responsible for setting up and carrying out ocular surveillance programs. At the least, he should give laser workers a complete ocular examination before they begin their assignment or employment. This should include a distance and near central visual acuity examination, both corrected and uncorrected, an Amsler grid examination, and an ophthalmoscopic examination of the fundus, with special attention to the fovea (any and all anomalies of the fundus should be meticulously recorded). A similar examination should be carried out at the termination of the assignment or employment. Annual ocular examinations are not considered necessary; however, anyone working with lasers who has an ocular complaint or claims to have been injured by a laser should be examined and the complaint evaluated.[21]

As stated at the beginning of this chapter, vision plays the most important role in data gathering for man. So much so that anything affecting his vision will be significant for the aviator. The flight surgeon and aeromedical examiner who care for the aviator and attempt to increase his effectiveness should pay special attention to the aviator's vision and visual system.

Instantaneous, clear vision assures us of receiving uncluttered and accurate visual data into our mental computers. The integrating and processing of this information after its reception is in the domain of the central nervous system and is enhanced by training and education of the aviator. If inaccurate or incomplete visual information is received, however, we are almost assured of failing to perform the task. With the time element for decision making becoming ever-shorter in modern aviation, there is added impetus to look carefully at the visual system.

This chapter has examined the physical, physiologic, medical, and bioengineering aspects of vision. With visual selection and enhancement by visual aids, the aviator's visual range has been extended, thus giving him more time for reaction and decision making. After selecting the aviator with exceptional visual capabilities, it is important to employ the techniques for maintaining and protecting his vision and visual apparatus so that he enjoys a full flying career. Ophthalmology and the other visual sciences are now complex scientific specialties. This chapter, however, has attempted to give information and data in a manner that is understandable and useful for all physicians.

REFERENCES

1. Office of Director of Air Service: Aviation Medicine in the Army Expeditionary Force (AEF), Washington, D.C., Government Printing Office, 1920.
2. Duke-Elder, S.S.: System of Ophthalmology. Vol. V: Ophthalmic Optics and Refraction. London, Henry Kimpton, 1970, p. 81.
3. Moses, R.A.: Adler's Physiology of the Eye, Clinical Applications. St. Louis, C.V. Mosby Co., 1981, pp. 545–561.
4. Pitts, D.G., and Tredici, T.J.: The effects of ultraviolet on the eye. Am. Ind. Hyg. Assoc. J., 32:235, 1971.
5. Campbell, F.W., and Maffei, L.: Contrast and spatial frequency. Sci. Am., 240(6):30–38, 1974.
6. Randel, H.W. (ed.): Aerospace Medicine. 2nd Ed. Baltimore, Williams & Wilkins Co., 1972, pp. 594–595.
7. Aircraft Instrument and Cockpit Lighting by Red or White Light. Conference Proceedings No. 26. Advisory Group for Aerospace Research and Development (AGARD)/North Atlantic Treaty Organization (NATO), Springfield, VA, October, 1967.
8. Mims, J.L., III, and Tredici, T.J.: Evaluation of the Landolt ring plaque night vision tester. Aerospace Med., 44:304–307, 1973.
9. Pitts, D.G.: Visual Illusions and Aircraft Accidents. SAM-TR-67-28, United States Air Force School of Aerospace Medicine, Brooks Air Force Base, Texas, April, 1967.
10. Procedures for Testing Color Vision. Report of Working Group No. 41, Committee on Vision. National Research Council, National Academy of Sciences. Washington, D.C., National Academy Press, 1981.
11. Welsh, K.W., Vaughan, J.A., and Rasmussen, P.G.: Aeromedical implications of the X-chrome lens for improving color vision deficiencies. Aviat. Space Environ. Med., 50:3:249, 1979.
12. Wulfeck, J.W., et al: Vision in Military Aviation. WADC Technical Report 58–399, Wright Air Development Center, Wright-Patterson Air Force Base, Ohio, November, 1958.
13. Provines, W.F., Kislin, B., and Tredici, T.J.: Multiple Images in the F/FB-111 Aircraft Windshield: Their Generation, Spatial Localization, and Recording. SAM-TR-77–32, United States Air Force School of Aerospace Medicine, Brooks Air Force Base, Texas, December, 1977.
14. Tredici, T.J.: Screening and management of glaucoma in flying personnel. Milit. Med., 145:1, 1980.
15. Epstein, E.L., Shacklett, D.L., Tredici, T.J., and Houck, R.J.: Idiopathic central serous retinopathy (choroidopathy) in flying personnel. Aerospace Med., 43:1251–1256, 1972.
16. Tredici, T.J.: Role of orthokeratology: A perspective. Ophthalmology, 86:698, 1979.
17. Rowsey, J.J., and Balyeat, H.D.: Preliminary results and complications of radial keratotomy. Am. J. Ophthalmol., 93:437, 1982.
18. Welsh, K.W., Miller, J.W., and Shacklett, D.E.: An acceptability study of photochromic lenses. Optometric Weekly, 21:16–21, 1976.
19. Byrnes, J.A., Brown, D.V.L., Rose, H.W., and Cibis, P.A.: Chorioretinal burns produced by an atomic flash. Arch. Ophthalmol., 55:351, 1956.
20. American National Standards for the Safe Use of Lasers. ANSI Z136.1—1976. New York, American National Standards Institute, 1976.
21. Air Force Occupational Safety and Health (AFOSH) Standard 161–10. Health Hazards Control for Laser Radiation. Washington D.C., Department of the Air Force, May 30, 1980, pp. 23–24.

Chapter 16

Otolaryngology in Aerospace Medicine

H. H. Hanna and C. Thomas Yarington, Jr.

If God had intended for man to fly, He would have provided him with wings.

Anonymous

In this chapter, otolaryngologic abnormalities related to aerospace medicine will be considered under the major headings of examination, clinical conditions, and implications of surgical procedures. Only anatomic and physiologic considerations pertinent to flying will be discussed. General aspects of assessment of hearing and vestibular function will be presented. Clinical conditions directly related to flying essentially will be limited to those entities that result from the mechanical effects that exposure to environments of changing barometric pressures has on gases trapped in various cavities of the head. Barodontalgia is included, although the exact mechanism of symptom production is not known and trapped gases may or may not be involved. Abnormalities not directly related to flying but having aeromedical significance will be discussed, as will the aeromedical implications of otologic and rhinologic surgical procedures.

EXAMINATION

Anatomic and Physiologic Considerations Pertinent to Flying

External Auditory Canal

The size and configuration of the external auditory canals vary considerably from person to person and even from one side to the other in the same individual. In general, the canal proceeds medially in a slightly anterior and superior fashion and at about its midpoint inclines somewhat inferiorly to reach the eardrum. This configuration is the basis for the need to pull the pinna posteriorly and somewhat superiorly to facilitate visualization of the eardrum. Some individuals have essentially a straight outer ear canal, and in others the apparent hump inferiorly is quite marked (Fig. 16–1). In many individuals, a bony prominence anteriorly overhangs the anterior portion of the annulus of the eardrum (Fig. 16–2). One of the primary

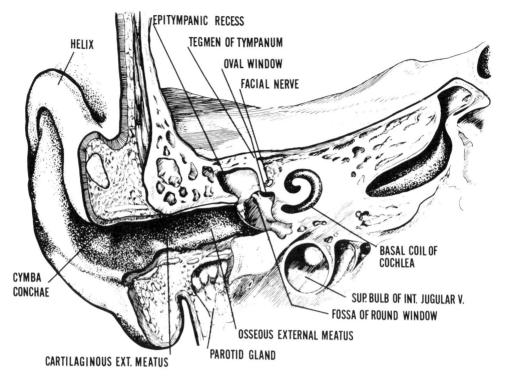

Fig. 16–1. Curved section through the external auditory meatus, tympanic cavity, cochlea, and pyramidal part of the temporal bone, right side. (After Jackson, C., and Jackson, C.L.: Diseases of the Nose, Throat and Ear. Philadelphia, W.B. Saunders, 1959.)

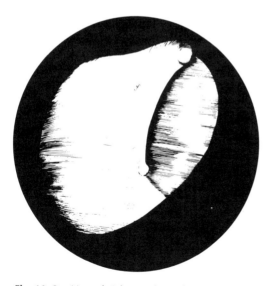

Fig. 16–2. Normal right ear drum showing the bony prominence (anterior canal wall) overhanging the anterior portion of the annulus.

aeromedical considerations is that the external auditory canal configuration be compatible with earplugs. Experience has shown that the majority of aircrewmen can be fitted; however, it is not uncommon for an individual to require different sized plugs for his ear canals. The disparity is usually no greater than one size difference. Our experience at the United States Air Force School of Aerospace Medicine (USAFSAM) has been that approximately 14% of candidates for such ear protection will require a different size plug in each ear. An equally significant aeromedical consideration is that the examiner must be able to visualize a sufficient amount of the eardrum to be able to check for satisfactory performance of the Valsalva maneuver and for the presence of significant findings on the eardrum (e.g., manifestations of acute barotitis media or an ear block).

The Valsalva maneuver is one way to

ventilate the middle ear cavities unphysiologically. The individual inhales, closes his nose with thumb and index finger on the nasal alae, and then exhales with his mouth closed. Positive pressure quickly builds up in the nasopharynx. The exhalation effort is augmented until the pressure in the nasopharynx becomes great enough to open the eustachian tubes and ventilate the middle ear spaces. When air enters the middle ear, the eardrum moves laterally and may remain distended for a while. Ventilation of one or both ears is readily perceived by the patient, who will generally mention that one or both ears "popped." The physician can verify ventilation of the middle ear by observing the eardrum while the patient performs the Valsalva maneuver.

Exostoses and osteomas occur in the inner half or bony portion of the outer ear canal. Exostoses are much more common and usually present as smooth, rounded, bony prominences of varying size along one or both of the suture lines joining the tympanic portion of the temporal bone to the squama and mastoid posteriorly and the squama and zygomatic process portion anteriorly. In rare cases, exostoses will attain sufficient size to preclude adequate visualization of the eardrum and may also limit access to the eardrum (e.g., cleaning and medicating the ear canal as in acute otitis externa). When exostoses are large enough to be clinically significant, surgical removal is indicated. An osteoma has the same clinical significance as exostoses; however, these benign tumors are much less frequent.

Middle Ear Cavity

The primary aeromedical consideration of the middle ear cavity is its role in barotrauma. In this consideration, the middle ear should be regarded as a rigid-walled cavity, even though its lateral partition, the tympanic membrane, is a thin structure normally consisting of an external layer of thin skin, an intermediate layer of elastic tissue, and an inner mucosal layer. As long as the eardrum remains intact, however, it is not capable of distending enough to accommodate any appreciable amount of pressure and thus functions as a rigid wall. The amount of pressure change (either positive or relatively negative) that the normal eardrum will tolerate varies; however, any time the pressure differential exceeds 100 mm Hg the eardrum may rupture.

Eustachian Tube

The eustachian tube extends from the lateral wall of the nasopharynx to the anteroinferior part of the middle ear space. It has two primary functions: (1) to ventilate the middle ear space; and (2) to drain the middle ear space. The primary aeromedical consideration is the role that the eustachian tube plays in the ventilation of the middle ear. The posterior third of the eustachian tube is a bony channel that is always open; the anterior two-thirds is a membranocartilaginous structure that is normally closed and opens physiologically only with swallowing, yawning, or working the lower jaw, any action that causes the tensor veli palatini and levator veli palatini muscles to contract. The action of the tensor veli palatini muscle is more important in opening the auditory tube than is the levator veli palatini muscle (Fig. 16–3). The structure of the anterior two thirds of the eustachian tube is such that it functions essentially as a one-way flutter valve. The lumen of the tube is a vertical slit that is normally closed (Fig. 16–4). Air under pressure in the middle ear space will readily pass through to the nasopharynx, but if the air pressure in the tympanic cavity is less than the pressure in the nasopharynx, the eustachian tube will remain closed unless it is opened physiologically or by one of the unphysiologic maneuvers (e.g., the Valsalva maneuver or politzerization).

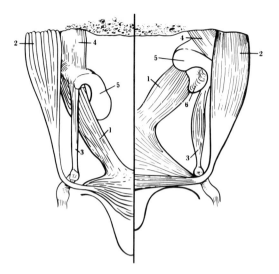

Fig. 16–3. The action of the tubal muscles. On the left side of the figure the tube is at rest, and on the right side of the figure the tube is illustrated during swallowing. The levator veli palatini (1) pulls the soft palate up, back, and lateral to help close the nasopharynx and to elevate and help rotate the tubal cartilage (5). Forward rotation is checked by the superior tubal ligament (4). Medial fibers of the tensor veli palatini (3) pull the hook of the cartilage (5) downward and dilate the tubal lumen (6), thus opening it. Lateral fibers of the tensor (2) tense and elevate the soft palate. (After Proctor, B.: Anatomy of the eustachian tube. Arch. Otolaryngol. 97:6, 1973.)

Nasal Cavity

In man, the nasal cavity is the preferred route for inspired air, and the nose performs three basic functions in preparing inspired air for the lungs: cleansing, humidification, and warming. Cleansing is accomplished by two means. Larger particles are screened out by the vibrissae, or hairs, in the anterior nares, and smaller particles, including bacteria, are trapped on the mucous blanket and swept by ciliary action posteriorly into the nasopharynx and then into the "common gutter," or oral pharynx. Inspired air is humidified, if necessary, by mucus, which is largely provided by glands located in the middle turbinates. If warming is required, this is accomplished by the inferior turbinates, or "radiators," which contain many submucosal venous sinusoids. These turbinates enlarge when subjected to cold air, thus reducing the airway and providing for longer contact of the air with the turbinates. This mechanism is the basis for nasal stuffiness commonly noted when one leaves a warm house in the wintertime and encounters the cold outside air. These functions of humidification and warming are under autonomic control; in essence, the amount of mucus in the nose and the size of the turbinates, primarily the inferior turbinate, vary constantly in response to the degree of dryness and temperature of the inspired air.

Adequacy of the nasal airways is critical in flying; any significant obstruction can result in an inability or decreased ability to conduct ventilation via the preferred route with loss of the cleansing, humidifying, and warming actions of the nose. Adequate nasal airways become even more important if oxygen is required for any appreciable period because oxygen in aircraft systems is very dry. If the aircrewman resorts to mouth breathing, the air is humidified at the expense of the oral, pharyngeal, and laryngeal mucosa, which can rapidly lead to dryness and irritation in these areas, as well as thickened residual secretions. Also, adequate nasal airways are required for optimum ventilation of the paranasal sinuses and middle ear cavities.

Paranasal Sinuses

The paranasal sinuses are rigid-walled cavities that communicate with the nasal cavity by way of ostia. These openings must be patent when the cavities are subjected to changing barometric pressures or abnormal conditions may be produced within the sinus, usually a relatively negative pressure, which can lead to pathologic changes. Normal pressure changes across sinus ostia are very small, and considerable time is required for the air in one of the larger sinuses to be replaced. With this relatively inefficient ventilation, it is critical for the sinus ostium to be unob-

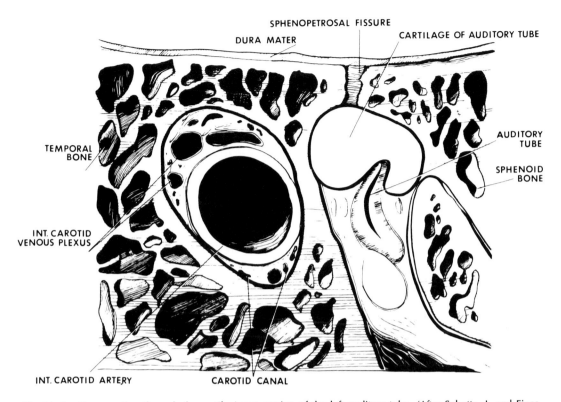

Fig. 16–4. Cross section through the cartilaginous portion of the left auditory tube. (After Sobotta, J. and Figge, F.H.: Atlas of Human Anatomy. Vol. 3. Hafner Press, NY, 1974, p. 185.)

structed, particularly when unphysiologic pressure changes are encountered.

The normal sinus lining is a thin, ciliated mucoperiosteum. Mucus glands are normally limited to the region of the ostium. Drainage is affected by both ciliary action and gravity in the frontal, ethmoid, and sphenoid sinuses; in the maxillary sinus, the location of the ostium is high on the medial wall, creating a "water bottle" effect, and drainage is dependent on ciliary action. In all of the sinuses, ciliary streaming always leads to the ostium. A sinus can renew its mucous coat in 5 to 10 minutes; the journey from the farthest corner of the most distant sinus to the pharynx takes about 20 minutes. Patency of the ostium is also critical for adequate clearing of secretions from the sinus cavity.

The close proximity of the roots of the maxillary dentition, particularly the mo-

lars, to the floor of the maxillary sinus may have aeromedical significance. Development of a relatively negative pressure in a maxillary sinus during descent from altitude may be interpreted as being of dental origin. Conversely, a pathologic process in a maxillary molar tooth (e.g., pulpitis and periapical abscess) may extend to the sinus cavity.

Pharynx

The pharynx can be divided into the nasopharynx, oropharynx, and hypopharynx (or laryngopharynx). The most aeromedically significant part is the nasopharynx because it contains the pharyngeal end of the eustachian tube in its lateral wall. The mucosa of the nasopharynx contains a significant amount of lymphoid tissue, which may respond to viral and bacterial invaders and lead to edema, which can compromise tubal function.

The velopharyngeal sphincter, which closes off the nasopharynx from the oropharynx, is also significant in flight. Competency of this sphincter is essential for proper deglutition and speech. Also, normal function of this mechanism is required for accomplishment of politzerization, an unphysiologic means for ventilating the middle ear space.

Larynx

The larynx has respiratory, sphincteric (protective), and phonatory functions. The main respiratory effect is the valvular action provided by variation in the size of the glottis. This influences intra-alveolar pressures and the interchange of oxygen and carbon dioxide. Sphincteric actions include protection against the aspiration of food and fluids, as the larynx is closed during the second stage of deglutition; tussive and expectorative functions, as the cough reflex requires tight closure of the larynx; and fixation of the chest for effective movement of the shoulder girdle and for efficient action of the abdominal muscles. In its phonatory role, vibration of the vocal cords generates sound, which is modified into speech by certain supralaryngeal articulators, mainly the lips, teeth, and tongue. Production of a voice that is adequate for radio communication is essential, and any laryngeal abnormality that affects this capability is aeromedically significant.

Functional Assessments

Hearing

The hearing of an aircrewman presenting for aeromedical evaluation should be assessed both clinically and audiometrically.

The clinical evaluation of hearing should consist of physician observation of the patient, with attention to any obvious difficulty in communicating. If the patient was referred for hearing loss, the examiner may wish to deliberately vary the intensity of his speech and to note the effect of depriving the patient of visualization of his lips while talking. This may reveal considerable dependence of the patient on lip reading. During examination of the patient, tuning fork tests should be done. These should consist of the Rinne test (comparison of air conduction with bone conduction) and the Weber test (test for lateralization with the fork placed in the midline). A 512-Hz tuning fork should be used. Results of the fork tests should be correlated later with audiometric findings.

Audiometry should be carried out by an audiologist or a fully trained technician utilizing a sound-attenuated booth and equipment that is in proper calibration. All patients should have as a minimum evaluation the determination of thresholds for pure-tone, air-conducted stimuli at the following frequencies (Hz): 250, 500, 1000, 2000, 3000, 4000, 6000, and 8000. If there is a significant hearing loss at 1000 and/or 2000 Hz, then a 1500-Hz evaluation also should be done. The threshold for bone-conducted sound should be determined for any frequency from 250 through 4000 Hz in which the air-conduction (AC) threshold is not within normal limits (up to 25 dB at any frequency). If there is a significant loss by AC in one or both ears, the bone-conduction (BC) thresholds can be utilized to determine whether the loss is conductive, sensorineural, or combined. If the BC thresholds are, in general, equal to the AC thresholds, the hearing loss is sensorineural; if the BC thresholds are within normal limits, the hearing loss is conductive. In a combined loss, the BC thresholds will lie somewhere between normal and the AC thresholds. In most aircrewmen, pure-tone audiometry will be adequate for the clinical evaluation of hearing loss, including determinations made for hearing conservation purposes. If indicated, additional audiometric procedures may be accomplished; these include speech audiometry, impedance audiometry, various so-called "site-of-lesion" tests intended to aid the clinician in differentiating an end-organ or hair-cell lesion from a nerve-fiber lesion, and certain special procedures such as auditory brain stem responses (ABR). A detailed discussion of all of these additional procedures is beyond the scope of this chapter; however, the procedures that are utilized most frequently at USAFSAM will be mentioned.

Speech audiometry should probably be requested for any patient with a significant pure-tone deficit, particularly if the pure-tone loss is unilateral. Speech audiometry consists of the speech reception threshold (SRT), which is determined with a suitable list of tape-recorded bisyllabic, vowel-rich words, and the discrimination score, which is determined with a suitable list of tape-recorded phonetically balanced (PB), consonant-rich words. The SRT is expressed in decibels and usually should correlate within 5 to 10 dB with the pure-tone threshold average for the primary speech frequencies (500, 1000, and 2000 Hz). The discrimination score is expressed in percent; the subject is given 50 words, and 2% is deducted for each word that is not repeated correctly. These words are presented at an intensity level well above the pure-tone threshold to minimize any sound transmission factors and determine, as accurately as possible, the true cochlear reserve. In general, patients with normal hearing, conductive loss, and mild sensorineural loss have good discrimination, which is defined as 90% or better. With cochlear impairment, the discrimination score will decrease as involvement of the speech range increases. An individual with high-tone loss only may have good discrimination. Lesions that involve the eighth cranial nerve usually produce more severe decrements in discrimination than do cochlear abnormalities.

Impedance audiometry primarily measures the functional compliance of the sound-conducting mechanism in the middle ear (middle ear transformer or imped-ance-matching mechanism). Because this instrument can demonstrate sudden changes in impedance of the middle ear mechanism, contraction of the stapedial muscle, the "stapedial reflex," in response to an appropriate stimulus can be recorded along with the intensity of the stimulus that is required to elicit the reflex. The acoustic reflex is normally present and can be elicited by stimuli below 100 dB in intensity. The most useful frequencies are 500, 1000, and 2000 Hz. The acoustic reflex is absent in conductive losses, which usually are easily determined; however, the acoustic reflex also may be absent or its threshold may be elevated or it may exhibit abnormal decay when there is a lesion that involves the eighth cranial nerve. Accordingly, the acoustic reflex may be useful in evaluating patients with unilateral findings that suggest nerve involvement.

A number of "site-of-lesion" tests are available to the clinician who may be confronted with the need to determine whether hearing loss and other otologic manifestations (e.g., tinnitus) are due to involvement of the inner ear (cochlear) or to some pathologic process of the eighth cranial nerve (neural). Most of the tests are based on demonstrating the presence or absence of a phenomenon that is known to be either cochlear or neural in origin. One cochlear manifestation that may be employed is recruitment. Recruitment may be demonstrated in suitable subjects by the alternate binaural loudness balance test. A neural manifestation that can be utilized in the differential diagnosis is the phenomenon of adaptation or tone decay, which may be demonstrated by several tests; the version generally preferred at this time is the suprathreshold adaptation test, originally described by Jerger and Jerger.[1] This version involves stressing the auditory system with intensity and has been shown to be more reliable than threshold techniques. Other tests are based on the difference limen phenomenon—the smallest difference in intensity that can be perceived by the patient; the test most commonly used is the short-increment sensitivity index. Individuals with cochlear disorders are able to hear 1-dB changes in intensity, whereas a person with normal hearing or a neural lesion usually cannot detect these changes in intensity. Another test that is useful in differential auditory diagnosis is based on the observation that the ability to discriminate PB words may break down at high-intensity levels in the presence of a nerve lesion. Such a patient may score well at 40 dB above threshold but do significantly poorer when the intensity is increased. This decrease in discrimination is referred to as the "rollover" phenomenon; that is, at high intensity levels, the discrimination score rolls over to a lower level. This test is usually called the performance-intensity functions for phonetically balanced words. As emphasized by Jerger and Jerger,[1] it is wise to obtain a battery of tests rather than rely on any one test.

A special audiometric procedure developed in the mid-1960s by Jewett and colleagues[2] is based on recording waveforms that are produced centrally during the first 10 milliseconds after exposure to a suitable auditory stimulus such as a click. Because this electrical activity is of very low voltage and is projected against ongoing brain activity, an averaging computer is required to record these auditory brain stem responses (ABR). A wave pattern is produced that consists of waves I through VII; however, the most clinically useful parameters are the intra-aural wave I to V interval and the interaural wave V latency difference. Lesions involving the eighth cranial nerve, usually an acoustic neuroma, may produce prolongation of the I to V intervals, which also may produce a significant increase in the interaural wave V latency. ABR has proven to be a very useful procedure in otolaryngology, primarily in the evaluation of unilateral otologic findings that suggest a cerebellopontine angle lesion. In any one patient, the test battery employed should be determined by consultation with an otolaryngologist.

Vestibular Function

Vestibular function usually is not specifically evaluated unless the patient has a history of vertigo or relates a complaint suggestive of an abnormality in the vestibular system. If assessment of vestibular function is indicated, it should be accomplished both clinically and by appropriate tests.

The clinical evaluation of vestibular function should include observing the patient for the presence of spontaneous nystagmus and testing for positional nystagmus. The Dix-Hallpike maneuver should be carried out while the physician observes the patient's eyes for nystagmus. This maneuver is the combination of a definite stimulus and the assumption of a certain head position. The patient, who is sitting up on the examining table, is briskly placed in the supine position with the head lowered about 30° below the horizontal plane and rotated so that one ear is down. After allowing the patient to rest for 5 minutes, the stimulus is repeated with the head rotated to the opposite side. A "typical" response is characterized by a brief latent period of a few seconds followed by rotary or horizontal-rotary nystagmus, which is accompanied by subjective vertigo. The nystagmus and vertigo also will be brief, usually lasting 5 to 10 seconds. If nystagmus and vertigo occur, the stimulus should be repeated after a 1-minute rest, and the response will be reduced or absent, which confirms that it is fatigable. An "atypical" response is the production of nystagmus without one or more of the other features. In a normal individual, this maneuver will produce neither nystagmus nor vertigo. A typical response is indicative of an end-organ or peripheral abnormality; an atypical response is a nonspecific finding.

The cranial nerves should be checked and coordination and balance assessed. The inability to walk in tandem fashion is usually indicative of a cerebellar disorder but also may be seen in unilateral labyrinthine disease. In the Romberg test, in which the patient stands erect with feet together and arms at the sides, closing the eyes eliminates visual input and can result in two of the three orientation mechanisms becoming inoperative. If the patient falls, there is disturbance of proprioception due to dorsal column involvement. The "sharpened Romberg" test, in which the patient's feet are placed in tandem rather than side-to-side, is a significant modification of the Romberg test.[3] This modified test is more sensitive and may be positive in labyrinthine abnormalities.

Vestibular function testing should be as complete as possible. If facilities permit only a simple cold water caloric test, this should be done. Ideally, appraisal of the status of the vestibular system by calorization should include both cold and warm stimuli, the bithermal technique, and the results should be recorded by electronystagmography (ENG). The suppressive effect of visual fixation can be eliminated by recording with the patient's eyes closed. In addition to caloric stimulation, the ENG usually records for ocular dysmetria and visual tracking, gaze nystagmus, spontaneous nystagmus, optokinetic nystagmus, positional nystagmus, response to the Dix-Hallpike maneuvers, and fixation suppression of calorically induced nystagmus. Responses to caloric stimulation are hand-scored and then converted to percentages of unilateral weakness and directional preponderance according to the method of Jongkees and Philipzoon.[4]

At USAFSAM, vestibular function testing includes stimulating the system physiologically with harmonic or sinusoidal acceleration at frequencies from 0.1 to 0.16 Hz, one octave apart, at a maximum velocity of 50 degrees/sec. Eye movement analysis yields primary measures of phase and left-right asymmetry, or labyrinthine preponderance.[5]

It is important for the clinician to keep vestibular function tests in their proper perspective. An ENG, regardless of how elaborate the equipment may be, does not make diagnoses; the ENG may provide the physician with findings that must then be correlated with the patient's history and physical examination in an effort to make as specific a diagnosis as possible. Either unilateral labyrinthine weakness or no response is a significant finding and usually indicates a peripheral abnormality. Directional preponderance is a nonspecific finding that may not be clinically significant. A vestibular spontaneous nystagmus and positional nystagmus are nonspecific findings. The "typical" Dix-Hallpike response is consistent with a peripheral disorder, but an atypical response is nonspecific. Calibration overshoot, abnormal visual pursuit or tracking, gaze nystagmus, optokinetic asymmetry, and failure of fixation suppression usually indicate a central abnormality. Phase shifts in response to harmonic acceleration cannot identify unilateral involvement; in general, peripheral abnormalities cause shifts at the low end (0.1 Hz) of the stimulus spectrum; central involvements can cause shifts at both low and high frequencies or even across the entire spectrum. Harmonic labyrinthine preponderance may be toward the involved side (irritative) or away from the involved side (depressed). Neuromas consistently show the picture of depression; with central abnormalities, the preponderance is usually the depressed type and is greater at the higher frequencies.

CLINICAL CONDITIONS

Conditions Related to the Flight Environment

External Otitic Barotrauma

The term external otitic barotrauma refers to injury to the lining of the external ear canal due to the creation of an airtight space between an object in the outer ear canal and the eardrum. Earplugs, such as those used for protection against aircraft noise, tightly impacted cerumen, or any other foreign material may produce a seal in the ear canal and entrap air. During descent, the pressure of this entrapped air may become relatively negative with respect to ambient pressure. Because of this mechanical effect, the outer layer of epithelium of the tympanic membrane and/or that of the inner aspect of the external canal wall may be sucked away from the underlying tissue to form hemorrhagic areas beneath the epithelium. If these areas become large enough, hemorrhagic bullae may be formed. The primary manifestation is pain and is most likely due to stripping of the epithelium from the underlying bone. Small subepithelial hemorrhages usually require no specific treatment. If large hemorrhagic bullae have formed, recovery will be more rapid if the blood is evacuated with a syringe and needle or by means of a small incision.

No one should be subjected to barometric pressure changes if the external auditory canal is completely obstructed in any manner. Earplugs and similar devices should be vented in some manner to permit pressure equalization to take place, or some provision for rapid removal should be made such as a loop of string through the tab on an earplug that is long enough to be accessible to the aircrewmen with the helmet in place. Various earplugs have been worn by United States Air Force personnel during flight operations in various aircraft for several years. Experience has shown that in most aircrewmen these earplugs do not form an airtight seal in the ear canal because in the overwhelming majority of instances, external otitic barotrauma does not occur, even with rapid descents. This fact was verified by a study at USAFSAM that was carried out in an altitude chamber.[6] External otitic barotrauma has occurred occasionally, and

even these relatively rare instances can be prevented if the crewmember is alert and responds to the early symptoms of barotrauma. It is not necessary to remove the plug completely; all that is required is that the plug be moved laterally enough to break the seal.

Barotitis Media (Aerotitis Media)

Barotitis media can be defined as an acute or chronic traumatic inflammation in the middle ear space that is produced by a pressure differential between the air in the tympanic cavity and mastoid air cells and that of the surrounding atmosphere. A classic description of this entity was published by Armstrong and Heim in 1937.[7] The middle ear space in this context should be regarded as a rigid-walled cavity that communicates with the nasopharynx by way of the eustachian tube, which acts essentially as a one-way flutter valve that favors the release of pressure from the middle ear to the nasopharynx but not the reverse. Ascent produces a relatively positive pressure in the tympanic cavity as the pressure of the atmosphere becomes progressively less. This positive pressure usually is readily equalized because the air can pass easily through the eustachian tube to the nasopharynx. The pressure change is greater at lower altitudes because the air is denser. This relatively positive pressure in the middle ear may be perceived by the individual as a slight fullness in the ear, which usually can be relieved readily by swallowing. On descent, however, a different situation exists. The eustachian tube remains closed unless actively opened by muscle action or high positive pressure in the nasopharynx. If the eustachian tube opens, any existing pressure differential is immediately equalized. If the tube does not open regularly during descent, a pressure differential may develop. If this pressure differential reaches 80 to 90 mm Hg, the small muscles of the soft palate cannot overcome it, and either reascent or an unphysiologic maneuver is necessary to open the tube.

Barotitis media, which is frequently referred to as an "ear block," results from failure of ventilation of the middle ear space on changing from low to high atmospheric pressure, that is, descent. The most common cause is swelling of the nasopharyngeal end of the eustachian tube, which is usually due to an acute upper respiratory tract infection. Edema secondary to allergic rhinitis may be an etiologic factor. Ignorance of the necessity for swallowing at frequent intervals during descent in an aircraft also may be a significant contributory factor. Most individuals engaged in diving receive adequate indoctrination before actual operation, whereas many individuals who fly, particularly those who do so in commercial aircraft, may not be properly indoctrinated. The ability to recognize the early pressure changes incident to beginning descent and to adjust the intervals between swallowing to meet the demands of the rate of descent comes only with flying experience; however, preflight indoctrination is certainly valuable. The rate of descent is also a significant factor. This fact has been recognized for many years by commercial airlines; their descent rates are usually quite gradual, generally less than 400 fpm, whereas descent rates in military aircraft are often much greater, frequently several thousand fpm. The use of oxygen during flight increases the likelihood of barotrauma because oxygen delivered from an aircraft's oxygen system is usually quite dry and may irritate the mucosa of the upper respiratory tract. Also, the absorption of oxygen by the middle ear and mastoid mucosa contributes to the relatively negative pressure in those cavities. When oxygen absorption is the primary factor in the development of a pressure differential, the term delayed barotitis media may be used. Personnel who fly in jet aircraft that are equipped with a system that delivers 100% oxygen throughout the flight are

most likely to develop this type of ear block. The absorption of 100% oxygen, however, usually must be combined with the infrequency of swallowing that occurs during sleep to produce a pressure differential sufficient to cause symptoms. Individuals who operate aircraft equipped with this type of oxygen system are aware of this possibility and will try to keep their ears well ventilated following the termination of a flight. However, if a flight is completed in the late evening hours or during the night and the individual retires a short time later, a significant pressure differential may develop during sleep because of the combined factors of oxygen absorption and infrequent swallowing. Once the pressure differential develops, the situation is similar to that which occurs due to failure of ventilation of the eustachian tube. Sleeping during descent in an aircraft can lead to an ear block, again due to the infrequency of swallowing while asleep.

Pathologic changes in the middle ear vary with the magnitude of the pressure differential between the tympanic cavity and the ambient air pressure and with the length of time the pressure alteration acts on the tissues before equalization takes place. For practical purposes, the pressure differential results in a partial vacuum in the middle ear space that produces retraction of the tympanic membrane and engorgement of the blood vessels in the eardrum and middle ear mucosa. In mild ear blocks, pathologic changes may be limited to these effects. If the pressure differential is great enough and persists long enough, a transudate usually forms, which may be serous, serosanguineous, or even hemorrhagic. In rare cases, with the development of a severe pressure differential, the eardrum may rupture, the break usually occurring in the weakest area or in an area previously damaged by an earlier pathologic process. Formation of a transudate is the more frequent occurrence. Once fluid accumulates in the middle ear space, tension on the eustachian tube is relieved, and this is followed by reinflation of the middle ear space, manifested by bubbling, and eventual resolution of the process.

Symptoms also vary with the magnitude of the pressure differential and the speed with which it develops. In minimal barotrauma, symptoms usually are limited to mild ear pain, a feeling of fullness in the ear, and mild conductive-type hearing loss. A low-pitched tinnitus may be noted. With this category of involvement, symptoms usually disappear fairly quickly and completely soon after the middle ear space is ventilated. With moderate degrees of pressure differential, all symptoms are increased in intensity. If a transudate occurs, the patient may notice sensations due to fluid movement as his head position is changed or during the act of swallowing. In severe barotrauma, particularly if the pressure differential develops relatively quickly, the pain may be so great that it will actually be incapacitating. The hearing loss usually will be greater and the tinnitus louder. Vertigo may be experienced with severe barotrauma; this is uncommon but significant because it may be disabling. The exact mechanism for the production of vertigo by reduced pressure in the middle ear is not known; the labyrinth is evidently stimulated by the pressure change that is applied to the oval and round windows. If the tympanic membrane ruptures, pain and other symptoms usually subside fairly quickly. Clinical findings also vary with the degree of pressure change and the length of time the condition has been present when the patient is seen. Development of a relatively negative pressure in the middle ear space produces retraction of the eardrum, with prominence of the short process of the malleus and what is referred to as "foreshortening" of its long process. Vascular engorgement produces injection and hyperemia of the eardrum, which is most marked peripherally and along the long process of the malleus. Hemorrhagic areas may be seen in the eardrum, again most likely along the long process of the malleus or in the drum periphery. These tiny hemorrhages also occur throughout the middle ear mucosa but usually cannot be seen. The formation of a transudate may be manifested by a middle ear that is full of serous fluid or by an air-fluid interface in the form of a relatively straight line (that shifts with changes in head position) or by bubbles. A hemorrhagic transudate will produce a hemotympanum. Perforation of the tympanic membrane may occur at any point, usually at the weakest area in the eardrum and possibly at the site of an earlier perforation or an atrophic scar.

The usual audiometric finding is a conductive-type hearing loss. In the earlier stages, before any transudate develops, the low frequencies are primarily affected due to increased stiffness of the conduction system. If transudation occurs, the stiffness is lessened and, the mass of the conduction system is increased, which is reflected in less involvement of the lower frequencies and increased involvement of the higher tones. This hearing loss is usually mild, unless hemorrhage occurs in the tympanic cavity, which can produce a greater loss. Fork tests are consistent with a conductive hearing loss.

The diagnosis in most cases should not be difficult and is based primarily on a history of pain and hearing loss developing during or immediately following descent in an aircraft. Retraction of the tympanic membrane and tiny hemorrhages into the substance of the eardrum, as well as serous or perhaps serosanguineous fluid in the middle ear space, aid in establishing the diagnosis. The differential diagnoses should include serous otitis media, acute and chronic otitis media, external otitis, and myringitis bullosa. An adequate history of barotrauma and the characteristic eardrum findings should aid in differentiating barotitis media from the other entities.

Therapeutic measures should be divided into two general categories: (1) inflight measures that can be employed by aircrewmen; and (2) therapeutic measures that the physician may employ when he sees an individual who has sustained an ear block.

The primary in-flight measure is the performance of the Valsalva maneuver as soon as a feeling of fullness is noted in either ear. If the individual has a nasal decongestant (such as 0.25% phenylephrine or Neo-Synephrine) with him, the nose should be sprayed. This procedure is best accomplished by spraying each side initially and then applying a second spray a few minutes after the initial application has had time to take effect. The second application has a better chance of reaching the nasopharyngeal area and shrinking the mucosa around the tubal orifice. If the ear cannot be ventilated by the Valsalva maneuver, a return to higher altitude should be carried out promptly if operational conditions permit. The ear should then be ventilated and a gradual descent carried out while the individual performs the Valsalva maneuver frequently.

If the aircrewman presents to the clinician with an ear block, management should be based on the clinical findings. If there is no evidence of transudation, an attempt should be made to ventilate the ear. Politzerization usually will be required because the Valsalva maneuver will not be effective; otherwise, the individual would not have developed an ear block in the first place. Either the Politzer bag or a source of compressed air may be used. The nose should be sprayed well with a decongestant solution; maximum shrinkage of the mucosa should be attained. For the bag method, the olive tip is placed in one nostril, the nose is compressed between the physician's fingers, and the patient is then instructed to say "kick, kick, kick" while the bag is squeezed, thereby increasing the pressure in the nasopharyngeal cavity to the point at which the eustachian tube will be

opened and the middle ear space ventilated. If compressed air is used, the pressure is turned down to 4 or 5 psi, and a suitable empty spray bottle that will take a nasal tip, such as a DeVilbiss nebulizer, is used to deliver the air to the patient's nose. It may be necessary to increase the pressure gradually several times until air enters the middle ear; however, the pressure should not be greater than 5 or 6 psi. If politzerization cannot be accomplished at this pressure level, it is not likely that increasing the pressure further will result in success. If the ear cannot be ventilated by having the patient say "kick, kick, kick," the procedure may be repeated while having him swallow a small amount of water during the application of the air. An effort must be made to synchronize delivery of the air with the second phase of deglutition, at which time the velopharyngeal sphincter is closed. The patient can be relied on to verify that the middle ear has been inflated. If necessary, however, the physician can use a Toynbee tube to auscultate the involved ear while air is being blown into the nasal cavity. If air enters the middle ear in any significant quantity, it usually can be heard. If desired, one physician can apply the air to the nasal cavity while another physician observes the eardrum directly for evidence of ventilation. It should be borne in mind that successful inflation of the ear does not necessarily mean immediate resolution of the ear block. If there has been significant trauma to the eustachian tube, simply ventilating the ear will not reverse the process. The one type of ear block in which ventilating the ear may effectively terminate the process is a delayed ear block due to oxygen absorption from the middle ear space because, in this variety of ear block, little or no trauma has occurred to the eustachian tube. If politzerization is initially successful, it may be necessary to repeat this procedure for several days until eustachian tube adequacy is reestablished.

If transudation into the middle ear space

has occurred by the time the patient is first seen, no attempt should be made to ventilate the ear. The formation of fluid usually eliminates any persisting pressure differential and relieves any pain, and the patient's primary complaint will be the feeling of fullness in his ear and the mild hearing loss. He should be started on conservative therapy, consisting of both topical and systemic decongestants. It is a good practice to combine the systemic decongestant with an antihistamine. When the eustachian tube begins to open, as manifested by bubbles behind the eardrum, resolution of the process may be hastened by politzerization. As soon as the patient can perform the Valsalva maneuver, however, politzerization can be discontinued.

Regardless of the condition in which the patient presents for treatment, therapy must be continued until the process has completely subsided and the eustachian tube and middle ear are functioning normally. It is imperative that an aircrewman be grounded for this period and that he not be returned to flying duties prematurely.

Hemotympanum should be managed conservatively. Considerable time, up to several weeks, may be required for blood to clear from the middle ear space. Myringotomy should be avoided if possible. The only absolute indication for myringotomy would be the need for an aircrewman to return immediately to flying duties for some compelling operational reason. Myringotomy will not restore the eustachian tube to functional status, but it will open the middle ear space and prevent further trauma to the eustachian tube and relieve ear symptoms.

Perforation of the tympanic membrane should be treated conservatively. The ear should be kept dry and the patient followed on an outpatient basis. If healing is not well under way by the end of 2 weeks, local measures, such as cauterizing the margins and installing a paper patch,

should be considered and would probably require referral to an otolaryngologist.

It cannot be overemphasized that the management of barotitis media is essentially conservative. It must be borne in mind that the mucous membrane of the upper respiratory tract is delicate and that nothing should be done that could possibly augment the existing trauma. Catheterization of the eustachian tube orifice is never indicated. This procedure would only further traumatize the eustachian tube and undoubtedly prolong the disorder.

Recurrent barotitis media is essentially the problem of chronic eustachian tube obstruction, which is usually secondary to a pathologic process in either the nose or nasopharynx. The most common causes are hypertrophic lymphoid tissue in the nasopharynx, allergic rhinitis, and chronic sinusitis. Lymphoid tissue deposited submucosally along the anterior two thirds of the eustachian tube (Gerlach's tonsil) may be hyperplastic. Occasionally, deflection of the nasal septum may be a significant factor. Treatment should be directed at the primary problem and may be either medical or surgical. In an occasional patient, no apparent cause for the chronic eustachian tube obstruction can be found, and hyperplastic submucosal lymphoid tissue along the anterior two thirds of the tube may be suspected. An effective way to reduce this hyperplastic tissue is external irradiation. The entire length of the eustachian tube can be treated in this manner, whereas radium applicators are mainly effective at the tubal orifice in the nasopharynx. Of course, radiation therapy should be reserved as a last resort.

Alternobaric Vertigo

Alternobaric, or pressure, vertigo should be regarded as a type of barotrauma in which symptoms result from the effect of expansion of trapped gases within the middle ear space. The exact mechanism by which vertigo is produced is not known; however, the role of positive pressure in the middle ear is generally accepted. The production of vertigo implies stimulation of the vestibular system, probably through an intact oval window. The increase in pressure due to failure to ventilate the middle ear on ascent is gradual and, in most instances, is not enough to produce vertigo; however, the addition of a sudden pressure increment caused by the performance of a forceful Valsalva maneuver can be sufficient for vestibular stimulation. Minimal residual eustachian tube edema secondary to a resolving upper respiratory tract infection can make ventilation of the ears on ascent difficult, requiring a more forceful Valsalva maneuver than is usually necessary.

Alternobaric vertigo is probably fairly common in pilots of high-performance jet aircraft capable of a rapid rate of climb. The role that pressure change plays is corroborated by the higher incidence of alternobaric vertigo in divers because pressure changes are much greater in an aqueous media. In 1957, Jones[8] reported an incidence of 10% in 190 pilots; in 1966 Lundgren and Malm[9] reported an incidence of 17% in 108 pilots. The understandable reluctance of pilots to report symptoms of this type makes it reasonable to assume that this entity is more common than is generally realized.

In most instances, the history is fairly typical. The aircrewman, most often a pilot flying a high-performance jet aircraft, usually relates the sudden onset of vertigo following the performance of a forceful Valsalva maneuver to relieve a feeling of fullness in one or both ears. This vertigo usually occurs on ascent, but it has been described on descent following a particularly forceful Valsalva maneuver.[10] The vertigo is characteristically brief, ordinarily lasting a few seconds. The individual usually feels perfectly normal as soon as the vertigo clears. Whether this brief episode of vertigo actually compromises flight safety is determined by the opera-

tional circumstances and the experience of the individual concerned, but that it is capable of so doing is obvious.

The management of alternobaric vertigo is essentially prevention. This implies a continual process of education for aircrewmen in which the common nature and hazard potential of this condition are emphasized. The admonition not to fly with a cold cannot be overemphasized. It is reasonably safe to assume that the most common reason for having difficulty ventilating the middle ear is residual eustachian tube involvement from an acute upper respiratory tract infection. Aircrewmen most likely to encounter this condition should be advised to clear their ears more frequently during climb-out and avoid the necessity for a forceful Valsalva maneuver.

The aeromedical significance of alternobaric vertigo is obvious; it is capable of producing sudden incapacity in flight. The fact that it may be of brief duration does not negate its significance, nor should one assume that it may not occur at a critical time in flight. In the operation of high-performance, fighter-type jet aircraft, all aspects of flight are critical, and several seconds are sufficient for an unsafe operational condition to develop. That alternobaric vertigo is relatively common must be realized by aircrewmen and should be emphasized on a continuing basis by flight surgeons.

Barodontalgia

Barodontalgia, or aerodontalgia, is a toothache that is provoked by exposure to changing barometric pressures (during actual or simulated flight).

In 1937, Drefus[11] first reported pain in a tooth that occurred in flight at 1800 m; he later relieved this pain by pulpectomy. In World War II, many episodes of odontalgia occurred during flight and were referred to as aerodontalgia. It was relatively uncommon, 1 to 2% in most series, but in many instances was severe enough to compromise mission success. Barodontalgia, the preferred term at present, has persisted as an aeromedical problem, although the incidence has remained low (e.g., less than 1% of altitude chamber reactions in calendar year (CY) 1964 and 1965, as shown in Table 16–1).

The precise mechanism for pain production in barodontalgia has not been determined; however, exposure to reduced atmospheric pressure is obviously a significant factor. This exposure to reduced barometric pressure is evidently a precipitating factor, with disease of the pulp the primary cause. Pressure changes do not elicit pain in teeth with normal pulps, regardless of whether the tooth is intact, carious, or restored. In his classic review on the effects of changes in barometric pressure, Adler[12] classified symptoms as due either to trapped gases or evolved gases, and he placed barodontalgia in the trapped gas category primarily because symptoms frequently appear at altitudes well below those considered necessary to produce evolved gases. Orban and Ritchey[13] concluded that the mechanism had to be the liberation and expansion of gases from the blood and tissue fluids; however, they were able to demonstrate empty, bubble-like spaces in only 6 of 75 teeth that they studied. Air trapped under restorations has been suspected of producing tooth pain, but experimentally produced air bubbles under dental restorations followed by exposure to reduced barometric

pressure did not result in symptoms. Other possible factors have been considered. Studies have found that low temperatures were not significant and have eliminated radial acceleration as a possible factor. Also, detrimental effects from the use of oxygen in flight have not been identified. Disease of the pulp appears to be the significant dental factor, and the initiation of symptoms is probably due to a circulatory disturbance. The pulp organ is unique in that it is encapsulated in a nonyielding structure. It contains a complicated vascular system, including metarterioles and precapillaries. Circulation to the pulp is a very delicate and sensitive system, which can be injured by tooth trauma. For reasons not fully understood at this time, a damaged pulp can react to reduced atmospheric pressure and produce pain. This reaction appears to involve edema, which can lead to necrosis. In some patients, gas may form by the action of enzymes on necrotic pulp tissue.

Strohaver[14] advocated the differentiation of barodontalgia into direct and indirect types. In the direct variety, reduced atmospheric pressure contributes to a direct effect on a given tooth; in the indirect type, dental pain is secondary to stimulation of the superior alveolar nerves by a maxillary barosinusitis. Direct barodontalgia is generally manifested by moderate to severe pain, which usually develops during ascent and is well localized, with the patient frequently able to identify the

Table 16–1.   Distribution of Altitude Chamber Reactions (%)

Symptom	52,113 United States Air Force Trainees—1964	49,603 United States Air Force Trainees—1965
Aerotitis	8.730	8.660
Abdominal gas pain	1.960	1.850
Aerosinusitis	1.590	1.860
Bends	0.310	0.300
Barodontalgia	0.230	0.300
Chokes	0.003	0.008
Neurologic symptoms	0.002	0.000
Other	0.780	0.670
Total	13.605	13.648

From Flight Surgeons Guide. Air Force Pamphlet 161-18. Department of the Air Force, U.S. Government Printing Office, Washington, DC, Dec. 17, 1968.

involved tooth, whereas indirect barodontalgia is a dull, poorly defined pain that involves the posterior maxillary teeth and develops during descent.

Certain generalities may be useful in establishing the diagnosis of direct barodontalgia. Posterior teeth are more frequently involved than anterior teeth, and maxillary teeth are affected more often than mandibular teeth. Teeth with amalgam restorations are more likely to be involved than unrestored teeth, and recently restored teeth are particularly susceptible. The character of the pain is useful in determining whether the pulp involvement is acute or chronic; however, in an individual patient, this degree of diagnostic precision may not be possible. If pain occurs during descent, indirect barodontalgia due to barosinusitis should be strongly suspected. The patient should be asked which tooth or teeth he suspects, and then the physician should inquire about the approximate age of any restorations in the suspected area, as well as any history of previous unprovoked pain and any sensitivity to heat, cold, sweets, or pressure.

Examination should include the estimation of the age of restorations in the suspected area, exploration for caries or defective restorations, percussion of any suspected tooth, and the patient's response to application of electrical stimulation and/or ice and heat. Appropriate radiographs of the suspected teeth should be obtained, with the understanding that a negative radiograph does not rule out pulpitis.

Management should include the removal of any restorations that are clinically or radiographically defective. Any carious lesions should be curetted, with particular attention paid to exposed pulp horns. Zinc oxide and eugenol base may be very useful if the pulpal condition is reversible. If irreversible pulpitis is found, endodontic treatment should be carried out, or the tooth should be extracted. Reex-

posure to altitude in a chamber can be employed to confirm a doubtful diagnosis or to determine the effectiveness of therapy. If indirect barodontalgia is diagnosed, the patient should be referred to an aeromedical specialist for treatment.

Strohaver[14] pointed out that the incidence of barodontalgia has apparently decreased since World War II, possibly due to better dental care for flyers and improvements in cockpit and passenger compartment conditions (particularly pressurization). To date, barodontalgia has not been a problem in space flight because astronauts operate in a pressurized cabin and are not exposed to the spectrum of pressure changes that are encountered in flights in modern aircraft. Direct barodontalgia can be largely prevented by high-quality dental care, with an emphasis on the slow and careful treatment of cavities and the routine use of a cavity varnish. Pulp-capping materials should be employed in deep preparations due to the possibility of a nonbleeding pulp exposure. Occlusion should be perfected to where it is not self-damaging. Flying duties should be restricted for 48 to 72 hours after dental treatment involving deep restorations to allow time for the dental pulp to "quiet down" or stabilize. Obviously, regular dental examinations are essential for aircrewmen; any dental problem that might predispose the crewmember to barodontalgia should be corrected and the development of symptoms prevented.

Barosinusitis

Barosinusitis can be defined as an acute or chronic inflammation of one or more of the paranasal sinuses produced by the development of a pressure difference, usually negative, between the air in the sinus cavity and that of the surrounding atmosphere.

In 1878, Burt documented the experience of Cezanne, who had noted bleeding from the nose and throat in his employees doing caisson work. The first detailed description of sinus barotrauma was made by Marchoux and Nepper in 1919; they described the results of their experiments in a decompression chamber and applied their conclusions to the operation of aircraft. They pointed out the increasing likelihood of this problem as the pilot approaches the runway, at which time he requires maximum use of his faculties to accomplish a safe landing. In the mid-1940s, Campbell published several papers on the effects of barotraumatic changes on the sinuses, including his demonstration of the formation of submucosal hematomas in the frontal sinuses of dogs.

The United States Air Force chamber flight data in Table 16–1 show the relative incidence of barosinusitis. According to these data, barosinusitis is much less common than barotitis media, the latter occurring four or five times as often. This general incidence is borne out by the frequency with which each occurs in flight operations.

A paranasal sinus is a rigid-walled cavity that directly or indirectly communicates with the nasal cavity or nasopharynx by way of an ostium. During ascent, air in such a cavity moves out by way of the ostium until equilibrium is attained at altitude. During descent, air moves back into the sinus cavity until equilibrium is again reached at the earth's surface. This movement of air out of and back into the sinus cavity is not perceived and does not produce any symptoms. Abnormal conditions may alter or even prevent this free flow of air from the sinus and produce symptoms and pathologic changes. The larger sinuses are more often involved than are the smaller ones. Sinuses having small-caliber tubal structures as exits, such as the frontal sinus with its nasofrontal duct, are more likely to be involved than sinuses with relatively larger orifices. The frontal sinuses are most often involved, with the maxillary sinuses next. Involvement of the ethmoid and sphenoid sinuses is possible but is rarely seen.

The free movement of air out of and back into a paranasal sinus may be impeded or blocked by pus or mucopurulent material covering its ostium or by redundant tissue or an anatomic deformity. If mucopurulent material covers the ostium of the sinus, the relatively positive pressure that develops during ascent can cause air in the sinus to bubble through the exudate, and no symptoms will result. On descent, however, the development of a relatively negative pressure within the sinus cavity may suck the material into the sinus ostium and sinus cavity. In the case of the frontal sinus, with its rather long and frequently tortuous nasofrontal duct, thick mucopurulent material can obstruct the duct and create a sinus block. Also, the mucopurulent material can contaminate the sinus cavity and result in a purulent sinusitis. When an ostium of a sinus is obstructed by swollen or redundant tissue or by an anatomic deformity, a one-way flap or ball valve may be produced. During ascent, the flow of air out of the sinus cavity will push the "valve" away from the opening, and the pressure will be equalized at altitude. On descent, however, the relatively negative pressure inside the sinus pulls the tissue into the ostium, forming an airtight seal and producing a sinus block.

The production of a relatively negative pressure inside a sinus cavity results in space-filling phenomena. The most common of these are swelling of the mucous membranes and/or transudation of fluid either into the cavity of the sinus or beneath the sinus mucosa. When sufficient space is filled to equalize the pressure differential, the valve mechanism is released and recovery begins. In mild and moderate degrees of sinus barotrauma, vascular engorgement and generalized submucosal edema occur. With more severe trauma, mucosal detachment and submucosal hematoma may develop.

The symptoms of barosinusitis are usually proportional to its severity and may vary from a mild feeling of fullness in or around the involved sinus to excruciating pain. Pain can develop suddenly and be incapacitating. The pain is thought to be produced by the submucosal accumulation of blood dissecting the mucoperiosteum from the underlying bone. There may be some tenderness over the involved sinus and also some bloody discharge from the nose.

Sinus barotrauma should be differentiated from acute purulent sinusitis. A history of pain over one or more of the paranasal sinuses during or shortly after exposure to a barometric pressure change usually simplifies the differential diagnosis. In the more severe cases, the patient usually describes the onset of pain as quite sudden and severe. In less severe cases, the pain may be described by the patient as having developed slowly after return to ground level. Exacerbation of symptoms after a return to ground level may be due to an increase in the relatively negative pressure within the sinus following the absorption of oxygen from the air trapped in the sinus (because oxygen is readily absorbed transmucosally). Bleeding from the nose during or after exposure to barotrauma strongly suggests sinus involvement. Radiographs are the most valuable diagnostic aid. The standard sinus radiographic series in most institutions consist of stereo-Waters, lateral, and submentovertex projections. Radiographs do not differentiate any contributory forms of preexisting disease or an anatomic abnormality from the results of barotrauma. The usual finding is mucosal thickening, which may be localized or so generalized and severe that it simply produces an opaque sinus. An air-fluid level also may be demonstrated. These are nonspecific findings that must be correlated with the history. If hematoma is present, it is usually found in the frontal sinus and presents as an oval density varying from a few millimeters in diameter to practically complete occupancy of the sinus cavity. Hematomas may be single or multiple, unilateral or bilateral.

In milder cases, the involvement is usually self-limited, with resolution taking place within a few hours to a few days. In the more severe cases, the clinical course may run from a few days to as long as a few weeks. Complete resorption of a submucosal hematoma may take several weeks. If secondary infection occurs, a severe purulent sinusitis may result from the lower resistance of the traumatized tissues and/or the excellent culture medium afforded by the transudate in the sinus cavity. This transudate, whether it is serous or serosanguineous, is usually sufficiently space-filling to relieve the pressure differential, thereby releasing the flap or ball valve and alleviating the pain.

Treatment should begin at the first sign of barosinusitis and consists of returning to the altitude at which the block occurred, spraying the nose well with a decongestant solution, and then slowly descending to ground level. This treatment may or may not be possible depending on operational conditions and may not be at all feasible in a combat situation. If the patient is first seen at ground level, an altitude chamber might be available at some installations in which he could be returned to altitude. From a practical standpoint, this procedure is rarely necessary. Active treatment is usually limited to those procedures that relieve pain, promote drainage from the sinus cavity, and offer protection from infection. Oral analgesics usually are sufficient. The patient's nasal mucosa should be thoroughly decongested with a topical agent, and he should be given a supply of the same along with a systemic decongestant. The application of heat, preferably in the form of hot packs, is usually helpful. If the maxillary sinuses are involved and significant pain persists, any relatively negative pressure in the sinus cavity can be promptly relieved by cannulating the sinus cavity. This procedure should be done through the inferior meatus; the region of the natural ostium should not be instrumented. Cannulation of the frontal sinus is not recommended; if the frontal sinus must be entered, it should be by an external approach. An adequate course of an appropriate antibiotic can be prescribed to prevent secondary infection.

In most patients, barosinusitis can be managed conservatively, and uneventful recovery is the rule. It is imperative that an aircrewman remain grounded until he is fully recovered and his nose and paranasal sinuses are functioning normally. A simulated flight in an altitude chamber may be required if there is any doubt as to whether the aircrewman is fully recovered and ready for return to flying duties.

The most important preventive measure that should be emphasized by physicians on a continuing basis is that aircrewmen should not fly when they have an upper respiratory tract infection. Any intranasal condition that could affect ventilation of the paranasal sinuses should be corrected such as a significant septal deviation.

Total cabin pressurization would prevent the occurrence of barotrauma; however, this cannot be anticipated in the foreseeable future. Partial pressurization decreases the rapidity of the fluctuations of barometric pressure, as well as their magnitude. The cabin altitude of commercial aircraft usually does not exceed 2700 m; consequently, little barosinusitis is experienced in commercial aviation. In military aviation, pressurization is used primarily to increase performance parameters. Obviously, in military operations, aircrewmen are subjected to greater barometric pressure changes because military aircraft are capable of much greater rates of ascent and descent.

Abnormalities With Aeromedical Significance

Otitis Externa

The acute diffuse variety of otitis externa is most common and usually results from wetting the outer ear canal. There may be sufficient pain and tenderness to preclude wearing a helmet or headset until the involvement has cleared. Also, the use of earplugs and earmuffs will not be possible in the presence of inflammation of the external auditory canal.

In a crewmember with recurrent otitis externa, an effective preventive measure is to dehydrate the outer ear canal after each wetting from swimming, shampooing, or showering with a solution of ethyl alcohol (95% is best, but 70% is usually adequate and is more readily available).

Perforation of the Tympanic Membrane

The tympanic membrane is the most important part of the middle ear mechanical transformer, which largely compensates for the impedance to sound that is created by an air-fluid interface due to air in the middle ear and fluid in the inner ear. This impedance-matching mechanism essentially offsets this loss of energy, and its primary factor is the ratio of the area of the tympanic membrane to the area of the footplate of the stapes (approximately 14:1). Sound is concentrated at the oval window. Also, the eardrum is part of the preferential route for the conduction of sound to the oval window. This is essential for maintaining proper phase relations, which are necessary for adequate stimulation of the organ of Corti in the cochlea. Obviously, an intact tympanic membrane is essential for the optimum accomplishment of these functions.

The tympanic membrane also seals the middle ear from the external auditory canal, which, in turn, communicates with the external environment. Perforation of the eardrum makes the middle ear vulnerable to contamination by way of the external ear canal and can lead to infection of the middle ear, which may be recurrent or even become chronic. A crewmember's performance can be compromised, particularly during operations in the field. Tympanostomy tubes have the same implications as other perforations. These tubes will provide a bypass for a malfunctioning eustachian tube, but this temporary measure is unacceptable as a definitive solution for tubal incompetence. A tympanostomy tube may become obstructed or displaced or be the route for contamination of the middle ear. These are unacceptable risks in flying personnel. The primary tubal problem must be resolved and continuity of the eardrum restored for the crewmember to continue on active flying status.

Vertigo

Vertigo has great aeromedical significance because it is capable of producing sudden incapacity that can compromise flight safety. Obviously, the flight surgeon must differentiate pathologic vertigo from spatial disorientation, or "pilot's vertigo," and alternobaric vertigo. A detailed history is the physician's best tool for accomplishing this differentiation.

Pathologic vertigo involves a false perception of movement or orientation in space. Vertigo is usually due to a peripheral vestibular abnormality, but it may be central in origin, which increases the likelihood that a serious condition is present.

Peripheral vertiginous entities include Ménière's disease, benign positional vertigo, labyrinthitis (toxic, serous, and infectious), post-traumatic vertigo, and perilymph fistulas. Cerebellopontine angle lesions rarely produce typical vertigo because the lesion is slow-growing and central compensation develops as the end-organ is deafferentated by the enlarging mass. Central causes of vertigo include vertebrobasilar insufficiency, vascular accidents, multiple sclerosis, epilepsy, migraine, neoplasms, and head injury.

The primary aeromedical implication of vertigo is the possibility of recurrence with sudden incapacitation. If the patient's history and findings are reasonably consistent with a fairly well-known entity,

disposition can be made with some confidence.[15] A crewmember with Ménière's disease should be permanently grounded because recurrence of vertigo is probable, and the interval between episodes is unpredictable. Conversely, an aircrewman with viral involvement of the vestibular system, either viral labyrinthitis or vestibular neuronitis, can be returned to flying duties after he has fully recovered. If benign positional vertigo or post-traumatic vertigo is suspected, a period of observation may be very helpful in deciding whether a return to flying duties should be recommended. If a perilymph fistula is confirmed by tympanotomy and the leak is sealed, with clearing of the vertigo, return to flying duties can be considered, although an aircrewman should probably be regarded as at greater risk for recurrence than nonflying personnel. All central causes of vertigo should be considered as disqualifying for flying duties except certain head injuries, after which return to flying duties may be possible following an adequate period of observation provided no neurologic symptoms exist.

Anosmia

Inability to perceive odors has obvious safety implications in that various substances, such as fuel vapors, lubricants, or smoke, may be present in the aircraft and go unnoticed by the pilot or other crewmembers. This may be less significant in aircraft where an oxygen mask is worn throughout the flight because the aircrewman would probably note only odorants in the oxygen system. In bomber and cargo aircraft, where crewmembers do not wear oxygen masks throughout the flight, olfactory capability is a significant alerting mechanism, and the loss of this sense through injury or disease will affect flying safety. An aircrewman who notes a diminution in his ability to smell or the complete loss of the faculty should receive a thorough medical evaluation to elucidate the causative factors and determine whether the abnormality is amenable to treatment. The impact of any persisting olfactory impairment on the patient's aircrew status should be determined.

Allergic Rhinitis

Allergic rhinitis is a common medical problem that can make an aircrewman more liable to barotrauma because nasal congestion and discharge are frequent manifestations. Antihistamines are effective in many patients with nasal allergy; however, because sedation is a common side effect, aircrewmen should be cautioned about the regular use of these drugs. Any crewmember with significant allergic rhinitis should probably have an allergy evaluation, and if significant sensitivities are found, he can be started on a hyposensitization program that is compatible with his continuation on flying status. Another therapeutic option that can now be considered is the inhalation of an intranasal steroid. The indicated agent is beclomethasone dipropionate; in the dose range recommended for intranasal use, no significant depression of adrenal function has been noted.[16] This agent may be very useful in the control of symptoms in certain patients with nasal allergy. Patients with allergic rhinitis should be strongly advised to avoid the use of intranasal decongestants because dependence on one of these preparations may ensue, with the development of rhinitis medicamentosa, which would clearly be disqualifying for flying duties.

Nasal Polyposis

The presence of nasal polyps clearly makes an aircrewman more vulnerable to sinus barotrauma and should be regarded as disqualifying for flying until the polyps are removed and any contributory condition is controlled. In some patients, polyps will be secondary to allergic rhinitis; however, in many patients, no relationship between nasal allergy and nasal polyps can be found. Evaluation of a patient with

nasal polyposis should include radiographs of the paranasal sinuses because ethmoid and/or maxillary sinus involvement also may be present. Small polyps may regress with medical management, the control of allergies, or a short course of a systemic or intranasal steroid; however, large polyps usually require surgical removal. Any coexisting sinus involvement also should be appropriately treated. The importance of adequate follow-up must be appreciated; nasal polyps have a strong potential for recurrence, and subsequent removal or removals may be required.

Vasomotor Rhinitis

Vasomotor rhinitis should be regarded as an autonomic dysfunction in that the basic mechanism consists of accentuation or exaggeration of normal vasomotor and secretomotor activity. A sympathetic-parasympathetic imbalance results, with peripheral vasodilatation, edema, and hypersecretion. The most common etiologic factor is stress; therefore, the vulnerability of aircrewmen in the highly demanding flight environment is obvious. In some individuals, physical factors of the environment (e.g., temperature and humidity changes) may be operative. Most patients complain of nasal congestion or rhinorrhea or a combination of the two symptoms. Shifting nasal obstruction is characteristic of this disorder; typically, one side of the nose will be obstructed for varying periods of time. Nasal drainage is usually described as clear or mucoid; it may be primarily posterior (postnasal drip) or anterior (frequent nose blowing) or both. Various therapeutic measures may be tried depending on the primary symptom and its severity. Antihistamines and systemic decongestants may be beneficial, but the use of these drugs may require grounding the aircrewman. Patients with vasomotor rhinitis frequently employ topical decongestants, which are readily available over the counter, and may develop rhinitis medicamentosa. Steroids are very effective; topical steroids are preferred, and beclomethasone dipropionate is the drug of choice. In some patients, the careful intermittent use of this preparation may be very beneficial. Most patients, including aircrewmen, must simply learn to live with their nasal problem. This "reality therapy"[17] is accepted much better if it is presented with a detailed explanation of normal nasal physiology and the aberrations present in vasomotor rhinitis.

Vasomotor rhinitis should be regarded as possibly disqualifying for flying duties unless it is mild and unlikely to limit flying activities. As indicated above, the possibility of interference with ventilation of the paranasal sinuses should be considered, as well as the propensity for self-medication with topical decongestants and the increased likelihood of developing rhinitis medicamentosa. If treatment is successful and significantly improves nasal function and the therapy is compatible with flying duties, aircrew duty may be resumed. Fortunately, most patients with vasomotor rhinitis have mild symptoms that can be tolerated without specific treatment other than explanation and reassurance.

Acute Sinusitis

Generally, acute sinusitis is an acute medical problem that requires grounding until the condition has cleared. Many patients regard headache as a manifestation of sinusitis; however, localized pain and tenderness are more reliable indicators of paranasal sinus inflammation. The importance of obtaining appropriate radiographs in the evaluation of an individual with sinus complaints cannot be overemphasized;[18] radiographs are the most valuable diagnostic modality and should always be requested, not only for immediate diagnosis but also as a basis for follow-up. At USAFSAM, a routine Water's radiographic projection was performed on everyone presenting for aeromedical eval-

uation and a 4% incidence of asymptomatic maxillary sinusitis was found.[19] The same incidence was found in a nonflying control group, so this condition is not related to flying per se. It was concluded that in many individuals, maxillary sinusitis often occurs asymptomatically and will evidently resolve without specific therapy. It also was concluded, however, that if relatively asymptomatic maxillary sinusitis is demonstrated radiographically in an aircrewman, appropriate treatment should be instituted and resolution confirmed by follow-up radiographs because normal function of the paranasal sinuses is essential in flying. Therapy should include an adequate course of an appropriate antibiotic and both topical and systemic decongestants. In choosing an antibiotic or chemotherapeutic agent, the physician should consider that the bacteria that most frequently cause acute sinusitis are the pneumococcus, Hemophilus influenzae, and various anaerobic bacteria.[20] Good therapeutic agents include ampicillin or amoxicillin, erythromycin-sulfisoxazole, trimethoprim-sulfamethoxazole, and cefaclor.

The maxillary sinus is most frequently involved by an inflammatory process, followed by frontal sinusitis, whereas ethmoid and sphenoid sinus involvement are relatively uncommon. Most patients with maxillary sinusitis can be treated on an outpatient basis; however, in an individual with frontal sinusitis, the possibility of significant complications warrants consideration of hospitalization unless resolution is prompt.[21] In all cases of diagnosed paranasal sinusitis, treatment should be followed by radiographic reevaluation to ensure resolution, and those patients whose condition is not resolved by appropriate medical measures should be considered for surgical intervention before being returned to flying duties.

Laryngitis

The primary aeromedical implication of laryngitis is impairment of the crewmember's ability to communicate effectively by radio, intercom, or against background noise in aircraft compartments, thus creating a significant hazard for the afflicted crewmember as well as other crewmembers in other than single-seat aircraft.

Acute laryngitis is usually viral in etiology, and the laryngeal involvement is frequently associated with other signs of an acute upper respiratory tract infection. Treatment consists of resting the voice and symptomatic measures for the accompanying upper respiratory tract infection. The importance of voice rest should be emphasized to ensure compliance and preclude prolonged grounding. Whispering should be prohibited. Smoking also should be discontinued during the period of voice rest. If the patient does not respond promptly to these measures, referral to an otolaryngologist for further evaluation is mandatory. Obviously, chronic or recurring hoarseness should be promptly evaluated by an otolaryngologist.

The management of acute airway problems secondary to inflammation or foreign body obstruction in aircrew who are isolated for long periods of time is important. Laryngeal intubation requires special equipment and training in its use. An instrument has been devised for use by relatively inexperienced individuals, and intubation training should be considered for aircrews who may be subjected to long-term isolation, as in space operations.[22]

Maxillofacial Trauma

Maxillofacial trauma may constitute a significant problem in air evacuation. Flight crews must be knowledgeable in the care of patients with injuries in this area.[23] The possibility of injury to the cervical spine should be considered and evaluated with an appropriate radiograph. Adequate initial measures, including tracheotomy for control of the airway, and essential inflight maintenance of the airway are paramount.[24] The treatment of fractures usu-

ally can be deferred to the specialty center; however, if the teeth are placed in interdental fixation, rubber bands should be used rather than wire, and the patient must be provided with scissors for the prompt release of the fixation in the event that vomiting ensues.

IMPLICATIONS OF SURGICAL PROCEDURES

Otologic Implications

Mastoidectomy and Tympanoplasty

Persistent perforations of the tympanic membrane should be closed to protect the middle ear from external contamination via the outer ear canal. This is the primary aeromedical implication of a type I tympanoplasty or myringoplasty. This premise assumes more significance when the aircrewman does not have medical care readily available and may be exposed to potential extrinsic hazards, as in combat situations involving bailout or ditching and water survival. A persistent perforation, including tympanostomy tubes, should not be regarded as an acceptable solution for an aircrewman with compromised eustachian tube function; a flyer should be able to ventilate his middle ear adequately with an intact eardrum under the stresses of flying.

Other types of tympanoplasty and mastoid procedures may be considered collectively from an aeromedical point of view, excluding auditory acuity (which should be assessed separately) and violation of the oval window area. The primary consideration is that any air-containing space must communicate with the nasopharynx through openings that are adequate to assure pressure equalization under the stresses imposed by flying, with no positive pressure buildup during ascent and no relatively negative pressure development during descent. In addition to no air-conditioning pockets without adequate openings, a sufficiently functional eustachian tube is important. The resolution of this condition can be assessed with a medical altitude chamber flight postoperatively after allowing adequate time for the maximum contraction of scar tissue; six months is advisable, assuming that the ear is dry.

Any surgical procedures on the middle ear/mastoid area must not involve the oval window area if continuation on flying status is a consideration. Any surgical activity in the oval window area can increase the likelihood of perilymph fistula formation, with the possibility of acute vertigo and sudden incapacitation.

Stapedectomy

Stapes procedures, stapedectomy being the most common, are directed precisely at the oval window area and, as indicated above, result in a situation in which the likelihood of the spontaneous formation of a perilymph fistula is increased. Following removal of the stapes, the oval window is sealed by a very thin membrane. Considerable accumulated experience has established that this membrane is more vulnerable to stresses than is the stapedial footplate with its annular ligament. These stresses may be applied from within (explosive), in the form of surges of increased cerebral spinal fluid pressure transmitted via the cochlear aqueduct, or from the middle ear side (implosive) due to changes in air pressure in the middle ear.[25] Perilymph fistulas are now known to develop in apparently normal individuals;[26] therefore, the increased likelihood of this significant complication occurring following stapedectomy is apparent. Obviously, this consideration becomes even more pertinent when the aircrewman is operating a modern, high-performance jet aircraft.

Removal of Acoustic Neuromas

The acoustic neuroma is a benign tumor; therefore, if one is completely removed without any significant complications other than hearing loss, the situation is essentially analogous to a "one-eared" pilot, and continuation of flying duties is possible if a good seal is obtained without any postoperative cerebrospinal fluid leak. The individual will compensate for the loss of the labyrinth; the hearing loss usually will be total and permanent. At USAFSAM, we have established a precedent for returning pilots with severe to total hearing loss in one ear to flying duties, assuming that no significant facial weakness results that might compromise eye function or the wearing of an oxygen mask.

Rhinologic Implications

Nasal Septoplasty and Rhinoplasty

Nasal septoplasty can result in significant improvement of nasal airway patency. Because adequate airways are a requisite for flying duties, any significant septal deflection should be corrected as soon as possible. In a candidate for pilot training, this correction should be done prior to beginning training. If the examining physician is uncertain as to the functional significance of any intranasal abnormality, the patient should be referred to an otolaryngologist for evaluation and recommendations.

Rhinoplasty primarily is a cosmetic procedure; however, reduction of a nasal hump or correction of some other significant abnormality of the external nose can result in a better fit for an oxygen mask.

Nasal Polypectomy

As previously indicated, nasal polyps may be disqualifying for flying due to the increased likelihood of sinus barotrauma. Insofar as the polyps are concerned, however, adequate removal will qualify an individual for return to flying duties. The frequent association of nasal polyps with allergic rhinitis also should be considered. In addition, the importance of adequate follow-up cannot be overemphasized. Nasal polyps have a strong tendency to recur, and follow-up by an otolaryngologist is essential to determine whether the treatment regimen is effective. If recurrence is noted, the aircrewman should again be advised that the polyps should be removed and any medical management reappraised.

Sinus Surgery

Current otolaryngologic opinion strongly supports a conservative approach to sinus surgery. Radical procedures with meticulous removal of all mucosa are avoided except in ablation of the frontal sinus for chronic recurrent infection. Because the maxillary sinus is most frequently involved by inflammatory processes, it is the sinus usually involved in aeromedical considerations. The value of the creation of an antrostomy in the inferior meatus should be fully appreciated. This procedure frequently will be curative for recurrent or chronic maxillary sinusitis, and it has no limiting effect on an individual's ability to fly. This opening can be made transnasally, but many surgeons prefer a sublabial antrostomy (Caldwell-Luc) approach for better visualization of the sinus cavity and the creation of a large, competent, and permanent nasoantral window.

The frontal sinus is most frequently involved in barosinusitis, and this condition requires consideration of procedures designed to improve ventilation of this sinus. Unfortunately, any procedure that involves enlarging the nasofrontal communication predisposes to late cicatrization, with reduction or closure of the nasofrontal duct. The only conservative procedure that should be considered is removal of the intersinus septum (creating a common cavity) for recurrent unilateral frontal barosinusitis. For recurrent bilateral frontal barosinusitis, total obliteration of the frontal sinuses can be done, but it must be borne in mind that ablation of every vestige of mucosa is essential to preclude repneumatization of the sinus. This

surgery is extensive for this continuation on flying status and is usually performed for persistent frontal sinus infection.

REFERENCES

1. Jerger, J., and Jerger, S.: A simplified tone decay test. Arch. Otolaryngol., 102:403–407, 1975.
2. Jewett, D.L., Romano, M.N., and Williston, J.S.: Human auditory evoked potentials: Possible brain stem components detected on the scalp. Science, 167:1517–1518, 1970.
3. Fregly, A.R.: Handbook of Sensory Physiology. Vol. VI, Part 2. Berlin, West Germany, Springer-Verlag, 1974.
4. Jongkees, L.B.W., and Philipzoon, A.J.: Electronystagmography. Acta Otolaryngol. (Suppl.), 189:1–111, 1963.
5. Wolfe, J.W., Engelken, E.J., and Kos, C.M.: Low-frequency harmonic acceleration as a test of labyrinthine function: Basic methods and illustrative cases. Trans. Am. Acad. Ophthalmol. Otolaryngol., 86:130–143, 1978.
6. Stork, R.L., and Gasaway, D.C.: Evaluation of V-51R and EAR™ Earplugs For Use in Flight. USAFSAM-TR-77-1. United States Air Force School of Aerospace Medicine, Brooks Air Force Base, Texas, 1977.
7. Armstrong, H.G., and Heim, J.W.: The effect of flight on the middle ear. JAMA, 109:417, 1937.
8. Jones, G.M.: Review of Current Problems Associated With Disorientation in Man-Controlled Flight. Flying Personnel Research Committee 1021. Great Britain, Royal Air Force, October, 1957 (restricted).
9. Lundgren, C.E.G., and Malm, L.U.: Alternobaric vertigo among pilots. Aerospace Med., 37:178, 1966.
10. Brown, F.M.: Vertigo due to increased middle ear pressure: Six-year experience of the Aeromedical Consultation Service. Aerospace Med., 42:999, 1971.
11. Drefus, H.: "Les dents des aviateurs." L'Odontolgie, 75:612–613, 1937.
12. Adler, H.F.: Dysbarism. USAFSAM Aeromedical Review 1–64:6, 1964.
13. Orban, B., and Ritchey, B.T.: Toothache under conditions simulating high-altitude flight. J. Am. Dent. Assoc., 32:145, 1945.
14. Strohaver, R.A.: Aerodontalgia: Dental pain during flight. Med. Service Dig., 23:35, 1972.
15. Lindeman, R.C.: Acute labyrinthine disorders. Otolaryngol. Clin. North Am., 12:375–387, 1979.
16. Harris, D.M., et al.: The effect of intranasal beclomethasone dipropionate on adrenal function. Clin. Allergy, 4:291–294, 1974.
17. Pogorel, B.S.: Vasomotor rhinitis and nasal dyspnea. ENT., 56:261–272, 1977.
18. Yarington, C.T., Jr.: Emergency problems involving sinusitis. Aviat. Space Environ. Med., 50:80–82, 1979.
19. Hanna, H.H.: Asymptomatic sinus disease in aircrew members. Aerospace Med., 45:77–81, 1974.
20. Gwaltney, J.M., Jr., Sydnor, A.S., Jr., and Saude,

M.A.: Etiology and antimicrobial treatment of acute sinusitis. Ann. Otol. Rhinol. Laryngol. (Suppl. 84), 90:68–71, 1981.

21. Yarington, C.T., Jr.: Sinusitis as an emergency. Otolaryngol. Clin. North Am., 12:447–454, 1979.

22. LeJeune, F.E., Jr.: Laryngeal problems in space travel. Aviat. Space Environ. Med., 49:1347–1349, 1978.

23. Yarington, C.T., Jr.: The initial evaluation in max-illofacial trauma. Otolaryngol. Clin. North Am., 12:293–301, 1979.

24. Linscott, M.S., and Horton, W.C.: Management of upper airway obstruction. Otolaryngol. Clin. North Am., 12:351–373, 1979.

25. Goodhill, V.: Traumatic fistulae. J. Laryngol. Otol., 94:123–128, 1980.

26. Fee, G.A.: Traumatic perilymphatic fistulas. Arch. Otolaryngol., 88:477–480, 1968.

Chapter *17*

Neuropsychiatry in Aerospace Medicine

David R. Jones and James L. Perrien

For a pilot, flying is never dangerous, for a man must be a little bit insane or under the press of duty to willingly remain in a position that he truly considers dangerous. Airplanes occasionally crash, pilots are occasionally killed, but flying is not dangerous, it is interesting.

RICHARD BACH, *Stranger to the Ground*

Aeromedical practitioners have a specific approach to the selection and care of flyers that differs from conventional health care delivery. Their focus on health maintenance applies to psychiatric concerns as well as somatic concerns. An operational flight surgeon must deal with the mental aspects of aviators' health when deciding who is qualified for flight training. The physician must assess the adequacy of psychologic defenses against anxiety about the natural dangers of flying and must decide when to ground and when to restore to flying duties. Much of our information in this field derives from military sources and is worth reviewing.

Specific mental health factors were not considered in the earliest pilot selection standards. A directive from the Surgeon General of the United States Army in 1912 did not mention psychiatric matters at all, although it did call for the rejection of any applicant with such psychophysiologic afflictions as chronic digestive disturb-ances, constipation, or "intestinal disorders tending to produce dizziness, headache, or to impair his vision." The United States Naval letter issued later that year echoed these prohibitions, adding that "any candidate whose condition shows that he is inclined to any excess that may disturb his mental balance or to alcoholism should be rejected."[1]

Flight surgeons quickly recognized the importance of psychologic influences on a flyer's performance. One of the first textbooks of aviation medicine contained nine chapters. Two, entitled "The Psychology of Aviation" and "The Aero-Neuroses," were devoted to mental and emotional matters.[2] "The Aero-Neuroses" dealt with the problem that we now call "fear of flying," which the author ascribed either to the strain of learning to fly or to involvement in an aircraft accident. "Nervous breakdowns have been noted since the early days of flying," he wrote, 15 years after the Wright brothers first flew. "In fact, they may be classed as an occupational neurosis [in] a comparatively new occupation, namely: flying."

Aircraft have come far, but flyers enclosed in titanium alloy are much the same as those borne on wings of fabric. Aeromedical practitioners understand the need for selection criteria that consider motivation as well as ability. Flyers are sought who are not merely sound of mind but who also have coping skills suited to the particular stresses and dangers of flight. It is known that adults are not unchanging in their adaptation to the stresses of life but that time and experience will alter their methods of responding to such stresses. Thus, the understanding of the psychologic makeup of the successful aviator must include considerations of personality style, motivation to fly, ability to fly, and adult personality growth patterns.

Once selected and trained, the flyer faces not only the stresses of aviation but also the normal stresses of everyday life. Wings on the chest do not protect against acute stress reactions, psychophysiologic disorders, or depression. The skilled physician must be prepared to recognize a variety of psychopathologic disorders and to make the required judgments about when to fly and when to ground. Psychiatric treatment may exceed the capabilities of many aeromedical physicians, just as may ophthalmologic or orthopedic treatment, but few mental health professionals can judge as well as the personal aeromedical practitioner when an aviator is ready to return to unrestricted flying duties.

Aeromedical practitioners in civilian practice face particular challenges in regard to mental health. Unlike their military counterparts, who function within a unitary health care system, civilian physicans may not have easy access to complete medical records. Psychiatric or stress symptoms occurring in flying or nonflying job environments may not easily be brought to the physician's attention by su-

pervisors or colleagues. The many informal contacts and even the opportunity to care for the flyers' families may not be practical or possible. Thus, civilian practitioners must develop a sharp clinical instinct for indirect and nonverbal clues to disorders arising from stress or from psychiatric symptoms, especially those with clear aeromedical implications.

This chapter will discuss the psychiatric aspects of aerospace medicine, the aeromedical aspects of psychiatry, and the neurologic function of the aviator.

PROFILE OF THE AVIATOR

Everyone knows what a military pilot is like: steely eyed, granite-jawed, an overgrown adolescent who can party till 4 A.M., slip into a clean uniform, and show up at 6 A.M. ready to "kick the tires, light the fires, brief on Guard, and the first one in the air gets the lead!" A stereotype about the personalities of aviators exists, to say the least, but flyers are quite diversified. Some, for example, are women. Still, something is distinctive in the way a successful aviator deals with life, an intangible factor that the experienced flight surgeon recognizes. Civilian pilots are even more diverse, yet have an essential sameness about them. Acknowledging the difficulty of capturing this essence in words, we will discuss some aspects of the "normal" aviator.

Personality

Personality describes the ways that people interact with situations and other people. These adaptations are generally developed by midadolescence and tend to change slowly, if at all, through the years. For example, the neat and careful teenager is likely to be neat and careful all his life.

It is likely that no occupation has attracted as many studies of its participants as has flying. Beaven[1] mentioned control of the imagination, confidence, patience, and especially a strong motivation to fly as important characteristics of successful aviators during World War I. Christy described the balance necessary between various factors such as rigidity and flexibility.[3] In other words, the flyer should be careful about such things as necessary checklists but also should be able to deal imaginatively with unforeseen situations or emergencies. As Christy pointed out, a good pilot who is mature, well motivated, and self-confident would probably succeed in any chosen profession or undertaking.

Fine and Hartman[4] studied 50 successful military pilots in detail, using both psychiatric and psychologic data. They defined the "model military pilot," contrasting these characteristics with flyers known to have failed and with characteristics reported in astronauts (Table 17–1). A similar report refers to the typical United States Air Force aviator as possessing an above-average intelligence, a matter-of-fact view of life, and a preference for action over introspection in dealing with stress.[5] This latter finding is of particular importance because exaggeration of such a tendency may lead a pilot who is frustrated to act out those frustrations in inappropriate ways (drinking or impulsive physical action) rather than thinking the problem through in a deliberate manner.

A study of 105 superior jet pilots noted that these men had a particular self-confidence, desire for challenge and success, and strong identification with their fathers, many of whom were also military flyers. These energetic and optimistic men tended to be firstborn or eldest sons. They tended to make life choices on a consciously rational basis, being willing to take risks only when a consideration of the odds led to a high chance of a successful outcome. They were curious, restless, in-

Table 17–1. Adaptive Personality Traits in Flyers

Conditions for Expected Failure or Adaptation (Grounding or Patient Status)	Typical Adult Adjustment (Modal Military Pilot)	Conditions for Expected Superior Adaptation (the Test Pilot or Astronaut)
Failure to succeed at a goal	Alloplastic; self-sufficient; short-range goal	More ambitiousness with success
Restriction from flying; retirement	Achievement; novelty; responsibility	Opportunity for a life-style that synthesizes these needs
Ambiguous situations (particularly social); inconsistency of background with current task	Terse; direct; non-intellectual; emotionally avoidant	Exceptional consistency of background and task
Less well endowed intellectually or physically	Bright-normal intelligence; perceptual, motor skills, courage, and energy	Outstanding endowment; better social or economic conditions while growing up
Physical illness; instability of background while growing up; neurotic predisposition	Excellent physical health; lack of neurotic symptoms	Freedom from neurotic conflict
Insoluble personality conflict at work	Unconflicted relationships with men	Work with teams of similar job-oriented men
Too much emotional stimulation; failure in family stability	Anxiety when too close to women	Marriage to self-contained women; good family functioning; easily explained absences from home
Unavoidable confrontation with inner emotional life	Relative inflexibility for drive reduction	Better capacity for emotional introspection
Irresponsibility or lack of social sanctions for hostility	Well-controlled unconscious hostility; tendency to act out	A nonhostile but aggressive assignment
Exceptionally strong limitations	Self-image; creative; intellectual limitations	Advanced education; a broader range of interests
Unavoidable confrontation with self-limitations	Low tolerance for personal imperfections	Much recognition and approval, for lifelong success

Adapted from Fine, P.M., and Hartman, B.O.: Psychiatric Strengths and Weaknesses of Typical Air Force Pilots. USAFSAM Technical Report 68-121. United States Air Force School of Aerospace Medicine, Brooks Air Force Base, Texas, 1968, pp. 131–168.

volved in many projects, and had high energy levels. They made friendships easily, but these relationships were rarely deep or intense. They preferred not to be dependent on other people but to keep interpersonal distance.[6]

The new flight surgeon will quickly begin to realize the diversity of personalities represented among successful pilots. Nevertheless, an appreciation of their similarities will begin to emerge. With experience, a flight surgeon will be able to feel whether a given individual thinks and acts like a flyer, a clinical instinct that is particularly valuable in assessing applicants for flight training. This perception is especially true in the case of military aviators, upon whom most of the data in the literature is based.

Motivation

Successful flyers have been identified as intelligent, energetic, competent, action-oriented men and women whose obsessive-compulsive personality style is usually flexible enough to adapt to novel situations. What motivates such a person to fly?

Motivation is the psychic force or energy that moves a person to satisfy a yearning or to attain a goal. Although the distinction may be a bit artificial, it is useful to consider these two aspects of motivation as the emotional component and the cognitive component.

Emotional Component

Most studies of the emotional aspects of flying motivation have been carried out in the context of the treatment of fear of flying. Bond[7] worked with fliers of the Eighth Air Force in World War II and noted that his patients' flying careers seemed to be based on deep-seated aggressive urges, with the aircraft perceived as a symbol of power that became an extension of the self. Indeed, pilots speak of feeling as if "the plane is a part of me" when describing the point at which flying

becomes a natural action. As with riding a bicycle, this unity, once achieved, is never lost. Pilots who return to the cockpit after a 10-year absence find that their hands "remember" what to do.

Human infants, like the young of other mammals, are born with an instinctive fear of falling. Children overcome this fear through life experiences such as learning to walk, playing on swings, or climbing trees and by engaging in other activities that increase their confidence in their ability to control their environment. A child's pleasure in mastering his body and environment may extend into powerful fantasies of flying, which is perceived as the ultimate freedom and mastery. Mythical figures from Apollo to Peter Pan to Superman have had the power of flight. Modern children learn at a young age that this power is available to them through the airplane. In their classic book, *Men Under Stress*, Grinker and Spiegel[8] describe "this super toy, this powerful, snorting but impatient machine" that enables a human to escape the usual limitations of time and space. Those who interview prospective student pilots frequently hear, "I've wanted to fly for as long as I can remember," that is, since before 5 years of age. Such an expression of a lifelong dream of flying signals a strong, deep-seated, and emotional attraction to flight.

An unhealthy or neurotic motivation to fly may have equally deep roots. A need to compete with or to overcome symbolically a father figure through such an aggressive activity carries with it the unconscious risk of danger should the effort succeed: such individuals may become increasingly anxious as they move toward the attainment of their goal. Others may have a neurotic need to prove themselves by undertaking dangerous activities. Such unhealthy motivational roots should be considered during the selection process and will be discussed further in the section on examination.

Cognitive Component

In contrast to those who have wanted to fly all their lives, many applicants express their interest in less emotional and more practical terms, such as, "As long as I was coming into the Air Force through ROTC (Reserve Officer's Training Corps), I thought I might as well try to be a pilot, since they get promoted faster." Frequently, the genesis of interest in such people is the result of conscious, logical decisions made in mid- or late adolescence, when career choices are considered. A career in aviation offers concrete rewards: the pay is good, the working conditions are reasonably pleasant, prestige is attached to such a career, and one certainly travels. In the military, the flyer has distinct career advantages over the non-flyers. Such realistic elements are a definite consideration and must not be ignored in a search for purely subconscious factors.

For example, some men applied for Unites States Air Force ROTC in the early 1970s to avoid being drafted from college into the Army and then applied for flying training to enhance their careers in the Air Force. Although this primary motivation to fly was purely cognitive, some of these men have decided to stay in the Air Force until retirement and have had wholly successful flying careers.

Ability

Along with motivation, the other neuropsychologic characteristic of a good pilot is the ability to handle aircraft. This ability requires a central nervous system free of significant injury or disease. Flying today is a complex activity and requires at least normal intelligence. In fact, United States Air Force flying personnel have intelligence quotients that average 123. Intelligence alone is not enough, however; the aviators also must possess good manual dexterity, a finely tuned organization of perceptual inputs, the ability to attend to important stimuli selectively and to tune out those judged to be extraneous, and the ability to reason quickly and clearly, especially when under acute stress.[9] Much research effort has been put into the development of psychologic tests that will measure these abilities, research which continues to this day. In general, the tests of ability will have been given to the candidate for military aviation before he ever sees the flight surgeon, and those individuals who fail these tests already will have been eliminated for further consideration. No such tests are given the civilian applicant, and it is left to the instructor pilot to weed out those who are so clumsy, inflexible, or ruminative in their responses to the sudden demands of aircraft control that they are unable to adapt to the novel situations that confront them. The application of flying skills must be flexible, rapid, decisive, and correct; nothing less will do.

Normal Adult Growth Patterns

Once selected and trained, flyers' attitudes toward flying may change. Young aviators generally have a total preoccupation with their newfound skills. No matter what the original topic of their conversation, it ends with flying. Any lingering fears generally have been overcome by the sheer delight of mastery of the sky. Youthful enthusiasm, along with a denial of the very real dangers, leads to a period when the new pilot may be dangerous because of inexperience and a failure to recognize all of the hazards that may occur. With time, however, comes experience. New factors also may intervene. Young pilots may be married by their late 20s and may have children. Responsibilities grow, and other interests compete with aviation for the flyer's attention and energy. Some fellow aviators have been killed in crashes, and every pilot has had a close call or two. The truth of the adage "there are old pilots, and there are bold pilots, but there are no old bold pilots" becomes clear.

During his 30s, a flyer generally becomes increasingly conservative, priding himself on his professional approach to flying. Physical health is generally good; a strong background of experience has developed, and the more cautious approach to the demands of the aircraft shows that youthful recklessness has been left behind. As time passes, other interests—career, promotion, family, preparation for years to be spent in areas not involving flying—may surpass the once all-consuming interest in flying. Should physical illness cause grounding, aviators in their mid-40s and beyond may greet the news with less disappointment than would their younger colleagues.

EXAMINATION TECHNIQUES

We have noted already that the psychologic aspects of the selection of prospective student pilots generally involve matters of innate ability or motivation. Tests assessing the ability to learn to fly usually are not considered a part of the medical examination, except in the unusual instances where the inability is due to a neuropsychologic deficit such as dyslexia. Flight surgeons are, however, charged with the responsibility for assessing the quality of the motivation of the would-be pilot. Because all of the information in the literature and almost all of the clinical experience is with male military applicants, this section will deal mainly with their assessment. Similar data on applicants for civilian training and on female applicants are almost nonexistent.

That part of the Federal Aviation Administration (FAA) regulations that deals with psychiatric standards makes no reference to the motivation to fly but addresses only psychopathologic conditions and alterations of consciousness. This approach is generally appropriate because a civilian pilot may stop flying whenever motivation or interest wanes. The aeromedical examiner should be alert to evidence of a desire to fly arising from

pathologic roots, however, such as counterphobic urges, which might lead to dangerous flying habits. These tendencies will be identified here.

The military requires a more detailed evaluation of psychologic factors. In each branch of the service, the appropriate regulation requires a psychiatric-style interview to evaluate the applicant's emotional stability and to assess motivation. This evaluation is in addition to any inquiry concerning significant psychopathologic conditions and requires the examiner to make an affirmative statement about the applicant and not just to assure that nothing negative is present. The United States Navy refers to this as the psychiatric examination. The United States Army and Air Force label this specialized interview the Adaptability Rating for Military Aeronautics (ARMA).

Interview Techniques

Everyone who flies has to deal with an initial fear. Flying is qualitatively different from other forms of transportation in that man is instinctively apprehensive about it. A real danger is involved. Military flying is more dangerous than civilian flying. Fighters are more dangerous than transports. Night flying is more dangerous than day flying. Flying in combat introduces even more dangers. One might reasonably assume that the basic, healthy way to deal with such fears is not to volunteer to fly in the first place. The aeromedical examiner, therefore, must find out how the applicant deals with the realities of the dangers of flight.

First, the examiner must identify those applicants with frank psychopathologic conditions. Table 17–2 compares briefly the psychiatric standards of the FAA and the three military services. One should note that the services add flying standards to the basic standards already applied to all those seeking entry into the service. These basic standards seek to eliminate all

Table 17–2. A Comparison of Military and Civilian Psychiatric Standards

Psychologic Factor	United States Army	United States Navy	United States Air Force	Federal Aviation Administration
Psychosis	+*	+	+	+
Personality disorder	+	+	+	+
Specific symptoms†	+	+	+‡	0
Substance abuse	+	+	+	+
Psychotropic medications	0	0	0	+
Adjustment reactions	+	0	+	0
Examiner's judgment	+	+	+	+
Fear of flying§	+	0	+	0

*+ means a disqualifying finding.
†Includes enuresis, somnambulism, nightmares, severe insomnia, tics, habit spasms, stammering, or psychogenic amnesia.
‡Original examination only; thereafter, a reason for administrative grounding unless a symptom of a psychiatric disease is present.
§Administrative action taken unless the fear is a part of psychiatric disease.

applicants with significant psychiatric disease.

Many of the additional flying standards may not appear at first glance to have any direct bearing on an individual's fitness to fly. For example, enuresis or somnambulism would not intrinsically affect a pilot who is presumably awake in the cockpit. One of these symptoms, however, may herald a significant personality disorder or may be the only evidence of an unsuspected seizure disorder. Similarly, prolonged nervous tics (nail-biting, hair-eating, or habitual grimacing) may lead the astute examiner to discover a history of significant psychopathology. Few would argue against the significance of such findings.

The assessment of motivation, however, requires different clinical skills, those of directive and nondirective interviewing. These skills cannot be taught in a textbook but must be learned in contacts with real patients or applicants, preferably under supervision. The art is one of gently helping an applicant who is by nature action-oriented to discuss feelings and fears. At times, direct questions are in order: "Was there anyone in your life who was as interested in flying as you are?" At other times, indirect methods apply: the understanding nod that elicits more detail, the timely "Can you tell me more about that?"

A good source for further discussion of these methods is the section on interview techniques in *The Psychiatric Interview in Clinical Practice*.[10]

Early flight surgeons gave rigidly structured interviews, seeking the answers to 40 or so specific questions. Modern techniques call for a more flexible approach, allowing the examiner to follow promising leads. At a minimum, the flight surgeon should allow 30 minutes to talk with the applicant about his interest in flying and how it came about.

One might begin by putting the candidate at ease in the office; asking how he became interested in flying is a good opener. Has he flown? Do other family members fly? Has he had flying lessons? Is he in the Civil Air Patrol? How did he like flying? Have there been any problems such as airsickness? If so, did it continue? (If it continued past three or four flights, one might inquire into other forms of motion sickness.) Now one may ask a more open-ended question: "What do you think it will be like to fly in the Air Force?" See if the answer is reasonable and the expectations realistic. What experience does he draw on for this? How does he feel about the dangers of flying? Again, is the answer reasonable? What do his parents or wife think of the danger of flight? What about combat flight?

If the examiner challenges the pilot applicant about the dangers of flying, the answer may be a mixture of rationalization and denial, sometimes including fantasy. Such answers might be, "you can get killed just crossing the street," or "you can always bail out if things get bad," or even "I never really think about it very much." Occasionally, one encounters an answer that may project anxieties about flying onto other people such as, "I know it worries my mother, but she never says anything about it to me." Because the mother is not available to interview, the examiner is left to decide whether the anxieties really belong to the mother or to the applicant.

From this point, the examiner may easily ask about the candidate's family background. Be alert to his father's expectations: it is common to find a son—especially an eldest son—whose flying is in response to his father's desires, especially if the father is an active or retired military flyer. This motivation is not necessarily bad, but one should look carefully to see whether the applicant is truly interested in flying or merely reflecting the father's desires. A good question to ask is, "What will you do if you get turned down for flight training?" One young man, the son of an Air Force colonel, relaxed, smiled broadly, and told the examiner with great animation about his real interest, music. Past history can then be gone over lightly. Examine past interests, achievements, and tendencies toward activity or passivity. Did he follow through on things or quit easily? Did he work after school? How did he socialize? Was family discipline strict, loving, or lax? What sort of trouble did he get into? What were his achievements?

While talking, watch the candidate. How is his social poise? Every candidate may be a little tense, but most candidates should loosen up fairly quickly: everyone likes to talk about himself. One study of the ARMA found only two specific cor-

relations of the interview with later flying ability: past history of positive achievements and social poise during the interview.[11] Be alert for nervous habits that emerge in the stress of the interview: scratching, wiggling around, tics, speech disturbances, blushing, poor eye contact, or mumbling.

As a subjective cue, one should attempt to see this youngster in a flight suit down at the squadron. Does he look and talk like a pilot? Operational flight surgeons get to know many successful pilot's backgrounds and have a clear picture of their personalities. The applicant should remind the flight surgeon of known successful flyers.

The astute examiner is aware of his reactions to the applicant: such perceptions can help to categorize the applicant. One should be careful of identifying with him ("how could I disappoint such a nice fellow?"). It may be the dependency needs of the applicant that elicit such protective feelings. Similarly, one should not disqualify an applicant who is somewhat negative about the examination if it really represents independence on his part. In moderation, this is an asset for a pilot, a quality with which every flight surgeon is familiar.

Formal Testing

Some formal psychomotor testing is done as a part of the selection process for student military aviators, but it is done separately from the medical examination, and the results are not easily available to the flight surgeon. One may generally suppose that the examinee's presence in the office is evidence of passing this portion of the evaluation process. This testing does not include clinical psychologic tests; these will be administered only if the flight surgeon requests them as a part of a further mental health examination that is obtained for clinical reasons.

A word of caution is in order about the clinical interpretation of such tests. Psychologic tests are standardized against the general public and are generally reported in terms of the presence or absence of overt psychopathologic conditions. The norms used at the United States Air Force School of Aerospace Medicine (USAFSAM) for successful pilots are sometimes significantly different from those of the rest of the population. For example, "average" intelligence is defined as being between 90 and 110 on common intelligence quotient tests. United States Air Force flyers average about 123 because of the selection process that chooses them. Pilots generally score higher on the 4 (psychopathic) and 9 (manic) scales of the Minnesota Multiphasic Personality Inventory than do average nonflyers. This score reflects their high energy level, independence, and tendency to use action to reduce stress. The clinician with questions about the interpretation of such results may wish to consult a mental health professional who is specifically familiar with the application of the results in a flying population.

Civilian applicants for flight training receive no such screening on routine examinations. The examiner dealing with such applicants should be particularly attuned to evidence of marginal psychiatric or neuropsychologic functioning (dyslexia or subtle choreoathetosis, for example) that may interfere with safe flying.

Referral for Specialist Evaluation

When the examiner is in doubt about the mental health or capabilities of an applicant, consultation is in order. The application of specific test norms to pilots has already been discussed. Similar considerations apply to requests for psychiatric evaluation. Generally, psychiatrists are concerned with the detection and diagnosis of frank psychopathologic conditions. Aeromedical practitioners must carefully explain requests to assess such matters as the health of the candidate's motivation to fly or to evaluate an applicant with such symptoms as persistent

somnambulism for underlying psychiatric disorders. Not all mental health professionals are fully aware of the purposes and parameters of flight physical examinations, and the wise aeromedical examiner will take the time and make the effort necessary to ensure that the consultant understands the purpose of the consultation. Even in the military, the consultant may answer with a rather brief note indicating only freedom from gross disease without addressing the health of the genesis of the applicant's desire to fly or the question of significant symptoms of anxiety.

A complete consultation should reflect a clear understanding of the reason why the consultation was requested, a statement about the development of the applicant's interest in flying (if this information was sought), a review of pertinent familial, developmental, and social factors, a mental status examination, a summary, a diagnosis (if applicable), and pertinent comments concerning disposition and recommendations. The mental status examination is the mental health equivalent of a physical examination and should include comments about the applicant's appearance and behavior, speech, mood, emotional tone (affect), intellectual function, sensorium (clarity of mental processes: memory, concentration, calculations, reasoning ability, and capacity for abstract thought), and thought content and processes (associative processes, morbid preoccupations, freedom from hallucinations or delusions, and adequate judgment and insight). Such a complete evaluation and report is particularly necessary if the examination must be sent forward to a higher military or civil agency for approval.

CLINICAL CONDITIONS OF CONCERN

Fear of Flying

Fear of flying is a term coined during World War II that originally referred to the mixtures of fear and anxiety seen in the combat theaters. In the United States Air Force today, the term fear of flying connotes unreasonable fear or anxiety that develops in trained aviators who are free of other emotional symptoms. Thus, fear of flying is a symptom and not a disease.

Fear, the emotion that we feel in the face of a real and immediate danger, is the emotional equivalent of pain. Both fear and pain warn us to withdraw from danger: fear at the instinctive level and pain at the somatic reflex level. A conscious act of will can overcome both fear and pain, at least for a while. For example, an individual may be fearful about his first dive off the high board, and yet he conquers this fear and dives, discovering that the danger is not as real as he thought it was. Most individuals also can learn to control their reaction to the pain of an injection and tolerate needles in their flesh with some degree of equanimity.

The primitive fear of falling has been overcome in most, if not all, military aviators. The initial physical examination and its accompanying inquiry into the prospective pilot's perceptions of the dangers of flying have, it is hoped, eliminated those with pathologic or inadequate defenses against these dangers. Those remaining should react to this perception with the usual mix of denial, rationalization, and healthy fantasy.

Once flight training begins, the fantasies about flight become realities. A few student pilots may drop out of flight training because they cannot maintain their defenses against the dangers of flight that are now real and immediate. Their fear may take many forms: as an overt apprehension that interferes with the progress of training, as a disabling psychophysiologic symptom such as headache or airsickness, or as a rationalized self-initiated elimination in which the applicant simply declares that he was not cut out to be a pilot. In the United States Air Force, such fear openly expressed during flight training is grounds for disqualification under the

heading "manifestations of apprehension." This disqualification is handled in a nonpunitive manner, with the student pilot generally being disenrolled from training and reassigned to a nonflying position. Civilian student pilots, of course, may merely stop their lessons.

Once the flyer completes flying training, it is assumed that he has successfully adapted to flying and has demonstrated healthy, mature defenses against whatever instinctive or primitive anxieties may be aroused by flying. From this point on, the United States Air Force handles openly expressed fear of flying in a different manner. An aviator who admits to disabling anxiety about flying is evaluated for any psychiatric disease. If none is found, he is declared physically and mentally fit to fly and then must meet an administrative flying evaluation board for disposition. This disposition may be as mild as reassignment to a nonflying job or as severe as a recommendation for dismissal from the service. A previously well-adapted aviator who becomes fearful thus has an additional conflict to face that arises from the knowledge that the Air Force may take punitive administrative action if his fears are openly admitted. In addition, organizational pressure and peer pressure may be exerted on such a flyer to continue flying and to overcome the fears by himself.

United States Army flight surgeons handle aviators who become fearful about flying in much the same way. The United States Navy takes a somewhat different approach. Such flyers may be evaluated at the Naval Aviation Medicine Institute at Pensacola, Florida. If no overt mental illness is detected and if the aviator affirms his fear of flying and is not amenable to treatment, he is designated physically qualified but not aeronautically adapted. Thus identified, he is reassigned to nonflying duties.

The flight surgeon may be caught in the middle between an aviator who wants to stop flying and the organization that requires him to continue. The briefly worded regulation is clear and apparently inflexible, reducing fear of flying to a single decision: is the disposition to be medical or administrative? In fact, the circumstances of various flying situations and the complexities of human emotions and behavior interact so that every case of fear of flying seems unique to the flight surgeon who must deal with it. Perhaps the simplest instance would be the flyer who develops a pure phobia to flight, a straightforward medical diagnosis. This condition is distinguished by its free-floating, primitive anxiety, which is generally considered unreasonable, its symbolic nature, and its ego-dystonicity, the psychiatric term that means that the aviator dislikes the fear and wants to be rid of it.

An F-4 weapons systems operator became increasingly anxious about low-level flying, although he could do any other sort of flying without difficulty. His anxiety was heightened if the pilot were younger than he. He finally became so anxious that he found himself holding on to his ejection handle while flying low-level missions, at which point he reported to his flight surgeon. It became apparent that the anxiety about flying with a younger pilot symbolized his need to perceive the pilot as a father figure, which was not possible when the pilot was younger than he. His symptoms were ego-dystonic in that he hated this feeling of fear and wanted to be rid of it so that he could enjoy his flying. Such phobias can be treated by behavioral means such as systematic desensitization, in which the flyer first learns to relax on cue and then is exposed to progressively closer contact with the feared situation within a brief period. Such a flyer, once cured of his phobia, may be given a waiver and returned to full flying duties, as happened in this instance.

Other aviators may become acutely fearful after a brush with death or the loss of a friend in an aircraft accident. In such situations, some flyers may be returned to flying by an aeromedical practitioner who uses a crisis intervention approach, giving the aviator a chance to express his feelings of anger, sadness, and guilt openly in an accepting environment, mutually exploring the realities of the situation, and helping the flyer to rethink the decision to fly

or not to fly. It is our impression, although we have no hard data, that the success or the failure of the flight surgeon or therapist in this situation may depend on the strength of the flyer's subconscious motivation and whether it originated in an early, primitive joy of mastery or arose from a later, less emotional, and more cognitive decision that "flying looks like a good career." Certainly, other current stressful factors, such as family or work problems, may contribute to the feeling of apprehension about flight. If these factors can be identified and successfully dealt with, the situational anxiety may subside and the flyer will return to the cockpit.

One is most likely to be able to help such a flyer conquer his anxieties and return to flying if he sees this as a desirable outcome. One may form a therapeutic alliance with a fearful flyer who wants to be rid of the fears but not with a fearful flyer who does not want to be helped. The physician should help the flyer find out what is wrong and explore all possible solutions. Insisting that the aviator work toward a return to flying duties puts one in an adversary position and is likely to fail. If the flyer agrees that the fear is a problem that needs exploration, examining that fear and looking for possible solutions is an acceptable therapeutic goal. Once this is done, the question of whether the aviator should fly again may be considered. If the flyer is not interested in exploring the symptom, however, and if there is no mental or physical disease present that would be disqualifying, one may only return the flyer to the squadron as physically and mentally fit to fly, with a recommendation for appropriate administrative action. This problem seems to be unique to military flying because civilian aviators may simply quit whenever they wish.

Some of the most difficult situations arise when the anxieties manifest themselves, not as a conscious fear of flying, but as psychosomatic symptoms. In such instances, the aviator will ask for help with the symptoms that prevent him from flying. He will not have any anxiety about flying itself but will discuss the symptoms mainly in terms of their preventing him from flying. Of course he wants to fly, he says, but these headaches (or abdominal pains or low back pains) bother him so much in flight that he is just not safe. Most aeromedical practitioners take a purely somatic approach at first, ruling out specific illnesses. Finding no physical explanation for the symptoms, the physician may then begin to consider that anxiety about flying is the basis for the problem. Three observations may help to identify this unconscious anxiety. First, the flyer will tend to describe the symptoms in terms of their effects on his flying. The experienced flight surgeon will quickly notice the difference in emphasis from that of the usual flyer, who tends to minimize this aspect of his illnesses. There is a clear difference between a flyer who comes in complaining about his backache and a flyer who comes in repeatedly complaining that his backache is so severe that he won't be able to fly today. Second, the aviator may express no particular anxiety about the possible illness causing the symptoms. One pilot expressed it: "I only worry about having the headaches when I'm flying." He was not concerned that his severe headaches might signal some underlying illness. Third, one may ask such a flyer, "Will you fly if (or "when," to be more positive) we get rid of your headaches?" The unconflicted flyer, without hesitation, will respond in the affirmative. The aviator who is conflicted about flying will pause, or equivocate, or otherwise signal reluctance, either verbally or nonverbally. When this question was put to the pilot with headaches, he paused, and finally answered "yes" in a very unenthusiastic tone. When told that he did not look very happy about this, he replied that he was not, repeating that he was worried about the effect of headaches on his flying. Although the flight surgeon may be sure that there is a basic anxiety about flying in such instances, the flyer is not conscious of it and will deny it. A medical disqualification based on the symptoms may be the most suitable disposition in refractory cases.

Fear of flying may present a somewhat different problem among nonmilitary professional flyers. It is generally regarded as basically a medical problem and may even be grounds for disability retirement action if it is severe enough and is not responsive to psychotherapeutic intervention. Although an individual presenting with fear of flying may have symptoms that are basically those of anxiety, one must not overlook the role of some secondary gain factor in intensifying the symptoms or in complicating the therapeutic process. Financial recompense and the chance to move from flying into fields of endeavor perceived as more attractive may be powerful gain factors, both in the military and in civilian life.

No problem in aviation medicine is more difficult to deal with than fear of flying. The flight surgeon who can deal with it gracefully is indeed a master of the art.

Adjustment Disorders

An operational aeromedical practitioner will probably see more adjustment disorders (stress reactions) than any other sort of mental health-related condition. These disorders vary considerably in the mode of presentation and in intensity and may occur in response to any sort of life stress. An event that one person accepts with equanimity may be dreadfully upsetting to another, the difference depending on the adequacy of coping mechanisms and particular vulnerabilities. Clearly, adjustment disorders may affect any sort of flyer: civilian, commercial, or military.

The third edition of the Diagnostic and Statistical Manual of Mental Disorders (DSM-III) defines an adjustment disorder as " a maladaptive reaction to an identifiable psychosocial stressor." By strict definition, such a disorder should be a departure from the individual's usual response to life stresses. The reaction occurs within 3 months of the stress and results in either social or occupational impairment or in symptoms beyond those ordinarily seen in such situations. Stressors may, of course, occur in groups ("a run of bad luck") or may be recurrent.

Adjustment disorders may take several forms. Depressive symptoms may predominate in one form, symptoms of anxiety in another. Some individuals, especially the young or the immature, may act out their distress by abusing alcohol, fighting, reckless driving, or flying violations. Others may become withdrawn. Obviously, some individuals may show a mixture of these symptoms.

Depressive symptoms may include disturbances in sleeping patterns or appetite. Self-esteem may be diminished, and the flyer may report feeling "down" or "blue." Inquiry will usually reveal a lack of energy or initiative, a loss of usual sexual interest, and perhaps an increase in minor physical complaints. Feelings of guilt (justified or unjustified), irritability, pessimism, or helplessness also may be revealed. One should always inquire after suicidal ideas or equivalent thinking ("I'd just like to chuck it all in," or "I'd like to get in my car and drive away—I don't care where").

Symptoms of anxiety are somewhat different. The flyer may report feeling uneasy or fearful, with no clear idea why this should be so. Autonomic symptoms may predominate: pounding heart, air hunger, dry mouth, digestive upset, tremulousness, a lump in the throat. In some instances, there may be attacks of real dread, as though an indefinable but fearful "something" were about to happen. These panic attacks may be so intense as to be disabling.

Some aviators are particularly apt to react to stress with inappropriate actions. Alcohol abuse is likely to be involved: "I was so upset I just went out and got loaded." Most of us are familiar with the person who acts out his emotions behind the wheel of an automobile. The alert clinician will listen carefully to aviators who report that a fellow flyer is flying poorly—taking chances, not as sharp, not up to his usual standards. Knowledge of a recent life stress in such instances should lead to an interview with the flyer involved, either in a formal medical setting or informally. The flyer who takes out his feelings on his aircraft is an accident looking for a place to happen!

Management of adjustment disorders is fairly simple in some instances, but the help of a mental health professional may be needed in other situations. An accurate review of recent life events usually will uncover the stressor: family disruption, job stress, financial reversal, sexual complaint, or other recent change. Once the stressor is acknowledged, the physician may explore the flyer's reaction to it, explaining the connection with the symptoms if the flyer is not already aware of it. Stressful life experiences occur to everyone; the ways one copes with stressful situations determine if the outcome is adaptive or maladaptive.

Some aeromedical physicians will feel comfortable exploring with the flyer the means used to cope with the crisis, explaining what is happening and strengthening healthy coping mechanisms. A nonjudgmental and sympathetic listener who encourages the patient to express his feelings, is reassuring, provides explanations, and give realistic advice may be all that is necessary in some of the milder cases. Grounding the flyer may be in order, especially if the symptoms are distracting. Medications should be used sparingly, if at all, and should be directed at clear target symptoms for a brief time only. The use of the benzodiazepines (Valium or Librium) for depressive symptoms should be strictly avoided because these antianxiety agents make depressions worse. If a flyer's situational reaction calls for medication, consultation with a psychiatrist is desirable.

Chronic or Delayed Stress Reactions

Post-traumatic stress disorders may be acute, beginning within 6 months of the trauma and lasting less than 6 months, chronic, lasting more than 6 months, or delayed, occurring more than 6 months after the trauma. The trauma is defined as an event that is psychologically damaging and is beyond the range of everyday human experiences. Such stressors include combat, natural or man-made disasters, rape, torture, or severe captivity or hostage experiences. The disorder evoked may include reliving the experience through flashbacks (brief dissociative states) or through nightmares. Emotional numbing may occur in response to real-world situations such as the inability to experience joy, pleasure, or intimacy. The individual may lose the ability to use concentration or memory fully, may have a hyperalert startle response, may feel guilty about surviving, or feel irrational anger at those who did not survive. Other reactions include irritability, insomnia, and difficulty in attending to the ordinary affairs of life. Symptoms may be intensified by exposure to events that are reminders of the trauma. Thus, survivors of an air disaster may become unbearably anxious when required to fly again. Conventional wisdom dictates that a person who has had a terrifying experience should face the circumstances of that experience again as quickly as possible to give the lie to the fantasy that the trauma will inevitably recur. One flyer who had escaped death in a crash by the merest of margins remarked after his next flight, "The thing I was most afraid of was that I'd be afraid. As soon as I took off and found that I wasn't afraid, I relaxed." This works in many instances but not in all. When such disorders do occur, they should be treated by mental health professionals.

Anniversary reactions are more common in flyers than in the population at large.[12] Marsh and Perry[13] reported anniversary phenomena in 11 of 360 carefully investigated aeromedical psychiatric consultation patients. Characteristically, the flyer will report symptoms of depression or anxiety with no clear-cut connection to recent life events. Careful inquiry into past history may yield a traumatic event occurring almost exactly 1, 2, 5, 10, or 20 years previously. Alternately, there may be a history of some tragic event—usually death—occurring to the same-sex parent or a parent-figure at the same age as the flyer's present age. At times, the event may be repressed, and the history is only elicited from another family member. Several times we have explained this concept to a flyer and asked him to check with other family members and had him return to report with some emotion that he didn't know why he forgot the death of this person who was so important to him. Such an emotional response almost certainly indicates psychologic paydirt: the traumatic event that is buried because it is too painful to bear, the emotion surfacing a year or more later as free-floating anxiety or depression. Deaths of friends in aircraft accidents may well be handled in this manner, repressed because they are too threatening. Usually, simple explanation and the chance for the patient to express his feelings will be sufficient treatment. Psychiatric consultation should be sought if symptoms persist.

Substance Abuse

Substance abuse is an exceedingly complex question and was discussed in Chapter 13, "Aircrew Health Care Maintenance." Aviators may abuse alcohol in response to stress, especially because it is somewhat sanctioned by others in the flying milieu. About one out of six civil aircraft accidents involves alcohol abuse. Pursch[14] has written humorously and realistically about the social situations that are used to excuse drinking: births, deaths, arrivals, departures, promotions, passovers, and so on. Alcohol abuse complicates many psychiatric conditions and must be carefully assessed in every situation.

As a general rule, we offer the following counsel. Nothing excuses alcohol abuse. It is maladaptive behavior that may quickly become an addicting disease. Alcoholics Anonymous (AA) has the best record in dealing with alcohol abuse. As the aviator participates in AA (or other rehabilitation activities), he must be put on notice that one slip will end his flying career. This rule must be enforced. Some individuals will not believe and will test the system. Their fate—certain and unmistakable dismissal—will let others know that the rules will be enforced. This procedure is the successful industrial approach: offer help and do not tolerate alcohol-degraded performances.

Drug abuse is simply not compatible with flying. More details are available regarding support to the airline captain in Chapter 25.

Personality Disorders

Personality disorders are particular traits or styles of interaction with others that are so marked, so maladaptive, or so lacking in flexibility that the individual suffers personal distress or is significantly impaired in social interactions or occupational functioning. This distress or impairment may begin in adolescence and will generally continue throughout the adult years, perhaps diminishing in late middle age. People with personality disorders are frequently regarded as eccentric, difficult to get along with, or merely unpleasant, without a diagnostic label being considered. The maladaptive features that mark the individual's relationships with others should be considered diagnostic of a true disorder when they are found to be typical of function in many areas of life over a period of years rather than being found only in circumscribed relationships or on a temporary basis.

These personality traits may be unpleasant to the individual, traits that he wishes to be rid of, or they may be regarded as adaptive and useful, even in the face of evidence to the contrary. Treatment is particularly difficult in this latter instance because the individual is comfortable with this method of relating to others and sees no reason to change. Such traits are called ego-syntonic. Traits regarded as undesirable by the individual are called ego-dystonic. It follows that a therapist has a better chance of forming a therapeutic alliance with an individual whose symptoms are ego-dystonic than with one whose symptoms are ego-syntonic and who generally will have been referred for treatment somewhat against his will.

Those personality disorders likely to be encountered in flyers will be discussed in the following sections. A fuller discussion may be found in any standard psychiatric text or in the DSM-III.

Paranoid Personality Disorder

The behavior of the individual with a paranoid personality disorder is marked by a thorough mistrust of others, a continuing and unjustified suspiciousness, and an unusual sensitivity to real or imagined slights. Suspicions are maintained even in the face of evidence that would convince an ordinary person that they were groundless. These people are alert for threats, tend to avoid blame for anything, and are regarded by those who know them as secretive, jealous, and thoroughly unpleasant. They argue, are always alert for the slightest insult, exaggerate disagreements, counterattack with vigor, are prone to legal action, and are quick to criticize but unable to accept criticism. They are uncompromising, hostile, stubborn, and do poorly in cooperative efforts. Such individuals are not psychotic; that is, they do not harbor underlying delusional systems nor do they have hallucinations. They may adapt very poorly to the enforced closeness of a military squadron. Such people are distinctly different from the usual aviator, who is more friendly, comfortable to converse with, and sociable. Treatment is extremely difficult because these individuals are threatened by the closeness necessary in a therapeutic relationship.

Narcissistic Personality Disorder

The person with a narcissistic personality disorder has an inappropriate sense of self-importance and a continuing need to be the center of attention. An unrealistic overestimation of personal abilities may occur, which is particularly dangerous in the flying environment. Ambitions and fantasies of achievement may be unrealistic and may be pursued with inappropriate energy and an insensitivity to the needs of others, who may be exploited and devalued. Thus, "the great one" expects others to smooth the way and to provide instant admiration while receiving nothing in return. Self-esteem, although overblown, is likely to be fragile under stress. A major failure, perceived or real, may lead to a significant depression that requires therapeutic intervention. Most successful flyers have narcissistic traits of independence, "cocky" self-assuredness, and a sense of being able to handle anything but not to the degree of arrogance and insensitivity displayed by people with a narcissistic personality disorder.

Antisocial Personality Disorder

Antisocial personality disorder has been known in the past as psychopathic or antisocial character and behavior disorder. Its onset in midadolescence heralds a lifetime of conflict with authority, lying, cheating, sexual promiscuity, and substance abuse. It is much more common in males and may arise in part from a chaotic childhood. Some evidence indicates that genetic influences also are important. A history of truancy, serious misbehavior in school, delinquency, fighting, lying, sexual misconduct, theft, vandalism, lack of responsible function as a parent, inability to work consistently, lack of acceptance of social norms, impulsivity, recklessness, or daring behavior should arouse the suspicion of the concerned flight surgeon. Such people may be superficially charming but are constantly in trouble. As flyers, their lack of dependable, predictable, and safe behavior, their impulsivity, their willingness to lie about anything, and their abuse of others make them poor risks to complete mission assignments safely. This condition is essentially untreatable.

Borderline Personality Disorder

As its name implies, the borderline personality disorder is difficult to diagnose because it represents instability in several areas, presenting different aspects at different times. The individual may vary between idealizing friendship and baseless rage, leading to shifting interpersonal conflicts. Moody and uncertain, such a person has difficulty with loneliness and boredom. Brief episodes of frank psychosis may occur. He lacks a firm sense of identity and has difficulty maintaining consistency in relationships with others. Suicidal gestures or irrational, self-mutilating actions may occur. Although such a person may be chosen for flight training, it is unlikely that he could maintain the consistent high level of performance and the close interactions with the instructors necessary to complete the training.

Compulsive Personality Disorder

Individuals with a compulsive personality disorder find it difficult to relate warmly to others. Their superficial perfectionism, expressed as careful planning, list-making, and scheduling, actually interferes with the accomplishment of tasks. Stubbornly insistent on "doing it my way," their moralistic dedication to their work excludes pleasure from leisure activities or cooperative relationships. Indecision is another indication; such people may be so afraid of making a mistake that they become immobilized by choices and are unable to establish realistic priorities. Like those with borderline personality disorders, these individuals are unlikely to succeed in the trying environment of flight training. Those who do succeed may have increasing difficulty in using compulsive behavior to control their anxiety, especially in the sometimes unpredictable world of the flier. Decompensation, if it occurs, may take the form of depression, phobias, or panic attacks.

Passive-Aggressive Personality Disorder

Individuals with passive-aggressive personality disorders express their resistance to the desires of others through covert opposition such as stubbornness, forgetfulness, chronic tardiness, poor work, inefficiency, or dawdling. Such behavior frequently elicits anger and frustration in associates, both in the occupational arena and in social settings. The frustrating behavior continues in spite of counseling, persuasion, or threats. Because it expresses hidden aggression, this behavior may be particularly disruptive in a group or organizational setting. In the flying environment, such a disorder might be expressed as a pattern of ineffective performance accompanied by lame excuses, grumbling, and obstructionism, with "the other guy" always blamed for the flyer's own shortcomings.

Psychophysiologic Disorders

Regardless of his specialty, every physician is aware of the influences that psychologic factors have on somatic diseases. Far from being "all in your head," these conditions may involve the body to a life-threatening degree. For example, peptic ulcers and asthmatic attacks may be lethal. Regional enteritis and ulcerative colitis are somatic conditions that are clearly affected by environmental stimuli mediated through emotions. Some patients affected by such ailments are aware of the connection between life stress and physical symptoms; other patients remain forever skeptical. Two psychosomatic complaints are of particular interest to the practicing flight surgeon: syncope and airsickness.

Syncope

Loss of consciousness in a flyer may have immediate and fatal consequences at worst. Because loss of consciousness is a neurologic event, the central nervous system must be carefully evaluated. The cause also may be of cardiac origin, such as an embolus or an arrhythmia. Less dangerous, at least from a general health point of view, are those losses of consciousness ascribed to an acute and self-limited loss of blood pressure, which are called vasovagal syncope, or "fainting." Psychologic factors also may be associated with low G tolerance.

Sledge and Boydstun[15] have reviewed the pertinent literature as it applies to aerospace medicine and have presented their own analysis of 24 patients seen at USAFSAM for vasovagal syncope. Upon investigating the life circumstances of these patients and comparing them with nonsyncopal controls, these authors found that those who had fainted reported considerably more difficulty in their work situation and less job satisfaction than those who had not fainted. Further, the events immediately preceding the faint almost always involved some sort of a threat, physical or social, against which the flyer felt unable to defend himself. Unable to fight or flee, the flyer becomes totally helpless by losing consciousness, thus, in a sense, giving up to the threat.

Classically, such events occur when the flyer is to have blood drawn, undergoes a minor surgical procedure such as electrodesiccation of a wart, or is required to see a motion picture about first aid. These circumstances are so commonplace that "fainting at the sight of blood" is a cliche. Tense social circumstances are not as commonly acknowledged but may be found in many instances of vasovagal syncope.

A high-ranking officer was entertaining an even

higher-ranking guest in his home. He had served oysters and had eaten one that he found was bad, too late to avoid swallowing it. Later, engaging his guest in a farewell conversation at the door, he felt nauseated. He did not want to excuse himself to vomit so near the end of the evening because his guest was only moments from leaving. Fighting back the nausea, he became weak and sweaty and fainted.

In this instance, the flyer felt bound by social amenities not to acknowledge his strong visceral urges but was helpless to stop them. A less-inhibited individual would have stated the truth of the matter and excused himself.

> A flyer was watching a training film on first aid when he became aware of strong defecatory urges. He fought them back because he was seated in the middle of the row and did not want to inconvenience everyone by crowding past to go to the bathroom. Finally, as the urges became stronger, he stood up to go to the bathroom and fainted. Later, he related that he had been upset by the sight of blood since the first time he saw his father castrating pigs. He had fainted twice before, each time in circumstances where he had felt the need to use the bathroom and was ashamed to admit it: once in class and once in the Air Force examination station where he had been told not to urinate until he got to the laboratory. This flyer had a strong sense of personal danger when confronted with blood. He also was extremely inhibited about his excretory functions. The combination of defecatory urges and of seeing blood was, for him, a uniquely intolerable threat.

In such cases, there is no immediate threat to flying safety as long as the flyer can take action when threatened. It is possible to teach flyers to avoid the feeling of powerlessness by showing them alternative behaviors. For example, such individuals may learn to demand to be allowed to lie down before blood is drawn. Simply knowing that they do not have to put themselves passively into the hands of the technician, but that they may retain power over the situation by controlling some aspect of it may be enough to alleviate the perceived threat.

Theoretically, such a flyer might be exposed to blood in the cockpit if a fellow flyer were struck by a bird coming through the windscreen or by shell fragments in a combat situation. This situation would pose no syncopal hazard because of the urgent need for corrective action in either circumstance. There would thus be no feeling of enforced passivity and no psychologic need to "leave the scene" through syncope. We have discussed with several syncope patients how they felt and reacted to real and bloody accidents; each time, the flyer was able to cope with the situation through action and did not faint.

Airsickness

Airsickness is a complex interdisciplinary subject, already discussed from the neurosensory point of view in Chapter 11. Psychologic elements clearly enter into instances in which the chronically airsick student aviator does not accommodate after continued exposure to flying. Some military student pilots become so conditioned by repeated airsickness that they are nauseated on the ground by the smell of jet fuel or the smell of the compounds used to clean their oxygen masks or even by the sight of the aircraft on the flight line. They become so anxious about the possibility of getting sick again and washing out of flight training that this anxiety itself contributes to their airsickness. This sort of anxiety also may affect civilian student pilots.

Several treatments are available to airsick student pilots. Two medication combinations may be tried: dextroamphetamine, 5 mg, and scopolamine, 0.5 mg, orally 1 hour before flight or promethazine hydrochloride (Phenergan), 25 mg, and ephedrine, 25 mg, orally 1 hour before flight. It is wise to try the first dose on the ground to guard against any idiosyncratic reaction that might pose a danger in the air. These combinations must be used only when the student pilot is accompanied by an instructor pilot. If one of the combination of medications effectively controls the symptoms, the student flyer may be able to accommodate to the novel and conflicting sensory inputs of flight after six or so flights and will then no longer need the medication.

A recent addition to the therapeutic possibilities is the behind-the-ear disk of 0.2 mg of scopolamine (Transderm-V), which leaks into the circulation over 3 days, possibly furnishing protection against motion sickness. It is reported to produce fewer side effects and to be about as effective as oral medication. This treatment has not been systematically tested in military fliers as of this writing.

USAFSAM has been testing a biofeedback-mediated behavioral modification procedure for selected, highly motivated flyers with chronic airsickness. This intense course of therapy is given 2 hours per day for 2 weeks. The flyers are given cross-coupled biaxial Coriolis stimulation by a revolving, tilting chair while electronically monitoring surface skin temperature and sweat rate. In lay terms, they are taught to remain warm and dry instead of becoming cold and clammy. When first reported, the technique had been successful in returning 16 of 19 airsick aviators (84%) to duty.[16] At present, 39 of 51 such flyers (76%) are successfully flying again. The disadvantages to this experimental technique are the special equipment required and its time-intensive nature. When further developed, it may become more widely available. Similar work by Cowings and associates[17] suggests the possible application of this technique to avoid the space sickness encountered by many astronauts during prolonged weightlessness.

Anxiety Disorders

Approximately 2 to 4% of the general population suffers from a clinically significant anxiety disorder at some time. This group of disorders includes anxiety either as the primary symptom or as a feeling experienced in specific situations. In the older literature, these disorders are referred to as neuroses or neurotic reactions. Phobic disorders, anxiety states, obses-sive-compulsive disorders, and stress disorders are included in this category.

Phobic Disorders

Phobic disorders are characterized by primitive anxiety experienced as fear of a situation or object. This feeling is recognized by the person as excessive or irrational, and it is ego-dystonic (i.e., he would like to be rid of it). These elements were discussed in the earlier section entitled "Fear of Flying." One such condition is agoraphobia, the fear of being alone or in public places where a panic attack or other incapacitation might leave one helpless. This fear usually results in increasingly restricted activities. Another condition is social phobia, a fear of situations that could potentially expose one to public ridicule such as fear of public speaking. A variety of simple phobias concern common objects or situations such as cats, snakes, heights, darkness, or cockroaches. In each case, the individual realizes that the anxiety is groundless or exaggerated, but the anxiety seems to be beyond cognitive control. When flying situations or aircraft are the objects of phobia, the treatment may be complicated by the fact that true dangers are involved, and the therapist must acknowledge them. Nevertheless, even the most risky military flying is felt to be reasonably safe by those involved in it, or they would not continue. As the quotation at the beginning of this chapter observes, they find it interesting.

Much of the general public, however, finds flying more frightening than interesting. Various surveys indicate that 15 to 20% of the American public is somewhat afraid to fly, if not clinically phobic about aircraft. For those dedicated nonflyers who wish to overcome their fear of airline flying, a number of behavior modification programs are available, some sponsored by commercial airlines.[18]

Panic disorders are attacks of pure terror occurring without reason in otherwise unremarkable circumstances not involving physical exertion or any true danger. No specific stimulus may be identified, as would be possible with a phobic disorder. Somatic symptoms may include dyspnea, palpitations, a sensation of choking, dizziness, vasomotor flushing or chills, trembling, or sweating. A fear of going crazy or behaving uncontrollably also may be present. Physical causes should be considered—hormonal or endocrine disturbances, for instance. In studies of patients with anxiety or panic disorders, some 40% have been found to have mitral valve prolapse, a percentage out of proportion to the 5 to 7% of individuals found to have this condition in the general population.[19] The reason for this association is not known but may involve an inborn dysautonomia. Such attacks occurring in flight would interfere considerably with a pilot's ability to fly safely.

Obsessive-Compulsive Disorders

Many flyers, particularly navigators, are informally referred to as being obsessive or compulsive. Such traits may be quite adaptive in flying, especially where adherence to standard procedures or checklists helps to maintain safe flight conditions. The obsessive-compulsive disorders are a grotesque magnification of these useful human characteristics. Obsessions are persistent, recurrent impulses, ideas, or images that the individual experiences as involuntary and nonsensical, if not outright alien to his way of life. They may be violent or sexual in nature. Compulsions are behaviors that are repeated in a purposeful way while serving no useful purpose. Omitting these rituals results in intolerable tension or anxiety, even if it is not clear what evil may befall the sufferer in consequence. These rituals may distress or effectively cripple the individual, and yet they must be carried out: washing one's hands dozens of times each day to avoid any dirt whatsoever is a common example. Flyers may experience mild anxiety if they do not recheck an item once

or twice, but they rarely become neurotically obsessed with elements of flight. Such strange urges and behaviors are obviously incompatible with safe flying.

Affective Disorders

Affective disorders also could be termed disorders of mood and include both depression and pathologic elation (mania). Because depression is a reasonable human reaction to a variety of circumstances, most physicians are already familiar with it.

Depression

In this spectrum of psychiatric disorders, the physician is most likely to encounter depressive symptoms, especially presenting as minor physical complaints that persist or bother the patient in a medically inexplicable way. Faced with a flyer whose headaches, backaches, dizziness, or malaise seems to have no physical basis, especially in an individual whose past record reveals no physical complaints or who has previously been stoic in the face of real illness or injury, the prudent aeromedical practitioner will inquire about changes in patterns of sleeping, eating, sexual desire, and general mood. Perceived difficulty with concentration and memory, loss of usual self-assuredness, an unaccustomed sense of despair about the future, or an unreasonable sense of guilt or worthlessness are positive indications of depression. Psychiatric consultation and treatment are in order. A full-blown depression may be associated clearly with a significant loss in a person's life, or it may occur for no obvious reason. Symptoms may include a change in eating habits: most depressed individuals lose their appetites and some overeat grossly. The flyer may complain of multiple vague or minor physical problems or symptoms. A loss of sleep or oversleeping may be a means of escaping the painful world. Activity may be slowed down or speeded up in an agitated way. Usual activities will seem joyless and uninteresting, and the individual may cry easily. Sexual drive may be considerably diminished, and the person will feel unable to concentrate or to remember with the usual clarity. Unjustified feelings of guilt, remorse, worthlessness, sinfulness, and self-reproach appear. Escapist thinking ("I just want to get away from it all") or frank suicidal ideation may be expressed. In depressions of psychotic proportion, delusions of things done or not done would, if true, be cause for the feelings the sufferer has. In such instances, behavior may become bizarre or neglectful.

We want to add a particular word of warning here. Many physicians do not distinguish clearly between the symptoms of anxiety and those of depression. In some people, clinical depressions include an overlay of anxiety and agitation, and the underlying depression may not be recognized. If the symptoms of anxiety are treated with the benzodiazepines (Valium, Librium, Dalmane, Ativan, and others), the depression may be made worse. If medications are to be used in such patients, they should include antidepressants, given in proper doses for a proper length of time by a physician skilled in their use.

Suicide

Suicidal potential should be considered when dealing with any patient who has emotional complaints, especially if depressive features are present. The vegetative signs of depression should alert the flight surgeon to the possibility of suicide: disturbed eating or sleeping patterns, loss of concentration of energy, diminished libido (sexual feelings), or loss of enjoyment of life. Some demographic information may be of help in assessing the potential for suicide in a given individual. Suicide is more likely in individuals who are unmarried, older, Protestant, belong to the lower socioeconomic classes, those with insomnia, alcohol abusers, homosexuals,

those who live alone, and those who are unemployed. Individuals who have recently lost someone close are more at risk, as are those who have had a relative or close friend commit suicide. Although women attempt suicide about twice as often as men, men succeed twice as often as women. Certainly, one should attend carefully to any mention of suicide by a flyer; suicide by intentionally crashing an aircraft is unusual but by no means unheard of.

Mania

Manic episodes are not as commonly encountered, and, because the individual may well find these episodes pleasant, they may be first reported by someone else. The mood of the manic individual is elated or elevated or may be predominantly irritable. Symptoms may include tireless activity with no time or need for sleeping, eating, or ordinary activities; there also may be overweening self-esteem and involvement in multiple, novel, and often unwise activities. These endeavors may have a strong potential for personal or financial disaster, which the individual will not recognize. The elation may have an infectious quality to it but may quickly turn to unwarranted anger if the person is thwarted. Incessant planning and activity may occur in business, social, religious, political, and sexual ventures, accompanied by inappropriate sociability; for example, telephone calls made to anyone in the world at any hour. Grandiosity may predominate: spree-spending, dangerous driving, flamboyant or intrusive behavior, loud and pressured speech, and incessant joking. Flight of ideas may occur, with easy distractability, sometimes internally generated, so that the individual appears to interrupt himself, causing disorganized speech and even incoherence.

No one would fail to recognize such mania in full bloom. The hypomanic states are less extreme and may be perceived as great good spirits occurring in a person who is usually more reserved. One's clinical suspicions should be aroused by pressured speech and behavior, decreased sleeping, inflated self-esteem, loss of usual inhibitions, heedless hypersexuality, physical restlessness, irritability, and inappropriate actions as a change from usual behavior.

Occurring alternately and severely, mania and depression comprise the disorders formerly known as manic-depressive and now termed mixed bipolar depressive disorder. In a lesser degree, without disordered thinking, such a condition is termed a cyclothymic disorder.

Psychotic Disorders

Disordered thinking is the hallmark of psychotic disorders: hallucinations (false perceptions), delusions (real perceptions misinterpreted because of false beliefs), bizarre thinking, autistic or idiosyncratic patterns of pseudologic, and loose associations are examples of psychotic thinking. Regardless of its cause, functional psychotic thinking that occurs in the absence of toxic or metabolic causes is generally cause for permanent disqualification from flying. Functional causes include schizophrenia, manic-depressive psychosis, paranoia (irrational grandiosity or ideas of reference), or an acute situational reaction of psychotic proportions.

Organic psychoses may result from a wide variety of causes, including neoplasms, injuries, toxins, drugs, alcohol, metabolic or endocrine disorders, or infections. The existence of an organic brain disorder requires removal from flying. Consideration for a return to flying status depends on a variety of factors, but the flyer should be clearly safe to fly and free of any specific risk of recurrence, seizure disorder, or significant neurologic dysfunction before such action is taken.

TREATMENT AND REHABILITATION

Psychotherapy

Simply listing some of the treatment modalities available for people with emotional disorders gives the aeromedical practitoner a feeling for the bewildering variety of choices for the flyer who needs help. Treatment may be given individually or in groups. The therapist may be a psychiatrist, psychologist, social worker, or clergyman. He may be a classic psychoanalyst (and there are many schools here: Freudian, Jungian, Adlerian and others) or may use psychodynamic psychotherapy. Then there are behavior modification, transactional analysis, gestalt therapy, biofeedback, rational-emotive therapy, family therapy, marital therapy, and the newer, fringe therapies: rolfing, est, primal screaming, rebirthing, and others. Few psychiatrists can speak authoritatively about all of these therapies. In such matters, the referring physician is best served by contacting local professional associations or societies and by talking with trusted colleagues. One certainly must help the patient avoid unethical practitioners and charlatans.

One also must consider the goals of therapy. The psychiatric consultant who is asked to evaluate a person's fitness to fly may well be faced with a defensive, somewhat hostile patient who wishes only to be cleared for flying status. The goal of the therapist may be to help the patient reach a better adaptation to life, whereas the goal of the flyer may be to return to flying. These goals may not always coincide, especially if the patient sees the therapist as an impediment to his flying, a person who is denying the sought-after goal. Such issues should be settled early in the therapeutic process; it may be best that the therapist should be someone other than the psychiatric consultant who evaluates flying status.

Medications

Psychotropic medications are not compatible with active flying duties, both because of their primary and secondary effects and because any flyer whose emotional distress requires medication should not fly until that distress is relieved.

Antianxiety Medications

The benzodiazepines are widely used to allay anxiety and also as sedatives. Two commonly used compounds are diazepam (Valium) and chlordiazepoxide (Librium). Both may be given orally or intravenously; intramuscular administration should be avoided because the lipid solubility of these drugs leads to unpredictable absorption rates and uneven therapeutic effects. The biologic half-life of diazepam is 20 to 50 hours, and the half-life of chlordiazepoxide is 6 to 30 hours, so several days should be allowed after completion of a course of medication before flying is resumed. These medications should not be used in patients who have symptoms of depression along with anxiety because they may deepen a depression. Flurazepam (Dalmane) is widely used for nocturnal sedation. The half-life of its active metabolite may extend to 65 hours, so repeated doses have a cumulative effect. Temazepam (Restoril) has a half-life of 10 hours, and oxepam (Serax) has a half-life of about 8 hours; these drugs may be desirable where quick clearance is desired.

Barbiturates have been used for sedation in the past, but their potential for abuse and for suicidal overdose makes them less desirable than the benzodiazepines.

Antidepressant Medications

Tricyclic antidepressants are the medications most commonly used to treat depression. In general, these medications must be taken for about 2 weeks at a therapeutic level before clinical effects are noted. The side effects, mainly anticholinergic and sedative, begin immediately and thus tend to interfere with compliance because the patient initially feels even worse than before. Desipramine (Norpramin, Pertofrane) has the fewest anticholinergic effects. If no antidepressant effect is noted after 3 weeks, blood levels of the primary drug and its metabolites should be obtained to assure adequacy of the dosage. Tricyclic antidepressants should be used with care in patients with known cardiac disease, and potentially suicidal patients should be given only 2 or 3 days' medication at one time.

The other major antidepressant medications are the monoamine oxidase inhibitors (MAOIs). These are powerful medications and should be employed only by those skilled in their use. Patients receiving these drugs should be carefully instructed to avoid foods with tyramine because ingestion of such foods and absorption of the tyramine, a catecholamine precursor, may lead to a hypertensive crisis. Such crises also may result from the concomitant use of sympathetic amines such as ephedrine, phenylephrine (Neo-Synephrine), or phenylpropanolamine (Propadrine). A hypertensive crisis may be treated with a slow intravenous infusion of phentolamine (Regitine).

Neuroleptics or Major Tranquilizers

The neuroleptic drugs or major tranquilizers now includes several families, including the aliphatic, piperidine, and piperazine phenothiazines, with which many physicians are already familiar, thioxanthine derivatives, butyrophenones, and some of the newer agents. Physicians who need to use these medications generally become familiar with one member of each group; intragroup differences are minor. Because the clinical indications for these medications usually include psychotic thinking or a major emotional disturbance, their use in a flyer should automatically indicate a psychiatric consultation.

Lithium Carbonate

Lithium carbonate is primarily used to treat bipolar affective disorders, usually manic in nature, and may be of some use in a subgroup of schizophrenic patients. Management requires a very careful attention to blood levels, sodium intake, and the state of hydration and should be undertaken only by a physician experienced in such measures. Toxic effects may involve the cardiac, renal, or central nervous systems. Physicians requiring detailed data should consult the current psychopharmaceutic literature.

Behavioral Techniques

Behavior therapy is based on experimental observations of animal and human behavior and on modifications of those human behaviors that therapist and patient agree are causing problems. Feelings and thoughts also may be changed when behavior is modified.

Psychotherapists today have a variety of behavioral techniques available. Many of these techniques are discussed superficially in lay magazines and popular psychologically oriented paperback books. Thus trivialized, they sound so simple that the casual reader may feel like an instant expert. Anyone who has approached a true psychopathologic condition this simplistically has probably encountered a maze of hidden agendas and subconscious resistances that seemed utterly inexplicable. Several of these techniques, however, may be useful in treating some of the problems a flight surgeon may face, and these methods will be discussed briefly in the following sections. They should not be undertaken by those unskilled in their application.

Relaxation

Perhaps the most familiar relaxation training was developed by Jacobson.[20] This technique consists of strongly contracting various groups of muscles and then slowly relaxing them so that, by contrasting the contracted and the relaxed feelings, the subject learns to relax even further. With training and practice, the subject may learn to become quite relaxed very rapidly, simply by willing himself to do so. Other techniques involve the visual imagery of quiet scenes, repeating relaxing phrases, and abdominal breathing techniques.

Biofeedback

Biofeedback uses electronic monitoring to give the subject digital or analog information about physical states that are otherwise only dimly perceived. Frontalis muscle tension, fingertip sweat rate, and peripheral skin temperature are frequently measured in this manner. With instantaneous information about any changes, the subject can learn by trial and error to control these functions and thus lower his state of autonomic arousal. This technique is frequently helpful in avoiding tension or vascular headaches, aborting airsickness, controlling other disorders of muscle tension, and enhancing relaxation.

Systematic Desensitization

Systematic desensitization was made popular by Joseph Wolpe.[21] This method consists of learning a relaxation technique and then applying that technique while being gradually but progressively exposed to a phobically feared object or situation. This method has been successfully incorporated into the treatment of flying phobias in would-be airline passengers and also has been used in a few military flyers with success. The subject must be motivated to change because this therapy requires close and intelligent cooperation between therapist and patient.

COMBAT FLYING

Considering the movies, books, and anecdotes arising from combat flying, one may recall Robert E. Lee's remark to General James Longstreet at the battle of Fredericksburg: "It is well that war is so terrible—we should grow too fond of it!" Solo aerial combat is probably second only to knightly jousting as a source of romantic fantasy. As judged from personal accounts, it is exhilarating but exhausting and is as wearing in its own way as warfare on the ground. Certainly, the chronic fatigue and stresses caused by combat flying in bombers and transports have been investigated by several psychiatric authorities.

The books by Bond[7] and Grinker and Spiegel[8] about their experiences in World War II are basic texts for anyone interested in anything deeper than a superficial discussion of this topic. One must keep in mind that the flyers of those days were usually high school graduates or college students who volunteered either from patriotic motives or to avoid being drafted into the ground forces. They were given relatively brief training and were quickly sent into combat. Missions were not necessarily undertaken in an area of air superiority, and, especially in bombers, casualities might be in hundreds per mission. Gann describes the "over the Hump" operation of transports in the Himalayas, when 32 men were lost in four crashes during one rather routine day of noncombat flying.[22]

Such heavy losses did not occur in the United States forces in Korea or in Vietnam, but the descriptions of the wear of combat flying are similar. Sleep disturbances, nightmares, anxiety symptoms, irritability, loss of sense of humor, social withdrawal, and other changes from the usual personality are the hallmarks of incipient battle fatigue in both aviators and soldiers. Irregular work-rest-sleep schedules add circadian upset to the mental strain of facing death daily and to the physical fatigue intrinsic in any flying schedule. The flight surgeon who has to support a flying unit in a combat situation can do a number of things to help lessen, or at least delay, the attrition of flyers from battle fatigue.

Environmental Factors

The basic amenities must be as well provided as possible. Sleeping facilities should be quiet and somewhat removed from the flight line. These quarters should be soundproofed and climate-controlled, so that flyers' sleep may be undisturbed. If flying operations are going on around-the-clock, as they frequently do, good sleeping quarters are particularly important. Meals should be nourishing, attractive, and easily obtained at any hour. The flyers should have easy access to showering facilities and to a source of clean laundry. Attention of base authorities to matters such as these is not only important in the physical comfort of the flyer but also serves as tangible evidence of the unity with which the base supports the combat mission. "Nothing's too good for our boys in combat, and that's what we give 'em" was a sarcastic tag line heard in Vietnam whenever another shortage occurred. Like much gallows humor, it disclosed true feelings about the perceived lack of support. We heard complaints from nonflyers about pilots sleeping in air-conditioned and soundproofed quarters, but pilots who could not sleep in the daytime because of heat and noise were certainly less than completely ready to fly night missions. This attention to physical comfort was not coddling; it was just good common sense.

Personal Factors

Today's military flyers, as we have noted previously, tend to be older, better educated, and more experienced as a group than those written about by past authors. If our experience in Vietnam was any indication, most will approach combat situations with that attitude that the United States Air Force refers to as "professional": that they are there to do the job for which they have been trained. Identification with a unit regarded as competent and professional is an important factor in overcoming any feeling of personal inadequacy in a combat situation.

Studies of infantry soldiers have identified the feeling that "only I am frightened" as contributing to battle fatigue in that the individual feels that he alone has the cognitive and autonomic sensations of fear. Frank discussion of these feelings by the flight surgeon or, more to the point, by the squadron commander help allay the perception of any individual that he is the only frightened man in a band of heroes. The clear message should be that it is normal to be aware of one's fears and that the unit will tolerate such fears without question as long as the individual performs his duties. Stated simply, it is acceptable to feel fear and to talk about fear, but it is not acceptable to act afraid in combat.

Battle fatigue is based on true physical fatigue, as well as on the struggle between the natural instinct to avoid danger and the will to face it in order to do one's duty. Thus, those responsible for scheduling flights should provide time for sleep; four hours' uninterrupted sleep per 24 hours is the irreducible minimum. Flyers should have 1 or 2 days off every week or two and a longer break every few months, if at all possible. Experience of flight surgeons in previous wars and in Vietnam concur in the observation that flyers on a rest and recreation break ("R and R") get much recreation and little rest; it is a good idea to have 1 or 2 days off the flying schedule after the flyer returns from R and R to allow him to catch up on sleep before he resumes flying.

Alcohol consumption generally rises in a combat zone. One can preach about it endlessly, but unit discipline is probably the strongest weapon in avoiding situations of excessive drinking and too-short rest periods before flying. Otherwise, the old rule of "12 hours between bottle and throttle" is extremely hard to enforce. Although it is not always sufficient aeromedically, it does have the virtue of being easy to remember. The flight surgeon should help the squadron and flight commanders establish such a rule as a strict squadron tradition, enforced by peer pressure as well as by fiat.

The brain and the mind occupy the same part of the body. A disorder occurring anywhere in the body, in peace or in war, may have major mental health implications, and so the distinction between neurologic and psychiatric disease is basically artificial. Alcoholism has psychic and somatic components, as do sudden loss of consciousness, epilepsy, brain injury, fatigue, and multiple sclerosis.

The wise aeromedical physician will keep mental health factors in mind when dealing with conditions labeled neurologic and will keep organic factors in mind when dealing with conditions labeled psychiatric.

NEUROLOGIC DISEASE IN THE AVIATOR

Disease of the nervous system can be as mild as psychophysiologic tension headaches or as severe as such degenerative central nervous system disorders as Huntington's chorea. In general, patients presenting with severe neurologic disorders are disqualified from further flying. Milder and frequently encountered transient neurologic deficits, however, may present a considerable problem in disposition, and prolonged vigilance is required for these conditions. The more commonly encountered problems associated with the determination of fitness for flight will be discussed in the following sections. These problems include head injury and post-traumatic sequelae, the role of the electroencephalogram as a predictive tool in epilepsy, transient loss of consciousness, headache, and multiple sclerosis.

As can be seen from Table 17–3, back pain and radiculopathy, as well as vertigo, are common reasons for neurologic referral. Significant radiculopathy is an obvious cause for flyer disqualification. Questions of back stability are best referred to neurosurgical or orthopedic consultants because these specialists are primarily responsible for operative

Table 17–3. Neurophysical Conditions Evaluated at the United States Air Force School of Aerospace Medicine During a 6-Month Period

Condition	Number Evaluated (out of 80 patients)	Duty Not Involving Flying Recommended
Headache	12	3
Head injury	17	5
Severe	8	
Moderate	1	
Mild	8	
EEG Abnormalities	5	3
Loss of Consciousness	13	8
Vasovagal	3	
"G" Related	2	
Unexplained	5	
Seizure	3	
Back pain	6	2
Vertigo	5	1
Alcoholism	5	1
Parkinson's Disease	1	1
Hydrocephalus	1	1
Visual Obscuration	1	1
Neuro-bends	1	1
Transient Ischemia	1	1
Electrocution	1	1
Narcolepsy	1	1
Multiple sclerosis	1	1
Special examinations	9	0

intervention in these cases. EMG is a valuable tool as it allows one to determine whether radicular signs and symptoms represent true radiculopathy or, more commonly, referred pain from ligamentous structures.

Peripheral vertigo is most frequently encountered, and can best be dealt with by the otolaryngologist. Central vertigo does occasionally represent seizure aura and should arouse suspicion in patients who have no peripheral cause for paroxysmal vertigo.

Head Injury

Several authors have made great contributions to the study of post-traumatic epilepsy after open and closed head injury. Although other post-traumatic sequelae, such as vertigo, headache, diplopia, and so forth, are certainly possible after head injury, they generally begin soon after injury. The determination of the risk of post-traumatic epilepsy presents the greatest difficulty to both the uninitiated and seasoned flight surgeon because it can begin months or years later. Jennett[23] has provided an in-depth study of closed head injury, which is by far the most frequently encountered category of head injury in the flying population. He has devised a series of post-traumatic risk tables. Other authors have taken Jennett's statistics and have devised a statistical best-curve fit to the logarithmic post-traumatic decay curve. This purely statistical approach is certainly attractive but allows some underestimation of risk when patients with prolonged (greater than 7 days) loss of consciousness or post-traumatic amnesia are considered.[27] Annegers and colleagues[24] published a study from the Mayo Clinic that is quite attractive because of the population considered as well as the quality of follow-up. These authors divide head injury into "severe" (brain contusion, intracerebral or intracranial hematoma, or 24 hours of either unconsciousness or amnesia), "moderate" (skull fracture or 30 minutes to 24 hours of unconsciousness or amnesia), and "mild" (briefer unconsciousness or amnesia). The risk of seizure development in the severe category was 7.1% in the first year and 11.5% when considered over a 5-year period. Similarly, after moderate head injury, the risk was 0.7 and 1.6%, respectively. Mild head injury resulted in little risk over that encountered in the general population. An important point to recall is that these are statistics of incapacitation based on the normal population and not in a chronically fatigued and intermittently hypoxic and stressed flying population. These conditions frequently occur in the combat and high-performance aircraft arena.

These studies can form a guideline for the consideration of return to flying duty as well as consideration for flight training. Risks of 1 to 2%, although above the incidence of seizures in the general population, are probably similar to the risk of incapacitation from cardiovascular disease in the general population and are considered acceptable.

Electroencephalogram

The electroencephalogram (EEG) and its potential role in predicting pilot reliability has been of interest for several decades. The EEG has played a stormy role in pilot candidate selection and pilot retention studies because it is subject not only to individual variation but also to interpretative variation. Some authorities have used grading systems to rate electrical abnormalities in terms of their severity, but severity has always been a problem when clinical correlation is required. Robin and colleagues[25] compiled and reviewed the records of asymptomatic, noninjured, pilots with severe EEG abnormalities and found a 5% incidence of sudden incapacitation from seizure occurrence. Other authors have quoted higher risks, but these have usually been due to inclusion of the mentally retarded in the study population. Another problem arises with waveforms such as the psychomotor variant, 14/6 spike, small sharp spikes (benign epileptiform transients of sleep), or the wicket temporal pattern. These patterns have been considered epileptiform in nature by some researchers, whereas others consider them variants of uncertain clinical significance. These patterns occasionally are associated with poorly understood vegetative signs such as headaches, syncope, and dizziness and, in some cases, psychiatric symptoms. With such a wide range of clinical variation, the only comment that can be made is to use caution when these "normal variants" are present in symptomatic patients.

The Mayo Classification System for EEG abnormalities has gained wide acceptance and is a useful tool. Spike and sharp waves that do not fit the well-known normal variants are of clinical concern. Theta dys-

rhythmias, on the other hand, can be quite difficult to grade as they are so state dependent. EEG interpretation is best left to well experienced electroencephalographers who have at their disposal trained technicicans and recording facilities where meticulous care is taken in artifact identification and elimination as well as in electrode application.

Loss of Consciousness

When loss of consciousness is encountered in pilots, the possibility of a cardiac or epileptiform abnormality immediately comes to mind. History is the most useful tool in determining the underlying pathophysiology.

Syncope is frequently preceded by a period of faintness, during which the patient is pale, diaphoretic, weak, and may complain of nausea. Loss of consciousness is slow in syncope, and subsequent injury from a fall is uncommon. Syncopal episodes usually take place in a standing or sitting attitude and occur in a setting of pain, emotional shock, or threat (injections, venipuncture, description of medical procedures, or patient involvement in their own medical procedure). Vomiting may follow the episode. Brief clonic twitches or tonic stiffening may accompany the episode but usually are quite different from and less intense than the forceful contractions of a grand mal seizure.[26] Focal signs are uncommon.

Seizures, on the other hand, are associated with a rapid loss of consciousness (LOC) or rapid march of aura or prodrome. The patient is rarely pale, as with syncope, and signs of autonomic prodrome are usually absent. Urinary and fecal incontinence frequently occur in seizures and are accompanied by forceful tonic spasms. Tongue biting, eye deviation, postictal confusion, and soreness, as well as a family history of epilepsy frequently accompany seizures. Frequent attacks during the day and attacks in the supine position also should suggest seizure.

Syncope may be acceptable if it occurs in the presence of pain, venipuncture, or severe emotional upset. In this circumstance, syncope is thought to represent dysfunction due to extreme autonomic outflow (vagal).

Syncope is occasionally seen in debilitated individuals after a long period of bed rest; here, the mechanism is probably one of orthostatic hypotension. These patients rapidly regain their postural autonomic reflexes as the acute illness subsides, and their risk of future syncope is low.

Micturition is occasionally a setting for syncope, particularly in the older or debilitated person who arises to void during the night. The consideration of "older or debilitated" may seem inappropriate to the pilot population, but pilots frequently find themselves debilitated from alcohol. The hangover is a frequent setting for neurologic events, and alcohol withdrawal can be a particularly fertile time to see convulsive activity in previously normal individuals.

Cardiovascular causes of syncope should always form the foundation of any evaluation of central nervous system dysfunction.

One should not overlook altered states of primary brain metabolites, such as occur with hypoxia, anemia, hypoglycemia, and decreased carbon dioxide secondary to hyperventilation, in the evaluation. Hematologic, biochemical, and blood gas screening usually suggests these causes if they are operative.

Transient cerebral ischemic attacks (TIAs) should be considered, especially when the patient is above 30 years of age. These attacks presage possible serious sudden incapacitation and represent the early sign of treatable stroke. Migraine is an important differential diagnosis that must be kept in mind in these cases because angiography is occasionally a devastating event in migrainous patients. Recent developments in noninvasive ultrasonographic investigation of the ca-

rotid arteries hold great promise in evaluating the potential TIA patient with suspected carotid atheromatous disease. When positive, these studies often can justify a more invasive approach when only nonspecific signs are available by the history and physical examination. Computer tomographic (CT) studies in these patients are usually normal and often are positive only after a subsequent devastating event has occurred.

Extracranial vascular insufficiency (vertebral, carotid) may be the cause of restrictive cerebral blood flow whether it be of intrinsic restriction (atheromas, giant cell arteritis) or thromboembolic. Doppler studies are frequently useful in extracranial blood flow determinations. The erythrocyte sedimentation rate, although nonspecific, remains a useful test when temporal arteritis is suspected. Recent evidence seems to indicate, however, that some patients may have normal erythrocyte sedimentation rates with histologic evidence of giant cell arteritis.

Diffuse arteriolar constriction from hypertensive encephalopathy is occasionally encountered as a cause of syncope. Emergent care forms the basis of treatment, and hypertension usually is discovered early in the patient evaluation.

Conversion reaction can be quite a problem unless this entity is considered. Although usually a diagnosis of exclusion after a thorough medical evaluation, one should consider this disorder after determining that cardiovascular and neurologic examinations are normal. Hysterical seizures and syncope can be evaluated with an experienced electroencephalographer in a recording session using mild suggestion. Frequently, the patient will produce the symptoms during the recording period and not infrequently patients look for the opportunity to display them to an experienced observer. This entity is more frequently encountered in the more emotionally immature individual, and a female predominance is observed.

Finally, one should not forget cataplexy as an important cause of postural loss of tone. Cataplexy may occur alone but usually is part of a larger narcolepsy, cataplexy, hypnagogic hallucinatory complex. Research in this area is intriguing, and the sleep disorders are becoming better defined with the appearance of sleep laboratories in some parts of the country and the recognition of sleep disorders by more clinicians. Patients with narcolepsy make sudden transitions from wakefulness to rapid eye movement (REM) sleep. The accompaniments of REM sleep also occur, including loss of postural tone and dreaming. Frequently, patients experience vivid dreams while postural tone is maintained; these are referred to as hypnagogic hallucinations. At other times, patients may lose postural tone without sleep. This is referred to as a cataplectic episode, or cataplexy. These conditions are usually precipitated by strong emotions.

The laboratory diagnosis of narcolepsy and cataplexy is unfortunately difficult. Sleep latency was thought to be reduced in these patients, but as research continues, this parameter is losing its former importance. At present, the diagnosis is based on history.

Treatment is often successful with combinations of tricyclic antidepressants and amphetamines. Both of these agents suppress REM sleep periods but recovery adequate for a return to flying seldom occurs. Needless to say, the use of these medications is incompatible with flying.

A further note of caution should be made considering paroxysmal cerebral events as a cause for loss of consciousness. The previously discussed temporal lobe variants occasionally have syncope or postural loss of tone associated with them, although the association is often debated. These waveforms should be kept in mind as a further key to understanding syncope in a setting of nondiagnostic cardiac evaluation and a normal neurologic examination.

Headache

Headache has been a common plague of mankind throughout the centuries. In addition to its role as an annoying factor, it presents some unique problems from an aeromedical point of view. Grossly, headache can be divided into tension, or muscle contraction headache and vascular headache. Although this division is probably overly simplistic, it provides a framework in which to discuss the subject.

Headache labeled as tension is best described rather than named. These headaches are usually frontal and/or occipital in location and occur as an aching or tight band-like sensation. Position and its effect is important information to seek because these headaches are usually unaffected by head position or events that tend to increase intra-abdominal or intrathoracic pressure such as coughing, sneezing, or straining. Tension headaches are frequently exacerbated by stress and long periods of vigilance and sometimes disappear quite rapidly when the stress-producing event is avoided or completed. Aspirin is frequently helpful, but the trip to the medicine cabinet may remove the individual from the stressful situation and, thus, is an act of avoidance, which may be as helpful as the aspirin itself. These headaches are usually thought of as mild, but devastating degrees of mental slowing occur when these headaches are severe.

Vascular headaches, on the other hand, are usually positional and intra-abdominal or intrathoracic state-dependent. The patient may complain of photophobia and exacerbation of pain with loud noise. Relief is usually slow in coming as compared with the tension or psychophysiologic headache. Frequently, a patient may complain of a combination of a tension headache followed by a mild or severe vascular component. In our experience, this combination syndrome is by far the most frequently encountered.

A special variety of vascular headache frequently arises with visual neurologic prodrome preceding the headache. This classic migraine variety usually has some family history and a unique responsiveness to beta blockers, ergots, and methylsergide. Migraine also may be preceded by other neurologic prodromes such as aphasia, hemiparesis, hemiparesthesias, or hemianesthesia, to mention only a few. These atypical or complicated variants are much less frequently encountered and occasionally may result in permanent neurologic residua.

Cluster headache, or Horton's cephalgia, is an interesting clinical syndrome worth mentioning because of its frequency and its devastating potential aeromedically. These headaches frequently start with severe, boring pain in one eye associated with conjunctival injection and nasal lacrimation. The headaches are severe and, unlike migraine, have been known to cause patients to beat their heads against the wall for relief. Many individuals are totally incapacitated. Fortunately, the headaches are brief, lasting only minutes to hours. The attacks may occur on a daily basis and persist for weeks and months. Suddenly, as fast as they appeared, they disappear, perhaps never to return or to return again in a predictable or unpredictable period of time.

This brief review of headaches is not intended to form a background for medical practice but rather to suggest important areas for aeromedical consideration. Tension headaches, although usually considered benign, can and occasionally do incapacitate flyers by slowing mentation and retarding their ability to concentrate. This condition obviously can lead to devastating results. On the other hand, migraine, particularly common migraine without neurologic prodrome, can be only a mild annoyance and not interfere with vigilance at all. The point to understand is to evaluate "functional impairment" during the headache and not to practice

routine grounding at the mere mention of the word migraine. The physician, however, should keep in mind that the usual medications used to treat these conditions, excluding aspirin, represent a hazard to flying.

Cluster headache, as alluded to previously, is a particularly devastating syndrome, and a considerable time without flying should elapse to allow assessment of the cluster pattern.

Headache syndromes, pharmacologic therapy, psychiatric substrates, and the art of care form a division of neurology that is fascinating and clinically rewarding. The reader is referred to the many excellent neurologic texts for further help.

Multiple Sclerosis

Multiple sclerosis (MS) is an elusive disease with so many faces that its place in the differential diagnoses of most central nervous system disorders is well deserved. The problem that seems to arise most often is an isolated occurrence of optic neuritis with a normal neurologic examination. Estimates of the risk of future multiple sclerosis development vary but may approach 15%. A distinctively different risk is that of sudden incapacitation, which is quite low and allows flyers with resolved episodes of optic neuritis to return to flying with little concern for flying safety.

Although this chapter has not dealt in depth with the diagnostic evaluation of the neurologic diseases so far considered, MS can hardly be thought of without some discussion of diagnosis. A specific lab test for MS, although desperately needed, does not exist. Patients with MS have some immunologic markers that are occasionally useful.

Some patients with MS have spinal fluid oligoclonal protein elevation. These protein elevations also are found in other neurologic conditions, such as subacute sclerosing panencephalitis and neurosyphilis, and evaluations of exclusion usually begin when oligoclonal proteins are sought. Spinal fluid myelin basic protein also is present in some patients with MS but is usually considered an acute phase marker of the disease.

The computer tomographic (CT) scan has added some to the clinician's diagnostic ability in MS, but this test is usually positive only after the diagnosis already has been established by the history of multiple episodes separated in time and space.

Evoked responses are quite useful when another lesion is sought in a single early episode of suspected MS. By combining visual, auditory, and somatosensory recording, the neuraxis can be quite extensively studied using a few sensory modalities. Although these studies do not necessarily provide accurate localized information, they do provide evidence of slowed conduction over diffuse pathways, which adds considerably more information when the diagnosis is in doubt.

Table 17–3 summarizes the neurologic diagnoses and aeromedical dispositions seen at USAFSAM during a 6-month period. These patients were seen because an aeromedical determination could not be made at the local base level and thus represent a selected population.

We have not attempted to provide rules and regulations regarding the neurologic evaluation of the flyer because hard and fast rules do not exist. The important point to consider is the inherent safety of the aviator and the risk of incapacitation in his flying role.

REFERENCES

1. Beaven, C.L.: A Chronological History of Aviation Medicine. The School of Aviation Medicine, Randolph Air Force Base, Texas, 1939.
2. Anderson, H.G.: The Medical and Surgical Aspects of Aviation. London, Oxford University Press, 1919.
3. Christy, R.L.: Personality factors in selection of flight proficiency. Aviat. Space Environ. Med., 46:309–311, 1975.
4. Fine, P.M., and Hartman, B.O.: Psychiatric Strengths and Weaknesses of Typical Air Force Pilots. SAM Technical Report 68-121. United States Air Force School of Aerospace Medicine, Brooks Air Force Base, Texas, 1968, pp. 131–168.
5. Jennings, C.L.: The use of normative data in the psychological evaluation of flying personnel. In Psychiatry in Aerospace Medicine. Vol. 4. International Psychiatry Clinics. Edited by C.J.G. Perry. Boston, Little, Brown and Co, 1967, pp. 37–52.
6. Reinhardt, R.F.: The outstanding jet pilot. Am. J. Psychiatr., 127:732–735, 1970.
7. Bond, D.D.: The Love and Fear of Flying. New York, International Universities Press, Inc., 1952.
8. Grinker, R.R., and Spiegel, J.A.: Men Under Stress. Philadelphia, Blakiston, 1945.
9. Sledge, W.H.: Aerospace psychiatry. In Comprehensive Textbook of Psychiatry. 3rd Ed. Edited by H.I. Kaplan, A.M. Freedman, and B.J. Sadock. Baltimore, Williams & Wilkins Co., 1980, pp. 2902–2914.
10. McKinnon, R.A., and Michels, R.: The Psychiatric Interview in Clinical Practice. Philadelphia, W.B. Saunders Co., 1971.
11. Rafferty, J.A., and Deemer, W.I., Jr.: Statistical Evaluation of the Experimental Adaptability Rating for Military Aeronautics (ARMA) of World War II. United States Air Force School of Aviation Medicine, Randolph Air Force Base, Texas. Project No. 21-02-097, Report No. 1, Aug. 1948, and Report No. 2 (Factor Analysis), Aug. 1949.
12. Perry, C.J.G.: Psychiatric support for man in space. In Psychiatry in Aerospace Medicine. Vol. 4. International Psychiatry Clinics. Edited by C.J.G. Perry. Boston, Little, Brown and Co., 1967, pp. 197–222.
13. Marsh, R.W., and Perry, C.J.G.: Anniversary reactions in military aviators. Aviat. Space Environ. Med., 48:61–64, 1977.
14. Pursch, J.A.: Alcohol in aviation: A problem of attitudes. Aerospace Med., 45:318–321, 1974.
15. Sledge, W.H., and Boydstun, J.A.: Vasovagal syncope in aircrew: Psychosocial aspects. J. Nerv. Med. Dis., 167:114–124, 1979.
16. Levy, R.A., Jones, D.R., and Carlson, E.H.: Biofeedback rehabilitation of airsick aircrew. Aviat. Space Environ. Med., 52:118–121, 1981.
17. Cowings, P.S., Billingham, J., and Toscano, W.B.: Learned control of multiple autonomic responses to compensate for the debilitating effects of motion sickness. Ther. Psychosomatic Med., 4:318–323, 1977.
18. Forgione, A.G., and Bauer, F.M.: Fearless Flying. Boston, Houghton Mifflin Co., 1980.
19. Kantor, J.S., Zitrin, C.M., and Zeldis, S.M.: Mitral value prolapse syndrome in agoraphobic patients. Am. J. Psychiat., 137:467–469, 1980.
20. Jacobson, C.: Progressive Relaxation. Chicago, University of Chicago Press, 1938.
21. Wolpe, J.: The Practice of Behavior Therapy. 2nd Ed. New York, Pergamon Press, Inc., 1973.
22. Gann, E.K.: Fate is the Hunter. New York, Simon and Schuster, 1961, pp. 265–271.
23. Jennett, W.B.: Epilepsy After Non-Missile Head Injuries. 2nd Ed. London, Heinemann Medical Books, 1975.

24. Annegers, J.F., et al.: Seizures after head trauma: A population study. Neurology, 30:683–689, 1980.
25. Robin, J.J., Tolan, G.D., and Arnold, J.W.: Ten-year experience with abnormal EEGs in asymptomatic adult males. Aviat. Space Environ. Med., 49(5):732–736, 1978.
26. Lin, T.-Y., et al.: Convulsive syncope in blood donors. Ann Neurol., 11:525–528, 1982.
27. Feeney, D.M., and Walker, A.E.: The prediction of posttraumatic Epilepsy. Arch. Neurol., 36:8–12, 1979.

Chapter *18*

Further Significant Medical and Surgical Conditions of Aeromedical Concern

Royce Moser, Jr.

Our health can be no better than the knowledge and skills of the physicians to whom we entrust it.

JOHN F. KENNEDY

The physician evaluating individuals with the conditions discussed in this chapter will find it necessary to apply the same basic criteria for qualification for flying duties as were discussed with regard to the other conditions considered in chapters elsewhere in this text. In essence, these criteria are that there be no hazard to the individual's health, to flying safety, or to mission completion if that person participates in flight activities. All three considerations are of concern for military and commercial crews and passengers, but the first two are of primary interest in general aviation.

In determining whether these criteria are met, the practitioner must consider both the significance of the underlying condition and the effects of any required medication or other treatment. Tragedy has occurred when a flight surgeon caring for a pilot was concerned only about possible side effects of a prescribed medication and did not consider compromises due to the medical problem itself. Because the medication produced no demonstrable side effects and was, therefore, thought to be "safe" for a flyer, the physician qualified the pilot to fly. Although the medication did not produce any problems, it only partly alleviated the symptoms. The pilot was distracted by the residual symptoms during a critical phase of flight and a fatal crash resulted. Of course, the physician caring for flyers must always determine whether a medication may produce a hazard if the patient is qualified for flight while taking the drug. Allowing a person to fly with a minor problem not expected to cause problems while prescribing medication with side effects such as drowsiness or similar unacceptable results can obviously set the stage for disaster.

The following discussion of some of the more typical conditions aerospace medicine practitioners will have to evaluate is not all-inclusive. Consideration of these specific conditions will assist the practitioner in managing patients with other medical and surgical conditions of aeromedical significance.

571

HEMATOLOGIC CONSIDERATIONS

Oxygen Transport

As was discussed more extensively in Chapter 5, oxygen is carried in the blood in physical solution and in combination with hemoglobin. The amount of oxygen in solution depends on Henry's Law. At 38° C and an arterial oxygen pressure of 102 mm Hg, each 100 ml of blood carries 0.306 ml of dissolved oxygen. Of far more significance is the amount of oxygen carried by hemoglobin. Each gram of normal hemoglobin will combine with 1.34 ml of oxygen. Thus, if a person has 15 g/dL of hemoglobin, each 100 ml of blood theoretically could carry 20 ml of oxygen (1.34 × 15) through the hemoglobin mechanism. Due to the admixture of fully saturated blood coming from the lungs with undersaturated blood which passed through anatomic or physiologic dead spaces in the lungs, arterial blood is approximately 97% saturated. As a result, the amount of oxygen carried by 15 g of hemoglobin is closer to 19 ml/100 ml of blood.

At the tissue level, 5 to 6 ml/dL of oxygen are consumed at rest. The returning venous blood is approximately 75% saturated with oxygen and the venous PO_2 is 40 mm Hg. Because of the shape of the oxygen dissociation curve, even slight reductions in the PO_2 at the tissue level will result in the release of significant additional oxygen, so a reserve does exist to meet additional demands for oxygen.

Due to its significance in oxygen transport, any reduction in effective hemoglobin concentration is of aeromedical concern to either a crewmember or passenger. This reduction may, of course, be due to actual blood loss, as in the case of acute or chronic hemorrhage. Reduction also may effectively occur when available hemoglobin, even if present in "normal" concentrations, is not able to carry the usual amount of oxygen. Carbon monoxide exposure is one such situation. Be-

cause of the greater affinity of carbon monoxide for the hemoglobin molecule, small amounts of inhaled carbon monoxide can prevent the normal transport of oxygen in an individual with a normal hemoglobin concentration who is inspiring air with a normal PO_2. In other instances, a hemoglobin abnormality may prevent the red blood cells from carrying a normal amount of oxygen. Again, an effective anemia exists even though the hemoglobin concentration may be within normal limits.

Aeromedical Concerns in the Anemic Patient

Whatever the cause, a reduction in effective hemoglobin concentration can significantly affect the amount of oxygen available for tissue metabolism. If, for example, hemoglobin is reduced to approximately half the normal value at 7 mg/dL, only 9.4 ml/dL of oxygen is carried by hemoglobin if the blood is fully saturated. Even if the tissue PO_2 level drops to 30 mm Hg, only 40%, or approximately 3.8 ml/dL of oxygen, is released to the tissues. If the body's oxygen requirement remains constant, cardiac output would have to increase, in accordance with the Fick principle, to meet the body's oxygen demand. Although such compensatory mechanisms can offset significant hemoglobin reductions, the reserve remaining to compensate for any additional demands is reduced. With exercise or heavy physical work, the oxygen requirement may increase twentyfold. In an individual who is compromised by anemia, sufficient additional compensatory reserves may not be present, and the exertion may precipitate the abrupt onset of symptoms. If the inspired PO_2 is reduced at the same time the exertion requirements occur, the situation could rapidly become critical. Obviously, just such a situation could occur in an anemic crewmember during a rapid decompression.

Because of the importance of compensatory mechanisms, the aerospace medicine practitioner evaluating an anemic patient who is contemplating a commercial flight must determine whether pathologic processes are affecting those compensatory capabilities. It also should be noted that patients with chronic anemias are more likely to have adjusted to the reduced hemoglobin than patients with acute anemias with similar hemoglobin levels. In general, an individual who is asymptomatic during mild exertion at ground level will not experience symptoms during a routine flight in a commercial aircraft.[1] If the passenger's compensatory capabilities are significantly compromised, however, the relatively slight reductions in PO_2 that occur in commercial flights could produce symptoms. If even an apparently compensated individual has a hemoglobin level of 50% of normal or less, a blood transfusion before flight or oxygen administration in flight may be necessary.[2]

In developing recommendations for an anemic traveler, the physician should consider both the duration of exposure and the cabin altitude. Prolonged exposure to reduced PO_2 increases the probability that the anemic patient who is marginally compensated will develop symptoms. Should the anemic patient smoke cigarettes during a flight, the oxygen-carrying capacity of hemoglobin may be reduced by as much as 15% due to the inhaled carbon monoxide. The practitioner also must note that the provision of supplemental oxygen in flight to prevent or control symptoms may be progressively more difficult the longer the flight. Unless additional arrangements are made prior to the flight, many airlines can provide only a limited supply of oxygen. This supply may not be sufficient for continuous use during a long flight. In advising the patient or flight attendants whether and when to use supplemental oxygen, the physician should emphasize that cyanosis may not be a reliable indication of significant hypoxia in an anemic patient. Approximately 6 g/dL of hemo-

globin must be deoxygenated for cyanosis to be manifest. In some anemic patients, it may not be possible to recognize cyanosis because all oxygen cannot be removed from the hemoglobin, even though the tissues may be hypoxic. As a result, several grams of hemoglobin per deciliter will remain oxygenated, and there may not be sufficient deoxygenated hemoglobin to produce cyanosis.

Sickle Cell Disease and Trait

Naturally, the physician providing a recommendation concerning flying also will be concerned with determining the cause of the anemia. Ascertaining the cause is essential to provide proper therapy and make an informed recommendation regarding flying. In one particular hemoglobinopathy, sickle hemoglobin (Hb-S), the differential diagnosis is of particular concern to the flight surgeon because exposure to reduced PO_2 can directly affect the ability of the red blood cells to carry oxygen. Sickle hemoglobin is due to alterations of the beta polypeptide chains of the hemoglobin molecule. Individuals with hemoglobin mixtures SS, SC, S-thal, SD, and SF have sickle cell disease. Those heterozygous people who have Hb-S and a normal hemoglobin (A, A_2) have the sickle cell trait. In sickle cell disease, the patient demonstrates a hemolytic anemia and, particularly during intercurrent infections, may experience hemolytic crises and tissue infarctions. When the blood PO_2 of patients with sickle cell disease falls below approximately 60 mm Hg, the erythrocytes become deformed in a sickle shape and rigid. The loss in elasticity prevents some cells from passing through some blood vessels, producing an effective increase in viscosity. As the viscosity increases, the blood flow is reduced further, increased hypoxia results, and more cells sickle. This vicious circle produces more blood vessel blockage and tissue infarction and crises.[3]

Because the alveolar PO_2 at 3048 m is

approximately 60 mm Hg and the tissue level would be below this level at lower altitudes, some physicians would not recommend passenger flight for patients with sickle cell disease unless oxygen were readily available.[4] Other practitioners would recommend avoiding air travel altogether if possible.[2] Because of the risk of a hemolytic crisis on altitude exposure, individuals with sickle cell disease should not be qualified for crewmember duties.

In contrast to sickle cell disease, the individual with the sickle cell trait may be completely asymptomatic. Overall life expectancy is the same as that for HAA individuals, and Hb-AS erythrocytes do not sickle until the oxygen tension is much lower than that required for Hb-SS erythrocytes. Although a recommendation regarding flying can be made with some assurance for patients with sickle cell disease, the situation is much more complicated for a patient with the sickle cell trait. Hemolytic crises and even sudden death have been reported in individuals with the sickle cell trait who were exposed to relatively low altitudes.[5] The investigators often reported the onset of symptoms after a period of exertion at altitude. Many of these reports, however, are anecdotal in nature and not all included hemoglobin electrophoretic studies to confirm the presence of Hb-S. In some cases, other hemoglobin abnormalities were present as well as Hb-S. Although some investigators recommended that no individual with the sickle cell trait fly, a national study group noted that such individuals should not be restricted from flight duties unless they were a pilot or copilot.[6] A number of countries accept individuals with the sickle cell trait for both commercial and military flight duties. Until 1981, the United States military restricted people with the sickle cell trait from flight training, service as an aircrew member, or attendance at the Air Force Academy in Colorado Springs, CO. The latter restriction was because the facility is located at over 1524 m, and symptoms had been reported after exertion at field training sites at comparable altitudes.[5] In 1981, this policy was changed, and individuals with the sickle cell trait can now be qualified to attend the Air Force Academy. In addition, candidates with the sickle cell trait can be accepted for flight training according to standards established for the services. In the Air Force, applicants who have 41% or less Hb-S will be accepted for such training. Simultaneously, a program was developed for the medical monitoring of Air Force individuals with the sickle cell trait in an effort to provide a definitive answer concerning any possible complications caused by altitude exposure.

GASTROINTESTINAL DISORDERS

Gastroenteritis

Gastroenteritis is a frequent problem of both crews and passengers. It has been cited as the leading cause of in-flight incapacitation in aircrews.[7] Fortunately, the incapacitation is usually not so abrupt that the crewmember cannot either pass the controls to another crewmember or land before symptoms reach their peak. Prevention is of paramount importance, and both crews and passengers will benefit by considering and applying the basic principles of sanitation. One of the most common afflictions of travelers is the so-called "traveler's diarrhea." The consumption of raw vegetables in salads, undercooked meat or fish, or shellfish is associated with particularly high attack rates of this malady. Although a variety of agents have been implicated in this condition, strains of enterotoxigenic Escherichia coli are a leading cause. Giardia also has been implicated frequently, and campylobacter also may produce gastroenteritis. Less frequently, more virulent pathogens, such as Entamoeba histolytica or Shigella species, are the causative agents. Therapy for these conditions previously included such antimotility or antispasmodic agents as diphenoxylate hydrochloride (Lomotil) or paregoric. More recently, however, it has been determined that these agents may prolong the duration of some of the conditions and increase the risk of complications. For example, the duration of shigellosis has been shown to be prolonged with diphenoxylate hydrochloride.[8] Similarly, the tendency for salmonella to invade the bloodstream may be enhanced by antimotility drugs.[9] Bismuth subsalicylate (Pepto Bismol) appears to be effective in treating some cases of traveler's diarrhea. Its use is often inconvenient, however, because a large quantity must be taken. Doxycycline has been effective in preventing diarrhea in Peace Corps workers when given in an initial dose of 200 mg followed by 100 mg/day for 3 weeks.[10] This drug has been shown to be particularly effective against certain strains of enterotoxigenic Escherichia coli. The use of these agents as prophylaxis is still questionable, however, because it appears that, although protective against E. coli pathogens, they may increase susceptibility to more serious invasive enteric pathogens.[11] Such considerations underscore the necessity for proper hygiene as the first line of defense against the onset of traveler's diarrhea.

In evaluating a patient with such symptoms, it is imperative that the practitioner obtain an adequate history, including travel and diet history. It is, of course, possible to return from a foreign country to a residence in the United States during the incubation period of a serious gastroenteritis infection. For example, one patient seen in consultation developed diarrhea several days after his return from the Far East. He was treated symptomatically through two recurrences over a 4-week period by a practitioner who neglected to obtain a history of either the recent travel or the fact that the patient had consumed fresh salads and seafood while overseas. While being treated with diphenoxylate hydrochloride, the patient collapsed and became semicomatose. He responded to intensive life-support measures, and subsequent evaluation disclosed systemic Entamoeba histolytica infection, with three separate liver abscesses. After prolonged therapy, the patient eventually resumed his normal activities. The development of the serious complications, however, could perhaps have been prevented by early recognition of the fact that he was at increased risk as a result of his recent sojourn overseas.

Peptic Ulcer

Peptic ulcer disease will be seen frequently by the aeromedical practitioner. Crewmembers who respond to treatment can be considered for a return to flying duty. Currently recommended criteria in the United States Air Force include freedom from symptoms, healing demonstrated by radiography or endoscopy without residual spasm, irritability, or duodenitis, absence of a continuing need for medications, absence of a continuing need for specialized or frequent feedings, absence of esophageal varices, erosive gastritis, hiatal hernia, or other complicating epigastrointestinal conditions, and the flyer's demonstrated understanding of the factors that affect recurrences and complications.[12] As indicated by this last requirement, patient education and involvement in any treatment program are essential components of a therapy plan for this condition. In achieving an effective education program, the practitioner must ensure that the patient is aware of both the possibility and manifestations of complications as well as the symptoms of a recurrence. Of particular aeromedical concern is the possibility of gastrointestinal hemorrhage due to ulcer disease. Hemorrhage may present, of course, as the initial manifestation of disease in up to 25% of cases. It also may pose a hazard to the flyer who has been treated for ulcer disease with a previous bleeding episode because of the significant risk of a recurrent bleeding episode. In addition to the fact that serious bleeding may occur without warning symptoms, the chance of incapacitation is increased in a flyer who works in even the slightly hypoxic environment of commercial flight. If the flyer is required to perform stressful duties or is exposed to low ambient Po_2 during an emergency, the chances for incapacitation are further increased. Changes in stool color, weakness, palpitations, or any other symptoms suggesting a bleeding episode should prompt the patient with a history of ulcer disease to seek immediate attention from the flight surgeon if the counseling and education efforts of the aeromedical practitioner have been effective.

Gastrointestinal Hemorrhage

Gastrointestinal hemorrhage in a flyer poses a challenging problem for the aerospace medicine physician. In addition to managing the acute problem, the practitioner must make every effort to determine the site of the bleeding. Endoscopic examination during the bleeding episode has been particularly valuable in making this determination. If the practitioner can demonstrate that bleeding is from gastritis due to excessive alcohol ingestion or the use of medications such as aspirin, it is presumably possible to prevent a recurrence by avoiding such insults. With appropriate patient cooperation, it would then be possible to recommend a return to flying duties. If the bleeding source is a peptic ulcer, however, the picture is more complex. In such situations, the practitioner has to determine whether the individual is likely to have a recurrence. Various authorities have reported different rates of recurrence of gastrointestinal bleeding in individuals who have had a prior bleeding episode due to peptic ulcer disease. For example, the reported recurrence rate of bleeding for medically treated patients ranges from approximately 7 to 51% and from 4 to 27% for surgically treated patients.[13] The success rate among different

surgical modalities varies as well, and the lower recurrence rate, from 4 to 10%, has been reported for patients treated by vagotomy and pyloroplasty.[13] Although controversy does exist, such findings indicate that surgery may be appropriate for pilots who have bled from a peptic ulcer before unrestricted qualification for flying duties is recommended. Naturally, an appropriate period of observation after surgery is necessary to evaluate the effectiveness of this treatment before recommending a return to flying duties. If a crewmember is restricted to transport or similar aircraft, recommendation for a return to duty may be appropriate without surgery if the source of bleeding was positively identified by endoscopy, no bleeding has occurred during a 6-month observation period, the ulcer has healed completely on endoscopic examination, and a complete gastrointestinal radiographic series is normal.

Hiatal Hernia and Gastroesophageal Reflux

Hiatal hernia disease may be either symptomatic or an incidental finding detected in conjunction with other evaluations. Symptoms due to gastroesophageal reflux may occur without demonstrable hiatal hernia disease, as well as in association with the condition. In evaluating such patients, it is imperative that the practitioner rule out more serious causes, especially cardiac disease. If, after such an evaluation, symptoms are attributable to gastroesophageal reflux, either with or without hiatal hernia disease, it may be possible to control the symptoms completely with standard treatment procedures such as smaller meals, no food 3 hours before retiring, avoidance of aggravating foods and alcohol, weight loss, and elevating the head of the bed. Patients who respond completely with no recurrence on such a program can be recommended for flying duties. In more severe cases, long-term medication therapy, including antacids and bethanechol, may be necessary. In chronic reflux esophagitis, surgery may have to be considered. Patients requiring chronic therapy to control symptoms cannot be recommended for military crew duties.[12] If symptoms are controlled, these individuals can fly as passengers. As an item of interest, United States Air Force crewmembers with previous hiatal hernia disease underwent altitude chamber flights before being qualified for flying duties to determine whether gas was being trapped in the hernia. No significant trapping was observed, and altitude chamber exposure is no longer required as part of the evaluation of crewmembers with this condition.

Functional Diarrhea

Patients with chronic or intermittent diarrhea may require extensive treatment programs. Specific diagnosis is often difficult, and treatment may not be completely successful. Individuals with functional diarrhea or irritable bowel syndrome may actually be manifesting a specific food intolerance. If this particular agent can be identified and removed from the diet, it is possible that such individuals may be able to return to flying duties. In other instances, periodic treatment with agents to expand stool bulk may be successful in preventing or controlling symptoms. If such programs are not successful, however, or if follow-up reveals worsening of the condition, these patients may have to be removed from crewmember duties due to the incapacitating nature of the problem. Their ability to fly as a passenger depends on the current status of the disease and response to therapy.

Inflammatory Bowel Disease

Individuals with Crohn's disease or ulcerative colitis may undergo extensive evaluation and treatment before a definitive diagnosis is made. Although these individuals can safely fly as passengers when these conditions are in remission or

have responded to therapy, such patients generally cannot perform duties as a crewmember. Regrettably, a symptom-free period of months or even years does not mean that the individual will not have problems while flying. The long duty hours, schedule disruptions, unusual foods, and other physiologic stresses that flight crews experience appear to be associated with exacerbations in individuals whose conditions were previously considered to be under control. Exacerbations could not only jeopardize flying safety and mission completion but, if they occur at a foreign location without adequate medical aid, could also present a very real threat to the individual. Because of such considerations, crewmembers with either Crohn's disease or ulcerative colitis are usually permanently suspended from flying duties in the military services.

Hemorrhoids

As in other occupations with prolonged sitting, disruption of sleeping and eating schedules, dehydration, poor nutrition, and similar stresses, flying appears to be particularly associated with hemorrhoids. It also appears possible that exposure to G forces may aggravate any tendency toward this condition. Although standard treatment procedures are appropriate for an acute problem, a definitive program to increase the bulk in the diet and hydration may be necessary on a long-term basis to preclude the recurrence of this condition. As in the other medical conditions previously considered, it is essential that the practitioner conduct the necessary evaluation to ensure that symptoms, including any bleeding, are due only to a benign condition and not to a more serious condition such as an underlying malignant tumor.

Other Gastrointestinal Considerations

Patients who have recently undergone intestinal surgery may experience significant pain due to trapped gas if exposed to reduced atmospheric pressures. In addition, sutures could rupture on exposure to such reduced pressures. In accordance with Boyle's Law, appropriately modified to reflect the fact that gases in the body are saturated with water, intestinal gases can expand over 50% at an altitude of 3048 m and over 100% at an altitude of 5468 m. Passengers recovering from intestinal surgery usually should not fly for 2 weeks after surgery, and those individuals with a history of gastrointestinal hemorrhage should defer flying for 3 weeks after the surgery. With respect to returning crewmembers who have undergone abdominal surgery to duty, time recommendations vary depending on the practitioner. In general, crewmembers are restricted from duty until wound healing is complete and full functional return of the affected area has occurred.

Patients with ileostomies and colostomies may fly as passengers after healing is complete. Patients, however, should take extra bags with them when flying because the expansions in the intestinal tract at altitude can produce significantly increased flow and require more frequent bag changes.

GENITOURINARY DISORDERS

Renal Lithiases

Urinary calculi are a significant problem for aviators and passengers. Although such calculi are responsible for approximately one hospital admission per 1000 individuals per year in the United States, the true incidence is considerably higher. Dehydration is associated with prolonged flights, and requirements to perform crew duties in hot environments can further aggravate the dehydration. As a result, the incidence of stone formation may be increased by flight operations. Although some stones can pass with minimal symptoms, others produce severe pain, which can rapidly become incapacitating. Whether in a crewmember or a passenger, the abrupt onset of such pain due to stone passage may require diversion to the nearest air field with medical facilities. The situation can rapidly become critical if the condition occurs in a single pilot of an aircraft.

On occasion, asymptomatic calculi are incidentally discovered in a crewmember during routine evaluation. In such a situation, the aviator's physician has to determine whether the individual should be qualified for continued flying duties. In the United States Air Force, the presence of a retained calculus in the parenchyma or collecting system of the kidney is grounds for disqualification from flying duties. Requalification is possible if the stone is passed, excretory urography reveals no congenital or acquired anomaly, renal function is normal, and any underlying metabolic disorder that could have led to stone formation has been excluded. Waivers are considered for individuals with a stone in a location where passage is not likely, such as a staghorn calculus or a calculus in the parenchyma. The only options previously available to Air Force crewmembers with stones that had the potential to pass, however, were waiting for unpredictable spontaneous stone passage or major open surgery to remove the stone. In 1974, a technique for closed endoscopic manipulation of small, asymptomatic renal stones was developed by Air Force physicians. Patients are first studied to rule out any metabolic or renal disorder. Manipulation is attempted only if the stone is 5 mm or less in size. The procedure involves the use of a ureteral catheter, through which flexible wires are passed to grasp the stone. The stone is then removed with the assistance of these wire grips. The overall success rate has been 65% with very low morbidity.[14] The flyer may then be returned to flying duties if follow-up studies do not demonstrate any residua or changes in the prior normal renal and metabolic status.

Proteinuria

Although most individuals excrete less than 50 mg of protein every 24 hours, some normal people pass considerably more after exercise or prolonged standing. Individuals in this latter category who apply for commercial or military flight training can pose a management problem for the aeromedical practitioner. Although the proteinuria may only represent benign orthostatic proteinura, it also may be the manifestation of significant kidney disease. If there is no significant excretion of protein during a prolonged period of bed rest, urinalysis is otherwise normal, and both renal function and anatomy are normal, the practitioner may recommend qualification. Because the proteinuria possibly represents early kidney disease, even though all the qualifying criteria are met, long-term follow-up on an annual basis is warranted.

OBSTETRIC-GYNECOLOGIC CONSIDERATIONS

Pregnancy

For a number of years, physicians were hesitant to recommend that a pregnant woman fly as either a passenger or a crewmember. Although part of this hesitancy was due to concerns about possible complications during the flight, much of the reluctance was because of fears that hypoxia might produce malformations of the fetus or cause abortions. It has subsequently been determined, however, that the fetus normally lives in an environment where the arterial partial pressure of oxygen is much reduced from that of an adult. The fetus is able to tolerate this environment because fetal oxyhemoglobin is able to deliver all necessary oxygen to the developing tissues. Thus, the normal fetus at sea level has a PO_2 of 32 mm Hg in its umbilical cord arterial blood and 10.6 mm Hg in the cord venous blood.[15] This is in sharp contrast to the PO_2 of approximately 100 mm Hg in the arterial blood of the mother and of 40 mm Hg in the mother's venous circulation. If the mother is breathing a PO_2 equivalent to 2438 m, her arterial

PO_2 drops to 64 mm Hg, but the fetal PO_2 drops only from 32 to 25.6 mm Hg. Even at this level, the maternal arterial oxygen saturation is still approximately 90%. Further assisting the fetal circulation in the delivery of oxygen during such mild hypoxic stress is the fact that the oxygen dissociation curve for fetal hemoglobin differs from that for mature hemoglobin. As a result, the fetal hemoglobin is more fully saturated at lower PO_2 levels than is the mother's. Also, with the change in pH resulting from any hypoxic stress, the dissociation curve shifts to increase oxygen delivery. Thus, the fetus appears able to withstand the hypoxia of a commercial flight. This impression is confirmed by recent findings that birth weights at high altitudes are essentially normal for gestational age.[16] This finding is in contrast to earlier findings that suggested that infants born to mothers living at high altitudes (3000 m) were small for gestational age. The earlier reports, however, did not adequately control for various factors that could affect birth weights, such as variations in the management of pregnancy, and preexisting conditions that could affect birth weights.

Different gestation times have been recommended for the cessation of flight duties by a pregnant crewmember. Recent reports have recommended that commercial crewmembers terminate flying at the thirteeth week, with 20 weeks' gestation as the limit for flight duties.[15] This recommendation is based both on concern over the ability to perform necessary duties and the increased possibility of injury due to the unavailability of adequate restraint systems, particularly during an emergency situation.

With respect to pregnant passengers, authorities also vary in their recommendations. Some experts rely on the judgment of the patient's own physician. Other authorities believe that pregnant passengers generally should not be accepted on flights if they are beyond the thirty-fifth week of gestation unless the flight is short.[2] In such short flights, it may be appropriate to accept patients through the thirty-sixth week. Certainly, both the duration of the flight and possibility for care at an enroute stop must be considered in providing a recommendation for a patient during the later stages of pregnancy.

Menstrual Cycle

Groups of flight attendants in different airlines have been studied in an effort to determine whether flying significantly affects the menstrual cycle. The irregular flight schedules, shifts in circadian rhythm, diet changes, and similar events could reasonably be expected to have an impact on the psychophysiologic factors affecting the menstrual cycle. Although these studies have demonstrated various changes in the cycles of some attendants, it has not always been possible to relate these changes solely to flight activities. One study demonstrated increased irregularity and dysmenorrhea in flight attendants when they first began flying.[17] With increased flight experience (6 years in the referenced study), however, these disorders tended to subside and the cycles to return to normal. This improvement was not due to age changes because individuals who ceased flying again experienced increased irregularity. These findings led the investigators to postulate that flight duties in themselves had less effect than did the stress associated with a job change—in this instance either beginning or ceasing work as a flight attendant.

Studies also have suggested that stewardesses flying transmeridian routes are prone to have irregular menstrual cycles.[18] In general, the irregularity consisted of prolonged cycles, and the investigators noted the possibility that the changes were due to disruption of the circadian rhythm. The investigators used isolation units to study the effects of time-zone changes on stewardesses. They could not demonstrate consistent changes in the group exposed to time-zone changes, however, when compared with a control group.

Stewardesses on another airline noted changes in their menstrual cycle after they began flight duties.[19] Thirty-nine percent reported either the development of menstrual disorders or aggravation of previous disorders as they commenced flight duties. The most frequent problems encountered were hyperpolymenorrhea, dysmenorrhea, or increased irregularity. Neither age nor sexual activity appeared to influence the development of or increase in menstrual disorders. The investigators also found that a large proportion of these women, 38%, experienced pelvic discomfort or congestion after prolonged flights, which could perhaps be attributed to the prolonged times the attendants spend upright or seated.

Although the various studies of the effect of flying on the menstrual cycle have demonstrated changes associated with flying, it is difficult to relate the changes to flying per se. Investigators have emphasized the need for further research to delineate the causes and mechanisms of the observed changes in the menstrual cycle. Overall, it would appear that the changes reflect the impact of the demands and stresses associated with flight duties on the delicately balanced hormonal system involved in menstrual cycles. As might be expected, the impact apparently subsides as the individual adjusts to these demands. At this time, there is no clear evidence that flying duties produce any long-lasting adverse effects on the menstrual cycle of crewmembers.

Acceleration Forces

United States Air Force female crewmembers have participated in acceleration studies on centrifuges for a number of years. An incidental observation during these studies was that exposure to forces up to $+9\,G_z$ did not produce any uterine problems. Nor were adverse effects reported during menstruation. Isolated instances of stress incontinence were reported in some subjects during high G loads and with anti-G suit inflation. Because pregnant women were excluded from these studies, it is not possible to define any possible deleterious effects of acceleration forces in this group.

ENDOCRINE AND METABOLIC ABNORMALITIES

Diabetes Mellitus

The spectrum of diabetes mellitus can extend from mild abnormalities of glucose metabolism detected only on screening examinations of blood to severe forms requiring intensive long-term therapy to prevent episodes of coma and, eventually, death. Although an individual requiring daily supplemental insulin cannot be qualified for flight duties, people with milder forms of the disease may be able to perform flying duties safely. Similarly, some passengers with diabetes mellitus may experience no difficulty during long flights, whereas flying may place other diabetics in a life-threatening situation.

Before considering recommendations for such individuals any further, it is perhaps appropriate to stress the necessity of confirming the diagnosis in patients with milder forms of the disease before recommending qualification or disqualification. Glycosuria only indicates the need for further evaluation and is not diagnostic. The standard test for evaluating the condition is the glucose tolerance test, but it also can be a misleading diagnostic tool. Although the need for effective carbohydrate loading (e.g., 150 g of carbohydrate for at least 3 days before the test) has been documented,[20] glucose tolerance testing is still accomplished without such a preparation. Of particular concern to the aerospace medicine practitioner is the fact an "abnormal" determination may be a false-positive result. Further evaluation could disclose that the abnormal result was due

to fasting, some other physiologic factor, or a different disease state.

Unless detected, a false-positive determination can result in a recommendation for disqualification for flying duties that can affect an individual's career and job opportunities for life. For example, on rare occasions, combat military crewmembers have been unnecessarily disqualified for a period of weeks because of a false-positive glucose tolerance test. Proper investigation, including a repeat glucose tolerance test after appropriate carbohydrate loading, revealed the spurious nature of the first determination, and the flyers were returned to duties.

Diagnosis of actual diabetes may be made by the Fajans and Conn criteria, Public Health Service criteria, World Health Organization criteria, or similar criteria. Some individuals with definite abnormalities can be considered for a return to flying duties. In the United States Air Force, a flight surgeon can recommend continued flying duties for a flyer with a confirmed abnormal glucose tolerance test if the blood glucose levels, as measured by the Somogyi-Nelson, O-Toluidine, AutoAnalyzer, glucose oxidase, or hexokinase methods, are no greater than 120 mg/dL fasting and 140 mg/dL 2 hours postprandial. Such a recommendation is contingent on the absence of any evidence of end-organ disease, no evidence of ketoacidosis, no signs or symptoms of hyperglycemia or hypoglycemia, and no use of any medication, particularly oral hypoglycemic agents. It should be noted that it has been found possible to return the blood glucose levels of some patients with levels above 140 mg/dL to an acceptable level through a weight reduction program alone. Some authorities might argue that individuals with an elevated glucose tolerance test have an increased tendency toward diabetes, and any deficiency in preparation for the test or weight elevation merely unmasked this tendency. Although it is appropriate to follow such patients to rule out the subsequent development of diabetes, it is not necessary to suspend trained aviators if subsequent tests disclose no abnormalities. One of the more satisfying aspects of the practice of aerospace medicine is watching a previously disqualified crewmember attain acceptable blood glucose levels solely through weight control. Although such aviators require periodic follow-up to ensure they do not develop more significant glucose elevations, their return to flying status benefits both them and their operational organization. The International Civil Aviation Organization (ICAO) and some airlines will allow consideration of the use of oral antidiabetic agents if their use is compatible with safe aircraft operation or air traffic control duties. Final decision in such instances is left to the appropriate national or military organization. In ICAO countries, the return of flyers using such agents is generally restricted to selected cases involving private pilots or air traffic controllers.

In considering candidates for crewmember training, both family history and current status are significant. A family history of diabetes in both parents places an individual in a prediabetic group at increased risk of developing diabetes. Intermittent glycosuria with abnormalities on glucose tolerance testing may place the patient in a "latent" or "chemical" diabetes category. These applicants also may have an increased chance of developing diabetes. Consequently, it may be appropriate to disqualify such individuals for military or commercial training rather than place them in an expensive training program for a career that has a higher-than-average risk of being terminated due to a medical disqualification. Applicants for private pilot training could be qualified with appropriate follow-up by the examiner.

Although the use of insulin generally precludes an individual from crewmember duties, numerous airline passengers do require this therapy. These individuals

may tolerate even long flights without problems. A required diabetic diet can be obtained on many airlines, and the passenger can carry the necessary insulin on the flight. The irregular meal schedules, fatigue, circadian rhythm shifts, difficulty in obtaining proper medical care for many medical problems, emotional stresses, and similar factors associated with flying can affect insulin requirements and dosage schedules, however. Compounding the problem are difficulties replacing medication, syringes, or needles that are damaged or lost in baggage transfer. Because of these factors, it is recommended that diabetic patients consult their physician before undertaking air travel to ensure that necessary adjustments to the dosage schedule are planned and any required arrangements for medication replacement are made.

Thyroid Disorders

Thyroid disorders can be similar to diabetes mellitus in presenting difficult diagnostic challenges to the practitioner. Certainly, tests for L-thyroxine (T4), 3,5,3-triiodo-L-thyroxine (T3), thyroid-stimulating hormone (thyrotropin, or TSH), the binding globulins, and other aspects of thyroid function have markedly assisted in the diagnosis of abnormalities. The manifestation of disease can be varied, however, and so many complaints can be attributed to any demonstrated abnormality that the physician faces a significant challenge in considering and then diagnosing the disorder, particularly in its earlier or milder forms.

Once the abnormality has been diagnosed and appropriately treated, the diagnostic tests used to uncover it are also of marked benefit in determining whether an aviator can return to flying duties. A patient with hyperthyroidism can be considered for a return to flying activities if treatment has produced a euthyroid status, as determined by appropriate endocrine studies, and there is no evidence of end-organ disease. In addition to cardiovascular effects, ophthalmopathy, myopathic problems, or evidence of a central nervous system disorder are of particular concern in evaluating a flyer with a history of hyperthyroidism.

Treatment of hyperthyroidism may result in clinical hypothyroidism. Whether spontaneous or as the result of hyperthyroidism therapy, adult-onset hypothyroidism does not necessarily require permanent suspension from flying duties if treatment has produced a euthyroid condition. Again, the practitioner must ascertain whether there is any evidence of cardiovascular or other end-organ disease. If the condition did not result from the treatment of hyperthyroidism, a central nervous system disorder must be ruled out. If no complicating factors are present and the patient has attained a euthyroid condition, a recommendation to return to flying duty may be considered. The use of long-term thyroid therapy does not preclude a return to flying duties. Naturally, in either situation, the practitioner must observe the patient for a sufficient period to ensure that a stable euthyroid status has been achieved and that there are no side effects from any required thyroid replacement therapy. Depending on the circumstances involved, this observation period may last several months.

Gout

Elevated uric acid levels may be associated with the typical symptoms of gout or may be detected fortuitously during a routine screening examination. Although the patient may present with a uric acid renal stone, the more usual manifestation is acute arthritis, typically in the first metatarsophalangeal joint. Because gout may involve multiple joints, as in rheumatoid arthritis, radiographic examinations may not be diagnostic. Uric acid levels also can be misleading, and the detection of negatively birefringent monosodium urate crystals in joint fluid is considered to be the hallmark of the disease. The aerospace medicine physician must not only be concerned with the diagnostic challenge of this condition but also determine what treatment program is appropriate for the patient with symptoms, as well as for the individual who has only elevated serum uric acid levels. If the patient is an aviator, the physician must then make the appropriate aeromedical recommendation.

An elevated uric acid level may be due either to the overproduction or underexcretion of uric acid. This distinction is of more than academic interest because it can play a significant role in determining which type of therapeutic agent to use if treatment is indicated. Making the distinction is complicated by the fact that some commonly prescribed therapeutic agents can affect the serum acid levels. Thus, aspirin in small doses, the chlorothiazides, some other diuretics, acute alcohol ingestion, and ethambutol will reduce the renal excretion of uric acid. If such factors are excluded, a patient can be considered an overproducer if more than 600 mg/day of uric acid is excreted after a 5-day period of restriction of dietary purines. These patients can be treated by attempting to inhibit uric acid production with an agent such as allopurinol. The majority of patients with elevated uric acid levels are underexcreters. These individuals can be managed with a uricosuric agent, such as probenecid, unless renal function is impaired, with a creatine clearance of less than 80 ml/min, tophaceous tophi are present, the patient excretes over 700 mg/day of uric acid on a regular diet, or uric acid nephrolithiasis occurs.[21]

Although the above treatment programs can be effective in caring for symptomatic patients with elevated uric acid levels, a number of individuals with asymptomatic hyperuricemia do not require therapy. In evaluating these patients, it is first necessary to ensure that the finding is not due to medication or underlying conditions such as a malignancy. Once such etiologic possibilities are excluded, the examiner must then consider whether treatment is warranted. Although considerable controversy exists, the treatment of asymptomatic elevations of uric acid may be deferred unless symptoms occur, the patient has a strong family history of renal disease, renal lithiasis, or gout, or excretes over 1000 mg/day of uric acid.[22] It should be noted that some patients with asymptomatic elevated uric acid levels who meet the criteria for treatment may respond to simple dietary control and weight loss alone.

If treatment with medication is initiated in a patient with either symptomatic or asymptomatic uric acid elevations, a return to flying duties should be deferred until a response to the treatment, as well as the absence of side effects, is demonstrated. Once the uric acid level is controlled and there is no evidence of gout complications or undesirable effects from any required medication, the physician may recommend a return to flying duties. If the elevation is an incidental finding in an asymptomatic patient and none of the criteria for treatment exist, the examiner may recommend continued flying duties.

MALIGNANT TUMORS

General Considerations

Many individuals with a history of a malignant tumor can fly safely as passengers or crewmembers. Others could pose a serious risk to themselves or others, even though there is no evidence of a tumor recurrence. The aerospace medicine physician must consider a number of factors in attempting to decide between the alternative recommendations concerning flying. Some items that have proven to be valuable in developing an appropriate recommendation for a particular patient are considered in the following sections.

Tumor Classification

The more virulent forms of a tumor may place the individual at increased risk of recurrence. Because the more aggressive neoplasms may express themselves sooner, however, the physician may be able to categorize a recurrence-free patient as "cured" sooner than would be possible if the tumor were not so virulent. It may thus be appropriate to recommend a return to flying duties sooner for the patient with a history of a more serious type of malignancy than for the patient with a less serious form. Such action would reflect the fact that if the patient survives, the risk of recurrence drops to an acceptable level faster than it does for a more slowly growing tumor, where a more prolonged period of observation is necessary to rule out recurrence.

Staging at Diagnosis

Spread of the tumor beyond the primary site obviously increases the risk of recurrence. For many tumors, however, local extension does not carry the severe prognosis that evidence of spread to more distant sites does. Microstaging also may provide information of value in defining the risk of recurrence. In melanoma, for example, microstaging by the methods of Breslow and Clark can aid in predicting both regional lymph node metastases and prognosis.

Method of Treatment

Once the type and staging of a malignant tumor are known, it is usually possible to define the expected effectiveness of the particular treatment regimen that was applied. In evaluating the patient, it is important to consider not only the effect of the treatment of the malignancy but also the impact on the physical and mental functioning of the patient. Radionecrosis, hormone imbalance, restricted use of an extremity, or similar results from therapy have the potential to restrict the patient from crewmember duties as completely as recurrence of the malignancy.

Current Therapy

The flight surgeon evaluating a crew-member for a possible return to status after treatment of a malignant tumor must evaluate the current therapy. Both the effectiveness of the therapy and the existence of any side effects have to be ascertained. Therapy may include long-term or periodic chemotherapy as well as medication to compensate for the necessary side effects of treatment. For example, hormone therapy may be required permanently after testicular, thyroid, or ovarian surgery. It may be possible to return the patient to flying duties on chronic maintenance therapy if there are no deleterious side effects and the therapy restores the individual to an essentially normal state.

Recurrence

Overall, the risk of recurrence decreases as the time without a recurrence increases. It is difficult, however, to use standard mortality tables to determine the earliest point when the risk of recurrence falls to an acceptable level to recommend flying duties. Conrad and colleagues[23] analyzed United States Air Force experience regarding cancer treatment and survival in an effort to provide information the flight surgeon could use to recommend return to flying. These investigators analyzed a series of Air Force patients with malignant tumors to develop techniques to help predict the chance of tumor recurrence. One technique is the hazard function. This technique defines the risk of developing a recurrence within the immediate future for all individuals who have survived to the beginning of a given time period. This is not the percentage of the entire patient population but only of that proportion which had been recurrence-free until the start of a given time period. The examiner can apply this information as a hazard rate to predict when the risk of recurrence has fallen to an acceptable level to recommend return to flying. The physician could, for example, decide that an acceptable hazard

rate was 5%, which means that only one patient in 20 who has survived recurrence-free to that point in time will develop a recurrence. Using hazard function information for that specific malignancy, the practitioner can thus determine how long a period of time is required before the patient reaches an acceptable level of risk. These techniques are more useful than the usual survival rates because the survival rates include patients with recurrences who are still alive. Consequently, survival rates cannot be used to predict recurrences. Hazard function information also can be used to predict the onset of symptomatic recurrence in conditions where the disease, although not cured, is in remission for a prolonged period.[24] Hodgkin's disease is one such condition. In some forms of the disease, a patient may be symptom-free for several years after therapy with a risk of symptomatic recurrence of less than 5%. In later years, the risk of recurrence increases, and the individual may require increased monitoring to detect new activity. Although the patient may have to be disqualified if a symptomatic recurrence occurs, the flight surgeon could have safely allowed the aviator to fly during earlier, low-risk years.

Site of Recurrence

The physician also has to determine whether a recurrence will be heralded by warning signs or symptoms or whether the first indication of complication may be abrupt incapacitation. Obviously, aeromedical disposition would be different if there were a significant risk of sudden incapacitation than would be the case if there were gradual progression. Even a recurrence hazard rate of less than 5% may be unacceptable for tumors where the initial sign of spread is a seizure or other form of abrupt incapacitation. Lung carcinoma, for example, is the most common metastatic tumor of the brain, and the physician may well choose to defer a return to flying duties for these patients even after the recurrence risk was less than would otherwise be acceptable.

Current Physical and Mental Status

A person who is treated for a life-threatening malignancy may experience long-lasting mental as well as physical effects. A residual physical defect can be evaluated in the same manner as it would be in an individual without a history of malignant tumor. The evaluation of mental trauma and effects is more difficult. Many patients experience the same acute emotional trauma at the time of initial diagnosis as do patients with confirmed terminal illnesses. Subsequent to the psychologic trauma resulting from the diagnosis, the patient undergoes the strain of waiting for the results of studies for metastasis. Then the patient awaits the outcome of the treatment program. Throughout these periods, the patient is continually concerned about whether a new symptom or finding represents recurrence. Changed relationships with family members or friends can add to the stress. In some patients, the emotional aspects can be overwhelming, even in the absence of objective evidence of recurrence. Such stresses can result in drastic action, and an "accidental death" in a patient with a known or suspected recurrence may actually be suicide. Because of such considerations, it is imperative that the physician ascertain both the mental and physical stability of a patient being considered for a return to flying duties. Even passengers must be similarly evaluated because disaster could result if a patient with actual or only suspected extension of a malignancy decided to take drastic action during a flight.

Specific Tumors

Germinal Cell Tumors of the Testes

Germinal cell tumors of the testes are among the more common malignant tumors in older males in the military. They can be classified by cell type using Dixon and Moore criteria and staged according to Whitmore's formulation. Conrad and colleagues[25] analyzed 551 cases of such tumors and determined the hazard rate for different combinations of type, stage, and treatment. For example, the hazard rate for recurrence falls to less than 5% after 1 year for teratocarcinoma (Dixon-Moore type IV) stage A (tumor confined to the testis and adnexa). Depending on the function of the other testis, lifelong testosterone replacement therapy may be necessary. Treatment may include lymphadenectomy, which can produce varying degrees of lymphedema. Should a teratocarcinoma of this type and stage recur, it would not be expected to produce incapacitation. Considering these factors, a recurrence-free patient with type IV, stage A tumor seen 1 year after definitive treatment could be considered for a return to flying duties. Return would be contingent on the absence of significant lymphedema or any other physical problem, serum hormone studies demonstrating adequate testosterone replacement, and an appropriate mental status.

Melanoma

Melanoma demonstrates the need to evaluate the possibility of abrupt incapacitation. Moseley and colleagues[26] evaluated 712 patients with this disease. Lesions were classified according to body site and staged to reflect spread from the primary site. When possible, microstaging using the techniques of Clark and Breslow was accomplished. Melanoma is known to metastasize to the brain, doing so in approximately one third of the cases. The brain, however, is not always the first site of metastases in this malignancy. These investigators found that the brain was the first site of recurrence in only 8% of stage III (disseminated melanoma) patients. In addition, the metastasis presented as a catastrophic event, such as a stroke or seizure, in only 1.6% of stage III patients. The risk of a catastrophic event dropped to 0.6% for the entire group of patients. Conrad and colleagues[23] studied 604 patients with melanoma, out of whom 184 had recurrent disease. Thirty-one percent of these patients had a brain metastasis, and central nervous system symptoms were the first evidence of recurrence in 7% of the 184 patients with recurrent disease. No catastrophic event occurred without prior symptoms in this study. The hazard rate for recurrence varied with tumor location and staging. For example, the hazard rate decreased to less than 5% in 3 years for head or neck lesions with negative lymph nodes but did not reach this level for 5 years for lesions on the trunk with negative lymph nodes. Considering the results of such studies, it is possible, if no other physical or mental contraindications exist, to recommend a return to flying duties for selected patients with a history of melanoma in spite of the possibility of metastasis to the brain. Conversely, if a patient has extensive disease, it may be appropriate to recommend against even passenger flight because of the risk of a seizure.

ORTHOPEDIC DISORDERS

Fractures, Sprains, and Dislocations

Although passengers can fly with an arm or leg cast, crewmembers must be able to perform their functions unencumbered. Further, theyusually must have normal function of the musculoskeletal system to accomplish the myriad of tasks involved in flight activities. In general, a crewmember who has experienced an orthopedic injury should not be qualified for a return to flight duties until the injured part has regained essentially normal motion and muscle strength. In addition, no residual discomfort or pain should be present at rest or during exertion that could restrict required activity. For example, a pilot may have a normal range of motion after an ankle injury but be unable to apply nec-

essary brake pressure due to residual pain. A flight attendant with apparently normal range of arm motion may not be able to operate emergency equipment because of residual muscle weakness or pain restriction. Such examples emphasize the need to ensure that the crewmember with a "healed" injury is in fact fully qualified for a return to duty. They also demonstrate the need for the aerospace medicine physician to have detailed knowledge of the crewmember's duties to make appropriate recommendations.

In still other instances, some obvious residual defect in strength or motion will exist in spite of excellent care. Again, the evaluating examiner needs to have sufficient knowledge of the crewmember's tasks to determine whether return to flying is appropriate. In evaluating patients with and without residual defects, the physician may find it beneficial to evaluate the patient in the actual work place. Monitoring a patient throughout a simulated flight has uncovered previously unsuspected problems that could compromise flying safety or the individual's well-being.

Another consideration in evaluating a postinjury patient is whether there is any predisposition to further injury in the flight environment. For example, a patient seen at the Aeromedical Consultation Center of USAFSAM had experienced a cervical spine fracture during a dive into a pool. He received prompt attention, and the paralysis he initially experienced due to spinal cord compression gradually subsided. He eventually regained essentially normal function and applied for flight training. The healing process had resulted in a marked angulation of the cervical spine, however. If the applicant were to participate in operational flying and had to eject, the very real possibility existed that the ejection forces could produce a fracture and even transsection of the spinal cord. Consequently, even though his musculoskeletal function was acceptable, the individual had to be disqualified for military flight duties.

A similar concern about the possibility of increased liability for reinjury was studied in crewmembers who had experienced a compression fracture during an ejection and then subsequently had to eject again.[27] In open ejection-seat aircraft, the T-10 to L-2 vertebrae are most frequently injured, usually as a compression fracture, during ejection. The compression fractures typically heal without difficulty, and the flyers return to flying duties. The review of crewmembers with this history who were involved in a subsequent ejection did not reveal any increased risk of additional fractures during the later ejection.

It is necessary to analyze the geometry of applied forces in analyzing injuries resulting from ejections. As mentioned, the lower thoracic and upper lumbar vertebrae are typically injured in open ejection seats. In ejections involving the crew-escape module of the FB-111, however, the T-4, 5, 6, and 7 vertebrae were most frequently affected. Investigation revealed that these vertebrae were affected because the geometry of the application of forces was altered due to positioning caused by preejection retraction of the inertia reel and positioning during ground impact of the module.[28] Action was initiated to modify the support and restraint system in an effort to prevent those injuries.

Back Pain

One of the more frequent conditions evaluated in family practice is back pain, and this problem is common to flyers, as well. Prolonged sitting, on occasion in seats without properly designed support, may cause initial or recurrent low back pain in passengers or crewmembers. The problem may be aggravated further for aircrew who have to wear personal equipment, including parachutes, and remain strapped in place throughout a long flight. These and similar stresses result in frequent patient visits to the flight surgeon

for the evaluation and treatment of back pain.

In evaluating a complaint of back pain, the examiner, of course, must rule out such disorders as renal lithiasis or malignant tumors. In some patients, the physician may detect significant disk disease, which can only be corrected by surgery. In most patients, however, the symptoms are due to mechanical derangement of the spine, often caused by faulty sitting or standing posture or improper use at work. Obesity and lack of exercise also may contribute to mechanical symptoms. The evaluation and treatment of this group may be complicated by the very studies obtained to rule out a more serious cause. For example, lumbosacral spine radiographs may demonstrate degenerative changes. Both the physician and the patient may then attribute the symptoms to these changes. It is known, however, that similar changes are present in a large proportion of otherwise normal individuals without any history of back pain. Consequently, it is possible that the changes seen in a particular patient are unrelated to the symptoms of that patient. Such possibilities are of concern in the long-term management of the patient. The acute symptoms may respond promptly to a standard treatment program, including bed rest with a firm mattress or bed board, heat, analgesics, and muscle relaxants. If the patient and practitioner believe that the symptoms are the inevitable consequence of back disease, they may feel there is no way to prevent future episodes. If, however, the practitioner decides all or most of the symptoms have a muscular etiology, the patient can be strongly encouraged to begin a program of regular low back exercises and proper use of the back in an effort to prevent a recurrence of the pain. A similar situation exists for those patients who have had surgery for an actual herniated nucleus pulposus or other spine disorder. Again, these patients may naturally attribute any subsequent back pain to the earlier surgery. As a result, they do not begin a program that may be successful in preventing future symptoms.

Back pain also may be a vexing problem for the practitioner because of the well-recognized fact that a patient may consciously or subconsciously use the complaint to avoid an unpleasant duty, for compensation, or for some other reason. This can result either in complaints when no symptoms actually exist or in exaggerations of the amount of discomfort present. The astute physician may be able to demonstrate the emotional or malingering basis of the complaints. Techniques such as accomplishing straight leg raising without pain by extending the legs while the patient is seated may convince both the physician and the patient that no further treatment is required. In other situations, particularly when the actual symptoms are exaggerated, demonstrating the actual cause of the pain is more difficult. Numerous evaluations and consultations may be necessary before a final appropriate disposition is accomplished.

Scoliosis

Scoliosis is an abnormal lateral curvature of the spine, with an associated lack of normal thoracic spine flexibility. The resultant change in the structure of the spine affects the response of the spine to both static and dynamic loads. As noted in the discussion of ejection injuries, the dynamics of force application have to be evaluated in an individual who is exposed to the stresses of flight. With increasing lateral curvature, the risk of symptoms and injury are increased if the individual is exposed to ejection or other high G forces. For example, one aviator with scoliosis experienced incapacitating back pain while experiencing 6.5 G in an F-4E aircraft. The pilot in the rear seat took control and landed. The patient could not exit the aircraft and had to be lifted from it by rescue personnel. The pain was at the point of maximum curvature of the spine where

old degenerative changes were present. Because of concern about the possibility of such incapacitation, current United States Air Force directives preclude flying duties for an individual with more than 20° of scoliosis as measured by the Cobb method.

Spondylolysis and Spondylolisthesis

Spondylolysis and spondylolisthesis appear to be manifestations of a fracture or cleft in the pars interarticularis of the vertebrae. In spondylolysis, there is no concomitant vertebral slippage. In spondylolisthesis, the vertebral body involved slips anteriorly on the vertebral body inferior to the affected vertebral body. These defects appear to reduce the ability of the spine to withstand the application of mechanical force. An increased incidence of back pain has been reported in patients with spondylolysis, and high G forces may produce symptoms in an individual with spondylolisthesis.[29] Such considerations preclude a recommendation for flying if the individual will be exposed to high G forces.

Klippel-Feil Syndrome

In contrast to the defects and slippage of spondylolisthesis, patients with the Klippel-Feil syndrome have fusion and deformities of the cervical vertebrae that result in restricted neck motion and, on occasion, symptoms of nerve involvement. This deformity also has been found in crewmembers experiencing pain after high G maneuvers.[29] The spine of patients with this condition is thought to be susceptible to fracture with relatively low G loads, and, as a consequence, individuals with this condition also should not be qualified for flying in situations where significantly increased G forces may occur.

Other Spinal Problems

Other conditions, such as Scheuermann's disease (rigid kyphotic deformity of the lower thoracic spine) and spondylosis deformans (occurrence of bony protuberances on the upper or lower ridges of vertebral bodies), also affect the ability of the spine to tolerate increased G forces. As a result, individuals with either of these conditions should be disqualified for flying duties in situations where they may be exposed to increased G forces.

OTHER CONDITIONS OF AEROMEDICAL SIGNIFICANCE

Sarcoidosis

Until relatively recently, aerospace medicine physicians usually recommended a return to flying duties for crewmembers who had sarcoidosis, provided certain criteria were met. These criteria included resolution, or at least prolonged stability, of any pulmonary adenopathy or infiltrates, normal pulmonary function studies, and the absence of any requirement for medications.

More recently, there have been disturbing reports of myocardial involvement at a rate far greater than previously suspected.[30,31] Sarcoid involvement of the heart has been reported in up to 27% of autopsies of patients with sarcoidosis.[32] Of particular concern to the aerospace medicine physician is the fact that such involvement can lead to conduction disturbances, arrhythmias, and sudden death. Indeed, sudden death has been reported in over 50% of patients with myocardial sarcoidosis.[33] Such a high frequency is found primarily in patients with more severe cardiac involvement who, as a result, usually had a history of cardiac symptoms. An increased incidence of arrhythmias and conduction disturbances, however, has been reported in patients whose myocardial involvement could only be demonstrated histologically.[32] The significance of myocardial sarcoidosis was recently demonstrated in a United States Air Force crewmember who was found to have pulmonary sarcoidosis during a routine periodic examination. Before evalu-

ation of the condition could be completed, he abruptly collapsed at his home and died. Autopsy studies demonstrated previously unrecognized sarcoidosis of the heart, and this condition was considered to be the cause of death.

Neurologic involvement also has been reported in sarcoidosis. Recent studies suggest that such involvement, although uncommon, is not the rare event once supposed. Although only limited autopsy studies are available and both peripheral and central nervous system involvement are grouped together, it appears that the nervous system may be involved in up to 5% of patients with sarcoidosis.[34] Of particular concern is the fact that neurologic abnormalities may be the first manifestation of the disease. Further, in those patients with neurologic symptoms, the more critical central nervous system involvement tends to occur early in the disease, whereas peripheral involvement is more often seen later in the chronic conditions.

Such findings resulted in extensive revision of the protocol for the evaluation of patients with sarcoidosis who were referred to the Aeromedical Consultation Center at USAFSAM. These flyers are evaluated by specialists in aerospace medicine, internal medicine, ophthalmology, neurology, and otolaryngology. In addition to the usual extensive laboratory screening studies, electroencephalogram, resting and exercise stress testing (treadmill) electrocardiograms, and abdominal and chest radiographs, the following are accomplished:

1. Holter monitor for 24 hours
2. Thallium myocardial scan
3. Gallium-67 citrate pulmonary and abdominal visceral scans
4. Skin testing with purified protein derivative tuberculin agent, mumps, and Monilia antigen
5. Coccidiomycosis and histoplasmosis serologic testing

6. Serum protein electrophoresis
7. 24-hour urine collection for calcium
8. Serum lactic dehydrogenase and creatine phosphokinase
9. Serum angiotensin I converting enzyme
10. Bronchoscopy with endobronchial and transbronchial biopsy only in patients with active disease in whom the diagnosis is in question

All crewmembers in whom the diagnosis is confirmed are disqualified for at least 2 years from the date when the diagnosis was established. Recommendations for flying duties are considered 2 years after diagnosis if the following criteria are met:

1. No use of anti-inflammatory agents
2. No disease activity, as evidenced by the following:
   a. No symptoms or signs of active sarcoidosis
   b. Normalization of adenopathy, including hilar adenopathy, radiographically. (Some gallium-67 citrate uptake into hilar nodes can be consistent with clinical inactivity.)
   c. Nonprogression of any pulmonary parenchymal infiltrates and no increase of gallium-67 citrate uptake into the infiltrates
   d. Stability of pulmonary function testing, especially of any restrictive components
   e. In general, normalization of significant supporting biochemical tests, such as serum and urine calcium, serum protein electrophoresis, erythrocyte sedimentation rate, and serum angiotensin convertase. Unrelated conditions of no aeromedical significance may cause minor abnormalities in some tests. Such abnormalities due to unrelated conditions will be delineated in the evaluations.

The criteria for permanent disqualification are as follows:

1. Bone or skin sarcoidosis
2. Posterior uveitis secondary to sarcoidosis
3. Cardiac involvement, as evidenced by such findings as AV block greater than first degree, significant arrhythmia (atrial, junctional, or ventricular ectopy greater than 10 beats/min or greater than 20% of the exercise heart rate or any paired ectopy), bundle branch block patterns, myocardial infarction, ventricular hypertrophy patterns, abnormal thallium scintigraphy or gallium-67 citrate uptake into the heart
4. Central nervous system involvement

Because of the increased concern regarding sarcoidosis, United States Air Force aviators who had previously been granted a waiver for sarcoidosis were reevaluated, according to the protocol delineated. Of the first 34 flyers reevaluated, six (18%) were diagnosed as having myocardial sarcoidosis. This frequency was in agreement with that reported in the literature (13 to 27%). The diagnosis of cardiac involvement was based primarily on a persistent filling defect on resting and exercise thallium scintigraphy. Two of the six patients also had defects on the gallium-67 citrate scans that matched those of the thallium-fixed defect. None of the six patients had cardiac symptoms, and it is noteworthy that only two patients still had bilateral hilar adenopathy. This finding is in accord with the suggestion by some authors that patients with myocardial involvement may not show other evidence of persistent or active disease.[33] Of concern is the fact that one individual so evaluated had normal scans 58 months after the sarcoidosis initially was diagnosed. One year later (approximately 70 months after the initial diagnosis), both his gallium and thallium scans were positive. Such findings have resulted in the recommendation for annual evaluations for any flyer with a history of sarcoidosis.

Dermatitis

Dermatitis is one of the leading causes of loss of time in industrial workers, and flyers may be affected similarly by skin disorders. Aviators may be exposed to dehydration during flight and then have to cope with increased temperatures, excessive humidity, and resultant marked perspiration during ground operations. Life-support and personal equipment, such as oxygen masks or parachute straps, can initiate skin reactions or further irritate an involved area of the skin. Prolonged operations with disruption of personal hygiene can set the stage for infection or other aggravation of an otherwise easily managed dermatologic problem. These complications may make diagnosis particularly difficult in spite of the usual scrapings, cultures, and other diagnostic procedures. As a result, appropriate therapy may be delayed. Of equal concern, dermatologic manifestations of an underlying systemic disorder may be so modified that the physician fails to diagnose the true cause of the skin condition. For example, aviators may be treated for a stubborn skin ailment over a period of months by different practitioners. Therapeutic failures may repeatedly be ascribed to aggravation resulting from flight operations before the actual cause, for example, an underlying diabetes mellitus, is diagnosed. Exposure to a variety of often exotic agents also may complicate diagnostic or therapeutic efforts. Many man-hours were recently expended in attempting to determine why flight attendants on one particular over-water commercial flight repeatedly developed an unusual dermatitis. Only after prolonged study was it found that the reactions were due to chemicals in the life vests the attendants used for demonstrations at the start of the flights.

In addition to making the diagnostic problem more difficult, flight duties also may foil treatment efforts or delay healing of the skin problem. The aggravating environmental factors and hygiene difficulties that made diagnosis a problem may likewise adversely affect therapy. In some instances, cure is possible only if the individual is removed from flight duties until healing is complete. Unfortunately, if the aviator has a chronic skin problem, such suspension may be for a prolonged period. In more severe situations, the crewmember may have to be permanently disqualified from flight duties.

Systemic therapy may be indicated for some conditions, and in many instances medication can be prescribed without prolonged disqualification from flying duties. Tetracycline may have to be used for a long period to treat severe acne. It is usually possible to recommend a return to flying duties for crewmembers receiving this medication after an appropriate observation period, approximately 4 weeks, to rule out any significant side effects.

In other situations, systemic medications may not be compatible with flying duties. It is usually appropriate to disqualify individuals on systemic steroid therapy from flying. This action not only helps prevent the onset of a complication at an en-route stop where only limited medical care may be available but also ensures that the physician will be able to evaluate the therapeutic response at the desired time. Systemic medications for fungal skin conditions also can preclude flight duties. Griseofulvin may be highly effective in controlling resistant fungal infections. This agent, however, has a number of significant side effects, including fatigue, dizziness, mental confusion, and impairment of performance of routine duties. Such effects obviously could be a significant hazard for an aviator. Because of this potential, United States Air Force policy precludes a crewmember from performing flight duties while taking griseofulvin.

As mentioned in the beginning of this chapter, it is not possible to consider all the medical conditions that can occur in flyers. It also should be recognized that the recommendations for even those conditions discussed cannot be considered absolute. The rapid progress in medicine will undoubtedly produce significant changes in the management of many conditions in the near future. The selected disorders are, however, representative of the more common problems that develop in aviators, and the principles of aerospace medicine used in evaluating and caring for patients with these conditions apply also to all other medical and surgical circumstances. Through the application of these principles, aerospace medicine physicians can develop appropriate treatment programs, including recommendations regarding flying, for the flyers they serve.

REFERENCES

1. Scott, V.: Anemia and airline flight duties. Aviat. Space Environ. Med., 46(6):830–835, 1975.
2. Green, R.L.: Carriage of invalid passengers in civil airlines. In Aviation Medicine. Edited by G. Dhenin, et al. London, Tri-Med Books Ltd., 1978.
3. McKenzie, J.M.: Evaluation of the hazards of sickle cell trait in aviation. Aviat. Space Environ. Med., 48(8):753–762, 1977.
4. Jones, F.R.: Haemoglobinopathies in relation to aviation. In Aviation Medicine. Edited by G. Dhenin, et al. London, Tri-Med Books Ltd., 1978.
5. Sears, D.A.: The morbidity of sickle cell trait, a review of the literature. Am. J. Med., 64:1021–1036, 1978.
6. Ad Hoc Committee on S-Hemoglobinopathies: The S-Hemoglobinopathies: An Evaluation of Their Status in the Armed Forces. National Research Council, National Academy of Sciences. Washington, D.C., National Academy Press, 1973.
7. Buley, L.E.: Incidence, causes and results of airline pilot incapacitation while on duty. Aerospace Med., 40(1):64–70, 1969.
8. DuPont, H.L., and Hornick, R.B.: Adverse effect of Lomotil therapy in shigellosis. JAMA, 226:1525–1528, 1973.
9. Kent, T.H., et al.: Acute enteritis due to Salmonella typhimurium in opium-treated guinea pigs. Arch. Pathol., 81:501–508, 1966.
10. Sack, D.A., et al.: Prophylactic doxycycline for travelers' diarrhea. Gastroenterology, 76:1368–1373, 1979.
11. Gangarosa, E.J., Kendrick, M.A., Lowenstein, M.D., Merson, M.H., et al.: Global travel and travelers' health. Aviat. Space Environ. Med., 51(7):265–270, 1980.
12. Air Force Regulation 160-43: Medical Examination and Medical Standards, No. 160-43.

Washington, D.C., United States Air Force Headquarters, 1979, (as supplemented).
13. Rayman, R.B.: Bleeding duodenal ulcer and the flier. Aviat. Space Environ. Med., 49(10): 1231–1234, 1978.
14. Novicki, D.D., and Ball, T.P., Jr.: Intrarenal stone manipulation in military aviators. Paper presented at the 53rd Annual Scientific Meeting, Aerospace Medical Association, 1982. Aviat. Space Environ. Med. (in press).
15. Scholten, P.: Pregnant stewardess—should she fly? Aviat. Space Environ. Med., 47(1):77–81, 1976.
16. Cotton, E.K., Hiestand, M., Philbin, G.E., and Simmons, M.: Reevaluation of birth weights at high altitude. Study of babies born to mothers living at an altitude of 3100 meters. Am. J. Obstet. Gynecol., 138:220–222, 1980.
17. Cameron, R.G.: Effect of flying on the menstrual function of air hostesses. Aerospace Med., 40(9):1020–1023, 1969.
18. Preston, F.S., Bateman, S.C., Short, R.V., and Wilkinson, R.T.: Effects of flying and of time changes on menstrual cycle length and on performance in airline stewardesses. Aerospace Med., 44(4):438–443, 1973.
19. Iglesias, R., Terrés, A., and Chavarria, A.: Disorders of the menstrual cycle in airline stewardesses. Aviat. Space Environ. Med., 51(5):518–520, 1980.
20. Air Force Regulation 160-12. Professional Policies and Procedures, No. 160-12. Washington, D.C., United States Air Force Headquarters, 1977.
21. Gordon, G.V., and Schumacher, H.R.: Management of gout. Am. Fam. Phys., 19:91–97, 1979.
22. Kelly, W.N.: Gout and other disorders of purine metabolism. In Harrison's Principles of Internal Medicine. 9th Ed. Edited by K.J. Isselbacher, et al. New York, McGraw-Hill Book Co., 1980.
23. Conrad, F.G., Rossing, R.G., Allen, M.F., and Bales, H.R., Jr.: Hazard rate of recurrence in patients with malignant melanoma. Aerospace Med., 42:1219–1225, 1971.
24. Conrad, F.G., Allen, M.F., Bales, H.R., Jr., and Rossing, R.G.: Hazard rate of symptomatic recurrence in Hodgkin's disease. Aerospace Med., 43(9):1020–1023, 1972.
25. Conrad, F.G., Bales, H.R., Jr., Allen, M.F., and Rossing, R.G.: Hazard rate of recurrence in germinal cell tumors of the testis. Aerospace Med., 43(8):893–897, 1972.
26. Moseley, H.S., Nizze, A., and Morton, D.L.: Disseminated melanoma presenting as a catastrophic event. Aviat. Space Environ. Med., 49(11):1342–1346, 1978.
27. Smelsey, S.O.: Study of pilots who have made multiple ejections. Aerospace Med., 41(5):563–566, 1970.
28. Kazarian, L.E., Beers, K., and Hernandez, J.: Spinal injuries in the F/FB-111 crew escape system. Aviat. Space Environ. Med., 50(9):948–957, 1979.
29. Kazarian, L.E., and Belk, W.F.: Flight Physical Standards of the 1980s: Spinal Column Consid-

erations. Aeromedical Research Laboratory Technical Report 79-74, AMRL, Wright-Patterson AFB, OH, 1979.

30. Fleming, H.A.: Sarcoid heart disease. Br. Heart J., 36:54–68, 1974.

31. Pettyjohn, F.S., Spoor, D.H., and Buckendorf, W.A.: Sarcoid and the heart—an aeromedical risk. Aviat. Space Environ. Med., 48(10): 955–958, 1978.

32. Silverman, K.J., Hutchins, G.M., and Bulkley, B.H.: Cardiac sarcoid: A clinicopathologic study of 84 unselected patients with systemic sarcoidosis. Circulation, 58(6):1204–1211, 1978.

33. Roberts, W.C., McAllister, H.A., Jr., and Ferrans, V.J.: Sarcoidosis of the heart; a clinicopathologic study of 35 necropsy patients (group 1) and review of 78 previously described necropsy patients (group 11). Am. J. Med., 63:86–107, 1977.

34. Delaney, P.: Neurologic manifestations in sarcoidosis, review of the literature, with a report of 23 cases. Ann. Intern. Med., 87:336–345, 1977.

Chapter 19

The Passenger and the Patient in Flight

Daniel H. Spoor

Aeromedical evacuation presents no problem so long as one remembers that man is adapted for life at or near sea level.

A. JOHNSON, JR.

The airplane has revolutionized virtually all aspects of life. In the past decade, aircraft travel has created a bit of a revolution or at least a major evolution in the transportation of patients by air. The ubiquity of air travel has generated questions for passengers and their physicians regarding the medical safety of this method of transportation. This chapter will provide principles and guidelines to physicians and flight surgeons regarding both the air transport of the patient and medical advice to the traveling public.

THE FLIGHT ENVIRONMENT

The flight environment is physically and physiologically different from man's normal habitat. These differences and their clinicopathologic implications make flying a challenge and sometimes a threat to the passenger and patient.[1,2,3]

Accelerative and Decelerative Forces

Accelerative and decelerative forces normally encountered in takeoff, landing, and maneuvers in general aviation and commercial aircraft are of no significance to the healthy individual other than the anxiety they may produce. For the seated passenger, these forces are either directed perpendicular to the abdomen and back or are head-to-foot force vectors of low magnitude produced in turns and are well tolerated. In a prone or supine patient, however, the landing and takeoff forces are in the long axis of the body and may be very significant.[4] In the patient whose head is toward the front of the aircraft and who has an unstable or compromised circulation, venous pooling on takeoff can cause a significant decrease in cardiac output. The aircraft attitude on climb-out further aggravates this condition as a consequence of the acceleration vector and the steep climb angle, thus creating a sustained reverse Trendelenburg position. A widely accepted rule in patient transportation is to position the patient with his head toward the rear of the aircraft. If there is any doubt about a given patient's sensitivity to this mild, sustained, headward acceleration, it can easily be countered by elevating his head and trunk.

Changes in Barometric Pressure

Barometric pressure decreases with increasing altitudes above sea level. The most familiar result of this change is "popping" or "clearing" of the ears, which equalizes the middle ear pressure. Gas volume expands as pressure decreases (Boyle's Law), doubling at 6000 m, where the pressure is halved. At cabin altitudes normally encountered in pressurized aircraft and in most unpressurized aircraft flights, these pressure/volume changes are not of great importance as long as air-containing body cavities are ventilated.

Barotrauma of the middle ear and paranasal sinuses is covered in detail in Chapter 16, "Otolaryngology in Aerospace Medicine," and only a few additional comments will be made here. The eustachian tube, normally closed, is readily opened by pharyngeal muscle action. The Valsalva maneuver will add active air pressure to this muscle action and is used by many experienced flyers. Flying with an upper respiratory tract infection is the usual cause of barotitis. But a "point of no return" can be reached, even with normal anatomy, at which the negative pressure in the middle ear cannot be overcome with maneuvers, and ear block or barotitis ensues. Sleeping while descending is a common cause because the sleeper does not readily sense the building ear pressure and also does not naturally swallow as often as when awake. Nursing infants should be fed or encouraged to suck on a pacifier to stimulate swallowing; chewing gum is adequate for most older children.

Topical vasoconstrictors and antihistamine/decongestant medications are advised when flying with an upper respiratory tract infection, or when chronic obstruction cannot be avoided. Persons who use nasal drops or sprays should be advised to use their medication 15 to 30 minutes before descent and definitely not wait for the first sensation of middle ear obstruction. "Before descent" deserves an additional caution: these preventive measures should be used when the cabin pressure starts to rise, an event that commonly occurs on commercial airline flights before actual aircraft descent begins.

If ear block develops in the passenger or patient, the immediate use of a topical vasoconstrictor may be of benefit and is worth trying. Many airline attendants and flight nurses are taught politzerization, forcing air into the middle ear with an external air pressure source while the patient swallows. This can be done using a rubber bulb designed for this purpose (Politzer bag), a bag-mask respirator, or, on most commercial aircraft, an emergency oxygen bottle-mask assembly. A common recommendation has been to ascend to an altitude above that at which the block occurred. Although sound, this is often impractical and may even be a safety problem with crowded airways and controlled airspace. A comatose, disoriented, psychotic, or uncooperative patient may require elective myringotomy before flight if transport by air is unavoidable.

The normal intestinal tract is relatively tolerant of gas expansion, and discomfort can be relieved by expelling flatus. Below 3300 m flight or cabin altitude, this gas expansion usually is not a problem unless compounded by gas-producing foods or gastrointestinal disorders. Normal abdominal gas expansion may cause considerable discomfort in the pregnant passenger, particularly in the last trimester of pregnancy.

Trapped gas anywhere in the body is a major problem and can have disastrous or fatal consequences. Disease, trauma, an invasive procedure, or surgery may cause trapped gas. In addition to gas trapped within the body, gas may be trapped around the body, as in pneumatic splints. Other pneumatic medical devices that may produce problems include cuffed endotracheal tubes, balloon bladder catheters, and aortic balloons. Such trapped gas must be eliminated, vented, or otherwise compensated for (e.g., by a pressurized cabin that prevents any altitude change). Certain specific conditions will be covered in more detail later in this chapter.

Hypoxia

The atmosphere contains 20.94% oxygen, and the absolute amount contained is a function of total atmospheric pressure. As one ascends to 3300 m, the partial pressure of oxygen falls; for all practical purposes, this is the range of primary importance to passengers and patients. Pressurized aircraft rarely fly at altitudes that produce a cabin pressure altitude higher than the equivalent of 3300 m, and the majority of unpressurized aircraft fly below that level. Physiologically, the body can compensate for altitudes of 3300 to 5000 m for a limited period of time. Above 5000 m, supplemental oxygen always should be used.

The term "indifferent stage" often is used to describe the hypoxia that may occur at altitudes up to 3300 m, but many individuals are not indifferent at all. Deeper respirations may be felt, particularly while in light sleep, and breathlessness may be noted on mild exertion such as walking to and from the lavatory in a commercial aircraft. Frequent flyers are accustomed to these sensations, but airline personnel and physicians must remember that not everyone is a veteran flyer. The first-time or very occasional flyer generally has some degree of anxiety about flying. This anxiety may be aggravated by mild symptoms of hypoxia and result in a distinctly uncomfortable, uneasy, or frankly agitated passenger or patient.

Compensatory mechanisms called into play in the presence of hypoxia include increased respiratory rate and volume, elevated heart rate and cardiac output, and the oxygen-hemoglobin transport characteristics often referred to simply as the oxyhemoglobin dissociation curve. Any condition that interferes with one or more of these compensatory mechanisms makes the person more sensitive to any decrease in oxygen tension.

Known disease in a passenger or patient must be considered and allowances made or precautions taken if necessary. For example, the patient with coronary artery disease and exertional angina should be specifically cautioned about avoiding exertion in the aircraft. This precaution appears obvious but should be further translated or expanded to include the restriction of fluid intake (particularly alcohol) to minimize required trips to the aircraft lavatory. Of equal significance to known disease is the threat of unknown disease: subclinical and compensated pulmonary or cardiovascular disease or undiagnosed gastrointestinal bleeding with secondary anemia are examples.

Pressurized Cabins, Altitude Restrictions, and Oxygenation

All aircraft with pressurized cabins can maintain a certain pressure differential. This varies with each specific aircraft model and is determined by the engineering design of the pressurization system. A sea-level or ambient ground-level cabin altitude can be maintained up to the flight level at which the maximum pressure differential of the system is equalled. Above that flight level, cabin pressure will rise as a function of the inside to outside pressure differential (ΔP).

Because airframes, pumps, valves, and seals age and wear, each airframe loses some pressurization capability with time. The actual or effective ΔP will thus be less than the predicted or original design capability. This difference generally is negligible, however.

The United States Air Force C-9A (DC-9) can maintain a sea-level cabin altitude to about 5500 m (Fig. 19–1). This is typical of large jet aircraft in commercial use, as well as executive jet aircraft. This capability is not indicative of the cabin altitude to be expected in normal flight profiles.

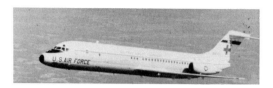

Fig. 19–1. Air Force C-9A transport. This aeromedical evacuation aircraft, a modification of a civilian airliner, is specifically designed to meet Air Force patient-carrying responsibilities (official United States Air Force photo).

Today, civil and military transport aircraft fly a profile that is determined by multiple considerations of distance, the best performance altitude, en-route weather, passenger comfort, aircraft safety, and optimum fuel economy. Pressurization systems consume energy and, therefore, are part of the total fuel costs. An aircraft capable of maintaining a 1300 m cabin altitude at 11,300 m altitude with a maximum cabin pressure differential may actually be flown with a ΔP that results in a 2300-m cabin altitude at that same flight altitude.

Medical recommendations for cabin altitude restrictions must be based on what a patient needs and how to meet these needs with a combination of supplemental oxygen and cabin altitude restrictions. Unnecessarily extreme restrictions force the aircraft to be flown at lower flight levels, thus putting the aircraft into bad weather and turbulence that otherwise could be avoided, increasing fuel consumption and flight time by virtue of slower airspeeds, and perhaps requiring an en-route fuel stop, which extends the total mission time.

Misuses or abuses of the physician-recommended cabin altitude restriction are common. A patient who is adequately oxygenated in Denver, Colorado (1700 m) or Albuquerque, New Mexico (2000 m) does not need a sea-level cabin on a flight to San Antonio, Texas but may well require a restriction to not exceed the cabin altitude of the point of origin.

A common problem that illustrates this

fact regularly occurred in the western Pacific with an emergency air evacuation request to move a neonate from the United States Army Hospital at Seoul, South Korea to the neonatal intensive care unit at Tripler General Hospital on Oahu, Hawaii. Often, this request included a sea-level cabin restriction. If an infant requires 100% inspired oxygen at ground level for adequate oxygenation, this request is appropriate. A C-141 can make this move with a sea-level cabin; however, it requires a flight altitude on the order of 6000 to 7000 m, the slower speeds increasing the travel time by nearly 2 hours and fuel consumption, requiring a refueling stop en route (Fig. 19–2). This well-intended sea-level cabin restriction may then affect the patient and the attendants by virtue of the extra landing and takeoff and the added total travel time, which can be as much as 5 hours.

In several years' experience with the United States Air Force worldwide aeromedical evacuation system, a 1700 to 2000 m cabin altitude restriction proved to be a magic number that ensured patient safety with a minimum impact on flight planning considerations in most cases. This rule of thumb was arrived at by assuming that ill patients do not have the same compensatory capabilities or tolerance to mild hypoxia as the healthy passenger because of obvious conditions such as anemia, cardiac disease, or pulmonary insufficiency. This assumption also was felt to be rational for anyone who was acutely or chronically ill. This empiric

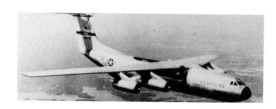

Fig. 19–2. Air Force C-141 transport. This aircraft can be rapidly retrofitted for aeromedical evacuation missions (official United States Air Force photo).

limit also correlates well with the conclusions of investigators at the British Royal Air Force Institute of Aviation Medicine after more than 20 years of experimental work.[5]

Another fairly obvious rule of thumb arrived at by experience is "when in doubt, add supplemental oxygen." An FIO_2 of 30 to 40% with a cabin altitude of 1700 to 2000 m allows for some leaks or losses in the delivery to the patient and still gives the patient a sea-level equivalent alveolar oxygen concentration.

The sine qua non in all difficult moves is a physician or flight surgeon who understands both the clinical needs of the patient and the capabilities and limitations of the aircraft and flight environment, serving as a consultant to the originating physician and balancing these often divergent factors.

Apprehension and Anxiety

Many individuals experience real apprehension or anxiety about flying. Some people are simply afraid to fly and, if they have the freedom to choose other options, either do not travel or use surface transportation. A widely known individual in this category is the former professional football coach and now television sports telecaster, John Madden. The majority of individuals do not have this freedom to choose an alternative method and are forced to fly because of various circumstances, such as the urgent need to travel a considerable distance in a short period of time, when occupational situations allow no other alternative. The plentiful statistics that testify to the safety of both general aviation and commercial aircraft travel do not make as strong an impression as the sensational news coverage attending a major aircraft accident.

Airline personnel are trained to recognize, expect, and deal with the anxious passenger. Doctors must not forget that patients also may be afraid to fly. Reassurance is of great benefit, but some passengers or patients with significant anxiety may require medication.

It is difficult to recommend any particular drug because the choices are wide and individual response is highly variable. Today, many people who become airsick easily are aware of this and know those medications that are effective for them. A recent addition to the wide spectrum of available drugs is transdermal scopolamine. Dramamine, Bonamine, dextroamphetamine-scopolamine combination, and others are effective, as are the classic antihistamines and a variety of tranquilizer preparations.

METHODS OF TRANSPORT

A variety of aircraft are in use worldwide for the movement of passengers and patients. Aircraft types generally can be viewed as single-engine and multi-engine, pressurized and unpressurized, and fixed-wing and rotary-wing. Single-engine and twin-engine unpressurized aircraft make up the largest group of general aviation aircraft; however, the number of executive and commuter, multi-engine, pressurized aircraft is increasing significantly. Rotary-wing aircraft (helicopters) are usually unpressurized; however, a new growth segment of the industry is the pressurized, "executive," turbine-powered helicopter. Commercial aircraft or those used in scheduled airline service are almost exclusively large, multi-engine, pressurized, turboprop or purejet aircraft.

Larger aircraft are less affected by turbulence, are less noisy, and the pressurized cabin offers significant comfort advantages to the passenger and the patient in the control of both cabin altitude and temperature. Features present in scheduled airline travel generally may apply to charter and airtaxi operations, with the exception that the amenities are fewer, and in some instances there may be no cabin attendant.

Commercial Airline Transportation

A paucity of data is available on the frequency and variety of passenger medical problems in commercial aircraft. Many anecdotal observations and experiences are well known to frequent travelers. Chapter 24, which discusses airline medical operations, provides some information for civil aviation. It also should be noted that there is only a limited system for reporting such data in military aviation.

The advent of jet aircraft that fly above most turbulence has greatly decreased the problems of airsickness, but it still occurs. Clinical problems of a more serious nature than airsickness also occur on commercial airlines and run the gamut from anxiety to heart attack and sudden death. The American Medical Association Commission on Emergency Medical Services has estimated that 46 to 47 persons die in flight each year in the United States.[3]

Cabin attendants on commercial aircraft are trained to recognize and cope with common and expected maladies but have minimal medical emergency training or supplies and equipment. At present, commercial airlines in the United States are only required to carry the first-aid supplies necessary to treat minor injuries occurring as a direct result of air travel. Consequently, these kits are for the most part composed of Band-Aids, bandages, and splints. A growing trend both in this country and internationally is to carry a more comprehensive emergency medical kit to be used by a physician-passenger in the event some serious medical problem occurs.

Passenger Accommodations

Major air carriers and airports are well equipped to accommodate the elderly, disabled, or ill passenger with a variety of assists for transportation within the airport terminal and getting on and off an airplane. The cardinal rule here is plan ahead. If forewarned, airlines can make provisions, but last-minute "shows at the gate" with a passenger requiring total boarding assistance may result in a missed flight.

Many patients are transported by scheduled commercial airlines and, again, preparation and advance notice are mandatory. A common airline practice is to accommodate stretcher patients in the first-class section by removing two to four seats (one to two seat pairs). This practice usually results, not unexpectedly, in a basic billing or fare scheduled based on four first-class seats.

Most commercial carriers are neither willing nor logistically able to transport a patient who requires extensive medical paraphernalia such as drainage tubes and bottles, suction, or electronic equipment (intravenous pumps or cardiac monitors). Nor are airlines required to carry a patient who might be considered offensive to other passengers. Virtually none have onboard therapeutic oxygen systems, but many airlines can provide or accept a carry-on oxygen supply if arranged well in advance. The Federal Aviation Administration (FAA) has stringent rules regarding oxygen bottles and other carry-on medical equipment, and individual airlines may have rules of their own. It is best to assume that there will be no preexisting clinical capability, and lead time will be needed to make everything work. (Don't forget connecting airline flights!)

Military Aeromedical Evacuation

The frequently cited first use of aeromedical evacuation was in 1870, during the siege of Paris, when casualties were evacuated by balloon.[2,3] The United States Army Air Corps used aircraft equipped to evacuate casualties in World War I, but an organized military patient air evacuation system did not exist until midway through World War II. The "air evac" value of the helicopter first became evident during the Korean War and was further expanded and widely utilized in southeast Asia. United States Air Force short-haul and long-haul fixed-wing air evacuation system likewise expanded during these same years, and in 1975, the United States Air Force Military Airlift Command became the single manager for aeromedical evacuation for the Department of Defense. By charter and doctrine, the ground combat forces retain responsibility for battlefield evacuation.

In 1943, 173,500 sick and wounded were evacuated from overseas to the United States; in 1944, 545,000 were transported, and at war's end in 1945, the rate reached 1 million/year. The deaths during transport decreaased throughout this period from 6/100,000 individuals in 1943 to 1.5/100,000 persons in 1945.[6]

The death rate for wounded in World War I who lived long enough to get to medical care was 8.5%. During World War II, this rate dropped to 4%; during the Korean War, this rate was approximately 2%, and during the Vietnam War, this rate was 1%.[6,7]

All improvements in the mortality rate cannot be attributed solely to air evacuation because many major advances were made in medical and surgical care, but rapid transportation by air with effective medical care en route certainly was a major factor. Not quantitative but perhaps even more important is the fact that the air evacuation system prevented overloading of the medical care facilities in the war theater.

Aircraft

Military air evacuation techniques always have been based on the inherent logistic facts of wartime that aircraft flying cargo (bombs and bullets) to the war zones are what must be used to evacuate patients on their return trip, or back-haul. Consequently, various systems or subsystems of medical personnel and medical equipment have been designed to refit the cargo aircraft for its air evac role. The C-131A Samaritan, introduced into service in 1954, was the first single-purpose aircraft in the United States Air Force inventory for aeromedical transportation, with built-in patient care features such as a therapeutic oxygen supply. This was followed in 1968 by the acquisition of the Mc-Donnell-Douglas C-9A, which was totally designed as a single-purpose air evac aircraft.

Today, the United States Military Airlift Command operates an extensive worldwide network of people and aircraft providing peacetime, routine, and emergency movement of patients within and between overseas areas and the United States (Fig. 19–3). Medical policy and management are exercised from the United States Air Force Surgeon General through the Command Surgeon, Military Airlift Command to the Deputy Commander for Aeromedical Services, 375th Aeromedical Airlift Wing (AAW), which is headquartered at Scott Air Force Base in Illinois.

This structure includes two United States-based and two overseas-based squadrons of medical personnel and over 30 similar units of the Air Force Reserve

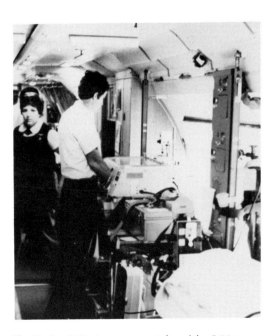

Fig. 19–3. Patient management aboard the C-9A transport. A flight nurse is attending a premature infant being carried in a portable incubator (official United States Air Force photo).

and Air National Guard. This system operates regularly in peacetime, providing a necessary service to the military personnel of all the services stationed around the world. The primary reason for these peacetime operations is to provide the training and experience necessary to maintain a wartime capability. The system is capable of responding to national and international catastrophes on a moment's notice, as was the case of the Jonestown, Guyana massacre and the Lebanon terrorists' attack on the peace-keeping forces.

The aircraft utilized in this Air Force system are the McDonnell-Douglas C-9A within the Pacific and European theaters and the CONUS and the Lockheed C-141 for the strategic or long-haul routes between overseas and the United States. The backbone of the tactical wartime system, the Lockheed C-130, is also used in some areas and circumstances.

Other military air evac operations include the United States Army Military Assistance in Safety and Traffic (MAST) helicopter units and elements of the Aerospace Rescue and Recovery Service. The MAST system is probably the single most important stimulus to the growth of community helicopter air ambulance systems.

Policy and Doctrine

The United States Department of Defense (DOD) is prohibited by law from competing with private industry, and this fundamental precept underlies the existing DOD and Air Force rules on the use of the military air evacuation resources in response to the many civil requests for assistance. A key determination to be made in every case is whether civilian commercial air ambulance service is available and adequate. If it is available and adequate, policy and public law dictate that these civilian resources should be used instead of the military. Genuine medical need and not merely convenience also must be present.

When a civilian or non-DOD beneficiary is moved in the military aeromedical evacuation system, reimbursement is generally required. Depending on the circumstances, the actual dollar amount arrived at may be based on actual flying hour costs or more often, a fare basis. In the latter case, the standard used, assuming the patient is a stretcher or litter patient, is the previously mentioned commercial airline system of charging four first-class fares; to avoid the competition rule, the government billing then adds $1.00.

These recurring requests for military assistance are not easily dealt with because other considerations come into play. Is the commercial air ambulance service available and adequate in terms of equipment, personnel, and aircraft capability and adequate in timeliness? Also, while the request for air evacuation may meet all the necessary criteria, is the patient stable enough to withstand the move? These are frequently judgmental issues without clear black and white definitions and/or answers. The requester is frequently dismayed or even outraged that such questions and deliberations are involved.

With the continued growth in the air ambulance industry, including national and international operators, final decisions more frequently support the private sector rather than the use of military resources.

Air Ambulance Service

The air ambulance industry has grown exponentially in the past decade. This growth has been driven by a number of factors. The military experience in general and in southeast Asia in particular demonstrated the value of rapid air transport of the injured to definitive care facilities. Advances in medical care, with the concentration of centers of expertise such as in neonatology and trauma centers, created a greater need for safe transportation. The United States Army MAST program provided an additional stimulus. Australia, a land of vast distances and a scattered population, probably deserves credit for being in the lead in integrating the airplane into the health care delivery system by taking routine and emergency health care to the patients as well as using aeromedical transportation to transfer patients to centers of care.

Today, there are many first-rate private air ambulance companies as well as community-operated systems. There are also individuals who equate "air ambulance" to nothing more than having an airtaxi operator's license and an airplane.

Standards

In the United States at present, there are no federally mandated air ambulance standards. An attempt was made to embody air ambulance standards in FAA regulations; however, this proposal was met with a storm of protest and died a political death in 1978. Indiana has enacted comprehensive rules and regulations pertaining to air ambulance operations and is the first state in the United States to do so.[8] Other states will surely follow Indiana's lead.

The air ambulance industry has not stood still, however. Major first-line companies have banded together and set a "standard" by precept and example, most notably the Association of North American Air Ambulances.[9] In addition, the American Medical Association, the Aerospace Medical Association, and other professional groups also have proposed standards and criteria.

Such peer-group pressures are effective. Another source of pressure comes from an educated professional community that asks for and demands certain standards of care. These consumer-derived standards are perhaps the most effective of all. Lastly, as of this writing, at least two cases in the courts also may affect the setting of standards for the air ambulance industry.

Type of Aircraft

Many air ambulance systems utilize the helicopter primarily for local area services

and generally are limited to a 1-hour flying time radius of operations (Figs. 19–4 and 19–5). This can translate to a 100 to 200 mile radius of coverage. Virtually all of these helicopters are unpressurized aircraft simply because of the costs and mission profiles. The turbine-powered, pressurized helicopter is a relatively new arrival in the helicopter market, and the capital investment required and costs of operating this aircraft will limit its attractiveness in commericial ventures.

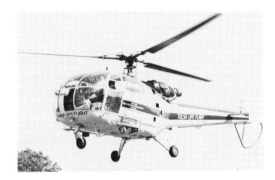

Fig. 19–4. A community helicopter ambulance used for emergency patient transport.

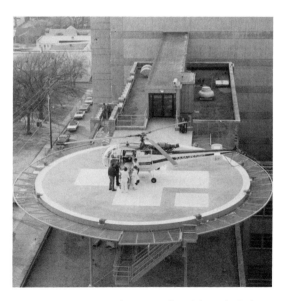

Fig. 19–5. A patient being transferred from the Tulsa Life Flight helicopter to Hillcrest Medical Center in Tulsa, Oklahoma. Frequently, hospitals have built helipads on or immediately adjacent to the medical facility to expedite patient transfer.

Helicopter transport of accident victims to hospitals can reduce patient mortality rates to less than half of those reported for similarly injured patients who are transported by ground ambulance. When similar injuries are considered, the airlifted patient experiences a 25% less mortality rate. To achieve such spectacular results, it is imperative that the equipment and personnel delivered by helicopter and accompanying the patient to the hospital are appropriately trained for this demanding task. Further, appropriate continuation of care must be guaranteed at the receiving institution if the use of the helicopter is to achieve its optimal potential.

Fixed-wing aircraft in air ambulance services are as varied as they are in general aviation. Many short-haul systems utilize single-engine or twin-engine unpressurized aircraft, and, again, costs are primary considerations to the operator. The geography of the terrain also may dictate light aircraft with short takeoff and landing capabilities such as in the intermountain western United States, Alaska, and Australia, where landing strips are often short, rough, and surrounded by natural obstacles. At the other end of the spectrum is the company offering coast-to-coast service in pressurized jet aircraft, the Lear Jet being a common example.

Costs

Local community systems and some regional services are primarily driven by community need and may have partial or total community and government subsidization. Consequently, the ultimate cost to the patient may range from nothing to a fee based on partial operating costs to a charge based solely on economics, that is, operating costs plus some amount of profit.[10,11]

The cost to the patient will certainly vary depending on the sophistication of the system, the number and type of attendants required, and the patient's needs for special medical equipment. This could be a few hundred dollars for a local-area helicopter mission to thousands of dollars for coast-to-coast jet air ambulance service. A recent example involved the move of a comatose stroke patient who required suction and oxygen from Houston to San Antonio, Texas. The quoted fare from a top-quality company for a twin-engine pressurized aircraft that provided all the necessary equipment and a qualified nurse-attendant was $1500.

Medical Attendants

Medical attendants should be provided by the air ambulance operator. In the major companies, these are often highly trained intensive care unit or coronary care unit nurses who have had additional training in flight physiology and patient care in the air. Major companies also will have full-time or consultant physicians who are both clinically expert and can fulfill the flight surgeon's role.

ASSISTING THE PATIENT

General Considerations

There are few, if any, absolute contraindications to moving a patient by air. Patients with acute myocardial infarction, pneumothorax, cerebral air embolism, and central nervous system dysbarism can be moved relatively safely with proper planning, personnel, medical equipment, and the right aircraft.

Improvements in medical care, somewhat synonymous with increasing technologic sophistication, also relate to the centralization of advanced medical institutions. This raises the demand for more patient transfers because the standards of care rise and the centers capable of meeting these higher standards are fewer and farther apart, for example, neonatal intensive care units, burn centers, coronary care units, and organ transplant centers.

The major questions that must be faced and answered include: Is the risk to the patient in being transferred less than the risk of not being moved? Is the patient adequately stabilized? Are the benefits of the move real, and do they justify the clinical and fiscal costs? Is the move medically necessary or being driven by nonmedical, emotional, or family based concerns?

These considerations may seem elementary, but one personal experience stands out that will illustrate the importance of some of these questions. The patient was a 13-year-old girl who had sustained 90 to 95% second- and third-degree burns and had pulmonary complications. The Air Force was asked to move her from a major, well-stafffed general hospital to a midwest burn center. Part of the attending physician's rationale was that, although her chances for survival were not good, she had the best chance in a burn center. She was hypotensive, had little renal output, and, with the pulmonary burns, could not be adequately oxygenated in spite of all the best measures. After a consultation with the attending physician, the receiving physician, the air evac physician, and a physician at the United States Army Burn Center, there was general agreement that an immediate move was not medically indicated nor was it in the best interests of the patient. A transfer would be planned if and when the patient could be stabilized.

The attending physician needs to be cautious when faced with pressures or demands to transfer a patient for essentially nonmedical reasons. An example is the tourist who has a myocardial infarction while on a vacation trip, and the family wants the patient moved back home. Perhaps the move can be arranged with minimal risk, but even minimal risk may not be justifiable when the care required and being provided is the same in Honolulu, Hawaii as in Milwaukee, Wisconsin.

Transport Concerns

Mode of Transport

The mode of transport is generally dictated by what is locally available because there are many major air ambulance companies with regional, national, and even international capabilities. In general, a patient will need at least the same provisions for care en route as is being provided at the hospital of origin such as oxygen, suction, intravenous tubes, and drainage bottles. Likewise, the medical attendant requirements will be at least as demanding.

A small, general aviation, unpressurized aircraft may be adequate in terms of distance and weather en route, but medical attendant and medical equipment requirements may dictate a larger aircraft. If cardiopulmonary resuscitation (CPR) is a potential en-route emergency, this will require an aircraft with adequate cabin room.[11] The medical indications for a transfer also may dictate speed and a long-distance flight. These conditions usually will mean utilizing a commercial air ambulance company that has larger jet aircraft.

Equipment

If a commercial air ambulance company is being used, all equipment needs must be made known to the operator and the equipment's availability and suitability verified. If the originating hospital is providing equipment, special care and effort must be taken to ensure that the equipment will work on the airplane. Most aircraft have 28 V direct current and 110 V/ 400 Hz power, but 120 V/60 Hz power, which most hospital-based equipment requires, is a rarity. If battery-powered equipment is used, the power supply must be sufficient for the entire trip. Spare batteries are generally a good idea and are absolutely essential if needed for critical life-support equipment.

The amount of oxygen required should be calculated and then doubled. Plastic intravenous bags should be used instead of glass bottles, which can become hazardous missiles in turbulence. Pressure pumps or intravenous infusion pumps should be available because most aircraft cabins do not have sufficient height for adequate gravity flow.

A valid rule or approach to planning is to assume that "Murphy's Law" will be functioning. Every possible contingency must be thought of and accounted for in supplies and equipment: "if you might need it, take it." This approach includes having all potentially necessary connections and adaptors for such items as ventilators.[11,12,13]

Coordination

The receiving hospital and attending physician must be fully aware of the evacuation plan and be prepared. Ground transport at origin and destination must be available and adequate to fully support the patient, equipment, and transport team. If the attendants who accompany the patient are not going the full route, that is, to the receiving hospital, the originating and receiving physicians and the air ambulance must make sure before the fact that all needed preparations have been made.

Records

All pertinent medical records should travel with the patient. In addition, there must be adequate documentation of the en-route phase—a complete record of treatment given and medication used.

CONSIDERATIONS FOR THE AEROMEDICAL TRANSFER OF PATIENTS WITH SPECIFIC CONDITIONS

Cardiovascular Disease

As has been indicated earlier, all care and treatment considerations that were needed at the hospital of origin are needed during transport. Whether the patient has a myocardial infarction, valvular heart disease, or some other cardiovascular disorder, if oxygen was required on the ground, it will be needed in the air, and the percentage of supplemental oxygen should be increased or "titrated" upward

to give the same oxygen concentration at the en-route cabin altitude that was used at the originating hospital. If the patient did not require supplemental oxygen, adding it should be strongly considered, particularly if the cabin altitude will be above 1400 m.

If there is any question of cardiopulmonary resuscitation being required en route, the patient should be placed on a CPR board before the flight. This will be uncomfortable for the patient, but having it in place will pay handsome dividends if CPR is needed. The medical attendant should be qualified to treat cardiac arrhythmias and have the necessary medication to control this condition.

Pulmonary Disease

Untreated pneumothorax is an absolute contraindication to movement by aircraft unless there is no respiratory compromise and the cabin altitude can be maintained at the ambient altitude of the point of origin. By far, the safest approach is to insert a chest tube. All chest tubes should have a Heimlich valve or other one-way valve assembly to prevent the retrograde flow of air into the chest.

Chest tubes should not be removed just before flight. Otherwise, evacuation should be delayed 72 hours after removal if possible, and a chest radiograph should be obtained 24 hours prior to flight. Glass-bottle drainage systems should be replaced with unbreakable plastic containers. Systems for this purpose are commercially available.

Chronic obstructive pulmonary disease patients require careful individual evaluation, with a tailoring of altitude and supplemental oxygen to maintain preflight conditions.

The transport of adults with acute respiratory failure is a major undertaking and is encountered more frequently today because of the recognition that specialized respiratory intensive care centers can greatly reduce morbidity and mortality.

This type of move is best managed by a highly trained and experienced team.[13] The physical space needs of such a team generally require a relatively large aircraft. Adequate stabilization of the patient prior to movement is of absolute importance. Cuffed endotracheal tubes will need frequent adjustment because ambient pressure changes, unless a self-compensating tube is used.[14] Given an adequately prepared and stabilized patient, blood gases en route are generally not needed.[13]

Anemia

The patient who is acutely anemic because of hemorrhage or hemolysis will require the continuation of blood transfusions en route as well as supplemental oxygen. Many chronically anemic patients are moved by air, and generally they do well if their hemoglobin is 8.5 g/dL or higher. Supplemental oxygen may be required in these patients, particularly on long flights or on flights with a cabin altitude above 1400 m. In patients with hemoglobin values below 8.5 g/dL, supplemental oxygen should be used routinely. Patients with sickle cell disease should be maintained on an F_{IO_2} equal to that of their point of origin.

Burns

The two single most important considerations in the burn patient are adequate assessment and stabilization.[15] Assessment is critical because resuscitation formulas are based on percentage of total body surface and the depth of burn. This calculation, in turn, determines the volume of fluids to be given in the first 24 hours and becomes a critical factor in stabilization. Commonly, the extent of burn in adults is overestimated, leading to overhydration and incipient or even frank cardiac failure and pulmonary edema. Infants and children are just as frequently underestimated as to the extent of burn. The presence or absence of pulmonary burn is likewise all-important, and all too often

the survivable surface burn is fatal because of pulmonary burn. A preflight chest radiograph is important as part of the assessment regarding pulmonary burn and particularly important if a subclavian line has been put in or attempted because of the risk of pneumothorax.

Stabilization includes adequate airway patency, ventilation, and oxygenation, as well as adequate fluid resuscitation. In addition to intravenous lines, the patient should have a nasogastric tube in place because gastric distension and ileus are common.

Gastrointestinal Concerns

The special considerations regarding gastrointestinal conditions relate to trapped gas and gas expansion with altitude. Anxious patients tend to swallow air. This action could predispose to nausea and vomiting, which is not desirable in a patient with recent gastrointestinal surgery. Following abdominal surgery, pockets of air may remain in the abdominal cavity. For this reason, a general recommendation is that patients not be transported by air until 24 to 48 hours after the surgery.

Trapped gas in an ileus, hernia, or volvulus can expand, producing pain, and also may compromise the circulation in the bowel. For this reason, it may be prudent to delay the transport of patients who have had bowel anastamoses until intestinal motility has returned. When these conditions are present or if there is any doubt, a nasogastric tube with suction is indicated. Colostomy patients need to be advised to expect more frequent bowel movements because of gas expansion and be provided with extra bags.

Orthopedic Situations

As a general rule, all casts should be bivalved, unless, in the opinion of the attending orthopedic surgeon, bivalving would jeopardize the fracture. This is not necessary in the case of an injury in which sufficient time has elapsed to be confident of no vascular compromise from wound edema. I have met many orthopedic surgeons who are skeptical about possible tissue swelling at altitude and the concern for bivalved casts. There is a dramatic and tragic illustrative case report in the literature, however, where this phenomenon led to bilateral leg amputation in a child who was transported by commercial airliner from the United States to South America on the sixth postoperative day.[3]

Swinging weights for traction are dangerous in an aircraft because the weights are potential missiles and, even if restrained, can bounce in turbulence and produce painful and possibly damaging jerks on the limb. A relatively simple solution is a bungee cord traction or spring tension. Air splints should not be used because of gas expansion. A newer type of "apneumatic" splint is available that is filled with plastic pellet material, molded to the limb, and becomes essentially rigid when evacuated. This should not be a hazard from gas expansion; however, some air will remain, will expand, and may weaken or lessen the rigidity.

Stryker frames are recommended for spine fractures and spinal cord injury patients. The "Wedge Stryker" should not be used because it cannot be secured to the floor of the aircraft with standard tie-down spacing; the "modified wedge" is acceptable. Stryker frames also should be shipped as a complete unit because not all parts are interchangeable with other frames.

Vibration in the aircraft can be particularly disturbing to the fracture patient, and this is especially true in helicopters. The frequency and amplitude characteristics of helicopter vibrations are distinctly different and can potentially cause fracture movement and displacement. In the case of vascular injury and repair, casts should be windowed over the site of the repair in addition to being bivalved. This windowing will allow immediate access to the repair site in the event of hemorrhage.

Neurologic Concerns

Patients with increased intracranial pressure and cerebral edema should be given supplemental oxygen to eliminate even the mild hypoxia present at reduced altitude. Cabin altitude should not exceed 2000 m. Brain injury patients may be exceedingly sensitive to footward acceleration on takeoff if transported with their head toward the front of the aircraft. If at all possible, these patients should be positioned with their head toward the rear.

Intracranial air is potentially disastrous regardless of whether it is from a penetrating injury, surgery, or diagnostic studies. If such a patient must be moved, a pressurized aircraft is necessary, and the cabin altitude should not exceed the ambient field level pressure at the point of orgin. The presence of a cerebrospinal fluid leak from the nose or the ear is sometimes a contraindication to air transportation. The primary concern is that cerebrospinal fluid will be forced out on ascent and air and bacteria will be forced into the cranial vault on descent. One solution is a pressurized cabin and maintaining the cabin altitude at the altitude of the point of origin. That solution is "no solution" if the patient is being moved from high altitude to low altitude, for example, from Colorado Springs, Colorado to San Antonio, Texas. In that instance, the attending physicians must be made aware of the aeromedical concerns and make the final decision.

A theoretical concern is that patients with a seizure disorder may be susceptible to having a seizure precipitated by the mild hypoxia encountered in flight. Supplemental oxygen to maintain the ground-level–equivalent inspired oxygen will eliminate that concern.

Psychiatric Situations

Psychiatric patients are just as prone to anxiety about flying as nonpsychiatric patients; consequently, sedative or tranquilizing medications should be ordered for the flight if indicated. Any patient who required locked-ward precautions prior to transport should be moved as a stretcher patient, be specifically sedated or otherwise medicated for the flight, and be restrained.

Physicians and air evac personnel tend to be reluctant to insist on patient restraints, but this is misplaced sympathy. A violent patient on an airplane can have serious or even disastrous consequences in an incredibly short period of time. Subduing a violent patient is difficult in the best of hands and circumstances, and an aircraft in flight is the worst time and place.

Air Embolism and Decompression Sickness

Patients with air embolism or decompression sickness, whether from diving, flying, or surgical misadventure, are "trapped gas time bombs." They may be disastrously ill, and air transportation is frequently called on to move the patient to a hyperbaric treatment facility. The two important aeromedical concerns are 100% oxygen en route and a cabin altitude control.

The 100% oxygen establishes a Po_2 differential to encourage nitrogen washout and may aid ischemic areas throughout the body. This is, of course, no substitute for compression therapy. A pressurized aircraft is mandatory unless faced with a short-distance move in an unpressurized aircraft that is immediately available versus a wait of several hours for a suitable pressurized aircraft. If faced with this dilemma, consultation with an expert in hyperbaric medicine should be obtained. The ideal solution is a pressurized aircraft that can maintain point-of-origin or destination field level pressure, whichever is lower.

High-Risk Pregnancy

Early identification of the high-risk pregnancy and elective transfer is clearly the best for mother, child, and the transport system.[16] Unfortunately, the pregnancy may not be high risk until the membranes rupture prematurely or there is early onset of labor. There is also a reluctance on the part of many women to accept an early elective transfer because of the impact on the family unit.

If there is no active labor or other complicating factors, the transfer of the high-risk obstetric patient presents little in the way of problems and is of no particular risk to the mother or the infant. A cabin altitude restriction to 1600 m may be recommended to avoid uncomfortable abdominal gas distension in an abdomen already filled with a uterus. If there is any question of placental insufficiency, supplemental oxygen should be considered.

If there is active labor, therapeutic efforts to stop or delay the labor should be used unless otherwise contraindicated, and a physician should accompany the patient.[16] An obstetric delivery pack should be included along with any special equipment required by the physician.

Neonates

Neonatal transport has become a highly specialized type of patient evacuation by ground and air. The necessity of such transport has been driven by the development of neonatal intensive care units and the recognition that these units can significantly decrease infant morbidity and mortality.

The approach used in the United States Air Force aeromedical evacuation system is similar to that found in many metropolitan areas in the United States and in other countries: first moving the neonatal transfer team to the patient for optimum assessment and stabilization and then transfer of the infant in a controlled-environment life-support system.[17,18]

All factors in the transport of a critically

ill neonate are vital, and the two most important factors are temperature control and adequate oxygenation. These factors present significant difficulties if special transfer units are not available. A standard hospital incubator is better than no incubator at all and can be aided by keeping the aircraft cabin at as high a temperature as possible.

An aircraft with a pressurized cabin is preferred both for better temperature control and to minimize barometric pressure changes. Cabin altitude restrictions should be carefully determined based on the infant's oxygen requirements and the opposing factors related to the flight itself, that is, the minimum safe altitude for the route of flight, the aircraft's pressurization capability, and time, distance, and fuel requirements.

Absolute assurance of compatibility must exist between the equipment needed and the aircraft to be used, as well as the availability and sufficiency of oxygen and electrical power. Equal attention must be given to the same factors in the transportation links at each end of the total move, from hospital to aircraft and aircraft to neonatal intensive care unit.[4,17,18]

FUTURE PROSPECTS

Today, we see what will be growth patterns for the future: air evacuation systems supporting specific needs and increasing specialization and sophistication. Community short-haul systems will proliferate, particularly in metropolitan areas driven both by centralized trauma units, neonatal intensive care units, and other specialty units, and city growth that outstrips surface road capacities. As these commercial ventures grow, they will create a larger market for specialized medical equipment designed for aeromedical use rather than fixed hospital use. This market exists today and will increase. This same market demand will see more specialized aircraft designs with built-in patient care features. Lastly, there will be a market for

the aeromedical physician to advise and counsel and above all to ensure that patient needs, insofar as possible, come first.

REFERENCES

1. Johnson, A., Jr.: Treatise on aeromedical evacuation: I. Administration and some medical considerations. Aviat. Space Environ. Med. 48:546-549, 1977.
2. Johnson, A., Jr.: Treatise on aeromedical evacuation: II. Some surgical considerations. Aviat. Space Environ. Med. 48:550-554, 1977.
3. Parsons, C.J., and Bobechko, W.P.: Aeromedical transport: Its hidden problems. Can. Med. Assoc. J., 126:237, 1982.
4. Reddick, E.J.: Aeromedical evacuation. Am. Fam. Phys., 16:154-159, 1977.
5. Ernsting, J.: The 10th annual Harry G. Armstrong lecture: Prevention of hypoxia—acceptable compromises. Aviat. Space Environ. Med., 49:495-502, 1978.
6. Department of the Air Force. Office of the Surgeon General: Concise History of the United States Air Force Aeromedical Evacuation System. 1976-626-850/379. Washington, D.C., Government Printing Office, 1976.
7. McNeil, E.L.: Airborne Care of the Ill and Injured. New York, Springer-Verlag, 1983.
8. Johnson, J.C.: Medical care in the air. Ann. Emerg. Med., 10(6):324-327, 1981.
9. Bare, W.W.: Air Ambulance Standards for Association of North American Air Ambulances. 116 West Church Road, Blackwood, New Jersey, 08012, Association of North American Air Ambulances, 1982.
10. Cooper, M.A., Klippel, A.P., and Seymour, J.A.: A hospital-based helicopter service: Will it fly? Ann. Emerg. Med., 9:451-455, 1980.
11. Gilligan, J.E., et al.: Retrieval of the critically ill in south Australia: A coordinated approach. Med. J. Aust., 2:849-852, 1977.
12. Safar, P., Esposito, G., and Benson, D.M.: Ambulance design and equipment for mobile intensive care. Arch. Surg., 102:163-168, 1971.
13. Harless, K.W., et al.: Civilian ground and air transport of adults with acute respiratory failure. JAMA, 240:361-365, 1978.
14. Stoner, D.L., and Cooke, J.P.: Intratracheal cuffs and aeromedical evacuation. Anesthesiology, 41:302-306, 1974.
15. Pruitt, B.A., Jr.: The burn patient: I. Initial care. Curr. Prob. Surg., 16(4):1-55, 1979.
16. Brown, F.B.: The management of high-risk obstetric transfer patients. Obstet. Gynecol. 51:674-676, 1978.
17. Colton, J.S., Pickering, D.E., and Colton, C.A.: Evaluation of a life-support module used for air transport of critically ill infants. Aviat. Space Environ. Med., 50:177, 1979.
18. Roy, R.N., and Kitchen, W.H.: NETS: A new system for neonatal transport. Med. J. Aust., 2:855, 1977.

Section *IV*

Operational Aerospace Medicine

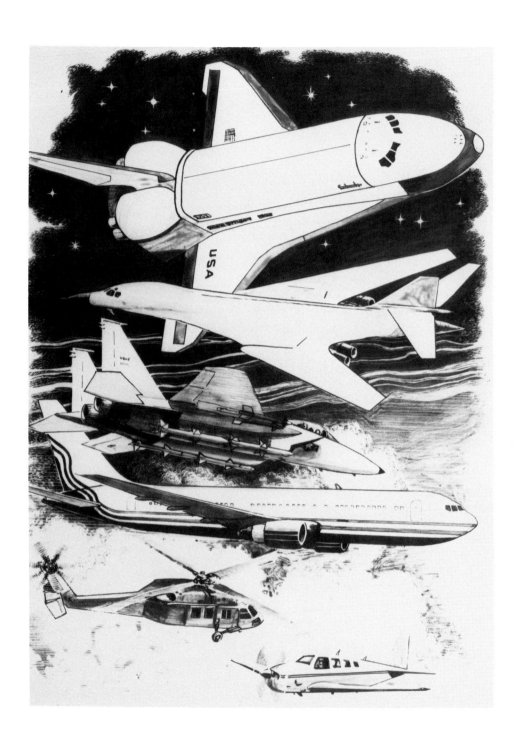

Section *IV*

Operational Aerospace Medicine

Supporting the flyer normally requires more than an office consultation. The physician who is unaware from observation and personal experience of the joy, demands, and stress of flying is ill prepared to deal professionally with the full spectrum of aeromedical issues. For the flight medical examiner or flight surgeon, the halls of the hospital become the runways of the airport. The excitement and tension of the surgical suite has its counterpoint in the exhilaration of flight, and the expectation of the delivery room is paralleled in each new experience that reaches beyond terra firma.

Like an expensive diamond, flying has many facets. Whether vocational or avocational, an airman is normally challenged by only a portion of the flight envelope. He may never need worry about hypoxia while flying his ultralight or, alternatively, may be faced with all the demands on his flying skill and physiologic limitations when orbiting the earth. Flight operations vary greatly, depending on the purpose of the flight; however, the physician needs to be knowledgeable about those operational activities he intends to support. Private flying ranges from soaring in a sailplane to flying high-performance jet aircraft. Commercial aviation may include agricultural flying, cargo transport, air ambulance activities, and, of course, passenger services, ranging from the small commuter airlines to the international air carriers. Military operations provide the greatest professional challenge to the flight surgeon because all aspects of the specialty come into play. Each branch of the armed forces has specific features to its air operations, and these features are delineated in the appropriate chapters. Although the numbers of individuals fortunate to go into space are small, the interest is great, and the physician lucky enough to work in the space program is frequently

613

involved in the scientific frontier of aerospace operations.

SUGGESTED READING LIST

1. Benford, R.J.: Doctors in the Sky. Springfield, Illinois, Charles C. Thomas, 1955.
2. Billings, C.E., Wick, R.L., Jr., Gerke, R.J., and Chase, R.C.: The Effects of Alcohol on Pilot Performance During Instrument Flight. Federal Aviation Administration Office of Aviation Medicine Report No. AM-72-4, U.S. Government Printing Office, Washington, D.C., 1972.
3. Booze, C.F., Jr.: An Appraisal of Federal Aviation Administration Frequency of Examination Requirements. Oklahoma City, Oklahoma, Federal Aviation Administration Civil Aeromedical Institute, 1975.
4. Caidin, M., and Caidin, G.: Aviation and Space Medicine. New York, E.P. Dutton, 1962.
5. Collins, W.E.: Performance Effects of Alcohol Intoxication and Hangover: Ground Level and at Simulated Altitude Federal Aviation Administration Report No. FAA-AM-79-26. U.S. Government Printing Office, Washington, D.C., 1979.
6. DeHart, R.L.: Biomedical Aspects of Soviet Manned Space Flight. Washington, D.C., Defense Intelligence Agency, 1975.
7. Dhenin, G. (ed.): Aviation Medicine. London, Tri-Med Books Ltd., 1978.
8. Dietlein, L.F., and Johnston, R.S.: U.S. manned space flight: The first twenty years. A biomedical status report. Acta Astronautica, 8(9–10): 893–906, 1981.
9. Engle, E., and Lott, A.S.: Man in Flight. Annapolis, Maryland, Leeward Publications, 1979.
10. Esch, A.F., and Albers, W.R.: Outline of Procedures for FAA Aviation Medical Examiner Participation in Aircraft Accident Investigation. Jamaica, New York, Federal Aviation Administration Office of the Regional Flight Surgeon, Eastern Region, 1961.
11. Gazenko, O.G., Genin, A.M., and Yegorov, A.D.: Summary of medical investigations in the U.S.S.R. manned space missions. Acta Astronautica, 8(9–10):907–917, 1981.
12. Institute of Medicine, National Academy of Sciences: Airline Pilot Age, Health and Performance. Washington, D.C., National Academy Press, 1981.
13. Klein, K.E.: Significance of Circadian Rhythms in Aerospace Activities. Agardograph 247. North Atlantic Treaty Organization, NTIS, Springfield, VA, 1980.
14. McCormick, E.J.: Human Factors Engineering. New York, McGraw-Hill Book Co., 1970.
15. McFarland, R.A.: Human Factors in Air Transport Design. New York, McGraw-Hill Book Co., 1946.
16. Military Standard: Human Engineering Design Criteria for Military Systems, Equipment and Facilities. MIL-STD-1472C, U.S. Government Printing Office, Washington, D.C., 1981.
17. Mohler, S.R.: G Effects on the Pilot During Aerobatics. Office of Aviation Medicine Report AM-72-28. U.S. Government Printing Office, Washington, D.C., Federal Aviation Administration, July, 1972.
18. Moore, W.S., et al.: The medical aspects of army aviation. J. Aviat. Med., 26(4)286–291, 1955.
19. National Aeronautics and Space Administration: Foundations of Space Biology and Medicine. Washington, D.C., Government Printing Office, 1975.
20. National Aeronautics and Space Administration: Biomedical Results from Apollo (NASA SP-368). Washington, D.C., Government Printing Office, 1975.
21. National Aeronautics and Space Administration: Biomedical Results from Skylab (NASA SP-377). Washington, D.C., Government Printing Office, 1977.
22. National Institute on Aging: Report of the National Institute on Aging Panel on the Experienced Pilots Study. Bethesda, Maryland, Department of Health and Human Services, Public Health Service, 1981.
23. Neel, S.H., and Shamburek, R.H.: History of army aviation medicine. U.S. Army Aviat. Dig., 9(1):1:17, 1963.
24. Nicogossian, A., and Parker, J.: Space Physiology and Medicine. (NASA SP-447). Washington, D.C., Government Printing Office, 1983.
25. Parker, J.F., and West, V.R. (eds.): Bioastronautics Data Book. 2nd Ed. Washington, D.C., National Aeronautics and Space Administration, 1973.
26. Rose, R.M., Jenkins, C.D., and Hurst, M.W.: Air Traffic Controller Health Change Study. Office of Aviation Medicine Report No. AM-78-39, Washington, D.C., Federal Aviation Administration, 1978.
27. Stevens, S.S., (ed).: Handbook of Experimental Psychology. New York, John Wiley and Sons, 1951.
28. Tierney, R.K.: Forty years of army aviation. U.S. Army Aviat. Dig., 28(8):514–524, 1982.
29. United States Army: Crash Survival Design Guide. TR-71-22. United States Army Air Mobility Research and Development Laboratory, Fort Eustis, Virginia, 1971.
30. United States Army: Army Flight Surgeons' Manual. ST-105-8. United States Army Special Text. United States Army Aeromedical Center, Fort Rucker, Alabama, 1976.
31. United States Naval Flight Surgeons' Manual. U.S. Government Printing Office, Washington, D.C., 1978.
32. Van Cott, H.P., and Kinkade, R.G. (eds.): Human Engineering Guide to Equipment Design. Washington, D.C., Government Printing Office, 1972.
33. Wegmann, H.M.: Models to Predict Loads of Flight Schedules on Cockpit Personnel. Twenty-Ninth International Congress of Aviation and Space Medicine. Nancy, France, 1981.
34. Whitfield, C.L.: Alcoholism. Current Therapy, 1981. Philadelphia, W.B. Saunders Co., 1981.

Chapter *20*

Aerospace Medicine in the United States Air Force

John W. Ord

In the future, the limitations for optimal use of Air and Space may not be imposed by mechanical systems but by the physiological systems of man.

HARRY G. ARMSTRONG

The United States Air Force's aerospace medicine program began with World War I. The high loss rate of American pilots in Europe caused General Pershing to direct a medical board to travel to France to study and define contributing medical problems and to draft recommendations for their correction. The resulting recommendations formed the rationale for the establishment of an aviation medicine program. To provide the trained military surgeons to implement and conduct this program, a school for flight surgeons was established in 1918. The first 50 flight surgeons were authorized by the Army in that same year. Central to many of the recommendations were three elements: (1) aviator selection criteria; (2) health maintenance specific to the needs of the aviator; and (3) the development of aircrew protective equipment. These three elements remain vital constituents of today's Air Force aerospace medical program.

The 600,000 active duty men and women of the Air Force form a key ele-ment of our national defense posture. Of the 34,000 aircrew officers, 22,000 are pilots. Assigned to support these and other aircrew personnel are over 500 flight surgeons, 100 of whom are certified specialists in aerospace medicine. The United States Air Force program has the largest professional commitment to aerospace medicine found in the western world.

THE AIR FORCE MISSION

In the pursuit of our nation's defense, the United States Air Force has a vital, diverse, and challenging role. It maintains a strategic warfare deterrent by operating two legs of our nation's triad (long-range bombers [Fig. 20–1 and Fig. 20–2] and intercontinental ballistic missiles [ICBMs]) and provides military ground forces with air superiority and tactical air-to-ground front-line support capability. The Air Force operates a massive airlift force capable of transporting men and equipment worldwide and has embarked on a broad space program including operational

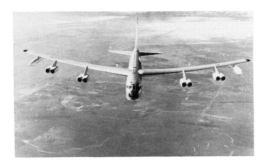

Fig. 20–1. B-52 "Stratofortress," currently the only operational strategic bomber in the Air Force (official United States Air Force photo).

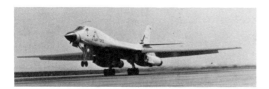

Fig. 20–2. B-1 strategic bomber. This aircraft is being developed to improve the technology and survivability of the nation's strategic force (official United States Air Force photo).

Table 20–1.   Number and Type of United States Air Force Aircraft

Type of Aircraft	Number
Bomber	363
Tanker	544
Fighter	3026
Reconnaissance	392
Cargo	828
Search and rescue	35
Helicopter	238
Trainer	1664
Utility	215
Total United States Air Force	7305
National Guard	1656
Air Force Reserve	458
Total available aircraft	9419

manned space systems. Table 20–1 summarizes the type and number of active Air Force aircraft.

The Training Mission

Each year, 1500 to 2000 young men and women enter undergraduate pilot training. A smaller number of individuals begin navigator instruction. Each of these students undergoes a preliminary flight phys-

ical examination and takes a written test to evaluate flying aptitude.

The physical examination is conducted by a flight surgeon. Unique to this examination is an extensive interview to assess the motivation and suitability of the candidate for aircrew training. The flight surgeon pursues the reasons why the candidate desires a flying career. During these inquiries, the physician assesses the psychosocial development of the candidate and focuses his attention on any history of susceptibility to motion sickness or episodes of unconsciousness. The physical standards for entry into pilot training are among the most demanding in the Air Force.

Table 20–2 illustrates that in the initial selection process approximately 15% of applicants are disqualified. Unusually qualified candidates who have only minor medical defects may be granted a medical waiver to permit further processing for possible selection for aircrew duty. Over the years, the medical reasons for disqualification have remained essentially the same. Historically, impaired vision and refractive errors have accounted for the greatest percentage of disqualifications. Other causes have included allergic and vasomotor rhinorrhea, excessive and substandard height, history of unconsciousness, and immature psychosocial development evident on the interview.

Once training commences, the candidate is again given a flying physical examination to ensure the adequacy and accuracy of the initial selection examination. This procedure is to ensure that the candidate will not be eliminated from flight training due to medical abnormali-

Table 20–2.   Applicants for Undergraduate Flight Training and Medical Qualifications

Factor	1979	1980	1981
Number of applicants	6737	8736	11,192
Medically qualified	5924	7554	9026
Granted medical waiver	367	523	982

ties that may not have been detected earlier or that have developed subsequent to the first examination. The rationale for the attention given the physical examination becomes clear when one realizes that the cost of undergraduate pilot training is $300,000 per student. Thus, to select an individual who is later eliminated for medical reasons is not only devastating emotionally to the individual but costly to the taxpayer.

One of the initial courses given students is physiologic training. This is an introduction to the stresses of flight and to the hazardous environment in which they will be working. An important feature of this training is the opportunity provided the student to experience the effects of hypoxia. The symptoms and their sequence of occurrence tend to be reproducible and unique to each student. The flight surgeon provides numerous hours of lectures and has the opportunity to interact with the students.

During the year of training, a percentage of students will be medically disqualified and fail to complete training. These numbers are small and reflect the excellence of the medical selection process in identifying medical defects prior to the student selection for training. Table 20–3 reviews the medical attrition rate for undergraduate pilot training for 4 consecutive years beginning in 1979. Chronic airsickness leads the specific causes for disqualification, followed by dysfunction of the eustachian tube, allergic and vasomotor rhinorrhea, and disorders of the musculoskeletal system. Sports injuries and motor vehicle accidents are the primary reasons for the musculoskeletal disorders occurring during training. In undergraduate flight training, medical attrition for all causes has averaged between 2 and 4% of the total number of students entering.

Students experiencing problems with airsickness may request assistance from the flight surgeon. It is the physician's responsibility to evaluate the problem thoroughly. Should there by no underlying cause other than the flight environment, the flight surgeon provides reassurance and, if necessary, supervises the limited use of medication for a prescribed period of time to permit adaptation. Should the student fail to overcome his symptoms, he is eliminated from training.

Following completion of primary training, the pilot or navigator is selected to enter training for a specific aircraft type. The designation is most often based on airmanship, with little consideration given to medical factors. As the demands are placed on the pilot by modern combat aircraft for increased cognitive abilities and adaptability to stress, there is a growing realization that aviation life sciences inputs are increasingly important in matching the pilot to the aircraft. The attributes needed by a pilot flying a low-level, high-speed, highly maneuverable A-10 mission (Fig. 20–3) or an air-to-air "dog fight" F-16 profile (Fig. 20–4) are different from those required of the pilot on a long-duration, tedious B-52 bomber mission or a short-haul, repetitive C-130 cargo flight. For example, visual correction may be tolerable in a cargo aircraft but could reduce the combat edge for a tactical mission. Asymptomatic mitral valve prolapse may be of little concern in selecting a KC-135 copilot but could result in serious cardiac arrhythmia when pulling G forces while maneuvering after a bomb run in an F-4. The flight surgeon, through his professional training and operational experi-

Table 20–3. Medical Attrition of Undergraduate Pilot Trainees (UPT)

	1979	1980	1981	1982
UPT	1755	1697	2355	2216
Requiring medical waiver	126	139	326	279
Medical attrition	28	38	79	105

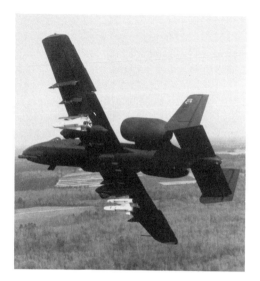

Fig. 20–3. A-10 attack aircraft. This airplane was principally designed as an antitank and close support aircraft (official United States Air Force photo).

ence, can make significant contributions in matching the man to the aircraft. The attributes that can be assessed biomedically are potentially as significant as airmanship or intellect.

The Airlift Mission

The airlift mission is the rapid transportation of military personnel and equipment anywhere on the globe. Strategic airlift employs large aircraft, such as the C-141, C-5 and KC-10 (Fig. 20-5), flying intercontinental, transoceanic, long-duration flights. The tactical element uses smaller cargo aircraft, such as the C-130 or C-7, conducting in-country, short-haul flights. The type of mission defines the aeromedical problems and issues to be addressed by the flight surgeon.

In the strategic airlift scenario, the crew is faced with fatigue, boredom, circadian rhythm desynchronization, in-flight feeding, and dietary disruption. The tactical airlift operation may involve numerous flights daily, often to poorly equipped airfields under marginal landing conditions with minimal hygienic standards, fatigue, environmental extremes, and noise. Use of the chemical defense protection suit may be required if the crew is in a combat area. The suit may compromise crew performance significantly and increase physiologic and psychologic stress.

The Tactical Mission

Military tactical airpower has two fundamental mission elements: assuring air superiority and providing air-to-ground

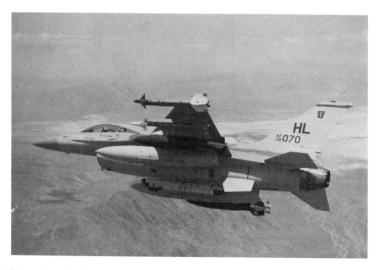

Fig. 20–4. F-16 fighter aircraft. This aircraft was designed as both an air superiority fighter and close support attack aircraft (official United States Air Force photo).

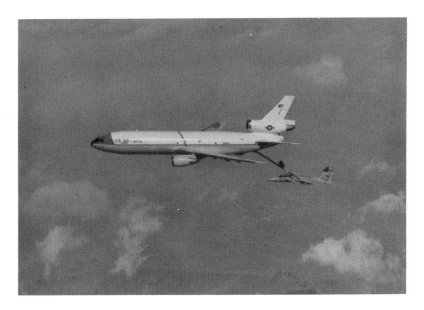

Fig. 20–5. KC-10 Extender aircraft refueling an F-15 Eagle (official United States Air Force photo).

interdiction and front-line support. The flight surgeon must be prepared to address the effects of the combined stressors that are inherent in the high-performance aircraft environment and that tend to reduce pilot effectiveness. High acceleration with rapid onset and extended duration can be exceptionally fatiguing and has the potential to impair vision and induce loss of consciousness. Sensory data inputs from inside and outside the cockpit have the potential for cognitive overload. Thermal extremes are common, and the intense threat from air-defense systems appropriately produces anxiety.

The Strategic Mission

The Air Force's strategic mission is accomplished from both airborne platforms and subterranean facilities. The B-52 and FB-111 constitute the major elements of the airborne strategic force. When operational, the B-1 will provide a major improvement in capability. The nature of the mission frequently requires aircrews to be on flight-line alert for immediate deployment. This procedure contributes to stress, which becomes amplified when airborne.

The flight surgeon, participating as an aircrew member, becomes intimately aware of these factors and the effects on the crew. Low-level, long-duration flight, involving precise navigation, frequent refueling, and constant threat in a combat environment are concerns for aeromedical support of these crewmen.

Missile crews in underground launch facilities also have specific stressors with which they must cope. Because of similarities in operational factors, missile crew medical support is the responsibility of the aerospace medical service. Boredom, isolation, and noise, as well as the possibility of radiation and toxic exposures, are some of the factors with which the flight surgeon must be prepared to cope.

Military Man in Space

The Space Command is responsible for the military man in space mission. Although still being defined, specific responsibilities and functions are more appropriate to a military organization than to a civilian space agency. Responsibilities in command and control, surveillance and observation, and testing and evaluation of military systems are potential activities for the military astronaut. The flight surgeon supporting this mission must be trained and well versed in the art and science of aviation medicine and, in addition, must be professionally competent in space medicine. He must be prepared to assist his crews in coping with the space adaptation syndrome (space sickness), problems of ergonomics and human engineering, galactic and solar radiation, cardiovascular and muscle deconditioning, bone demineralization, and the many problems involved with extravehicular activity.

THE AIR FORCE AEROSPACE MEDICINE PROGRAM

United States Air Force directives define succinctly the objectives of the aerospace medical program to be the promotion and maintenance of the physical and mental health of Air Force personnel and other persons for whom the Air Force is responsible. These objectives are to be attained by the application of the principles of flight medicine, preventive medicine, occupational medicine, and bioenvironmental engineering. The flight surgeon is charged with the primary responsibility for the conduct of this program. He is the coordinator of the team of specialists involved. In the Unites States Air Force, the operational systems that the flight surgeon supports include aircraft, missiles, and space vehicles.

Flight Medicine

Within the Air Force environment, flight medicine is that branch of health care that is responsible for the medical aspects of the selection and maintenance of flying personnel. The population served by this discipline is not limited to aircrew members but frequently involves all personnel who are directly involved in the support of aerospace operations, including all flying personnel, missile crewmembers, and air traffic controller personnel. Many flight medicine clinics expand their

medical role by incorporating other individuals, such as maintenance personnel, who support operational activities. It is not uncommon for the flight surgeon to become the "family physician" to the dependents of flying personnel.

The flight surgeon's responsibility is broad and includes a variety of activities integral to the maintenance of the health of flying personnel. These activities include providing periodic flight physical examinations, supporting flying safety activities, ensuring crew effectiveness, providing medical training regarding selfcare, conducting periodic aeromedical indoctrination on the hazardous environment of flight, actively participating in the squadron's flying activities or joining a crew in a missile launch facility, conducting a variety of medicomilitary activities, and encouraging participation in prospective health care programs. To accomplish these activities, the flight surgeon must spend a considerable amount of time outside the office. As in the case of any practicing physician, the flight surgeon must make ward rounds, but in this context the ward becomes the flight line or the missile launch facility.

In the Air Force, flight surgeons must be physically qualified to participate in aerial flight. Where possible, the flight surgeon is expected to fly frequently as a crewmember in the primary aircraft of the squadron. When multiseat aircraft are not available, the flight surgeon conducts his flying activities in designated support aircraft.

For 30 years, the United States Air Force has conducted a pilot-physician program. These physicians, who are qualified both as operationally current pilots and flight surgeons, have made significant contributions to advancing aerospace medicine. Currently, five to ten physicians are flying as operationally qualified military pilots. Their activities are deeply involved with flying safety, aircraft accident investigation, medical consultation to aircraft systems project offices for new aircraft, and evaluation of problems involving man-machine interfaces. Past experience has shown that one to five ex-military pilots rejoin the Air Force as physicians each year. From this pool, the cadre of pilot-physicians is drawn to meet high-priority Air Force requirements.

Environmental Medicine

Within the aerospace medicine program context, environmental medicine is concerned with preventive medicine, public health, and health education. Responsibilities for this phase of the aerospace medical program may rest with flight surgeons, veterinarians, and/or environmental health nurses. This function, in its broadest sense, has as its concern the health of the community. The immunization status of the population on the base, not only the military work force but civilian employees and dependents, is an area of interest. The public health control of communicable diseases, such as influenza, hepatitis, and diseases endemic in other parts of the world, is a responsibility of this program. The wholesomeness of food brought on base for serving military personnel, its preparation, and its storage are appropriate areas of interest. Issues of hygiene in such public places as swimming pools, barber and beauty shops, and food service concessions receive attention under this program.

The role of appropriate health education to encourage effective preventive health practices is a part of environmental medicine. Programs are conducted not only in the medical and dental facilities but also in educational and recreational facilities throughout the base. Special courses are conducted periodically to assist in weight control, physical fitness, smoking cessation, and nutrition.

Occupational Medicine

The objective of the United States Air Force occupational health program is to protect personnel, both military and civilian, from health hazards in their working environment. The department assists in the placement of personnel in jobs that the individual can perform effectively without endangering himself or others. Such placement advice is provided after due consideration of all the physical and emotional capabilities of the employee. The flight surgeon or occupational medicine specialist provides guidelines for physiologic monitoring of exposure to adverse environmental factors, requests hazard assessments, establishes diagnoses and makes disposition in occupational illnesses, and works closely with other components of the aerospace medical team toward optimizing the working environment for the employee.

Working closely with the physician is the bioenvironmental engineer. His primary responsibility is conducting the nonclinical portion of the occupational medicine program. The engineer supervises the assessment of the work environment and the implementation of controls for hazard abatement. It is the bioenvironmental engineer's responsibility to establish and conduct environmental monitoring programs to assess compliance with federal, state, and local pollution standards. The engineer becomes actively involved in international health activities as a monitor of quarantine programs associated with movement by aircraft of matériel across international borders. This department also maintains surveillance of potable water supplies and waste disposal systems. Engineering expertise is most needed in responding to accidents that could pose significant health hazards to the base and the community.

POSTGRADUATE MEDICAL EDUCATION IN AEROSPACE MEDICINE

Within the United States, the Air Force is the largest employer of professionally and paraprofessionally trained personnel in the field of aerospace medicine. To meet the demand for high-quality trained professionals, the Air Force conducts an extensive program in postgraduate education in the field of aerospace medicine. The scope of the program ranges from a primary course to a residency program for physicians, education and training for nurses and medical technicians in aeromedical evacuation, training for scientific personnel in the environmental hazards of flight, and training for engineers in the assessment of the environment.

The Primary Course in Aerospace Medicine

Approximately four times per year, 100 physicians arrive at the United States Air Force School of Aerospace Medicine (USAFSAM) at Brooks Air Force Base, Texas to begin their indoctrination and professional education as Air Force flight surgeons (Fig. 20–6). Their education process already has begun through the use of a self-paced advance study program that requires about 40 hours to complete. In the 8 weeks that they remain at USAFSAM, they will be exposed to and participate in

lectures, seminars, and workshops. They will receive training in aircraft egress, altitude chamber indoctrination, principles of survival, and fly in an Air Force jet trainer. The clinical skills of these physicians will be sharpened in those areas of particular interest to aerospace medicine such as ophthalmology, otolaryngology, and internal medicine. Throughout the course, one principle is stressed—an effective flight surgeon is above all an excellent physician. The training is devoted to the extra attention necessary to meet and solve the special problems of the flyer.

The training and practice in aerospace medicine involves three functional areas. The first area addresses flight and missile medicine, the most unique area for the majority of physicians coming into the field. The prospective flight surgeon must learn the processes of applying medical standards in the initial selection and follow-up evaluation of aircrew members. As in most phases of medicine, there are periodic examinations for the detection of unexpected disease and to prevent the onset or progression of chronic ailments. Emphasis is placed on the concept of careful eval-

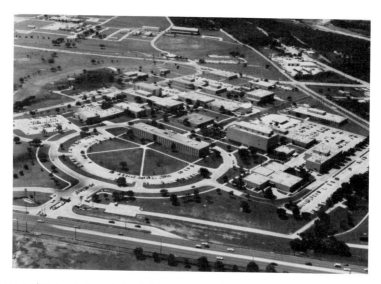

Fig. 20–6. The United States Air Force School of Aerospace Medicine, Brooks Air Force Base, Texas (official United States Air Force photo).

uation of minor complaints to maintain the pilot in optimum mental and physical health for fully successful performance of his flying duties. The second functional area receiving emphasis is the application of clinical medical specialties in aerospace medicine. Specialists in the fields of otolaryngology, ophthalmology, internal medicine and its subspecialties, neurology, and psychiatry have significant contributions to make in their areas of expertise in relation to the health maintenance of the flyer. The third functional area is the broad concept of environmental health. This concept involves the review of classic public health principles and the establishment of an appreciation of the responsibilities of occupational medicine. The various techniques of evaluating occupational hazards are discussed and the concept of protective measures introduced.

Successful completion of this primary course permits the physician to wear the wings of a flight surgeon. Not all flight surgeons are assigned primary duty in support of flyers or to operational flying units. Career Air Force physicians are encouraged to take the primary course in aerospace medicine to enable them to better support the Air Force mission regardless of their normal clinical and professional responsibilities. Since the conclusion of World War II, approximately 20,000 physicians have received primary aerospace medical training in the Air Force.

The Specialty of Aerospace Medicine

The specialist in aerospace medicine has made the career decision to receive extensive formal training in the field. The United States Air Force has requirements for over 100 specialists in aerospace medicine. To satisfy these requirements, the Air Force conducts the largest aerospace medicine residency program in the western world. Each year, 20 to 25 physicians enter the program. These residents in aerospace medicine (RAM) are men and

women who have had operational experience as flight surgeons and have now selected more extensive education in the field. The Air Force program also trains military physicians from other services, applicants from other federal agencies, and medical officers from allied nations. For convenience of management, the residency is divided into three phases.

Phase 1 is an academic year conducted normally at a university department of public health leading to a master's degree in public health. This year ensures that the flight surgeon receives appropriate postgraduate education in epidemiology, biostatistics, health care administration, and environmental medicine. This academic year provides a strong foundation on which to base future contributions to the field of aerospace medicine.

Phase 2 is conducted at USAFSAM. The RAM receives an extensive ground school and indoctrination program in an Air Force jet trainer and actively participates in the evaluation and disposition of problem aeromedical cases involving aircrew. The RAM participates in site visits to numerous operational Air Force Bases, industrial and manufacturing complexes, space training and launch facilities, and research institutions. The RAM also has the opportunity to pursue individual research interests.

Phase 3 is also conducted at USAFSAM, with additional field trips, including aircraft accident investigations, an opportunity to conduct special research projects, and participation in boards of inquiry and in staff assistance visits to base medical facilities. With completion of this phase, the RAM is ready for a challenging operational assignment, entering the research and development community, or participating as a policy maker in aerospace medicine at a Command or Headquarters.

Additional Professional Education and Training

To ensure that the broadest application of all aspects of aerospace medicine are applied to the aerospace medicine program, all other team members also are trained at USAFSAM.

Hyperbaric Medicine

Management of cases of air embolism occurring in aircraft or altitude chambers led the Air Force to initiate a hyperbaric medicine program. Located at key bases around the world, the Air Force has positioned small, one-patient hyperbaric chambers to be available if needed for the management of aviators' bends. More recently, these chambers have begun to be used to deliver oxygen under hyperbaric conditions as a treatment method for specific medical conditions. Technicians, physicians, and nurses are trained in hyperbaric medicine to operate these chambers. With a growing awareness in the medical community of the benefits of hyperbaric oxygen therapy, the Air Force has a dynamic program under way for the construction of hyperbaric centers at its major facilities. The training program at USAFSAM is geared to provide the experienced cadre of professionals and technicians to man these chambers as they become available.

Aeromedical Evacuation

Each year, approximately 300 nurses and technicians receive training in the management of patients to be transported in the Air Force international aeromedical evacuation system. Key to the training of these aeromedical crews is knowledge of the environmental factors of flight. Although aircraft such as the C-9 are designed for aeromedical evacuation, they are not, as has occasionally been intimated, true flying hospitals. These aircraft are patient transportation systems, and although sophisticated in their capability to support the patient, they are nevertheless aircraft generating acceleration forces, atmospheric pressure changes, noise, and temperature and humidity variations. These medical crews receive extensive

training in the management of the patient in such an environment.

Aerospace Physiology Training

Within the Air Force, the aerospace physiology training officer is the individual principally responsible for the indoctrination of student aircrew in the discipline of altitude physiology. The training of these officers and the technicians who support them is conducted at USAFSAM.

Bioenvironmental Engineering

The bioenvironmental engineer receives training in environmental assessment, hazard abatement, and employee protection at USAFSAM. These graduate engineers receive extensive firsthand experience as part of this educational program.

Preventive Medicine Residency

Similar to the RAM program, other physicians receive postgraduate training in general preventive medicine and occupational medicine at USAFSAM. These separate residency programs are conducted to satisfy Air Force requirements. The programs draw on the enormous potential for worldwide teaching experience in these fields that is available to the Air Force.

Allied Officer Training

Many of the courses described in the previous sections are attended by allied officers from throughout the free world. An advanced course for allied medical officers in aerospace medicine is offered yearly by the Air Force. This 6-month course is attended by 10 to 20 highly selected medical officers from friendly nations throughout the world. This advanced course is designed to provide the knowledge and experience necessary for the flight surgeon to return to his own country and become a leader in aerospace medicine. The course has many parallels to the USAFSAM portion of the RAM program previously described. It is usual for the senior leadership of a nation's Air

Force medical department to be drawn from graduates of this program.

AEROMEDICAL DISPOSITION AND WAIVER ACTION

The aeromedical disposition process begins when the applicant applies for flight training. When selected to participate in aerial flight, the individual has successfully completed the first element of a career-long physical assessment process. Subsequently, the aircrew member will receive periodic physical examinations varying in frequency and detail depending on his duties as a crewmember. Normally, these assessments find the aircrewman in excellent health, but occasionally medical abnormalities are revealed that require further evaluation and illnesses are experienced requiring intervention of the medical team. The disposition of these medical problems, whether found on physical examination or presenting as a clinical problem, must be evaluated with regard to job performance and safety.

Primary Care: Evaluation by the Flight Surgeon

When a crewmember presents for medical treatment or evaluation, the flight surgeon must decide whether the medical findings will jeopardize health, flying safety, or mission completion. Within the Air Force, it is normal practice to remove aircrewmen from flight duty when they are experiencing acute illnesses, have sustained injury, or require medication. During the periodic physical assessment, changes in examination findings may exceed acceptable norms. In such cases, the flight surgeon must make a disposition regarding the patient's ability to continue flying. In the vast majority of cases, the aircrewman is grounded only temporarily to allow sufficient time for the acute illness to subside or to clarify the significance of an abnormal physical finding.

Procedurally, the flight surgeon does not actually ground anyone. He serves as a consultant and staff officer to the flying unit commander and provides a recommendation that the aircrewman be removed from active flying status for a period of time. Such recommendations are rarely ignored.

Once the aircrewman has recovered from his acute illness, he returns to his flight surgeon for reassessment and for clearance to return to flying. Likewise, if the physical examination has revealed a minor abnormality outside the range routinely permitted for that physical condition, the flight surgeon will request a waiver from his higher headquarters for the medical problem. In both cases, the flyer is returned to duty. Periodically, the flight surgeon will be faced with a disease or physical finding requiring the assistance of consultants.

Secondary Care: Evaluation by the Consultant

Acute illnesses with a potential for serious sequelae or physical findings necessitating more refined evaluation require the flight surgeon to turn to his professional colleagues for consultation. Such consultative services may be available at his own medical facility or may require the aircrewman to go to a larger regional hospital or medical center for more extensive evaluation. From the aeromedical point of view, these evaluations have two goals. The first goal is to ensure that the medical problem is not complicated by engaging in aerial flight, and the second goal is to ensure that the medical condition will not compromise flying safety. With these two goals in mind, the flight surgeon arranges for the consultation and necessary evaluation.

The consultant's primary role is to evaluate the medical condition and to provide a diagnosis. The consultant physician may recommend treatment as appropriate or determine the frequency and scope of further evaluation. It is not the consultant's role to define the impact of the medical condition on the flying career of the individual. This remains the province of the unit flight surgeon who is directly responsible for the medical support of the aircrewman.

Once the consultation is complete, the flight surgeon initiates the appropriate disposition action, returning the aircrewman to his aeronautic duties, requesting waiver for an established medical condition, or advising the flyer of the incompatibility of his medical condition with continued flying. Periodically, the base flight surgeon will request evaluation and consultation from the Aeromedical Consultation Service of USAFSAM.

Tertiary Care: Evaluation at the United States Air Force School of Aerospace Medicine

The Aeromedical Consultation Service at USAFSAM was established to bring together experts in the major clinical specialties for the purpose of making recommendations regarding flyers whose aeromedical disposition is in question. Each year, 600 to 700 aircrewmen, predominantly pilots, are evaluated by the Aeromedical Consultation Service. Historically, in 80% of cases, the result has been a recommendation for a return to flying duties. The vast majority of those individuals arriving for evaluation are grounded at the time they are to be evaluated. These evaluations have enabled the Air Force to retain the invaluable experience of more senior aviators and to avoid the enormous cost that otherwise would have been incurred in training replacements.

The consultation center is staffed primarily by specialists with flight surgeon experience. It is common to have physicians professionally qualified both in aerospace medicine and in a clinical specialty assisting in the assessment of those being evaluated. To ensure the emphasis on aerospace medicine and the integrity of the operational flight medicine concept,

each patient is assigned to a flight surgeon who serves as his personal physician during the evaluation. The evaluations are extensive and take approximately 1 week to conduct. The problems most frequently seen are related to the cardiovascular system, central nervous system, and the visual system. Consequently, these are the strongest departments in the consultation center.

Not all patients are initially referred by their base flight surgeon. Some referrals are requested by the consultation center as a result of preliminary evaluations. This request occurs most commonly in the area of cardiology because USAFSAM reviews all electrocardiograms performed on aircrews throughout the world. Abnormalities revealed by these tracings may require further evaluation, and, consequently, the consultation center may request that the aircrewman be sent for assessment.

Once the evaluation is complete, an aeromedical summary is prepared and forwarded to the base flight surgeon who is responsible for the primary care of the aircrewman. It then becomes the flight surgeon's responsibility to determine the necessary action for disposition of the case. Because of the significant nature of the majority of cases seen by the consultation center, waiver by higher headquarters, including the Office of the Surgeon General, is frequently necessary.

Disposition by Waiver

When it has been determined that the event or the medical condition, although normally disqualifying, would not in fact compromise the health of the individual or flying safety, the flight surgeon may initiate action requesting a waiver. It remains the flight surgeon's responsibility to determine whether the condition of his patient is compatible with flying duties and, if so, to submit the appropriate waiver request. In many cases, the Major Air Command Surgeon has the authority to approve a waiver for history of an event or a medical condition. For potentially serious medical problems, the Air Force Surgeon General is the exclusive waiver authority. Aircrewmen who are medically disqualified but receive waivers for the disqualification frequently will be required to periodically undergo special medical assessments.

Within the Air Force, the waiver policy is dynamic. It changes with improvements in diagnostic capabilities resulting from advancements in medical technology and the prognostic estimations of modern epidemiology. For many years, it was Air Force policy that a pilot must be medically qualified to fly any aircraft in the Air Force inventory. Recently, a major change has occurred in the medical waiver policy for flying personnel. Waivers are issued in four major categories: (1) the aircrewman who is universally assignable; (2) the aircrewman who is limited to tanker, transport, bomber, and mission support aircraft; (3) the aircrewman who is limited to flying nonejection seat aircraft; and (4) the aircrewman for whom specific limitations are described.

By broadening the waiver window, the Air Force can expect to save between $50 and $60 million annually by avoiding the replacement training costs for aircrewmen who otherwise would have been lost from duty. This new waiver policy increases the responsibility of the flight surgeon to make the proper aeromedical disposition.

Not all aircrewmen receive a waiver for their disqualifying medical problems. Table 20–4 lists the causes for medical disqualification of pilots and navigators for 1980 and 1981 for which the Surgeon General has records, representing approximately 60% of those aircrew disqualified.

CENTERS OF EXCELLENCE SUPPORTING THE AEROSPACE MEDICINE PROGRAM

For half a century, the United States Air Force has had two institutions that have been keys to the quality of its aerospace medicine program. Founded by General Harry G. Armstrong prior to World War II, the Aerospace Medical Research Laboratory at Wright-Patterson Air Force Base in Ohio has maintained a continuing research program. The School of Aerospace Medicine at Brooks Air Force Base, Texas has maintained its preeminence in the fields of education, clinical evaluation, and research. Both of these institutions are under a single organization for management and program direction—the Aerospace Medical Division.

Air Force Aerospace Medical Research Laboratory

The Air Force Aerospace Medical Research Laboratory (AFAMRL) was established in the mid-1930s to resolve protective equipment deficiencies for aircrews flying open-cockpit pursuit aircraft. Through the years, this focus on equipment design has been the central thrust of AFAMRL. The development of oxygen equipment, cabin pressurization technology, ejection seat testing and evaluation, human engineering research, and noise and communications have been major long-term activities.

The staff of more than 300 scientists, engineers, and technicians at AFAMRL are currently involved in research organized in three primary disciplines: (1) the toxicologic study of the chemical compounds required to support operational and industrial Air Force needs; (2) man-machine integration as it relates to aerospace systems; and (3) biodynamics.

Toxicology

The research program in toxicology is designed to identify and quantify toxic hazards created by chemical agents characteristic of advanced Air Force systems and operations. Safe exposure criteria are developed for toxic chemicals that have the potential for adverse effects on personnel and the environment. Advanced analytic techniques are employed to study the environmental impact of these com-

Table 20–4. Causes For Medical Disqualification of United States Air Force Pilots and Navigators For the 2 Years From 1980 to 1981*

Diseases	Age Group			Total	Percentage
	20–29	30–39	40+		
Coronary artery disease	0	2	29	31	10%
Hypertension	0	7	23	30	10%
Degenerative spine disease	3	2	15	20	7%
Diabetes mellitus	0	6	8	14	5%
Asthma	3	4	6	13	4%
Headaches (migraine, other)	5	2	6	12	4%
Arrhythmias	1	4	5	11	4%
Abnormal ECG and/or ETT (treadmill)	0	0	10	10	3%
Peptic ulcer disease	3	0	5	8	3%
Syncope	1	4	3	8	3%
Alcoholism	0	3	5	8	3%
Obesity	2	2	4	8	3%
Abnormal EEG and/or seizure disorders	3	3	1	7	2%
Allergic rhinitis	5	1	1	7	2%
Sarcoidosis	2	4	0	6	2%
Ulcerative colitis	4	1	0	5	2%
Melanoma	2	1	1	4	1%
Peripheral neuropathy	1	1	2	4	1%
Chronic sinusitis	1	2	1	4	1%
Personality disorder	3	1	0	4	1%
Total	39	50	125	214	71%
Other diseases	14	35	41	90	29%
Total	53	85	166	304	100%

*Data abstracted from the United States Air Force medical waiver file by R.C. Whitton.

pounds and to clarify the modes of toxic action of a compound in biologic systems. The data derived from these studies provide guidance to Air Force product developers and users to ensure safe operations. Effort is continuing to evaluate a number of new in vitro and in vivo screening methodologies for compounds with mutagenic, teratogenic, and oncogenic potential. Major studies have concentrated on hydrazine, jet fuels, and metallic slurries.

Man-Machine Integration

Conducting modern warfare, particularly against numerically superior forces, demands that Air Force research and development programs design systems and equipment for maximum effectiveness. The human operator is often simultaneously the critical component and the limiting factor of manned systems. High-performance aircraft, low-level, high-speed flight, and high-density threat environments combine to provide a severe chal-

lenge to effective mansystem performance. This challenge necessitates the development of revolutionary methods of reconnaissance, target acquisition, rapid data processing, decision making, and effective command and control. The AFAMRL conducts a major program to develop the technology for advanced visual display systems. These efforts concentrate on display and control systems that optimize the interface of systems operators to flight control, navigation, and command and control subsystems. This work has enhanced pilot capabilities through the development of new head-up and head-down display systems. Other aspects of this research address the critical questions of systems automation, that is, the allocation of decision making and control functions to the operator or to the onboard computer, the types of display information, stress effects, work load control, effective human communications, and appropriate man-machine interaction. Critical to evaluating the effectiveness of the application of these technologies is the development of methods to quantify the work load imposed on the aircraft operator. Both subjective and objective methods are under development to improve the ability to quantify work load and, more significantly, to prevent overload.

Biodynamic Research

Mechanical forces are imposed on the crewman in the day-to-day operations conducted by the United States Air Force. These forces include sustained and transient acceleration and deceleration, aerodynamic deceleration, vibration, impact, and noise. For successful mission accomplishment, it is essential that the effects of these forces be controlled to acceptable levels in terms of human tolerance and safety. Research in the areas of noise and direct mechanical forces emphasizes effective performance and safety in the operational flight environment. Another application of biodynamics technology is in the reduction of morbidity and mortality resulting from ejection from disabled high-performance aircraft.

Noise produced in the Air Force environment impairs performance and can affect health. Voice communication problems are critical in tactical air operations. Research is ongoing to reduce these difficulties. The objective is to establish specifications and parameters that will ensure voice communications effectiveness in high-noise–level environments. For the communities surrounding air bases, noise as an environmental quality issue becomes a concern. Technology has been developed by AFAMRL to permit Air Force organizations to satisfy environmental noise assessment requirements stemming from the National Environmental Policy Act of 1973. Appropriate noise assessment technology must be available also to meet the requirements of the Air Installation Compatible Use Zone (AICUZ) program.

The AFAMRL provides the Air Force expertise in the bioeffects of mechanical force resulting from impact or alternating force fields (vibration). The research and development activities are typically associated with performance enhancement, crew comfort, and safety. With the use of the dynamic environmental simulator, a multidimensional centrifuge, the laboratory conducts complex, real-time, simulations of air-to-air and air-to-surface combat engagements to define the effects of acceleration on pilot performance. Research is then directed toward developing technologies to reduce any performance decrements.

The AFAMRL represents a national resource with regard to both its scientific expertise and its sophisticated flight environment simulation devices. Consequently, other federal agencies, such as the Department of Transportation and the National Aeronautics and Space Administration, turn to this laboratory for support of their research requirements. The laboratory also accomodates both Army and Navy aeromedical research needs.

United States Air Force School of Aerospace Medicine

From its origin in support of medical requirements for the fledgling Air Force in World War I to research supporting the space shuttle orbiter, USAFSAM has been at the forefront of aerospace medical research and development. As noted previously, the USAFSAM fulfills clinical aerospace medical practice and education missions in addition to its research and development role. This execution of Air Force programs in research and development, education, and medical support in the same institution has been highly successful because of the synergistic effect and cross utilization of the professional staff. Clinicians involved in aeromedical assessment of problem medical cases fulfill a significant teaching role in the educational program. The epidemiologists not only teach but define research requirements to be pursued by other elements of the school. Training of flight nurses and technicians in aeromedical evacuation has delineated shortfalls in patient support requiring the research and development of new equipment. The USAFSAM research and development program is divided into three disciplinary categories.

Clinical Sciences

The value to the Air Force of highly skilled aircrew members increases in direct proportion to the increasing complexity and cost of new aeronautic and space systems. It is critical, therefore, that accurate and specific medical selection criteria be applied in choosing candidates for flight training, that the best possible medical care be given to the fully trained aircrewmember, and that prevention of disease and the refinement of medical retention criteria be optimized to increase the career life expectancy or "cockpit longevity" of the Air Force Flyer. The process of evaluating an aircrewman in the Aeromedical Consultation Service contributes to a growing data base enabling the clinical specialist, with increasing precision, to establish the significance of a medical finding to aerospace flight. Crucial to much of the effort conducted in this research program is the differentiation of normal from abnormal findings in asymptomatic, generally healthy aircrew. It has become clear that medical findings in this population may have a very different significance from that related to hospital treatment populations.

Research is conducted and techniques developed to enhance aircrew performance. Biofeedback has been successfully employed in the treatment of aircrew suffering from chronic airsickness. Visual corrective devices that are compatible with the aerospace environment have been developed. The evaluation of the use of soft contact lenses by aircrew of high-performance aircraft is such an effort. Research is ongoing to identify the psychophysiologic characteristics that may predict pilot performance in high-performance aircraft. This research will contribute to the criteria for the selection of pilots for specific types of flight vehicles and missions.

Advanced Crew Technology

Research programs under this discipline are pursued to ensure the protection, readiness, and effective utilization of aircrew in advanced and future aeronautics and space systems. The multistress environment of flight is simulated by the use of altitude chambers, thermal stress-generating devices, motion-based flight simulators, and a human centrifuge. Advanced life-support systems, including oxygen systems, breathing and filtration masks, acceleration protection equipment, altitude protection systems, and personal thermal stress protection systems are the products of the research and development efforts.

Another research program has as its objective the prevention of aircraft accidents caused by human error. A data base is being generated that will include actual accidents, near mishaps, and data concerning flight systems and operations. This data base is being structured to provide the ability to analyze actual accidents and to predict situations that could lead to accidents and, therefore, to the capability to control and eliminate human-factor–related accidents.

Medical systems requirements for safe and effective transportation of patients by air in peacetime and wartime require research and development and operational testing of new airborne medical equipment. This is accomplished in the advanced crew technology research and development program.

Radiation Technology

The biologic effects of all forms of electromagnetic radiation, including lasers, radio frequency emitters, directed energy beams, and sources of ionizing radiation, are addressed by this disciplinary effort. Technology documents are developed defining personnel hazard assessments, safe separation distances, performance estimates, and nuclear radiation hazard environments. Research is conducted to determine the bioeffects of both continuous wave versus pulsed radio frequency radiation generated by radar systems. Biologic dosimetric methods, the effects of electromagnetic radiation, and the mathematical modeling of the environmental impact of various energy generators are other important elements of this research thrust.

For the foreseeable future, the Air Force's principal operational commitment will be to aeronautic rather than space systems. Hardware technology will continue to impose greater demands on the operator both in terms of environmental stresses and in the area of performance and the integration of cognitive information processing with decision making and systems control. The Air Force aerospace medical program will continue to be expected to meet the challenges: to select quality flight crewmen, to ensure their protection in the flight environment, to optimize their interactions with the flight vehicle systems, and to maintain and extend their longevity in their profession.

Chapter 21

Army Aviation Medicine

N. Bruce Chase and Robert J. Kreutzmann

If military history teaches us anything, it is that victory goes to the side that can best maneuver its forces and use its firepower to close with and destroy the enemy.

Unknown

From a few Sikorsky R4-Bs in 1944 to a fleet of over 8000 United States Army rotary-wing aircraft in 1982, helicopters have provided mobility of men, matériel, and firepower unequalled in the annals of military history. In the civil sector and in other military forces around the world, the helicopter has served in missions ranging from air ambulance to offensive gunships. The phenomenal success of the helicopter in a multitude of missions results from its ability to move quickly from place to place without the need for large, fixed facilities or interference from intervening terrain. From oil platforms in the oceans to mountaintop rescue and from aerial command posts to nap-of-the-earth (NOE) tank killer, the helicopter has proved itself to be one

of man's most useful and versatile products of technology. There are few areas of technology where the interface between man and his machine is more important than in rotary-wing aviation. The helicopter pilot's ability to assimilate and integrate information, control the aircraft and its subsystems, and endure an unfriendly environment are often stretched to the absolute limit. The flight surgeon's role in selecting personnel who will perform well in that environment, in maintaining their health and performance, and in reducing the hazards of the environment is critical. Each facet of military and civil helicopter aviation has its own unique set of man-related problems that must be solved effectively by aeromedical personnel if man, machine, and mission capabilities are to be preserved. With increasingly sophisticated aircraft and increasing dependency on those aircraft, the aeromedical aspects of rotary-wing aviation have grown from a scarcely noticeable beginning many years ago to a full-fledged although not

The authors wish to thank other senior members of the Society of United States Army Flight Surgeons for their contributions to this chapter: P. Elroy Jenkins, M.D.; Dudley R. Price, M.D.; Ronald R. Rossing, M.D.; David J. Wehrly, M.D.; Clarence R. Collins, M.D.; Nicholas E. Barreca, M.D.; and Bennett G. Owens, Jr., M.D.

formally recognized, component of the specialty of aerospace medicine.

Army aviation medicine faces the challenge of supporting worldwide air, terrestrial, and sea operations. Army aviation forces are assigned to units deployed around the world and are exposed to environmental extremes, exotic diseases, parasitic infestations, high terrestrial elevation, chemical and toxic agents, noise, vibration, and other stresses common to aviation. The Army aviator often lives in the vicinity of unit ground soldiers and is, therefore, subject to the same diseases unless meticulous preventive medicine principles are strictly adhered to. Military flight missions include everything from the wearing of bulky chemical protective gear during NOE flight in a tropical environment to night flight in isolated and distant mountain terrain during bitter cold winter operations. The Army aviator must know the limitations of both the aircraft and himself under these highly varied conditions to enhance both safety and military effectiveness.

Advances in technology and the associated communication, navigation, target acquisition, and weapons system management have increased aviator work load levels. The effective use of sophisticated visionics equipment requires exceptional visual acuity and ocular motility. Nap-of-the-earth flight with night vision goggles under adverse weather conditions demands the utmost levels of skill, training, and mental acuity. The burdens of chemical, toxic, and laser protective equipment add significantly to the combined stresses the Army aviator endures.

The Army flight surgeon must enhance human dimensions to the fullest by carefully integrating the principles of preventive, occupational, behavioral, and clinical medicine. He must apply his knowledge of these principles to the aviator's environment and equipment and to the total threat the aviator faces, which ranges from disease to enemy doctrine.

The Army flight surgeon's knowledge of scientific, medical, aviation, and military disciplines must be applied throughout a total mission spectrum to achieve peacetime safety and combat readiness. To this end, the Army flight surgeon must be observant, inquisitive, action-oriented, and must work in concert with his unit, staff, and professionals of many other disciplines.

HISTORY OF ARMY AVIATION

Once the transition from the Army Air Corps to the United States Air Force had begun, the Army continued to need limited, organic, direct support aviation. On June 6, 1942, following feasibility tests conducted in 1941, the War Department approved organic, fixed-wing aviation for field artillery. Flight training began under Air Corps supervision for a few field artillery lieutenant and staff sergeant pilots headed for assignments overseas. The first operational use of small, fixed-wing aircraft began on November 9, 1942, when three L-4 Grasshoppers (Piper Cubs) took off from the aircraft carrier U.S.S. Ranger to adjust artillery fire during the invasion of North Africa. Subsequent missions performed by small L-4 and L-5 aircraft included the adjustment of artillery, mortar, and naval fire, reconnaissance, photography, message drop and pickup, guiding patrols through dense jungles, supply of isolated units, and courier missions. Army aviation continued to support forces throughout World War II in both the European and Pacific theaters.

The initial demands for organic Army aviation were for observation and short utility missions by small, fixed-wing aircraft. The subsequent technologic development and growth of rotary-wing flight later was to fill the Army's need for rapid evacuation of wounded from confined areas, rapid insertion of troops and supplies on short notice, and tactical support.

The current Army helicoper fleet of 8250 aircraft began on April 20, 1942, when Igor Sikorsky successfully demonstrated the XR-4 prototype helicopter. By January, 1943, the YR-4B helicopter was undergoing tests as an air ambulance. Procurement and deployment soon followed, and on April 23, 1944, the first rotary-wing combat medical air evacuation was begun in the China-Burma-India theater. Air ambulance applications in Korea and the added tactical applications in Vietnam proved the versatility and military importance of the helicopter. By overflying impassable terrain and landing at unimproved sites, helicopters dramatically reduced response time from days to minutes for resupply, evacuation, and other missions. The military applications of helicopters have steadily grown, so that now almost every combat division has become heavily dependent on rotary-wing aviation.

Fixed-wing aircraft have been important to the Army, but after reaching a peak of over 3000 aircraft in the mid-1960s, Army fixed-wing aircraft have been steadily replaced by the helicopter. Of 8821 Army aircraft today, only 571 fixed-wing aircraft remain in the inventory. Because the helicopter now dominates Army aviation, this chapter will concentrate on the application of aeromedical principles to rotary-wing flight.

HISTORY OF ARMY AVIATION MEDICINE

The June 6, 1942 order establishing Army aviation made no provision for specialized medical support. Because the United States Army Air Forces (USAAF) were part of the Army, specialized aviation medicine support to liaison pilots and other pioneer Army aviators was provided by the USAAF facilities and personnel. When the United States Air Force formed its own medical service in 1949, most trained Army aviation medicine personnel transferred to the Air Force. In 1950, Lieutenant Colonel Rollie M. Harrison was the

Army's only practicing aviation medical officer.

Until March, 1951, Lieutenant Colonel Harrison conducted the Army aviation medicine program at Fort Sill, Oklahoma. Medical problems encountered during the early months of the Korean War by isolated Army aviation units operating in forward areas underscored the need for organic Army aviation medicine support. In March, 1951, Major Spurgeon H. Neel (Major General, Ret.) became the first Army physician to complete the Air Force basic aviation medicine course at Randolph Air Force Base, Texas. He immediately applied aeromedical principles to the helicopter aeromedical evacuation of casualties during the Korean war. The growing importance of Army aviation led to the formation of an aviation medicine section in the Office of The Army Surgeon General and publication of the first Army Medical Standards for Flying in 1952. The Army began its own abbreviated aviation medicine training program in 1953 at the Medical Field Service School at Fort Sam Houston, Texas; however, this program was short-lived because of reduced funding at the close of the Korean War. By 1954, a separate military occupational specialty was established for aviation medicine. Completion of a recognized course in aviation medicine was made a requirement for award of the new designation.

Army flight training was moved from Fort Sill to the newly established Army Aviation School at Fort Rucker, Alabama, in 1954. Colonel William H. Byrne became the Aviation School Flight Surgeon in 1955 and became involved in programs to minimize aviator fatigue. During the same year, flight status for aviation medicine officers was authorized, and the first official publication of *Army Aviation Medicine* was issued. By September, 1955, there were 28 Army aviation medical officers actively engaged in the practice of aviation medicine. Distinctive wings for Army aviation medical officers were authorized in 1956. A majority of the 150 Army physicians trained as flight surgeons between 1956 and 1961 were trained by the Air Force. In July, 1960, Fort Rucker was formally recognized as a third-year (Phase 3) training site for residents in aerospace medicine. On July 6, 1962, The United States Army Aeromedical Research Unit (now the United States Army Aeromedical Research Laboratory [USAARL]) was established at Fort Rucker under the command of Lieutenant Colonel John D. Lawson.

As the importance of aviation to the Army in the field continued to grow and as United States involvement in the Vietnam War expanded, the need for flight surgeon training in the Army became apparent. In 1964, the Department of Aeromedical Education and Training (DAET) was established at Fort Rucker as a part of the United States Army Aviation School, with Colonel Neel as the director. The department graduated the first class in 1964 and expanded to graduate over 130 flight surgeons per year from 1966 to 1969.

In January, 1970, the first *Army Flight Surgeon's Manual* was published by the United States Army Aviation School. This publication, a two-volume text, covered classic aeromedical subjects but, more importantly, also prepared the student flight surgeons for their expected responsibilities as field combat surgeons and preventive medicine specialists in Vietnam. This manual served as an important asset for Army flight surgeon training, as a reference for the practicing flight surgeon, and as a source of information for the aircrewman.

Aeromedical instruction for student and graduate aviators began in 1971. Early support for this essential training was given by North Atlantic Treaty Organization (NATO) Standardization Agreements requiring the aeromedical instruction of aircrew. The new subjects were received with enthusiasm by the aviators, who recognized their importance to peacetime safety

and combat readiness. The Army's first altitude chamber for aviation training became operational in 1970 and was used by DAET to demonstrate the use of aircraft oxygen systems and the effect of hypoxia. Medical Service Corps officers with backgrounds in physiology have joined ranks with the flight surgeons to continue this valuable aeromedical training of aircrew.

In April, 1974, The United States Army Health Services Command approved reorganization of Lyster United States Army Hospital, Fort Rucker Medical Department Activity, and the Aviation School's Department of Aeromedical Education and Training into a consolidated medical command known as the United States Army Aeromedical Center (USAAMC). The DAET became the Army Aeromedical Activity within the Aeromedical Center.

After the Vietnam War, serious shortages of physicians occurred following the loss of mandatory military service. Despite severe constraints, Army aviation medicine programs were kept alive through the hard work and dedication of those who remained. By 1980, a resurgence occurred in aviation medicine training. A major milestone was reached in August, 1980, when 3 weeks of TH-55A helicopter flight training through solo were added to the flight surgeon course (Fig. 21–1).

The Army is currently training approximately 100 flight surgeons each year in

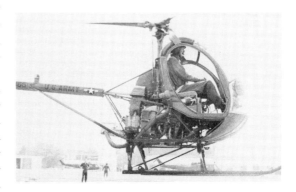

Fig. 21–1. First TH-55 solo flight by a student Army flight surgeon (official United States Army photo).

the basic course, and physicians are entering the postgraduate medical training program in aerospace medicine at the rate of five or six per year. This training will now extend the best aviation medicine to the aviation unit.

AEROMEDICAL CONCERNS OF ROTARY-WING FLIGHT

The helicopter has introduced new and unique aeromedical challenges. Most aspects of rotary-wing flight are similar to those of fixed-wing flight; however, some significant differences are evident. Use of the helicopter in the combat environment as a weapons platform and transport vehicle adds a substantial number of points for consideration.

Helicopters are similar to fixed-wing aircraft for many aspects of psychologic stress; however, unlike fixed-wing aircraft, the helicopter is basically an unstable platform, cannot be trimmed to fly itself, and must be under active control during all phases of flight. Until the recent introduction of the UH-60 Blackhawk, few helicopters have been equipped with automatic piloting equipment or flight directors, thus increasing pilot work load during instrument flight to significant levels. Army helicopter pilots often fly extended hours during challenging NOE profiles, climatic extremes, and difficult tactical missions. All of these considerations are highly important for the physician in dealing with problems of aircrew fatigue.

Disorientation

Disorientation, an already troublesome problem of aviation, is aggravated by three characteristics of helicopter flight: hovering flight in all directions, low-level flight with reduced visibility, and the inherent instability of the helicopter platform. Flight operations at night, under marginal weather conditions, and with or without night vision goggles increase the chances of disorientation.

Although fixed-wing aircraft may slip in a turn and a low-speed aircraft may even achieve negative ground speed in a strong head wind, these do not compare with the helicopter's ability to travel sideward, rearward, or vertically. These motions cause relatively few problems under good visual conditions but are significant when visual cues are reduced. Most flight instruments used on helicopters were initially designed for fixed-wing aircraft and respond poorly to helicopter maneuvering at low speeds. Disorientation also can occur when helicopters are hovered over terrain covered with snow, sand, or loose dirt that is picked up by the rotor wash, leading to loss of visual reference by the pilot. The sudden change from visual to instrument references, combined with the unreliability of both human sensory perception and instrument indications during hovering, can lead to disorientation and a subsequent accident. New horizontal situation indicators and cathode ray tube displays (CRTs) have been developed and help alleviate this problem. Also, aircrew education, avoidance of the situation, and aircraft stability augmentation systems (including an automatic hover mode) hold the greatest promise for reducing this problem. Strong aeromedical and aviation training programs remain the most important defensive measures for disorientation.

Vision

Vision has taken on a special significance during search operations, low-level and NOE flight, and the use of visionics for the identification of targets and the firing of ordnance. During NOE flight, the aircraft is flown only a few feet above (and sometimes beneath) obstructions, with frequent changes in airspeed and heading. Exceptional vision and flying skill are required to choose the best tactical route of flight and avoid obstructions. Wire strikes are a prevailing danger in NOE flight. Careful selection of aircrew with good vision, training of aircrew concerning visual limitations and scanning, and the use of ancillary clues (e.g., where there's a pole, there's a wire) are all within the role of a flight surgeon to help reduce this type of hazard. Various wire-cutting devices are currently being tested on the Army's OH-58 observation helicopter. In these systems, hardened steel rails mounted on the leading edges of the aircraft deflect cables into cutting devices mounted on both the roof and bottom of the aircraft. This system further reduces the inherent hazards of low-level flight.

The requirement for an around-the-clock capability in both military and civilian helicopter operations has generated the need for night flight. Initial efforts were directed primarily at making the best use of unaided night vision: protecting vision during the day, scanning for use of off-center (scotopic) vision at night, and utilizing red cockpit lighting. The visual illusions common to night flying also apply to helicopters. Low-level flying is much more hazardous at night because obstructions like wires are often obscured, and visual references may suddenly be lost due to inadvertent entry into clouds or to blowing snow or sand during hover. Disorientation with flight over water or mountainous terrain is more apt to occur at night.

Enhancement of night vision by various night vision devices is now routine in Army aviation. The Army has proceeded through several generations of night vision goggles and aircraft-mounted night vision devices. Night vision devices generally tend to provide less resolution, constricted fields of view and depth of field, seriously reduced cues for perception of distance, and inadequate color differentiation. The night vision goggles commonly used today by the Army aviator were initially developed for use by ground forces. These vision goggles give only a 40° field of view, give a maximum visual acuity of 20/50, and require manual focus for near viewing inside the cockpit. A proposed

modification of the night-vision goggle faceplate will allow peripheral scanning and under-the-goggle near vision of the instrument panel (Fig. 21–2). The new aviators' night-vision imaging system will give improved image resolution. The helmet mounting will allow peripheral vision, view of the cockpit, and the wearing of spectacles. Because night-vision goggles disrupt dark adaptation, view of the instrument panel is somewhat compromised with standard red instrument lights. Also, the image-intensifying system of the night-vision goggles is more sensitive to the blue-green wavelength spectrum. A need for blue-green instrument lighting is recognized. Future aircraft are expected to have both red and blue-green lighting options for dual compatibility.

Environmental Control

Helicopters traditionally have been equipped with minimal environmental

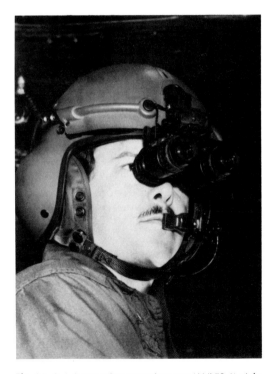

Fig. 21–2. Army aviator wearing new (ANVIS-6) night vision goggles (official United States Army photo).

control systems and cabin insulation of marginal adequacy. As a result, aircrews are often subjected to environmental temperature extremes that affect comfort, endurance, performance, and safety.

Cold Weather Operations

The Army aviator often must fly with cold-weather clothing designed to be worn on the ground. Current vapor barrier boots are usually too bulky to operate the anti-torque pedals, arctic mittens are too bulky to operate small switches, and large parkas interfere with movement, vision, and emergency egress. Although it is hazardous to fly in isolated winter climates without adequate winter clothing, the bulky nature of such clothing can compromise the fine control movements necessary for safe flight. Experience, education, and patience are all required for winter operations while better solutions are sought.

Cold environmental temperatures present many other operational challenges for the deployed aviation unit. Oil seals often crack and leak, requiring increased maintenance. Cold temperatures may triple the time to accomplish even the simplest maintenance work. Supercooled fuel presents a cold injury hazard should it come into contact with exposed skin. Hypothermia can result in psychologic degradation and apathy, leading to impaired flight performance and maintenance errors. Cold-weather operations must always include the prospect of winter survival. The flight surgeon must be especially observant for signs of difficulty in those personnel involved in winter operations.

Hot Weather Flying

The climb to altitude in fixed-wing aircraft brings welcome relief in hot climates. The non-air–conditioned helicopter flying near the ground subjects the aircrew to significant heat stress. The problem is compounded by synthetic flight suits and other life-support equipment, especially current chemical protective gear (Fig. 21–3). Forced water intake is one method used by aviation units during hot weather operations to avoid dehydration hazards.

Noise

Balloonists and glider enthusiasts are the only aeronauts who feel that silence is golden. For all others, the absence of sound in the aerial environment is an unwelcome and ominous sign that the flight may be about to terminate. But the sounds of engines, transmissions, and rotors have a way of being excessive and of facilitating detection by an enemy force. Noise generated by most rotary-wing aircraft is very significant because of the combined effect of engine, transmission, and rotor-blade activity. Each aircraft tends to have a particular part or system that generates the majority of noise at each crew site. Noise spectra for many aircraft not only exceed the damage risk criteria by a wide margin

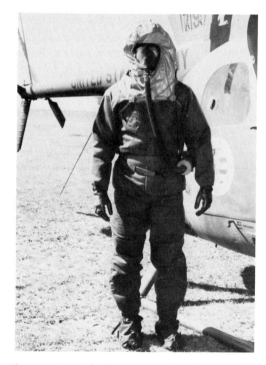

Fig. 21–3. Standard United States chemical defense ensemble, shown without the protective vest, which would normally be worn with it (official United States Army photo).

but also can exceed the limits of many hearing protective devices and communication systems.

Helicopter noise can be reduced at its source by improving gear design (i.e., the use of polished helical gears), shrouds to enclose noisy components, and insulation. Acoustic blankets are used inside most helicopters. Individual protection is the main method of protecting the aircrew.

Vibration

In recent years, the ubiquitous symbol of Army aviation has been the UH-1, better known as the Huey. A hallmark of the Huey, known to everyone who ever listened to or rode in the aircraft is the low-frequency (11 Hz) vibration of the semirigid see-saw–type two-bladed rotor system. Low-frequency vibrations produced by many helicopters are as low as 5.4 Hz, with respective octaves to 50 Hz. Resonance with body structures at certain frequencies produces a more pronounced effect than nonresonant frequencies. Disturbances in dynamic visual acuity, speech, and fine muscle coordination result from vibration exposure. Most aviators tend to adapt to the vibration; however, difficulties with back pain and premature intervertebral disk disease have been reported and are under study at USAARL. Attenuation through improved helicopter seat design is one method of reducing objectionable vibration.

The vibration spectrum is altered by changes in the number of blades used in the main rotor system. Although the most commonly used utility, observation, and gunship helicopters in the Army today all have two-blade main rotor systems, newer replacement aircraft will have four main rotor blades, with resultant changes in characteristic vibration patterns and vertical amplitude. Tests of all of these aircraft indicate that their vibration spectra are less likely to cause problems than the older, two-bladed aircraft.

Rotary-Wing Aircraft Accidents

In-Flight Escape

One of the primary concerns in rotary-wing flight is escape from disabled aircraft. The usual low-altitude flight profiles and the potential hazard of the rotating blades discourage the use of parachutes. Several escape systems have been designed that employ rocket extraction or ballistic ejection systems combined with rotor-blade jettison; however, the future use of such devices is uncertain. The penalties in useful load, cost, possibility of malfunction, and inherent dangers of aircrew ejection or blade jettison in the proximity of other aircraft offsets many of the advantages. The "ride-it-in" philosophy will probably continue in helicopter aviation and continue to underscore the need for crashworthiness and survivability, in addition to the importance of proficiency in autorotation. This approach also has the advantage of salvaging the aircraft and its cargo.

Midair Collision

The maneuverability of the helicopter in all directions and aircraft density in many tactical scenarios increase the risk of midair collisions during military maneuvers. The tips of most helicopter blades move at tangential velocities approaching Mach 1; any contact with other structures usually results in blade damage, causing intense vibration incompatible with aerodynamic or structural integrity. Fatality rates with midair helicopter collisions are high. Many midair accidents have occurred under conditions of good visibility; therefore, the flight surgeon and safety officer must continually concentrate on problems of channelled attention, limitations of peripheral vision, and on the value of effective visual scanning. The educational effort must extend to air traffic control personnel.

Crash Injury Effects

In contrast to the typical longitudinal crash pattern of fixed-wing aircraft, the helicopter tends to impact vertically, often at relatively low forward speeds. Rotor blades and mechanical components are often thrown great distances and can cause serious injury if they penetrate the cockpit. The transmission and other heavy mechanical components are frequently torn from their mountings and found distant from other aircraft structures. New Army helicopter design criteria call for structures to sustain separate acceleration loads of $+20\ G_x$, $+18\ G_y$, and $+20\ G_z$.

Injury Patterns

Spinal injuries and basilar fractures of the skull are often associated with the high-magnitude $+G_z$ acceleration forces of helicopter impacts. Basilar skull fractures account for the most serious injuries sustained by the aircrew of the rotary-wing aircraft. Compression fractures of the spine often occur in the T-10 to L-2 region. Impact injuries in newer helicopters (UH-60) have been markedly reduced through crashworthy design to protect the cabin area and provide uniform deformation of structure through load-limiting devices. For example, the pilot seats employ telescoping legs that deform at a uniform rate on impact and reduce the peak amplitude of high-magnitude G forces experienced by the seat occupant. Troop and gunner seats are suspended from ceiling-mounted steel cables that limit high-magnitude forces by stretching and bending (Fig. 21–4). Such refinements provide protection to the fifth through the ninety-fifth percentile person in crashes with an up to 12.8 m/sec vertical descent speed.

Another problem unique to helicopter accidents is the intrusion into the cockpit or cabin area of the main rotor system or transmission on impact. This intrusion often has resulted in destruction to both the aircraft and the human occupants. The use of new materials to strengthen com-

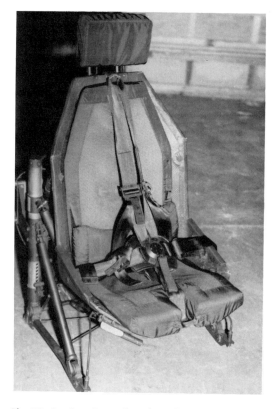

Fig. 21–4. Experimental crashworthy troop seats developed in a joint United States Army Aeromedical Research Laboratory (USAARL) United States Army Safety Center (USASC) project, circa 1972–1976 (this was the first seat to utilize ceiling-mounted, shock-absorbing devices). The ideas incorporated in this seat were later used in the Blackhawk (UH-60) production aircraft (official United States Army photo).

ponents and mountings, the elimination of the long rotor mast, and the relocation of aircraft systems have helped to alleviate this problem.

Postcrash Fires

For years, the postcrash fire was one of the greatest causes of fatality and disability in an otherwise survivable helicopter accident. The thin aluminum skins of helicopter fuel cells tended to rupture easily, resulting in a large fuel vapor cloud that ignited rapidly on contacting hot engine components, sparks, or electrical sources. The resulting 1150°C inferno allowed only a few critical seconds for the uninjured aircrew to escape. Thermally resistant flight clothing (polyamide Nomex flight suits and gloves), leather boots, and helmets with face visor greatly improved the chances of escaping a postcrash fire without serious burn injuries. Extensive research at USAARL led to the development of biodynamic standards for the protective helmet and fire-resistant materials used by Army aircrew.

Crashworthy Fuel Systems

A major thrust in the 1960s was to find a suitable postcrash fire prevention device for helicopters. Although fuel solidification, honeycomb tank fillers, and ignition inerting methods were evaluated, the neoprene-impregnated nylon cloth tanks with breakaway valves proved to offer the most economical and effective protection. In 1967, a UH-1 helicopter equipped with nylon tanks and breakaway valves was crashed by remote control. There was no fuel spillage or subsequent fire. Crashworthy fuel cell retrofit of the Army helicopter fleet began in the early 1970s and is now complete. As accident data of Army aircraft equipped with the new crashworthy systems were analyzed, the results exceeded all expectations. Crashes through 1982 showed a thermal injury and fatality rate of zero as compared with 40% in helicopters having conventional fuel systems. This success underscores the need for the combined efforts of aeromedical and aeronautic engineering disciplines.

Civil Helicopter Aeromedical Concerns

Except for the tactical combat considerations of military aviation, the civilian aviator faces many of the same problems as the Army helicopter pilot; however, a significant difference occurs in the degree to which the civilian pilot is protected against adversity. The use of protective helmets, fire-resistant flight clothing, and crashworthy fuel systems is by no means universal in civil flying due to economic, useful load, and performance considerations. Should a crash occur, the results may be more devastating to a civil pilot and his passengers. In military aviation, an extensive support system provides a high degree of safety surveillance through multiple systems of inspection, including aviation resource management surveys, operational readiness and safety evaluation, and general inspections. These are all done to monitor aviator selection, training, equipment, maintenance, and unit operations. Each pilot undergoes an annual check ride, must take a written examination and flight physical examination, and must meet flight currency requirements. Equivalent programs are not necessarily conducted in the civil aviation sector because of economic or other constraints. What has proved cost-effective in military helicopter aviation, however, could as well save lives and costly equipment in the civilian sector.

ARMY AVIATION MEDICINE PROGRAM

Army aviation medicine is preventive in concept, environmental in nature, and military in orientation. Stringent selection standards help prevent accidents by providing aircrew who have no known medical or psychologic problems that would predispose them to accident causation. These standards are paralleled by a major effort to preserve the health of the selected aircrew population. The aviation medicine specialty deals with the full range of psychophysiologic problems of personnel who must function well in an essentially hostile environment. The military orientation of the program means that mission considerations are of paramount concern. This approach is often in contrast to the disease-oriented and patient-oriented medical practice of most physicians.

Nature of the Program

The Army aviation medicine program includes (1) the establishment and administration of medical standards for flying duty; (2) the clinical care of aviation personnel, with particular reference to aeromedically significant problems; (3) a care of the flyer program that is aimed at reaching maximal individual and unit effectiveness; (4) aeromedical advice to commanders in the control of aviation assets; and (5) the development of policy, procedures, concepts, and matériel for the employment of aviation medicine in support of Army aviation.

Aviation medicine is a critical service needed to support approximately 14,000 officers and 18,000 enlisted aviation personnel at nearly 100 worldwide locations. The unit-level flight surgeon who practices the basic and specialized skills of aviation medicine is the keystone of the Army's aeromedical support program. Army flight surgeons are deployed around the world, assigned directly to aviation units or to fixed hospital facilities. The practice of Army aviation medicine parallels that of the sister services in only a few locations where large numbers of pilots are located such as Fort Rucker, Alabama, and Fort Campbell, Kentucky. Other Army aviation assets are widely scattered, with units ranging in size from an aviation company (less than 50 pilots) down to utility flight detachments of only two pilots. The Army flight surgeon, therefore, often practices alone as opposed to his Air Force and Navy colleagues, who usually practice under the supervision of an aeromedically experienced Chief of Aerospace Medicine or carrier Senior Medical Officer. Many Army physicians in clinical specialties have previously been unit-level flight surgeons at some time in the past and function in a supportive role to the new unit-level flight surgeon.

Residency-Trained Flight Surgeons

The residency-trained flight surgeons are the individuals who make Army aviation medicine policy, train new flight surgeons, oversee medical fitness for flying, conduct aeromedical research, and serve as aviation medicine staff officers, command surgeons, and medical unit com-

manders. The success of aerospace medicine as a career specialty in the Army is striking. From the first resident in 1957 up through 1982, 70 officers have entered the program. Only four residents have dropped out of training and only nine have resigned from active duty. Four of the latter are now on duty with other services and two are in reserve components. The total federal service retention rate for Army aerospace medicine specialists exceeds 90%.

The total number of active Army physicians practicing aviation medicine is approximately 130. The reserve components have 120 more flight surgeons. Together, they care for nearly 20,000 pilots.

When assigned to an aviation medicine position, the Army flight surgeon is responsible for conducting the aeromedical program. Examination of aviation ersonnel is intended to identify changes in health status that could impact on mission effectiveness within the aviation environment. Clinical aeromedical care is provided for Army aircrew in settings ranging from small flight-line clinics to well-staffed flight surgeons' offices in Army hospitals. Where possible, the flight surgeon also coordinates or actually provides care for the aircrewman's family.

Because the Army flight surgeon cares for an aviation force often deployed with ground soldiers, the threats of physical and climatic extremes, injury, disease, and psychologic stress must all be dealt with. When the stresses of demanding operational flight are combined with the other combat and aviation stresses, the importance of unit-level aviation medicine support becomes critical. A close bond must be established between the flight surgeon and his unit. Often, the flight surgeon must live, work, and sometimes even fight alongside his aviators.

PROFESSIONAL TRAINING OF THE ARMY FLIGHT SURGEON

The mission of the Army aviation medicine professional training program is to advance the science and art of aviation medicine, promote the professionalism of the flight surgeon, and teach the application of scientific and medical principles to the aircrewman for achieving maximal combat readiness and peacetime safety.

The Army Aeromedical Activity (AAMA) is the proponent for the Army's professional education program in aviation medicine. The program is an accredited, comprehensive, and postgraduate level program. Educational, clinical, and operational support to Army aviation are provided by AAMA. The Office of the Surgeon General has delegated the following missions to the Army Aeromedical Activity:

1. Professional education leading to designation as a flight surgeon
2. Training of aircrewmen in aviation medicine principles
3. Physiologic training of medical and aircrew personnel
4. Continuing medical education programs for medical and aircrew personnel
5. Aeromedical review and disposition of flight physical examinations; to include flight-training applicants, aviators, aircrewmen, and air traffic control personnel
6. Worldwide aeromedical consultation and in-flight evaluation for determination of medical fitness
7. Operation of an aeromedical data repository and epidemiologic studies
8. Aeromedical consultant advisory panel
9. Clinical aviation medicine support
10. Clinical research and development
11. Coordination with the United States Army Medical Research and Development Command for selected research topics

The Department of Education and Training of AAMA conducts both professional education courses for flight surgeons and aeromedical training of aircrewmen in the following areas:

1. Army flight surgeon course (7 weeks, three times each year, 100 students)
2. Army aviation medicine orientation course (2-week course, twice each year, up to 20 students)
3. Army operational aeromedical problems course (1-week CME course, 100 flight surgeons)
4. Aeromedical and physiologic training of initial entry rotary-wing (IERW) students (21 hours, every 2 weeks, 2600 students)
5. Aeromedical and physiologic training of graduate aviators participating in transition and qualification courses (12 to 20 hours, every 2 to 4 weeks, class sizes of 5 to 12 graduate aviators)
6. Safety programs delivered by the unit flight surgeon, who often uses training materials distributed by the Army Aeromedical Activity

Throughout the Army flight surgeon course, the students are exposed to the expertise of a faculty composed of specialists in aerospace medicine, specialists in other clinical disciplines, and experienced aviators. Emphasis is placed on unit-level operational medical requirements through the use of seminars and student presentations of aeromedical problems. The designation of Army flight surgeon and the Army flight surgeon silver wings are awarded to the physician-student who successfully completes the course.

Course Content

The course provides intensive instruction in applied cardiology, internal medicine, otorhinolaryngology ophthalmology, psychiatry, neurology, orthopedics, urology, dermatology, and aviation pathology. The subjects of altitude physiology, acceleration, oxygen systems and life-support equipment, and aviation toxicology are related to operational needs and are presented in a series of detailed lectures. Special emphasis is placed on the stresses of flight, including disorientation, fatigue, vibration, noise, and perceptual overload. Physical fitness, health education, and preventive medicine principles are reviewed. Considerable emphasis is placed on the performance of the flying-duty medical examination and aircrew selection process and on the associated administrative requirements. The students receive experiential training in spatial disorientation, color vision, night vision, and dark adaptation. They undergo ejection seat qualification, night flight and night vision goggle training, flight simulator orientation, and hypobaric chamber training with hypoxia and rapid decompression. They also receive instruction in aerodynamics, navigation, meteorology, aircraft systems, cockpit design, and restraint systems. The United States Army Safety Center staff provides lectures and practical experience in accident investigative techniques during the course, which prepares the students for their role as participants on the accident investigation team (Fig. 21–5).

Flight Training

The students receive flight instruction in the TH-55A helicopter, including solo flight, in order to experience the stresses, demands, and hazards of the aviation environment and gain the perspective of a pilot contrasted to that of a passenger. During flight instruction, the student is exposed to a comprehensive flight training schedule and trains alongside primary-level student Army aviators. The credibility of the flight surgeon has been strongly enhanced by the addition of this flight training phase to the Army flight surgeons' course.

Orientation Course

A 2-week orientation course is conducted to introduce Air Force- or Navy-trained flight surgeons to the Army and the special requirements of unit-level support. Special emphasis is given to Army aviation medicine administrative requirements, the flying-duty medical examination, night vision goggle and nap-of-the-earth (NOE) missions, noise, vibration, stress, fatigue, and the Army aviation medicine program. Following completion of the orientation course, the flight surgeon is awarded the designation of Army flight surgeon and is authorized to wear the Army flight surgeon badge.

Aerospace Medicine Residency

Specialty training in aerospace medicine is available to all Army flight surgeons through either the Air Force or Navy residency training programs. A minimum of 1 year of field duty as a unit-level flight surgeon is required prior to acceptance into the postgraduate training program. Both the Air Force and Navy programs lead to board eligibility and certification as a specialist in aerospace medicine by the American Board of Preventive Medicine. The first year of training is at a civilian school of public health and leads to a master's degree in public health. The second year is at the United States Air Force School of Aerospace Medicine, Brooks Air Force Base, Texas or the Navy Aerospace Medical Institute, Pensacola, Florida. The aerospace medicine specialist has a virtually unlimited opportunity for interesting assignments to operational positions requiring a broad knowledge of military and aviation medicine. The aerospace medicine specialist is a valuable asset in operational medicine. The specialty provides the flight surgeon with excellent opportunities to achieve leadership and management positions.

MEDICAL SELECTION PROCEDURES FOR AIRCREW

The flight surgeon is the key element in the selection of the aviator and other aviation personnel. Personnel are selected for Army aviation based on administrative

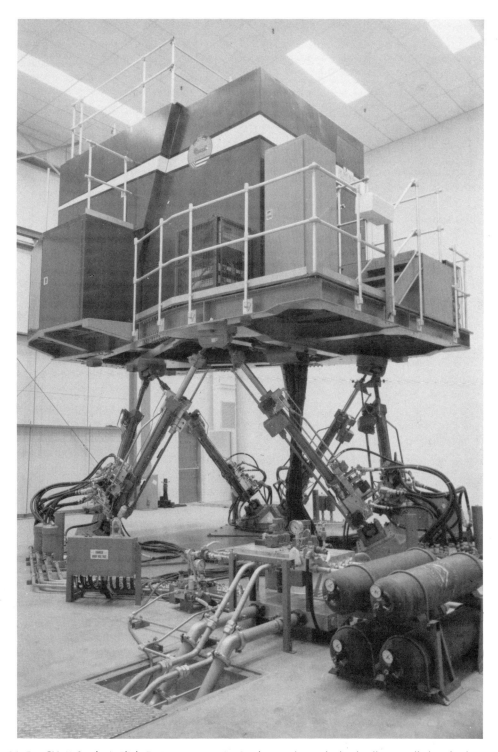

Fig. 21–5. CH-47 Synthetic Flight Training System (SFTS). This simulator is hydraulically controlled, with telescoping legs, which allows the platform to tilt in response to control movements (official United States Army photo).

and medical standards that are designed to maximize aviation potential, aircrew effectiveness, and flying safety. Training aircrew members is costly, and the Army must be conservative in its selection of applicants for initial training.

Personnel applying for Army flight training first take a Flight Aptitude Selection Test (FAST). Those individuals who score successfully on this test are next interviewed by a field-grade officer Army aviator to assess motivation, background, and potential. The final step is the completion of an initial flying-duty medical examination, which is performed by a flight surgeon at a medical facility of the armed forces.

The initial physical is designated Class 1 for Warrant Officer Flight Training and Class 1A for commissioned officers. These examinations and standards are identical, with the exception of slightly more lenient visual acuity and refractive error tolerances for Class 1A. Class 2 standards apply to subsequent annual flying examinations and initial and annual air traffic control (ATC) and flight surgeon examinations. Class 3 standards apply to aviation mechanics, crew chiefs, and aerial observers.

Reports of all Class 1, 1A, and 2 examinations are reviewed at the Army Aeromedical Activity, Fort Rucker, Alabama and are categorized as either medically qualified or disqualified. Subsequently, this information is transmitted back to unit commanders. Class 3 examinations are reviewed and disposition made by the local flight surgeon. Flight physical examinations are reviewed against specific standards that have been developed through research and clinical experience. These standards are found in Army regulation 40–501.

Aeromedical Training of the Army Aviator

All aviators attending courses at the United States Army Aviation Center (USAAVNS) are given either initial or refresher instruction in aeromedical sub-

jects. Aeromedical instruction uses a combination of lecture and participatory methods to reinforce the information being presented. This instruction is designed to develop an awareness of scientific and medical information necessary for safe and effective flight.

The most basic medical information is presented to the fledgling aviator during a 3-hour aviation medicine orientation prior to the first flight. This orientation includes the proper fitting and wear of personal protective equipment. The emphasis of this class is to inform the student of the effects on man of the aviation environment.

The necessity for Army aviators to understand altitude physiology is often questioned by the beginning student. Once he has been taught the effects of altitude on the body, a demonstration of these effects is given during a flight in the hypobaric chamber. During this flight, the validity of the training is apparent when night visual acuity wanes at altitude and when each student identifies his own symptoms of hypoxia and sees its effect on others.

The effects of life stresses, substance abuse, sleep deprivation, and their contribution to aviator fatigue are another important block of instruction. This instruction assists the students in recognizing stressors and encourages them to seek help when necessary.

Noise as a serious problem in Army aviation is dealt with by educating the aviator on its origins, its effects, and how to combat it. By acquainting the aviator with the frequency range and decibel level of noise in specific Army aircraft and with the use of personal protective equipment, the incidence of hearing damage has been substantially reduced.

As with altitude physiology, the relevance of acceleration, or G, forces is often not initially apparent to the Army aviator. The instruction presented is designed to acquaint the aviator with the effects of acceleration and its application to Army aviation. The effects of high-magnitude acceleration always have been recognized in crash injury protection. With the advent of third-generation helicopters, the importance of knowing the body's reaction to low-magnitude acceleration and methods of minimizing its effects are becoming more important. These new helicopters impose substantial G-loading in routine operational flight profiles. The mission-need statement for the UH-60 (Blackhawk) is for $+3$ G_z and -0.5 G_z whereas that for the AH-64 is $+3.5$ G_z.

One of the most important classes taught aviators in the aeromedical block involves spatial disorientation and illusions of flight. The role of the perceptual apparatus in maintaining orientation in flight is discussed, to include types of disorientation that can be experienced. A comprehensive lecture is given to ensure student understanding of human limitations arising from misperceptions originating from the visual, vestibular, and proprioceptive systems. Practical exercises in a Barany chair and experience with certain visual illusions reinforce this lecture. This instruction provides an opportunity to experience the powerful conflicting sensations that can affect a student in flight and provides methods to avoid or minimize disorientation.

Instruction in night vision is presented just before the student begins night flight and night-vision goggle training. By delaying this instruction, the student enters the first period of night flying with a better knowledge of the physiology, anatomy, and limitations of the visual process. The lecture is reinforced with practical exercises that demonstrate vision limitations and illusions.

Most aviators return to the Army Aviation Center for graduate flight training several times during their aviation career. At these times, refresher training in aeromedical subjects is always a part of the curriculum. For the aviator who does not return

to Fort Rucker, a transportable training packet is provided by the Army Aeromedical Activity for use in annual aeromedical refresher training. The unit flight surgeon and safety officer utilize this material to aid in accomplishing this vital training.

AEROMEDICAL CONSULTATION

An important mission of Army aviation medicine is to determine medical fitness for flying duty, combat effectiveness, and longevity of useful service. A frequent problem is the aeromedical disposition of the experienced aviator who is found to have a disqualifying condition but who appears physiologically suitable for continued flight duties. Experience has shown the value of keeping the senior aviator in the cockpit with a medical waiver despite the presence of certain disqualifying medical conditions provided that mission completion, safety of flight, and the individual's health will not be compromised. Proper aeromedical disposition is essential for this to be realized and can only be achieved through the simultaneous application of both aeromedical and military aviation principles.

A full medical evaluation usually is required when an aviator is disqualified from flying duties. A waiver recommendation may then be made as indicated by the clinical findings and past aviation history. The evaluation generally is performed by the unit flight surgeon, who frequently uses specialty consultation from local or regional medical resources. The medical findings, comments from members of the individual's unit, pertinent aviation records, and recommendations of the unit flight surgeon are forwarded to the commander of the United States Army Aeromedical Center (USAAMC), as action agent for the Surgeon General for the determination of individual fitness for flying duty. Each case is reviewed by the Aeromedical Consultant Advisory Panel (ACAP), which is comprised of aerospace medicine specialists of senior rank and experience, flight surgeons who possess additional training in traditional clinical medical specialties, and two senior aviators appointed by the Commanding General, USAAMC. Following approval by the commander of the USAAMC, the ACAP recommendations are forwarded to the United States Army Military Personnel Center for final action. If a waiver is granted, it is usually valid for a specific period of time and may even place limitations on the scope of aviation duties to include the requirement that the aviator be accompanied by another fully qualified pilot. Annual renewal of the waiver is generally contingent on a repeat medical evaluation that demonstrates stability of the condition.

Medical conditions frequently arise for which adequate local medical evaluation is not feasible and, therefore, require specialized aeromedical evaluation. These cases may be sent for evaluation to the aeromedical Consultation Service at USAAMC. The Air Force Aeromedical Evacuation Service is often used to transport individuals stationed overseas to Fort Rucker for evaluation. Any individual on flying status may be referred to Fort Rucker for aeromedical consultation by the unit flight surgeon, command surgeons, or the Commanding General, United States Army Health Services Command. Each case is then carefully reviewed by the ACAP for appropriate aeromedical disposition.

Fort Rucker is a unique and valuable location for the Aeromedical Consultation Service. The invaluable experience of senior aeromedical specialists on the staffs of the USAAMC, USAARL, and United States Army Safety Center (USASC) is frequently applied during consultation. Research scientists, technicians, data analysts, and sophisticated hardware are available to assist in each evaluation as necessary. In addition to a comprehensive medical study, a complete flying performance evaluation may be undertaken. All aircraft currently flown by the Army along with corresponding standardization instructor pilots are present at the Aviation Center for the in-flight testing portion of the aeromedical consultation (Fig. 21–6). New-generation synthetic flight training simulators are also available for use in aeromedical consultation. These simulators have six degrees of freedom for realistic sensory stimulation, have both IFR and VFR flight modes, and are driven by sophisticated computers capable of delivering objective grading from specific flight profiles.

Another important mission of the Aeromedical Consultation Service is to collect clinical epidemiologic data on a prospective basis. These data are stored in the aeromedical data repository and serve as a scientific basis from which to recommend aeromedical disposition and changes to medical policy and regulations. The Aeromedical Consultation Service is expected to expand its scope in the near future to become actively involved in prospective experimental research protocols of aeromedical significance. Studies involving the natural history of disease processes and their effects on aviation performance will be undertaken.

THE FUTURE OF ROTARY-WING AVIATION MEDICINE

The helicopter matured with the medical evacuation of patients during the close of World War II, through the Korean War, and, finally, in Vietnam. Casualties were

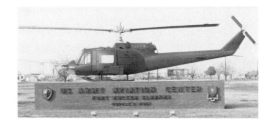

Fig. 21–6. UH-1 Iroquois (Huey) greets visitors to Fort Rucker, Alabama, home of the United States Aviation Center (official United States Army photo).

saved by rapid transport to hospitals where systematic and definitive care was given by teams of specialists. This same service was later offered to many civilian communities in the proximity of military installations through the Military Assistance to Safety and Traffic (MAST) program authorized by Congress in 1975. Many civil helicopter ambulance services have offered similar services to rapidly transport patients to medical centers for definitive and highly specialized care.

Modern technology, coupled with the definitive emergency care available at medical centers and larger hospitals, has drastically altered previous mortality and morbidity statistics for many diseases and categories of trauma. This advanced technology must be utilized early in the patient's course to be effective; thus, the helicopter is ideally suited to transport critical patients to medical specialists and their equipment. Recent examples of this include victims of head trauma, where the early employment of computerized tomographic (CT) scanning leads to early and definitive surgical treatment. The individual who suffers spinal cord injury may benefit from hyperbaric oxygen therapy, which is only available at a few locations. Emergency coronary artery surgery has recently averted myocardial infarction and loss of the myocardium following the onset of preinfarction angina.

These and other important medical advances will be available to many through helicopter transport systems. The aviation medicine specialist will play a critical role in the planning, design, and operational aspects of the aeromedical rescue and transport of critical patients. The general medical orientation of most aviation medicine specialists will prove highly valuable for these needs; however, those with additional clinical specialties will add critical and specific information to a growing body of aeromedical knowledge.

The Army is making a major commitment to vertical lift aircraft to satisfy the needs for mobility and firepower over large and diffused battlefields, for logistic support, and for the evacuation of casualties. This emphasis has led to intensive research and development efforts to field larger, faster, and highly maneuverable helicopters, represented by the Army's UH-60 and AH-64 (Figs. 21–7 and 21–8). The new third-generation helicopters are capable of extended ranges, carry large useful loads, and approach or exceed the cost and complexity of many jet fighter aircraft. The pilot of these and future Army helicopters will find himself seated in a cockpit of an aircraft capable of $+3$ to $+4$ G_z and -0.5 to -1.0 G_z and equipped with complex armament for air-to-air and air-to-ground combat. Image intensifiers integrated with weapons and aircraft instrument presentations, highly accurate navigation systems, electronic countermeasure equipment, and devices to counter microwave and laser energies will all be used by the aviator during combat flight to enhance effectiveness and counter the threats. Filtered positive pressure environmental control systems to counter chemical and toxic threats and an onboard oxygen-generating system for night and mountain operations also will

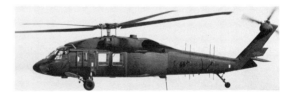

Fig. 21–7. The UH-60 Blackhawk has the capability of carrying an 11-man infantry squad, fully equipped (official United States Army photo).

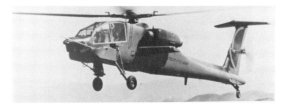

Fig. 21–8. The AH-64 Apache advanced-attack helicopter (official United States Army photo).

be present in the new aircraft. Required NOE flight will make a significant demand on the aviator. Human engineering with automation of flight control, weapons, communication, countermeasure, and weapons systems will be employed wherever possible to reduce work load and capitalize on human capabilities. Simulators and automated training devices will reduce training costs; however, investments in aircraft and crew will be substantial.

Army aviation will likely undergo greater specialization, resulting in increasing specific requirements for aeromedical support. The unit flight surgeon will apply specific medical and scientific information to support training and specific mission requirements to help the commander achieve optimal combat effectiveness.

Because rapid technologic growth has outpaced the ability of man, aviation medicine must concentrate on the develop-ment of information systems to correlate performance with measurable physical and psychologic guidelines. Flight surgeon involvement in research, development, and the acquisition of new aviation systems will achieve the best man-machine interface. The flight surgeon's close involvement in combat doctrine development will help counter chemical, toxic, biologic, and electromagnetic energy threats. Medical expertise critical to the research and development of protective equipment, systems, and techniques will protect the aviator and maintain optimal performance. Preventive medicine principles will become ingrained in the aviation force to meet the challenges of a worldwide mission. The multifaceted contributions of the Army flight surgeon will maintain aviation safety and combat readiness to meet tomorrow's challenges and help Army aviation live up to its motto: ABOVE THE BEST!

Chapter *22*

Naval Aviation Medicine

R. Paul Caudill, Jr.

From depths of sea to ends of space,
the limits of the human race
Are still, as once in days of yore,
of flesh and spirit, little more.

R. PAUL CAUDILL, JR.

The challenge of the practice of aviation medicine in the environment of the oceans of the world is unique and stimulating. Although military forces have aviation units that serve at sea, the environment of the oceans is by no means the exclusive domain of the military. The characteristics of life at sea are in many ways similar for both the military member aboard his ship or the individual serving aboard a merchant vessel or on a deep-water oil rig. Although missions and purpose may be vastly different, the details of daily life in a restricting, artificial environment are strikingly similar. The challenges posed to the practitioner of aviation medicine are many. In the United States Navy, the practice of aviation medicine is spreading gradually to every corner of the Navy's operations afloat. Nearly every vessel of the Navy is now aviation-capable, able to receive and launch rotary-winged aircraft. The broad knowledge of preventive medicine is an essential part of the aviation medicine practitioner's armamentarium; the complexity of shipboard environments leads to professional challenges not immediately apparent to the individual who has never served at sea. Knowledge of the aviator must include knowledge of the environment, both in flight and at rest. The concepts and precepts of the practice of aviation medicine at sea in the military environment translate directly into the work of the civilian aviation medical specialist. The support of the work of corporations involved in transportation and commerce at sea and in the exploration and extraction of the oceans' resources also demands knowledge of the work place. Aviation medicine in the environment of the oceans is a demanding and intriguing discipline (Fig. 22–1).

HISTORY OF NAVAL AVIATION MEDICINE

The history of aviation medicine in the United States Navy is interwoven with the history of aviation medicine throughout

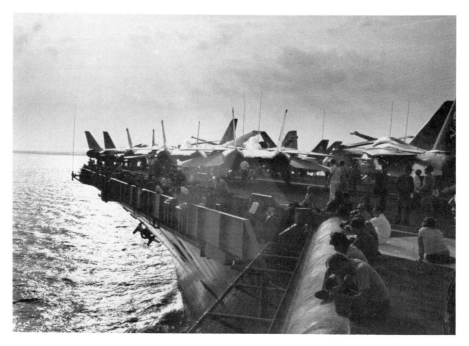

Fig. 22–1. Men and machines at sea in a floating city present an infinitely variable pattern of challenge to the practitioner of aviation medicine (official United States Navy photo).

the United States and the world. As the energies of mankind were intermittently involved in military pursuits, not all of those activities were to the detriment of humanity. Many of the scientific advancements that were forged under the clouds of war or rumors of war found their ultimate and most beneficial expression in peaceful applications; those expressions of the scientific achievement of mankind have benefited the people of all nations. The United States Navy has made its share of worthy contributions to the art and practice of aviation medicine worldwide.

The Early Years

The first awakening of aviation medicine in the United States Navy took place in October, 1912. The first physical standards for prospective naval aviators were established in the Bureau of Medicine and Surgery Circular Letter 125221. Over the years that followed, 1912 to 1921, the Navy Medical Department had no formal training program for medical personnel

serving those involved in aviation. By 1919, the Army had established a formal course in aviation medicine at its Central Research Laboratory, and on November 8, 1921, five Navy medical officers were ordered to report to the Army's School for Flight Surgeons at Mitchell Field, Long Island, New York. One year later, the Bureau of Medicine and Surgery established the Aviation Medicine Division, and one of the graduates of the April, 1922 class became the first chief of the Aviation Medicine Division.

During the 1920s and 1930s, naval aviation medicine began its early growth in earnest. Flight surgeons trained during those early years were often assigned, after training, to organizations other than those in aviation facilities, and their work was not always accomplished with ease.

In 1927, one class of eight students graduated from a program established at the Naval School of Medicine in Washington, D.C. For several years thereafter, no additional flight surgeons were trained. Between 1935 and 1939, an additional 20 Naval flight surgeons were trained at the Army's school, then located at Randolph Field, Texas. After their Army training, Naval flight surgeons reported to the Naval Air Station, Pensacola, Florida for additional training and flight indoctrination. Pensacola was called "the cradle of Naval aviation" and was to become the true birthplace and home of aviation medicine in the Navy.

In 1938 to 1939, the Bureau of Aeronautics of the Navy established a program to provide flight training to four flight surgeons per year, leading to a formal designation as naval aviator.

During those early years, the Aviation Medicine Division in the Bureau of Medicine and Surgery was staffed only by a single medical officer and one clerk. By the late 1930s, approximately 50 Naval flight surgeons were serving with aviation commands ashore and afloat. They provided aeromedical support to 300 personnel in naval aviation (Fig. 22–2).

Still, no Navy school was established to train aviation medical personnel. Neither funds nor facilities were available for aviation medical research, nor were Naval flight surgeons engaged in formal Navy research programs. The interest was there, however, and work began through the efforts of a few Navy aviation medical research pioneers, but formally structured programs were not yet available within the Navy.

World War II

On November 8, 1939, the President of the United States declared a limited state of emergency because of the threatening conditions throughout the world. On November 29, 1939, a school for Naval flight surgeons, the School of Aviation Medicine, was organized at the Naval Air Station in Pensacola. Funds for the school were provided by the Bureau of Aeronautics. The first class of students was in place by the end of November, 1939, initially completing a course designating them as aviation medical examiners. The first class of designated Naval flight surgeons graduated on November 30, 1940. Nearly 4000 Naval flight surgeons have been trained since that beginning.

Also in 1939, the first steps toward a formalized Navy aviation medicine research program were completed. A Naval

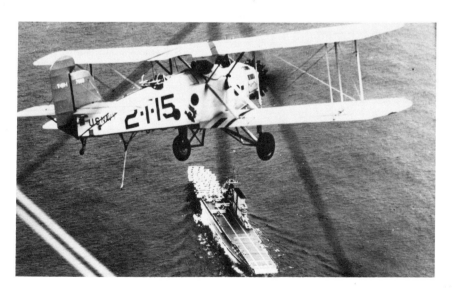

Fig. 22–2. Early carrier aviation. A T4M-1 circles the USS Saratoga (CV-3) prior to landing (official United States Navy photo).

flight surgeon was assigned to initiate the Navy's aviation medicine research effort.

World War II led to tremendous expansion in every aspect of aviation medicine within the Navy. By the end of that war, the aviation medicine service of the Navy had more than 1200 medical officers and flight surgeons in service. They staffed an aircraft carrier force of over 100 ships. They serviced all Marine Corps aviation units in the Pacific theatre. Naval flight surgeons experienced a death rate two and one-half times greater than any other group of naval medical officers in the combat areas.

Within the Bureau of Medicine and Surgery, the Aviation Medicine Division grew in response to the demands of the war. Extensive programs in aviation candidate selection, physical and psychologic screening, and aviator training were developed. More than 50 psychologists and many physiologists and other scientists were added to the aeromedical organization, paralleling the rapid growth in physician members.

Program growth occurred at the School of Aviation Medicine at Pensacola, as courses for training aviation medical technicians, low-pressure chamber technicians, and medical personnel involved in air-sea rescue were initiated.

The research effort in Navy aviation medicine began in earnest during that period. Early studies concerned the selection and training of personnel, problems of vision, and other problems of aviation physiology. In December, 1941, psychologists and statisticians were added to the staff to carry on the selection and training studies. Subsequently, the aviation medicine research section was transferred to the Bureau of Medicine and Surgery as the research branch of the Aviation Medicine Division. Throughout World War II, the objective of naval aviation medicine research was to improve flight safety, human efficiency, and the selection and training of aviation personnel.

Early research endeavors begun years before the beginning of World War II had seen studies accomplished in acceleration and its effects on aviation personnel; acceleration studies had been in progress as early as 1932. Much work was done concerning protective clothing, diet and hydration, motion sickness, decompression sickness, spatial orientation and visual illusions of flight, effects of altitude and oxygen deprivation, development of oxygen equipment, the effects of various pharmacologic agents on flight, vision, and other areas of concern.

In 1940, the "Thousand Aviator Study" was begun in the United States Navy. Initiated by distinguished military and civilian scientists of the Harvard Research Group, the study was sponsored by the Civil Aeronautics Authority, the National Research Council, and the United States Navy. It was and is a long-term study of more than 1000 members of the naval aviation community, who initially were students and instructors in naval aviation at Pensacola, Florida.

Throughout World War II, an active exchange of cooperation took place with Great Britain and Canada. Many universities, civilian institutions, and scientists joined in the work to advance the art and science of aviation medicine.

Following World War II, as the world attempted to return to peaceful pursuits, the United States Navy returned to peacetime status. The School of Aviation Medicine continued to produce Naval flight surgeons, although at a rate far below that of the war years. In addition, the school was granted new status. For the first 7 years of its existence, the school had operated as a part of the Naval Air Station, Pensacola, Medical Department, with no other official status. On October 15, 1946, the school was made an official entity within the Naval Air Basic Training Command. It was formally recognized as the United States Naval School of Aviation Medicine and Research.

In the late 1940s, the development of aircraft escape systems continued within Navy research and field facilities. By 1949, ejection seat training was being provided to fleet pilots. In addition, the Aviation Medical Accelaration Laboratory was established at the Naval Air Development Center, Johnsville, Pennsylvania. Its mission was to study human performance in environments of accelerative change.

Progress in the 1950s

By 1951, the School of Aviation Medicine had established formal classes for aviation physiologists, and in January of that year, the first class was brought aboard.

Another landmark for Navy aeromedical education occurred in July, 1951 when the School of Aviation Medicine became an official Navy command. In that same year, the first repeat examinations of the "Thousand Aviators" were accomplished.

In July of 1955, the School of Aviation Medicine was approved by the American Board of Preventive Medicine as a site for 2 years of formal residency training in aviation medicine. This action took place only after much effort on the part of many of the leaders of aviation medicine in the Navy Medical Department and with great cooperation from specialists outside the Navy.

The Special Board of Flight Surgeons was established in 1956 by the chief of Naval Air Training. Convening at the School of Aviation Medicine, the Special Board of Flight Surgeons became the touchstone for the evaluation of difficult cases in aviation medicine. Its purpose originally was to provide prompt review of the qualifications of aviation trainees and to speed up the processing of those not qualified to continue in that training. From that original charter, the Special Board of Flight Surgeons expanded its scope to cover the evaluation of difficult cases of members of the aviation community, line, and staff, whenever the sit-

uation warranted such careful deliberation. The Special Board of Flight Surgeons has convened regularly in the more than 25 years since its establishment. It expertly evaluates the physical qualifications of naval aviation personnel to accurately assess their suitability for further aviation service.

The evolution of the Navy's aviation medicine center continued in 1957. Through the commissioning of the Naval Aviation Medical Center at Pensacola, the Navy Medical Department combined under a single command the clinical, training, and research efforts of the School of Aviation Medicine and the Naval Hospital at Pensacola. Elsewhere in the aviation medicine establishment in the Navy, studies continued in acceleration, ejection systems, altitude and spaceflight simulations, and spatial orientation studies.

The Navy's involvement in the space program was extensive. In the late 1950s and early 1960s, the Navy was involved in primate research in support of the space program; and Navy aviation medical personnel were involved in high-altitude balloon flights, which provided information on the development and use of full-pressure suits for aviation and space travelers.

The 1960s and 1970s

By 1964, the Navy had established a Coriolis acceleration platform and vestibular research unit at the School of Aviation Medicine, and research in vestibular function proceeded steadily.

In May, 1965, the Navy dedicated and entered new and much needed facilities for the School of Aviation Medicine. Later that year, the school was renamed the United States Naval Aerospace Medical Institute.

Further organizational changes led to the consolidation of research functions within the newly named Naval Aerospace Medical Institute. In 1970, the research component of the Naval Aerospace Medical Institute was officially designated a subordinate unit of the Institute as the Naval Aerospace Medical Research Laboratory (NAMRL). Subsequent Navy Medical Department organizational changes saw the research functions of the Institute reassigned to the newly established Naval Medical Research and Development Command and the Institute assigned organizationally to the Naval Health Sciences Education and Training Command.

The 1980s

Another organizational shift occurred in 1981, when the Naval Aerospace Medical Institute was assigned status reporting directly to the Bureau of Medicine and Surgery, and its mission was broadened to include other tasks in support of the operating naval forces.

Throughout the reorganization and changes that have characterized the last 20 years, the various components of the naval aviation medical community have worked to continue the progress of the past. Marked progress has been made in every field, from the work of the flight surgeon to that of the aerospace physiologist, the aerospace experimental psychologists, and the host of superb civilian scientists and technicians serving throughout the Navy's aviation medical support establishment. The past is but the prologue.

RESEARCH IN NAVAL AVIATION MEDICINE

The center of research in naval aviation medicine is the Naval Aerospace Medical Research Laboratory (NAMRL) located in Pensacola, Florida. Colocated with the Naval Aerospace Medical Institute and having the same history, NAMRL shares some physical facilities but has its own extensive physical plant and mission base. It is a command subordinate to the Naval Medical Research and Development Command within the Medical Department of the Navy.

Today, the Navy's aviation medical research program is broad-based. Although

numerous aviation medical research endeavors are going on in a variety of commands throughout the Navy, the principal focus of effort is within NAMRL.

The work of the research laboratory is divided among five departments, each of which manages subordinate divisions of related function. The departments include: applied aeromedical sciences, sensory sciences, bioenvironmental sciences, human performance sciences, and veterinary sciences. Rounding off the department structure is a sixth department, an administrative department that provides the various administrative, operating services and facilities management, fiscal, supply, and research support services.

NAMRL maintains a continuing flow of scientific reports providing detailed information concerning the ongoing work accomplished. Staff members of NAMRL actively support the education and training missions of the Institute and provide lecture and laboratory support for special groups involved in advanced aeromedical education.

PROFESSIONAL TRAINING

The Naval Aerospace Medical Institute is the foundation of the Navy's operational, clinical, and educational aviation medicine programs (Fig. 22–3). A continually evolving entity within the Navy Medical Department, the Institute is the direct descendant of the original School of Aviation Medicine. In response to the direction established by the Bureau of Medicine and Surgery, a number of functions vital to the Navy's aviation mission are currently assigned to the Institute, as follows:

1. Education and training of aeromedical personnel
2. Maintenance and administration of various programs for the selection of aviation personnel
3. Medical review of aviation candidate qualification

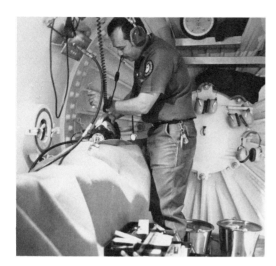

Fig. 22–3. A diving medicine technician readies a patient for decompression therapy at the Naval Aerospace Medical Institute chamber (official United States Navy photo).

4. Aviation candidate entrance physical evaluation
5. Physical qualification and waiver procedures fleetwide
6. Aeromedical consultations and the Special Board of Flight Surgeons
7. Initial flight physiology training of aviation candidates
8. Development of curricula, programs, and training procedures for physiologic training units

The foundation of the Navy's current aeromedical effort is the education and professional training provided to those individuals who will serve in the Navy's aviation support roles. Initial training in aviation medicine for all entering aeromedical personnel is provided by the Naval Aerospace Medical Institute. The following programs exist to provide aeromedical education and training:

1. Student flight surgeon curriculum
2. Residency in aerospace medicine
3. Student aerospace physiologist curriculum
4. Student aerospace experimental psychologist curriculum
5. Aviation medical officer curriculum
6. Student aviation medicine technician curriculum
7. Student aerospace physiology technician curriculum

These programs, managed by the Training Department of the Institute, draw on the total resources of the Institute for their execution.

Physician Training

Student Flight Surgeon Training

The initial course of training for physicians in aerospace medicine takes place at the Institute. The curriculum is a 24-week course that provides a unique background for the naval physician who is beginning a period of service in aviation. The Navy course prepares the student flight surgeon for duty in the Navy operational environment. Both Navy and Marine Corps units are called on to serve with forward units aboard ship and are deployed all over the world. Fleet Marine Force units may operate independently of fixed, well-staffed medical facilities, particularly when operating outside the United States. Therefore, the Navy flight surgeon is expected to have a high degree of expertise in the practice of aerospace medicine. The curriculum provided at the Naval Aerospace Medical Institute is tailored to provide that professional competence.

First, because Naval flight surgeons serve closely with line naval and fleet Marine Force units, great care is taken to give the entering physician some background in naval customs and traditions. A grounding in the organization, management, and operations of the United States Navy is provided. Thus, the Naval flight surgeon is, it is hoped, spared the culture shock of entering the military aviation environment without previous acclimatization. Such careful military indoctrination facilitates the aeromedical professional's work with military peers: it enables the physician to understand the true nature of the military aviator's work place and to share in the tasks of that work place as a participant and shipmate rather than as an observer.

After the introduction of the student to the environment in which future service will take place, a rapid transition to more personal issues takes place. Every entering physician must complete course requirements in basic survival skills, and training and practice are provided in both land and water survival. It is logical that individuals bound to serve in a naval environment be at least minimally acquainted with water survival. To that end, definite physical performance requirements are levied in water survival. Once those skills are mastered, advanced training is provided. As water survival skills are mastered, the student is trained in emergency egress from both single-cockpit underwater "dunker" trainers and multiplace underwater helicopter escape trainers. The training is rigorous and enables the candidate to experience and understand the demands imposed in the water survival environment.

Concurrent with other portions of the training, the physician-students receive training in the aviation physiologic training unit, undergoing indoctrination in simulated altitude training ascents in a multiplace trainer, including hypoxia demonstrations and hands-on instruction in the use of various personal support devices. Ejection seat dynamic training is provided, as is training in night vision and spatial disorientation.

A major segment of the course is devoted to studies of the environmental physiology of flight. Many hours of didactic instruction are dedicated to studies of the physiology of the human body in the flight environment. The course addresses the demands, stresses, and hazards imposed in the flight environment. The effects of environmental stresses on the various systems of the human body are studied, with particular emphasis on flying safety.

The course continues into a detailed series of lectures and clinical instructional encounters; the physician is introduced to traditional medical subjects as they relate to the unfamiliar environment of flight. Detailed didactic instruction is provided in otorhinolaryngology, ophthalmology, neurology, psychiatry, internal medicine, and cardiology and special short courses of instruction in urology, dermatology, and orthopedics. Special clinics are held in the major fields to introduce the student to the application of the theory studied in the didactic setting. Considerable emphasis is placed on the application and practice of these traditional disciplines not only in the flight environment but also in the military, deployed environment when consultations with highly trained specialists may not be possible. The training is provided in the anticipation that the Naval flight surgeon frequently may be called on to act in an environment in which there is no backup and no reinforcing support. The high level of detail provided in the training is to that end.

Strongly interwoven into the curriculum is environmental and preventive medicine. A broad range of topics of preventive medical concern are presented to the student. From communicable diseases worldwide to the epidemiology of occupational and industrially encountered disease, the course structure is designed to prepare the student for future duties in many environments.

Finally, the student is introduced to the flight environment through a period of actual flight indoctrination in the Naval Aviation Training Command. For a period, the student is committed full-time to studies in the flight environment, living alongside student naval aviators and participating in an introduction to flight training experience. Some students who demonstrate skill and application and who are physically qualified are allowed to solo in

Navy training aircraft. The principal effort of the indoctrination period, however, is to give the student a clear and firsthand understanding of the flight process, environment, and its inherent stresses and hazards. The experience simultaneously tempers the student through understanding and gives him a degree of credibility to carry to the Naval aviation unit that, as flight surgeon, he will ultimately support.

Throughout this course, the student is under the tutelage of clinical specialists, fleet-experienced physicians, and military and civilian scientists and professionals in the disciplines of medicine, physiology, psychology, and the various military disciplines. They are exposed continually to the integration of traditional medical and academic disciplines and the aviation environment. Well-schooled in the demanding experience of Navy and fleet Marine Force environments, the instructors are able to pass an invaluable body of information to their students.

At the completion of each portion of this demanding course, the student is examined for successful completion of the physical, academic, and flight indoctrination requirements. When the student has completed all requirements successfully, the designation of Naval flight surgeon is awarded, and the gold wings of a Naval flight surgeon are presented. The new flight surgeon is then sent to serve with the fleet.

Aerospace Medicine Residency Training

For flight surgeons who desire to pursue a career path in aviation and aerospace medicine, the Navy offers an aerospace medicine residency program. The program is offered at the Naval Aerospace Medical Institute in Pensacola and leads to eligibility for examinations and certification as a specialist in aerospace medicine. The basic requirements for specialty board eligibility are those imposed by the American Board of Preventive Medicine.

The special concern of the Navy program is tied to the role of the Navy aeromedical specialist in the deployed environment, both ashore and afloat. The middle-career Naval flight surgeon normally serves as Senior Medical Officer aboard an aircraft carrier, the largest of the Navy's ships. In that environment, one often likened to a floating city and airport, the Naval flight surgeon is the manager of a large and well-equipped medical department. For the embarked community of 4000 to 6000 personnel, the medical department is charged with the delivery of health care, the practice of aviation medicine, and the total management of a complex program of preventive, occupational, and industrial health. Thus, the Navy's residency in aerospace medicine encompasses all aspects of the American Board of Preventive Medicine's requirements, augmenting those requirements with specific Navy training.

Although it is not immediately apparent, the medical department of the aircraft carrier is the referral center for all ships in company during periods of forward deployment. Preventive medicine expertise becomes as essential as clinical competence in such an environment. Again, the special requirements of preventive medicine, mastered by the resident in aerospace medicine, are essential to the health of the task group of carrier and ships in company. It is better to provide strong preventive programs to maintain health than to be forced to intervene, treat, and perhaps evacuate in cases of illness, toxicity, or injury.

The Navy's aerospace medicine residency includes Navy sponsorship of an academic year leading to the completion of requirements for a master's degree in public health or its equivalent. As many graduates of such years of study have learned, the basic grounding in health and public administration, statistics, epidemiology, and other special health care studies is essential to the well-grounded preventive medicine specialist. Such knowledge and skills are especially valuable to the Navy physician and flight surgeon serving with deployed units.

In addition, the Navy offers 2 years of study at the Naval Aerospace Medical Institute. During those 2 years, the resident is given advanced and careful indoctrination in clinical specialty applications in the Institute's clinics. Advanced skills are developed in the various clinical disciplines, as the resident learns to refine his diagnostic and therapeutic skills and his experience.

The following special courses and field trips are provided:

1. Annual scientific meeting of the Aerospace Medical Association
2. Operational aeromedical problems course, United States Air Force
3. Aircraft crash survival investigators' school, Arizona State University
4. Alcoholism seminar for physicians, Naval Hospital, Long Beach, California
5. Aerospace pathology course, Armed Forces Institute of Pathology, Washington, D.C.
6. Hyperbaric medicine course, Naval Diving School, Washington, D.C.
7. Nuclear weapons effects course, Bethesda, Maryland
8. Chemical biologic warfare course, Aberdeen Laboratories, Maryland
9. Emergency management of severe burn cases, Institute of Surgical Research, Fort Sam Houston, Texas
10. Emergency medicine and trauma rotation, Baptist Hospital, Pensacola, Florida

The residents participate actively in the course of instruction provided to student flight surgeons and are periodically assigned special tasks in support of local and operational units.

The Navy's residency in aerospace medicine provides the Navy with a steady flow of broadly trained aeromedical experts who are as capable in general preventive,

occupational, and industrial medicine as they are in their specialty discipline. This breadth of training and experience makes them uniquely qualified to assume roles of leadership and management in the Navy's demanding environments ashore and afloat, at home and deployed.

Aerospace Physiologist Training

In the years that have passed since the first physiologists began their work in aviation medicine, the milestones reached and passed have been legion. Today's Naval aerospace physiologist is a highly trained professional officer of the Navy Medical Department. The aerospace physiologist is entrusted with a broad range of tasks, serving both in the Medical Department and in a variety of billets, from direct-line support to research, in Medical Department and line commands. Aerospace physiologists occupy positions of leadership and responsibility, not only as the administrators and managers of aviation physiology training units but also as aeromedical safety officers, experts in personal and life-support equipment for aviators, environmental physiology experts, and highly competent investigators and managers in a variety of fields related to the safety of the aviation member in the environments of earth, sea, sky, and space.

The initial Navy training in the specialty of aerospace physiology is provided at the Naval Aerospace Medical Institute. At the successful conclusion of all course components at the Institute, those student aerospace physiologists who have completed the requirements move on to join their student flight surgeon classmates for naval flight indoctrination. In the training squadron environment, the student aerospace physiologist undergoes another kind of testing, experiencing the flight environment and testing skills and industry as students in the cockpit of Navy training aircraft. Those students who are qualified physically and academically and who demonstrate aviation competence may be allowed one solo flight. Again, to solo is not a course goal; the goal is the demonstration of the ability to understand and grasp the principles of both the aircraft and the human system in the act of flight (Fig. 22–4).

Upon the successful completion of all course requirements, the student may be designated a Naval aerospace physiologist and be awarded the physiologist's wings of gold.

Aerospace Experimental Psychologist Training

Psychologists have served naval aviation with distinction since the early years of Medical Department involvement with candidate selection. In the early years, when the staff of psychologists came aboard, no one could have foreseen the role psychologists were to play in naval aviation.

Today, aerospace experimental psychologists in the Navy fill assignments in research commands, in training and operational commands, and through the entire breadth of Navy aeromedical operations. Psychologists are members of highly trained accident investigating teams, participating in both accident prevention efforts and in accident investigation. Involved in the whole spectrum of aviation research, they provide skilled and expert contributions to the efforts of the naval aviation team.

At the Naval Aerospace Medical Institute, the initial training of psychologists begins. Already highly trained by virtue of their graduate degrees, the psychologists must undergo the metamorphosis required to make them both competent naval officers and experts in naval aeromedical matters. Thus, they enter, with their physician and physiologist classmates, the basic Navy indoctrination, proceeding to studies in basic aviation environmental physiology. They complete the didactic experience in operational medicine, which

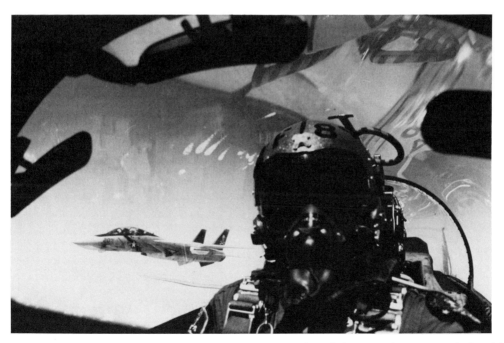

Fig. 22–4. Naval aviation physiologists and aerospace experimental psychologists work to improve the lot of the aviator in the modern high-performance aircraft. Personal flight equipment, life-support systems, and cockpit ergonomics are continuously studied and improved to increase aircrew performance in high-technology flight environments (official United States Navy photo).

introduces them to preventive medicine, sanitation, communicable diseases, toxicology, drug and alcohol abuse, crash survival investigations, and a variety of related topics. Thus prepared with a basic aeromedical and a naval indoctrination, they then embark on a curriculum structure for their particular career path.

Studies to which the student aerospace experimental psychologist is introduced include the following:

1. Contemporary problems in aerospace psychology
2. Human sensory and information-processing capabilities
3. Human factors engineering
4. Performance measurement
5. Personnel selection
6. Training systems
7. Research and contract organization and management
8. Aviation accident prevention and aircraft accident investigation

During the course of study, each student selects a pertinent investigation topic and conducts research under the supervision of a scientific investigator. The project concludes with a written report.

Upon the successful completion of the course requirements at the Institute, the student psychologist joins physician and physiologist classmates for naval flight indoctrination.

When all course requirements are complete, the successful student may be designated a Naval aerospace experimental psychologist and awarded the psychologist's wings of gold.

MEDICAL SELECTION PROCEDURES FOR AIRCREW

Within the Navy, aircrew members are selected by the line. The selection process is based, in part, on advice contributed by the Medical Department. The selection process contains a number of steps, each of which contributes a portion of the information on which the final decision for selection or nonselection is based. When an individual applies for admission to the Navy flight program, while still a civilian or in the Navy in a nonaviation unit, initial evaluation is begun. The candidate is requested to take a battery of aptitude tests that provide an index of the individual's potential for success as an aviation program candidate. Those tests are scored in the field by recruiters involved in the aviation application process; the scores are subsequently validated by the Operational Psychology Department of the Naval Aerospace Medical Institute. If the aptitude tests give a favorable picture of the applicant's potential, certain other nonmedical considerations are evaluated, including such factors as past life history and educational experience.

Initial Physical Evaluation

Included among subsequent studies completed in the field is a physical examination. This first physical examination may be performed at any of a number of examining facilities. The completed physical evaluation is forwarded to the Bureau of Medicine and Surgery, where it is reviewed. If the first physical examination indicates a healthy potential candidate, recommendation for approval is forwarded to the line from the Navy Medical Department.

The Preentry Evaluation

If all the various indicators are positive, the individual candidate is brought to the Naval Aviation School's Command at Pensacola. While there, prior to entering training, the candidate has a final physical examination at the Naval Aerospace Medical Institute. At this time, a meticulous flight physical examination is accomplished, and the candidate is provided any needed consultations or special evaluations. In most cases, the Institute's specialty clinics are capable of providing the needed expert evaluation. The Institute then provides a final recommendation to the Commanding

Officer of the Naval Aviation School's Command, and the candidate either enters training or is reassigned.

Physical Standards

The physical standards used to select candidates for naval aviation programs are the outgrowth of years of cumulative experience of naval aviation medicine and the work of individuals dedicated to research in aircrew selection. The standards are altered as experience, knowledge, and circumstances require. Standards are promulgated primarily through the manual of the Navy Medical Department but may be augmented with special guidance through naval notices, messages, and instructions. Because the standards are based on the best knowledge at the time of implementation, they are subject to change as new information is considered.

The Navy is fortunate that all aircrew candidates for officer courses receive their initial training at Pensacola. This fact has enabled the concurrent focusing of a highly skilled cadre of aeromedical experts at the Naval Aerospace Medical Institute who can provide the finest and most informed evaluations of candidates for naval aviation programs. The cumulative experience gained by the examiners simultaneously expands both their skill and insight. A highly accurate and consistent examination method has been developed. Both candidates and naval aviation are well served by the process.

Pitfalls in the Examination and Selection Process

Experience at the Naval Aerospace Medical Institute indicates that the most common pitfalls in the physical selection process occur in the early periods of evaluation. Pitfalls are typically of two sorts: (1) obtaining an accurate history; and (2) assessing the state of the candidate's eyes and vision. Other failures are generally random in type and occurrence.

Obtaining the History

In the Navy experience in candidate examination, examiners sometimes encounter applicants who tend to minimize their past medical histories. Minimization can be as minor as omitting a history of a few early childhood episodes of motion sickness, or it can be as major as omitting the history of anaphylaxis after an insect bite or denying the past occurrence of a grand mal seizure. On rare occasions, candidates have been encountered who would deliberately falsify documents to achieve their goal of admission to flight training. The examiner responsible for the initial screening of aviation applicants has, at best, a difficult task. Often, candidate examinations are only one of many types of evaluation the examiner must perform in a given day. Many other demands are made of the examiner's time. To establish rapport with a candidate and accurately explore and assess the candidate's past medical history is a time-consuming task, one that is not usually affordable to a busy or harrassed examiner. The confluence of candidate reluctance and examiner preoccupation can result in a false reading at the initial screening point, leading to subsequent disappointment and frustration of the candidate and cost to the referring organization.

Assessing Vision

The second source of frequent difficulty in early candidate processing is in the examination of candidates' vision. In examining facilities so diverse in mission and staffing as those providing initial military aviation candidate evaluation, it is not surprising that there are some difficulties in the evaluation of vision.

Examiners are often unaccustomed to the realities of the encounter between aviation applicants and their examiners. Unstudied Navy experience indicates that, whenever it is possible, candidates will establish a "gouge" or "crib" concerning eye examinations. Information concerning the charts and tests will be passed from candidate to candidate. Sympathetic examiners or technicians will occasionally coach a failing candidate, allowing the individual to "pass," not realizing that such an action ensures later disqualification and greater disappointment. The precise and correct administration of vision tests will ensure that subsequent candidate disqualification and related candidate frustration and disappointment do not occur.

The principal caveat for indivduals charged with performing entrance physical examinations of aviation candidates is this: aviation candidate entry examinations are not routine. In the military aviation environment, taxpayers and the government expend many hundreds of thousands of dollars in selecting and training aviation candidates. Their investment should be made in those best qualified. Selecting the truly best qualified is not a routine process.

NAVAL AEROMEDICAL CONSULTATION

Primary Care

Within the naval aviation establishment, the primary care of aircrew members is provided by individuals trained in aviation medicine at the Naval Aerospace Medical Institute. Those individuals may be flight surgeons, aviation medical examiners, or aviation medical officers, depending on the level of training they have achieved. The primary care network extends through every aviation-related facility within the Navy, whether clinic ashore or sick bay afloat; it includes facilities that provide support to aviation units of the United States Marine Corps.

Secondary and Tertiary Care

More sophisticated and complex care is provided within the Navy Medical Department's Regional Medical Center hospitals and clinic facilities by individuals trained in the many specialty and subspecialty disciplines. At the completion of pe-

riods of care, as the patient recovers and is considered for a return to duty, decisions regarding that return are made.

Return to Flight Status

Local Decisions, Medical Boards, and Limited Duty

A decision is first made regarding the individual's general fitness for a return to duty in the Navy. If the patient is not yet fully fit to return to full duty in the general sense, a limited duty status is provided for the individual by a special administrative procedure, the Medical Board. While an individual is serving on limited duty in the United States Navy, the individual may not serve on flight status. Once the limited duty period is resolved and if the patient is returned to full duty, a decision regarding a return to flying is made. That deliberation is made by the flight surgeon of the aviation unit or the medical facility supporting that aviation unit.

Local Board of Flight Surgeons

If there is any question about fitness for duty involving flying, a Local Board of Flight Surgeons may be convened. Through this mechanism, several flight surgeons consider the case and all pertinent information and make a recommendation in the case. That recommendation is then passed to the Bureau of Medicine and Surgery for endorsement. In an uncomplicated case, positive or favorable endorsement by the Bureau results in an immediate return to flight status. In other cases, upon the recommendation of the Local Board of Flight Surgeons or at the direction of the Bureau, the individual is recommended for a Special Board of Flight Surgeons. Upon approval and endorsement by the higher authority, the patient is ordered to Pensacola, Florida for evaluation by the Special Board of Flight Surgeons.

Special Board of Flight Surgeons

The Special Board of Flight Surgeons convenes within the Naval Aerospace Medical Institute. Because of the staffing of the Institute, it is possible to convene a board of highly trained aeromedical specialists with representatives from many disciplines. Available to the Board are specialists representing psychiatry, psychology, neurology, otorhinolaryngology, ophthalmology, optometry, internal medicine, aerospace medicine, cardiology, and other disciplines. Most of these individuals have had extensive experience as Naval flight surgeons. In addition, specialists in other disciplines are available on call from the Naval Aerospace and Regional Medical Center nearby. Aerospace physiologists and experimental psychologists are also available to the Board. Consultants from the Naval Aerospace Medical Research Laboratory participate, both as expert consultants and as flight surgeon participants in the Board process.

Patients appearing before the Special Board of Flight Surgeons undergo a week of careful study. They are evaluated by each of the specialty disciplines represented within the Institute. At the end of the week of studies, the Special Board of Flight Surgeons convenes formally. The case is presented and deliberated, a decision is reached, and recommendations are passed to the Bureau of Medicine and Surgery and to the Naval Manpower and Personnel Center.

Review by Higher Authority

After the deliberations of the Special Board of Flight Surgeons are completed and recommendations and reports forwarded to higher authority, the patient has the right to appeal or request consideration at a higher level. That may take place through the convening of a Board of Senior Flight Surgeons in Washington, D.C. The option is rarely elected by higher authority.

The Aeromedical Recommendation

All decisions reached by flight surgeons in the Navy are submitted to line commanders as recommendations. The process of grounding of an aircrew member with an acute disease, for example, is in the form of a recommendation to the cognizant commanding officer, who must make the final decision concerning whether to accept the recommendation. No flight surgeon in the Navy has the authority to unilaterally ground an aircrew member; grounding is recommended to the line commander.

Other Consultations

Other sorts of aeromedical consultations occur with great frequency at the Naval Aerospace Medical Institute. Phone calls and letters are received from units afield with great regularity, and consultants within the Institute respond with practical advice and counsel. On occasion, at the request of units afield, individual patients are sent to the Institute for consultation.

The Thousand Aviator Program

The "Thousand Aviator Program" is a project now in progress at the Naval Aerospace Medical Institute and is carried out as a part of the Institute's clinical and consultative services. Its initial phase began in 1939, when the Committee on Selection and Training of Civilian Aircraft Pilots of the National Research Council received funds from the Civil Aeronautics Authority. The intent was to plan and supervise research on the human portion of aviation. In 1940, the Council included military aviation; the United States Navy joined the study, and "The Pensacola Study of Naval Aviators," or the "Thousand Aviator Program" began.

The 1940 portion of the study took place under the guidance of such distinguished scientists as McFarland and Graybiel, Hoagland, Davis, Forbes, Phillips, Gates, Peckham, Bennette, Wilson, Channell, and Webster. More than 1000 aviators and aviation candidates were examined. The initial thrust of the study was to explore the value of psychologic and physiologic testing of applicants for flight training to develop and apply measures that would enable the rapid selection of candidates who were truly promising for flight training.

A large body of data was accumulated on the subjects of the study. After World War II, those who reviewed the earlier work were aware that the large data base was an invaluable source of information as a foundation for a prospective study of the aging process. With this in mind, the first subsequent follow-up study took place in 1951. Investigators included Graybiel, Packard, and Graettinger; their intent was to estimate the physical status of the group of men 10 years after the original studies were accomplished. Cardiovascular status, morbidity and mortality rates, and the effects of the aviation experience were to be reviewed and comparisons made with the results of the 1940 and 1941 studies.

The nature of the disease processes being reviewed and the unique aspects of the population under study led to the natural conclusion that a long-term follow-up would be valuable. That indeed took place, with further reviews occurring in 1957, 1963, and 1969; subsequent studies have been accomplished in the last 10 years. The process has been an intermittent one because of funding and sponsorship issues. The study, however, is now assigned to the Naval Aerospace Medical Institute, where it is ongoing under leadership well acquainted with its origins and long-term purposes.

AVIATION MEDICINE AT SEA: CARRIER MEDICINE

The First Principle: Interdependence

At sea, as in the air, the first principle underscoring all activities is that of inter-dependence. Just as members of the aeronautic team of pilot, navigator, engineer, loadmaster, mechanic, and flight-line airman work together to make manned flight successful, at sea every member of the embarked crew works to ensure the safety and security of every other crewmember. No act occurring aboard a ship occurs singly. Every act occurs in the context of the sea and its unrelenting demands. As individuals working in the confines of deep-ocean oil exploration rigs have discovered, the demands of the sea are as immutable as the demands of the air. To compromise or to fail is to invite disaster. Thus, in the seaborne environment, the aircrew extends its membership to include the members of the vessel or platform on which they serve. All are interdependent. The mechanic tending the freshwater production devices affects the health of the aircrew; the aviation mechanic tending the rotors of the helicopter can directly affect the safety of every member of the crew of the small vessel to which the helicopter flies.

The preventive, occupational, and epidemiologic skills mastered by the practitioner of aviation medicine become of concentrated value in the seaborne aviation platform environment. From gigantic, nuclear-powered aircraft carrier to ordinary merchant vessel, from patrol vessel to industrial oil exploration rig, the environment demands from each person its due; each member of the operating team is interdependent on the skills and will of others also embarked. The aviation medicine practitioner brings unique skills that are well suited to the environment at sea, whatever the vessel. Those skills are well grounded in the understanding of interdependence.

Living at Sea: Crew Support and Hotel Services

Hotel services is the term used frequently in the United States Navy to refer to those facilities and activities aboard ship that support the basic life activities of the crew. Such services include living and berthing spaces, food services, personal services, entertainment, and so on.

Every crewmember of a vessel at sea must have a clean and safe place in which to relax and rest. Standards vary depending on the mission of the vessel and the status of the crewmember, but the underlying requirements are the same, The living area must be properly controlled for ventilation, humidity, and temperature and be free of odors and toxic materials. It must be comfortable and clean and be maintained in a tidy and hospitable manner. It must have easily accessible escape avenues and offer its occupants a degree of personal security. Linens, mattresses, and pillows must be clean and well maintained. Lighting must be satisfactory for activities therein, and there must be provisions for the emergency lighting of escape routes. Individual sleeping areas are needed, with secure space for storing personal clothing, gear, and valuables.

Bathing and toilet facilities must be constantly maintained and monitored. Sanitary facilities require manual cleaning. Most mechanical devices in the end fail to provide an adequate level of cleanliness. The human eye and hand are the ultimate weapons in the attack on soil and odor. Many times, the odors and soil encountered in certain areas are not the result of design or plumbing failures but rather are the result of the inadequate application of basic cleaning techniques.

The aviation medicine specialist aboard a ship or platform must make visits to the living areas a part of his daily routine. Disorder in living spaces and failure in the delivery of hotel services can strongly influence the performance of those who support the aviation team aboard.

Living spaces must be monitored for hazards similar to those found in the working environment. Noise is a particular problem in some vessels; it is difficult for crewmembers to obtain adequate rest in spaces that are in close proximity to noisy shipboard or industrial work. Adjustments must be made to allow crewmembers to obtain adequate relaxation and rest free from the stress of noise. Fumes, vapors, and airborne infiltrates are also of concern. Ventilation systems must be meticulously maintained to ensure their efficiency and the effectiveness of their filtration systems.

Health Care Delivery at Sea

Isolation

In some respects, health care delivery at sea is identical to onshore health care. In other ways, it is radically different. Few shorebound practitioners would consciously choose to deny themselves access to high-level, skilled technical support in unrestricted volume on short notice. The practitioner at sea frequently stands alone in an environment in which help or consultation may be far away or unobtainable. Therefore, every aspect of the practice of the aviation medical specialist at sea is colored by this reality; the specialist works alone or in a small team of professionals in an environment of professional isolation, dependent on his own skills, and interdependent for his personal survival and that of his patients on the will and skill of his shipmates. In the end, the most demanding of situations exists. When the threat and danger are greatest, help is least accessible and obtainable. With that reality, the practice of aviation medicine at sea takes on a singular urgency.

Planning

All planning that takes place centers on the basic premise that in daily operations and in the first stages of emergency, the practitioner has only the vessel's basic resources. Those resources, human and material, are the result of planning, staffing, and decision making that take place before and during normal operations. To obtain augmentation and assistance in an emergency or to evacuate to safety requires dependence on planning and most frequently on the availability of suitable outside assistance. Planning must include what to do when assistance cannot be obtained.

Finally, even in modern times, the practitioner cannot overlook the basic dangers inherent in operations at sea. There is no escape from the challenge posed by the sea.

Principles of Operations

Before beginning practice in a seaborne vessel or on an ocean platform, the practitioner must first assess the environment and the mission. Whether the setting be civilian or military, the practitioner must understand the environment and the challenges it represents. This understanding is accomplished through a review of the directives and instructions already existing, through conversations with those experienced in operations in the new environment, and through careful personal study of the environment. As experience is gained, the integration of information from these and other sources will allow the practitioner to become increasingly effective.

The dispersion of resources is essential in any seaborne setting. Emergencies that deny access to some areas of the ship or platform may deny the medical support personnel access to a portion, or all, of their resources. Therefore, there must be some degree of dispersion of resources. Although daily medical support activities may take place in a single, well-defined area, the capability to provide emergency care in other sites about the ship must be provided. In military vessels, multiple sites may be absolutely essential. An old Navy principle is "the rule of thirds." It is considered highly desirable to divide all supplies into thirds and disperse them widely throughout the vessel. Thus, an emergency in the forward part of the ship would not necessarily cause the loss of all

of a particular item; similar stocks of supplies amidships and aft still would be available.

Portability of supplies is another useful principle. If one is facing the possibility of emergency, planning for that should include methods of moving supplies from point to point. If one's ship were vulnerable to disasters and large numbers of casualties might be expected, provision for moving adequate amounts of supplies should be established. Methods of stowing supplies in accountable, easily moveable, and secure containers should be provided.

Planning for emergencies, with appropriate staff and crew training, is essential to readiness for disaster. In every seaborne environment, the potential for a complicated emergency is enormous. If planning is thorough and meticulous, almost no disaster is unmanageable. Even the absolutely overwhelming emergency can be conceptualized and some orderly method of dealing with overload devised.

Redundancy in equipment is desirable but not always affordable or provided. Redundancy in training, however, is always possible. For every job that must be accomplished by the aviation medical and ship's medical support unit, cross training of personnel should be accomplished. Loss of one or more individuals in a disaster should not bring the medical support unit to a standstill. If personnel are trained and cross trained, work can go on. Training should be carried out as a continuing process and bring the highest possible level of skill to assigned personnel. Military experience has taught that, in welltrained units, the loss of key staff personnel need not mean unit collapse. Work may slow down and the level of possible care decrease somewhat, but work need not stop. Cross training and redundancy in training are crucial to that process.

Routine Health Care

In nearly every shipboard or industrial platform environment, space is dedicated to the delivery of health care. Traditionally called sick bay, the space, its size and equipage, and its staffing are decided by the size and mission of the platform or vessel. In the sick bay, the conduct of daily medical activities goes on, and the practice of a very direct form of preventive medicine occurs. The care delivered through the sick bay must go beyond basic "sick call" and care of the sick and injured. Its extent must be determined by the extent of industry and activity aboard the vessel, by its crew and mission, and by the potential for danger it faces.

On an aircraft carrier of the United States Navy, the activities of the medical department and sick bay are numerous. From the delivery of daily care to the sick and injured to the provision of dozens of types of physical examinations, the work goes on day and night. The technical capability of these facilities depends on the size of the physical plant. The largest ships include laboratory and radiographic facilities of significant capability and competence and provide a wide range of diagnostic tests and studies to practitioners aboard the ships.

Larger vessels have their own preventive medicine sections, which maintain the thrust of a variety of programs in industrial and occupational health. In addition, those other traditional preventive medicine programs of sanitation and food service monitoring, immunizations, and epidemiology and disease outbreak control continue. On some of the largest ships, these programs use automated data processing systems that provide program support.

Programs carried out by the medical departments of vessels today include many that, in 1970, were not considered in vessels at sea. In those days of the dawning of preventive medicine endeavors afloat, asbestos, heat stress, radiation health, and noise hazards were the principal focus of shipboard programs. Today, literally dozens of specialized occupational health programs exist, many of which require special physical examinations, periodic health screening, and detailed recordkeeping and reporting to higher authority.

The monitoring of environmental hazards today requires a great deal of the time of skilled technical personnel. Inherent in this monitoring process is the necessity for familiarity with the operating environment, that is, the physical layout of the ship and its maze of compartments.

The increase in attention to external environmental considerations has led to the implementation and installation of programs and systems to avoid the dumping of waste into the oceans. Sewage systems today are being retrofitted to older ships, with the resulting ability to avoid environmental pollution of rivers, harbors, and oceans. The presence of complex sewage collection and holding systems, however, poses unique hazards in the closed environment of the ship. Preventive medical and mechanical maintenance monitoring is required on a continuing basis.

Emergency Health Care Delivery

Emergencies at sea, whether from combat or from accident or misadventure in peacetime, are often fearsome events. The confining nature of the environment prevents easy escape. The equipment for dealing with the emergency is frequently restricted to that which planners had the foresight to provide and no more. Escape avenues from the vessel may be nonexistent. Finally, disasters commonly occur when weather and sea conditions prevent easy evacuation. If aircraft are involved, the evacuation is even more complex because of the risks associated with such operations at sea. Thus, a medical or surgical emergency or multiple casualty situation at sea is a severe test.

The aviation medicine practitioner must carefully assess the threat environment for potentially hostile and harmful substances and forces. Plans must then be formulated to deal with those sorts of events that can be imagined.

Special problems to be anticipated in a ship at sea include the loss of electrical power, freshwater supplies, and waste disposal systems. Medical and surgical care may have to be delivered from a most primitive base of operations, and the plans must anticipate that. Loss of electricity and freshwater can prevent the use of radiographic facilities, laboratory functions, and access to sophisticated surgical equipment and techniques. Portability of supplies must be ensured to allow flexibility.

In every situation in which disasters may occur, a plan for handling large numbers of casualties must be developed. Once a plan is staffed, it should be drilled in detail, observed, critiqued, and redone.

Plans for evacuation must be made, including methods, communication, supplies escorts, and routes. If rafts or lifeboats are included, supplies for those must be planned and accounted. Once put in place, maintenance of the emergency supplies must be assured. During normal operations, any medical supplies left anywhere without adequate security may be pilfered. Security is an absolute necessity.

Occupational and Environmental Medicine

Te practice of occupational and environmental medicine in the environment aboard the ship or platform at sea is highly demanding and complex. With no relief from the immediacy of the presence of threats presented by the environment, work must be done with continuous care.

The accurate and total assessment of the hazards of the working environment must be accomplished. Care must be taken to include an accurate appraisal of synergistic factors at work in the environment that increase or alter the nature of the hazards in the work place. Once again, there is no possible way a practitioner can know the work place without being out and about

in it. Staying in the sick bay or medical department will not allow proper insight to evolve. Time must be spent studying the environment, and the practitioner must personally experience and identify the effect of the work place on its occupants. In some vessels with small staffs, daily work may seem to preclude daily trips into the ship's work places. The practitioner must make time, however; even a few minutes a day, taken regularly, will rapidly add up to hours of experience.

The appropriate use of specialists in environmental and occupational subspecialties is often indicated. The military services provide scientific and technical support personnel in a variety of disciplines for consultation. These individuals provide knowledge and insight gained in long study of vector control, toxic environmental hazards, epidemiology, heat stress, sanitation, and a host of other areas of problems that occur aboard ship.

Launch and Recovery

Some of the most visible and dramatic acts of the naval aviator's career take place from the deck of the carrier. A place where modern tactical aircraft are hurled by steam catapults into the air, accelerating in seconds to flight speed, the flight deck is a place of inherent danger (Fig. 22–5). The forces involved in launch and recovery of aircraft are great. To decelerate from flight speed to a full stop in the length of a deck landing area requires energy-absorbing mechanisms, airframes, and flight techniques of great complexity.

The process of launch and recovery involves radical forces acting on the human system in stressful ways. The launch process, whether at day or night, may induce disorientation sufficient to disable an unskilled or unhealthy pilot or crewmember. Similarly, the return to the deck of the carrier extracts its own particular toll. The pilot must fly a precise pattern, using visual cues to establish a final lineup and descent rate. Clarity of thought must par-

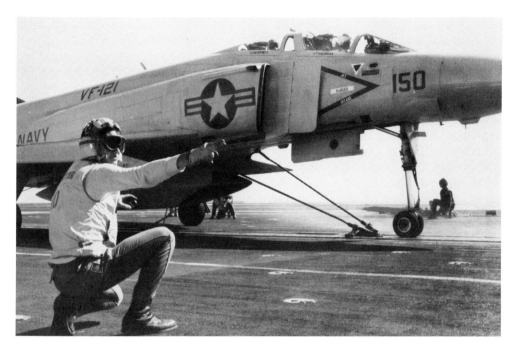

Fig. 22–5. Launch and recovery. Catapult launches impose physiologic stress and sensory illusions on aircrew members. Simultaneously, members of deck crews work against environmental extremes and significant occupational hazards (official United States Navy photo).

allel clarity of vision. Reflex skills must be at their sharpest levels.

During the launch and recovery phase of carrier operations, flight crews must be at their best, and support personnel on deck and below decks must also be sharp and ready. Many hands participate in the successful launch of an aircraft from a carrier; other hands similarly influence the aircraft's recovery. The pilot's fate does not rest on his own skills alone.

It is the duty of the practitioner of aviation medicine living in the shipboard environment of a carrier to see that all members of the team are fit for duty. Many hands work to build a successful launch and recovery; none can be neglected.

AIRCREW AT SEA: SMALL PLATFORMS

The aircrew serving at sea in small detachments is faced with special problems. The smaller the unit to which the aircrew is attached, the more isolated the assignment may be; the more isolated the as-

signment, the more likely that experienced aeromedical support will not be available. Living accomodations may not be as conducive to sound rest as those on larger, aviation-oriented vessels. In ships not accustomed to providing for aircrew members, a thorough understanding of the need for adequate rest and relaxation may not be present. In some units, quarters provided for aircrew may be the least desirable aboard and thus not provide the most restful environment. Health maintenance of aircrew may be provided by individuals not familiar with the precepts of aviation medicine. In such cases, aircrew members themselves are faced with participating in their own care with regard to decisions about flight. Optimally, all medical personnel supporting aircrew in small vessels should have access to advice and counsel in problems regarding the health of flight crewmembers. The work environment provided the aircrew must be adequate to the task at hand. Both flight crew and maintenance personnel must have the space and equipment required for their various tasks. The space issue is frequently a critical one and is most advantageously addressed through careful planning in advance of the deployment.

Small unit operations frequently impose heavy mission demands on embarked aviation personnel. It is easy for aircrew members and maintenance personnel to be tasked heavily, leading to unusual fatigue and stress (Fig. 22–6). When no backup units are available and missions must be carried out, the personal pressure of feelings of duty and command pressure to get the job done are present. Aircrew in such environments thus have a special problem with which to deal.

AIRCREW STRESS

Disorientation

Disorientation in flight is a problem that is a particular enemy of the aircrew at sea. Flight operations in the extremes of daylight, morning and evening, and in darkness at sea pose their own problems. With poor weather, decreased visibility, and heavy seas added to that flight environment, the aircrew is faced with a great challenge. Adding low-level operations over pitching decks on which a variety of lights may be visible may lead to disorienting sensations against which the aircrew must be on guard constantly. Strong skill development in instrument flight and great reliance on in-flight teamwork between pilot, copilot, and crewmember can reduce some of the hazards inherent in this situation.

Survival

It is important for aircrew members living aboard a vessel at sea to learn basic skills of seamanship and survival at sea. Therefore, each crewmember should participate in drills and classes that teach members of the crew to survive in difficult situations at sea such as fire, collision, and

heavy weather. Crewmembers should have a working familiarity with the ship's survival tools, firefighting equipment, damage control gear, and boats and rafts. Most basic of all is the skill that allows the aircrew to move about the ship without visible clues. Escape from berthing and work spaces without lights or other clues is a skill each member of the crew should develop.

Diet

Aircrew of ships at sea face special problems in obtaining their meals. Although aircrew on larger ships are frequently served by special kitchens (galleys) that cater to those involved in irregular flight hours, smaller ships may not provide such services. Thus, it might be easy for flight crews involved in heavy operations to fail to obtain regular meals. Again, advance planning and understanding with members of the ships' crew will reduce the frequency of improper or missed meals.

Fatigue and Intoxicants

Operational pressures in small unit operations may involve a fast pace of duties, leading to fatigue and numbing indifference. Each aircrew member and maintenance member must be constantly on guard against the effects of fatigue and boredom. In addition, if flight operations take place against a background in which alcohol is available and used, great care must be taken to ensure adequate "bottle to throttle" times for those in control of aircraft and similarly adequate time for maintenance personnel to be absolutely free of the aftereffects of any indulgence. The best physiologic state for the individual involved in any aspect of aviation, whether crewmember, maintenance personnel, communicator, or controller, is an intoxicant-free state. That is, no intoxicants of any kind can be used safely, and no hangovers or residue of their use can be tolerated. The use of illicit drugs and intoxicants of any kind is strictly contrain-

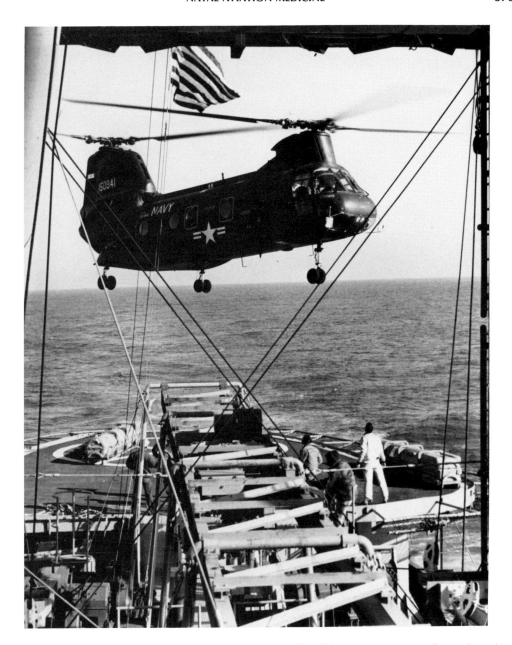

Fig. 22–6. Aircrew at sea: small platforms. Vertical replenishment of small ships requires precision flying in hazardous proximity to ships' structures. The aircrew must be in optimal mental and physical condition for such duty. (official United States Navy photo).

dicated. Prescription drugs should be administered and used only with thorough understanding of their effects and side effects in light of the work at hand. Operational pressures should never allow compromise of these principles.

Exercise

Exercise is important to flight crews. Prolonged sedentary activity and access to generous caloric supplements can cause declining physiologic conditioning.

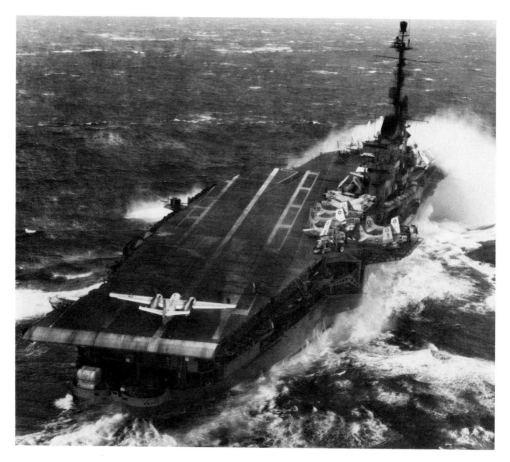

Fig. 22–7. The aircraft carrier in rough seas presents crewmembers with a demanding launch and recovery environment. Hazards of pitching decks and water over the bow make flight operations most difficult (official United States Navy photo).

Therefore, aircrew and maintenance personnel should be encouraged to maintain an active personal exercise program. In confining environments, it may not be possible to accomplish many of the exercises practiced ashore; however, compensating forms of exercise are available and offer their own advantages in physical fitness and cardiovascular conditioning. Many ships have small integral exercise facilities that allow workouts. Larger vessels may have enough deck space to allow jogging. A principle to always remember is that aboard ship there are no soft places to fall. Falls almost always result in some sort of injury. Therefore, during exercise and in normal movement about the ship,

individuals should take great care to move with deliberate sureness and care. Even in exercise, planning should allow the exercise to take place with a minimum risk of injury to the participant.

Boredom

The aircrew at sea must always deal with the ancient nemeses of the seaman, boredom, familiarity, and indifference to the hazards present. The flight environment under the most normal shorebound circumstances demands the total attention and care of the members of the aviation team. To add to that normally demanding situation the complications inherent in operations at sea makes the process vastly more complex. Maintaining flight proficiency during long periods of shipboard confinement is difficult; when skills are not razor sharp, flying from small decks pitching in bad weather requires the aircrew's greatest attention and skill (Fig. 22–7). Boredom and complacency must not be allowed to further decrease the aircrew's proficiency.

Aerospace medicine in the naval environment is among the most challenging tests of the practitioner's art and his science. It is also among the most rewarding for the successful flight surgeon. Many of the professional challenges of the future in space medicine are but extensions of those currently experienced by the Naval flight surgeon at sea.

Chapter *23*

Civil Aviation Medicine

Stanley R. Mohler

The commonplace of the schoolbooks of tomorrow is the adventure of today, and that is what we are engaged in.

JACOB BRONOWSKI

The air transport industry, including the airrame manufacturers, the airlines, general aviation, and a myriad of supporting activities of every variety, has become a major force in the nation's, as well as the world's, economy and industry. The original lead established by the United States with the introduction of the DC-2/DC-3 series aircraft in the 1930s has never been relinquished. Every year, the aviation industry contributes over $50 billion to the gross national product and provides employment for over 1 million individuals. Approximately 80% of the free world's civilian transports were manufactured in the United States.

Today in the United States, public air carriers have become a primary long-haul mover of people. It is estimated that 85% of long-haul public carrier transportation is by air and that 95% of international travel is by air. The scheduled airlines move nearly 300 million persons per year, the equivalent of moving the entire United States population from one place to another. Of equal significance has been the enormous growth of general aviation, the private, corporate and business fleet, which is now carrying 100 million people both domestically and internationally.

Significant aeromedical factors are involved in civil aviation. These factors will be discussed with a particular emphasis given to their application to general aviation. These factors represent a combination of specialized aeromedical knowledge, general medical information, and, as importantly, common sense.

The practitioner engaged in civil aviation medicine must be receptive to new concepts and data developed from research, aircraft accident investigations, and direct clinical experience. Professional and ethical concerns must bridge the chasm between obligations to the aviator and obligations to the public safety.

SCOPE OF CIVIL AVIATION MEDICINE

Aeromedical support to civil aviation is complex due to two primary factors. First, aeronautic systems range in complexity from balloons, gliders, and ultralights to large jumbo and sleek supersonic commercial jet transports (Figs. 23–1 and 23–2). Second is the diversity of education, training, experience, sophistication, and health status of the aviator flying these systems.

Airline Operations

Within the United States, 2500 airline aircraft belong to more than 30 airline carriers and fly over 2800 million miles annually. The long-term trend in the number of passengers carried continues to increase. It has been estimated that by 1990, 3050 airline aircraft will carry 420 million passengers within the United States each year.

Worldwide, nearly 8000 airline aircraft are in operation, providing air transport service to over 600 million passengers. These aircraft log over 700,000 million passenger-miles per year.

The captain (pilot-in-command) of these aircraft must have an airline transport pilot certificate and a Class 1 medical certificate. The first-officer (copilot) and flight engineer positions require a commercial pilot certificate and a Class 2 medical certificate. On March 15, 1960, the then Federal Aviation Agency imposed a controversial upper age limit of 60 years on pilot-in-command and copilot duties aboard airline transports. The limit was not applied to flight engineers because there was no stated justification for doing so.

Since the promulgation of this rule, it has been the subject of continuing scrutiny and controversy. The Federal Aviation Administration (FAA) defends the age 60 rule as necessary to protect the public from age-related performance decrements in pilots, contending that such deterioration cannot be measured dependably. On the other side, persons who oppose the rule (and many are physicians) say it is discriminatory, because it is based on age alone and does not consider the individual's ability to do his job; arbitrary, because there is no scientific basis for choosing age 60; and unnecessary, because it is now feasible to measure individual performance and estimate the risk of incapacitation.[1]

Air Taxi and Air Commuter Operations

In 1980, air taxi and air commuter operations carried 13.1 million people, usually utilizing aircraft at the smaller end of the passenger capacity scale (4 to 60 passengers). The continuing growth of this segment of aviation is forecast by the aviation authorities. Many of the aircraft used in this type of passenger transport are designed for short field operations and include rotary-wing helicopters (Fig. 23–3).

Aircrew members of these aircraft must have at least a commercial pilot certificate

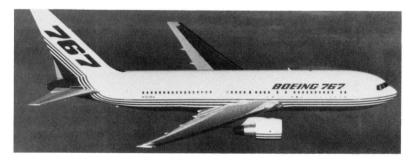

Fig. 23–1. The Boeing 767 airliner contains advanced technology design features. It is certified by the Federal Aviation Administration for a flight deck crew of two, a result of diminished crew work load through the extensive use of automation. The supercritical wing airfoils and the two-engine configuration provide fuel-efficient operations. The Boeing 767 can carry 211 passengers and has a maximum range of 5200 km (photo courtesy of the Boeing Company).

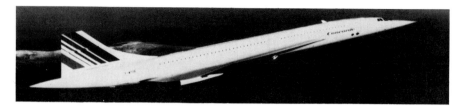

Fig. 23–2. The Mach 2 supersonic transport (SST) Anglo-French Concorde has halved the flight times from Europe to the Americas (it is also used on Europe to mid-East runs). It carries up to 140 passengers and can cruise at an altitude of 20,000 m. At a weight in the range of 171,000 kg, or 376,000 pounds (190,000 pounds of this weight is fuel), it can carry a payload of 11,400 kg. Due to the continuous sonic-boom "carpet" produced during supersonic flight, the Concorde confines speeds of Mach 1 and above to overocean segments when flying between Europe and the Americas (photo courtesy of the British Aerospace Corporation).

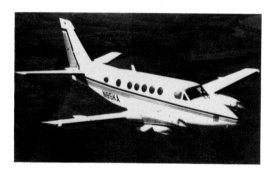

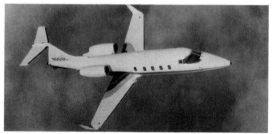

Fig. 23–4. The Lear Model 55 represents the latest design in corporate jet technology. The aircraft is capable of cruising at 16,000 m with a maximum range of 3600 km. It can carry ten passengers with a crew of two. The wing incorporates the winglets, developed by NASA, that markedly increase aerodynamic efficiency (photo courtesy of the Gates Learjet Company).

Fig. 23–3. The Beechcraft King Air B-100 is a turbo-prop corporate, freight, air taxi, or commuter aircraft that has a passenger capacity of eight plus a crew of two. It is fully equipped with anti-ice equipment and can operate in virtually any kind of weather (photo courtesy of the Beech Aircraft Company).

and a Class 2 medical certificate. No upper age limit applies to these aircrew members.

Corporate and Business Flying

Businesses of all sizes are finding the use of small and, at times, large aircraft a useful adjunct in meeting their executive travel needs. The aircraft operated may range from single-engine or twin-engine propeller aircraft through turboprop and small turbojet aircraft (Fig. 23–4).

Corporate pilots may be corporate officers or, more often, career pilots. No upper age limit applies to these crewmembers. When flying for hire, the crewmembers require a Class 2 medical certificate and a commercial pilot certificate. Occasionally, a corporation may operate certain of its

aircraft as a revenue-generating activity in charter operations.

Aerial Application

Agricultural spray operations include the application of insecticides, weed control chemicals, defoliants, fertilizers, fire control substances, sterile male screwworm fly larvae, and other materials. Many of the chemicals used are very toxic and most can cause illness and death. Crashes have occurred as a result of impairment caused by exposure to these substances.

Aerial application flying, also referred to as "crop dusting," or "top dressing" in New Zealand and Australia, is governed by FAA regulations. Operators must demonstrate a knowledge of the chemicals they use, including their purposes and toxic aspects. Many of the aircraft used in these operations are specifically designed for the purpose (Fig. 23–5). The aircraft are more maneuverable, have significantly more powerful engines, and have a crash-resistant cockpit area. Other special design features may include wire cutters on the landing gear struts to sever any power or telephone lines that are inadvertently struck. The pilots must have a commercial pilot certificate and a Class 2 medical certificate when flying for hire. No upper age limit applies.

A few of the major categories of toxic substances used in aerial application are discussed in the following sections to provide a better understanding of their toxic potential.

Organophosphate Insecticides

Insecticidal and mammalian toxic effects in the organophosphate insecticides are derived from the inhibition of acetylcholinesterase enzymes in the nerve cells, as is the case with parathion. Symptoms may include nausea, vomiting, sweating, salivation, visual disturbances, bradycardia, and respiratory cessation. Death may follow. Pilocarpine-like pupillary constriction is ordinarily present, but dilated pupils also may be found.

Washing the contaminated areas with

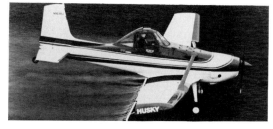

Fig. 23–5. Modern agricultural aircraft constitute the most efficient spray planes to date. The Cessna Husky can carry 920 L of liquid for dispersal. Rates of dispersal range from less than 1 L/acre to more than 20 L/acre. The cabin has air conditioning, and the aircraft can be equipped with external lights for night spray operations. "Automatic flagmen," little flags dropped at the end of each swath, can be used to improve the precision and efficiency of spraying (photo courtesy of the Cessna Aircraft Company).

soap and water is the first treatment, followed by atropine for symptomatic relief, if necessary, and pralidoxime (2-PAM) for cholinesterase enzyme reactivation.

Plasma cholinesterase enzyme measurements are useful as indicators of exposure during the spraying season. Heparin is the desired anticoagulant for the freshly drawn blood samples because other anticoagulants may inactivate the enzyme.

Carbamate Insecticides

The symptoms, signs, and course of poisoning by carbamate insecticides are similar to, but do not last as long as, those of the organophosphates. A representative carbamate is tetraethyl pyrophosphate (TEPP). Carbamates also produce motor paralysis. Atropine is used for symptomatic treatment. Pralidoxime is ineffective.

Red blood cell cholinesterase enzyme measurements may be used to assess the degree of exposure. Again, heparin is the desired anticoagulant for the blood samples.

Chlorinated Insecticides

Because of increasing restrictions on their use, chlorinated insecticides (e.g., DDT, Dieldrin, Aldrin, Endrin) are now rarely used by aerial sprayers in the United States. The toxic symptoms derive from central nervous system effects, including convulsions. Intermediate-duration barbiturates (amobarbital [Amytal], pentobarbital) are used in treatment. The intermediate barbiturates help assure that the stimulant effect of the pesticide is not exceeded by the depressant effect of the barbiturate.

Chlorinated Herbicides

Broad leaf plants are especially susceptible to the chlorinated herbicides. These chemicals cause growth stimulation, including the production of bizarre plant configuration and plant death. Toxicity is low in humans. During the Vietnam War, herbicides were often disseminated by aircraft, and these chemicals have served as a focal point for a wide range of medical complaints alleged by veterans of that war.

To investigate the alleged health effects of these compounds, often referred to as Agent Orange, and the highly toxic compound, dioxin, that contaminated the herbicides, the United States Air Force is conducting an extensive epidemiologic study of the aircrew associated with its aerial application. Although combat troops on the ground may have come in contact with the herbicide, by far the highest level of exposure was experienced by the aircrew flying the spray missions.

Nitrophenols

Nitrophenols produce ovicidal, acaricidal, and insecticidal effects. This group of chemicals also has herbicidal effects. In some cases, these substances are used as defoliants. Signs of poisoning include excessive sweating, thirst, euphoria, and subsequent fatigue. Immediate treatment for contamination is to wash off the chemicals with soap and water. No antidote exists.

Paraquat

Paraquat is a potent irritant to the skin, although it is not readily absorbed. Oral intake of small amounts causes severe damage to the mouth, throat, and esophagus, followed by pulmonary edema, pulmonary hemorrhage, and renal toxicity effects. There is no antidote.

Chemical Log Book

An advance relating to aerial application flight safety has been developed in the Soviet Union: the chemical log book.[2] Each agricultural pilot in the Soviet Union maintains a chemical log book, an entity separate from the flight log book. The chemical log records the specific chemicals used during aerial application flights plus the times of exposures. This log is especially valuable to the attending physician should symptoms or signs of illness develop.

Recreational Flying

In the United States, there are an estimated 190,000 recreational aircraft and 700,000 active general aviation pilots. These pilots may own their own aircraft, belong to flying clubs, or rent aircraft. The pilots need have only a Class 3 medical certificate, which, in the case of student pilots, may be a combined student/pilot medical certificate. The certificate is valid for 2 years, the lower age limit is 16 years and there is no upper age limit on these pilots. The subjects of hypoxia, pressure changes, and disorientation are included in the instruction given to all general aviation pilots. The written examination for the pilot certificate includes questions on these subjects. Because of the importance of the material, aeromedical practitioners need to take the opportunity to review with their pilot populations these physiologic concerns. Periodically, situations will arise where pilots will be misinformed regarding their own limitations or those of the equipment they use. For example, a recent publication circulated among hang-glider enthusiasts advocated flights to 6096 m without oxygen. Such misinformation could lead to fatal mistakes. The physician must assist in providing sound and rational advice to the flyer.

The spectrum of recreational flying continues to expand. The small, fixed-wing, single-engine aircraft is by far the most common aircraft used in flying for fun, with over 200,000 registered (Figs. 23–6 and 23-7). Gliding is a popular sport. These delicate, long-wing, powerless aircraft have achieved altitudes requiring supplemental oxygen and may remain airborne for many hours in long-duration flight. Each year, the skies near Albuquerque, New Mexico become filled with multicolored "gum balls" as hundreds of hot air balloons participate in mass ascension.

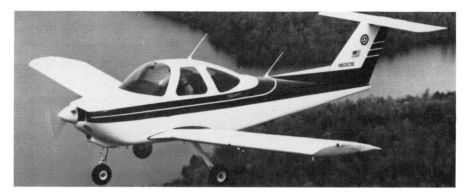

Fig. 23–6. The Beechcraft Model 77 Skipper, a two-seat training plane, reflects a typical light plane design of the late 1970s. It has a 115 hp Lycoming engine and cruises at 105 knots. An inertia-reel shoulder harness is provided for each seat (photo courtesy of the Beech Aircraft Company).

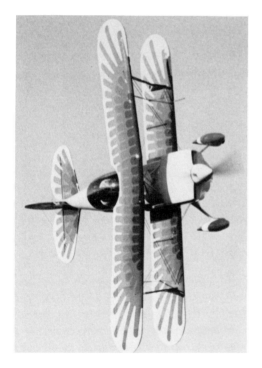

Fig. 23–7. The Cristen Eagle II is a top two-seat aerobatic aircraft. Introduced in the 1970s, it is capable of maneuvers in excess of +9 Gs and −6 Gs. It can perform any conceivable aerobatic maneuver, including multiple inverted snap rolls, multiple turning tail slides, prolonged inverted spins, knife-edge flight, and Lomcovaks (photo courtesy of Christen Industries).

Hang-glider flying and parachuting are both recreational activities with growing numbers of participants. The ultralights do not presently require a FAA certificate, nor must the pilot be certified. These very small aircraft must weigh less than 70.3 kg and carry 6.8 kg or less of fuel (Fig. 23-8).

Pilot Medical Certification Exceptions

At the minimum, civil pilots require the medical and pilot certificates necessary for the type of flight operations conducted. In the case of United States glider and balloon operations, self-proclamation of health status is all that is necessary. Public safety is the concept underlying medical certification. In 1979, over 800,000 civil airmen held certificates (Table 23–1). Approximately one third of these aviators held instrument flying qualifications (Table 23–2).

Persons who do not meet one or another of the medical standards subsequently may become certified through the waiver route (the FAA concludes that there are compensatory factors in the pilot requesting reconsideration that safely allow medical certification), the exception route (the FAA decides that in a specific case, the condition, although disqualifying by regulatory provisions, is no longer a safety hazard), or the judicial route (the National

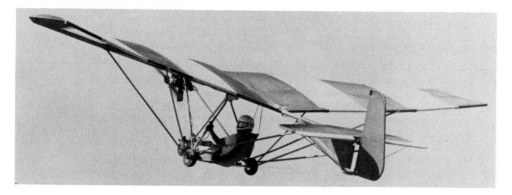

Fig. 23–8. The Weed Hopper C is an ultralight aircraft available in kit form. It can be assembled in 1 day and requires no Federal Aviation Administration aircraft or pilot certificate. Ultralight flying is today's fast-growing homologue of the pre–World War I era, with its Wrights, Curtiss, Stinsons, and Bleriot pioneer aviators. The Weed Hopper cruises at 48 kph. Takeoff and landings are at 40 kph (photo courtesy of Weed Hopper of Utah).

Table 23–1. Certificates Held in 1979

Type of Certificate	Number
Pilot	*814,667*
Student	210,180
Private	343,276
Commercial	182,097
Airline transport	63,652
Glider (only)	6796
Helicopter (only)	5218
Nonpilot	*377,213*
Engineers	36,679
Navigators	1994
Control tower controller	25,232
Aircraft mechanics	237,611

Table 23–2. Civil Airmen Medical Certifications*

Medical Certification	Number of Airmen Certified
Class 1	50,982
Class 2	194,448
Class 3	535,985
Total	781,415

*Total airmen certified as of December 31, 1980.

Transportation Safety Board or the courts overturn a prior medical certificate denial based on appeal information supplied by the plaintiff, frequently consisting of expert medical testimony by front-line physicians emphasizing modern medical advances in diagnosis and treatment).

In issuing a waiver, the FAA may base the decision on a "Statement of Demonstrated Ability." This statement is obtained by the requesting pilot, who may have paraplegia, monocular vision, color vision deficiency, hearing losses, or other impairment, following a satisfactory demonstration of performance to an inspector of the FAA. The inspectors have protocols for dozens of conditions that arise in this connection from time to time. Pilots with the following conditions have been individually certified on appeal: replacement heart valve, coronary bypass surgery, cerebral fluid shunt, chronic or paroxysmal atrial fibrillation, and a cardiac pacemaker.

Aircraft Certification

The design, performance, and operational safety characteristics of an aircraft are determined by the FAA from data supplied by the manufacturer or obtained by flight tests. Table 23–3 provides data illustrating the progressive increase in civil aircraft.

The categories of airworthiness include fixed-wing airline aircraft (5670 kg and over) and general aviation aircraft. Rotary-wing aircraft and lighter-than air categories also are specified.

A complex body of regulations has evolved regarding civil aircraft certification and operations progressively augmented each time new aircraft are developed. An infinite series of cabin altitude versus time profiles are physically possi-

Table 23–3. Civil Aircraft Registered in the United States, 1976 to 1980

Type of Aircraft	1976	1977	1978	1979	1980
Fixed-wing	195,537	203,947	223,924	237,280	244,025
Turbine-powered	7263	7738	8681	9586	10,603
Turbojet	4395	4623	5055	5479	5869
Turboprop	2868	3115	3626	4107	4734
Piston-powered	188,274	196,209	215,243	227,694	233,422
Multi-engine	22,906	23,545	26,293	28,118	29,126
Single-engine	165,368	172,644	188,950	199,576	204,296
Rotary-wing (includes autogyros)	6391	6855	7688	8380	9012
Turbine	1888	2196	2659	3032	3509
Piston	4503	4659	5029	5348	5503
Gliders	2972	3284	3610	3808	3909
Blimps	6	6	6	10	11
Balloons	975	1189	1561	2038	2453
Total	205,881	215,281	236,789	251,516	259,410

ble between 2438 m, the upper allowable routine cabin altitude in United States civil airline operations, and the maximum cruising altitudes of civil aircraft. Selected key altitudes, for civil aviation certification and operational purposes are as follows (given in feet as used in regulatory documents):[3]

8000 feet (2400 m)—cabin altitude provides a blood oxygen saturation of approximately 93% in the resting individual who does not suffer from advanced cardiovascular or pulmonary disease. After suffering a hypoxic experience, this is the ceiling altitude to which an individual should be returned for physiologic compensatory mechanisms to effectively reoxygenate the body. Operationally, this altitude has been prescribed as the altitude above which passenger oxygen must be available in specified amounts.

10,000 feet (3000 m)—cabin altitude provides a blood oxygen saturation of approximately 89%. After a period of time at this level, the more complex cerebral functions, such as making mathematical computations, begin to suffer, and night vision is markedly impaired. Crewmembers must use oxygen when the cabin pressure altitudes exceed 3048 m (10,000 ft).

12,000 feet (3600 m)—the blood oxygen saturation falls to approximately 87%. In addition to some mathematical computation difficulties, short-term memory begins to be impaired, and errors of omission increase with extended exposure. Oxygen must be used by each crewmember on flight duty and must be provided for each crewmember during the flight when the cabin altitude is above 3600 m in consideration of these physiologic findings.

12,500 feet (3750 m)—the use of oxygen is required by the flight crew of unpressurized aircraft beginning at altitudes above 3750 m (the crew can fly for about 30 minutes without oxygen between 3750 and 4200 m, a compromise zone to let, for example, a mountain be "crested"). The blood oxygen saturation is 87%.

14,000 feet (4200 m)—the blood oxygen saturation is approximately 83%, and all persons are impaired to a greater or lesser extent with respect to mental functions, including intellectual and emotional alterations. Thus, at a 4200 m cabin altitude, oxygen will be provided for at least 10% of the passengers in recognition of the marginal physiologic aspects of this altitude and the decompensations experienced by a variable proportion of the general population.

15,000 feet (4500 m)—this altitude gives a blood oxygen saturation of approximately 80%, and all persons are impaired, some seriously. The FAA regulations provide that oxygen be available for 30% of the passengers between a 4200- and 4500-m cabin altitude. Above a 4650-m cabin altitude, oxygen must be available for all passengers because all persons are seriously impaired beyond this cabin altitude.

20,000 feet (6000 m)—the blood oxygen saturation is 65%, and all unacclimatized persons become torpid, increasingly stuporous, and lose useful consciousness in about 10 minutes. The time of useful consciousness (TUC) is determined generally from the time breathing oxygen is lost from the respiratory tract with reference to an initial safe level to the time when purposeful activity, such as the ability to don an oxygen mask, is lost. Although for most persons the TUC at 6000 m is about 10 minutes, some individuals may stretch this to 20 minutes and a few to 30 minutes.

25,000 feet (7500 m)—this altitude and all those above it produce a blood oxygen saturation below 60%. A TUC of about 2.5 minutes exists at this altitude. Above 7500 m, the rate of occurrence of bends (nitrogen bubble evolution and embolism) increases as a threat following decompression. If an airline pilot leaves a duty station above 7500 m, the other pilot must have an oxygen mask in place to protect against problems should a decompression occur.

37,000 feet (11,100 m)—the TUC is approximately 18 seconds. Provision of 100% oxygen will produce approximately 80% blood oxygen saturation. As this altitude is exceeded, the oxygen begins to leave the blood unless positive-pressure oxygen is supplied. A draft standard covering this altitude was prepared at the time when the United States was developing its own supersonic transport (SST). With the demise of the United States SST program, the standard was not put into the regulations, but it has been used as a guide in approving the British-French SST Concorde for operations in the United States.

45,000 feet (13,000 m)—the TUC is approximately 15 seconds, and positive-pressure oxygen is of decreasing practicality because of the increasing inability to exhale against the oxygen pressure.

Certain executive jet aircraft have been certified to a 51,000-ft (15,300-m) altitude (Gates Learjet). Specific service histories and rational analyses showing a high degree of pressure vessel integrity (that portion of the aircraft hull designed to hold atmospheric pressure higher than the outside), a low probability of catastrophic or major pressurization failures, and certain in-place emergency procedures in the event of a decompression or pressurization problem form the basis for this certification. The civil airline aircraft having the highest certified cruise altitude is the British-French SST Concorde (60,000-ft, or 18,000-m, range).

MEDICAL FACTORS IN GENERAL AVIATION ACCIDENTS

The three major factors in fatal general aviation accidents are (1) mixing alcohol with flying (15%); (2) conducting unwarranted, low-level, maneuvers that satisfy some emotional need that overrides logic (30%); and (3) penetrating known adverse weather beyond the pilot or aircraft capabilities (40%); many such accidents are due to an emotional drive to reach the destination. The remaining 15% of the fatal accidents include carbon monoxide poisoning from heater leaks (about 12 cases per year), drug impairment of the pilot (several dozen cases per year), in-flight heart attacks (about four to six per year), and a miscellaneous group, including in-flight incapacitation due to renal colic. General aviation accident rates are presented in Figure 23–9.

Pilot suicides through flying into a bar, church, school, or other structure or geographic area occur several times per year. Strictly speaking, these are not accidents and are not used in accident rate computations by the National Transportation Safety Board.

Two or three hypoxia accidents occur each year, including decompression and loss of consciousness by those on board. Two such hypoxia cases follow.

On January 11, 1980, a Cessna 441 departed Shreveport, Louisiana, in the evening for Baton Rouge, the pilot and one passenger on board. The pilot notified air traffic control at about 2130 hours that bad weather had been encountered. He requested an eastern routing, and the flight was cleared to 7010 m. The controllers, however, subsequently noticed that the aircraft continued climbing beyond the assigned altitude. As the flight proceeded to the east, it continued to climb. It was tracked along its northeast route, and two Air Force planes were scrambled from Seymour-Johnson Air Force Base in Goldsboro, North Carolina. These aircraft picked up the Cessna shortly after midnight, 15 miles west of Raleigh, North Carolina at 12,000 m flying at a speed of 410 kph. Fuel exhaustion occurred over the Atlantic at 12,300 m. The Cessna began a spiraling turn and struck the water.

Investigators concluded the Cessna was on autopilot and that its occupants had become incapacitated from hypoxia, with hypoxic death occurring several minutes thereafter. The incapacitation was thought to have occurred when the aircraft was climbing near 7010 m.

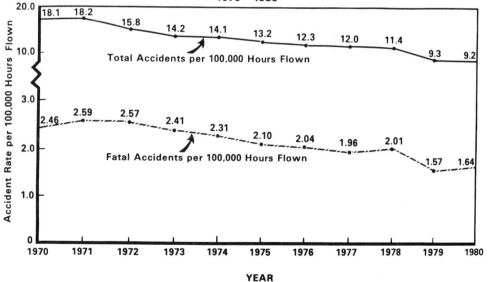

ACCIDENT RATES PER 100,000 HOURS FLOWN
U.S. GENERAL AVIATION
1970–1980

Fig. 23–9. General aviation accident rates have consistently improved over the years. This illustration covers the period between 1970 and 1980. More effort is necessary to ensure that the aeromedical factors related to fatal and nonfatal accidents can be more adequately addressed within the pilot population.

Four months earlier, on September 25, 1979, a Beech King Air 200 departed Stansted Airfield, England at 1341 hours in order that the left seat pilot could receive a checkout. After a few practice landing approaches, the aircraft received clearance to climb to 9144 m. Nothing further was heard from the aircraft, which flew across the English Channel toward France at an altitude of 9144 m.

A British Nimrod intercepted the King Air and followed it along. No radio contact could be established. In addition, a French Air Force Mirage flew close to the King Air and observed the flashing warning lights in the cockpit indicating that the cabin altitude was above 3810 m. Fuel exhaustion brought the aircraft down to a crash near Nantes, France at 2035 hours.

Investigators found that both pilots had been wearing oxygen masks and concluded that a practice decompression had gone wrong in that oxygen had not flowed into the masks. The time of useful consciousness at 9144 m is about 30 seconds, and the crew apparently did not recognize the early symptoms of hypoxia and thus did not initiate an emergency descent.

It was concluded that both pilots had lost consciousness during a practice decompression followed by subsequent death in situ.

Evidence was found that an incorrect connection of mask assembly pipes and flight deck bulkhead supply points had possibly existed. The oxygen supply pipe bayonet may have been incorrectly inserted in its socket, resulting in failure of depression of a valve necessary for oxygen flow. The bayonet may appear to be inserted properly but not actually be so. Further complicating the above situation are two oxygen control handles that may be confused in an emergency in that one handle has a manual override for the passenger system that can be selected accidentally when the pilot wants the other handle. If this happens, oxygen would not be delivered as desired. These are factors for preflight consideration and have aeromedical importance.

SPECIFIC CIVIL AVIATION MEDICINE TOPICS

Alcohol

The euphoria produced by the consumption of alcohol is an extreme hazard to persons who fly while under its influence. Judgment is modified in the intoxicated state, and the pilot may attempt maneuvers that he would not undertake while sober.

In addition to its euphoric effect, alcohol tends to promote a narrowed span of attention, producing visual and concentration fixation effects. The time of concentration may be shortened, leading to a flight of ideas and a false sense of well-being. With increasing levels of intoxication, coordination becomes impaired and drowsiness occurs. All of these changes are incompatible with safe pilot performance.

Actual in-flight studies with pilots having varying blood levels of alcohol have shown that levels as low as 0.04% (40 mg/dl), three standard alcoholic beverages for the average person, markedly impaired pilot performance on instrument landing system (ILS) approaches.[4] Laboratory studies have revealed performance degradations at levels below the 0.04% level.

Federal Aviation Regulation 91.11 provides that no person may act as a crewmember of a civil aircraft (1) within 8 hours after the consumption of any alcoholic beverage; (2) while under the influence of alcohol; or (3) while using any drug that affects his faculties in any way that could be unsafe. A consideration regarding this regulation is that the crewmembers must be alert to the detrimental effects of hangovers, effects that can last 24 to 48 hours after consuming alcohol, especially consumption in amounts exceeding one or two standard drinks.

Drugs

The two main considerations in regard to the adverse effects of a drug on an aircrew member are whether the drug impairs judgment and whether it impairs alertness. Some drugs may exert these effects directly or may bring about these effects through emotional, sleep-disturbing, or physiologic actions. In addition, drugs that degrade vision, impair coordination, or interfere with elimination functions are incompatible with safe flight, as are drugs that lower the crewmembers's tolerance to in-flight G forces.

For purposes of civil aviation, drugs may be catergorized as follows:

1. Flight duties are normally permitted when taking the drug (e.g., aspirin, candicidin, ascorbic acid, ethynodiol, and phenacetin).

2. Flight duties are permitted if the flight surgeon (aviation medical examiner) or the Federal Aviation Administration gives permission (e.g., ampicillin, chloroquine, metronidazole, oxytetracycline, and pyrimethamine).

3. Flight duties may be approved by the Federal Aviation Administration (e.g., allopurinol, benzthiazide, chlorthalidone, propranolol, and thyroid preparations).

4. Flight duties are not permitted until the drug is discontinued and cleared from the body (clearance time of three times the drug's half-life) (e.g., amobarbital, buclizine, codeine, glutethimide, prednisolone, and tripelennamine).

5. The condition for which the drug is taken precludes flight duties (e.g., bishydroxycoumarin, bretylium tosylate, digitoxin, diphenylhydantoin, insulin, nitroglycerine, and tolbutamide).

6. The adverse effect of the drug precludes flight duties (clearance time of five times the drug's half-life) (e.g., amphetamine, carbamazepine, chlorpromazine, diazepam, doxepin, hydralazine, meperidine, and reserpine).

7. The drug is either illicit or is disapproved by the Food and Drug Administration (e.g., cocaine, heroin, LSD, and marijuana). Disapproved drugs include azaribine, and triparanol.

A great deal could be said concerning the placement of specific drugs in the above scheme. Judgment by competent aeromedical and pharmacologic authorities must be applied, allowing maximum benefit to the pilot with no adverse effect on safety. Research results and accident data are valuable aids in arriving at decisions concerning specific drugs. Of special concern are the potential side effects of the drug.

Aerobatics

Civil sport aerobatic activities can result in pilot G_z axis accelerations in excess of $+7G$ and -5 G. During aerobatic training, pilots are taught methods of countering the adverse effects of G forces.

Some fatalities occur each year that are apparently related to the loss of consciousness during positive G_z maneuvers. On occasion, these accidents are attributed to pilots who undertook aerobatics while ill or anemic. Fatalities have been attributed to the loss-of-consciousness effect of sequentially conducting a powerful negative G_z maneuver $(-3 G_z)$ followed by a powerful positive G_z maneuver.[5] This latter sequence results in a transient desensitization of the carotid and aortic sinus blood pressure reflexes during the negative G_z maneuver, with a delay in activation of the reflexes during the immediate positive G_z maneuver. Unconsciousness at the 7 to 9 o'clock position is very apt to occur. The solution to avoiding the unconsciousness is to perform the positive G_z maneuver first and then immediately undertake the negative G_z maneuver (Fig. 23–10).

The Vertical "8"

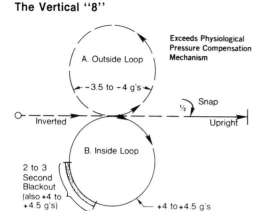

Fig. 23–10. This diagram is cast in the Aresti system for portraying aerobatic maneuvers. To perform the vertical 8, an aircraft enters inverted horizontal flight (left dashed line). An "outside" loop is performed (the head is to the outside with the blood consequently centrifuged cephalad) followed by a lower "inside" loop (the head is to the inside with the blood centrifuged toward the feet). The loop is completed in the inverted portion, and recovering to upright is achieved by a half-snap roll. Desensitization of the carotid pressure sensors during the top loop results in a sluggish response during the 7 to 9 o'clock position in the bottom loop, resulting in hypotension and the high likelihood of loss-of-consciousness for several seconds. Conducting the top loop as a (+)G loop followed by a (−)G loop does not result in a blackout.

Civil aerobatic pilots who regularly perform at air shows or in periodic competitions develop amazing tolerances to imposed G forces, illustrating significant increases of physiologic adaptation. This tolerance is rapidly lost after a few months of nonaerobatic flying. Unlike military aircraft, most civilian aerobatic aircraft are not equipped to handle G-suit inflations; hence, no anti-G gear is worn.

Fatigue

The circadian oscillator is located in the suprachiasmic area of the brain, and by its cyclic alteration in alertness, it can produce degradation in performance levels if work is attempted during the low phase of the cycle.[6] Accumulated sleep deficits can move the work cycle toward the low phase and play a powerful role in decreasing pilot alertness during flight. Pilot education on the above phenomena is a corner-

stone of air safety. Fatigue is significant to single-pilot operations involving less experienced pilots, as well as multicrew airline operations.

The key scheduling factors contributing to the development of aircrew fatigue are multiple night flights, multiple time-zone displacements, flights departing 24 hours after an evening arrival, and multiple takeoffs and landings. Additional aggravating factors include departure delays of several hours that require pilots to lounge about airports, in-flight malfunctions, emergencies, adverse weather, or other factors that markedly increase work load. In aerial application flying, the required low-level maneuvers, long hours, and chemical exposures promote the onset of fatigue.

The worst aircraft accident in aviation history occurred between two Boeing 747 aircraft on March 27, 1977 at Los Rodeos Airport, Santa Cruz de Tenerife, Tenerife, Canary islands (583 fatalities).[7] The Spanish investigators, assisted by United States and Dutch specialists, found that relatively recent changes in Dutch flight-time regulations removing the captain's flexibility regarding discretionary duty time extensions contributed to the cause of the accident. A number of significant safety lessons can be derived from this accident for flight surgeons and those who are working in the area of air safety.

The specific incident leading to the above catastrophe was a terrorist bomb explosion in the terminal of the Las Palmas Airport, the original destination of the two aircraft. Because of the explosion, incoming aircraft were diverted to Los Rodeos Airport, about 60 statute miles away.

KLM 747 PH-SUF arrived at Los Rodeos Airport at 1338 hours and was parked at the end of the taxiway. Other aircraft arrived, including a Pan Am 747 (N1736) at 1415 hours. This airplane was parked near the KLM 747. Because of the small ramp size and the number of aircraft that landed, the Pan Am aircraft was blocked from taxiing to the runway by those behind it and by the KLM aircraft. The passengers were kept on board both aircraft.

Cockpit voice recorder data from the two aircraft reveal that the captain of the KLM aircraft was very concerned that the diversion and delay would bring about a violation of the Dutch flight-time limitations in effect. These regulations were very rigid, did not allow judgmental extensions by the captain, and carried severe penalties for those who exceeded them (including loss of license). The phrases, "Yes, that would mean imprisonment" and "Yes, then you are hanged from the highest tree" occur during the KLM cockpit discussions. The captain elected to refuel (55,000 L) on Tenerife so that after flying to Las Palmas, the departure for the return flight to Amsterdam could be made with a minimum delay (no refueling). A crewmember states, "I can do without Las Palmas." The discussions also note concern about the airport weather: "Hurry, or else it will close again complete."

The Pan Am crew became upset with the refueling decision by the KLM crew because it delayed the former's departure by an hour, the result of the slow refueling process. This is revealed in the cockpit voice recorder data. Discussions of "ready for the sack" also took place. Las Palmas was the crew change point for this flight.

At 1650 hours, the KLM crew received engine start-up clearance. Shortly thereafter, the Pan Am crew received clearance. As the aircraft taxied, light rain and fog developed over the runway, with runway visibilities dropping to 300 m. The temperature and dew point held at 14° and 13°C, respectively.

The aircraft taxied down runway 12 in trail, the KLM crew aware that the Pan Am aircraft was behind them. The tower controller could not see the two aircraft due to the fog. He cleared the KLM aircraft to the end of the runway for a 180° turn in order that the KLM departure on runway 30 could be expedited. The runway is 3400 m long and 45 m wide. The Pan Am air-

craft was directed to turn left from the runway on taxiway C-3, "the third taxiway." The turnoff was tricky for large aircraft because it was a 90° turn. An ambiguity problem occurred, however, in that the "third taxiway" from the aircraft was actually taxiway C-4, keeping the Pan Am aircraft on the runway for a longer time.

At 1705 hours, the KLM crew were given the departure clearance to Las Palmas, which was read back by the crew. The crew reported at 1706 hours that they were in a takeoff position. The Pan Am crew immediately informed the tower, "We're still taxiing down the runway." The tower requested, "Report the runway clear."

At 1706 hours, one Pan Am crewmember said to another, "He's anxious, isn't he" (referring to the KLM captain). The reply was, "Yeah, after he held us up for an hour and a half, that ***." (*** stands for profanity.) "Now he's in a rush," the other crewmember said. The captain then said, "There he is—look at him—***—that, that *** is coming!" A crewmember said, "Get off! Get off!" The impact then occurred, tearing off the top of the Pan Am 747. The aircraft then began burning as the emergency escape procedures were activated.

The KLM crew could not see the Pan Am aircraft due to the fog. A brief discussion had occurred concerning whether the Pan Am 747 was clear of the runway, and the KLM captain concluded that it must be. The fog was worsening, the runway center-line lights were not working, and the flight-time limits reviewed by high-frequency radio with KLM headquarters were running out if the departure did not occur soon (the crew would not be able to fly the Las Palmas to Amsterdam return flight, disrupting the schedules and passenger and crew plans).

Still within the 1706 time frame, the KLM initiated takeoff (cockpit voices in Dutch, translated to English as follows):

> 1706:32—KLM crewmember: "Isn't he off then?"

1706:34—KLM captain: "What do you say?"

1706:34—KLM crewmember: "He is not off, that Pan American?"

1706:35—KLM captain: "yes, well!"

1706:43—KLM copilot: "V One." (This is the go-no go decision speed.)
1706:47—KLM captain: "Oh god-damn!"
1706:49—sound of impact

The KLM aircraft lifted off the ground and struck the top of the Pan Am aircraft, burst into flame and fell back to earth, and everyone on board was killed (14 crew and 234 passengers). Of the 396 persons on board the burning Pan Am aircraft, 9 crew-members and 326 passengers died. The total dead were 583.

The investigators concluded that the KLM captain took off without clearance and did not interrupt takeoff on learning that the Pan Am aircraft was still on the runway. When asked by his flight engineer if the Pan Am aircraft had left the runway, the captain had replied emphatically, "Yes."

The investigators concluded that the following were major reasons for the accident:

1. A growing feeling of tension as the KLM captain's problems mounted (strict flight-time limitations)
2. Deteriorating weather conditions
3. Two transmissions occurring simultaneously, blocking for the KLM captain the Pan Am transmission, "We are still taxiing down the runway"
4. Certain language problems, in which the KLM copilot stated, "We are now at takeoff." This was misunderstood by the tower controller, who had not granted takeoff clearance
5. The communication confusion between the tower and the Pan Am crew about "the third intersection" being the C-3 or C-4 intersection (a minor point because the Pan Am crew twice advised that the aircraft was still on the runway)
6. The unusual traffic congestion leading to short cuts allowing taxiing down runways

Flight surgeons who work with crew-members, airline companies, and controllers can actively participate in preventive activities in regard to the above factors. These include a continued assessment of flight-time limitations and how changes can affect future operations. Conducting educational programs for crewmembers concerning emotional factors and the effects of fatigue is important. The comprehensibility of communications, including the tendencies under stress to "hear" or perceive what one wants to hear, should be emphasized. The slogans, "when in doubt, reassess" and "if you are in a hurry, you are in danger," apply to the above mentioned disaster, aviation's worst accident.

The present United States flight-time regulations do not incorporate any circadian component, although physiologic indices exist that can be applied in scoring specific flight schedules for their fatigue potential.[8,9] Application of the indices has been slow to evolve, but one can forecast their increasing use as the general knowledge regarding fatigue and circadian rhythms increases.

Flight Attendants

The medical aspects of flight attendant work have emerged relatively recently as a significant added dimension in aerospace medicine. Beginning May 15, 1930, when United Airlines' predecessor, Boeing Air Transport, hired the first eight stewardesses, and into the 1960s, United States flight attendants were predominantly young, petite, white females. If the flight attendant became overweight, married, or pregnant, she almost always was terminated by the airlines. Sprogis versus

United Airlines (1970) and other cases settled the marriage issue. The Civil Rights Act of 1964 and the Age Discrimination in Employment Act of 1967, plus many legal suits brought by flight attendants, have led to the elimination of virtually all of the old restrictions arbitrarily imposed by marketing-oriented airline managers. Today, approximately 50,000 people of diverse sex, race, and age groups (the potential upper-age limit is 70 years) work for the airlines as flight attendants.

Flight attendants are the front line of passenger safety when aircraft disasters occur, serving a critical role in the accomplishment of emergency evacuations. Accidents may happen on land or water, near airports or in remote locations. Flight attendants are also the primary in-flight providers of emergency aid to passengers should illness, injury, or aircraft decompressions occur.

Among the environmental factors that are significant to flight attendant health and well-being are the need for fresh air flow, absence of gaseous or particulate contaminants (including cigarette smoke and other pollutants), absence of ozone (or quantities below 0.1 ppm by volume), temperature and humidity control, circadian rhythm scheduling, and adequate nutrition, layover facilities, and rest periods. The work environment requires energy expenditures in the range of 3 to 5 mets. Flight attendants with normal, uncomplicated pregnancies can fly on many airlines into the third trimester. They also can fly with well-controlled diabetes and with a prior history of epilepsy if the condition is controlled by medication. Turbulence injuries and accident impact and fire injuries are potential occupational hazards.

The aeromedical practitioner has the opportunity to assist in the assurance that flight attendants are provided adequate support medically, operationally, and environmentally to accomplish a quality job.

Age

Age, race, and sex traditionally have been limiting factors on the range of work activities available to a given individual. Modern concepts and medical progress in understanding, diagnosis, and treatment (prodded by legal actions) have progressively whittled these limitations to a few rearguard areas.

It is now known that the normal aging process is a developmental continuum, proceeding along a species-specific time line. Graying hair and lost hair are genetically determined changes of no consequence to flying abilities. In similar fashion, wrinkling of the skin and changes due to years of exposure to the elements are inconsequential.

The progressively extending visual near point occurring in most persons in the 40s can be fully refracted and is, therefore, of no significance to aviation activities. Acquired chronic diseases, especially those related to cardiovascular risk factors, may be significant. These diseases occur in individuals who have lived long enough for the chronicity aspect to develop, but the diseases are not a part of the normal aging process, as demonstrated by the many persons who maintain low risk factors, and reach an advanced age of 80 years or more without these diseases appearing. Medical screening and performance tests are available for individual health assessment irrespective of age, race, or sex.

The significant factors in regard to safe pilot performance are (1) ability to perform; (2) freedom from impairing disease; and (3) motivation to fly.[10] Age, race, and sex are not indicators of a pilot's competency. Analyses of observed versus expected accidents in commercial and airline transport pilots from 1978 to 1979 reveal that beginning in the 30s age bracket, fewer accidents actually occur per 1000 pilots than is the case with younger pilots. Maturity, experience, and increased judgment are key factors in the improving safety record accompanying increasing age. In 1981, the median age of United States Boeing 747 captains was 58 years. The figure for the Lockheed 1011 was 58; the McDonnell-Douglas DC-10 was 57; the Air Bus A-300 was 56; the DC-8 was 54, the B-707 was 52; the B-727 was 50; the DC-9 was 48; and the B-737 was 47. The wide-body, advanced, jet aircraft are flown by the senior, most experienced captains in their late 50s. The overall safety record of these aircraft reflects the direct correlation between air safety and increasing judgment and experience accompanying normal, healthy aging.

Accidents per 1000 pilots-in-command for civilians having commercial or air transport pilot certificates are shown in Table 23–4. As is the case with automobile accidents, increasing maturity and experience (concomitants of the aging process) are positively correlated with a decreasing accident incidence (more than twofold decrease from the teenage period to the late 50s and older). Some critics have decried the absence of precise exposure data, but this aspect is not critical to pilot safety because each pilot-in-command determines the risk to which he is exposed; deliberate penetration of thunderstorms, intentional, unwarranted, low-level maneuvers, and flight under the influence of alcohol or drugs are all related to immaturity and impulse control problems. As with automobile accidents, about 90% of aircraft accidents result from operator error.

Improved screening methods for significant diseases in pilots are increasingly available, as is better understanding of the role of cardiovascular risk factors in disease causation. A growing movement is developing to abolish all upper-age limits in regard to pilot duties. This movement is impelled further by the remarkable increase in health and longevity in the United States population. The average length of an individual's life is currently in the neighborhood of 73 years and is rapidly moving toward a healthy 85 years. The implications for the continued productive employment of aircrew members are clear, as is the role to be played by the

aeromedical specialist under these circumstances.

Mental Functions

The main requisites for safe pilot performance are sensory accuracy, cognitive capacity, including judgment, motor efficiency, and emotional stability, and drive. All of these elements can be evaluated either in the clinic or through flight performance. The two accident reports that follow fall into the realm of mental dysfunction.

A United McDonnell-Douglas DC-8 passenger flight experienced complete fuel exhaustion at night on December 28, 1978 over Portland, Oregon.[11] Ten persons on board received fatal injuries in the deadstick landing that followed. Investigators determined that the pilot had not properly monitored the fuel supply because his attention had been diverted by a landing gear malfunction. The investigators also felt that the first officer and the flight engineer did not fully appreciate the development of a critically low fuel state. They concluded that these two crewmembers should have been more alert to the status of the fuel supply and should have been more assertive in communicating the developing problem to the captain.

The attitude indicators failed on a night flight in a Transamerica Lockheed L-188 near Salt Lake City, Utah on November 18, 1978.[12] The turn needle and directional heading indicator remained functional, but the captain became spatially disoriented when he attempted to integrate unreliable attitude information and the information from the other instruments. The large turboprop aircraft entered a typical graveyard spiral and broke up in flight, killing the three crewmembers. Insidious failures of critical flight instruments still remain a major hazard in flight activities, as demonstrated by this accident. A mental state of alertness to possible partial failures of flight instruments is necessary if

Table 23–4. Pilot Age and Accidents*

Age	Active Pilots— 1978	Active Pilots— 1979	Number of Accidents Observed— 1978	Number of Accidents Observed— 1979	Number of Accidents Expected— 1978	Number of Accidents Expected— 1979	Accidents Per 1000—1978	Accidents Per 1000—1979
16–19	374	468	8	7	3	4	21.4	15.0
20–24	10,839	11,839	167	160	92	90	15.4	13.5
25–29	26,102	25,755	312	294	220	196	12.0	11.4
30–34	45,011	44,606	414	359	379	341	9.2	8.0
35–39	41,742	42,520	321	309	352	324	7.7	7.3
40–44	35,270	35,031	236	209	297	267	6.7	6.0
45–49	28,012	29,585	214	191	236	225	7.6	6.5
50–54	19,660	18,803	164	149	166	143	8.3	8.0
55–59	22,499	23,073	131	123	190	176	5.8	5.3
60+	12,205	14,069	71	72	103	107	5.8	5.1
Total	241,714	245,749	2038	1873	2038	1873		

*Pilots-in-command having commercial and air transport certificates; general aviation accidents.
From the National Transportation Safety Board and Federal Aviation Administration Statistical Handbook, U.S. Government Printing Office, Washington, D.C., 1978 to 1979.

recognition and proper actions are to be taken.

Civil Protective Equipment

The basic protective equipment available in civil aviation relates to the nature of the aircraft, the flight mission, and the minimal standards for this type of equipment.

Gliders, agricultural aircraft, aerobatic aircraft, and most airline aircraft have been equipped with shoulder harnesses since the 1960s. Only since the late 1970s have other newly manufactured general aviation aircraft required shoulder harnesses, and there are even exceptions to this.

It can be forecast that approximately half of the annual general aviation accident fatalities can be prevented by the simple expedient of using a proper shoulder harness-seat belt-restraint system.

"Delethalized" instrument panels and controls have helped to prevent fatalities in general aviation, but much more remains to be done, including protection against pyrolysis and heat from fire.

The requirement for protective equipment aboard airline aircraft is extensive and depends, in part, on the routes flown. Water survival equipment is, of course, necessary for prolonged overwater flights. For general aviation aircraft, the requirements are not as extensive. Most single-engine private aircraft fly without oxygen equipment. If the owner wishes to fly at altitudes requiring oxygen supplementation, however, inexpensive portable oxygen systems are available. Most aircraft now carry emergency radio beacons that activate should a crash occur. Many private pilots equip their aircraft with emergency equipment, that is, water, first-aid kit, survival kit, and food. The aeromedical specialist can provide assistance to those airmen wishing to prepare such an emergency kit for carrying aboard their aircraft.

International Civil Aviation Medicine

Civil aviation activities among the world's countries are coordinated by the International Civil Aviation Organization (ICAO), a component of the United Nations. Recommended standards and practices are developed, and member nations, virtually all countries, either adhere to these standards or file "exceptions." The United States has more general aviation activities and pilots than all of the rest of the world combined and has perhaps filed more exceptions to the ICAO standards than any other nation. This is felt by many to reflect the progressive actions in the field of general aviation historically taken by the United States.

The Future and Civil Aviation Medicine

The trend in medical certification in the United States is to move away from arbitrarily fixed standards toward a more functional approach. For example, the present standards call for binocular vision, but 5000 one-eyed civil United States pilots have been certified based on individual performance capabilities.

Pilots with missing limbs have received medical certificates based on a Statement of Demonstrated Ability, as demonstrated in the flight environment. Paraplegic pilots have been certified, with limitations requiring the use of a specially equipped aircraft. Airline pilots have been recertified with prosthetic replacements for part of the leg. One pilot has been returned with bilateral artificial hip joints.

Pilots with hearing losses have been certified, with the requirement that a hearing aid be worn. Aphakic pilots have received certification contingent on wearing proper contact lenses. More than 500 recovered alcoholic airline pilots have received medical certification by exemption, a process involving inpatient treatment, cessation of intake of all alcoholic beverages, and the institution of a periodic follow-up program (Table 23–5).

In the United States, pilots also have

Table 23–5. Overview of Medical Rejections, Reconsiderations, and Exemptions—1980 Medical Certifications

Condition	Number
FAA Rejected Medical Certifications for Medical Causes, Including Cases at Various Appeal Levels Within the FAA	
Medical history rejections	62,116
Visual rejections	126,620
Blood pressure or pulse problems	18,304
Other medical problems	136,242
Hearing problems	28,901
Total	372,183
Medical Certifications Based on Reconsideration Appeals to the Federal Air Surgeon	
Eye	23
Ear, nose, and throat	1
Respiratory	2
Cardiovascular	64
Abdominal	10
Neurologic	46
Psychiatric	22
Bone/joint	1
Miscellaneous	22
Total	191
Medical Exemptions Petitions Granted or Denied by the FAA	
Eye	1
Cardiovascular	86
Neuropsychiatric	107*
Miscellaneous	3
Total	197

*Includes a significant number of recovering alcoholic airline pilots.

been returned to commercial flight duties (airline captain, corporate pilot) following coronary bypass surgery on appeal to the National Transportation Safety Board. The same return to duty by airline pilots has been accomplished in Canada. As medical research develops new understanding of disease, new diagnostic techniques, and new treatments, a marked individualization of medical certification for those having various conditions is predicted. It is anticipated that all arbitrary upper-age limits will give way to individual assessments of functional capability and freedom from disease when the desire to continue flying exists.

A possible direction for the civil medical standards and certification process is the elimination of the mandatory denials due to medical history. This action leaves the individual determination of certification essentials to decisions by the FAA based on the currrent health and functional status of the applicant (special issuance procedures). Consideration will be given to the probability that no significant change in medical status is likely to occur within 2 years from the date of certification, the longest potential duration of a medical certificate not otherwise time-limited.

Among the key medical issues for the next decades in civil aviation medicine are the following:

1. The quantification of crew work load levels at specific flight phases (including sensory, cognitive, and motor elements)
2. The management of crew fatigue, including scheduling aspects related to multiple night flights, transmeridian desynchronization, 24-hour layovers following night arrivals, and multiple takeoffs and landings
3. Biomedical assessments of flight display characteristics, emphasizing the increasing replacement of mechanical instruments by cathode ray tube displays (CRT) and other electronic optical instruments, including flat panel dot-matrix displays (Fig. 23–11)
4. Institution of programs that deal with pilot fitness and behavior, medical standards, and exceptions to these standards
5. Further research and pilot education programs on the acute and long-term alcohol and drug effects on crew performance
6. Refinement of the understanding of in-flight environmental factors, including G forces, hypoxia, and spatial disorientation
7. An air traffic control system that will be increasingly automated, further removing the human controllers

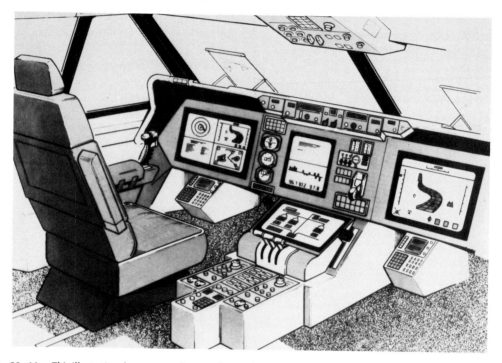

Fig. 23–11. This illustration demonstrates how modern technology can simultaneously simplify and improve displays for future airline aircraft. Available to the crew is a head-up windshield and a cathode ray tube (CRT) display that projects a "pathway in the sky," enabling the pilots to easily follow either inertial coordinates or external electronic navigation beams to a specific point. Virtually all necessary operating data can be called up for display on the CRTs. A side control replaces the traditional yoke, giving a superior view of the instrument panel (courtesy of the Lockheed Georgia Company).

from the pilot/air traffic controller interactions

8. Improved accident investigation methods, leading to a better understanding of the underlying causes of accidents so that preventive programs can be enhanced

9. Improved aircraft accident survivability, including impact attenuation, crash fire minimization and control, and improved emergency escape systems

New generations of civil aircraft will contain increasing levels of automation and will extend current limits of aerodynamic envelopes. The hypersonic transport, flying several times the speed of sound at altitudes in the 60,000-m range, is projected to provide a 3-hour flight from New York to Australia. Civil aerospace medicine physicians must increasingly incorporate in their work new biomedical advances so that these advances can be applied in preventing human failure in flight activities.

REFERENCES

1. Institute of Medicine: Airline Pilot Age, Health, and Performance. Washington, D.C., National Academy Press, 1981.
2. Mohler, S.R.: Agricultural aviation medicine in the Soviet Union. Aviat. Space Environ. Med., 51:515, 1980.
3. Mohler, S.R.: Physiologically Tolerable Decompression Profiles for Supersonic Transport Type Certification. Office of Aviation Medicine Report AM-70-12. U.S. Government Printing Office, Washington, D.C., Federal Aviation Administration, July 1970.
4. Billings, C.E., Wick, R.L., Gerke, R.J., and Chase, R.C.: The Effects of Alcohol on Pilot Performance During Instrument Flight. Office of Aviation Medicine Report AM-72-4. U.S. Government Printing Office, Washington, D.C., Federal Aviation Administration, 1972.

5. Mohler, S.R.: G Effects on the Pilot During Aerobatics. Office of Aviation Medicine Report AM-72-28. U.S. Government Printing Office, Washington, D.C., Federal Aviation Administration, 1972.

6. Klein, K.E.: Significance of Circadian Rhythms in Aerospace Activities. Agardograph 247. National Technical Information Services, Springfield, Virginia, North Atlantic Treaty Organization, 1980.

7. Spanish Government: Accident Report, Fatal Collision, KLM Boeing B-747 (PH-SUF) and Pan American Boeing B-747 (N1736), Los Rodeos Airport, Tenerife, Canary Islands, March 27, 1977.

8. Federal Aviation Administration: Flight-Time Limitations. Subpart Q, Domestic Air Carriers; Subpart R, Flag Air Carriers; Subpart S, Supplemental Air Carriers and Commercial Operators.

Federal Aviation Regulations 21, Title 14. U.S. Government Printing Office, 1982.

9. Wegmann, H.M.: Models to Predict Loads of Flight Schedules on Cockpit Personnel. Twenty-ninth International Congress of Aviation and Space Medicine, Nancy, France, 1981.

10. Mohler, S.R.: Reasons for eliminating the "age 60" regulation for airline pilots. Aviat. Space Environ. Med., 52:445, 1981.

11. National Transportation Safety Board: Aircraft Accident Report, United Airlines, Inc., McDonnell-Douglas DC-861, N8082U, Portland, Oregon, December 28, 1978. NTSB-AAR-79-7. U.S. Government Printing Office, Washington, D.C., June 7, 1979.

12. National Transportation Safety Board: Aircraft Accident Report, Transamerica Airlines, Inc. Lockheed L-188, N859U, Salt Lake City, Utah, November 28, 1979. NTSB-AAR-80-11. U.S Government Printing Office, Washington, D.C., August 26, 1980.

Chapter 24

Aviation Medical Support to Airlines

Roy L. DeHart and Charles C. Gullett

When meditating over a disease, I never think of finding a remedy for it, but, instead, a means of preventing it.

LOUIS PASTEUR

Throughout the world, airlines provide for the aviation medical needs of their aircrews and for the industrial medical care of their other employees by a variety of methods. The majority of the large airlines have chosen to develop their own departments of aviation and occupational medicine, and most of the remaining airlines obtain medical support by contract or other arrangements with aviation medical practitioners.

Within the United States, there are over 60 airlines, ranging from large corporate giants to regional and commuter air service companies. Combined, these airlines carry over 265 million passengers flying approximately 200,000 million passenger-miles (Fig. 24–1). The industry is responsible for the direct employment of nearly 341,000 workers with an annual payroll exceeding $10,230 million. Among these employees are 37,000 flight deck and 53,000 cabin crewmembers.[1] The health maintenance of such a major industry is primarily the domain of physicians trained in the field of aviation medicine.

THE EVOLUTION OF CIVIL AVIATION MEDICINE

The airline industry has changed gradually over the past 50 years. A review of this evolution is useful in understanding the variations that exist in today's airline medical organizations. In the early days of the airline industry, the personnel officer was the first to recognize the need for medical support. These medical needs were twofold: medical evaluation for the selection of new employees, especially flight personnel, and on-site first aid for job injuries. These needs usually were fulfilled by sending the applicant to a local physician for a physical examination and hiring a nurse to operate a first-aid facility in the maintenance building. As the industry grew, the needs increased in magnitude and complexity. In the transition, the next step was frequently employing a consulting physician, first part-time and then full-time. The medical responsibilities began to broaden to include job placement examinations, periodic special examinations to monitor personnel in critical jobs, job

DOMESTIC PASSENGER SERVICE
U. S. SCHEDULED AIRLINES

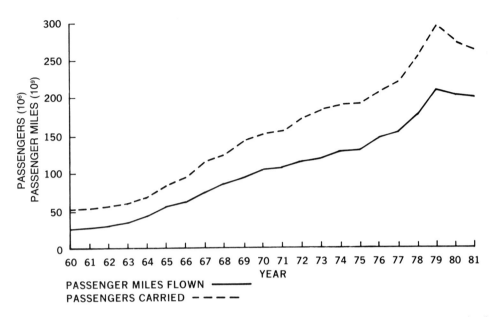

Fig. 24–1. Domestic passenger service for United States scheduled airlines, 1960–1981, by passenger miles flown and number of passengers carried.

safety, including human factor and environmental health, aircraft accident investigation, and consultation on group and workmen's compensation insurance. As a result of this beginning, many airline medical departments became a part of the personnel department. Occasionally, such an organizational structure was found to be less than optimal and new organizational arrangements were tried.

One of the first airlines to hire private physicians to support the selection and health maintenance of aircrew was Pan American. In 1928, this airline employed private physicians to examine its flying crews. Early in its history, Eastern Airlines employed physicians on a fee-for-service basis in various cities along its route structure to accomplish preemployment and flight examinations and to care for injuries or illness involving passengers or employees. In 1936, Eastern Airlines appointed Dr. Ralph N. Green, a former Army pilot

and the first United States physician to attain military flight status, to develop a medical service for its flight crews. In 1931, American Airlines began to provide medical care for its pilots. Qualified physicians and part-time consultants provided this service. In 1940, the airline established its first medical office and selected as its first medical director Dr. Edward C. Greene. United Airlines appointed Colonel Arnold D. Tuttle, a retired Army flight surgeon, to be its first medical director, and in 1938, United Airlines opened a completely new and specially designed medical center to house all the necessary facilities for a sophisticated airline medical department.

As medical departments were developing in the United States, Canadian airlines began establishing their own medical departments. In 1937, Dr. Kenneth Dowd was named airline medical director for Trans Canadian Airlines.

Many of the leaders in the field of aerospace medicine were actively involved in the development of airline medical departments, for example, doctors Eric S. Lilgencrantz, Ross McFarland, and John Tamisiea. Other early names associated with the medical support to airlines were Dr. W. Randolph Lovelace and Dr. Jan H. Tillisch.

In 1944, airline medical physicians formed their own professional society—the Airline Medical Directors Association. In 1956, airline medical directors from throughout the world came together to form the International Academy of Aviation and Space Medicine. Their annual congress has met at major capitals worldwide.

The rapid technical developments during and immediately following World War II brought about the need for more specialized training for the airline physician. Airplanes were becoming more sophisticated as they flew faster and higher, and materials used to make and maintain such equipment became more exotic and hazardous. The cost of operating an airline became increasingly expensive, especially those costs related to flight training, crew salaries, and insurance and retirement programs. This cost of operation led to the need for the aeromedical specialists trained to the standards established by the American Board of Preventive Medicine.

ORGANIZATIONAL STRUCTURE FOR AIRLINE MEDICAL SUPPORT

One of the unique features of medical practice in the airline setting is the considerable concern for the public's safety and the possibility of liability resulting from activities and decisions in connection with practicing aviation medicine. Regardless of the structure through which aviation medicine support is provided, it is imperative that the physician never lose sight of his obligations to public safety. Airline medical departments also must be sensitive to the fact that flight crewmembers are regulated by a federal regulatory agency, the Federal Aviation Administration (FAA), where medical fitness is a concern of that agency's regulatory responsibilities.

Self-Contained Medical Departments

It is common to find the airline medical department located in the corporation's major headquarters. For the larger airlines, it is standard practice for a considerable portion of the medical resources to be concentrated at the home office. Regional medical offices also may be established and house at least one physician and additional paraprofessional and support personnel. They are normally located at one of the major hubs of the airline route structure where aircrews are domiciled. This location provides the aircrew ease of access to medical services. One major airline has centralized its medical resources and uses its system to bring the employee to the physician. In acute medical situations, consultants have been identified throughout the United States who can support the medical needs of the aircrewman. In determining the medical services structure within a corporation, a cost-benefits analysis would be appropriate.

Titles and organizational level can be a significant influencing factor in obtaining or sustaining a program or in making decisions within a company. Some airlines overcame the difficulty by designating the medical department as a separate, high-level department reporting directly to the president of the airline. The chief physician in such a structure carries the title of Corporate Medical Director or Vice President of Medical Services. Such formalized medical departments were being set up just prior to the outbreak of World War II.

Contractual Services

Other airlines have elected not to develop a medical department within their own corporate structure but rather to rely on a contractual arrangement. In these situations, it is common for the airline to turn to a nationally recognized clinic such as Mayo, Lovelace, or Kelsey-Seybold for the necessary medical support. Each airline must, in turn, weigh the benefits of this arrangement against those of developing their own medical department. At times, it proves to be less convenient to both the employee and the airline to use a separate clinic. Further, the clinic may be unable to adjust to corporate needs as expeditiously as the airline company might desire. Such an arrangement, however, does reduce the potential for conflicts of interest regarding the employee's health status. Another advantage to this arrangement is that senior consultants frequently are readily available as members of the clinic staff.

Contingency and Fee-For-Service Arrangements

Among the smaller airlines, medical support commonly is provided through a contingency arrangement with a private practitioner or simply on a fee-for-service basis. Physicians knowledgeable in the field of aviation medicine or aerospace medical specialists are often available near the nation's major airports. Smaller airlines turn to these physicians for medical support requirements. This procedure is frequently an acceptable alternative in view of the routine nature of the services required. These same physicians may provide en-route medical support to even the major airlines. The availability of their services at or near airports can be particularly attractive.

FUNCTIONS OF AN AIRLINE MEDICAL DEPARTMENT

The functions of a medical department within an airline corporation depend on the size and complexity of the corporation. For this discussion, the focus will be on a major airline's medical department. Many activities, programs, and services can be

required and quickly move the scope of the medical services from aviation medicine to occupational medicine to the broadest spectrum of preventive medicine. Such services would include those necessary for the selection and health maintenance of both flight deck and cabin crews, aircraft maintenance personnel, aircraft servicing personnel, counter and administrative personnel, and the executives. Typical services available to the employee are as follows:

Preplacement assessment

Periodic medical examination

On-the-job illness and injury treatment

Counseling services

Health hazards screening

Health and safety educational activities

Employee assistance for substance abuse

Work hazard assessment

Consultative services

Preplacement Assessment

The preplacement assessment is tailored to the specific position the prospective employee will be expected to fill. The degree of sophistication of this assessment is divided between two categories: aircrew and all other.

Aircrew Preplacement Assessment

The success of the airline is in large measure dependent on adequate flight crews to operate the aircraft. It is to the airline's advantage to select aircrew who can reasonably be expected to maintain their medical standards throughout their working lives. Consequently, the preemployment assessment of pilots is rigorous and designed to ensure that, as a minimum, the aircrew members can reasonably be expected to retain their FAA first class licenses. Most airlines, however, carry this examination far beyond the minimum screening examination required for certification. The medical assessment is generally designed to be sufficiently sophisticated to identify defects or medical conditions that, although not currently disqualifying, could reasonably be expected to progress toward more significant disease. Further, many of the assessment procedures are designed to reveal preclinical disease. These assessments often include neuropsychologic test batteries to define the personality structure of the individual.

Historically, the airlines have drawn the majority of their flight deck personnel from the military; therefore, the candidate will frequently have proven academic credentials, demonstrated leadership skills, and will have 2000 or more flying hours. He will have satisfactorily met the medical standards for commissioning in the armed forces, as well as the more stringent standards required for pilot training. It is not surprising, then, that the majority of airline pilot candidates come to the preemployment physical assessment in an unusual state of good health. Because of the excess of applicants for available positions in recent years, it has not been necessary for the airlines to consider employment of any but the healthiest individuals. This, however, has not always been the case, and the medical standards for employment required by a particular airline company during any specific year depend primarily on supply and demand. Nevertheless, the aviation medical specialist frequently will play a key role in the employment decision of airline crewmembers.

Nonpilot Preplacement Assessment

In the preemployment assessment of all other employees, the medical examination usually is not as stringent. It should be recalled, however, that there are categories of prospective employees, such as flight attendants, crane operators, and motor vehicle operators, who also should be medically evaluated against established health standards. There may be other categories of employees who require a license, with medical qualification as a precondition to their employment. One of the features for most flight attendants that should not be overlooked is the need for a food handler certification issued by a public health authority. Employees entering the administrative, clerical, or reservation category may require nothing more than a health history to satisfy preemployment assessment. Special attention should be given to the musculoskeletal system and to establishing an audiologic baseline in individuals seeking placement in heavy industry or maintenance.

In the 1950s, flight attendants aboard United States airlines had a job expectancy of approximately 2 years. Nearly all flight attendants were female, young, and unmarried. In the three decades since then, major changes have occurred in the social expectations of society and in federal legislation addressing employee discrimination. Flight attendants are now of both sexes, capable of working until the age of 70, may be married, and, in fact, may serve in the cabin while obviously pregnant. It is appreciated by all associated with airline operations that the flight attendant is the primary cabin safety factor during in-flight or ground emergencies. The absolute minimum number of flight attendants for a given flight and their distribution within the cabin of the aircraft during takeoff and landing are specified by regulations. Currently, it is estimated that 50,000 flight attendants are employed by United States air carriers. Preventive medicine, health promotion programs directed toward flight attendants have been outlined by Alter and Mohler.[2] Basically, the concerns are the same as those that must be addressed by the aviation medicine specialist when dealing with flight deck crews. Unfortunately, the application of preventive medicine and health promotion programs to the occupation of flight attendant has lagged behind the progress of medical and engineering sciences. The airlines medical department must provide a realistic and needs-specific program directed to the requirements of these cabin personnel.

In a number of corporation settings within the United States, it is becoming standard practice to require a candidate for a high executive position to undergo an extensive medical examination, including cardiac stress testing. The type of evaluation and sophistication of the assessment is frequently established by the medical department, with the approval of corporate management. Thus, the aviation medicine practitioner not only is responsible for conducting such an assessment but, more importantly, may be the individual who establishes its need and scope.

Periodic Medical Examinations

Periodic medical examinations are normally done on pilots, flight attendants, and corporate executives. The degree to which other employees are afforded the opportunity for periodic health assessments depends on the individual airline. The flight crews are normally the only employee group for whom the frequency of the examination is set without consideration for age. For all other categories, the examination will be scheduled periodically based on the individual's age at the time of examination. A schedule that has been found acceptable in some industrial settings would begin the periodic assessment at age 30, with repeat examinations at 35, 40, 43, 46, 49, and 52 years of age and each even-year anniversary thereafter. The components of the periodic assessment are determined by the category of the employee. Again, it should be pointed out that the physician generally is not only responsible for conducting such assessments but for establishing their periodicity and scope.

Periodic Medical Assessments of Pilots

The airline medical departments provide a system of preventive health maintenance for their flight deck crews. This system may demonstrate the presence of early disease, and by initiating ameliorative programs, the crewmember who might otherwise have lost his medical category and thereby his livelihood is salvaged. In addition to the periodic assessment required by the airline and conducted by their medical personnel, the pilot possessing a Class 1 medical certificate must undergo a medical examination by an FAA-designated senior medical examiner every 6 months. This regulatory requirement is periodically reviewed, and a growing body of evidence supports a reduced frequency for a more thorough examination.

In 1960, the designated aviation medical examiner (AME) system was established for the purpose of identifying medical examiners to perform assessments on all civil airmen required by regulation to hold a valid FAA medical certificate. Currently, it is permissible for the airline aviation medical physician to conduct the FAA-certifying examination provided the physician is a senior medical examiner.

With respect to medical examinations conducted by AMEs, there are several areas of interest. Because a commercial airline pilot may turn outside the company for the periodic medical examination, several considerations weigh in choosing a particular physician to conduct the medical examination. These considerations include such factors as cost, availability, convenience, and the reputation of the examining physician. In this particular circumstance, one must be cautious in judging the elements that establish the physician's reputation. Unlike a patient seeking a physician who may be best able to diagnose and treat a medical condition, it is conceivable that an airline pilot would seek a medical examiner who is less precise and detailed in the examination and cavalier in the history-taking. The pilot may mistakenly judge it an advantage to have a less thorough medical examination because it lessens the possibility of medical conditions being identified that could compromise the medical certificate. This statement is not meant to imply that most pilots would seek such a superficial examination but is simply meant to alert the aviation medical specialist to that possibility and to remind the specialist that the selection of medical examiners is not a chance occurrence.

Thirty-three percent of the designated senior AMEs examined 87% of the Class 1 certificate holders in 1971.[3] Further, the majority of the pilots of the smaller scheduled air carriers were examined by fewer than five physicians. Within airlines, those pilots who occupy the copilot and engineer positions are only required by federal regulation to meet the requirements of a valid Class 2 medical certificate. In reality, the majority of these pilots maintain a Class 1 certificate.

Within the airline corporate structure, the aviation medical practitioner walks a tightrope. On one side is his commitment to the corporation, public safety, and federal law. On the other side is his ethical obligation to the patient (the employee) and the representative body (the union). This situation calls then for a delicate balance between services primarily designed to benefit the flight crewmember and those actions that must be taken in compliance with the regulatory requirements. In the air carrier industry, one specific article is common in contracts between the aircrew and the airline: no medical information obtained by the airline medical department will be released to the regulatory agency without the expressed written permission of the involved aircrew member. Further, pilots will be deemed to be medically fit as long as they possess a current, valid FAA medical certificate. A potentially explosive situation is created in which the airlines, through their more thorough examinations, may become aware of a medical condition that is not known to the FAA. Actions taken by the medical department or the operations division of the airline to prevent a pilot from flying as a result of a disqualifying defect are subject to the established grievance procedures in the contract. The medical practitioner is again reminded that the FAA Class 1 examination is neither sophisticated nor extensive, and it does not require provocative or stress testing or the use of high-technology procedures or facilities. The examination is performed by a senior medical examiner in the privacy of an office with a stethoscope and is dependent on the conscientiousness of both parties with regard to history and physical assessment.

Nonpilot Periodic Health Assessment

The scope and periodicity of nonpilot health assessments are normally determined by the airline medical personnel. Factors that come to bear on the decision are the age of the employee, employment category, the degree of risk or stress related to the job, and the cost-benefits of such assessments. It is important that the philosophy of periodic assessments not be confused with the need for periodic biologic monitoring as a result of the work environment. The periodic medical examination is designed to focus on particular organs that are susceptible to disease over time and have as a goal reducing the significance of the effects of impairment from diseases common to the population. Periodic biologic monitoring focuses on body systems that may be susceptible to harm from stressors within the work environment and are unique to the conditions of the employment rather than to the population as a whole.

Job-Related Illness and Injury

A corporation has both a legal and moral obligation to ensure emergency care, follow-up, and, if necessary, rehabilitation of any employee injured under conditions of employment. Fortunately, the more common injuries are readily cared for within a first-aid setting. Serious injuries could well require immediate evacuation of the employee to a major medical center for stabilization and appropriate care. The medical department arranges for the provision of such care throughout the entire airline system and, where numbers of employees dictate, provides the facilities and personnel to satisfy these requirements. The airline is faced with the full spectrum of occupational hazards, although some hazards are obviously more prevalent than others. One of the major flight-line occupational hazards is noise. Consequently, an airline medical department must ensure that procedures are established to identify employees who are experiencing noise-induced hearing loss early enough to take preventive measures. The medical department must work closely with safety and maintenance personnel to ensure that employees have available and use noise protection devices. Numerous other physical hazards, including heat, radio frequency radiation, and ionizing radiation, are constituents of the work environment. Because the airline serves as a common carrier, the potential exists for the employees to be exposed to toxic chemicals, isotopes, zoonosis, and plant products.

Occupational illnesses are often subtle and readily can be confused with common medical conditions. A high index of suspicion on the part of the examiner is frequently the key to the diagnosis. Because of the character of airline operations, the kind of insult or hazard that could result in the manifestation of illness is nearly unlimited. In an airline medical department, little purpose is served by subdividing the medical practice into aviation and occupational medicine. In fact, the full spectrum of the components of both are at work. Fortunately, the principles of both aviation and occupational medicine have

their foundations in preventive medicine, and a physician trained in the discipline can serve both fields well.

The employee returning to work following an illness usually is not of major concern. It is common practice to restrict an employee, when necessary, to various aspects of his employment to ensure that recovery is rapid and not complicated by the stresses of the job. For flight crews, this is far more difficult. Because of the potential extremes in the environment of flight, it may not be appropriate to return an otherwise essentially healthy individual to work. For example, a cabin attendant who is pregnant may find her agility and mobility in the in-flight environment of an airline cabin becoming compromised during the fifth to sixth month of pregnancy and could be medically disqualified for further flight duty until several months post partum. Under identical medical circumstances, a pregnant employee working the reservation desk or in management may function quite effectively without undue hazard to herself or the fetus until near term. A moderately severe cold that would prove only an inconvenience to a mechanic would result in the temporary grounding of an aircrew member.

Counseling Services

The medical department's counseling service has two focuses. The first approach involves those services provided to the employee, who derives direct benefit to himself or to members of his family. This type of counseling is frequently provided to an employee seeking reassurance or further explanation of a situation that he doesn't fully understand and does not feel comfortable in pursuing further with his private physician. The employee may be seeking advice regarding health maintenance activities such as a dietary regimen for weight control, assistance in understanding his recently diagnosed hypertension, advice regarding fitness regimens, or recommendations on health services available in the community. These same questions may be asked by the employee but with reference to members of his family. With all the media attention to potential hazards introduced into the home from the work place, he may request reassurance or clarification.

A second major focus of counseling is directed at supervisors and management. The concern here is mainly an employee with a medical problem who needs to be helped to cope with the stresses this problem brings into the workplace. The focus of these counseling activities often centers on personality aberrations of or substance abuse by the employee. The aviation medicine specialist is doing a disservice to management if he fails to encourage employees to avail themselves of his expertise in dealing with these sorts of problems. Generally, the medical practitioner is the staff member best trained to advise on the employee whose behavioral change is stressing the work environment.

Advice should be offered, whether asked or not, to the supervisor of an employee returning to work following a major health crisis. Employees returning following serious trauma, loss of a loved one, recovery from a myocardial infarction, or a diagnosis of cancer are examples where assistance to the supervisor may be helpful.

Health Hazard Assessments

A medical department has many reasons for establishing a program of health hazard assessments for the airline employees, including compliance with federal law or regulatory requirements, compensation costs, union demands, insurance considerations, and altruistic motivations of the company. Such a program that is pervasive among the airline companies is the hearing conservation effort. This program is designed to identify methods of reducing noise generation and individuals susceptible to hearing loss in the high-noise environment of aircraft opera-

tions. Another program focuses on individuals who potentially are exposed to toxic chemicals and require periodic biologic monitoring that consists of both physical examination and specific blood and urine chemistry analyses. Other periodic assessment programs may be established for those employees who potentially are exposed to ionizing or nonionizing radiation, hazardous vibration, or a variety of toxins and additional physical hazards.

Such assessments fulfill only a part of the obligation of a company to the health and welfare of its employees. Parallel to the biologic monitoring is an entire system of work-site monitoring efforts. Environmental engineers, industrial hygienists, and technicians assess the noise profile and noise hazard areas, measure the adequacy of ventilation in paint shops and fueling stands, monitor both ionizing and nonionizing radiation fields with dosimeters, and assess with other monitors a variety of hazards within the work environment.

Other aspects of a selective health screening program are those activities periodically conducted for the benefit of the employee. The medical staff may choose to mobilize its resources in parallel with a national drive to focus on a particular medical affliction. For example, screening services might be made available to the entire employee population for conditions such as hypertension, diabetes, pulmonary disease, or glaucoma.

Educational Activities

The airline medical department has an obligation both to management and to the employee to publicize the services that are available. In addition, the medical department frequently is required to publicize specific health or safety information throughout the corporation. For example, a recent hearing survey may have indicated the need for a greater emphasis on the use of hearing protection or an industrial accident may highlight the need for emphasis on the use of eye protection. Appropriate educational programs go hand in hand with periodic health assessments and special health screening programs and are far more effective when accompanied by appropriate educational media attention. One recent example of a satisfactory combined health screening and educational program conducted by an airline was related to colon cancer.

Employee Assistance Programs

The more progressive airlines have moved to establish employee assistance programs for those individuals who have found their lives altered due to substance abuse. Although many forms of abuse are dealt with within these programs, ranging from prescription drugs to illicit drugs, the drug of greatest abuse among airline employees, including flight crews, is alcohol. In developing programs to address this very sensitive issue, it is necessary to gain the support of many different constituencies. The medical department will need the commitment of all levels of management, support from employee organizations, commitments from trade associations outside the airline, and, not infrequently, a working arrangement with a regulatory agency. Once it is agreed to proceed with such a program, an extensive educational effort must be undertaken to advise all employees and to remove any aspects of a witch hunt. In this medical program more than most, it is perception rather than reality that will determine the success of case finding. The success of the Airline Pilots Association in addressing this issue is provided in greater detail in Chapter 25, "Aeromedical Rehabilitation and Health Promotion for Civilian Professional Aircrew."

Even giving the benefit of the doubt to airline companies, it can be reasonably expected that 5 to 10% of employees will have a substance abuse problem of some magnitude. Unfortunately, many of these employees are among the most effective and productive of the work force, and their value eventually will be compromised unless effective employee assistance is provided. In the industrial setting, the problem drinker generates excessive costs—three times the company average in terms of absenteeism, accidents, and illness benefits. It is difficult to calculate other costs that may be of greater magnitude, including the loss of the experienced employee, friction in the work group, lowered morale, inefficiency, waste of supervisory time, bad decisions, damage to customer and public relations, and, when dealing with a flight deck crewman, a potential compromise of public safety.

For an effective substance abuse program, the airline should commit to and publicize a number of principles. Recommended corporate policy regarding substance abuse should (1) recognize substance abuse as a health problem affecting the employee's job performance; (2) recognize the need for early identification and treatment of substance abuse to maximize the recovery rate; (3) make the company's health benefits programs, including sick leave and group insurance benefits, available for employees participating in an approved treatment program; (4) ensure that identification of an abuser per se is not cause for termination; (5) avoid the appearance of a moral crusade under the substance abuse rehabilitation program; and (6) recognize that the airline will not dictate its employee's social habits.

Once recovery has begun, the employee, with the support of the airline, often will turn to a community-based support organization. One of the most effective support organizations is Alcoholics Anonymous. By using such an organization, the recovering abuser has a broad-based support system, including the medical department of the airline, the philosophy of the company, coworkers, or the union, the home, and the community.

For the recovering alcoholic pilot, provisions are made for a return to the cockpit following evidence of satisfactory progress in a recovery program. The Federal Air Surgeon is willing to consider a petition once adequate information is available to establish that recovery is progressing. It should be emphasized, however, that recovery is defined as total abstinence from alcohol. In the case of a recovering alcoholic, a return to social drinking is not classified as recovering. It should be noted that a slip occurring soon after discharge from an alcohol rehabilitation facility is not all that rare and would not necessarily preclude a return to flying status provided the aircrewman followed a successful course of recycling treatment. It is reassuring to all associated with airline operations to witness the high recovery rate of pilots entering the alcohol rehabilitation program.

Health Hazard Inspection of the Work Environment

One of the more challenging activities of an airline medical department is describing and understanding the potential hazards of the work place to the workers. For the aeromedical specialist, the initial step to understanding the environment is an indoctrination tour of the company. Because of the nature of airline operations and the shift work of many employees, it is necessary to visit each shift because different activities are frequently conducted in response to the flight schedule. The flight service ramp is a dynamic environment, with numerous individual operations going on simultaneously but, again, all activities are coordinated with the flight schedule. While aircraft taxi, ground service vehicles are moving about as service personnel move over, around, and in between the vehicles. Noise is ubiquitous. Weather conditions vary. Oil and fuel are everywhere and at times are mixed with deicing solution. Food service is loading at one end of the aircraft while the sanitary

systems are being serviced at the other end. All of this is complicated by the press of time and the competitive environment.

In the maintenance hangars, nearly every industrial process from painting to degreasing and from welding to engine tear-down can be found. Eye, ear, and respiratory protection is frequently required.

For the aviation medical specialist, one of the most exciting working environments to visit is the operational flight deck. A full appreciation for the work load and performance requirements of the aircrew will only come after in-flight observations in a variety of flight conditions. Flying in all types of weather, both day and night, is necessary to make one truly appreciate the skill and talent of the typical airline flight deck crew.

After being oriented to the work place, the physician is better able to make sound recommendations regarding environmental health surveys. Such recommendations normally are made in consultation with an industrial hygienist or technician. Frequently, the physician who sees an occupationally induced illness will recommend an environmental survey of that particular work place to determine the appropriate corrective measures. Having visited the work place, the physician is much more sensitive to the potential for specific categories of occupational illness for a particular employee. Further, the physician can make a more rationale recommendation regarding the degree of work restrictions for a convalescing employee returning to work but yet not fully recovered.

Consultation and Advice to Management

The airline medical department has an opportunity to serve management in a far wider role than simply by its clinical activities. This consultative role may range from international health activities to aircraft accident investigation.

Health and Sanitation

For those United States air carriers operating in the international air carrier system, the medical department must be up to date regarding disease incidence and prevalence in the regions of the world served by the airline. It will be necessary to establish and maintain the immunologic status of aircrews and to ensure appropriate prophylaxis for diseases such as malaria. Crews must be educated in ways of reducing the potential exposure to foodborne diseases and in awareness of the hazards of hepatitis, tuberculosis, and other contagious diseases. It is appropriate that a member of the medical staff visit the various domiciliary sites throughout the international route structure. Necessary health care must be provided for in the same way that such care is provided in the domestic setting. It is the responsibility of the medical department to ensure the competency of the local physician who is to care for the aircrew.

Although the subject of international sanitation is covered by various regulatory agencies, the airline medical department should have some established methods to validate such standards periodically. Inspection of food service facilities providing local support to the airline is an obvious responsibility. Such inspections should stress sanitation, including food and water sources, refrigerative storage, and insect and rodent control. The source of potable water and the way it's handled should be inspected and tested.

The medical department periodically should review the insect control methods employed by the airline. Although disinsection is also a subject of international health regulations, options are available to the airline, and the aviation medical physician should make sure that the most effective methods available are being employed while creating minimal inconvenience to the air traveling public.

Human Factors

Working closely with the engineering department, the aeromedical physician can provide expert advice on human fac-

tors in aeronautic systems. During the upgrading of aircraft or the purchase of new equipment, the opportunity occurs to ensure that human factors are considered and optimized. Aircraft cockpit instrumentation has been undergoing a revolution and currently is capable of presenting nearly any dynamic information desired in a vast array of formulations via a number of cathode ray tube displays (CRT) or flat-plate displays. The physician should be prepared to advise on the selection of such instrumentation with regard to alphanumerics, character size, color rendition, brightness, and impact to overall aircrew work load.

The flight deck crew may request consultation regarding the use of sunglasses, visual corrective devices, including contact lenses, and other issues related to the visual environment of the cockpit.

Within the human factors arena, one area is exceptionally sensitive between management and the union. This area relates to optimizing the work-rest cycle with regard to aircrew duties. Management's desires and requirements, as voiced through operations, may have significant counterpoint among the flight crew, including both cabin and flight deck personnel. Although regulatory requirements have been established, considerable leeway for implementation is left in the hands of airline management. The medical department can provide sound scientific advice and assist in selecting the optimal solution for scheduling crew duty.

A specialist in aerospace medicine is expected to provide consultation to management on a variety of human factors related to airline operation. Additional concerns are situations resulting from the environmental flight conditions at altitude. Such issues as the quantity, flow rates, and types of oxygen equipment to be provided both in the cabin and on the flight deck are issues where the medical specialist can provide advice. In dealing with the subject of hypobarics, advice can be provided regarding the pressurization differential, the reliability of the system, and planning contingency operations in case of rapid decompression. Other altitude-related factors include the potential for industrial radiation exposure to both cabin and flight deck crews. This issue becomes a concern with high-altitude flying aircraft such as the supersonic transport and the occasional wide-body jet routinely flying above 13,000 m, where measured radiation levels from solar flare and cosmic bombardment can produce hazards. Generally, the question is one of chronic exposure based on industrial standards for the working life of the crewmember; thus, the energy of radiation received, duration of exposure, methods of dosimetry, and procedures for protection are areas for recommendation and consultation.

Human factors related to ground escape by passengers in an emergency ground egress scenario are subject to medical advice. Medical input to training is often helpful with regard to emergency escape, use of onboard oxygen equipment, number, location, and content of onboard emergency first-aid kits, type and number of smoke masks, and other aspects of emergency aircraft operation.

Other factors related to the aviation environment, such as sudden descent in turbulence, ozone contamination of the cabin air, and the issues of diurnal work-rest cycles related to flying safety, provide a challenge to the airline medical director.

Aircraft Accident Investigation

The initial steps in any accident investigation begin well before the actual event. It is important that the airline medical director and his staff consider the improbable and develop procedures for handling a multitude of challenges that will arise when an aircraft is involved in a serious accident. It is important to ensure that emergency equipment, facilities, and personnel are available at airports serviced by the airline. The medical director should

be aware of the procedures at these major airports in case of an on-field accident or an off-field catastrophe.

Once the event has occurred, the physician assumes some part of the responsibility in coordinating and monitoring the treatment and disposition of survivors. Concern is directed toward both crew and passengers. Once the press of the emergency has subsided, the physician must then turn to the difficult task of informing the family and friends of those aboard the aircraft. It is important that an airline representative be available to answer questions and when possible to allay concern. In the situation where deaths occur as a result of the accident, the airline medical department will be asked to assist in the identification of the deceased. Such activities must be coordinated with the National Transportation Safety Board (NTSB) and the local medical authority, whether it be the coroner's office, the sheriff's department, or the local justice of the peace. Frequently, resources are not available at the accident site to provide the necessary forensic support, and the airline may find it necessary to bring professionals with this experience to the site.

Among the many agencies involved in an aircraft accident investigation, the NTSB is charged with the primary investigative responsibilities. Medical personnel from the airline may be requested to provide assistance to the investigative effort, but more probably these individuals will be involved in dealing with circumstances and situations peculiar to airline operations. If it becomes evident that human factors are involved in the accident, the medical department will wish to work very closely with airline operations to reduce the probability of similar events recurring within the airline. Once the immediate ramifications of the accident have been resolved, a time will come when the medical director will be asked to assist the airline's legal department in handling the inevitable litigation that will arise from the accident. Scientific and expert medical advice can provide invaluable assistance in developing the airline's legal position. It should be pointed out, however, that such legal advice does not prevent the physician from being requested to participate at the direction of the NTSB in their investigative procedures. It would not be uncommon for the medical records of the crew in the accident aircraft to be subpoenaed as part of the investigative procedures and for the physician to be asked to appear and testify relative to those records.

PASSENGER AND CARGO SERVICES

The obligation of a common carrier to receive and transport passengers and freight without discriminating in the choice of accommodations has come down from the common law of medieval Europe. The travel and transportation of goods in those early days was considerably more hazardous, and the merchant was dependent on the carrier. Thus, it was decided that the carrier was liable for damages if he refused to accept goods for transport. The logical development was to extend this obligation to passengers as well. Consequently, from the beginning of the establishment of our judicial system, it has been recognized as the duty of a common carrier to accept and carry without discrimination those who offered themselves as passengers. The carrier also was charged with the responsibility to transport its passengers safely to their destination. This extraordinary responsibility has served society well, despite the revolutionary changes that have occurred in the modes of transportation. It is a long way from the sailing ship to the palatial ocean liner, from ancient caravans to the modern passenger train, from the oxcart to the automobile, and from the stagecoach to the airliner of today.

Passenger Services

Services provided the typical airline passenger range from adequate to opulent.

The passenger is reasonably secure in the belief that he will travel from his point of departure to his destination in a safe and timely fashion. The airline will make a reasonable effort to ensure his comfort and will diligently try to satisfy all reasonable requests. Efforts are made to cater to the needs of the young and the aged and to provide for the physically handicapped. It is considered the law, however, that one who is so mentally or physically infirm as to be unable to care for himself or who may become a burden on his fellow passengers or demand medical assistance may be refused transport. Should an infirm passenger be voluntarily accepted, his inability to care for himself having been made evident to the airline prior to or at the time of his acceptance, a greater duty and responsibility are placed on the carrier. This section does not address those passengers who, in fact, are patients and require aeromedical transportation because this was covered in Chapter 19, "The Passenger and the Patient in Flight." If the passenger becomes ill or helpless after having started the journey, it is considered the duty of the carrier to extend reasonable and necessary help to him until suitable provisions can be made. This duty may require that the passenger be removed from the aircraft and left at a suitable place until he is well enough to resume his journey or obtains other appropriate aid. A carrier's duty to other passengers cannot be overlooked, however, in observing the rights of any individual traveler. If a passenger's conduct or condition is such as to render his presence dangerous or offensive to fellow passengers or create a serious annoyance or discomfort to those passengers, it is the duty of the airline to remove him. These general guidelines have been tested extensively in the courts.

One example of a court's decision is in the case of Casteel versus American Airlines, Inc. This case involved an initial acceptance to carry a passenger who was known to be very ill with tuberculosis and was subsequently removed because his condition worsened en route. The courts concluded that the nature of the business and the machine made it almost necessary that the court sanction a reasonable discretion in these matters on the part of the operator and that their judgment, if exercised in good faith and on reasonable grounds, should be accepted prima facie as justification. The Civil Aeronautics Passenger Rules Tariff is quite specific on the carrier's rsponsibilities, rights, and liabilities.

Transporting the Ill Patient

To accommodate a stretcher patient, several commercial airline carriers have developed unique and convenient stretcher kits that fit essentially all aircraft without the necessity of removing seats. These kits are located strategically at several airports along the flight route and are ready for quick installation. The seatbacks are designed to fold down into the arms of the seat, and a stretcher platform is then secured over these folded-down seats adjacent to the windows. A foam rubber mattress is placed on top of the platform to make a more comfortable bed. The seats on the aisle are available for the patient's attendant, who must accompany any stretcher passenger. To provide privacy, curtains can be attached to the overhead storage compartment and surround the four seats containing the stretcher. It should be evident, however, that transportation of this type is not without some considerable expense because this requires paying for four first-class seats. It is obvious that prior arrangements must be made with the airline.

It is not uncommon for an airline medical director to be consulted regarding the possible transportation of an ill passenger. In the majority of cases, arrangements can be made for the adequate and safe transport of the passenger. Provisions can be made for special diets and for medical oxygen. If it is not possible to load the pas-

senger via the standard ramp, or mobile lounge, arrangements can be made for a forklift or an elevating truck bed. Passengers with orthopedic apparatus who can not board through the normal passenger door frequently can be boarded using the galley entrance.

In-flight Medical Incidents

One major airline reports experiencing approximately 1500 to 2000 in-flight medical incidents per year. This number represents about one incident per 10 million passenger-miles flown. Despite the potential of serious illness developing during flight, the incidence has proved to be quite low. Nevertheless, airlines do make nonscheduled landings to obtain either emergency medical aid for an ill patient or to seek consultation about and relief of non-life–threatening symptoms. Experience has shown that these diversions occur once per 2 million passengers carried, or once per approximately 3000 million passenger-miles flown. Preplanning by the potential passenger and, when in doubt, consultation with the airline medical department can minimize untold developments occurring in flight. Deaths occurring in flight from natural causes have likewise proved to be infrequent events and can be expected to occur approximately once each 2 to 3 million passengers flown. The same airline reports further that there were a total of 287 injuries in 1 year, in which 5.8 million passengers were carried 5650 million passenger-miles. During the same time frame, the number of illnesses reported in flight totaled 342. (Tables 24–1 and 24–2).

There is a periodic interest in requiring air carriers to provide a more extensive first-aid kit on board than is currently required by federal regulation. Currently, the airline is required to have suitable equipment available to treat injuries likely to occur in flight or in minor accidents and provided in a quantity appropriate to the number of passengers and crew accom-

Table 24–1. Passenger Injury Experience For a Major Air Carrier

Type of Injury	Number
Contusions/sprains	*238*
Inside aircraft	118
On steps	91
In terminal	10
Struck by objects	11
Struck by seat belt buckle	8
Burns	*29*
Spilled food	25
Exploding matches	3
Fuel in eyes	1
Lacerations	*13*
Dental injury	4
Ear injury	3
Total	287

Table 24–2. Passenger Illness Experience For a Major Air Carrier

Type of Illness	Number
Cardiovascular	124
Respiratory	87
Neuropsychiatric (including 25 cases of airsickness)	55
Gastrointestinal	28
Eye, ear, nose, and throat	26
Other (Diabetes, Dermatologic, Orthopedic)	22
Total	342

modated in the airplane. These provisions have been further expanded by FAA interpretation to recommend specifically that each kit should be dust-proof and moisture-proof and contain only materials that meet federal specifications and should contain as a minimum the following: adhesive compresses, bandage compresses, rubber bandages, triangular bandages, ammonia inhalants, burn ointment, antiseptic swabs, tape, limb splints, and scissors.

Many international airlines carry medical kits that are to be opened only by proper medical personnel in the case of a serious in-flight medical emergency. It has been proposed that airlines in the United States should carry as a minimum a kit with equipment and supplies to aid in the treatment of heart attack, allergic reactions, seizures, diabetic comas, choking, and bleeding. Bills introduced by Con-

gress also would recommend providing liability immunity for the airline physician or flight crew providing emergency care. Supplies in such a medical kit should include stethoscope, blood pressure cuff, digitalis, nitroglycerin, epinephrine, and plasma expanders.

A counter argument put forward by the airlines and the FAA is that emergencies requiring such medical support seldom arise. Should such an emergency occur, it would be necessary for someone trained in medical resuscitation to be on board the aircraft and, of course, for an airline representative to determine, while aloft, the appropriate training or credentials of the individual who may come forward to provide assistance. Dr. F.O. Hemming of Canadian Pacific Air has stated that it is rather futile to call for a physician to handle in-flight medical emergencies and expect him to perform without appropriate equipment. On board 70% of their international flights there are one or more physicians, and the medical kits currently provided have been used on an average of 1.4 times per week. The kit's use is restricted to physicians because of the potent drugs it contains. The issue of proper security for the kits has been solved by this particular airline.[4] Air Canada has developed an on board medical kit for use by passenger-physicians. The contents are listed in Table 24–3. On the average the kit is used once per week somewhere in the system[5].

Cargo Service

The medical department will be expected to establish protective health standards for the carriage of dangerous or toxic cargo. Such cargos that are rather frequently carried in the cargo compartments of aircraft include radioactive materials, live virulent cultures for manufacturers and research laboratories, toxic gases, including carbon dioxide from the off-gasing of dry ice, and dangerous or diseased animals. The medical department needs to

Table 24–3.   Contents of the Doctor's Medical Kit Carried on Air Canada Aircraft

2	0.9% Sodium Chloride injection, USP 250 ml
2	5% Dextrose injection, USP 250 ml
1	Blood pressure manometer
2	Lastorel gauze bandages
2	Venipuncture kit: 21 infusion set, Merthiolate, gauze pads, roll tape, tourniquet, alcohol prep pak
1	Ventolin salbutamol inhaler
4	Adrenalin 1 mg (epinephrine) injection USP
2	SolmuMedrol 125 mg USP (methylprednisolone sodium succuinate)
2	Benadryl 50 mg (diphenhydramine hydrochloride) injection USP
2	Dextrose 50% 50 ml—500 mg/ml—USP
1	Intropin 200 mg—500 ml (dopamine hydrochloride)
2	Valium 10 mg (diazepam) injection USP
2	Aminophylline 50 mg/ml injection
3	Morphine sulfate injection 15 mg
2	Isuprel 5 ml hydrochloride (isoproterenol hydrochloride) injection USP
2	Atropine 0.6 mg/ml sulfate injection USP
2	Lasix 40 mg (furosemide) injection USP
2	Xylocard 100 mg (lidocaine hydrochloride) injection USP
2	Calcium gluconate 10% injection USP
4	Sodium bicarbonate 7.5% 50 ml injection USP
2	Sterile water for injection USP 10 ml
5	Nitrostat tabs 0.3 mg
1	Lifesaver tube
1	Emergency tracheal catheter 2"
1	Stethoscope
1	Solution administration set 2.4 m long with Y-injection site
1	Flashlight
1	Diastix–Glucose in urine tests
1	Cuticular surgical needle ⅜
1	Skin closures
1	3-0 Chromic Gut (Catgut Chrome) 45 cm Absorbable surgical suture, USP
1	Instrument set: Needle holder, scissors s/b, tissue forceps, gauze sponges
1	Needle–21 g 1½
8	Disposable syringes—(1) 1cc; (2) 3cc; (2) 5cc; (2) 10cc; (1) 20cc
2	Vinyl medical glove
1	Urinary catheter
1	Thermometer
2	Intracath
2	Fiorinal C capsules

be available to assist in making arrangements and to advise on the proper management of personnel and facilities involved in transporting potentially hazardous cargo. In the unlikely event that there is a misadventure resulting in spill or leakage, on-site medical support at the airport may be required to ensure the safe and proper clean-up and protection of personnel.

COST-EFFECTIVENESS OF AN AIRLINE MEDICAL DEPARTMENT

The resources necessary to support an airline medical department must compete with the other areas of expenditure on the airline's cost ledger. Because it is the nature of the airline medical department to provide long-range, tangible cost benefits, it becomes difficult to establish the cost-effectiveness ratio for these departments solely on the basis of short-term gains. Nevertheless, it is essential if one is to ensure the survivability of such departments to clearly demonstrate the cost-effectiveness to the airline profit motive. The medical program should not be considered as primarily a fringe benefit or an altruistic expression by the airline toward its employees. A viable, dynamic, preventive program conducted by the airline medical department makes smart business sense.

Few airline medical departments have accumulated and maintained records sufficient to establish a sophisticated cost-benefits analysis. One major exception was the medical department of Trans World Airlines (TWA), and these data have been reported by Anderson and Gullet.[6] In 1971, Kulak and colleagues[7] reported a study on in-flight airline pilot incapacitation. Age-specific incident rates of fatal and nonfatal causes of career termination for an 11-year period were compiled from members of the Airline Pilots Association (ALPA). When the rates of incapacitation were compared with national population norms, the pilots fared far better in all disease categories and in all age groupings, with the exception of younger pilots dying from aircraft accidents. The "healthy worker effect" was clearly evident in the rates derived from this study. Two other important points are evident in the review of this important epidemiologic investigation. First, it was possible to establish an expected incident rate for potential serious in-flight pilot failure, and second, the data provides a baseline to compare a dynamic preventive medicine program under airline medical sponsorship.

Based on these epidemiologic findings, the expected incident rate for in-flight failure was established for serious disease manifestations such as sudden coronary death or convulsive seizures. These estimates are presented in Table 24–4. As is evident, annual in-flight pilot incapacitation is estimated to be extremely low, and it would be difficult to justify an airline medical program purely on the premise of reducing these already low estimations.

The study conducted by Anderson and Gullett[6] addressed the long-term payback potential of a preventive medicine program for airline pilots. Over time, many airlines changed the emphasis of their traditional cockpit crew safety medical examinations to a more comprehensive program that stressed the principles of preventive medicine. Because of the enormous expenses incurred in pilot training and in disability programs, efforts were geared to ameliorate diseases that could be most effectively addressed by preventive measures. Aviation safety has remained an important consideration, but the emphasis clearly has shifted to one of economics. This approach has taken on even greater significance as the flight deck crew have grown older with the stability of the airline industry in the past several decades.

The medical director of TWA retained the authority to determine the eligibility for pilot disability benefits and whether the individual qualified for disability retirement status should the crewman inadvertently lose his medical certification. Consequently, the medical department has been able to maintain oversight and records on each incident of pilot disability occurring at the airline since 1948.

The study conducted by Kulak and colleagues[7] previously described and a subsequent study that was published as part of the report *The National Institute of Aging, Panel on the Experienced Pilot Study*[8] served as a comparison base for the TWA program.

The crew disability rate reported for the TWA pilots remained remarkably constant from 1962, averaging 7.9 pilots per 1000 man-years. This occurred during a period when the average age of the aircrew increased from 36 to over 46 years. The progressive decline in the age-adjusted disability rate at TWA was influenced most significantly by a drop in the rate of dis-

Table 24–4.   Estimated Probability of Pilot In-Flight Incapacitation

Age Group	Annual Events
30–34	1/58,000 pilots
35–39	1/36,000 pilots
40–44	1/16,000 pilots
45–49	1/9500 pilots
50–54	1/5500 pilots
55–59	1/3500 pilots

From Kulak, L.L., Wick, R.L., and Billings, C.E.: Epidemiological study of in-flight airline pilot incapacitation. Aerospace Med., 42(6):670–672, 1971.

Table 24–5. Estimated Cost Avoidance Associated With TWA Pilot Preventive Medicine Program

| Age | Pilot Wastage | | Net Gain | Cost Avoidance* (million dollars) |
	TWA Experience	Expected Experience		
35–44	22	27	5	3.5
45–54	28	53	25	13.0
55–59	49	71	22	9.8
Total	99	151	52	26.3

*Cost based on $200,000 per pilot in training and disability payments. From Anderson, R., and Gullett, C.C.: Airline pilot disability: Economic impact of an airline preventive medicine program. Aviat. Space Environ. Med., 53(4):398–402, 1982.

ability for pilots in the oldest age group, followed by a lesser drop in the 45 to 49-year-old and 50- to 54-year-old age groups. This decline in disability rates in the older age groups suggested a major influence from TWA's preventive medicine program. Undocumented reports from several sources suggest that those airlines not providing preventive medicine programs will experience disability rates significantly higher than has been the demonstrated case with TWA. When the baseline studies were compared with the TWA study, the age-adjusted rate of disability resulting from disease in TWA pilots was significantly better than those from ALPA-represented pilots (7.92/1000 to 10.92/1000, with P< 0.0005).

Comparison with the ALPA disability data supports the thesis that the TWA pilots became disabled at a rate significantly below that of other airline pilots. An appropriate assumption has been made that this difference is attributable to the comprehensive medical program.

To quantify the economic impact, a detailed analysis of cost benefits to TWA was developed and is summarized in Table 24–5. The preventive medicine program demonstrated the ability to reduce the disability of airline pilots by one-third while demonstrating a cost avoidance to the airline exceeding 6 million annually, with a yield-to-investment ratio of 6.1. It is difficult to establish the cost savings of a non-event that has been avoided; however, it is an economic reality that within a free enterprise system these economic factors must be determined. Excellent records, sound data, and sophisticated analyses conducted over time are required to establish cost-benefit ratios.

The medical departments of United States air carriers will be expected to meet numerous responsibilities in providing for the physical and mental health of personnel and to contribute to the economic well-being of the airline. A properly conducted and managed medical department will satisfy the expectations of the corporation by providing a professional aviation medicine service and at the same time assist the airline in conserving valuable resources. The physician trained as a specialist in aerospace medicine is best able to bring to bear the numerous disciplines necessary to manage and administer an airline medical department.

REFERENCES

1. Aerospace Facts and Figures, 1982/83. Washington, D.C., Aerospace Industrial Association of America Inc. 1982.
2. Alter, J.D., and Mohler, S.R.: Preventive medicine aspects and health promotion programs for flight attendants. Aviat. Space Environ. Med., 51(2):168–175, 1980.
3. Norwood, G.K.: Senior Aviation Medical Examiners Conducting FAA First-Class Medical Examinations. FAA-AM-71-38, U.S. Government Printing Office, Washington D.C., Federal Aviation Administration, 1971.
4. Hemming, F.O.: In-flight medical kits. Letters to the Editor. Aviat. Week Space Technology, 23 January, 1983.
5. Saint-Pierre, A.F.: Personal communications, 1984.
6. Anderson, R., and Gullett, C.C.: Airline pilot dis-

ability: Economic impact of an airline preventive medicine program. Aviat. Space Environ. Med., 53(4):398–402, 1982.

7. Kulak, L.L., Wick, R.L., Jr., and Billings, C.E.: Epidemiological study of in-flight airline pilot incapacitation. Aerospace Med., 42(6):670–672, 1971.

8. Report of the National Institute on Aging. Panel on the Experienced Pilot Study. Bethesda, Maryland, United States Department of Health and Human Services, U.S. Government Printing Office, Washington, D.C., 1981.

Chapter 25

Aeromedical Rehabilitation and Health Promotion for Civilian Professional Aircrew

Richard L. Masters

The Divine Hippocrates informs us, that when a physician visits a patient, he ought to inquire into many things, by putting questions to the patient and to bystanders. You must ask, says he, what uneasiness he is under, what was the cause of it, how many days he had been ill, how his belly is affected and what food he eats. To which I presume to add one interrogation more; namely, what trade he is of. . . .But I find it very seldom minded in the common course of practice, or if the physician knows it without asking he takes little notice of it.

BERNARDINO RAMAZZINI, 1700

Approximately 40,000 professional airline pilots in the United States are employed by some 45 air carriers. These carriers are classified by the Civil Aeronautics Board according to income as major, national, and regional carriers. The carriers also range in size, as measured by the number of pilots employed, from those employing over 5000 pilots to those with less than 25 pilots. Fewer than 50% of United States airline pilots work for companies employing a full-time medical director. Air carrier size generally is unrelated to the employment of a physician because large carriers may have no physician or may employ several physicians. Small carriers usually employ no physician, or they maintain a consulting relationship with a physician in the local community where the carrier is based. Hence, a significant number of professional airline pilots do not receive the services of a formal corporate medical department, making the provision of alternative specialty resources necessary. In terms of aerospace medicine specialty representation in private practice, these other sources have been insufficiently provided. The long-standing lack of aerospace medicine specialist support for many professional airline pilots has necessitated the development of resources through the initiative of the airline pilots' representative union (the Airline Pilots Association, or ALPA). This chapter outlines the scope of aeromedical problems facing professional airline pilots and the services provided by medical and other professional resources outside of airline medical departments.

AEROMEDICAL SERVICES

Needed and Provided Medical Services

Professional airline pilots constitute one of the few professions in which sustained good health is an absolute prerequisite for productivity and employment. The airline pilot not only must meet Federal Aviation Administration (FAA) periodic certification examinations but also is expected to maintain his health in a manner consonant with the highest level of air safety. When medical problems arise, the airline pilot must seek specialty evaluation, treatment, rehabilitation, and continuing care and then be prepared to undergo recertification evaluations. Pilots must seek medical services from various resources, especially if none of these services is provided by an airline medical department. Employers typically do not provide FAA periodic certification examinations but may assist pilots in special follow-up evaluations and referral to specialists in the event disqualifying conditions raise questions as to their continued eligibility for flying duties. Air carrier physicians do not routinely provide medical treatment but may assist in the referral of pilots to competent treatment resources and in the oversight of rehabilitation, continuing care, and monitoring. The pilot who does not have medical services provided by his airline must seek those services in the private market. How these services are provided, by whom, at what facilities, as well as quality and quantity, are proper matter for consideration. As with all medical care, the quality will vary from physician to physician and from health facility to health facility. Ideally, the aerospace medical specialist provides the major source of quality control. The number of such specialists, unfortunately, is limited.

Federal Aviation Administration Periodic Medical Certification Examinations

The FAA requires periodic medical certification examinations of all airmen who operate aircraft. The details and protocols of such examinations are specified in the applicable portions of the Federal Aviation Regulations (FARS). Detailed information pertaining to medical certification and to the requirements are contained in the chapter entitled "Federal Aviation Administration's Responsibilities in Aerospace Medicine." Periodic FAA examinations are designed to determine whether an individual meets FAA standards. The examinations are conducted by designated physician aviation medical examiners (AMEs), who are selected and trained by the FAA and who are geographically distributed throughout the United States. In addition, some AMEs are located overseas. The examinations are not designed to encourage or require the practice of preventive medicine because they constitute an examination of an individual's physical condition at a static point in time. Further, the FARs do not require that agency to practice preventive medicine. The AME is required to determine whether an airman meets the medical standards, and if so, that physician is empowered to issue the airman's FAA medical certificate. The results of the examinations are forwarded to the FAA, where they undergo further scrutiny to determine whether the decision made was consonant with the regulations. If the airman is qualified, his certificate remains in force for a specified period of time, and he merely is required to have future evaluations at established intervals. Airline pilots seek their FAA examinations from senior AMEs, physicians designated to perform Class 1 FAA physician examinations. AMEs assume varying degrees of responsibility for the pilots they examine. For example, some AMEs may feel that, acting as an agent of the federal government, they are required strictly to perform the examination and make no basic decisions if any disqualifying condition is dicovered. This minimal service often is inadequate, and the pilot may have to seek further evaluation elsewhere. Other AMEs will do what is necessary to get thorough specialists' evaluations and follow-up to ensure that the information presented to the FAA is as complete as possible. A recent study found the quality of physical examinations given by the FAA examiners to be uneven and recommendations were advanced both to improve the quality and to expand the content of examinations.[1]

Federal Aviation Administration Special Follow-up Evaluations

In the event that the AME or FAA physicians determine that some conditions may not be in accordance with the standards, special follow-up evaluations may be required. For example, a pilot having borderline hypertension and receiving treatment with diuretics may be allowed to fly but be required to have follow-up evaluations specifically directed at his blood pressure and cardiovascular health. Such evaluations may be requested by the AME, the pilot's personal physician, or a medical specialist. The determining factor here is the protocol for the follow-up evaluation, as well as which physician would be expected to provide the information to the FAA. As mentioned earlier, the information sometimes can be provided by the AME; at other times, specialists' follow-up evaluations are required at specified intervals.

Specialists' Evaluations

When a deviation from normal is detected, the pilot usually is directed to a medical specialist. The specialist provides information necessary for the AME and the FAA to make a determination as to whether the pilot meets the standards and, if not, whether the standards could be set aside in a particular instance without ad-

versely affecting flight safety. The full range of medical specialists are employed in these evaluations, but the most common medical specialties consulted are cardiology, ophthalmology, otorhinolaryngology, neuropsychiatry, and, to a lesser degree, the other specialties. The airline pilot usually cannot identify highly qualified specialists for a particular condition. Hence, the specialists in aerospace medicine should refer the airmen to appropriate high-quality specialists. Because the FAA must depend almost entirely on the quality of the medical reports submitted to it in determining an airman's continued eligibility for medical certification, a deficient, incomplete, or overly brief report serves neither the airman nor the interests of aviation safety.

Treatment

The full scope of medical specialty practice is brought to bear on various problems affecting the health of pilots. Again, the most commonly required treatment pertains to disorders of the cardiovascular system (including hypertension). The aim of treatment must be to restore the pilot to his premorbid condition and to ensure that his recovery returns him to a level of functioning that is fully consistent with the safe and efficient performance of his duties. Oversight of the health and specific medical problems of pilots is the proper responsibility of the specialist in aerospace medicine. He acts, in a narrow sense, as the generalist and ensures, through appropriate consultation, that the highest quality medical treatment is focused on complete recovery and/or rehabilitation. Specialists in aerospace medicine can play a very important role in the management of a given patient if they choose to be in charge of treatment, utilizing specialists for required areas. Usually, however, they play a somewhat different role, monitoring the treatment and the pilot's progress after having directed him to the highest quality resources. They can be helpful in explaining to the specialists the requirements for FAA medical certification, the requirements for return to work specified by particular air carriers, and any special needs in preparing the pilot for reconsideration and recertification. Often, they must take special precautions to ensure that the pilot continues after the normal course of treatment into the stages of recovery and rehabilitation necessary for a return to flying duties, which may not be recognized by the treating physician. The treating physician often may have one goal in mind, whereas the goal required of persons treating professional pilots may be quite different.

Rehabilitation

The aim of rehabilitation of a pilot cannot be limited. Rather, rehabilitation must be aimed in every aspect toward returning him to a level of optimal functioning consistent with his ability to return to duty. The importance of rehabilitation cannot be overemphasized because of the necessity, both economic and humane, to preserve and protect the professional capabilities of pilots. The costs of training an airline pilot are estimated to range between $250,000 and $500,000. It thus is not feasible to discard such highly skilled professionals as long as they can be rehabilitated and safely returned to their flying duties. In achieving the major aim of the reestablishment of full premorbid functional capacity, the flight surgeon must be guided by his comprehensive knowledge of job requirements, physical capacity, the aviation environment, and the details of man-machine interactions. Often , the professional airman finds himself in a situation in which guidance by specialists in aerospace medicine is required. Rehabilitation experts should rely on this background knowledge in individualizing the rehabilitation plan for optimal results. An example of this would be the situation in which the rehabilitation is directed toward a return of functional ca-

pacity, say, of an injured ankle. The orthopedist or the rehabilitation director may be quite satisfied if the person is able to walk, whereas a professional pilot must aim his rehabilitation at the point where ankle function is compatible not only with the use of rudder pedals under normal operating conditions but also under emergency conditions when power boost is lost. Factors such as these may be unknown to the treating physician and can provide delays and misunderstandings in the ultimate attempt to regain flying duties.

Continuing Care and Monitoring

Certain illnesses may require that a pilot undergo continuing care and that his condition be monitored for extended periods of time. For example, an individual who has been rehabilitated following a cardiovascular disability should be monitored periodically by specialists' evaluations. Reevaluations necessary to the continuing certification and qualification for flying duties must be timely, complete, and accurate. Certification decisions are affected by the ability of the FAA to ensure themselves of continued stability of the pilot's medical condition. This becomes especially critical in the special services area, notably alcoholism rehabilitation, and will be addressed later in this chapter.

Recertification Evaluations

Following prolonged illnesses or conditions resulting in decertification, the FAA, upon petition from the airman, will consider recertification. Such reconsideration is judged on the individual's state of health, appropriate treatment, and state of rehabilitation. The FAA requires complete information pertaining to the pilot's medical history and treatment, as well as documented evidence of recovery. Recertification judgments are based on the airman's ability to return to his cockpit duties free of any condition deemed detrimental to the safe performance of duties.

Final determination of certifiability rests with the FAA but must, of course, depend on accurate documentation submitted by the applicant's physician.

Other Evaluations

The professional airman's career is punctuated by various evaluations and physical examinations that are required for a number of reasons. For example, the professional airman frequently comes to air carrier employment from a background of military service and has undergone a number of physical examinations during his military career. Also, many air carrier pilots maintain their affiliation with Air National Guard and reserve units after their separation from active duty and incur additional physical examination requirements. Preemployment physical examinations are required for a number of air carriers. Some air carriers, however, simply will accept a pilot as physically qualified for the job if he is able to demonstrate that he can hold a Class 1 FAA medical certificate. Some carriers also require periodic physical examinations. Carriers also may require evaluations following long illnesses or when there is reason to believe that the pilot may not meet medical standards. Examinations to determine eligibility for medical disability, as well as for purposes of termination evaluations, inevitably are required. These evaluations are obtained from various resources, either at the direction of the requesting organization or at the selection of the individual airman. In the case of disputed claims, a neutral physician sometimes is selected to make the final determination. Often, disability determinations rest on the opinion of the pilot's personal physician, and he may be unfamiliar with the specific requirements of the airline environment. In cases where the pilot's physician believes that his patient is disabled, the company physician may feel otherwise. In most instances, final disability determination depends on the applicant fulfilling a certain specified set of procedures that are designed to be fair to the disabled pilot as well as to the providers of the funds that support disability payments.

Factors Affecting System Efficiency

Mechanisms for providing health care to professional airline pilots lack uniformity. Standardization may occur within a specific airline medical department, but there is, for all practical purposes, no uniformity between airline medical departments. For those carriers not having medical departments, there often is not even a foundation for establishing uniformity. Some air carriers adopt the physical standards of the FAA as their own; other airlines have physical standards that are applied by their medical departments, whereas still others may have physical standards that are unwritten or are interpreted by laymen. In the airline industry, there is little or no horizontal mobility between jobs. That is, the airline pilot working for one carrier is not free to seek employment from other carriers without great financial loss to himself and loss of seniority, to say nothing of the difficulty of getting a job with another carrier.

Some carriers have good disability insurance benefits available for pilots who lose their medical certificates. Other airlines have a less desirable plan, and still others have no medical disability insurance at all. Within the medical disability insurance programs, some carriers allow pilots to be retained on the disability rolls for certain periods of time so that, upon recovery, eventual return to flying status is possible. Few carriers require a pilot's removal from the seniority roll as soon as he begins to collect disability insurance.

Because airline pilots' careers are so directly affected by physical standards and various medical conditions, they have an understandable tendency to fear those individuals who make medical qualification decisions. Aerospace medicine has not escaped the general suspicion that has been borne of late by practitioners of occupational medicine, that is, the concern related to conflict of interest on the part of the professionals handling health matters. Pilots, too, often display this distrust. Although the FAA makes every effort to apply standards in a uniform fashion, they do operate under the principle that each case should be given individual consideration, and, therefore, the real or perceived uneven application of standards from case to case may occur.

A major factor affecting system efficiency is the lack of sufficient numbers of aeromedical specialists throughout the country. Very few aeromedical specialists have been trained, and very few are being attracted to the field; however, the need for these specialists is not diminishing. The sporadic disappearance of airline medical departments does nothing to diminish the need but shifts the burden to aeromedical specialists in private practice.

For a preventive medicine system to be effective, knowledge of the epidemiologic background of the population is needed. Hidden diseases within the population are possible and are a matter of continuing concern. The incidence and prevalence of disease within the population of airline pilots is difficult to determine. The systematic collection of such information is lacking. Airline medical departments may be reluctant to share data. FAA medical data lack closure information. For example, if a pilot takes an FAA examination one day, he conceivably could become ill the next day and never fly again because of that illness, but the FAA might never know about the illness. The FAA does not have a systematic follow-up program for detecting unreported disease, and the open-ended nature of their information system thus renders their "epidemiologic" evaluations incomplete. In a recent report, the National Academy of Sciences has pointed to this deficiency of systematic data collection and has recommended long-term remedies[1]

ADVISORY SERVICES

The unavailability and lack of uniformity of medical services for airline pilots caused the Board of Directors of the Airline Pilots Association (ALPA) to establish the position of Aeromedical Advisor in 1968. The ALPA represents approximately 33,000 professional airline pilots in the United States. The position of Aeromedical Advisor was established to provide advice and guidance to the president and national officers of ALPA and professional medical advisory assistance to the membership. Besides counseling the president and other national officers on all matters pertaining to the general health and welfare of the membership, the Aeromedical Advisor's office is also responsible for maintaining a liaison with the FAA and the awareness of technical and scientific advances in medicine and its various specialties as they pertain to problems in the flight environment, human factors, and related areas. Liaison also is maintained with airline medical departments where indicated. Any member of the ALPA may, upon request, receive advisory services from the office as a provision of his membership. A very important continuing function of the Aeromedical Advisor's office is to develop and encourage the practice of preventive medicine in its broadest aspects. The goals of this function are as follows:

1. Promotion of health education
2. Early diagnosis and treatment
3. Limitation of disability
4. Rehabilitation
5. Return to the cockpit where possible
6. Protecting, preserving, and lengthening the productive life and health of professional pilots

Preventive Medicine and Health Maintenance

Principles and Practice

Given the interdependent relationship between maintaining good health and preserving a career in aviation, there is ample motivation for the provision of preventive-oriented medical services. The official policy of ALPA is to provide for a broad preventive medicine program and to encourage the membership to maintain the highest levels of health. Ongoing efforts in these areas may fall short of total success; however, they must be pursued with vigor.

Services and Providers

Comprehensive programs involving a sound patient-physician relationship, accomplishing thorough preventive-oriented physical examinations, counseling and directing clients in preventive measures, and formal programs aimed at diminishing or deferring the impact of career-threatening diseases are scarce indeed. The handful of physicians who offer such programs around the country are too few. Besides the specific programs offered by ALPA in the areas of preventive cardiology and alcoholism prevention and rehabilitation, a few centers and practitioners offer a comprehensive type of service to pilots. Some pilots seek out the services only when they have a health problem; others may participate in the hope of preventing future disease. Perhaps providers would step forward to assume roles of comprehensive health care for professional pilots if the demand for such services were sensed.

Enhancing Participation and Effectiveness

Pilots must be educated about the importance and efficacy of preventive-oriented health maintenance programs. Although the usefulness of health maintenance programs that involve the use of periodic comprehensive physical examinations may indeed be questioned among the general population, there can be little doubt that their use in specific populations such as airline pilots is cost-effective. Given the high cost of pilot replacement and the impact of good health on air safety, it behooves both employers and employees to enhance participation in the programs. The development of programs is controversial, and the reluctance of pilots to participate in programs hangs largely on their fear of adverse FAA certificate action. The FAA may take the position that a finding is indicative of a disqualifying disorder. Because the professional pilot has no assurances that adverse findings would not disqualify him, he is reluctant to participate. Hence, regulatory concepts have a negative motivating effect on preventive health maintenance programs for professional airline pilots. If positive findings in a health maintenance physical were viewed as risk factors warranting more in-depth study rather than as disqualifying criteria, preventive programs and pilots' health would be served better. A broadened understanding of the importance and necessity of preventive programs may lead to accommodation between carriers, the FAA, and the various providers of medical service to professional pilots, resulting in the encouragement of effective preventive-oriented health maintenance programs.

Preventive Cardiovascular Program

ALPA's preventive cardiovascular program was begun in 1980 and is designed to intervene in the progression of debilitating heart disease in its membership and to effect the successful rehabilitation of members with cardiovascular disorders of such severity as to pose a potential or actual threat to their careers and/or longevity. Data collection will provide information pertaining to the health of professional airline pilots, forming a better reference source than general population studies. The actual incidence and prevalence of cardiovascular disorders in the professional pilot population are uncertain, but one previous study using estimates based on medical loss of license claims experience has pointed to a lower incidence of cardiovascular disease than that of the United States white male population.[2] It would not be unexpected that the incidence of heart disease in the pilot population would be lower, but what is interesting is that the figures show the relentless progression of the disease with age (Table 25-1). In fact, starting from a very low incidence, which can largely be accounted for by selection, the prevalence of the condition has almost approached that of the United States white male population by ages 55 to 59 (as represented by the Framingham study results).

Drug Abuse and Alcoholism

In my experience, the incidence of drug abuse in the professional airline population is practically nonexistent. For example, except for cases where polydrug abuse involving tranquilizers is seen in association with alcoholism, only one isolated case of drug abuse was seen in over 1100 medical cases in the past 2 years. Some use of marijuana and other drugs might be expected in the younger group of pilots, reflecting sociocultural attitudes, but it is not clinically manifested. The incidence of alcoholism in commercial aircrews is impossible to state precisely but is believed to be in the same general proportion as that found among white-collar and professional persons in the United States population.

Environmental Protection

Aviation Physiology

Adverse physiologic effects resulting from low humidity in aircraft cabin atmospheres, pressurization problems (including rapid decompression), and such matters as hypoxia are not the everyday concerns of the private practitioner. The airframe manufacturers and air carriers are much more directly involved in providing protection from such adverse effects. The flight surgeon's concern is to monitor these conditions for any changes in the frequency of incidents and to call these matters to the attention of the proper authorities.

Hazardous Cargo

The safe carriage of hazardous materials, including explosives, flammable substances, and biologic and radioactive materials is a matter of ongoing concern to the FAA, carriers, pilots, and passengers. Pilot committees follow this subject very carefully and encourage the enforcement of regulatory controls to protect both passengers and crew from undue exposure to hazardous substances. Specific FAA regulations involving the protective measures to be taken when such materials are transported are carefully monitored, but that task generally is outside the purview of the practitioner of aerospace medicine.

Atmosphere Agents

Ozone has been a cause of some concern both to passengers and crewmembers in

Table 25–1. Incidence of Coronary Heart Disease, ALPA and Framingham Study of White Males (Age-Specific Incidence Per 1000 Persons)

Age Group	Framingham Study	ALPA	Framingham/ALPA Ratio
29–34	2.93	0.151	19.40
35–39	2.44	0.678	3.60
40–44	5.16	2.050	2.52
45–49	7.23	4.460	1.62
50–54	12.70	8.740	1.45
55–59	19.80	15.900	1.25

Adapted from Kulak, L.L., Wick, R.L., Jr., and Billings, C.E.: Epidemiological study of in-flight airline pilot incapacitation. Aerospace Med., 42:670–672, 1971.

recent years. Complaints of symptoms by passengers and crew have led to FAA regulations that delineate the maximum allowable levels of ozone in cabin atmospheres. Also specified are certain preventive measures, including the use of onboard equipment to reduce ozone levels. A substance that may constitute hazardous cargo is carbon dioxide. Dry ice frequently is used in the shipment of perishables in the frozen state, and the amount of dry ice on board a given commercial airliner may be substantial. Airline rules generally require passengers to declare dry ice that is being checked in baggage and also limit the amount of dry ice that may be placed aboard an aircraft. Carbon dioxide, if released in significant quantity, could displace oxygen and enhance hypoxia.

Communicable Disease

Although flight attendants are more likely to be exposed to communicable diseases carried by passengers, pilots may be similarly exposed. In addition, aircrews may be billeted in areas of the world where they may be exposed to contagious illnesses; hence, aircrews must be informed regarding epidemic communicable diseases. Good hygiene and appropriate precautions in the consumption of local foods and liquids are important. Generally, the air carriers maintain careful surveillance of appropriate lodging and eating facilities and arrange to billet aircrews in inspected quarters. Primary preventive measures include proper inoculation and the use of antimalarial agents.

Ionizing Radiation

With the possible exception of the Concorde, the British-French supersonic transport, the exposure of pilots to ionizing radiation is within the limits provided under radiation health standards. No hard data confirm an increased prevalence or incidence of radiation-induced illnesses such as malignant tumors. Hence, no con-

crete information is available on which to support any standards different from those now in effect. Continued monitoring of the possible occurrence of increased or decreased amounts of radiation and associated morbidity or mortality is indicated.

Nonionizing Radiation

Microwave radiation is known to be a potential cause of cataracts and has been alleged to be a cause of numerous other maladies, none of which has been proven specifically. Monitoring sources of microwave radiation is important because airline pilots may accidentally be exposed to significant doses of microwave radiation if inadvertently caught in the beam of a radar device from either a stationary source or the nose cone of an airplane. Generally, radars are in the "off" mode when the aircraft is parked on the ground, but the radar occasionally is left on and continues to operate. In such circumstance, pilots performing their walk-around inspections or standing on the ground near the aircraft may be exposed to hazardous levels of microwave radiation. The Aeromedical Office has encouraged reporting such incidents so that baseline health evaluations may be conducted to facilitate the further study of any potential adverse effects. I and my colleagues also are studying the incidence of cataracts in airline pilots, but no data have yet been established that would lead to any supportable conclusions.

Crew Scheduling, Desynchronosis, and Fatigue

Few areas are more controversial than scheduling, especially as this may relate to the prevention or alleviation of fatigue and the prevention of the undesirable effects of desynchronosis. The exigencies of the air carrier business require some flights to begin and end at undesirable times; aircraft must be stationed at a given airfield so as to be available at a later time. Therefore, some crews will be scheduled to fly at night and in the early morning hours. There are scheduling situations in which fatigue could play a potentially serious role in the functional capability of the aircrew. The complexity of the scheduling system, plus the varying degree of compliance with the principles of crew-rest and nutrition, both on the part of carriers and aircrew, serve to complicate the problem further. No simple solutions exist. FARs have specified certain hours and duty times that may not be exceeded, but these regulations are over 30 years old and were developed prior to the initiation of the jet age. A recent FAA attempt to promulgate new rules was withdrawn and has been followed by still further proposals. The outcome is uncertain. Desynchronosis and fatigue have received increased emphasis in recent months, and studies are currently under way under the sponsorship of the National Aeronautics and Space Administration (NASA) to delineate the specific indicators of desynchronosis and methods that can be used to combat both desynchronosis and fatigue.

Human Factors

Cockpit Design

Although not of specific concern to the private practitioner of aerospace medicine or to the Aeromedical Advisor's office, the subject of cockpit design long has been a matter of serious deliberation by ALPA. Standing committees interact with the airframe manufacturers and the air carriers in an attempt to modernize and make more efficient the design of airframes and cockpits. Commercial airline cockpits have been designed in the past either for two or three operating crewmembers. In 1981, a Presidential Commission determined that future aircraft may utilize two crewmembers without detriment to flight safety. The capability of two pilots to operate highly advanced modern aircraft has been attributed to advances in control instrumenta-

tion and cockpit design, as well as to improved systems to assist pilots in their cockpit duties.

Human Error and Aircraft Accidents

Although no United States commercial air carrier jet accident has been attributed to pilot incapacitation, a large number of air carrier accidents have been attributed to human or pilot error by the National Transportation Safety Board (NTSB). Pilot error is a catch-all term that has very little meaning. In a NASA-sponsored study published in 1974, Kowalsky and colleagues[3] reviewed all commercial United States air carrier jet accidents from the first one in 1958 through 1970. Accident causation was analyzed by a complex matrix analysis technique, and numerous conclusions were drawn. A major finding of the study resulted in the recommendation that, since very little information is gained from posthumous evaluations of accidents, much more could be gained from the use of incident data and near-miss data.

Aircraft Safety Reporting System

In 1978, NASA inaugurated the Aircraft Safety Reporting System (ASRS) as a means of attacking the problem of human error in aircraft accidents. This highly innovative system provides, with FAA cooperation, a degree of immunity to those pilots who will report incidents and near misses in the operating environment. The ASRS concept is supported by the air carriers, the pilots' unions, and the FAA. Long-term analyses of data acquired in ASRS are ongoing and may well lead to a reduction of aircraft accidents. Although the commercial air carrier accident rate is commendably low, complacency must be shunned, and every effort must continue to reduce that rate to an even lower figure.

Regulatory Medicine

The FAA is charged by public law, among other things, to monitor the safety and provide for the conduct of air commerce. The Federal Aviation Act of 1958 enables the FAA Administrator to promulgate regulations to carry out these responsibilities. The Federal Air Surgeon functions under the authority of rules published in 1959 and revised periodically, which also establish the periodicity, content, and application of physical examination standards. Provisions are made for the setting aside of the standards in certain instances in which the medical condition of a pilot is such that he would not be felt to affect flight safety adversely if allowed to resume his duties. Details of the system, as described in Chapter 26, "Responsibilities of the Federal Aviation Administration in Aerospace Medicine," are complex and require careful evaluation and monitoring. Lack of perceived uniformity of enforcement is a significant issue. The Federal Air Surgeon must ensure that a pilot meets the medical standards; however, this does not mean that the Federal Air Surgeon is required or expected to provide guidance or assistance to pilots in the management of their medical conditions. Hence, pilots may be subjected to adverse decisions without guidance as to what can be done to correct the underlying medical condition or to prepare an appeal for recertification.

Regulatory Versus Preventive Dichotomy

A long-term effect of the regulatory process has been to diminish and nullify the favorable impact that preventive medicine could have in the field of aerospace medicine regarding air carrier pilots. Increasing frustration on the part of some disqualified pilots has led to petitioning for legislation to overturn some of the long-standing standards under which the Federal Air Surgeon has operated since 1959. Countering these moves and under the stimulus of court decisions that pointed to the need for more definitions in the standards, the FAA recently has published new rules under which certain

medical certification decisions will be made. In addition, a comprehensive review of all medical rules has been undertaken by a special committee under the American Medical Association. It is hoped that medical problems can be solved through the highest quality practice of aviation medicine and of the various medical specialties involved rather than having to resort to legal means to resolve medical certification issues.

Aging

Although the FAA established 60 years of age as the point beyond which an airline pilot could not act as a captain or first officer, this did not resolve a long-standing controversy. The rule is not a medical regulation, but many individuals feel that tests of the efficacy and validity of the rule should rest in the hands of the medical and scientific communities. Still unresolved, the issue has been subjected to intense study and is the focus of a comprehensive report by the National Academy of Sciences Institute of Medicine.[1] The Academy report did not establish a specific age as a cutoff point for functioning as an airline pilot; likewise, it was unable to establish sufficient evidence to recommend the discontinuation of the age-60 rule. A further exposition of the subject was advanced by a special committee of the National Institute on Aging of the National Institutes of Health.[4]

SPECIAL SERVICES

The term special services characterizes certain functions performed for professional pilots by or through the auspices of their representative organization. ALPA, for example, provides these services to its membership because they historically have been nonexistent in the private sector and, to some degree, in airline medical departments. Specifically, special services may include alcoholism prevention, intervention, referral to treatment rehabilitation, and return to duty activities required by virtue of the nature of the illnesses of alcoholism and drug abuse, as well as by the special requirements of FAA medical certification. Performance problems, neuropsychiatric abnormalities, domestic crises, and other psychosociologic factors having an adverse effect on pilot's careers also are dealt with under the umbrella of special services. Clearly, all problems of this generic subject area require an eclectic approach, bringing to bear the several disciplines of psychology, social counseling, and psychiatry in the evaluative phase, and dedicated treatment and rehabilitative specialists in the management phase of these conditions. Here, the flight surgeon may serve as the coordinating focus.

Alcoholism

Definition

Many acceptable definitions of alcoholism can be found in the literature. Most definitions bear considerable similarity to one another, and only three will be mentioned here. The American Medical Association's definition is that "alcoholism is an illness characterized by preoccupation with alcohol and loss of control over its consumption such as to lead usually to intoxication if drinking is begun; by chronicity; by progression; and by tendency toward relapse. It is typically associated with physical disability and impaired emotional, occupational, and/or social adjustments as a direct consequence of persistent and excessive use of alcohol.[5]" The National Council on Alcoholism's definition is that "alcoholism is a chronic, progressive and potentially fatal disease. It is characterized by tolerance and physical dependency, pathologic organ changes, or both, all of which are the direct or indirect consequences of the alcohol ingested.[6]" These definitions have basic parallels. The definition that is of greatest importance to pilots is the FAA's definition of alcoholism as "a condition in which a person's intake of alcohol is great enough to damage his physical health or personal or social functioning, or when alcohol has become a prerequisite to his normal functioning.[7]" Note that medical complications, aberrant behavior patterns, and disturbed social functioning are key elements of these definitions. Not all elements are necessary to the establishment of a diagnosis of alcoholism in a given individual, and their detection may be related to the severity of the illness, accuracy of the history, willingness of significant persons close to the suspected alcoholic to discuss the facts openly, and the comfort, knowledge, and understanding with which the physician approaches the case.

Impact and Prevalence

Alcoholism is at once a manifest and a hidden disease in our society. Long ignored or deliberately suppressed as a diagnosis, alcoholism has been understated both as a primary condition and as an underlying factor in associated conditions and known complications and concomitants of the disease. Estimates of prevalence in the United States population generally refer to problem drinkers, a generic term that includes alcoholics. A problem drinker is a person who drinks alcohol to an extent or in a manner such that an alcohol-related disability is manifested. There are an estimated 13 million problem drinkers in the United States. The economic and social costs to the nation are staggering. Besides an estimated alcohol-related death rate of over 200,000 persons per year (11% of deaths), costs for lost productivity, health and medical expenses, motor vehicle accidents, violent crimes, and social responses were nearly $43 billion in 1975.[8]

Etiology

A number of theories have been advanced regarding the possible causes of alcoholism. Psychodynamic models, pathophysiologic mechanisms, endocrine effects, genetic predisposition, sociologic models, and racial differences, to mention but a few, have been investigated. Although many theories are academically and philosophically attractive, none have proven to be founded on solid scientific grounds. Because the causes are unknown, no method of primary prevention is available. Hence, only secondary and tertiary mechanisms of prevention are applicable.

Pathophysiology

The effect of alcohol on the body is widespread. The gastrointestinal tract, liver, hematopoietic system, nervous system, and cardiovascular, musculoskeletal, and endocrine systems can be and often are adversely affected by alcohol. Cardiomyopathy, coronary artery occlusive disease, and atrial fibrillation, for example, are associated with heavy alcohol consumption. The hallmark effects of alcohol on the liver include alcoholic hepatitis and cirrhosis. Nervous system effects include peripheral neuropathy, a general depressant effect on the central nervous system, and, with long-term abuse, organic brain damage, which may be irreversible. Neoplasia of various organ systems is known to be increased in the alcoholic person.

Psychosocial Aspects

The deterioration in the psychosocial behavior patterns of the alcoholic person is generally relentless and progressive and has characteristic symptoms and signs that Johnson[9] feels are present in persons addicted to other chemicals. He delineates the progression to the universal alcoholic profile as a series of steps involving the learning behavior of the alcoholic person, increasing use and discomfort, waning feelings of self-worth, and ebbing ego strength through self-destructive and, finally, suicidal emotional attitudes. The well-known psychologic defense mechanisms of projection, rationalization, repression, and denial interact to contribute to a delusional memory system in which the alcoholic person is unable to understand what is happening to him and thus may not be able to seek help on his own.

Alcohol in Aviation

The consumption of alcohol followed by the operation of an aircraft is prohibited by FAA regulations. FAA rules prohibit aircraft operation under the influence of alcohol and specify an 8-hour period following alcohol consumption during which attempted aircraft operation would constitute a violation (FAR 91.11). In addition, air carriers have internal operating procedures that either parallel the FAA regulations or establish more stringent prohibitions. No known alcoholism prevalence studies have been conducted in the professional pilot population, but the rate is not markedly different in pilots than in other professionals. Although no commercial United States air carrier jet accidents have been attributed to pilot incapacitation, including intoxication, no alcohol-related accidents would be acceptable. In military aviation accidents, there persists a low but steady incidence of accidents in which alcohol or drugs are associated but not causative agents. Collins[10] reviews the literature concerning the performance of pilots under the influence of alcohol and documents by his own research specific performance decrements.

Industry and Federal Aviation Administration Attitudes Toward Alcoholism

INDUSTRY ATTITUDES. Few conditions in medicine are as socially sensitive as alcoholism. The stigmas attached to alcoholism are so thoroughly ingrained in society that it is easily understood why air carrier executives would want to avoid even the suggestion that their pilots might suffer from alcoholism. Given this concern, as well as the generally accepted public attitudes toward alcoholism as an untreatable mental illness or moral weakness, air carrier leaders formerly felt a sense of hopelessness in dealing with the condition and ignored, hid, or fired alcoholic pilots. To change these attitudes, some leaders in air carrier medical departments have worked quietly, although little effective action was taken elsewhere. Losses of lives and careers were the inevitable consequences in a majority of cases prior to the 1970s. Most importantly, no uniform approach impacted alcoholic pilots across the industry.

THE AIRLINE PILOTS ASSOCIATION ATTITUDES. Attitudes prevalent in the general public and airline management carried over to the leadership and membership of ALPA. That is, in addition to the general disdain and feeling of helplessness in dealing with the problem, "sweeping it under the rug" avoided for pilots the abhorrent consequences of public condemnation, as well as the equally abhorrent responsibility for destroying the careers of fellow pilots. Every pilot knew well that disclosure of alcoholism to the FAA meant mandatory and permanent denial of medical certification.

FEDERAL REGULATORY ATTITUDES. A 1976 FAA formal statement on alcoholism and airline flight crewmembers outlines their position on the disease and its management. It points out that: "An individual who has a medical history or clinical diagnosis of alcoholism does not meet the medical standards and may not act as a flight crewmember, unless an exemption to the medical standards has been granted. Between 1960 and 1971, there were eight petitions from air transport pilots for exemption from the alcoholism standard. None were granted. . . ."[11] Thus, all three major elements of the airline industry, the carriers, the pilots, and the regulatory agency, either implied or practiced attitudes that precluded the pilot from continuing his career even if his condition was treated.

THE UNDERGROUND SYSTEM. Given the prevalent attitudes outlined above, pilots with a history of alcohol abuse or alcoholism could turn only to covert methods of dealing with their problems. Those persons with knowledge of the problem in others often ignored it and, by so doing, silently condoned the activity, or they took action that almost certainly led to discharge or permanent medical disqualification. The risk of discovery haunted all concerned, and the dangers to flight safety were not remedied. Fear of discovery often prevented pilots from seeking help from qualified treatment resources, further decreasing the likelihood of arresting the illness. Even those pilots who arrested their illness through the effective methods of Alcoholics Anonymous were denied the ability to shed themselves of the cloak of secrecy. The persistence of the underground system was, in fact, locked in by societal attitudes and a punitive regulatory atmosphere.

Treatment

INTERVENTION. The alcoholic person's life can be described as being punctuated by crises. As the disease progresses, the person is beset with social problems (e.g., drunk driving arrests, legal entanglements), marital and family problems, and occupational threats. The alcoholic person is unable to cope effectively with the series of crises, and the downhill spiral continues. It is in these phenomena of repeated crises common to alcoholics that the best opportunity exists for assisting the victim and his family, concerned friends, and employers. Years of practical experience have led to the development of Johnson's principles of intervention.[9] The basic assumption is that the chemically dependent person can accept reality when it is presented to him in a receivable form. The goal of the intervention process, which involves several steps that must be followed carefully, is to have the alcoholic individual see and accept enough reality to admit the need for help. The technique avoids the pitfalls of failure and it works.

MODERN CONCEPTS OF TREATMENT. Ill-conceived approaches to the alcoholic person, including one-on-one confrontations by physicians, and construing alcoholism as a mental illness or a deficiency of moral character, are doomed to failure. Physicians who intend to deal with alcoholism in an effective manner must expose themselves to educational efforts to overcome the dearth of information they received in most standard medical school curricula. Careful preparation of family members and significant others in approaching the alcohol victim is important. The psychoanalytic approaches of insight-oriented or in-depth psychotherapy are felt to be contraindicated, and alcoholism must be treated as a primary illness.[12] A multidisciplinary approach is most likely to expose the broad symptomatology and dynamics of the illness and includes a team consisting of physicians, nurses, psychologists, social workers, and lay counselors with personal experience with Alcoholics Anonymous and group therapy. Family oriented treatment is a paramount consideration, and individualized after-care plans often comprise the essential elements of successful rehabilitation. Both inpatient and outpatient modes of treatment are available and, at least in the general population, appear to meet with similar success. In experience with air carrier pilots, however, the preferred treatment mode is inpatient, providing a structured approach and wider patient access to specialties to deal with any physical and psychosociologic complications or accompaniments of the illness. In all cases, the goal of treatment must be to reestablish the premorbid state and to take the steps necessary to assist the pilot in attaining long-lasting, total abstinence. A comprehensive program must be capable of meeting and dealing with relapses when or if they occur.

A Model for Industry Alcoholism Programs

EVOLUTION OF PROGRAM CONCEPTS. The attitudes of the public and the medical professions changed gradually from 1965 to 1975. It became recognized practice to utilize the motivational force of threat of job loss as a means of encouraging alcohol-troubled persons into self-help programs and into the professional treatment programs that were developing concurrently. With this development of so-called occupational alcoholism programs—later more commonly titled employee assistance programs—awareness of their efficacy spread. Some air carriers discreetly developed in-house programs, but, for the most part, no formal industry-wide methods evolved, and pilots remained underserved in a vital health care area. In 1972, the ALPA Board of Directors was apprised of the need for action, and in 1974, the ALPA Human Intervention and Motivation Study (HIMS) was begun with the assistance of government demonstration grant funds. The major aim of the HIMS was to encourage a nonpunitive atmosphere in which the combined forces of union, management, and FAA could cooperate to bring pilots needed assistance in obtaining careful evaluation, referral to competent treatment resources, recovery with comfortable sobriety, and rehabilitation and return to work. This aim has been achieved, but only because of the long-term cooperative efforts of all segments of the tripartite group. All parties conceded that the most important matter was the safe rehabilitation of pilots, and this required both ALPA and management foregoing some traditional but counterproductive stances in the disciplinary area. ALPA established peer identification systems because traditional day-to-day supervisory roles are absent in the industry. It also meant that a new stance and a change of policy was required by the FAA. The FAA first developed a policy allowing for recertification by exemption from applicable portions of FAR Part 67.[11] Then in May 1982, the FARs were ammended to abolish mandatory denial of recertification for alcoholism and to allow discretionary special issuance of medical certificates to certain recovered, abstinent applicants. The HIMS consists of three concurrent efforts—education, case management, and model program development. The majority of carriers whose pilots are represented by ALPA have formal alcoholism rehabilitation programs, often utilizing in-house professionals. Education of the membership, with seminars, mailings to all pilots, printed handout material, and the showing of films at recurrent pilot ground training classes has progressed. Management participation in training nearly matches pilot participation. FAA regulations carefully specify the conditions under which recertification is granted and which must be fulfilled continuously for a minimum period of 24 months through monitoring of the pilot by chief pilots, union representatives, and medical sponsors. Total abstinence is mandatory. As of January, 1985, approximately 600 exemptions had been granted by the FAA.

PROGRAM NEEDS. Carriers with medical officers and professional alcohol and drug abuse counselors have the on-property expertise to establish and carry out rehabilitation programs. Experience in intervention, evaluation, treatment referral, follow-up, monitoring of after-care, and continued observation of pilots returned to flying status are contributions of the medical department. Peer identification by trained pilots in cooperation with trained supervisors (chief pilots) will bring 70 to 80% of cases to the attention of the program personnel. The remainder are identified through proficiency problems and self-referral. Carriers not having medical services available must rely on ALPA medical resources or independent services having expertise with pilots.

MANAGING CONTINUING NEEDS. The re-

quirements for an industry-wide alcoholism rehabilitation program will assure the continued long-term cooperation between ALPA, air carrier managements, and the FAA. Education of pilots and management regarding the disease nature of alcoholism and systems available to deal with the problem is continuing. Refinement of techniques and ongoing quality control are vital to assure excellence of the programs. The development of a network of independent medical sponsors capable of handling the exigencies of pilot alcohol cases will be expanded. Even though these needs will require much time and effort, the inherent pressures of necessity will guarantee the perpetuity of these types of rehabilitative projects. The success or failure of such projects and of all aviation medicine services for pilots must depend in large measure on the motivation of dedicated physicians who recognize the needs without concern for rewards.

REFERENCES

1. Institute of Medicine, National Academy of Sciences: Airline Pilot Age, Health and Performance. Washington, D.C., National Academy Press, 1981.
2. Kulak, L.L., Wick, R.L., Jr., and Billings, C.E.: Epidemiological study of in-flight airline pilot incapacitation. Aerospace Med., 42(6):670–672, 1971.
3. Kowalsky, N.B., et al.: An Analysis of Pilot Error-Related Aircraft Accidents. NASA CR-2444. Washington, D.C., National Aeronautics and Space Administration, 1974.
4. National Institute on Aging: Report of the National Institute on Aging Panel on the Experienced Pilots Study. Bethesda, Maryland, United States Department of Health and Human Services, Public Health Service, 1981.
5. American Medical Association: Manual on Alcoholism. Chicago, American Medical Association, 1973.
6. National Council on Alcoholism: Criteria for the diagnosis of alcoholism. Am. J. Psychiatry, 129:127–135, 1972.
7. Federal Aviation Administration: 14CFR Part 67:13(d) (1) (i) (c), Department of Transportation, U.S. Government Printing Office, Washington, D.C., 1982.
8. Berry, R.E., et al.: The Economic Cost of Alcohol Abuse–1975. Final Report, Contract No. ADM 281-76-0016. Washington, D.C., National Institute on Alcohol Abuse and Alcoholism, 1977.

9. Johnson, V.E.: I'll Quit Tomorrow. 2nd Ed. New York, Harper and Row, 1980.

10. Collins, W.E.: Performance Effects of Alcohol Intoxication and Hangover at Ground Level and at Simulated Altitude. Federal Aviation Administration Report No. FAA-AM-79-26. Washington, D.C., Federal Aviation Administration, 1979.

11. Federal Aviation Administration: Alcoholism and Airline Flight Crewmembers. Washington, D.C., Letter of November 10, 1976.

12. Whitfield, C.L.: Alcoholism. Current Therapy, 1981. Philadelphia, W.B. Saunders Co., 1981.

Chapter 26

The Federal Aviation Administration Responsibilities in Aerospace Medicine

J. Robert Dille

If you are looking for perfect safety, you will do well to sit on a fence and watch the birds.

WILBUR WRIGHT

On May 20, 1926, President Coolidge signed the Air Commerce Act, which assigned federal government responsibilities in civil aviation to the United States Department of Commerce. A requirement for a physical examination for pilot licensure, which would not cost more than $5, was contained in a draft of proposed aeronautic regulations circulated for comments in August, 1926. Louis H. Bauer, M.D., was appointed the first director of the Medical Service on November 16, 1926, after then Secretary of Commerce Herbert Hoover obtained his release from the Army Air Service. Dr. Bauer promptly developed the first physical standards and examination frequencies; these were included in section 66 of the Air Commerce Regulations and became effective December 31, 1926. Dr. Bauer also designated the first aviation medical examiners (AMEs) in February, 1927, conducted 12 training conferences for them in 1929 and 1930, proposed district flight surgeons in 1928, studied (with Cooper) aircraft accident and training success correlation with physical deficiencies, and established procedures for practical flight tests and waivers before his resignation on November 26, 1930.

ORGANIZATION AND RESPONSIBILITIES

Federal Aviation Administration

The federal government's regulatory role in civil aviation, begun in 1926 under the Aeronautics Branch of the Department of Commerce, was transferred to an independent Civil Aeronautics Authority and expanded under the Air Commerce Act of 1938. The administrator's operational functions under the law included fostering civil aeronautics and commerce, establishing civil airways, providing and technically improving air navigation facilities for such airways, protecting and regulating air traffic along the airways, and surveying the existing system of airports to determine the recommended extent of federal participation in their development, construction, improvement, maintenance, and operation. The Civil Aeronautics Authority also was given regulatory powers regarding airline tariffs, airline business practices, investigation of accidents, determination of probable cause in each accident, and recommendations for accident prevention. These economic and accident investigation responsibilities were transferred to an essentially independent Civil Aeronautics Board (CAB) in 1940, and the accident investigation functions, for all types of transportation, were vested in the independent National Transportation Safety Board (NTSB) in 1975. The operational functions of the Civil Aeronautics Authority were placed under the Department of Commerce in 1940 in a new organization, the Civil Aeronautics Administration (CAA), and the list of responsibilities was gradually expanded to include licensing of pilots and other airmen, research, training, certain delegated aircraft accident investigation and safety regulation activities, certification of airports serving CAB-certified air carriers, airport grant-in-aid programs, and certification of the design, manufacture, and performance of every civil aircraft. These duties were performed by the independent Federal Aviation Agency beginning December 31, 1958 under the provisions of the Federal Aviation Act of August 23, 1958 and by the Federal Aviation Administration (FAA) under the Department of Transportation after the Transportation Act was signed on October 15, 1966.

To perform these functions for a system that includes approximately 715,000 active pilots, 290,000 active aircraft, and 16,000 airports in the United States, the FAA operates over 450 Airport Traffic Control Towers, 25 Air Route Traffic Control Centers, more than 300 Flight Service Stations, and over 19,000 total facilities in the National Airspace System, with about 50,000 personnel, half of whom are normally air traffic control specialists and an-

other one sixth of whom install and maintain the air navigation and air traffic control facilities. The country is presently divided into nine FAA regions (Fig. 26–1) and contains, in addition to the Washington, D.C. headquarters, the Mike Monroney Aeronautical Center in Oklahoma City, Oklahoma, the FAA Technical Center in Atlantic City, New Jersey, 34 General Aviation District offices, 16 Manufacturing Inspection District Offices, 49 Flight Standards District offices, nine Flight Inspection Field offices, ten Aircraft Certification Offices, 11 Air Carrier District Offices, and 18 Airport Field offices. Consolidation (particularly of Flight Service Stations) and some contracting out (especially of VFR Towers), as well as modernization, are likely under the 1984 National Airspace System plan.

Office of Aviation Medicine

The Office of Aviation Medicine, headed by the Federal Air Surgeon, is the principal FAA staff element with respect to the physical fitness of airmen and other persons associated with safety in flight, medical certification systems, the designated aviation medical examiner system, occupational health programs, aviation medical research, medical factors in civil aircraft accident investigations, aeromedical education, and biostatistical data for use in human factors evaluations. To accomplish these functions, the Office of Aviation Medicine is organized into Aeromedical Standards, Occupational Health, Biomedical and Behavioral Sciences, and Program Operations divisions.

Federal Air Surgeon

The Federal Air Surgeon provides professional advice and assistance to the Administrator and is delegated the authority to do the following:

1. Determine the medical qualifications of applicants for airman certificates and issue, to qualified applicants,

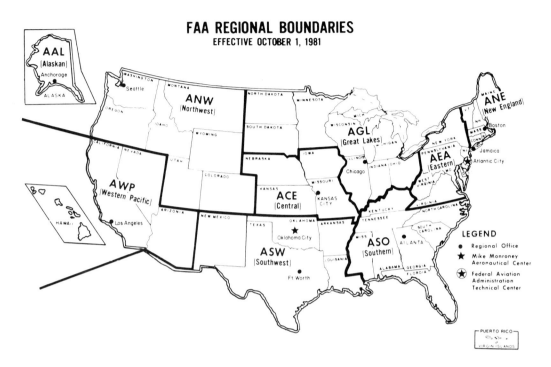

FAA REGIONAL BOUNDARIES
EFFECTIVE OCTOBER 1, 1981

Fig. 26–1. Federal Aviation Administration (FAA) regional boundaries.

certificates of medical qualification bearing such limitations as may be required in the interests of safety

2. Deny applications for certificates of medical qualification
3. Refuse to issue medical certificates to applicants who fail to provide requested additional medical information or to authorize the release of such information
4. Require medical reexamination or other investigation of the medical qualifications of holders of airman certificates
5. Designate or rescind the designation of aviation medical examiners (AMEs)
6. Reconsider, reverse, change, or modify the medical certificate actions of designated AMEs
7. Grant or deny airman petitions for

medical exemptions from the regulations

8. Issue notices of proposed rule making and hold public hearings in rule-making proceedings pertaining to the establishment of medical rules and regulations
9. Issue instructions for application by all agency medical officers, scientists, and professional persons engaged in FAA aviation medicine activities on technical procedures required to ensure compliance with medical standards, rules, regulations, and agency orders
10. Review and approve all aeromedical research projects or tasks

Aeromedical Standards Division

The Aeromedical Standards Division develops and recommends minimum medical standards for airmen and policies for medical certification activities, provides guidance for the AME and aeromedical education programs, makes recommendations to the Federal Air Surgeon on the disposition of referred airman medical qualification cases, and operates a system for processing airman appeal cases.

Occupational Health Division

The Occupational Health Division recommends minimum medical standards for agency air traffic control specialists, administers the Air Traffic Control Specialist Health Program, recommends procedures for the emergency treatment and physical examination of employees and for monitoring their work areas for environmental hazards, recommends and evaluates protective procedures, and develops agency medical criteria for airport disaster planning. Policy guidance is provided for the regions, a clinic at the Technical Center, and clinical and industrial hygiene activities at the Mike Monroney Aeronautical Center in Oklahoma City, Oklahoma.

Regional Flight Surgeons

Regional Flight Surgeons conduct and direct the Air Traffic Control Specialist Health Program, other employee health functions, AME designation and performance appraisal, aircraft accident investigation to determine human factors aspects, and some airman medical certification activities within their regions. They also regularly participate in the training of AMEs and airmen.

In July, 1928, Dr. Bauer had requested the appointment of district flight surgeons to instruct AMEs, visit them in their offices, and check on their performance. He continued his pleas for 2 years as the numbers of pilots and AMEs increased but to no avail. This probably influenced his decision to resign in November, 1930.

A district flight surgeon, Eldridge S. Adams, later to become a Medical Director, was assigned to Kansas City, Missouri,

in November, 1931, where he worked with AMEs in the western states. This office was closed in October, 1932 for economic reasons, however, and Dr. Adams returned to Washington, D.C. headquarters.

Regional medical officers were hired for New York City, Atlanta, Georgia, Chicago, Illinois, Fort Worth, Texas, Kansas City, Missouri, Los Angeles, California, and Seattle, Washington in 1946, with former Medical Director Adams, who was just out of military service, in the Los Angeles office. Regional medical offices were opened in Anchorage, Alaska in 1948 and in Honolulu, Hawaii in 1949, and these were the only two regions that retained medical offices when medical certification functions were recentralized in Washington, D.C., the nine regions were reduced to six, and all regional medical officer positions were eliminated, again for reasons of economy, in October, 1953. In 1954, the New York, Fort Worth, Kansas City, and Los Angeles offices were restaffed with physicians with a new title—Regional Flight Surgeons. Positions in Atlanta (1962), Boston, Massachusetts (1971), Denver, Colorado (1971), Chicago (1971), and Seattle (1972) were authorized and staffed later. Assistant Regional Flight Surgeons were added in 20 Air Route Traffic Control Centers beginning in 1970 to conduct the Air Traffic Controller Health Program. The Denver and Honolulu regional offices were abolished during fiscal year 1982.

Civil Aeromedical Institute

In October, 1965, the Civil Aeromedical Research Institute (CARI), the Aeromedical Certification Division, and Aeronautical Center clinical and industrial hygiene programs were combined into a new Civil Aeromedical Institute (CAMI). The Medical Examiner Training and Performance Branch was added and expanded, and the Georgetown Clinical Research Institute positions were transferred to CAMI during the next 2 years.

CAMI develops and conducts a system

for the medical examination and certification of civil airmen; medical research projects applicable to the mission of the FAA; an aviation medical education program for AMEs and civil airmen, including a national program for physiologic training at FAA, military, and National Aeronautics and Space Administration (NASA) facilities; an employee health program at the Aeronautical Center, an industrial hygiene program for the Aeronautical Center and five western regions; and aircraft accident investigation to determine predisposing medical factors, the presence of drugs, alcohol, and toxic chemicals in pilots, survivability, identification of victims, emergency evacuation problems, vehicle crashworthiness, and the adequacy of seats and restraint systems.

MEDICAL STANDARDS

The original civil airman medical standards were based on rather arbitrary military standards. Although lacking in detail, they were directed toward diseases with the maximum perceived risk to aviation safety, and they were fairly rigid. The regulatory agencies responsible for setting and enforcing these standards to ensure adequate safety also have been charged with promoting air commerce, goals that may conflict if medical standards are either too strict or too lax. Pressures from inside and outside of these agencies have been exerted, from the beginning, for the relaxation of medical standards to minimum and practical levels, less frequent examinations, waivers for many airmen with physical defects, and an appeal mechanism. Society has come, in time, to accept that absolute safety is not feasible or economically tolerable, that a level of safety is desired which is obtainable at reasonable cost, and that minimum standards and regulations should be set by the federal government. Pilot performance and the risk of sudden incapacitation now receive primary attention.

Development of Standards

Dr. Bauer developed physical standards for three classes of civil pilots during the last 6 weeks of 1926.

Effective December 31, 1926, private pilots were required to be free of any organic disease or defect that would interfere with the safe handling of an airplane under the conditions of private flying and to have visual acuity of at least 20/40 in each eye (less than 20/40 might be accepted if the pilot wore corrective lenses in his goggles and had normal judgment of distance without correction), good judgment of distance, no diplopia in any position, normal visual fields and color vision, and no organic disease of the eye or internal ear.

Industrial pilots were required to be free of any organic disease or defect that would interfere with the safe handling of an airplane and to have visual acuity of not less than 20/30 in each eye (although in certain instances less than 20/30 might be accepted if the applicant wore correction to 20/20 in his goggles and had good judgment of distance without correction), good judgment of distance, no diplopia in any field, normal visual fields and color vision, and no organic disease of the eye, ear, nose, or throat.

Transport pilots were required to have a good past history, sound pulmonary, cardiovascular, gastrointestinal, central nervous, and genitourinary systems, freedom from material structural defects or limitations, freedom from disease of the ductless glands, normal central, peripheral, and color vision, normal judgment of distance, only slight defects of ocular muscle balance, freedom from ocular disease, absence of obstructive or diseased conditions of the ear, nose, and throat, and no abnormalities of equilibrium that would interfere with flying.

Provisions were made for waivers by the Secretary of Commerce for trained pilots with disqualifying physical defects who apparently compensated adequately for their defects by experience. Dr. Bauer intended to limit waivers to trained pilots, but both congressional and industry pressure and the erroneous issuance of medical certificates to applicants with defects by AMEs contributed to the issuance of waivers to student pilots with disqualifying defects. Instructions were soon issued to AMEs to recommend waivers whenever appropriate, and practical flight tests with Aeronautics Branch inspectors were authorized to resolve doubts about the ability of applicants to compensate for static defects. Despite this increased leniency, Dr. Bauer and his assistant, Dr. Cooper, continually studied the success of pilots with physical defects and generally reported strong negative correlation between defects and training progression (licensure within 1 year) and safety.[1,2] They remained opposed to waivers.

In March, 1927, the requirements for student pilots were clarified when they were added to the private pilot class, which, like the industrial pilot class, was to be examined every 12 months. A new class, limited commercial pilots, was added with the same medical standards and examination frequency (every 6 months) as the transport pilots. By September, 1929, glider pilots were required to meet the physical standards for private pilots.

When the number of new student pilot permits fell in 1930, unreasonable medical standards rather than a depressed economy were blamed by many. Despite further studies that found poorer progress in training and a higher accident rate for pilots with physical defects, the standards were relaxed for student and private pilots. Dual-control permits were issued to applicants without a physical examination. Distant visual acuity standards were reduced from 20/40 to 20/50 uncorrected and to any acuity correctable to 20/30 in 1931. After all, improved aircraft cowlings and more enclosed cockpits lessened the

chance of prescription goggles being knocked off or askew by wind or prop blasts. Only diplopia that appeared within 45° of the straight-ahead line of sight, rather than any diplopia, was now disqualifying. In 1959, diplopia within 35° was allowed for first-class and second-class certificates, and there was no standard for third-class certificates. Diplopia was dropped from the physical standards altogether in 1961, but AMEs have been instructed to deny or withhold medical certificates for the condition.

The vision standards of 20/50 uncorrected and any acuity correctable to 20/30 were extended to amateur, commercial, and glider pilots—all but airline transport pilots—in 1934. The distant vision standard for airline pilots was reduced to 20/50 or better in each eye if corrected to 20/20 in each eye by glasses in 1938 and to 20/100 in 1965.

In 1937, the hearing standards for student and private pilots were lowered to perception of a whispered voice (in either ear) at 3 feet.

Depth perception requirements for first-class and second-class medical certificates were removed by an amendment in 1960.

Current Standards

Part 67

In 1959, the Federal Aviation Agency identified nine medical conditions with a high risk of sudden incapacitation and altered judgment that would constitute mandatory denial for any class of airman medical certificate: history or clinical diagnosis of a myocardial infarction, angina pectoris or other evidence of coronary heart disease, epilepsy, a disturbance of consciousness without satisfactory medical explanation of the cause, diabetes mellitus requiring insulin or other hypoglycemic drugs for control, psychotic disorders, drug addiction (later drug dependence), chronic alcoholism (later just alcoholism), and a character or behavior (later personality) disorder sufficiently severe to have repeatedly manifested itself by overt acts.

A summary of the medical findings for which AMEs are instructed to deny or defer the issuance of a medical certificate is presented in Table 26–1. Justification is debatable, but it is generally true that standards are more stringent with increased pilot responsibilities although not necessarily with increased aircraft performance.

A recent amendment to Part 67 permits the use of contact lenses, as well as eyeglasses, to satisfy the corrected distant visual acuity requirement for all three classes of medical certificates. Part 67 also provides the authority for special medical flight or practical tests, special medical evaluations, operational limitations, limited duration of certificates, and penalties for falsification of any application for a medical certificate or alteration or fraudulent duplication of a certificate. It further provides for delegation of authority to issue or deny medical certificates, a max-

Table 26–1.   Summary of Federal Aiation Administration Medical Standards for Pilots

	First-Class Medical Certificate—Airline Transport Pilot	Second-Class Medical Certificate—Commercial Pilot	Third-Class Medical Certificate—Private Pilot
Distant Vision	20/20 in each eye separately without correction or at least 20/100 in each eye separately corrected to 20/20 or better with corrective lenses (glasses or contact lenses)		At least 20/50 without correction, or, if poorer than 20/50, must correct to 20/30 or better with corrective lenses (glasses or contact lenses)
Near Vision	At least 20/40 with each eye separately, with or without correcting glasses		At least 20/60 with each eye separately with or without correcting glasses
Hyperphoria	Maximum of 1 diopter (D)		No standard
Esophoria and Exophoria	Maximum of 6 D of esophoria or exophoria		No standard
Color Vision	Normal color vision	Ability to distinguish aviation signal red, green, and white	
Audiometry	Maximum of 40 dB at 500 Hz; 35 dB in frequencies of 1000 and 2000 Hz, ISO	No requirement. Audiometry may be performed as a service to the applicant with his permission	
Hearing	Able to hear whispered voice at 6 m with each ear	Able to hear whispered voice at 2.4 m with each ear	Able to hear whispered voice at 0.9 m
Ear, nose, and throat	No acute or chronic disease of ear, mastoid, or problem with equilibrium; no unhealed perforation of eardrum		No acute or chronic disease of ear, including no problem with equilibrium
Pulse	At rest, maximum of 100 beats/min; maximum of 120 beats/min after exercise, returning to within 10 beats of resting pulse after 2 minutes		
Blood pressure	Maximum of 160/98 at age 50 and over	Maximum of 170/100	
Electrocardiogram	Required at age 35 and annually after age 40 (resting)	Not required if cardiovascular examination is normal	
Other conditions	Examiner must disqualify if the applicant has a history or diagnosis of diabetes mellitus requiring hypoglycemic medication; angina pectoris or other evidence of coronary heart disease that may lead to an infarction; myocardial infarction; epilepsy; alcoholism; drug dependence; disturbance of consciousness without satisfactory medical explanation; personality disorder manifested by repeated overt acts; or psychosis		

imum of 60 days after an AME issues a medical certificate for the FAA to reverse the issuance, requesting additional medical information, and examinations by senior flight surgeons in the armed forces.

Guide for Aviation Medical Examiners

Because the medical standards are not detailed, considerable guidance is necessary for the AMEs to perform the proper tests for the applicant's age and class of certificate desired using acceptable equipment and procedures and to decide whether to issue, deny, or withhold a medical certificate. A manual, *Guide for Aviation Medical Examiners,* intended for official use only, is provided to each designated civilian physician and to each military flight surgeon's unit performing FAA physical examinations. It contains administrative information, a list of acceptable vision testing equipment, recommended examination procedures, instructions for completing each item on forms, a list of medical conditions established by history or examination for which the AME will not issue a medical certificate, and a directory of FAA and NTSB field offices.

The dissemination of information to AMEs also is accomplished through seminars (attendance is required the first year after appointment and every 5 years thereafter), a Federal Air Surgeon's Medical Bulletin, special mailings when necessary, and a monthly column in the journal *Aviation, Space, and Environmental Medicine.*

Policies

Numerous internal policies supplement Part 67 and *Guide for Aviation Medical Examiners* and help considerably in operating the medical program. Most policies cover administrative procedures and are of little outside concern. They are of professional interest when they involve medical conditions (e.g., atrial fibrillation), acceptable medications (e.g., thiazide diuretics, lithium), permissible doses of certain medications (propranolol, metoprolol tartrate), waiting periods before certification (e.g., after myocardial infarction, coronary artery bypass surgery, loss of an eye), and required procedures for exemptions or for special issuance of medical certificates (e.g., angiography to demonstrate patency after bypass surgery). The policies are based on advances in medical science, research findings, consultants' opinions, NTSB decisions, court rulings, and, conceivably, legislation. Changes in policy are disseminated at staff medical conferences and documented in FAA Orders and in a Medical Guideline Letter system. Although nothing is classified about current FAA medical policies, they are not readily available outside of the agency. A student of medical standards and certification should contact an FAA flight surgeon for the rest of the story.

Review and Updating

Recommendations are received almost daily from airmen, attending physicians, pilots' organizations, and members of Congress to change—usually relax—medical standards. Studies by the General Accounting Office and the NTSB, on the other hand, usually have suggested the adoption of improved detection methods for diseases felt to be associated with decreased flying safety. Standards were extensively reviewed by a Federal Air Surgeon's Medical Advisory Council in 1964 and at the First Bethesda Conference of the American College of Cardiology in 1965.

The Eighth Bethesda Conference of the American College of Cardiology,[3] held April 25 and 26, 1975, again was devoted to airman medical standards, specifically the causes, clinical course, and possible risks of cardiovascular problems associated with aviation safety. Task forces have made recommendations on ischemic heart disease, cerebral vascular disease, hypertension, valvular heart disease, congenital heart disease, myocardial-pericardial disease, and arrhythmias.

In 1977, the FAA solicited a proposal from the American Medical Association for an authoritative document concerning the current state of knowledge about selected neurologic and neurosurgical conditions as part of a continuing review of medical standards, examination procedures, and certification decisions. Nearly 50 medical experts, mostly from the American Academy of Neurology and the American Association of Neurological Surgeons, participated in the study and in the preparation of the final report, which was published in 1979.[4]

Frequency of Examinations

The physical examination frequency for noncommercial pilots was extended to 2 years in 1933, returned to every year in 1942, and set again at every 2 years in 1945 (where it remains today). Commercial pilots had the frequency of their physical examinations extended from every 6 months to every 12 months in 1942 (where it remains today). Airline transport pilots were examined every 3 months from October 1934 until November 1937 following a pilot fatigue study. With the establishment of an 85-hour flight-time limitation, the more frequent checks were no longer felt to be necessary. Physical changes significant enough to affect certification were found in only two pilots during this 3-year period. In 1947, an advisory committee to the CAA administrator recommended the elimination of periodic examinations for student and private pilots. Medical Director William P. Stovall recommended the elimination of the periodic 2-year examinations for noncommercial pilots except for those with physical defects likely to progress, following an accident, for flying higher performance aircraft, for international operations to comply with International Civil Aviation Organization standards, and when felt to be indicated by a Regional Flight Surgeon. In 1956, the Civil Aeronautics Board recommended intervals of 2, 3, and 5 years for pilots under

40 years of age. In 1966, the Federal Air Surgeon proposed extending medical certificates for airline transport pilots under 50 years of age to 12 months together with more stringent electrocardiographic examinations.

Booze studied the frequency of examination requirements in 1975.[5] His conclusions included (1) a need for less frequent examinations for airmen less than 35 years old in view of the lower incidence of disease experienced by this group and the type of pathologic process most frequently occurring, but (2) greater emphasis on disease detection for airmen 60 years of age and older through a combination of increased examination frequency and additional ancillary testing.

In May, 1979, the Aircraft Owners and Pilots Association petitioned the FAA to extend the validity period for third-class medical certificates from 2 to 3 years without regard to an airman's age.

In 1981, a contract was awarded to Johns Hopkins University to reexamine the indicated frequency of airman physical examinations by using FAA data tapes. A proposed rule for less frequent physical examinations for private pilots under age 55 resulted. The American Medical Association is conducting an in-depth review of the scope and frequencies of airman medical examinations at the current (1983–1985) time. The question of the frequency of examinations has not been permanently settled.

MEDICAL CERTIFICATION

Aviation Medical Examiners

Designation

Dr. Bauer initiated a system of examination of applicants for civil airman medical certificates by specially designated physicians with the appointment of 57 interested physicians in 46 cities in February, 1927, 2 months after the first physical standards were established. The first airline pilot medical examiners were selected in 1935. Except for a period between 1945 and 1960 when any competent, licensed physician could examine student and private pilots, the medical certification system has depended on physical examination by designated AMEs.

Appointments and annual decisions on reappointment for domestic civilian AMEs are made by Regional Flight Surgeons based on qualifications, licensure, good professional standing, local need, proper equipment, and willingness to attend a seminar for orientation and training before appointment and every 5 years thereafter. Computer-generated performance reports, which show activity and administrative errors, are supplied by CAMI to assist with the reappointment decisions. An attempt is made to have an average of about one AME for every 100 airmen to achieve adequate convenience and choice for the airman, security for forms and other materials, maintained proficiency for the AME, and economy for the system.

Senior aviation medical examiners, who have the authority to give examinations for first-class medical certificates and to issue or deny first-class medical certificates in accordance with Part 67, are so designated by Regional Flight Surgeons based on seminar attendance, 3 years of acceptable performance, and, again, need in the area.

Some AMEs are also specially appointed to assist the FAA in the preemployment and annual physical examinations of air traffic control personnel.

The system has grown considerably from Dr. Bauer's initial 57 to about 7600 domestic AMEs, 320 international designees, and 520 military flight surgeon units. For the domestic AMEs, of all who apply for designation, 46% are or have been pilots, 18% are former military flight surgeons, and 78% have volunteered to participate in the aircraft accident investigation program as indications of

their level of interest. Many also participate in airman education activities. Many (55%) are in family practice, but all medical specialties are represented. Physicians in residency training, with closed practices, and in emergency medicine are not usually recommended for designation or retention of designation because of anticipated irregular accessibility to any airman and record retention problems. Continued appointment as an AME after a geographic move into one of these areas is not automatic.

Training

Training of designated civil AMEs was an integral part of Dr. Bauer's original plan, and at least 12 conferences were conducted in fiscal year 1930. Also, training of the AMEs was contained in the earliest proposals for regional medical officers in 1928 and in the duties of the earliest regional medical officer in 1931. Problems of staffing and funding ended these efforts.

The first of the present series of 3-day AME seminars was conducted at the Georgetown University Medical School from December 14 to 16, 1960. Despite poor weather, 49 of the 50 AMEs who were invited attended. Well over 200 of these popular and successful programs have been conducted. Approval for Category I American Medical Association (AMA) Continuing Medical Education (CME) credit was received in January, 1973, and American Academy of Family Physicians (AAFP) and American Osteopathic Association (AOA) credit also are now given.

A series of 5-day seminars was begun in April, 1969 at CAMI. These seminars place increased emphasis on instructional techniques, aviation physiology, aircraft accident investigation, pesticide poisoning, and research for the more active AMEs. Seminars frequently have been conducted in conjunction with the annual meetings of the Aerospace Medical Association and the Civil Aviation Medical Association.

Fees

Fees for civilian pilot physical examinations were set by the federal government for many years, but they have never been controlled by the FAA. They are paid to the examining physician by the applicants and vary considerably.

International Aviation Medical Examiners

The designation of AMEs in other countries is handled by the Manager of CAMI. They are all appointed initially as senior aviation medical examiners because their main purpose is to examine airline pilots who are flying aircraft of United States registry or who are United States citizens whose 6-month medical certificates expire while employed abroad or when passing through. The required seminar attendance may be waived for those with training in aviation medicine because of the distances, travel costs, and generally lesser volume of examinations conducted. Proficiency in the English language, which is required of both the physicians and their examinees, is of considerable concern with this segment of the certification system.

Military Installations

Military units, including the National Guard and the Reserve Forces, which have flight surgeons assigned and for which recognition is requested, are sent forms, supplies, and a designation number by CAMI. Here, too, no orientation or training is required, and, although clinical competence is not questioned, administrative errors have been frequent. At the request of the Surgeons General, military units are not authorized to issue first-class medical certificates.

Aeromedical Certification Branch

The Aeromedical Certification Branch of CAMI is the central screening facility and repository within the FAA for the collection, processing, adjudication, investigation, and analyses of medical data generated by the aeromedical certification program.

Medical certification criteria have changed dramatically in favor of the airman during recent years as a result of the evolution of aviation medicine and increased efforts in the area of aeromedical research. A primary function of the Aeromedical Certification Branch is to identify and provide substantive data support of current medical criteria in the furtherance of aviation safety, as well as to provide better service to the airman. For example, visual acuity requirements are more realistic, and contact lenses are now permitted.

Since 1927, the FAA and its predecessors have been charged with the responsibility for medical certification of all United States and some international civil airmen. Each airman must hold a current medical certificate of the appropriate class to validate any pilot certificate he may possess. As of January 1, 1985, about 715,000 active airmen were medically certified. Federal Aviation Regulations stipulate that physical examinations must be performed at 6-month intervals for air transport pilots, annually for other commercial pilots, and at 2-year intervals for private pilots. Medical certification has soared from an annual workload of approximately 14,000 applications during the first year of operation to 529,051 applications involving 800,000 active airmen during 1980. Current projections are for resumption of an average annual growth rate of 3% following a recent drop of about 100,000 airmen.

Processing of Applications

Physical examinations to detect medical conditions that could incapacitate or otherwise adversely affect pilot performance are given by the AMEs, and all reports of these examinations from throughout the world are forwarded to the Aeromedical Certification Branch in Oklahoma City,

Oklahoma. Reports are especially important on applicants who fail to complete an examination after finding they are disqualified, particularly by the medical history.

The Aeromedical Certification Branch mail room receives approximately 2200 applications for medical certification each day. Documents are sorted for routine or priority processing and are assigned medical identification (MID) numbers, which provide subsequent document control.

Coding personnel assign alphanumeric codes to medical and administrative data contained on the report of examination.

The coded examinations are sent to the Data Conversion Unit, where a typing function transfers the coded data onto a disk for computer input. Input is processed against several edit programs to assure a complete record. Records are further screened for significant deviations from established medical criteria and compared with previous findings. When a discrepancy is encountered, the computer creates a notification of the administrative or medical discrepancies, which require manual review.

The Medical Review Section medical record technicians review documents rejected by the computer. They are able to initiate corrective action or make the final certification decision in approximately 90% of these cases. The remaining 10% of cases involve technical medical problems that require manual review and adjudication by the Branch Manager and staff medical officers.

Review

Issuances and denials of medical certificates by AMEs can be reversed by full-time FAA medical officers, usually on review in the Aeromedical Certification Branch. Except for airmen with one of the nine conditions that require denial under Part 67, some will be completely cleared and others will qualify for special issue of a medical certificate until or after special medical or practical tests. A student pilot who is monocular may receive a medical certificate that is "valid for student pilot purposes only" until he takes and passes a practical flight test, at which time a Statement of Demonstrated Ability and a medical certificate free of limitations are issued. These are valid until the clinical condition deteriorates or until a higher-class medical certificate is sought. Pilots with defective color vision will carry a limitation of "not valid for night flying or by color signal control" until they take and pass a signal light gun test. Deaf individuals cannot fly in and out of an airport with a control tower, paraplegics require an aircraft modified with all hand controls, and others must wear appliances such as artificial limbs and hearing aids. The most frequent limitation, one that rarely requires a flight test and can be applied by AMEs if within set standards, is for corrective lenses; about 40% of airmen must wear them.

A time-limited certificate may be issued and/or periodic special medical tests may be required. These airmen are usually satisfied with the actions taken.

Until a federal court order issued on May 16, 1980 enjoined the Federal Air Surgeon from placing any limitation on the medical certificate of an airman which describes the flight functions that such airman may perform, functional limitations such as "second class privileges limited to flight engineer duties" occasionally were placed on medical certificates.

For about 1% of airmen, a final denial is issued or affirmed. Denial is more frequent for first-time applicants.

Airman Appeals Mechanisms

A prominent feature of the medical certification system is the provision of several mechanisms for the appeal of denial actions.

Reconsideration

For medical conditions other than the nine requiring mandatory denials, the

Federal Air Surgeon can be asked to reconsider the action. Several hundred airmen pursue this course of action each year; historically, about one-third are successful.

Exemptions

For applicants with a history or clinical diagnosis of myocardial infarction, angina pectoris, or other evidence of coronary artery disease, epilepsy, an unexplained loss of consciousness, diabetes mellitus requiring insulin or other hypoglycemic drug for control, a psychotic disorder, drug dependence, alcoholism, or a personality disorder with repeated overt acts, there are two avenues. They can petition for an exemption from the medical standards. Petitioners usually are asked to submit the reports of all, or even additional, medical evaluations. The complete records are reviewed by consultants and recommendations are made to the Federal Air Surgeon, who grants or denies the petition.

Several hundred airmen petition for exemptions each year, approximately 200 of whom are successful. Every mandatory denial condition except diabetes mellitus requiring insulin or other hypoglycemic drug for control has been exempted. A program for exempting and closely monitoring airline pilots with alcoholism has been very successful and is detailed in Chapter 25. Interestingly, nearly half of those who obtain exemptions never validate their grants for various personal reasons, including the cost of required periodic evaluations.

The 1980 court order previously referred to (*United States District Court for the Northern District of Georgia, in Delta Air Lines v. the United States, et al.,* Civil No. 78-445A) enjoined the FAA from issuing medical certificates to airmen possessing any of the absolutely disqualifying conditions enumerated in Part 67 and from exempting any airman from these provisions without a proper finding that such exemption is in the public interest. Clarification was made the following month, which permitted the reissuance of medical certificates based on grants of exemption issued before May 16, 1980. Several months were required to clarify "public interest," after which the exemption process was resumed, but now, more than ever, with individualized consideration that negates the use of form letters.

Special Issue of Medical Certificates

Effective May 17, 1982, the nine mandatory denial conditions were no longer excluded under the special issuance procedure, section 67.19, and applicants who did not meet the medical standards could now be considered expeditiously under this section instead of through the lengthy exemption process. This authority of the Federal Air Surgeon is delegated to the Chief, Aeromedical Certification Branch, Civil Aeromedical Institute, and to each Regional Flight Surgeon.

The entire certification and exemption process is reviewed periodically for possible changes.

Petitions to the National Transportation Safety Board

Within 60 days of receipt of a final denial letter, an airman may alternatively or concurrently petition the NTSB for a review of the denial of the application for a medical certificate. Basically, the question is whether the airman has the medical condition the FAA says he has.

In the event of an NTSB hearing on an airman's appeal of an FAA action taken within 60 days of the examination, the burden of proving qualification is on the airman. If the FAA action occurred 60 days after the examination, the burden of proof is on the agency. For this reason, timely receipt and review of applications where the AMEs have issued medical certificates is a major objective of the medical certification program.

FLIGHT SAFETY

Aircraft Accident Investigation

As with medical standards, aircraft accident investigations and observations to identify problems, reduce accidents, and increase survival in those that do occur can be traced to military aviation prior to the United States' entry into World War I. It has been said that the benefits of restraint systems and helmets were recognized after Lieutenant Selfridge's death in the world's first fatal accident in powered flight, which occurred on September 17, 1908 at Fort Myer, Virginia. Hap Arnold was photographed wearing his college football helmet shortly thereafter. Safety belts were installed. The cowl was cut out when it was observed that half of the injuries sustained in crashes were caused by the aviator's striking his head on the cowl; head injuries subsequently were practically eliminated. England, France, and Italy found 90% of aircraft accidents to be due to troubles in the flyer himself. The situation in civil aviation some 65 years later is disappointingly similar—the pilot is a causal factor in 80 to 90% of general aviation accidents, and upper torso restraints, which studies show could prevent 85 to 93% of serious injuries and deaths in survivable general aviation fatal accidents, have only been required since 1978 and only for front-seat occupants of newly built aircraft.

The NTSB is responsible for determining the primary cause and causal factors for each aircraft accident. Due to limited staffing, the NTSB has delegated a considerable portion of general aviation aircraft accident investigation to the FAA. The division of responsibility between NTSB and FAA generally has been based on fatalities. Most nonfatal accidents and the fatal accidents involving aerial application, home-built aircraft, and restricted aircraft have been delegated to the FAA, and the NTSB investigates all other fatal accidents—some as major investigations by a headquarters "Go Team" and the remainder as field investigations. The NTSB also has investigated selected injury accidents. An expanded NTSB program is planned that will investigate all accidents involving public confidence, property damage, and selected safety issues with accident prevention potential. Continuing oversight to maintain public confidence would be the basis for the investigation of all accidents involving commercial passenger service, newly certified aircraft, and midair collisions (where FAA air traffic control frequently becomes an issue). The expanded study of selected safety issues would include emphasis on human factors, crashworthiness, and survivability.

Medical assistance has been provided through the years by the FAA and AMEs, with some assistance from the Armed Forces Institute of Pathology and loaned military flight surgeons.

Reports of accident summaries, annual reviews of data, and special reports on a number of topics, including fire, emergency evacuation, and chemical oxygen generators, are quite valuable. Unfortunately, there is frequently a 2- to 3-year lag in their publication.

Pilot Causes and Factors

The NTSB determined the cause and causal factors in 3502 United States general aviation accidents that occurred in 1981. The pilot was a causal factor in 86.9% of 654 fatal accidents and 79.0% of all accidents. The most frequently cited causes or factors in 761 fatal accidents in 1978 were pilot-continued visual flight rules (VFR) flight into adverse weather conditions (19.71%), pilot failure to obtain or maintain flying speed (19.45%), spatial disorientation (11.56%), inadequate preflight preparation or planning (11.04%), and improper in-flight decisions (9.72%). The complete list adds to over 100% because multiple factors are frequently identified. An underlying reason for each improper action usually is not determined but may include inadequate training or inexperience, drug or alcohol impairment, carelessness, distraction, preoccupation, fatigue, and illness.

The NTSB has found that the pilot was a cause or factor in 86% of all aircraft accidents and 90% of the fatal accidents in a study of over 17,000 general aviation accidents involving propeller-driven, single-engine aircraft from 1972 through 1976.

The NTSB said it could not analyze fully the pilot factors in the accidents because of a lack of comprehensive data from the FAA. It is uncertain whether the 1978 data represent a significant sustainable improvement.

Attempts to improve FAA data collection and analysis continue with expanded forms, a training course for FAA medical officers and AMEs, and incorporation of medical accident data into the total safety information system to enhance analyses.

The numbers of specific medical or physiologic causes or factors in fatal general aviation accidents in 1978 included 88 cases of spatial disorientation, 48 cases of physical impairment, 45 cases of alcoholic impairment of efficiency and judgment, 14 cases of pilot fatigue, eight cases of pilot incapacitation, four cases involving the pilot's psychologic condition, three cases of carbon monoxide poisoning, two suicides, one heart attack, and one case of hypoxia.

Toxicology

In their 1961 Eastern Region outline of procedures for AME participation in aircraft accident investigation, Esch and Albers[6] called for crash-injury correlation examinations, autopsies, and blood samples for alcohol, carbon monoxide, and barbiturate determinations in all cases, including both fatalities and survivors, if possible. In 1964, Harper and Albers[7] attracted considerable attention when they reported that 35.4% of the fatal 1963 general aviation accidents that they studied

(158, or about one third) were positive for blood and/or tissue alcohol (over 14 mg/dL). The actual involvement of ethyl alcohol in accident causation has been difficult to determine. In the absence of an established blood level for impairment of pilot judgment and performance, state levels for operating motor vehicles under the influence of alcohol have been used for many years. For the determination of a realistic estimate of alcohol involvement in general aviation accidents and trends, the results from the CAMI accident toxicology program are probably the most useful. Specimens are received from about 60% of the fatal accidents now in this study, which was started in 1968. Blood alcohol levels greater than 40 mg/dL were found in 11.5% of the pilots killed in general aviation accidents from 1968 to 1971. The 8-hour rule (between drinking and flying) was effective December 5, 1970. The percentage of alcohol-related fatalities dropped to 7.1% in 1972 and to 6.1% in 1973, rebounded to 11.2% in 1974, averaged 8.6% for the 1974 to 1978 period, dropped to 5.7% in 1979, and rose to 6.5% in 1980 and 1981.

Medications also are routinely looked for and are present in about 6% of general aviation fatal accidents. Tissue levels are found in one fourth of these accidents (most commonly barbiturates, antihistamines, tranquilizers, and salicylates), but a causal role is difficult to determine and is rarely assigned. A reliable detection method for marijuana has only recently become available. The presence of medications occasionally alerts investigators to the presence of medical conditions that have been found to be causes or factors.

Plasma and red blood cell cholinesterase levels should be determined in pilots killed in aerial application accidents to determine possible organophosphate pesticide involvement as an accident cause and whether acute or chronic poisoning occurred. Low levels of cholinesterase are found in about one half of these pilots where self-medication with atropine and pralidoxime is common.

Carbon monoxide levels are also regularly determined. Levels above smoking levels in accidents without fire are found in one to three accidents each year. The manifold always should be examined for cracks in these accidents. The carbon monoxide level in an accident with fire can be used to determine the cause of death.

Fire carboxyhemoglobin levels of 30 to 60% were found in 16 victims of an air carrier landing accident with fire at Denver, Colorado on July 11, 1961. Placards for the location of exits and research to provide passengers with an uncontaminated air supply during evacuation were recommended. Smoke saturation of the cabin is estimated to have occurred in 2 to 2.5 minutes.

In another landing accident with fire at Salt Lake City, Utah on November 11, 1965, 43 individuals were overcome by dense smoke, intense heat, and flames or a combination of these elements before they were able to escape. Carboxyhemoglobin levels of 13 to 82% were found. Fuel line strength and location and B-727 landing speed were changed as a result. Thereafter, a flight attendant was stationed by emergency exits during takeoffs and landings. Research programs on fire toxicity, more crashworthy fuel tanks, jellied fuel, explosive exits, and filling the cabin with foam were initiated. Numerous toxic products of combustion, including hydrogen cyanide, hydrogen chloride, hydrogen fluoride, diisocyanates, ammonia, and acrolein, were identified, as well as carbon monoxide. Overkill levels of hydrogen cyanide and carbon monoxide were found within 2.5 minutes when cabin interior materials and jet fuel were burned; the systemic effects were found to be supra-additive, and the effects of dozens of other products of combustion became academic. The required maximum time for evacuation for new air carrier aircraft and new seating densities was reduced from 150 to 90 seconds.

Determination of cyanide levels in victims of fire accidents was started by CAMI after a takeoff accident in Anchorage, Alaska on November 27, 1970 in which 23 people died. Possibly lethal cyanide levels were found in 18 of the 19 blood specimens received. Similar carboxyhemoglobin and cyanide levels have been found in the few air carrier accidents involving fire that have occurred since then.

Work is progressing on antimisting kerosene and other fuel additives to reduce the occurrence of crash fires and on a combined hazard index to rate cabin interior materials for relative ignition, burning rate, smoke production, and toxicity of combustion products properties.

Other safety measures include cargo fire detection and suppression systems, improved cabin fire extinguishers, fireproof lavatory trash bins, and smoking restrictions. No smoke protection equipment has been adopted for passenger use, but improved equipment is available for crew use, primarily for in-flight smoke and fires.

Because the complete prevention of fires is unlikely and a problem of toxic products from the combustion of cargo, carry-on luggage, and occupants' apparel will remain, primary emphasis must continue to be given to rapid emergency evacuation.

Evacuation

Because of the importance of prompt emergency evacuation in an accident with fire, continuing attention is given to the training, placement, and protection of flight attendants, communication, emergency lighting and exit location, containment of carry-on items, aircraft attitude effects, special problems of handicapped passengers, and flow rates on spiral stairs, out exits, and down double-lane slides. A mathematical model has been investigated to calculate evacuation times with a large number of recognized variables to save the expense and occasional injuries of the required demonstration evacuations.

Ditching

Ditchings and survivable crashes in water of United States air carrier aircraft are rare. A ditching 30 miles from St. Croix, Virgin Islands on May 2, 1970 and a crash into Escambia Bay on an approach to Pensacola Regional Airport, Pensacola, Florida on May 8, 1978 are recommended for study by students of this subject. Provisions are made for such events with life vests, flotation seat cushions, life rafts, combination evacuation slide/rafts, crew training, and passenger briefings. Deficiencies in crew and passenger performance due to the infrequency of accidents have resulted in drownings. For a number of years there was little concern about the suitability and adequate retained buoyancy of flotation seat cushions. Inflatable life vests have been in use that failed some tests of donning and buoyancy, and some air carriers have obtained permission not to carry life rafts on some overwater routes.

Potential shark and hypothermia problems have received some attention, but no shark-related deaths and only extremely rare hypothermia incidents have been documented in United States air carrier accidents.

Decompression

Decompression at altitude and hypoxia from any cause are relatively rare events in civil aviation. Although a window-out decompression of an aircraft in 20 to 25 seconds is the usual assumption for training purposes, the chances of the actual loss of a windscreen, window, entry door, or emergency exit are remote. Turbine blades, a cargo door latch problem, a tire exploding in the wheel well, an explosive device, and, in one instance, a hijacker leaving by the rear ventral stair (which is no longer possible) are some actual causes of decompression. When decompression does occur, it is of paramount importance that the crew maintain useful function with adequate oxygen equipment and be prepared to use it properly in a surprising event. The classic case occurred in a wide-body jet at 11,700 m, 104 km southwest of Albuquerque, New Mexico on November 3, 1973. When a passenger went through a window, flight attendants in a lower level galley lost consciousness, and one attendant reportedly suffered permanent neurologic damage, some oxygen masks failed to deploy promptly, some passengers failed to pull the masks toward them to activate the flow of oxygen, and three oxygen generators were pulled from their mountings and activated, resulting in scorched seat upholstery and burned fingers. Subsequent studies[8,9] vindicated the solid oxygen generators from concerns about too slow a rate of onset of flow, determined that male and female flight attendants had the same time of useful consciousness, set 15 seconds as the maximum safe time for a flight attendant to reach an oxygen supply after the onset of decompression, and found an average time of useful consciousness of 32 seconds from the onset of decompression for active attendants, resulting in the advice to take care of themselves and not the passengers. As more and more general aviation aircraft fly above 7500 m, occasional problems are to be expected.

Crash Injury Correlation

Despite efforts for decades to collect crash injury correlation data in the field for general aviation accidents, the completion of detailed forms has not been adequate to permit analysis on a large scale as envisioned. Valuable observations have been made, however, by De Haven, Hasbrook, Snyder, Kirkham, and others, studied in the laboratory by Swearingen and Chandler, and adopted by the government and airline industry. Attempts are still being made by the FAA (through the Regional Flight Surgeons and AMEs) and the NTSB to improve the coverage of this part of aircraft accident investigation.

The value of upper torso restraint is now generally accepted. Authorities have disagreed about the need for dynamic testing of seats and restraint systems for many years. Standards have been written for infant and child restraint systems in aviation. A 25-g seat, found in agricultural aircraft, has been recommended by FAA medical scientists for all of general aviation but does not appear likely soon. NTSB figures can be used to show that aerial application has almost 1.5 times the accident rate for all of general aviation (16.44 versus 11.4 per 100,000 hours) but only half the fatal accident rate (1.01 versus 2.01 per 100,000 hours)—a factor of about 3; agricultural aviation has about 10% of all the general aviation accidents but only 3.5% of the fatal accidents—a factor of about 3; and 6% of agricultural aircraft accidents are fatal, compared with 18% of all general aviation accidents being fatal—again, a factor of 3.

Airman Education

One successful program not attributable to Dr. Bauer or to anyone else before the establishment of the FAA concerns educating airmen about the medical and physiologic factors of flight. Films, slide sets, exhibits, brochures, handbooks, lectures, demonstrations, material for flight instruction programs, and physiologic training, including chamber flights, are used to address safety problems. Spatial disorientation, a cause or factor in 11 to 17% of general aviation fatal accidents, is demonstrated in a popular exhibit and with about 90 portable Barany-type chairs in the hands of Accident Prevention Specialists from the General Aviation District Offices and CAMI education specialists (Fig. 26–2). The message is that disorientation is physiologic, no one is immune, and pilots should obtain an instrument rating, stay proficient, and believe the in-

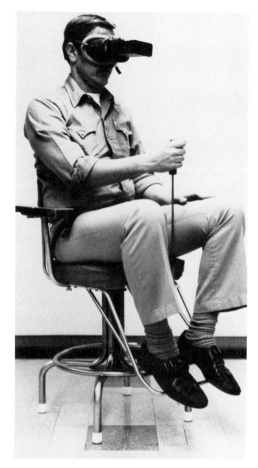

Fig. 26–2. An inexpensive, lightweight, portable Barany-type chair and a hood with blue fixation lights, which will hopefully reduce motion sickness, both designed at the Civil Aeromedical Institute (CAMI), are used to demonstrate spatial disorientation, the Coriolis effect, and nystagmus to pilots at aviation safety programs.

struments or else not fly without reference to a true horizon. Disorientation also is covered in brochures, handbooks, a film, lectures, research reports, and the physiologic training course. Because hypoxia is primarily a potential problem in civil aviation and rarely determined to be an accident cause, it is important that other, more critical safety issues also be discussed during physiologic training courses. About 4000 civilian pilots receive physiologic training each year at CAMI and at cooperating United States Air Force, Navy, and NASA chamber facilities. No operational requirement exists for this training; therefore, interest, not mission, determines who attends the course. Drugs, alcohol, vision, preoccupation, and physical and emotional problems are other common topics in the airman education program, which emphasizes preflight self-assessment for pilots as well as for aircraft to determine fitness to fly on a day-to day basis.

Cabin safety workshops have been conducted since 1975 to exchange research data and information on operational problems with cabin procedures instructors and union representatives from all major United States and several foreign air carriers. These widely acclaimed sessions have been fully attended with, at times, a 1-year waiting list.

Regulations

Only Part 67 of the Federal Aviation Regulations, Medical Standards and Certification, has been mentioned so far.

Part 61 sets requirements for medical certificates, the durations of medical certificates, and minimum ages for the various airman certificates (there is no age restriction for medical certification), prohibits acting as a pilot in command or as a required pilot flight crewmember anyone with a known medical deficiency or an increase of a known medical deficiency that makes the airman unable to meet the requirements of his current medical certificate, and contains the penalty for offenses involving narcotic drugs, marijuana, and depressant or stimulant drugs or substances.

Part 91 contains the requirements for the use of supplemental oxygen and safety belts, the 8-hour rule regarding alcohol consumption,and other general operating and flight rules for aircraft operating within the United States.

Part 121, regarding certification and operations for air carriers and commercial operators of large aircraft, sets requirements for crewmember emergency train-ing, minimum contents of first-aid kits, crewmember flight-time limitations for air carriers and commercial operators, and, under section 121.383, the "age-60 rule" (no certificate holder may use the services of any person as a pilot on an airplane engaged in operations if that person has reached his sixtieth birthday, and no person may serve as a pilot on an airplane engaged in operations if that person has reached his sixtieth birthday).

Alcohol and Drugs

Section 91.11 states that

1. No person may act as a crewmember of a civil aircraft
   a. Within 8 hours after the consumption of any alcoholic beverage
   b. While under the influence of alcohol
   c. While using any drug that affects his faculties in any way contrary to safety
2. Except in an emergency, no pilot of a civil aircraft may allow a person who is obviously under the influence of intoxicating liquors or drugs (except a medical patient under proper care) to be carried in that aircraft

Supplement Oxygen

The requirements concerning supplemental oxygen are in section 91.32 as follows.

1. *General—no person may operate a civil aircraft of United States registry*
   a. At cabin pressure altitudes above 12,500 ft (3750 m) up to and including 14,000 ft (4200 m) unless the required minimum flight crew is provided with and uses supplemental oxygen for that part of the flight at those altitudes which lasts more than 30 minutes
   b. At cabin pressure altitudes above 4200 m, unless the required minimum flight crew is provided with and uses supplemental ox-

ygen during the entire flight time at those altitudes

c. At cabin pressure altitudes above 15,000 ft (4500 m) unless each occupant of the aircraft is provided with supplemental oxygen

2. Pressurized cabin aircraft—no person may operate a civil aircraft of United States registry with a pressurized cabin at flight altitudes above flight level 250 (25,000 ft.; 8,300 m) unless at least a 10-minute supply of supplemental oxygen, in addition to any oxygen required to satisfy part 1 of this section, is available for each occupant of the aircraft for use in the event that a descent is necessitated by loss of cabin pressurization

Air Piracy

Aircraft piracy, hijacking, or "skyjacking" of United States aircraft to Cuba started in 1961, ceased for 3 years after President Kennedy signed Public Law 87-197 making aircraft piracy a federal crime, recurred in 1964, and became a serious problem in 1968 when there were 22 attempts to hijack United States aircraft to Cuba; eighteen of these attempts were successful.

In February, 1969, the FAA Task Force on the Deterrence of Aircraft Piracy was established, and Dr. Homer L. Reighard, the (then) Deputy Federal Air Surgeon, was appointed chairman. A system to reduce hijackings was developed that combined the use of a ferrous metal detector and a behavioral profile based on characteristics found in a large number of the hijackers. Three airlines began using the system at some airports within the first year. Federal sky marshals were hired, specially trained, and used on flights between 1970 and 1972. The record of hijacking attempts gradually improved, but only after a February, 1973 ruling that all passengers must be screened by a magnetometer and all carry-on luggage be searched

did air piracy in this country virtually cease.

AEROMEDICAL RESEARCH

Bauer and Cooper's studies of the effects of physical defects on flying ability were not conducted under a formal research program, but they did collect, analyze, present, and publish data for 1927, 1928, and 1929 that showed that accident and fatality rates were directly related, and that advancement to a higher category of license was inversely related to the presence and severity of physical defect.[1,2]

Bureau of Air Commerce Medical Director Roy E. Whitehead, M.D. (1933 to 1937) was a pioneer in the study of hypoxia, the adequacy of supercharging the cabin as a means of pressurization, and oxygen requirements for flight crewmembers and passengers. The historical impact of these studies, conducted in an altitude chamber at the National Bureau of Standards, has been nearly forgotten. After a presentation of the findings at the 1935 meeting of the Aero Medical Association, Dr. Harry G. Armstrong, who was working at Wright Field in Dayton, Ohio, wrote that Dr. Whitehead "has the honor of being the first to present what is most certainly to be the coming method of oxygen administration." Dr. Whitehead also reported finding no direct relationship between private flying aircraft accidents and the physical condition of the pilots.[10]

Internal Organizations and Programs

A Medical Science Station, headed by Dr. Wade H. Miller, one of the original AMEs, was opened in April, 1938 in Kansas City, Missouri to study pilot fatigue, minimum medical standards, and hypoxic effects in airline operations. Contracts were awarded to university and foundation laboratories to augment the in-house capabilities. Lingering controversy over studying airline pilot fatigue and the duplication of other laboratories' capabilities and problems of funding, however, caused the closing of the station in 1940.

Plans were made in 1941 for a Houston Medical Center to study medical standards, the detection of heart disease, environmental factors, including hypoxia, in light aircraft, and aircraft crashworthiness. World War II interrupted the full implementation of this program.

When the Civil Aeronautics Administration (CAA) Standardization Center in Houston, Texas was moved to the new Aeronautical Center in Oklahoma City, Oklahoma in 1946, an Aviation Medical Development Center was to be established as one part to test physical standards and to identify hazardous features in aircraft design. Critics pointed to existing military aviation medical research laboratories, but proposed CAA studies of civil airman standards, crash injuries, and survival were not being conducted elsewhere. A smaller Aviation Medical Branch did result, however.

John J. Swearingen joined the CAA in 1947 as chief scientist of the Aviation Medical Branch and directed crash injury and survival research for about 25 years. The branch was moved to Columbus, Ohio, in 1953 and renamed the Civil Aviation Medical Research Laboratory; returned to Oklahoma City in 1958, where, in 1960, it became the Protection and Survival Laboratory, Civil Aeromedical Research Institute and was incorporated into the Civil Aeromedical Institute in 1965. Despite the moves, small staff, and, at times, miniscule budget, numerous accomplishments paved the way for improved aviation safety. Human tolerances to impact and body kinematics were determined, and the information was provided to aeronautic engineers as evidence of the need for upper torso restraint systems and the use of padding and deformable materials in aircraft interiors. The first anthropomorphic crash test dummy was constructed in 1950. Seat tie-down and bottom failures were documented,

and 40-g seats and molded seat pans were recommended. Emergency evacuation procedures and equipment were evaluated. Protection from hypoxia, decompression, ditching, and fire and smoke also was studied. Ernest B. McFadden contributed a smoke protective hood, the round passenger oxygen mask, the aneroid-actuated passenger oxygen mask presentation, an adhesive oxygen mask for children, an infant flotation device, and a flotation test dummy before his retirement in 1978 (Fig. 26–3). Physical standards were not studied, however.

Georgetown Clinical Research Institute

On June 27, 1959, the Federal Aviation Agency proposed and on March 15, 1960 effected a rule that no individual who had reached his sixtieth birthday could be utilized or serve as a pilot on any aircraft engaged in air carrier operations—the Age 60 rule. The agency recognized from the outset the desirability of basing pilot retirement on a physiologic age rating rather than on chronologic age. Plans were promptly developed for a clinical research program to develop such a rating, and the Georgetown Clinical Research Institute (GCRI), headed by Arthur E. Wentz, M.D., was established at the Georgetown University Medical Center in Washington, D.C. in 1960. A contract was awarded to the Lovelace Foundation for Medical Education and Research to identify the criteria for studies that would provide the basis for a physiologic age rating. Special tests utilized at GCRI included pupillography, rheoencephalography, ballistocardiography, and the psychomet, a test that measured the speed and accuracy of subjects' reactions to visual signals. The Lovelace Foundation submitted their FAA contract report to the Public Health Service as a grant application and began a funded study with identical purposes—a physiologic age rating for pilots—in Albuquerque, New Mexico. By 1965, the FAA was accused of costly duplication of

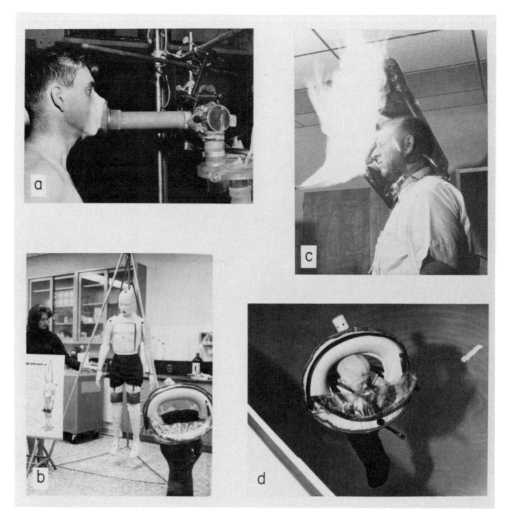

Fig. 26–3. Contributions to environmental protection by Ernest B. McFadden include a. the round passenger mask; b. an anthropomorphic flotation test dummy with controlled variable segment buoyancy and telemetry capabilities; c. a smoke and flame protective hood; and d. an infant flotation device.

Public Health Service-funded pilot aging research. This criticism, plus findings from another study that research facilities in Oklahoma City, Oklahoma were only one-third occupied, led to the closing of GCRI in 1966, transfer of the positions to CAMI, and deemphasis of aging research. No scientists made the move to CAMI. Data were turned over to the Public Health Service, but no useful physiologic age indices were developed from the abbreviated effort.

Civil Aeromedical Research Institute

A second medical research facility, the Civil Aeromedical Research Institute (CARI), was established in 1960 in Oklahoma City. Headed by Stanley R. Mohler, M.D. from 1961 to 1965, CARI incorporated the Civil Aviation Medical Research Laboratory as its Protection and Survival Laboratory, added biodynamics, biochemistry, physiology, neurophysiology, and psychology laboratories, and moved into a new 212,000-square-foot facility, custom designed for a staff of 350, at the Aeronautical Center in October, 1962. New, important research on air traffic controller selection, pesticide poisoning, spatial disorientation, drug effects, circadian rhythms, vision, hearing, fatigue, and cardiac rehabilitation was initiated, and close ties were established with the University of Oklahoma. The full-time research staff never exceeded 75, however.

Civil Aeromedical Institute

In late 1965, the Civil Aeromedical Research institute became the Aeromedical Research Branch of the Civil Aeromedical Institute, which also included medical certification and clinical branches. Within the Civil Aeromedical Institute, there was no lasting growth of the research program, and chronic funding problems persisted, but there was organizational and geographic stability, medical, statistical, and chamber support from other branches, a commitment to applied research, and ample opportunities to identify current safety-related problems in civil aviation. The latter was achieved by the increased scope of involvement in aircraft accident investigations, medical certification cases, collaborative research efforts, industrial hygiene surveys, and abundant user and field contacts through regular participation in FAA Academy operations inspector and Transportation Safety Institute accident investigation courses, cabin safety workshops, presentations at flight instructor and accident prevention clinics, AME seminars, visitors, and meetings and other activities of professional organizations.

An aircraft accident toxicology program, established in 1968, has been one of the best indicators of the incidence and trends of pesticide-, drug-, and alcohol-related fatal accidents in general aviation. Improved methods of specimen shipping and analyses were developed. A procedure to culture delayed, warm, or contaminated specimens for alcohol-producing bacteria was established. Testing for hydrogen cyanide and carbon monoxide in victims of air carrier accidents with fire was initiated, and this opened a whole new chapter in the determination of the toxicity of burning materials. Studies determined the relative toxicity from flaming and nonflaming combustion of about 100 materials found in aircraft cabins, homes, offices, and hotels. Times to incapacitation and to death were determined to estimate how long victims were capable of escaping. Extrapolation of data from rats to humans based on body weight and respiratory volume have been confirmed by available information from accidental fire victims. Research on combinations of toxic products and on whole fire effects is continuing. The ultimate objective is a combined hazard index that incorporates ignition, rate of burning, smoke production, and toxicity data for consideration in the selection of materials for aircraft furnishings.

A forensic anthropology unit has studied restraint system design, body measurements for improved anthropomorphic test dummies and models (including the first one for 6-month-old infants and upgraded dimensional data for 3-year-old and 6-year-old children), flight attendant size and strength, and improved victim identification techniques to assist in aircraft accident investigation efforts.

The addition of a pathologist further enhanced the scope of aircraft accident investigations, even in the crashworthiness, seat, and restraint areas where there had been long-standing interest and research. Several additional improvements in general aviation aircraft seating and restraint systems have resulted that are certain to improve survivability in accidents.

In the area of air carrier accident survival, improvements have been made in crew smoke protection, crew oxygen equipment, emergency evacuation equipment and procedures, and provisions for the carriage of handicapped passengers as a result of CAMI efforts. Ditching survival, child restraint, and passenger smoke protection are receiving attention at the time of this writing. The concept of a smoke protective hood with an added air supply has found wide application. The flotation test dummy and infant flotation device and studies of shark reactions to current flotation equipment have had limited adoption.

A multiple task performance battery has been used to obtain valid and consistent measures of complex performance with alcohol, several medications, altitude, heat, fatigue, crash dieting, time zone changes, and smoking withdrawal. It also has been used to explore psychomotor test methods for air traffic controller selection. Alcohol has been found to affect complex performance in a moving environment at a 27 mg/dL blood level. Congeners and hangover effects also have been evaluated in several other alcohol studies, but no practical significance has been found.

Studies have continued on aptitude, experience, and age factors in air traffic controller selection, and the adoption of recommended selection tests and a maximum entry age by the Civil Service Commission (now the Office of Personnel Management) has decreased attrition from the training program. Studies of validity and fairness of selection and training methods, including direct involvement in new radar training and computer-based instructions systems, continue at a pace that generates thousands of reports each year.

Other studies of air traffic controllers have concerned motivation, vigilance, and reported stress. Air traffic control was not found to be inherently more stressful than other occupations, but an efficient method was found to measure and display a relative indication of acute stress, chronic stress, neuromuscular activity, and total stress between facilities, shift rotation schedules, and different equipment by using urine samples.

Although GCRI was not successfully transformed into a clinical research branch of CAMI, studies of color vision

requirements and testing, contact lenses, speech audiometry, altitude tolerance with chronic obstructive pulmonary disease, alcoholism detection, sickle cell trait compatibility with flight, medication effects on pilot performance, and aircraft accident correlation with age, weight, vision disorders, and several static physical defects have been conducted in support of physical standards and policies.

A variety of environmental problems have been studied. The acute effects of ozone on cockpit and cabin crewmembers and on healthy passengers have been determined and the chronic effects estimated, and operational limitations have been established to limit exposures to safe levels. The effects of ionizing and microwave radiation have been studied, estimates of risk have been calculated, and a guide for acceptable loading of radioactive cargo has been prepared. Noise effects, including headset test tones in air traffic control facilities, have been calculated, and hearing protective devices have been rated.

Studies of accident, medical defect, age, and occupation correlations are regularly conducted using the aeromedical certification data base, which contains records on over 800,000 active airmen.

The results of FAA medical research are published in Office of Aviation Medicine (OAM) reports and usually in the open scientific literature. OAM reports and a biennial index are available from the National Technical Information Service, Springfield, Virginia, 22161 and, on a limited basis as long as a supply of extra copies lasts, from CAMI, AAC-100, P.O. Box 25082, Oklahoma City, Oklahoma, 73125.

Contract Studies

The FAA has sponsored relatively little contract medical research. For many years, $100,000 was requested in annual budget submissions to fund contract resolutions of problems that could not be solved within the FAA. Historically, however, the funds usually were needed to cover budget cuts and to help absorb pay raises, so few studies resulted. Of those studies conducted, four are deemed worthy of special mention.

A 1961 report by Blockley and Hanifan[11] and a 1965 report[12] and film by Barron and Cook have served as the bases for FAA medical staff opposition to increased operational altitudes for jet aircraft and relaxed requirements for crew oxygen use at these altitudes as long as decompression is felt to be possible. Results have still proved useful in a reexamination and possible tightening of requirements 20 years later.

Billings and colleagues' 1972 study[13] found that even 40 mg/dL of blood alcohol exerted decremental effects on the performance of instrument-rated pilots of simple (single-engine, fixed-propeller, fixed-gear) civil aircraft that were incompatible with flight safety at a time when 100 to 150 mg/dL blood alcohol levels, set by states for impairment of motor vehicle operation, were used to officially determine alcohol involvement in fatal aircraft accidents. A maximum blood alcohol level of 40 mg/dL for pilots and an implied consent provision to permit the determination of alcohol levels in pilots involved in nonfatal accidents have been proposed.

The most extensive contract effort was Rose and colleagues', 5-year study of air traffic controller health changes, which was completed in 1978.[14] Findings included in the 800-page report suggested that it was not so much what air traffic controllers were doing but the context in which they were doing it and the attitudes and feelings they had about their situation that influenced their risk for health changes. The largest single chronic illness condition among air traffic controllers was hypertension, but the interpretation of these findings was that, for individuals who are predisposed to developing hypertension by reason of a host of genetic and biologic factors, exposure to air traffic control work increases the risk or perhaps hastens the rate of the development of hypertension. About half the men in the study had at least one psychiatric problem, but most of these individuals did not receive professional treatment, and no other occupational group is known to have been studied using Rose and colleagues' criteria to permit comparison. A slightly increased risk for developing peptic ulcer also was found in the study population.

AIR TRAFFIC CONTROL SPECIALIST HEALTH PROGRAM

The Civil Aviation Act of 1938 required that control tower operators take and pass the same physical examination and possess the same medical certificate as commercial pilots. Despite growth of the system to include controllers in air route traffic control centers and flight service stations, the Federal Aviation Act of 1958 only continued the existing requirements for tower controllers and ignored the center and station controllers. At the request of the FAA, the Civil Service Commission established selection and retention physical standards for tower, center, and flight service station controllers in 1965. An air traffic control specialist (ATCS) health program was initiated by the FAA in 1965. Psychologic testing to demonstrate the absence of mental, neurotic, and personality disorders proved to be controversial and was fully implemented only after some proposed tests were dropped and the remaining test—the 16 Personality Factors, or 16 PF, test—was modified and revalidated. Beginning in 1970, Assistant Regional Flight Surgeons were hired in the air route traffic control centers, primarily to examine and treat ATCSs. Early studies reported a greater incidence and prevalence of coronary artery disease, hypertension, peptic ulcer, neuropsychiatric disorders, and diabetes mellitus in ATCSs, and an act providing for early retirement and for training in another field ("second career") was passed by Congress in 1972.

Claims for disability retirement rose significantly after this legislation was passed. Because of limited diagnostic testing in most claims for retirement or retraining and conflicting reports of analyses of available data, the true incidence and prevalence of possibly stress-related disease in this population probably will never be known.

New ATCS health program standards and procedures for selecting controllers and, most importantly, helping them to remain fit and on the job were published in 1980.

A comprehensive health information system was established by the Office of Aviation Medicine in the Washington, D.C. headquarters in 1981 to collect, for the first time, all available medical information on each ATCS. This system is collecting and analyzing data for a different population following the firing of about 11,400 ATCSs in August, 1981 for striking illegally.

PROJECTIONS

Despite increased costs and the effects of the strike by the Professional Air Traffic Controllers Organization (PATCO), an average annual growth of about 3% is forecast in the civil airman population. It is easy for those in aviation medicine in the FAA to conclude that all programs are essential and that, at the very least, they should be continued with adjustments for growth and inflation. Review of the history of federal civil aviation medicine in the United States can have a sobering effect, however. Under political and economic pressures, physical standards have been relaxed, less frequent physical examinations have been proposed and some changes adopted, field medical offices have been closed, educational programs have been discontinued, research programs have been abolished, the medical certification process has been crippled by reduced staffing, and the requirement for examinations by designated physicians

was suspended for about 15 years. Of late, one group has petitioned the FAA for less frequent physical examinations of private pilots, one federal court judge has dealt exemptions and operational restrictions a serious setback, and Congress has directed an independent study of the mandatory age-60 retirement of airline pilots. Although the needs are essentially unchanged, nothing is certain.

The FAA gradually has adopted more lenient medical standards and certification/exemption policies on alcoholism, visual acuity, contact lenses, and the use of medications, but there is continuing pressure to relax standards even further, examine pilots less frequently, and repeal the age-60 rule.

On the other hand, studies point out serious deficiencies in current examination procedures to detect coronary artery disease, alcoholism, psychiatric problems, reduced cognitive function, and glaucoma, to mention a few; a need for more frequent examinations for older pilots and more research on pilot aging; and increased dependence on the AME's examination to assure pilot fitness with recent reduction in airline medical staffs.

The tenets of Dr. Bauer are still true. The FAA medical program is still felt to be meeting responsibly a valid safety need. Now, as never before, however, there is a need to be objective, flexible, and economical in carrying out these responsibilities.

REFERENCES

1. Cooper, H.J.: The relation between physical deficiencies and decreased performance. J. Aviat. Med., 1:4, 1930.
2. Cooper, H.J.: Further studies on the effect of physical defects on flying ability. J. Aviat. Med., 2:162, 1931.
3. Eighth Bethesda Conference of the American College of Cardiology, Washington, D.C., April 25–26, 1975. Am. J. Cardiol., 36:573, 1975.
4. Neurological and neurosurgical conditions associated with aviation safety. Arch. Neurol., 36:731, 1979.
5. Booze, C.F., Jr.: An Appraisal of Federal Aviation Administration Frequency of Examination Requirements. Oklahoma City, Oklahoma, Federal

Aviation Administration Civil Aeromedical Institute, 1975.

6. Esch, A.F., and Albers, W.R.: Outline of Procedures for FAA Aviation Medical Examiner Participation in Aircraft Accident Investigation. Jamaica, New York, Federal Aviation Administration Office of the Regional Flight Surgeon, Eastern Region, 1961.

7. Harper, C.R., and Albers, W.R.: Alcohol and general aviation accidents. Aerospace Med., 35:462, 1964.

8. Busby, D.E., Higgins, E.A., and Funkhouser, G.E.: Effect of physical activity of airline flight attendants on their time of useful consciousness in a rapid decompression. Aviat. Space Environ. Med., 47:117, 1976.

9. Busby, D.E., Higgins, E.A., and Funkhouser, G.E.: Protection of airline flight attendants from hypoxia following rapid decompression. Aviat. Space Environ. Med. 47:942, 1976.

10. Department of Commerce Conference. J. Aviat. Med., 7:22, 1936.

11. Blockley, W.V., and Hanifan, D.T.: An Analysis of the Oxygen Protection Problem at Flight Altitudes Between 40,000 and 50,000 Feet. Final Report on Contract FA-955, prepared for the Federal Aviation Administration by Psychological Research Associates, Arlington, Virginia, 1961.

12. Barron, C.I., and Cook, T.J.: Effects of variable decompressions to 45,000 feet. Aerospace Med., 36:425, 1965.

13. Billings, C.E., Wick, R.L., Jr., Gerke, R.J., and Chase, R.C.: The Effects of Alcohol on Pilot Performance During Instrument Flight. Federal Aviation Administration Office of Aviation Medicine Report No. AM-72-4. Washington, D.C., Federal Aviation Administration, U.S. Government Printing Office, Washington, D.C., 1972.

14. Rose, R.M., Jenkins, C.D., and Hurst, M.W.: Air Traffic Controller Health Change Study. Federal Avaiation Administration Office of Aviation Medicine Report No. AM-78-39. Washington, D.C., Federal Aviation Administration, U.S. Government Printing Office, Washington, D.C., 1978.

Chapter *27*

Aircraft Accident Investigation

Robert R. McMeekin

Aviation in itself is not inherently dangerous. But to an even greater degree than the sea, it is terribly unforgiving of any carelessness, incapacity or neglect.

UNKNOWN

Aircraft accidents are not new occurrences. An accident badly damaged the front rudder frame of the Wright Flyer, cutting short the early flights of Wilbur and Orville Wright in the first successfully controlled, powered, and manned heavier-than-air machine near Kitty Hawk, North Carolina, on Thursday, December 17, 1903.

The first reported aircraft fatality in the United States occurred when the Wright brothers were demonstrating their standard Wright Type A Flyer to the United States Army Signal Corps at Fort Myer, Virginia, on September 17, 1908. When a crack developed in the starboard propeller of the Flyer, causing violent vibrations, Orville, who was at the controls of the aircraft, was unable to prevent the nosedive

and resulting crash (Fig. 27–1). First Lieutenant Thomas E. Selfridge, who was aboard as an observer, died as a result of a compound, comminuted fracture of the base of the skull suffered during the crash. An autopsy was performed, and Captain H.H. Bailey (Medical Corps, United States Army) determined the cause of death. An Aeronautical Board investigated to determine the cause of the crash.

Most people considered flying to be particularly dangerous in the early days of flight, and fatal aircraft crashes were not surprising. Transcontinental and Western Air flight no. 6, en route from Los Angeles to New York with intermediate stops in Albuquerque, New Mexico, Kansas City, Missouri, Columbus, Ohio, and Pittsburgh, Pennsylvania, crashed in dense fog near Millard, Missouri, on May 6, 1935. Few people would have taken notice of this crash, which killed five persons, except that Senator Bronson M. Cutting (R-New Mexico) was among those who died.

As a result of this crash, an outraged

The author gratefully acknowledges the valuable assistance of Lt. Col. Charles Ruehle, USAF, MC, Chief of the Armed Forces Institute of Pathology Division of Aerospace Pathology, and his staff, especially Lt. Col. Charles Springate, MC, USA, who located and shepherded many of the photographic negatives, illustrations, and references.

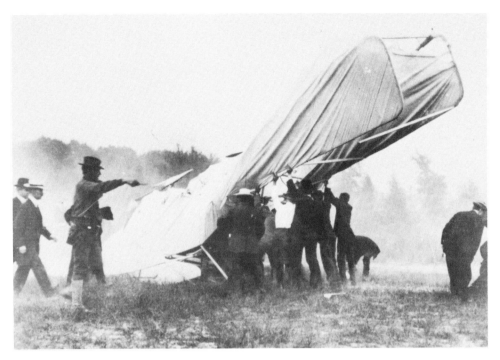

Fig. 27–1. Crash of the Wright Flyer at Ft. Myer, Virginia, on September 17, 1908 (Armed Forces Institute of Pathology photo).

Senate quickly authorized the Committee on Commerce:

> to investigate. . . [the Cutting crash]. . . and any other accidents or wrecks of airplanes engaged in interstate commerce in which lives have been lost; and to investigate. . . interstate air commerce, the precautions and safeguards provided therein, both by those engaged in such interstate air transportation and by officials or departments of the United States Government; and to investigate. . . the activities of those entrusted by the Government with the protection of property and life by [sic] air transportation, and the degree, adequacy, and efficiency of supervision by any agency of Government including inspection and frequency thereof.[1] . . .

This action established federal interest in aircraft accident investigations.

Although investigation into the mechanical causes of crashes progressed, it was not until the 1950s that the value of medical investigation of aircraft crashes became apparent. Several mysterious crashes of the jet-powered British Comets, a new generation of pressurized aircraft, led to medical investigations that marked the beginning of modern aerospace pathology. One Comet crashed on January 10, 1954 with 35 persons on board approximately 25 minutes after taking off from Rome, Italy en route to London, England. Another Comet crashed en route to Cairo, Egypt from Rome on April 8, 1954 with 21 persons on board. Both planes crashed at sea, and there were no indications as to the cause. Postmortem examination of the remains of the passengers and crew who floated to the surface allowed pathologists to determine that an explosive decompression had occurred. This structural failure resulted from insufficient hull strength to withstand the pressure differential between the cabin and the outside atmosphere at altitude.[2]

Until the development of jumbo airliners led to the potential for numerous fatalities associated with crashes, "mass disaster" meant up to 50 or perhaps 100 fatalities. Nevertheless, few people were prepared to comprehend the collision of two Boeing 747 jumbo airliners at Tenerife in the Canary islands on March 27, 1977, nor could they understand the problems that more than 580 fatalities presented (Fig. 27–2). This accident focused attention on the problems that aircraft accidents and other mass disasters can present.

There are a number of reasons to investigate aircraft accidents and incidents. The general public has a morbid curiosity about death. Certainly, a sudden occurrence such as an aircraft accident arouses public concern, and individuals have a pressing interest in the results of an aircraft accident investigation. Survivors of those who die in the crash are interested in obtaining adequate documentation to substantiate their claims for damages when they sue in the courts. The local government has an interest in ensuring the public health, safety, and welfare. It wants to be sure that no crime against the state or individuals has been committed and that there is no risk of infectious diseases. The federal government has many of the same interests as the local government. In addition, it has other interests such as the safe and efficient operation of interstate commerce. Investigators feel the pressure of all of these interests, but they must not forget that the primary purpose of aircraft accident investigation is to prevent future accidents, injuries, and fatalities. To achieve this goal, they must thoroughly investigate all injuries and circumstances of a mishap.

Although this chapter uses aircraft accidents to illustrate the techniques for the investigation of accidents, identification of the victims, and evaluation of injuries, the methods are in most cases directly applicable to accidents involving other modes of transportation.

ORGANIZATION OF THE INVESTIGATION

The development of a multidisciplinary team approach to accident investigation leads to coordinated efforts in the following general areas of interest:

1. Operations
2. Structures
3. Power plants
4. Human factors
5. Air craft systems
6. Witnesses
7. Air traffic control
8. Weather
9. Flight data recorder
10. Maintenance records
11. Evacuation, search, rescue, and fire-fighting

One or more team members are often assigned to each of these areas, but the actual composition of the accident investigation team always depends on the cir-

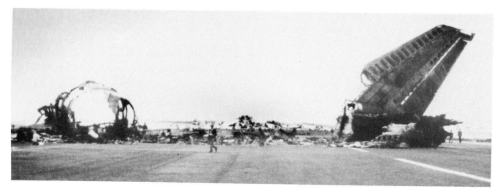

Fig. 27–2. Wreckage of two 747 airliners on the runway at Tenerife, Canary Islands, on March 27, 1977 (Armed Forces Institute of Pathology photo).

cumstances of the accident and the number of persons involved. For example, human factors teams generally consider the crashworthiness aspects of the investigation, with particular emphasis on organization, identification, injury tolerance, and analysis of injury patterns. The human factors investigation evaluates the cause of injuries received by the occupants and the psychologic or physiologic factors that may have contributed to the accident. These observations are the basis of recommendations for changes in standards for the physical examination of aircrew and pilot selection. They also lead to improvements in cockpit or passenger compartment layout and the design of seats, restraints, protective equipment, and escape mechanisms and pathways.

Phases of the Investigation

The immediate postaccident period may seem chaotic, and experienced investigators recognize the importance of the early development of an organizational plan that considers the following five general phases:

1. Preliminary evaluation
2. Data collection
3. Data analysis
4. Conclusions
5. Recommendations

The Joint Committee on Aviation Pathology (JCAP) prepared an outline of six steps for the pathologist to take when investigating fatal aircraft accidents. These steps are an adaptation of the five investigation steps listed above, and they are useful guidelines for any investigating physician. Although no rigid protocol can describe in detail how to investigate all accident types that a pathologist may encounter, JCAP recommends the following steps for the investigation of injuries sustained by the victims of a crash:

The first step in the investigation is for the pathologist to familiarize himself thoroughly with the type of aircraft—its internal structure, seating arrangement, ejection mechanism, and general layout and, if possible, to examine an intact plane of the type in question. An exact knowledge of the size, contour, and color of the objects that the pilot's body may have hit is extremely helpful in evaluating the injuries observed in and on the body. The pathologist should confer with pilots, engineers, and other experts who are familiar with the aircraft, parachute, ejection mechanism, and other equipment, to gain first-hand knowledge.

The second step in the investigation is for the pathologist to acquaint himself with all available information relative to the flight: the nature of the accident, severity of damage at the crash site, known factors about the weather, airfield, the health record and past performance of the pilot and his condition prior to and during flight, information regarding the passengers, the nature of any radio contact, and other pertinent information.

The third step in the pathologist's investigation consists of careful observations and written and photographic records of the position of the body and its relation to the total wreckage (or the parachute and other escape mechanism) and the conditions under which the body was found. The pathologist should examine carefully the pilot's protective helmet, clothing, shoes, and any other attachments. In the absence of the pathologist on the crash scene, these items should be left on the body as recovered. No article of clothing, harness, and so on should be cut or removed prior to inspection by the pathologist. The protective helmet and articles of clothing, shoes, gloves, and so forth, may reveal important information about the crash and may suggest defects in the design of the plane. Cytologic and ultraviolet light studies may offer helpful data.

The fourth step performed by the pathologist and his assistants will consist of meticulous examination of the exterior of the body and the viscera, with necessary close-up photographs and radiographs, and removal of properly selected tissue for chemical, toxicologic, and histopathologic examination. Special attention must be given to the detailed examination of all abrasions, lacerations, superficial and deep wounds. For example, a single small wound on the lateral or posterior portion of the lower legs may be strong evidence that ejection occurred but that the individual's feet were not positioned properly at the time. Photographing such wounds will be of great assistance in later correlation of the findings. Specimens of urine, blood, liver, kidney, and brain (unfixed) are best suited for the identification of poisons. For histopathologic examination, tissue sections from all organs, including the skin, bone, middle and inner ears, entire brain, spinal cord, entire heart and aorta, and organs showing significant lesions, should be preserved in 10% neutral formalin. These sections should include not only the diseased or traumatized area but also its margin and the adjacent normal area. In cases where a less than complete body is recovered, the examination of the remains should be carried out as conditions permit. It is essential to find as much of the body and internal organs as possible. The condition of the heart, brain, spinal cord, larynx, liver, skeletal muscle, and bone may well explain the cause of the crash.

The fifth stage in the investigation consists of microscopic study of the sections and chemical analysis for poisons. The pathologist must take special notice of the occurrence of vital processes such as vascular dilatation and the cellular exudation of early inflammation in the proximity of burns, contusions, etc.

The final step in the investigation is completed by summarizing the report of the accident and correlating it with the findings of the autopsy. The pathologists may participate in the proceedings of the Investigating Board.[3]

Preliminary Evaluation

Preliminary evaluation of the crash site, nature of the casualties, available resources, and the chain of events that immediately preceded the crash will save much of the investigator's time in the long run and will allow him to determine the most efficient course to follow. This early phase, which is easily underemphasized, is certainly the most important.

The investigator must become familiar with the type of aircraft, seating arrangement, restraint systems, structural arrangement, and personal equipment. He should examine an intact aircraft of the same type. If possible, this aircraft should be available for comparisons during examination of the wreckage.

Examining the cockpit of a similar aircraft may provide important clues. Comparison of details of the paint scheme of the crashed aircraft with the location of paint fragments found at the crash site may help in determining the kinematics of the occupant in the crash. Review of manuals for the operation of the aircraft and its systems, as well as information about the injury patterns and accident circumstances associated with previous crashes of the same or similar types of aircraft may also be helpful.

Data Collection

The initial phases of accident investigation involve gathering information about the circumstance of the accident and the casualties. The investigator begins collecting data to evaluate many factors; background information about the general health, emotional attitude, experience level, and training of the crew is particularly important. He should look for behavior patterns that might have led to errors of judgment or errors of action or reaction on the part of crewmembers, as well as for the presence of adverse physiologic conditions that might have impaired the crew. He should seek clues regarding the speed, direction, and attitude of impact, which will be helpful later in analyzing injury patterns.

The investigator must be particularly alert in obtaining all available information about the circumstances of the accident, ·and he must coordinate this information with other groups involved in the investigation. He should interview any witnesses because their observations may give clues about what occurred immediately prior to the crash. Even seemingly insignificant factors can be valuable to the human factors investigator in understanding the kinematics of the crash and in evaluating the causes of any unusual injuries. For example, severe turbulence associated with thunderstorms may explain the wreckage distribution following in-flight breakup.

Security at the crash site is important to ensure that no one alters the wreckage and its valuable clues as to the cause of the crash. Taking photographs and making diagrams is essential before anyone disturbs the wreckage. Well-meaning investigators often create problems by unintentionally altering crash sites. Nothing should be disturbed until someone photographs or otherwise documents the site. This, of course, assumes that survivors already have been evacuated from the site.

Adequate investigation requires careful documentation of the scene, and all participants in the investigation need to consider the final location of the debris. The investigator should note the exact location of various parts of the wreckage, the location and configuration of ground impact, the stopping distance of the aircraft, and the exact amount of crush of the aircraft structure and should record this information on a scaled diagram. The diagram should also note the location of the bodies. These notes will be helpful in the identification of bodies, estimation of crash forces, and determination of the sequence of events.

A thorough description of the nature and extent of each injury will also be helpful, and photographs, radiographs, and diagrams will be useful in documenting injuries. Careful examination to document preexisting disease and toxicologic studies to evaluate possible toxic substances or self-medication are also important.

Radiologic examination of the entire body, particularly the hands, feet, and vertebrae, is important. Radiographs often enable the investigator to determine who was operating the vehicle controls at the time of the crash or estimate the magnitude and direction of impact in high-speed crashes (Fig. 27–3A and B).

A complete autopsy examination of all fatalities is essential. Autopsies of fatally injured crewmembers may uncover preexisting disease, incapacitation, or the presence of toxic substances in aircraft. Autopsies of the passengers may speed their identification and allow correlation of the design features of the aircraft or peculiarities of the accident that are responsible for the deaths of some passengers and the survival of others.

Data Analysis

The investigator must diligently collect and evaluate the data. Having collected the facts, he must then carefully analyze the questions to be answered. Given properly posed questions and adequate investigation, most answers follow surprisingly easily. Although initial impressions as to the cause of an accident may be tempting conclusions, the investigator must not summarily dismiss any observation as insignificant. He must remain unbiased while conducting the investigation and be continually aware of possible new areas in which to pursue the investigation before forming conclusions. Each piece of factual information must be weighed as to its validity. The investigator must even suspect the witnesses' observations if they cannot be substantiated with factual information. Proper evaluation of the factual data that have been collected involves ruling out all other possible explanations.

Conclusions

After determining and evaluating the facts, the investigator must reach conclusions as to the cause both of the accident and the injuries received by the passengers and crew. Three of five important questions that Fryer proposed must be answered in the conclusion and recommendation phases:[4]

> Why did the fatally injured lose their lives?
> To what feature of the accident or of the aircraft can be attributed the escape of the survivors?
> Is there any indication that the main or any subsidiary causes of the accident might have been of a medical nature?

The conclusions should reflect the investigator's best opinions based on the available factual information. The cause of the accident or of specific injuries need not be proven beyond any shadow of doubt because the questions that require this degree of certainty are matters for the courts and collateral boards of investigation to determine. After defining substantiating facts, reasonable speculation is of definite value in deriving conclusions. A determination of "cause—undetermined" does nothing to advance the prevention of accidents and injuries.

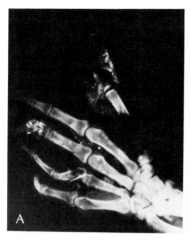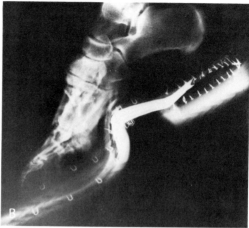

Fig. 27–3. Radiograph of hand *(A)* and foot *(B)* indicate that these were the extremities of the pilot, who was at the controls when this accident occurred (Armed Forces Institute of pathology photo).

Recommendations

The investigation is not complete until the investigator makes recommendations for changes that will prevent similar injuries and fatalities and, if possible, prevent the recurrence of the factors that caused the accident. The recommendations should address at least Fryer's[4] last two questions:

1. Would any modification of the aircraft or of its equipment have improved the chances of survival of those killed or reduced the severity of injury of the survivors?
2. Would the incorporation of such modifications have a detrimental effect on the chances of any of the survivors?

JURISDICTION

The jurisdiction to conduct investigations of deaths usually rests with the government of the territory in which the death occurs. Nevertheless, disputes occur at the state, national, and international levels over jurisdiction to conduct postmortem investigations, including autopsies of aircraft accident fatalities.

Jurisdiction for postmortem investigation at the international level is usually clear, if not entirely satisfactory, to the parties. According to customary international law, in the absence of a contrary agreement, a sovereign nation may establish whatever laws it chooses with respect to matters that are essentially within its domestic jurisdiction. One country cannot enforce its laws within the territory of another country, and the law of the country where an act is done wholly determines the character of the act. Treaties, conventions, and executive agreements resolve many of the problems that result from differences in laws among countries. The 1944 Chicago Convention provides for international participation by the state of registry in investigations of civil aviation accidents:

> In the event of an accident to an aircraft of a contracting State occurring in the territory of another contracting State, and involving death or serious injury, or indicating serious technical defect in the aircraft or air navigation facilities, the State in which the accident occurs will institute an inquiry into the circumstances of the accident, in accordance, so far as its laws permit, with the procedure which may be recommended by the International Civil Aviation Organization. The State in which the aircraft is registered shall be given the opportunity to appoint obervers to be present at the inquiry and the State holding the inquiry shall communicate the report and findings in the matter to that State.[5]

Effective international cooperation resulted when a major air disaster involving two Boeing 747s occurred in Tenerife in the Canary islands in 1977. United States representatives participated in the investigation, and the Spanish government permitted the removal of the fatally injured United States passengers from Tenerife to Dover Air Force Base, Delaware for identification.

Jurisdictional disputes also occur at the functional level between government agencies. The National Transportation Safety Board (NTSB), the Federal Bureau of Investigation (FBI), and the Department of Defense (DOD) are only a few of the United States agencies with interest in accident investigation. Although these interests may occasionally be diverse, personnel from the agencies are able to work together harmoniously. Statutes, regulations, and letters of agreement covering most situations clearly define the relationships between the various federal agencies.

Serious conflicts over postmortem jurisdiction occur most frequently between federal and state interests. In the United States, by virtue of the tenth amendment to the Constitution, the individual states retain jurisdiction over matters that federal legislation has not preempted. State laws regarding postmortem investigations differ considerably, and the official who authorizes postmortem examinations varies from state to state. Autopsy is available in some states only when this official suspects that a death resulted from unlawful means. Strong arguments maintain that this authority does not extend to fatalities resulting from aircraft accidents.

The United States military services, as well as armed forces from many other countries, recognize the importance of the pathologic investigation of fatal aircraft accidents, and they have published regulations requiring the postmortem examination of all fatally injured crewmembers. Civil jurisdictions, on the other hand, do not universally recognize this role of pathology, and investigators encounter major problems when fatal military aircraft accidents occur outside exclusively federal jurisdiction. Even when they acknowledge the federal interest, these civil jurisdictions consider it secondary to their own authority. The result is that many postmortem investigations of military aircraft accident fatalities are inadequate.

Adequacy of Investigations

Investigations of aircraft accident fatalities are inadequate or unavailable in certain circumstances because appropriate legislative authority is lacking. Approximately 90% of United States military aircraft accident fatalities occur in areas where the federal government has no authority to obtain postmortem information that may be essential to aviation safety and accident prevention and where many local officials refuse to fully cooperate with the military investigations.

The primary interest of coroners and medical examiners is in determining the cause and manner of death and seldom in collecting information concerning aircraft accident and injury prevention. The authorizing official or examining pathologist may have no interest in aircraft accidents and may have no knowledge, experience, or training in the techniques involved. These officials often conduct only an external description of the body, frequently omitting the microscopic and toxicologic examinations necessary to determine the presence of toxic substances in the aircraft and preexisting disease in the aircrew. Even when local officials have the authority to conduct complete autopsy examinations, they may elect not to perform them. In one instance, in answering a request for information about his investigation following a fatal aircraft accident, a coroner's pathologist responded that "according to local interpretation of state law, a coroner's autopsy precedes to [sic] the cause of death and is not an academic endeavor. When the cause of death is obvious in the gross autopsy, as in usually the case in aircraft accidents, microscopic examinations are not performed." In cases such as this, the military must depend on local civilian officials to conduct whatever examinations they deem advisable.

Even the presence of trained forensic pathologists with experience in investigating aircraft accidents does not ensure adequate examinations. Statutory authority often limits even these trained investigators in the scope of postmortem examinations. Most coroners and medical examiners do not have sufficient funds or staffs to permit the more than 2 man-days often needed for a thorough investigation. Situations where it is not clear who, if anyone, has jurisdiction are especially disconcerting because nothing is accomplished, even though everyone agrees that postmortem examinations are needed. In the above mentioned major air disaster involving two Boeing 747s at Tenerife, there were more than 580 fatalities, of which more than half were United States citizens. Three hundred and thirty-four of the 396 persons aboard the Pan American aircraft died. The jurisdiction of Spain to investigate the accident and of the United States to participate was clear under the provisions of the Chicago Convention. Logistics, however, necessitated the removal of the United States fatalities to Dover Air Force Base, Delaware, where easier access to communications facilities aided the identification process. Detailed postmortem examination could have determined the exact cause of death and why so few survived this ground collision, but no one established the jurisdiction to conduct complete autopsy examinations. Without these examinations, the investigation was incomplete. The state of Delaware could not give adequate authorization for postmortem examinations because the deaths did not occur in Delaware. The NTSB did not have jurisdiction because Spain was in charge of the investigation. Everyone

agreed that the investigations were necessary, but no one could cite a proper authority. The result was that the investigators used only those methods necessary to establish the identity of the bodies. Valuable information was lost that could have contributed to the furtherance of air safety.

Other cases of particular concern involve deaths of (1) personnel on board foreign military aircraft; (2) contractor and Department of Defense civilians who fly military aircraft; and (3) manufacturers' maintenance and test personnel who fly aircraft being constructed under contract for sale to the military and other federal agencies. If a fatal accident involving one or more of these persons as crewmembers occurs outside exclusively federal jurisdiction, the federal government must depend on the scope of local civil laws regarding autopsies. Even if local officials agree that postmortem investigations should be done, they cannot be conducted if the state laws provide for autopsies only in cases where it is suspected that death occurred by unlawful means.

Federal Interest in Aircraft Accident Investigation

Congress has expressed an interest in the investigation of aircraft accident fatalities. Congress determined that the federal government has an overriding interest in aviation safety and enacted legislation to ensure thorough investigations, including autopsies, of all civil aircraft accidents. The NTSB may conduct these autopsies regardless of provisions of local law unless the local laws pertaining to autopsies are based on the protection of religious beliefs:

> . . . In the case of any fatal accident, the Board is authorized to examine the remains of any deceased person aboard the aircraft at the time of the accident, who dies as a result of the accident, and to conduct autopsies or such other tests thereof as may be necessary to the investigation of the accident: Provided, That to the extent consistent with the needs of the accident investigation, provisions of local law protecting

religious beliefs with respect to autopsies shall be observed.[6]

A similar federal interest exists in military aircraft accidents where the economic effects and the impact on national defense are critical, but the authority of the NTSB does not extend to the investigation of accidents involving military aircraft only. Statutes authorize the United States Army and Air Force to conduct autopsies of persons fatally injured on board military aircraft when a fatal accident occurs on a military reservation where there is sole United States military jurisdiction. The military services recognize the importance of postmortem investigations of all fatally injured military crewmembers, and their regulations require autopsy examination regardless of where death occurred. Regulations give military commanders, like coroners, power to direct the performance of autopsies of aircraft accident fatalities involving military personnel.

A special division of the Armed Forces Institute of Pathology (AFIP), staffed by fully trained forensic pathologists with extensive aviation experience, investigates all fatal United States military aircraft accidents. The AFIP also provides consultation and pathology support to the NTSB and other government agencies. Active aviation pathology departments also exist in Germany, the United Kingdom, and other countries.

Preemptive Federal Authority

Federal, state, and local jurisdictions have legitimate interests in the investigation of aircraft accident fatalities. The difficult question is which interest prevails when more than one jurisdiction asserts its interest.

Exclusive Jurisdiction

The federal government has exclusive jurisdiction in the case of enumerated powers and when legislation expresses congressional intent to preempt the field.

The federal government also has exclusive jurisdiction over property of the United States, except to the extent that a state, when ceding land to the federal government, reserves jurisdiction or to the extent that Congress enacts legislation granting jurisdiction to the state. This means that an accident does not necessarily come under federal jurisdiction simply because it occurred on federal land.

Concurrent Jurisdiction

When federal and state laws conflict, federal law, under the supremacy clause and the preemption doctrine, supersedes state law. Even if federal and state laws do not conflict, federal law will prevail when Congress intends to provide complete federal regulation on the subject matter. Courts look to the classification of the subject matter in determining congressional intent, and state laws designed to protect the public health or safety of local citizens traditionally are subject to local regulation. Extensive federal legislation in the field is evidence of intent to preempt any state regulation. When the subject matter is of inherent national interest or when state regulation would be inconsistent with federal objectives, federal law prevails. The most consistently controlling factor, however, is the federal interest in uniform, national regulation of the subject matter. A court will balance the nature and extent of the burden against the purposes and merits of the state regulation. Because state coroner and medical examiner statutes protect public health and safety, courts probably will uphold those laws unless there is specific federal legislation such as the statute empowering the NTSB to investigate fatal United States civil aircraft accidents.

Conflicting Interpretations of the Law

Major problems occur when fatal accidents involving other than civil-registry aircraft occur outside exclusively federal jurisdiction. The NTSB does not have jurisdiction over these accidents. The NTSB may conduct autopsies on the remains of aircraft accident victims, but the NTSB authority applies only to accidents involving civil aircraft. The NTSB authority does not extend to military, prototype, or manufacturer's aircraft.

Military regulations permit commanders to authorize autopsies on the remains of military personnel who die in the military service while serving on active duty or during training, whether these personnel died on or off a military installation. The legal authority for this comes from Title 10 of the United States code and from the constitutional powers of the Service Secretaries, acting as the alter ego of the President, to prescribe rules and regulations having the force and effect of law on the administration of the service.

The extent to which these regulations apply to civilians or to military personnel where there are conflicting state laws is arguable. State law clearly governs investigations of sudden, violent, or unexpected death—except in situations where Congress has found an overriding federal interest and granted preemptory power, as in The Federal Aviation Act of 1958. The federal government's authority to investigate sudden, violent, or unexpected deaths of military personnel when they occur in areas of exclusively federal jurisdiction is also clear.

It is only arguable whether the federal government has the authority to conduct postmortem investigations in cases of civilian deaths that occur as a result of accidents involving military aircraft or involving experimental, prototype, or manufacturer's aircraft that are not of civil registry and are operating under an approved-type certificate or postmortem investigations of military personnel who die as a result of aircraft accidents occurring outside exclusively federal jurisdiction. Even if military regulations having the force and effect of law apply to postmortem examinations of military personnel on board the aircraft, these regulations apply to civilian crewmembers only if one may consider them part of "the land and naval forces." The authority of the NTSB does not apply because such an accident would not involve an aircraft of civil registry. If an aircraft manufacturer's employee dies in an aircraft that is still in test or production phases and before actual delivery to the military or assignment of civil registration number, a similar situation arises and autopsies may not be performed.

The possible concurrent authority of state officials is an issue, even if the military services have legal authority to conduct the autopsy investigations. Few state officials recognize claims of federal jurisdiction based merely on military regulations. Even if regulations grant commanders power to authorize autopsies of aircrew who die while serving on board military aircraft, other regulations require the approval of civil authorities before removal of the remains when death occurs at a place other than a military installation. The civil authorities usually require compliance with state laws regarding autopsies before granting approval. The extent of state examinations is generally sufficient to satisfy military requirements because of factors such as limited scope of civil law governing postmortem examinations, limited personnel, financial support, and equipment of local medical examiner and coroner systems, and political conflict. The nature of an autopsy is such that the first examination inevitably distorts or destroys the information that may be obtained during a subsequent investigation.

MASS DISASTERS

Identification of Victims

Investigating a mass disaster is a very complex task, and identifying the casualties is one aspect that can be particularly difficult if it is not approached in a systematic manner. Regardless of the nature of the disaster, be it natural, transportation-related, or other man-induced chaos, investigators participate as members of multidisciplinary teams to determine the cause, assign liability, and establish preventive measures for the future. Unfortunately, the other phases of the investigative process have received disproportionately more attention than has organization of the process of identifying casualties.

Many investigators know about identification techniques, but they have considered them as an isolated process and have not integrated them into the overall investigation. Typically, physicians, dentists, and other medical personnel are assigned tasks based on a preconceived disaster plan that they had no role in developing. The practical aspects of the identification process then usually develop on an ad hoc basis.

The seemingly simplistic nature of identification procedures is deceptive and perhaps explains why systematic organization of the entire process is seldom adequately addressed. The ensuing inefficiency produces conflicts among personnel and increases expenses, delays, and errors of identification.

The identification process is an essential element of an adequate investigation. Accurate identification of all fatalities incurred in an aircraft accident or other mass disaster is often the first step in determining where each person was located at the time of the disaster and what role they may have played in its cause.

Another obvious reason for identification is to allow families to recover the correct body for burial. Following some disasters, inexperienced people determined identity solely on the basis of the visual inspection of physical features, clothing, and items of personal effects such as jewelry and dog tags. They allowed families to claim portions of bodies even when no identifying characteristics were present, and when religious beliefs required

prompt burial, families were often quick to claim any body. Grieving during the emotional period following the death of a family member sometimes produced denial reactions, and families refused to accept definitive identification of their relative. Although visual inspection is usually more than adequate, possible litigation or insurance claims may hinge on documenting that the victim was, in fact, correctly identified.

The task of identifying disaster victims is not difficult if it is approached in a logical, meticulous manner. Separated into basic elements, the identification process involves (1) the collection of identifying information about the missing persons; (2) the observation of identifying features of the victims; and (3) the comparison of the two groups of information. Identification is impossible if any one of these three elements is inadequate.

Planning for the Unknown

The following discussion of the planning process is largely theoretical, rather than a step-by-step description of a plan. Each community must individualize its disaster plan after full consideration of the types of disasters that may occur.

The most serious drawback of any disaster plan is that no one can determine exactly where a disaster will occur. Although many high-risk areas can be identified, even with today's modern transportation technology, the possibility cannot be eliminated that an accident will occur in dense population areas. For this reason, planners often cannot properly select the necessary facilities until after the disaster has occurred and the investigators know the nature and number of casualties and the location, type, and severity of the disaster.

Regardless of these difficulties, predisaster planning can take place. In fact, predisaster planning must take place. Although successful investigation of disaster and identification of the victims may be possible without a plan, the job is much easier when everyone knows what his role is and what he must do. But unless the planners have already considered the theoretical aspects by planning, the necessary decisions usually cannot be made rapidly and correctly. Expedition of the identification process following the occurrence of a disaster will more than compensate for all the time spent on predisaster planning.

Planners may be able to follow certain guidelines when developing a pre-accident plan, but direct incorporation of someone else's plan usually is not possible without at least some modification to accommodate specific circumstances. The plan must reflect the risks, resources, and decision-making process unique to the community in question. A plan that could be used successfully in New York City, for example, may not be suitable for a small town of 3000 to 4000 individuals. The larger cities have more extensive resources to purchase equipment and hire full-time staffs, allowing them to respond more efficiently to a wider range of disasters. On the other hand, the larger cities have more bureaucratic channels that often make even the simplest decisions complicated. Even in the most carefully thought-out plans, some unique circumstance may arise that the planners did not anticipate.

Nevertheless, a facility that is prepared for the eventuality of a mass disaster will be able to cope on a larger scale than will the facility that has no organization or plan. The unprepared facility must organize rapidly after a disaster occurs and is likely to make mistakes that would not have been made had more time been available for preparation.

Initiating the Planning Process

The disaster investigation organizer or committee can benefit from reviewing the plans and experiences of other communities, even though the plans may not appear directly applicable. The next step is

a "brainstorming" session to see how many different possible disaster scenarios the planners can develop. The important questions are (1) what types of disasters might occur; (2) where might they occur; (3) what is the magnitude of the risk of occurrence; (4) how many casualties might occur; and (5) what resources will be available.

Type of Disaster

The initial consideration should be to determine what type of disasters might possibly occur in the geographic area encompassed by the plan. Reviewing past disasters may provide useful indicators of possible future events, considering that each city, county, state, or other geographic area has its own unique industries, topography, geography, and people. Denver, Colorado probably has little reason to be concerned with hurricanes, and Miami, Florida certainly has little reason to fear blizzards and driving snow. Cities in the midwestern and southern parts of the United States must be prepared for tornadoes, and Pacific coastal cities recall their disasters resulting from earthquakes. Cities along rivers need to consider flooding and boat and ship disasters.

Location of Disaster

Almost all cities, but especially those located near airports, must be concerned about aircraft crashes. Industrial explosions and other accidents must be anticipated near factories. Highways are an ever-present source of disasters.

Risk

A recurring feature of disasters is that they produce casualties. Having determined the type of disasters that the plan must anticipate, the next step is to estimate the likelihood of an occurrence with significant numbers of casualties. If an airport is nearby, how large are the aircraft that land there, how many people do they carry, and what is the safety record?

Casualties

Categories of casualties consist of persons who are killed, injured, or displaced from homes. The nature and severity of the disaster influences the number of persons to be found in each of these categories. Generalizations are difficult, but Lane and Brown[7] studied this problem in relation to 1086 aircraft accidents involving 34,369 occupants. They reported that no occupants were seriously injured in 82% of the accidents, that more than 50% of the occupants were seriously injured in less than 1% of the crashes, and that in most accidents (95%), not more than 25% of the occupants were seriously injured.

Resources

What a community will consider as constituting a disaster will be largely determined by the resources available to cope with it. Some communities would consider an automobile accident resulting in three or four fatalities a mass disaster, but some other cities could easily process 20 or more fatalities. Much depends on the exact circumstances of the accident. A city that would have no difficulty processing 20 fatalities from an aircraft accident that occurred at an airport might be totally incapacitated if the same accident and same number of fatalities occurred on a main street or involved a major administrative building such as that of the police or fire department.

Testing the Plan

Although no amount of planning can totally prepare a community, disaster drills are effective ways to test the plan before an actual disaster occurs.[8] The drill may point out weaknesses in the plan; seemingly insignificant details often turn out to be critically important when the actual disaster occurs.

Organizational Concept

Approaching identification of the victims of a mass disaster in a logical manner greatly simplifies the process and increases the efficiency and accuracy of identification. Recognizing the concept of the "3 C's"—command, communication, cooperation"—is fundamental.

Although the literature contains many accounts of specific disaster investigations, the organizational concept described here was developed as a result of participation by personnel from the AFIP in the investigation of many aircraft crashes and other disasters. These disasters have involved casualties varying in number from a single fatality to nearly a thousand deaths.

The organizational concept developed by the AFIP for identifying disaster victims is another application of the five distinctive phases of investigation: preliminary evaluation, data collection, data analysis, conclusion, and recommendation.

These five phases apply equally to the identification process and to the investigation in general, and all investigators need to know the importance of this flow in the identification process, complementing and not clashing with other working groups who are participating in the overall investigation.

The AFIP investigators retain flexibility within each of the investigative phases to allow general applicability. This flexibility of the process lends it to general application, and, in fact, recognition of this flexibility factor is the key to understanding the concept of mass disaster casualty identification.

The major emphasis of the AFIP mass casualty identification scheme is on quality control. This control consists of multiple checks during the phases of data collection and analysis, and the AFIP personnel attempt to confirm each identification by all available methods. The AFIP personnel also make an intensive effort to obtain complete antemortem records and descriptions as soon as possible, because they know that no identification will be possible without these data for comparison.

Preliminary Evaluation

The process begins with preliminary evaluation of the location and nature of the disaster, number of casualties, and availability of resources. Careful evaluations of these factors at the outset will allow effective structuring of the individual efforts and the most effective use of available resources.

Security

Security procedures to protect the disaster site are important. Looters can quickly strip all identifying evidence from the scene, and bodies and baggage are inviting targets. Some disruption of the site may be inevitable in the course of rescuing survivors, but beyond this initial stage, strict security measures should allow only trained investigators or other specially instructed personnel to enter the site. Disruption of the disaster site compounds an already difficult identification task, and uncontrolled access to the disaster site or to the investigation facilities can have disastrous effects on the outcome of the investigation.

Likewise, appropriate security measures must be taken at the investigative facility to prevent unauthorized entry. Suitable isolation may be necessary for family, news media, and other persons who have a legitimate interest in the investigation but whose presence may distract investigators and result in errors of identification. This consideration usually dictates selection of a site for the identification facility somewhere other than a centrally located public place.

Jurisdiction

The investigator should determine the legal aspects of jurisdiction to proceed with the investigation because many people have legitimate interests in actively participating in the investigation. Rescue teams are concerned with saving the lives of those who have been injured, and these efforts necessarily take precedence over other investigations. The fire department responds to extinguish the fire and investigate its cause. The police investigate possible wrongdoing, provide security, and control spectators. Many police, fire, and rescue teams may respond, and the question of who has primary jurisdiction may not be clear.

Medical examiners and coroners examine the fatally injured casualties to document the causes of death, detect possible infectious disease, and assist the police in detecting evidence of foul play. Representatives of the news media have an important role in reporting the circumstances of the event and communicating the extent of any continuing hazards to the community. Undertakers want to prepare the bodies as quickly as possible. The operator of the vehicle or industry involved in the disaster is interested in determining the cause, and relatives want to ascertain the status of missing family members. Attorneys help the potential plaintiffs and defendants determine their possible claims and liabilities. In the case of transportation disasters, representatives of various agencies such as the NTSB and the Federal Aviation Administration (FAA) also participate. The international nature of many disasters poses special problems for international relations.

These are only a few of the individuals and organizations that may have an active interest in the investigation, and the process must provide a framework for all interested parties to work together. Fortunately, even in another's jurisdiction, bona fide offers of assistance are seldom refused.

Leadership

Lack of consensus among the early arrivals as to who should be in charge is one of the greatest problems at the scene of a mass disaster, especially when all of the investigators are not participants in a pre-conceived plan. Many interdependent decisions must be made, and too many people attempting to assert command and give orders only increases the state of mass confusion.

Although each of the activities will have a leader, the various parties with interests must determine who will have primary control of the overall investigation. Selection of this "commander" is particularly important. His most important job is as a "front man" in dealing with outsiders, and, from a practical standpoint, the greater his standing in the community, the more effective he will be. He should have experience in identification techniques, but his direct involvement in the identification process is less desirable in larger disaster investigations. Rather than dealing with the technical aspects of the identification process, he must see that the needs of the identification personnel are promptly filled and that interruptions are prevented. He handles all inquiries from the press, families, undertakers, lawyers, and others and arranges for any support that the identification team needs.

The Headquarters Site

The investigator must establish a central headquarters to control and monitor progress in the investigation and to maintain necessary liaison. This headquarters must be easily accessible to transportation and communications, although it need not actually be within the identification facility. In many respects, investigators will find it advantageous if the headquarters is separate from the identification facility when it comes to dealing with press, families, and others whose presence may disrupt the identification process. Accommodations for eating and sleeping may be necessary.

The Identification Facility

As the investigators begin the process of finding a site to set up an identification facility, a number of considerations should come to mind. The facility should be convenient to the disaster site, and the problem of removing casualties should not be complicated by moves of great distances. The investigators will need to make repeated trips from the facility to the disaster site, and these trips may waste time unnecessarily if distances are too great or terrain is too difficult.

The facility must have adequate equipment or at least be located such that needed equipment can be installed quickly. Commercial power lines or portable/mobile electrical generators can provide adequate electricity to power lights and electrical equipment. Refrigeration may be needed to protect temperature-sensitive reagents and foods, and large refrigerated storage vans may be required to store the bodies prior to identification and release to next of kin. Workgloves, rubber gloves, pencils, clipboards, waterproof tags, plastic bags, sawhorses and plywood to construct examination tables, and heavy-duty plastic sheets to cover floors may be needed.

Although there are many reasons for conducting the identification process as near the disaster site as possible, other factors may be overriding. For example, the availability of refrigeration, communication systems, and other facilities are important factors the investigator must consider. The problem of working in a hostile environment also must be taken into account.

Given a choice, most investigators will opt to set up operations in a well-equipped headquarters that is selected, manned, and equipped exclusively for disaster investigations. Unfortunately, the location of disasters often cannot be foretold. Most communities cannot afford the luxury of a specially designated disaster headquarters and necessary associated facilities, and the number of fatalities in a disaster may far exceed the capacity of established morgue facilities. Frequently, the disaster investigation facility will have to be created after the disaster has occurred.

Communications

The establishment of an effective communications system should have high priority. The investigator must seek information from outside sources to correlate with identifying characteristics, and obtaining antemortem records and other information for use in identification may be impossible without adequate means of communication. The coordination of operations at the disaster site, hospitals, mortuary, headquarters, and other facilities also requires communications. Telephones are usually the most needed means, but radio communications may be needed, especially to the disaster site.

The investigator must consider public relations. Often, the success of disaster investigation depends on public support. In many instances, the local community can be of valuable assistance, particularly by providing lodging and mess accomodations, canteen facilities at the disaster site and headquarters, transportation, communications (radio, telephone, and runners), secretarial and clerical help, and general construction help and labor. The dissemination of adequate information requires attention to ensure that the public is aware of the continuing activities and of any needs for local participation. On the other hand, aside from problems of security, continuous and uncontrolled access to the facility by sightseers is not desirable.

To provide reasonable access for press representatives, who invariably have an interest in the causes and effects of the disaster, as well as the conduct of the investigation, the investigator should establish a special press area where the public relations group can provide regular scheduled briefings and other press releases can be made available.

Transportation

The investigator must consider transportation requirements. Injured persons need transportation to medical treatment facilities; bodies must be removed to a mortuary; personnel must be transported to and from the disaster site, mess facilities, and sleeping accommodations; equipment must be brought to the facility for installation; mail and other documents to aid in identification and treatment must be transported; and special requirements may exist for transportation of materials to specialized laboratories for analysis.

Personnel

Typically, communities are entirely unprepared for a disaster. Implementation of a previously designed plan can be the most important step taken when a disaster does occur. But even if the community has elaborate predisaster plans, people will not be just sitting around in well-organized disaster centers with all of the necessary equipment, poised and ready to go. Therefore, a critical element of any predisaster plan is notifying participants and giving them instructions as to what they must do.

The investigator must determine what personnel will be needed to cope with the emergency. He often must select appropriate personnel, equipment, and a work site on short notice and without direct knowledge of the nature and scope of the disaster. Extra attention at this point invariably simplifies subsequent tasks.

Fortunately, finding people who are willing to assist in the investigation is seldom a problem. Most people in a community will respond in any way they can. The more serious problem is finding sufficient professional staff in large-scale disasters.

Care and Feeding

Logistic problems must be solved if food is to be brought into the facility; likewise, transportation requirements are involved if the workers must leave the facility to find mess and sleeping accommodations. The facility should be selected with consideration to the comfort of the workers who will be using the facility. One cannot expect workers to function effectively under extremes of temperature or humidity. Adequate heat and ventilation must be provided, and mess and sleeping facilities may be required. The conditions under which the investigators must work often will influence the speed with which the problems can be resolved. The establishment of work schedules is necessary, especially in adverse climatic conditions. Errors made as a result of fatigue, hypoglycemia, or cold can delay the investigation far more than any possible time-saving from extended hours of work under adverse conditions. AFIP investigators have found that they cannot reasonably expect more than about 18 hours' effort from the workers on the first day and 10 hours on subsequent days without unacceptable errors being induced.

Inventory Control

A key factor in disaster victim identification is inventory control. An inventory system will greatly facilitate keeping track of each fatality and survivor. This control must begin with the first rescuer on the scene.

The problem of inventory may be attacked in a number of ways. One method is to establish an Inventory Group. The most effective method involves locating this group at the disaster site, triage area, morgue, hospitals, and holding area, and the central command post. The duties of the Inventory Control Group would be to see that all casualties were properly and securely tagged and not commingled. Further, they should keep a running inventory of exactly where each of the survivors is located, as well as in what stage of the identification process each fatality may be found.

Rescuers should remove only survivors unless immediate danger threatens further destruction and loss of the identifying features of the fatalities. When survivors are removed, they should be questioned to de-

termine their names and other identifying information in anticipation of the possibility that their conditions may suddenly deteriorate en route to the treatment or holding facility. This questioning is particularly important to avert the situation that occurs in large-scale disasters in which a complete list of missing persons is frequently unavailable, thus rendering the identification of fatalities more difficult.

All survivors are taken to the initial triage area, usually a medical facility, so they can be queried more completely as to their identity. After referral to a holding area, uninjured survivors can be questioned by investigators as to the cause of the disaster. Persons who are displaced from their homes must be accommodated in this area until other arrangements can be made, whereas others may be returned to their own homes. Injured survivors may be transferred to the holding area from the hospital after they have been treated.

Injured survivors, depending on the severity of injuries, should be transferred rapidly to a medical treatment facility. Care must be taken to ensure that haste does not interfere with inventory control. When more than one medical treatment facility is being used, it is not difficult to "lose" casualties. Investigators must know who is where. Casualties who die en route to or at the medical treatment facility must be transferred to the mortuary facility.

Much more care is necessary in the recovery of fatalities to preserve identification information. Valuable information that would be helpful in identification is often lost when recovery is unplanned and hastily performed. The exact location where the fatality was found must be recorded. In the case of mass disasters such as aircraft accidents, this record can conveniently take the form of a wreckage diagram indicating the recovery location of each of the bodies. This chart may provide helpful clues in the identification of family members. In the identification of crewmembers in an aircraft accident, knowing which bodies were found in the cockpit wreckage and, if possible, the description of the seats in which each body was found is helpful. Photographs should be taken of each body in place at the scene prior to disturbing the position of the bodies. Although these photographs are primarily of interest to those who are investigating the cause of the accident or the survivability aspects, they may also be useful in identification to detect any errors that may occur in the numbering of bodies. Obviously, for this to be valuable, the body number must be conspicuous in the photographs.

The investigator must consider how and where to store the bodies. Particularly important are the containers for the bodies, the means to preserve the bodies, and a system to allow organized retrieval of specific bodies. Body bags are not always readily available, especially in large quantities. In these cases, sheets, temporary coffins, or even shipping containers may be used.

Although the preservation of the bodies is important, the investigator needs to collect any tissues needed for chemical studies before chemical preservation is used. Refrigeration is perhaps the best method of preserving the bodies until the investigation is completed, although charred bodies do not have the urgent need for refrigeration. Refrigeration is particularly important in warm climates, and the investigators may need to rent refrigerated truck-trailers. Although the design of a typical truck-trailer will accommodate approximately 50 bodies, the inventory and retrieval process will be easier if fewer numbers are stored in each vehicle.

Keeping track of more than about 20 bodies at a time is often difficult, and assigning one person to keep track of each body whenever it is out of the storage area is one very effective quality control procedure. This person follows the assigned body as it proceeds through each stage of the identification process and keeps the labels and other paperwork in order.

Many times, rescue workers, in an effort to safeguard jewelry from looters, have removed personal effects from bodies and placed them in bags. Although this procedure may seem reasonable if the personal effects are placed in individual bags and labeled with the number of the corresponding body, the possibility still exists for errors in numbering. The situation in which two bodies have the same number readily illustrates the nature of problems that may be encountered. In any case, the identification investigator can only hope that the personal effects he did not personally observe to be attached or associated with a body were properly marked.

Collection of Identification Data

The second phase in the investigative process focuses on data collection. This is a particularly intensive period for personnel, and the effective direction of efforts will result in an uneventful and thoroughly successful investigation. Overcoming the initial inertia is one of the hurdles. People often seem to stand around waiting for something to happen, frequently not realizing that they are the ones who must take the first step.

Figure 27–4 shows the organizational flow of work that AFIP investigators usually follow in collecting and evaluating data. This protocol is not rigid, and I cannot overemphasize the importance of flexibility in applying any organizational scheme to specific situations. Frequent deviations may be necessary to accommodate specific conditions as operational or other requirements necessitate. Nevertheless, this order does allow logical progression in the typical case.

Who is Missing?

The investigator must accurately determine the answer to this question as early as possible. He must take immediate steps

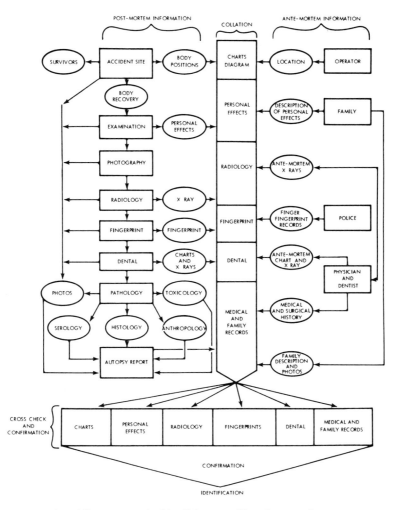

Fig. 27–4. Organizational workflow concept for identifying casualties of a mass disaster.

to obtain a list of persons believed to be missing and their last reported position. The identification methods he will use, the types of additional assistance that he may need, and the duration of the investigation depend on this list. Finding this information may be extremely difficult, especially in the case of natural disasters; in the case of aircraft accidents, however, this information should be available from the owner or operator in the form of crew-member assignments, flight manifests, passenger lists, and seating assignment charts.

Manifest lists of affinity groups usually are the easiest to determine accurately. For example, when a military aircraft crashes, a manifest, or list of persons on board the aircraft, will almost certainly be available. Unless a last-minute crew change occurred or passengers boarded the aircraft at the last moment without proper documentation, accurate information should be readily available from the flight operations department that dispatched the aircraft. Problems can occur, however; for example, following the crash of an aircraft presumed to have only eight persons on board investigators recovered 17 feet from the wreckage.

Without a preexisting list of persons suspected of being missing, the problem of identifying the disaster victims may be impossible. Disasters at airport, bus, or train terminals, hotels, and sports stadiums, circuses, and other entertainment events are only a few examples of situations where determination of who is missing is difficult. Almost every large medical examiner's office has had a body that remained unidentified until someone finally noticed that the person was missing and filed a missing persons report.

The problems are even more difficult when people use names other than their own when traveling. This immediately raises questions of illegal activity and foul play. These activities seem particularly prevalent in international travel, but they also occur in domestic travel.

Less sinister reasons are usually the case, such as when a large corporation makes travel reservations for one employee but at the last minute sends a different employee instead or when an executive sneaks off with his secretary for a holiday frolic. Even such simple errors as misspelled names on a manifest can pose serious problems in discovering the identity of the missing person.

Antemortem Information

After establishing a tentative missing persons list, knowledge of the general condition of the bodies gained during cursory inspections in the preliminary evaluation phase will allow investigators to pursue the antemorten information needed for comparison with postmortem observations. They may seek some types of information more vigorously than other types, although still recognizing that even the secondary information is important. Medical and dental records may be more helpful than fingerprint records and information about clothing and personal effects in the case of severely burned and charred bodies. On the other hand, in the case of children, medical and dental records may have less importance. This underscores

again the importance of the preliminary evaluation phase.

Positive identification can be made only by comparison of observed features with those previously observed and/or recorded. Someone must find records of uniquely identifying characteristics for each of the missing persons if they are to be identified positively. If the investigators cannot obtain this information, positive identification will not be possible. Investigators can ask various sources, such as the missing person's family, friends, employer, physician, and dentist, as well as law enforcement agencies, for information and records. They should make every effort to obtain as much identification information as possible as rapidly as possible.

An effective organization is essential to actively seek the required antemortem records, and numerous checklists of desirable identification information are available. Although many of the commercial air carrier operators have detailed questionnaires that can serve as useful checklists, the investigators should inform the interviewers of the specific types of information required for that particular investigation and remind them that the people they interview seldom appreciate the urgency of the request for information and the necessary detail. The immediate acquisition of complete antemortem data is essential if the identification process is to proceed with dispatch and, in fact, if it is to succeed at all.

Postmortem Information

The collecting of postmortem information actually begins with the first person at the disaster site. Although the bodies must, at some point, be recovered from the disaster site and transported to the mortuary facility where identification is to take place, under the best of circumstances the rescuers will leave the bodies in situ until the investigators arrive. Impressing the importance of this on rescue organizations should be part of any disaster plan.

Knowledge of the exact location of each body, its injuries, and its position relative to various parts of the wreckage and to other bodies can be helpful. Prior to removal of any body, the investigator should have someone photograph it, chart its location on a diagram of the disaster site, and apply an identifying tag. The investigator may be able to correlate the body locations with the duty positions of crewmembers or with passenger seat assignments as a preliminary identification procedure. It should be noted that identification by seat or duty assignment is merely a preliminary step and does not result in positive identification.

Fragmented bodies require special care in collecting, tagging, and identifying each fragment. Investigators must search the disaster site carefully to ensure that they have not overlooked any body fragments. Even small fragments of tissue may aid in identification; small fragments of dentition or printable skin may be the evidence needed to identify some of the casualties. In the example cited earlier, only eight people were missing following one crash, but investigators found body fragments that included 17 feet. Since no one knew of a ninth missing person, the entire process of identification was much more difficult and time-consuming than if some clue to the identity of the ninth missing person had been known.

Rescuers may not be able to recover all of the bodies in some instances, such as in disasters at sea. Investigators must then decide when to terminate further search efforts; they may have to resolve by other aspects of the investigation whether there may have been more victims than the persons reported missing and consider the possibility of foul play.

The following will provide the information required for the documentation of identity in most cases:

1. Color photographs of the body (clothed and unclothed)
2. Total-body radiographs (including all extremities)
3. Documentation of all scars, tattoos, deformities, operations
4. Documentation of body characteristics (hair and eye color, and so on)
5. Documentation of all clothing, jewelry, and personal effects
6. Dental chart
7. Fingerprints and footprints
8. Blood type
9. Anthropologic measurements and estimates of height, weight, body build, age, race, and sex

Initial Examination

Even though the initial screening examination of each body does not require much time, it frequently provides immediate clues to identity. The investigator should take particular care at this stage to correlate any associated injuries as he removes, photographs, labels, and describes clothing and personal effects. Although the personal-effects group will investigate these items further, the information about them should be noted and made available to the investigators of each successive work station. Dentures and other dental material are best left for subsequent examination and removal by the dental investigators.

Complete photographic coverage of this initial examination is important. Photographs of all aspects of the body, particularly specific identifying features of the face, ears, hands, feet, and tattoos, are especially helpful documentation, and the investigator should obtain them before and after removing clothing and personal effects. Additional photographic coverage should be available to document any noteworthy observations made at subsequent work stations.

Radiologic Examination

Radiologic examination has become an increasingly important identification tool.

Lichtenstein and colleagues[9] demonstrated its value in screening for foreign materials and identifiable structures, in comparing antemortem radiographic examinations, and in evaluating injury patterns. Obtaining comprehensive radiographs of the entire body frequently pays unexpected dividends. Occasionally, metal fragments from old traumatic injuries or war wounds will be demonstrated. In many cases, investigators can obtain further information concerning the circumstances of death and the nature of the forces involved from the interpretation of these radiographs.

The identification value of radiologic examination is greatest in instances in which the deceased is below the age of 25 years. In this age group, the interpretation of ossification centers and closure of the epiphyses can give a close approximation of the age of the individual. For these interpretations, the often overlooked radiographs of the hands and feet are essential.

Investigators can take advantage of travel time when they must travel long distances to the disaster site. When they will not arrive at the disaster site until after the bodies have been removed to mortuary facilities, they can save time by requesting that initial radiologic studies be obtained before their arrival. Dental and fingerprint consultation may also be requested during this travel period. The radiographs, dental charts, and fingerprint records will then be available for immediate review when the team arrives. Additional or complementary radiographs may then be obtained if necessary.

Fingerprints and Footprints

The next step in identification consists of examining the victim's hands and feet for the presence of printable surfaces. Fingerprint identification is the first method of choice for positive identification because it is one of the most accurate and reliable methods for the identification of unknown remains. Experienced investigators can examine fingerprints obtained from disaster victims and, using various coding methods, search the massive files that are kept at organizations such as the FBI in the United States. If records are immediately available, even the physician can make a preliminary comparison. Most countries accept fingerprints and footprints as positive proof of identification.

The use of fingerprints or footprints as means of identification depends on the availability of previous known prints for comparison. Employers, police, and other government agencies can often provide antemortem fingerprints for comparison. Hospitals may have fingerprints of mothers and hand or foot prints of children appearing on birth records. Inquiry during the preliminary evaluation phase should have revealed whether any of these antemortem records are available. Some countries keep no fingerprint records. Other countries have these records available only from convicted criminals. Many adults in the United States have fingerprint records available for comparison, but even the FBI's large file of records contains fingerprints of less than 25% of the population.

Even when no antemortem records are available, the investigator may still be able to obtain latent fingerprints from the missing person's home, office, or vehicle. Good latent prints are often on objects such as drinking glasses, mirrors, windows, and doorknobs. Satisfactory prints from only the palm of the hand may be on a drinking glass; the investigator must take prints of the entire hand for comparison in this case. The FBI Disaster Squad identified one or more victims through latent fingerprint impressions in the majority of the disasters in which they assisted. These techniques are not for the unskilled, but knowing that the techniques are available may greatly shorten the process of identification.

The forensic pathologist or other identification personnel may be able to accomplish many simple screening procedures because comparison of good quality antemortem fingerprint records with sharply defined postmortem impressions is not difficult. In most circumstances, however, the professional assistance of trained fingerprint experts from a local enforcement agency or military police is advisable in obtaining both prints and records.

Even in badly burned or decomposed bodies, satisfactory fingerprints for comparison can often be obtained by special techniques. Badly wrinkled or macerated fingers ("washerwoman skin") can often be restored to printable condition by the injection of a fluid such as saline. When burn-charring involves only the epidermis, scraping away the charred tissue may enable prints or photographs to be made of the underlying dermis. If the facilities to obtain prints are not available, the investigator may remove and retain the finger pads, fingers, or even the entire hand until prints can be made.

In the case of the badly fragmented body, the investigator must make a diligent search for fragments of printable tissue. In a recent, severe crash, following which the investigators could find only minute fragments of tissue, a ¼-inch square portion of skin from the thumb of the pilot was found inside the control stick. This not only served to identify the pilot but also indicated that he was probably attempting to control the aircraft at impact.

Dental Examination

Dental identification is probably the most widely used method other than visual recognition for the identification of unknown remains. Dental techniques for the identification of disaster victims have become increasingly important. More people worldwide have dental records than have fingerprint records.

Hill[10] described the dental techniques used by forensic odontologists in the United Kingdom for identifying aircraft accident victims. Morlang[11] described the organizational structure, technical procedures, and methods of documenting dental findings used in the United States. His system for computer-assisted comparison of the antemortem and postmortem records is particularly interesting. The computer program also allows comparison of other identification information such as age, race, sex, height, weight, hair and eye color, scars, blood type, and surgical implants.

The assistance of a dentist, particularly a forensic odontologist, will greatly facilitate dental charting and identification. The postmortem dental charting should show, as a minimum, the presence or absence of each tooth, the presence and exact location on the tooth of any restorations (fillings), in addition to the shape of the restorations, and the presence of cavities. In cases of extensive traumatic injuries, radiographs of the whole body that were obtained at an earlier station in the identification process may aid in the location of dental material that traumatic forces translocated elsewhere in the body.

The dentist can remove any dentures at this time for possible correlation with antemortem dental materials. Dentists often inscribe the person's name or other identifying information on artificial dentures, and in many other cases, they will recognize dental work that they personally performed or perhaps will recognize other characteristics of the person's mouth.

Severe head trauma often dislodges the maxilla, enabling it to be removed with only a scalpel. The dentist may need to remove the mandible and maxilla in some other cases for adequate exposure or further inspection, and if a body still remains unidentified at the completion of the investigation, he should remove and retain the teeth for possible subsequent identification. The technique for removing the teeth intact is simple. With a Stryker saw, the mandible and maxilla can be removed easily with the teeth undisturbed.

The widespread use of radiographic documentation of dental prophylaxis and the decline in the scope of fingerprint identification files are responsible for the great progress in dental identification techniques. Radiographs of teeth may be made to compare the shape of restorations, the location and extent of cavities, the shape of individual teeth and their root structure, or any preexisting abnormalities with antemortem radiographs. Comparison of the root structure of the teeth in antemortem and postmortem radiographs may establish identification even if no restorative dental work has been performed.

The introduction of dental radiographs into the identification process has eliminated the confusion that can follow when the dental chart does not accurately show the actual dental characteristics. In many cases, the dentist verbally transmits his observations to a technician, who records it on the dental chart. Many possible sources for errors exist in this system, and finding "left" recorded when "right" was intended or "buccal" recorded when the actual location was "lingual" is not unusual. The forensic odontologist can readily verify the correct positions by inspecting the radiographs.

Dental identification depends on the availability of antemortem dental records for comparison. As with fingerprint records, the dental records may not be immediately available. The investigator can save time by taking the radiographs and doing the dental charting of the victim while awaiting the antemortem radiographs and charts. Because dental records are not maintained in central, coded repositories as are fingerprint files, finding dental records depends on a reasonably accurate missing persons list. Using this list, the investigator should obtain all available previous records, including dental charts, radiographs, casts, and impressions. Even when the actual dental record

is not available, the missing person's dentist can provide the necessary information by telephone.

Victims who had dental work performed subsequent to the last known dental record create a difficult problem of identification. If a victim's dental record indicates that he has 32 teeth and no restorations, a victim whose third molars are absent would not seem to be a likely possible match without knowledge that the teeth were extracted subsequent to the date of the record available for comparison. The investigators must take great care to avoid eliminating possible identity matches by errors such as this, and comparison of more detailed anatomic observations of radiographs is usually helpful in avoiding these problems.

Postmortem Examinations

Pathologists discuss the radiographs with radiologists, review the antemortem records, and then perform thorough postmortem pathologic examinations at the next station. The radiographs may show surgical materials, contraceptive devices, or other items of personal effects that were overlooked previously, particularly in the case of burned bodies, and allow the pathologist to recover them for further examination. The postmortem examination should be thorough, and the pathologist should record all weights, measurements, and possible identifying features carefully and collect appropriate tissue specimens for possible toxicologic and serologic studies. The toxicologic examination of tissues or body fluids may reveal the presence of medications that the investigator can correlate with medical records to confirm identification. Anthropologic and histologic procedures may also be necessary for identification, but this requirement will depend on the availability of antemortem data for comparison. Because the pathologist frequently will not know until some later time whether antemortem data will be available, he should consider collecting appropriate measurements and specimens of bone and tissue.

Documentation of body characteristics may serve to further narrow the possibilities of the identity of the deceased. The value of separating tall from short persons is obvious, but investigators often overlook the possibilities for comparing hat size, sleeve length, neck size, waist, inseam length, and shoe size. Measurements that may be affected by postmortem effects on soft tissue must be interpreted with great caution, but they are nevertheless of value in the subjective evaluation of the victims.

Many people have unique identifying body characteristics as a result of exposure to the environment. Other body characteristics may not necessarily be identifying, but they may facilitate further categorization. Categorizing characteristics include surgical scars, such as from an appendectomy, circumcision, and pierced ears for earrings; and many tattoos and scars are unique.

The investigator may compare hair obtained from a pillow or comb in a person's home to head hair on an unidentified body. He may compare the characteristics of an ear with those in an antemortem photograph or fingernail clippings found in the home with fingernails on the body. The use of these techniques is less common, and they tend to be last-ditch efforts.

Anthropologic Observations

The direct observation of findings in skeletonized remains (i.e., without resort to the techniques of radiology) may be possible. The investigator can determine age, race, sex, and stature from the interpretation of skeletal remains. Even in intact bodies, the pathologist may excise the pubic symphysis by using a saw and examine the opposing faces of the pubic bones for the presence of "parturition pits," indicating a past pregnancy, or to determine age.

Personal Effects

Personal effects can provide clues to identity. These helpful materials may vary from specific information such as identification cards containing photographs and fingerprints to less specific items such as jewelry, clothing labels, and watches. Careful chain-of-custody throughout the identification process is important. Photographs are helpful for documenting each item, and the investigator can circulate the photographs among the identification groups or show them to relatives without having to handle the actual material excessively.

Laboratory Examination of Tissue

The investigator first examines the tissue grossly to determine its general appearance, texture, consistency, and the presence of any odor. This may allow him to determine whether the material is tissue and, if so, whether it is human and what part of the body it is from.[12] The pathologist may be able to determine whether materials found at the crash site are mammalian by examining them under the microscope. The erythrocytes of all species other than mammals have nuclei. Figure 27–5 illustrates the nucleated erythrocytes from tissue found at the site of an accident caused by a bird strike. Serologic studies may be helpful, and some of these are described in a later section.

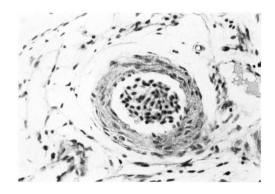

Fig. 27–5. Nucleated erythrocytes from bird-strike accident (Armed Forces Institute of Pathology photo).

The intensive effort during this data-collection phase is critical. With tissue, observations must be documented as quickly as possible before postmortem changes obscure them. The lack of suitable antemortem data for comparison will make much of the postmortem information useless, but the investigators risk incorrect identification of some of the casualties if they fail to document all possible identifying features.

Application of Identification Techniques

Certain techniques, such as the comparison of fingerprint and dental records, are more reliable and provide definitive identifications directly. On the other end of the reliability scale are such characteristics as height, weight, skin color, and hair color that may be subjective, difficult to measure, and are subject to change from time to time; however, even combinations of these subjective characteristics may provide reliable and, in some cases, the only identification. The "odd-man-out" method (described in the section entitled "Techniques") is a practical screening technique that can lead to identification in carefully selected instances even in the absence of identifying features. The careful application of these techniques and avoidance of the pitfalls will enable even the inexperienced investigator to collect valuable information to simplify and shorten the identification process.

Certainty of Identification

One issue in the course of the mass disaster identification process is how certain the identification of each victim must be. How positive are the investigators that they have made correct identifications? As a practical matter, in some disasters, where bodies are severely fragmented and burned or where little antemortem information is available for comparison, positive identification of all of the casualties may not be possible.

Hardly a person has not at some time seen an apparent acquaintance at a distance only to find on closer observation that the identification was incorrect. Perhaps this occurred because the physical resemblance of the suspected and actual persons was great or because the observer based his determination on limited information. An observer can seldom be certain about identification when he observes only a part of the whole. For example, the identification of known persons from the posterior aspects of the head is possible, but this identification is not usually as reliable as when the observer makes the identification after seeing the person's face. Hair length is no longer a reliable basis for distinguishing males from females.

The reasons for the certainty in identification are more than academic. Of course, the usual social and moral reasons are sufficient to pressure the investigator to identify casualties and return them to their families. In different societies, pressure may be expressed in a variety of ways. Some cultures are meticulous in their desire to identify all casualties with certainty; in other cultures, the pressure is more to release a body to the family before some religious deadline. In the latter circumstance, it often seems that the desire is for the determination of certainty of death rather than for the certainty of identity of each individual body. Some governments have issued individual death certificates on the basis of aircraft manifests and held mass burials when they presumed that all persons on board were dead.

Careless identification techniques can initiate a parade of horrors. The problems usually begin with insurance claims, survivors benefits, and other disposition of personal property. In one case, the haste in providing early identification and release of the body of a prominent political figure was for naught. Investigators had to have the body exhumed when it was dis-

covered that they had incorrectly identified it.

Cases of borrowed clothing and dog tags
have also occurred. The importance of
clearly understanding the distinction between definitive and supportive evidence
of identity is readily apparent.

An important question that the investigator must answer at the onset of the investigation is: How, with all of the various
methods of identification that are available, can I most efficiently achieve certainty of identification of these casualties?
Four general categories of procedures are
available: definitive, secondary, cumulative, and confirmatory. Obviously, any one
procedure may fall into more than one of
these categories, depending on the circumstances in which it is used.

Definitive Methods

The methods of identification that stand
alone as means of identification are definitive methods. Theoretically, these methods assume that one person, and one person alone, can have a particular set of
characteristics. As a practical matter, investigators can seldom, if ever, achieve
this degree of certainty. As a result, they
tend to settle for a degree of certainty of
identification on the basis that the probability of any other person having those
particular characteristics is low. Labels in
dental restorations that contain the deceased's name and identifying number are
examples of "absolutely" definitive methods of identification. Of course, even this
evidence is not 100% reliable, unless the
investigator is certain that the deceased or
the preparer had no motive to falsify the
identity, that no mistakes occurred in the
antemortem preparation of the labels or in
the postmortem examination process, and
that the antemortem records are correct.

All methods of identification involve
the comparison of observed characteristics
of the bodies with known or reported characteristics of persons missing or presumed
to be dead, and definitive identification of

a person occurs when investigators identify a sufficient number of objective features that belong to the missing person and
only to that person. Theoretically, two
people may have certain characteristics
that are similar enough to be identical for
all practical purposes. For this reason, the
investigator must assign a degree of probability to each method of identification.
The greater the number of identical characteristics found, the more certain the
probability that the identification is correct. For example, the probability is much
greater if 25 matching fingerprint or dental
characteristics are present than if the only
comparable feature is blood type A.

How many presumptive correlations are
necessary to approximate a definitive
identification? No set number applies un-
equivocally to all circumstances. Correlation of three characteristics such as
height, weight, and hair color usually will
not be as corroborative as the correlation
of the evidence of surgery and other scars,
congenital defects, and dental restorations. On the other hand, if only one of
the missing persons weighed over 150
pounds and if he happened to weigh 250
pounds, this might be a very significant
identifying characteristic indeed.

A high degree of negative correlation
may also be of great value in limiting the
number of persons under consideration.
For example, if investigators determine
that 20% of the victims have blood type
A, the missing persons known to have
blood types AB, B, or O are not likely to
provide a match.

Secondary Methods

Secondary methods of identification are
those methods which use characteristics
that could belong to more than one person
and which, therefore, do not by themselves give a high degree of probability of
certainty of identification. On the other
hand, in many instances, secondary methods that are considered by themselves to
have a low probability may, in fact, pro-

vide almost certain identification. Secondary methods are of the greatest usefulness when they are used in combination with the cumulative methods described in the following section. Examples of secondary materials and characteristics are age, sex, hair color, color and type of clothing, and so on. Secondary methods can give highly reliable results, but the positivity seldom approaches that of the definitive methods. The limited value of determining that the sex of an unidentified body is male when all of the missing persons are male is easy to appreciate; likewise, a similar determination is of little assistance when half of a large group of missing persons are male. On the other hand, the finding of a male body is highly significant when only one male is missing.

Cumulative Methods

Especially when using secondary methods of identification, the investigator needs to somehow increase the probability that identifications are correct. Using the cumulative methods to analyze several secondary characteristics, the combined probability of certainty of identification increases. In the hypothetic example in Table 27–1, finding a male body cannot result in definitive identification; similarly, finding an edentulous body cannot result in definitive identification. A male body could be either A or B, and and edentulous body could be either A or C. But by cumulating these findings, assuming that these four bodies do, in fact, represent these four missing persons, an edentulous male body can be only missing person A. Thus, methods that have an inherently low probability of definitive identification

Table 27–1. Example of the Cumulative Identification Method

Victim	Sex	Dental Data
Person A	M	Edentulous
Person B	M	Present
Person C	F	Edentulous

can be combined using cumulative techniques to provide certain identification.

Fingerprint identification is a widely used method of definitive identification, but this technique is actually an example of the cumulative identification methods. The theoretical possibility of any two persons having identical sets of fingerprints depends on the degree of cumulation used. Dental examination, another of the commonly used means of "positive" identification, also could be considered a cumulative method, and one could likewise calculate degrees of certainty of this identification method.

Confirmatory Methods

The use of confirmatory methods is another variation of the cumulative technique. For example, using the hypothetic situation described in Table 27–1, having identified body A using the cumulative methods, the investigator may find it possible to obtain definitive identification. Fingerprint or dental records may be available for comparison, or, in unusual cases, investigators may obtain latent fingerprints from the missing person's home for comparison.

Selecting the Identification Techniques

How is the investigator to select which of these methods to use in particular situations? The practical answer is that he must use every method that he reasonably can in every case. Even in the situation where definitive methods are readily available, the investigator must always be on guard against the possibility that there may be an error in the records or the observations.

Missing persons lists are frequently incorrect in at least some aspect. When dealing with commercial modes of transportation, these errors are almost a routine occurrence.

Errors may occur because of fraud or mistake; even criminal misconduct may occur. Certain errors may occur as a normal course of business and may not be detected without knowledge of the business practices. When using prenumbered forms for recording observations of the unidentified bodies, an observer can very easily record his findings on an incorrect form. When many bodies are involved, especially when identifying features are not readily apparent (as in severely burned bodies), observations may be correctly charted but from a different body. Clerks may file records in an incorrect folder or, when using wall charts, may place an X in an incorrect column.

How is the investigator to avoid the pitfalls that these errors can induce? He cannot entirely. He must always be alert to the possibility that errors may exist, and he must continually take steps to minimize the effect they will have on the overall investigation; he should take whatever steps are possible to detect their existence. He should be especially wary of methods that tend to remove a missing person from consideration too early.

From a practical standpoint, three general rules are helpful. First, do the best you can with what is available. Second, do the easiest things first. Finally, don't release a body before making definitive identification.

Data Analysis

Data analysis occurs in the third phase of the investigation, as working groups continue to evaluate the data they collected in the data-collection phase. The investigators who observed the postmortem findings are best suited to analyze the data, but substantially fewer people are necessary. Reducing the total number of personnel by 50% or more is usually possible at this stage.

Analyzing the data consists of integrating the information from the antemortem records and the postmortem observations. Of particular importance is organization of the techniques for recording, charting, and storing antemortem and postmortem data so that investigators can easily find the necessary information. The early installation of appropriate quality cntrol procedures and careful consideration of which identification techniques, such as spotting, mix-and-match, exclusion, or odd-man-out, will be most productive and will increase the efficiency of the data analysis process.

Quality Control

The antemortem records almost invariably contain some inaccuracies, and other errors will probably occur in the observing and recording of postmortem findings. Transposition of left and right occurs frequently in medical records, and estimating the height, weight, sex, or age of fragmented or severely burned bodies can be extremely difficult. Recognizing the probability of these errors caused by human frailty allows the investigator to plan to avoid the most serious pitfall, misidentification as a result of an irreversible error.

Early adoption and strict adherence to quality control procedures will minimize these errors. More than one observer should confirm each postmortem finding, and each of the working groups should reexamine observation notes from the preliminary examination and from other working groups. Each member of the working group should verify all of the postmortem evidence from a matching antemortem record before making an identification, and making this evidence available to all of the other working groups provides an additional measure of control. Rigid adherence to these seemingly tedious and often redundant procedures will save valuable time in the long run.

Morlang[11] described a computer program used to assist in the identification of victims of the 1977 Tenerife disaster, but few investigators have applied computer technology at other disasters. Converting the antemortem and postmortem data to an acceptable format for the computer requires substantial effort, and few investigators have been willing to invest the effort involved to set up a computer system when fewer than 25 to 50 casualties are involved. Opportunities to test these computer applications under actual disaster conditions are infrequent, and investigators have been unable to agree on a standard terminology to describe identifying characteristics that the computer will accept. Nevertheless, small, portable, yet powerful, computer systems are receiving increasing acceptance, and the logical nature of the procedures in the data analysis phase is ideally suited for their application in facilitating the scientific identification of disaster victims.

Techniques

The methods of analyzing identification data fall into four general categories. "Spotting" depends on investigators remembering characteristics observed at the postmortem examination when they encounter similar features as they review the antemortem records. The initial review of the records frequently reveals several obvious identities, and investigators may even correctly identify some victims whose postmortem characteristics were recorded incompletely, inaccurately, or perhaps not at all.

"Mix-and-match" consists of the logical manipulation of the records into groups that have characteristics in common. Selecting all of the casualties that have a particular characteristic in common, such as age, sex, or race, that have dental or fingerprint information available, or that have unique items or personal effects such as rings or watches will allow the investigators to focus their attention on more likely identification matches. They should prepare lists grouping these possible matches and make their lists available to all of the other working groups for possible confirmation. As this "mixing" occurs, identity "matches" may become apparent, but this preliminary match must not be the sole basis for positive identification.

Identification by "exclusion" is another data analysis technique, but investigators should apply it with great caution. Where two crewmembers are missing and investigators have positively identified one, the temptation is great to conclude that the second body found within the wreckage is the other missing crewmember. This conclusion may be correct in many instances, but it becomes infamously wrong when the missing persons list turns out to be incorrect. Investigators should avoid the temptation to regress to identification by exclusion when the identification process progresses slower than expected. They may need to reexamine the bodies or resort to other methods of identification.

The investigator may be able to identify some victims by a process of elimination if he is certain that all of the bodies have been recovered. If he is reasonably certain that the missing persons list corresponds to the identities of the recovered bodies, the problems of identification are much simpler. In this situation, the degree of certainty necessary to approximate a positive identification need not be as great. Identification by exclusion cannot occur, however, unless all of the bodies have been recovered and the list of missing persons is complete.

The exclusion techniques are also useful in other ways. Tables of exclusion are often helpful for the early categorization of identifying features by the mix-and-match method. Determination of sex is usually easy, and this may exclude a large number of possible missing persons from further consideration. The investigators can exclude person C on the basis of sex and person B by the presence of teeth, and the cumulation of these observations greatly increases the probability that the victim in the example in Table 27–1 is person A.

After first applying the best and most positive methods in attempting to identify victims, a few bodies without definite identifiable features may still remain. In these cases, methods that would not otherwise establish identification may be useful when investigators apply them to a large number of bodies using the odd-man-out technique to produce good evidence of identification. Mason[13] proposed the odd-man-out theory for the evaluation of distinctive injury patterns in reconstructing the cause and sequence of events in an aircraft accident. The logic process of Mason's injury analysis technique applies equally to the preliminary identification of fatalities, where it relies on the cumulation of observations or, in some instances, the absence of certain observations, and in some applications is an extension of the exclusion method of identification.

Initial screening examination of the bodies usually reveals that some of the bodies have characteristics for which the investigators will almost certainly discover comparison data. Pregnancy and the presence of a glass eye or an artificial limb are identifying data that identification questionnaires seldom seek, but finding this information can be extremely valuable. The presence of any one body with features different from all other bodies found in the wreckage sets the odd-man-out process in motion.

Simplification of the identification process by the odd-man-out method does not require that the characteristics be totally unique. If all of the passengers and crew were male except for one female flight attendant, the investigators could presumptively identify the only female body found as the female flight attendant. Investigators occasionally find an identifying feature that almost certainly must be unique—that only one person in the whole world could possibly have—and, unfortunately, will find nothing in any antemortem record of the missing persons to substantiate the characteristic.

Investigators must exercise great care to avoid eliminating a particular body or missing person from consideration prematurely on the basis of a characteristic that was not unique or that was described improperly. This caution applies especially to the application of the exclusion and odd-man-out methods.

Conclusion Phase

The conclusion phase begins when a working group makes a presumptive identification. Other members of the working group check the observations to confirm the presumptive match first and then refer the presumptive match to the other working groups, where confirmation will lead to preliminary identification.

The working group may be unable to reach a presumptive identity determination, but their list of possible matches may be helpful to another group. When a second group reviews the list, their observations may provide additional clues to focus on the identities. This aspect of the conclusion phase overlaps somewhat with the data-analysis phase.

Each working group examines all of the data. If they find no inconsistencies, the responsible senior investigator then reviews the observations that support the match before confirming the positive identification. The senior investigator should release no body before each working group reviews the identification data and he confirms their determination. Adequate records should reflect this observation and review process.

Recommendation Phase

The recommendation phase involves more than just identification. Usually, the investigator must prepare to make other recommendations as well. He must decide when to abandon search efforts for additional bodies or body fragments, especially in circumstances such as disasters at sea, where rescuers may be unable to recover all of the bodies; he must determine whether, particularly in the case of fragmented bodies, there may have been more victims than persons reported missing and whether continued searches for additional information will be productive. He also must provide other investigators with recommendations about whether to pursue any possibility of foul play as a cause of any of the casualties.

The investigator finally must determine what to do about any unidentified bodies or body parts that remain. He must thoroughly reexamine each of the body fragments to assure that he has not overlooked any clues to identity, and he may be able to match some of these fragments with previously identified bodies by means of blood type, injury patterns, or hair and fingernail characteristics. This problem is another reason for the investigator to take special care to document findings and maintain records throughout the identification process.

The investigator should thoroughly document the remaining body fragments using photographs, radiographs, diagrams, and written descriptions. Retaining mandibles, maxillas, and fingers will make subsequent dental and fingerprint comparison possible. The remaining body fragments should be retained for a reasonable period of time, the length of which will depend on the location and condition of the fragments and the likelihood of finding suitable antemortem information for comparison.

Whether to dispose of the remaining fragments or to bury them depends on the bulk of the tissue, whether identifying characteristics are present, and whether the investigation accounted for all of the missing persons. Burial of each unidentified body or all associated body parts in the case of fragments in individual, numbered sites will facilitate subsequent exhumation should the investigators discover additional identifying information.

INJURY PATTERN ANALYSIS

Determining the sequence of events in an aircraft crash is essential to any crashworthiness investigation, and injury pattern analysis focuses on that determination. Various combinations of injuries form certain characteristic patterns that relate to the sequence of events in the accident, and careful analysis of these patterns often explains otherwise obscure circumstances of an accident. Trauma, the environment, and preexisting diseases are the significant factors the investigator must consider.

Tolerance and Injury

The tolerance of each part of the body to injury varies considerably. The force may have no residual effect, may result in minor injury, or may produce irreversible or even lethal injuries. The ultimate consequences of force that amputates an arm are quite different from those of force that, when applied to the neck, results in decapitation.

Although man has a definable tolerance to injury, much confusion exists in the literature as to what constitutes an acceptable degree of injury. One controversy is over whether greater effort should be spent on preventing fatal injuries rather than less serious ones. The number of fatalities from crashes is relatively small compared with the number of injured casualties, and the total cost of treating the injuries is much greater than the cost of dealing with the fatalities. Accepting some fatalities may be the price paid to reduce more frequent and costly injuries.

The better approach gives equal consideration to the prevention of injuries and fatalities. Although evaluation of the injury tolerance issues may appear difficult, the investigator must avoid any first impulse, when confronted with fragmented bodies and wreckage, to conclude that survival would have been impossible.

Injury Pattern

An injury pattern is simply the enumeration of injuries that a victim sustained during or as a result of a crash. After he determines the specific event that caused each injury pattern, the investigator can prepare charts to use in comparing the pattern of injuries observed in one person with those seen in others. He can compare the injury patterns of casualties in the same aircraft accident or compare the injury patterns in one accident with injuries observed in another crash. Finding many burned bodies near an exit in an aircraft destroyed by fire suggests the malfunction of the exit, and bodies or parts of the aircraft located great distances from the main wreckage suggests breakup of the aircraft in flight.

The investigator must document each injury pattern carefully and correlate it to the circumstances of the accident. This information is essential to making any modifications that will prevent similar injuries in the future. Because few injuries are specific for aircraft accidents, the accident investigator may apply general forensic pathology techniques in interpreting the injuries.

A number of factors directly influence the specific injuries and patterns of injury. Decelerative forces, environmental factors,and the structural configuration of the aircraft produce injuries. Incisions, lacerations, fractures, thermal injuries, and interference with respiration are specific types of injuries, but the severity of each injury may range from minimal to fatal.

The most difficult problems facing the investigator are the determinations of (1) exactly when an injury occurred; (2) the nature of the force that produced the injury; and (3) whether the observed injuries are the result of the impact forces or an artifactual change induced by the post-crash environment. Did the injury occur before or after death or did it perhaps even exist before the crash occurred? How much force was required to produce the injury, and how was the force applied? Is the injury pattern misleading, being in fact something other than what it appears to be?

Injuries have misled investigators be-cause they erroneously appeared to be classic, diagnostic accident injury patterns when they were actually caused by entirely different factors or were artifactual. These preexisting injuries and artifacts are probably the most frequent cause of erroneous interpretations of injury patterns and the sequence of events in the crash.

Injury patterns and specific injuries are directly related to the following:

1. The magnitude, duration, direction, and pulse shape of the acceleration forces
2. The cockpit or passenger compartment configuration
3. The nature of the accident and subsequent occurrences
4. The occupant kinematics in the accident, particularly those relating to the restraint systems

Acceleration Forces

The magnitude, duration, direction, and pulse shape of acceleration forces affect the pattern of injuries and are major factors in determining injury tolerance. Certain levels of force produce one type of injury, whereas greater force may produce transient injuries. Still greater force may produce irreversible injury or even death.

Eiband[14] suggested that the magnitude of tolerable acceleration is inversely related to the duration of its application. Human volunteers tolerated acceleration forces of great magnitude for short periods of time. Colonel John P. Stapp experienced more than 45 -G_x on a rocket sled. Early ejection system experiments exposed human subjects to more than 25 +G_z, with vertebral fractures as the only resulting injuries.

Many people have survived apparently impossible circumstances of high-G deceleration such as falls of more than 300 m. The factors that contributed to survival in these cases are poorly defined, but perhaps the high velocity resulted in reduced pulse duration and increased tolerance.

By contrast, only 1 G in the $-G_z$ acceleration field may be fatal within a period of several hours. These two examples, representing the extremes of the acceleration scale, illustrate the complexity of the problems associated with tolerance to acceleration.

Cockpit or Passenger Compartment Configuration

The configuration of the compartment may restrict expeditious exit after the crash. The occupant may strike some part of the cockpit or passenger compartment and experience fatal injuries in what would have otherwise been a survivable accident. Loose objects set in motion by the crash forces may strike the occupant, or he may strike the fuselage or be crushed by it or by other objects in his immediate vicinity. The likelihood of injuries increases significantly if external objects penetrate the occupant space or if the space is crushed by the crash forces. Engine, transmission, and still-turning rotor blades may penetrate the occupant space and produce fatal injuries during helicopter crashes.

Nature of the Accident

The nature of the accident and subsequent events will explain many injury patterns. In general, the types of injuries seen in helicopter accidents are different from the injuries that result from crashes of fighter or large transport aircraft. This is due in large part to the differences in operational activities of each of these aircraft.

The nature of the accident and the sequence of events influence the character and severity of crewmember injuries following ejection from an aircraft. Bird strikes, in-flight explosion, striking part of the aircraft or ejection seat after exiting the aircraft, parachute-opening deceleration, or impacts during or after landing may produce similar injury patterns. The investigator must seek trace evidence such as paint scrapings or tissue fragments from suspected contact points to reconstruct the sequence of events.

Mason[12] suggested the odd-man-out theory for the evaluation of injuries. He compared injuries received by multiple fatalities in a single crash with those received by fatalities in separate crashes and looked for similarities in injury patterns. If the investigator finds dissimilar injury patterns, he must determine what the individuals with each injury pattern were doing that was different. Finding cabin crewmember injury patterns that are similar to passenger injury patterns suggests that the cabin was prepared for the crash, but dissimilar injury patterns would indicate that the occupants may not have anticipated the crash. The finding of leg fractures may explain why many occupants did not exit the aircraft, even though the fire may not have developed until many minutes after the crash.

Occupant Kinematics

Many factors influence the trajectory an occupant follows during a crash. The magnitude and direction of the acceleration vector, the shape of the acceleration pulse, the amount of crushable material in the aircraft, and the nature of the seat and restraint systems can vary the trajectory considerably and greatly influence the force applied to the occupant. The investigator must evaluate all of these factors carefully before reconstructing the occupant kinematics during the crash. Special techniques such as computer simulation may be helpful.

Various types of protective devices and equipment such as specially designed seats and other restraint systems, helmets, and protective clothing frequently modify injury patterns. Most protective systems have many components, and the failure or inadequate design of almost any of these system elements can exponentially increase the force applied to the occupant and lead to injury or death. If an attachment point of a seat to the basic structure fails, the occupant will feel an acceleration force of shorter duration but of much greater magnitude. Force magnification also occurs when the restraint system fails or, because of elasticity or plasticity, allows the occupant's motion to extend lethal areas outside the protective envelope.

Traumatic Injuries

Head Injuries

Head injuries are the most frequent cause of death in aircraft accident victims. These injuries often result when the unrestrained head, neck, and upper torso flex over a lap belt because they are unrestrained by a shoulder harness system. This allows the unprotected head, chest, and extremities to strike exposed structures, resulting in serious or fatal injuries.

The skull provides reasonable protection to the cranial contents, but impacts that damage the integrity of the cranial system or transmit the impact force to particularly sensitive areas are often fatal. Concentrations of impact force are particularly lethal, and designs that distribute the force greatly increase the magnitude of the impact the head can withstand.

Certain preventive measures can reduce, if not entirely prevent, these head injuries. Helmets can provide energy absorption and distribute the impact force; shoulder restraint systems can reduce the range within which the head could strike cockpit objects. Aircraft designers can avoid introducing possible injurious impact surfaces into the cockpit during the development phase.

Linear fractures of the skull tend to occur in the plane in which the force was applied. This has sometimes led investigators to believe erroneously that transverse fractures of the base of the skull, extending from ear to ear and across the sella turcica, could result only from a blow to the side of the head (Fig. 27–6). At least as frequent a cause of the transverse fractures, however, are blows to the bottom of

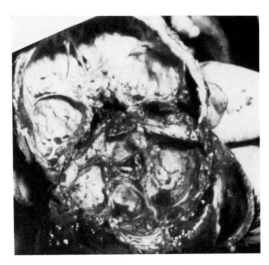

Fig. 27–6. Transverse fracture of the base of the skull (Armed Forces Institute of Pathology photo).

the skull, transmitted via the mandibular rami when the face impacts with an instrument panel.

Ring fractures, fractures around the circumference of the foramen magnum, may result from force transmitted up the spine in $+G_z$ impacts. Although this fracture pattern can occur from force transmitted from a blow to the top of the head, this possibility is rare. Because the center of gravity of the skull is forward of the spine, a blow to the top of the head tends to produce flexion, resulting in asymmetric application of force to the foramen magnum. This results in anterior cervical fracture and Jefferson's fracture (see section entitled "Spinal Injuries") rather than ring fractures.

Skull fractures tend to be subtle, and the investigator may not be able to see them without careful observation. He must meticulously remove the dura before concluding that no skull fractures are present. Blunt trauma of greater magnitude may produce eggshell fractures of the skull. Even more severe impact, especially when the upper torso is not restrained or when the upper-torso restraint system fails, results in partial or complete decapitation.

Head injuries will sometimes mislead

the investigator if he relies on examination of the strike envelope alone in considering the possible causes of the injuries. He should consider the possibility that collapse of the aircraft structure or impact with loose objects produced the injury. Figure 27–7 illustrates such a case. The pilot of a small, single-engine plane received fatal head injuries during the crash. Brain tissue was on the instrument panel, and investigators found imprints of the knobs and instrument dials on the pilot's face. The investigators did not believe that the pilot had an upper-torso restraint system available, and they suspected that this deficiency allowed his upper torso to flex forward and his head to strike the instrument panel, which resulted in the fatal head injuries. Examination of the cockpit of the wrecked aircraft, however, clearly indicated that the injuries resulted from the pilot's head being crushed between the instrument panel and the aft overhead cockpit bulkhead. This occurred when the aircraft fuselage buckled at impact.

Unusual head injuries may lead to erroneous conclusions, especially when the investigator is not fully cognizant of the circumstances of the accident. Figure 27–8 is a photograph of a crewman who walked into the tail rotor of a helicopter. Figure 27–9 illustrates a blowout fracture of the skull from increased intracranial pressure that resulted from steam production as the postcrash fire heated the skull.

Internal Injuries

Crash forces can damage the internal organs of the chest and abdomen by any of several mechanisms, and this damage may result in death if prompt medical and surgical assistance is not available. Because the internal organs are relatively unrestrained and are suspended only by attachments within the chest and abdomen, they move during the impact sequence in

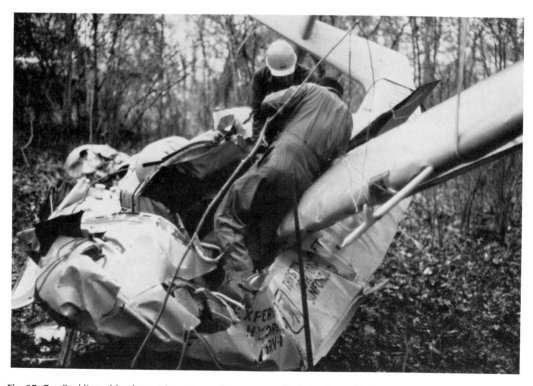

Fig. 27–7. Buckling of fuselage at impact as primary cause of injuries (Armed Forces Institute of Pathology photo).

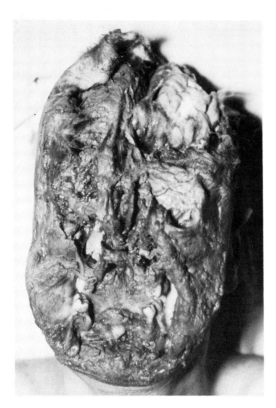

Fig. 27–8. Head injury as a result of walking into the tail rotor of a helicopter (Armed Forces Institute of Pathology photo).

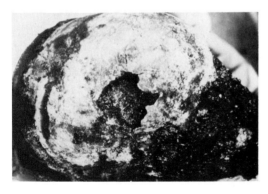

Fig. 27–9. Steam blowout fracture of the skull (Armed Forces Institute of Pathology photo).

a manner that may be quite different from the deceleration of the body as a whole. This frequently means that these organs are affected by decelerative forces that are much greater than other, more restrained body parts. Internal tears may be caused

by shearing forces applied as a result of differences in the mass of various tissues, and organ asymmetry may introduce torsional forces.

The direct application of force to internal organs as a result of penetration of the body cavities by external objects or as a result of impact with cockpit structures or seat belts can cause serious injuries. Overlying bony structures, such as the ribs and pelvis, provide a measure of protection to many of the internal organs, but other organs are more vulnerable.

The ribs, sternum, scapulae, and thoracic vertebrae, being bony structures, protect the organs of the chest. Application of about 2250 kg of force by a restraint belt may produce rib fractures. The jagged ends of the broken rib may lacerate the heart and lungs and even some of the abdominal organs such as the spleen, kidneys, and liver.

Approximately 13% of aircraft accident fatalities sustain significant cardiovascular injury. Missiles, broken ribs, or portions of the aircraft cockpit or controls may penetrate the chest and puncture the heart or major blood vessels. The heart or great blood vessels may burst as a result of being compressed between the sternum and vertebrae or from force transmitted from compression of the chest and abdomen. Once adequately designed cockpit enclosures, torso restraints, and head protection systems are in use, the tolerance of the cardiovascular system will determine the magnitude of the decelerative force that man can survive.

Tears of the aorta are frequent findings in aircrash fatalities who have little external evidence of injury, and the pathologist must carefully examine the heart and the aorta in situ and avoid introducing artifactual lacerations. Aortic rupture as an isolated finding is more common just distal to the left subclavian artery, but in cases of cardiac injury, 65% of the tears are in the ascending aorta just above the aortic valve. The origins of the subclavian and carotid blood vessels at the aortic arch provide relatively fixed attachment points for the heart and descending aorta, and even if a restraint system prevents significant movement of the upper torso, decelerative force may cause the heart and descending aorta to swing forward, like pendulums, during a crash. Because the heart is asymmetric (because the left ventricle is more muscular than the right ventricle), the deceleration may concentrate torsional forces and produce tears in the ascending aorta. Concentration of the shearing forces that result from the different deceleration rates of the heart and descending aorta from that of the aortic arch produces tears of the ascending and descending aorta near the insertions of the ligamentum arteriosum.

Blunt force applied to the abdomen can produce lacerations, tears, or rupture of the abdominal organs, and blunt trauma to the thorax or abdomen may rupture the diaphragm. Although both liver and spleen receive some protection from the rib cage, the liver is the more vulnerable of the two organs to impact injury. An improperly positioned or loosely fitted seat belt or a soft seat cushion may allow a seat occupant to slide under, or "submarine" beneath, the restraint system. This increases the frequency of spinal fractures and rupture of abdominal viscera.

Spinal Injuries

Examination of the spine provides the investigator with especially valuable information, particularly the evidence needed to determine the direction and magnitude of impact.

Vertebral fracture occurs frequently with vertical forces ($+G_z$) of greater than about 20 G. Compression fractures of vertebrae occur from the imposition of high $+G_z$ forces, especially in ejections from fighter aircraft or hard landings in helicopters. Two thirds of subjects sustain vertebral fracture at G levels greater than $+26$ G_z, but vertebral fracture can occur at

forces as low as 10 to 12 G, especially when the positioning of the spine is not entirely vertical. Multiple compression fractures in the same individual are unusual and seldom occur at levels less than $+35$ G_z.

G_y or G_x forces in excess of 250 to 400 G may produce shearing fractures of the vertebrae, especially in high-speed crashes (Fig. 27–10). The mass of the more dense vertebral end-plate, which is greater than the mass of the vertebra, may contribute to this injury pattern. When crash force is applied, this inertia creates much the same situation as can be shown by the elementary demonstration of inertia in which a book is placed on a piece of paper to illustrate that the paper can be removed without dislodging the book.

Pure compression fractures ($+G_z$), shearing fractures ($+/-G_x$ or $+/-G_y$), or Chance fractures ($-G_z$) are rarely seen. Most vertebral fractures result from combined

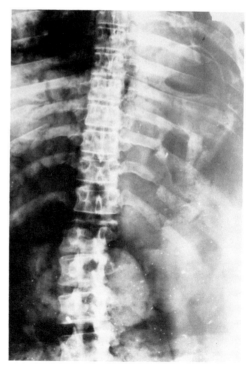

Fig. 27–10. Shearing fracture of vertebra (Armed Forces Institute of pathology photo).

x, y, and z force vectors but especially from the x-axis and z-axis. This causes a fracture pattern much like that which would be produced by a crowbar—with compression of the anterior portion of the vertebra and pulling apart of the posterior bony or ligamentous portions in tension (Fig. 27–11). This results because the force vector effectively places the fulcrum in the anterior portion of a vertebra.

Various crash circumstances may apply force to the neck and cervical vertebrae, causing fractures and dislocations. Windblast during ejection from an aircraft may cause the aviator's protective helmet to rotate and the edge of the helmet to strike the neck, much like a guillotine, causing fracture or dislocation of cervical vertebrae. Aircraft wiring and parachute lines entangling the neck are examples of mechanisms that result in "hangman's" fractures of the pedicles of the C-2 vertebra (Fig. 27–12). Impact to the top of the head may cause Jefferson's fracture, a fracture that consists of vertical splitting of the ring or lateral masses of the C-1 vertebra and lateral displacement of fragments of the vertebral body. Dissection of the anterior and posterior neck, followed by careful examination, is often helpful in these cases.

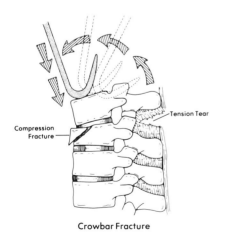

Compression Fracture

Tension Tear

Crowbar Fracture

Fig. 27–11. Mechanism producing a "crowbar fracture" of vertebra.

Injuries of the Extremities

Injuries to the extremities result from the flailing of unrestrained extremities and from impact with structures and are seldom fatal unless complicated by other factors. Excessive loss of blood may result from multiple injuries, and injuries of the extremities may prevent or impair escape from a hazardous postcrash environment.

Flailing of arms and legs during ejection from an aircraft may generate sufficient force to cause fractures. The flailing motion, much like that of cracking a whip, concentrates the force more distally, producing fractures of the tibia, fibula, radius, and ulna more frequently than of the femur and humerus. Femoral fractures may result from force applied by the anterior edge of the ejection seat.

Unrestrained extremities may contact aircraft structures within the strike envelope with sufficient force to produce injuries. The legs and arms may strike the instrument panel or a seat in front. "Dashboard femoral fracture" may result from the knee impacting with the instrument panel. Although extremity injuries are of little help in estimating the impact velocity and the parameters of the crash pulse, they may produce patterns that will indicate to the investigator exactly what structure the occupant struck.

Injury patterns of the hands and feet may provide good evidence of who was controlling the aircraft at the time of the crash, especially if other data, such as trace evidence, correlate with the patterns of injury. The best evidence of control is fracture of carpal, metacarpal, tarsal, and metatarsal bones, with associated patterned lacerations of the palms and soles of the hands and feet. Coltart[15] described "aviator's astragalus," fractures of the talar neck in pilots of aircraft with toebrakes. Fractures of the phalanges may be helpful indicators of control, but they are less reliable. Dummit and Reid[16] described unique tibial shaft fractures in helicopter

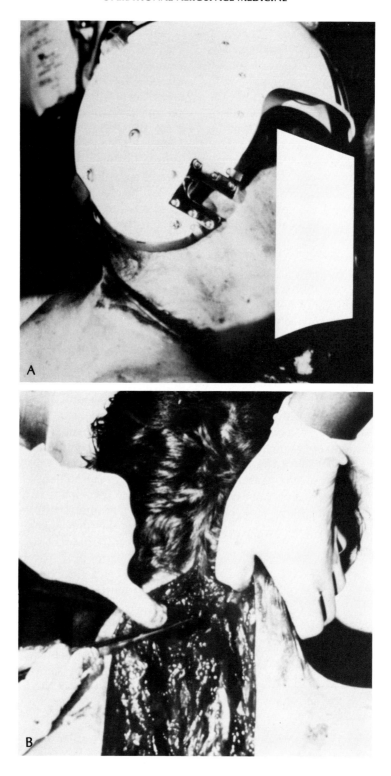

Fig. 27–12.   Cervical fracture resulting from entanglement with helmet microphone cord. *(A)* Anterior disection; *(B)* Posterior disection. (Armed Forces Institute of Pathology photos).

pilots. Similar tibial fractures also occur in pilots of other aircraft.

Environmental Factors

Environmental factors can contribute to the cause of an accident, can cause injuries, and can modify the appearance of injuries. Bird strikes, adverse weather conditions, hypoxia, fire, and water are some of the most significant hazards.

Bird Strikes

Each year, many aircraft collide with birds in flight. These collisions are significant problems, especially when they involve larger birds, supersonic aircraft, or the ingestion of birds into an engine.

Determination of a bird strike as an event is seldom difficult if investigators examine the wreckage carefully. Even in the most severe cases, they can find remnants of the bird. An ornithologist, on examining the feathers, bone, or other fragments of a bird, can often determine the species and sex and estimate its age and weight. Laboratory personnel can examine fragments of tissue microscopically for nucleated erythrocytes and can perform other serologic tests.

Weather

Turbulence, thunderstorms, and temperature extremes are examples of weather conditions that can influence the course of events in an accident. Turbulent weather conditions can produce in-flight breakup of the aircraft. If some of the occupants are thrown from the aircraft as a result, as in the case of the comet disasters, they will have different injury patterns, due to falling from altitude, than those who remained inside the aircraft.

Thunderstorms are a source of extreme turbulence, hail, and electrical activity. The cold temperatures at altitude and the lifting energy and moisture of thunderstorms combine to create hailstones up to several inches in diameter. These hailstones can damage lifting surfaces, cause engines to fail, and break windscreens. They also may be responsible for some abrasions and contusions in crewmembers following ejection in or near a thunderstorm. The effects of striking these hailstones is not as serious as the injuries inflicted on the crewmembers by the same extreme turbulent force that hurls hailstones thousands of feet into the air (Fig. 27–13).[13]

Many persons on the ground have died after being struck by lightning, but few similar deaths have occurred in occupants of aircraft. The electrical discharge passes primarily along the surface rather than through the center of a conductor. This "skin effect" diverts the electrical charge over the surface of the aircraft and protects the occupants except in a very few cases. Deaths have occurred in occupants of small planes and gliders, especially fabric-covered craft, that have passed directly in the path of a lightning discharge. Pinpoint burns of entry and exit, an arborization pattern of cutaneous erythema, and deposits from the arcing of electrical discharge along zippers and other metal objects among personal effects are evidence of a lightning strike.

Hypoxia

Hypoxia may occur suddenly, as in cases of rapid decompression at high altitude, or may be more insidious, as in prolonged flight at intermediate altitudes of 3000 to 4500 m. Information such as flight-planned altitude and radio transmissions provide key clues to suggest the incapacitation of crewmembers by hypoxia, and the laboratory determination of lactic acid in the brain will provide confirmation.

Fire

In-flight fires, impact "flash" fires, and postcrash fires produce characteristic patterns. In-flight fires produce streaming patterns of soot deposition, usually seen best on aircraft surfaces rather than on the

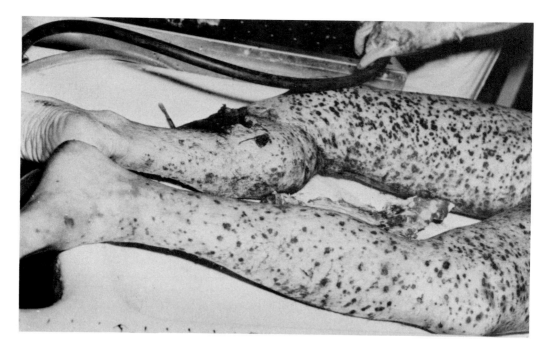

Fig. 27–13. Injuries resulting from impact with hailstones following ejection in a thunderstorm (Armed Forces Institute of Pathology photo).

bodies of the victims. "Flash" fires, as from the fireball of ignited fuel at impact, produce first- and second-degree burns of unprotected skin surfaces. The interpretation of injury patterns in the case of a postcrash fire is much more difficult.

Burn fatalities occur when occupants have insufficient time to escape because of the rapid onset and propagation of fire, when incapacitating injuries prevent them from exiting the aircraft, when exits are jammed or obstructed, when personal protective equipment is inadequate, or when rescue and fire-suppression efforts are ineffective. The investigator must answer the following key questions:

1. Was the victim alive at the time of impact?
2. Was the victim incapacitated by preexisting disease, medications, toxic gases, or fire injury before impact?
3. Were the burns received post mortem; that is, were fatal injuries sustained at impact, with the burns occurring after death?
4. Did death occur because the victim was unable to exit the aircraft because of injury, toxic gas, smoke, or problems with emergency egress systems before being overcome by smoke and fire?

The most difficult determination is whether burn injuries occurred after death, yet the answer to this question is often the most important. Whether the burns resulting from the postcrash fire or the injuries inflicted by the impact were more responsible for the occupant's death influences whether the investigator recommends improvements of egress systems and fire prevention or of seats, restraint systems, and structural design.

The occurrence of burn injuries in United States Air Force aircraft accident victims increased from 27.4% to 40.2% from 1953 to 1967, and injuries from fire as the primary cause of death increased from 6.7% to 17.0%.[17] Burns as the primary cause of death in United States Army aircraft victims also increased, from about 25% in 1957 to more than 40% in 1969, but the installation of a crashworthy fuel system on board Army UH-1 helicopters has virtually eliminated burn injuries as a cause of death in crashes of these helicopters. This is a dramatic illustration of the importance of the correct interpretation of whether burns occurred before or after death.

Laboratory determination of lactic acid levels in the brain and blood carboxyhemoglobin saturation may be of value in determining whether a crash victim was alive during the postcrash fire. The pathologist may also examine the respiratory system grossly for soot deposits and microscopically for a conclusive histologic response to combustion products of the fire.

Inexperienced investigators often conclude that fire-related postmortem artifactual changes were antemortem injuries. Heat-induced muscle contraction causes the body to assume a pugilistic attitude, as if the victim were protecting himself from the fire. The strongest muscle groups prevail, resulting in flexion of the hips, knees, and elbows but hyperextension of the neck. These heat contractions of muscles are frequently strong enough to produce bone fractures at the muscle attachment points. Rectangular bone fragments are characteristic in heat fractures of long bones.

Increased intracranial steam pressure that results from heating of the skull in a fire may produce "blow-out" fractures that appear similar to an impact injury. Finding bone fragments within the cranial cavity may help distinguish these fractures. Heating of the skull may also force blood into the extradural space, creating the appearance of extradural hemorrhage. Exposure of the skin to gasoline or other aviation fuels produces epidermolysis, skin bullae, and erythema, and the artifactual appearance of burn injury.

The investigator can usually relate the cutaneous burn pattern to protective equipment or to specific agents. Location of flare guns and oxygen bottles may provide clues to the cause of localized, severe burns. Extra thickness of clothing, such as pockets, belts, and waistbands, provide extra protection from burns.

Water

Postcrash survival in water is difficult. Drowning is a frequent cause of death following aircraft crashes into water, but the exact frequency is difficult to estimate. No one autopsy finding or laboratory test is diagnostic of drowning; the investigator must consider many factors before reaching this diagnosis, largely by excluding other diagnoses. Nevertheless, the correct determination of whether death occurred from drowning or from impact injuries is important.

A few of the external autopsy findings associated with drowning are a mushroom of froth in the nose and mouth and, occasionally, petechial hemorrhages beneath the conjunctiva. Prolonged exposure produces wrinkling of skin, so-called washerwoman's skin, but this finding may occur after death and is not an indicator of drowning. Internal findings include dilated blood vessels engorged with dark-red blood that does not clot, congested lungs with petechial hemorrhages, and hemorrhage into the temporal bones. Microscopic examination may detect diatoms in blood or tissues, but this finding is of little value without comparison with samples of the water from the crash site. Laboratory tests to compare the concentrations of various electrolytes in the blood from the left and right sides of the heart and to determine lactic acid concentration in the brain may be helpful, and these tests are discussed in the sections entitled "Blood Electrolytes" and "Brain Lactic Acid."

PREEXISTING DISEASES

Pilots are not immune to the wide variety of diseases that affect the general population. The literature contains reports of almost every imaginable disease process, from a congenital anomaly, cardiovascular disease, neoplasm, to infection, causing a crash; however, the selection criteria, physical standards, and frequent medical supervision of flight crews probably detect most preexisting disease before an acute catastrophic health condition occurs in flight. The accident investigator is more likely to encounter what most people consider minor disease processes.

Did the minor disease cause the accident? The investigator will want to answer this question. Minor diseases probably play a much greater role in causing accidents than most investigators have been willing to accept, and diseases that remain undisclosed at autopsy, such as epilepsy and cardiac arrhythmias, are of particular concern.

Detection of Preexisting Disease

Following an accident, the first suspicion that preexisting disease may be present often comes from examining the medical records of the crew. Examination of their medical records early in the course of the accident investigation, certainly prior to the autopsy examination, can be a valuable timesaving step. In fact, the documentation of some preexisting conditions may require special techniques that the pathologist would not usually employ, and if the medical records are not available until after he has completed the autopsy, the pathologist may be unable to identify a suspected preexisting disease.

A careful, complete autopsy usually will disclose any preexisting injury or disease that is present, but even when the cause of death appears obvious, the investigator must be alert for underlying preexisting conditions. Although the pathologist can easily detect most preexisting diseases by gross examination of the tissues, the discovery or confirmation of some conditions will require toxicologic or microscopic examinations. Histologic examination may be the only way to determine whether a contusion occurred days or weeks prior to the crash, during the crash, or after death. Pilot incapacitation has resulted from acute appendicitis, acute glaucoma, and Meniere's disease, but the investigator may not detect these conditions until he examines the histologic sections.

Significance of Preexisting Disease

The presence of preexisting injuries or disease can often be a source of confusion. Distinguishing acute from chronic disease processes is not always easy, and even a preexisting, long-standing disease process can precipitate an acute catastrophic event. Distinguishing between those disease processes that might have contributed to the accident and those that probably were entirely unrelated to the cause of the crash is especially important but often very difficult. The mere presence of preexisting disease does not mean that it was a factor in causing the accident. Investigators may have a difficult time proving that it was a cause, but the preexisting disease may have been a contributing factor in causing a "pilot error" or "cause—undetermined" mishap.

The most significant disease is one that goes undetected in the screening process, contributes in causing an accident, and remains undetected during the investigation process. Careful scientific analysis is necessary to find any previous disease and to distinguish merely incidental pathologic findings from disease entities causing disability of crewmembers.

Neurologic Disease

Review of aircraft accident investigation data has disclosed few cases attributed to neurologic disease. The AFIP files contain a few aircraft accident cases involving crewmembers with neurologic disorders such as Parkinson's disease, Meniere's disease, and space-occupying intracranial lesions, including pituitary adenomas and colloid cyst of the third ventricle.

Well-documented cases where investigators have shown epilepsy to be the cause of an aircraft accident are conspicuously absent, but incapacitation of professional pilots due to epilepsy has occurred in flight. The United States Air Force reported that 33% of 30 asymptomatic aircrewmembers who had abnormal electroencephalographic findings were involved in accidents or incidents or had a neurologically related clinical event. It also reported that 13% died in accidents.

Cardiovascular Disease

Cardiovascular disease in aircrew members is part of the normal aging process and is of major concern as a cause of fatal incapacitation and accidents. It is quite prevalent, even in the relatively young military population. Pettyjohn and McMeekin[18] reported the AFIP experience in reviewing autopsies of 6500 aircraft accident victims. Of these fatalities, 816 (13%) had preexisting, nontraumatic heart disease.

The literature contains numerous reports of pilots having heart attacks at the controls, but few crashes have occurred. The United States Air Force concluded that in-flight myocardial infarction is a rare event, after it found only two cases of confirmed and five cases of suspected in-flight myocardial infarction between 1962 and 1972. One international airline reported that only 17 of its pilots experienced health-related incidents between 1948 and 1972. Of the 13 incidents related to the cardiovascular system, only 11 were

coronary infarcts, and no crashes occurred.

This low incidence is consistent with the experience of other airlines. and the statistics may be quite accurate, considering the fact that most airlines have cockpit voice and flight data recorders. Nevertheless, the general flying public worries about the health of airline pilots who literally hold the passengers' lives in their hands. Most investigators reflect this concern.

Histologic examination of the heart is particularly helpful. The shearing forces of trauma (Fig. 27–14) and the coagulating effect of heat from fire may create lesions that appear grossly like coronary thrombosis. Careful microscopic examination of multiple sections may reveal the foci of myocarditis. Because these foci also occur in healthy people who die, they may be simply minor injury patterns representing the normal wear and tear of repetitive cardiac contractions. The investigator should evaluate the finding of myocarditis carefully with full consideration of all the facts associated with the accident.

The pathologist may occasionally encounter myocardial infarction associated with an aircraft accident, but trying to find evidence to prove early myocardial infarction, especially in the absence of coronary thrombosis, is especially frustrating. Although histologic examination may be helpful in estimating when the infarction occurred in relation to the times of death, the most optimistic histochemical tests purport to detect myocardial ischemia only as early as 30 minutes after onset, and this is of no value when a crash precipitously follows the acute myocardial event.

Sarcoidosis

Sarcoidosis is a relatively common disease that may cause sudden incapacitation and even death, but the incidence of clinical manifestations is low. Balfour[19] reported 16 cases of "sarcoid-like granulomas" in autopsies of 852 crewmembers,

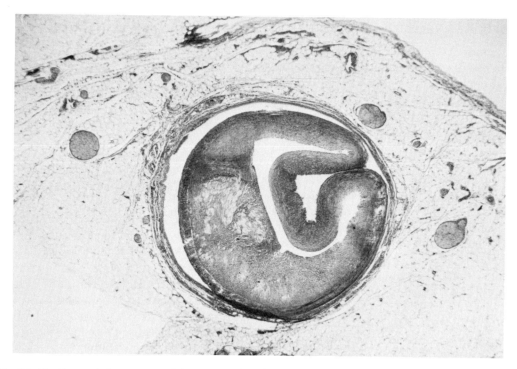

Fig. 27–14. Traumatic force separated the intima and media from the less dense adventitia, creating the artifactual appearance of coronary occlusion (Armed Forces Institute of Pathology photo).

although the reported incidence of clinical sarcoidosis in the United Kingdom is only about 3/100,000 inidividuals per year. Only one of his cases had cardiac involvement. Pettyjohn and colleagues[20] reported on 36 United States military aircrew members with clinical sarcoidosis. Thirty-three percent had evidence of cardiac involvement; four of the 36 individuals had significant cardiac abnormalities, and eight individuals had electrocardiographic abnormalities. These findings are higher than the generally reported incidence of 13 to 20%.

Although no evidence clearly establishes that sarcoidosis causes aircraft accidents or that aviation duties make aircrew members more susceptible to the lesions of sarcoid, investigators may be underestimating the importance of sarcoidosis as a significant etiologic factor in aircraft accidents. Figure 27–15 illustrates the case of a pilot with severe sarcoidosis with multiple organ involvement, includ-

ing the heart. Investigators concluded that the cardiac involvement probably resulted in incapacitation of the pilot. The injury pattern observed in the passenger suggested that the passenger and not the pilot was operating the controls at the time of the crash.

Infections

Infections of the upper respiratory tract, especially those involving the sinuses, occur frequently in aircrew members as a result of repeated barotrauma from ascending and descending during flight. These infections may lead to ear involvement, disturbances of equilibrium, and a subsequent accident. The frequency of "nonspecific but definitely abnormal" respiratory tracts in pilots of unexplained, single-seat, high-performance aircraft that crashed impressed Mason,[21] and he suggested that these infections may cause more crashes than investigators have been willing to acknowledge.

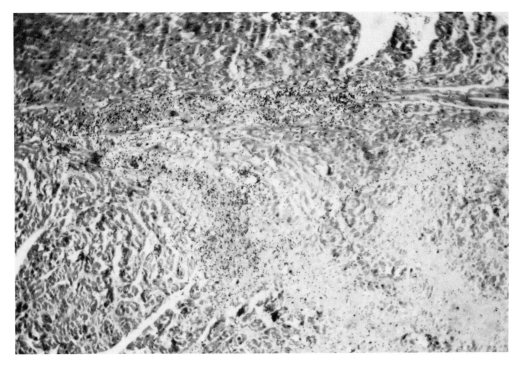

Fig. 27–15. Sarcoid granulomas in the heart (Armed Forces Institute of Pathology photo).

Tumors

The AFIP reported reviewing 6405 aircraft accident fatalities and finding 90 unsuspected tumors (Fig. 27–16). This number is impressive considering the following factors:

1. That the tumors occurred in crewmembers who were required to have a physical examination at least once each year
2. That the pathologists were able to obtain tissue for microscopic examination in less than 50% of the cases
3. That microscopic examination was present in less than 30% of the cases
4. That the microscopic examination in other cases was superficial

Alcohol, Self-Medication, and Substance Abuse

The ingestion of alcohol, prescribed or illicit drugs, self-medication with over-the-counter drugs, or even the excessive consumption of various food products can lead to impaired function of crewmembers.

Aircraft accident toxicology laboratories find that crewmembers ingest ethyl alcohol more than any other toxic substance. Of the unusually large number of aircraft accident victims positive for alcohol before about 1965, many were probably "positive" as a result of postmortem putrefaction or inadequate laboratory methods; however, even after the introduction of better collection and preservation techniques and gas chromatography, the incidence is still greater than 10%. Many positive results are still caused by postmortem decomposition with the resultant bacterial production of alcohol.

The United States Air Force reported that the ingestion of ethyl alcohol was associated with 28 of approximately 4200 aircraft accidents from 1962 through 1974.[22] The FAA reported that alcohol levels in 28 (13.9%) of 202 general aviation accidents were greater than 50 mg/100 g.[23] General aviation accidents in the United

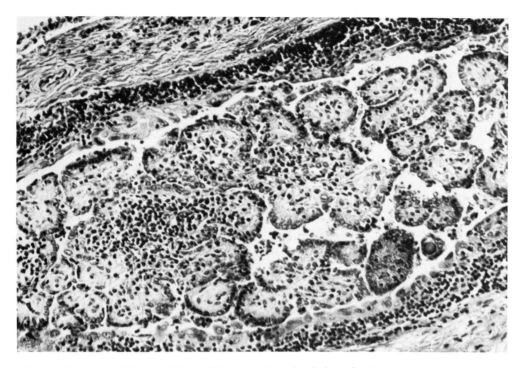

Fig. 27–16. Carcinoma of the thyroid (Armed Forces Institute of Pathology photo).

Kingdom during a similar period of a study, 1964 through 1973, resulted in positive alcohol determinations in 34 of 102 pilots; however, only 12 accidents (11.6%) involved alcohol ingestion before flight.

Table 27–2. Drugs Found Upon the Examination of 2326 Occupants of Aircraft Mishaps in 1983

Substance	Number of Occupants
Salicylates	109
Acetaminophen	61
Cannabinoids	54
Ethanol	51
Opiates	18
Chloroquine	6
Barbiturates	5
Amphetamines	2
Benzodiazepines	1
Chlorpheniramine	1
Cocaine	1
Diphenhydramine	1
Furosemide	1
Hydrochlorothiazide	1
Lidocaine	1
Phencyclidine	1
Total	**314**

The AFIP toxicology laboratory found the substances listed in Table 27–2 when they examined 2326 occupants involved in aircraft mishaps during 1983. Some of these substances (e.g., lidocaine) may have been used in resuscitation efforts by rescue personnel; other agents, such as the cannabinoids, would certainly be associated with drug abuse. The presence of drugs such as chloroquine probably represent cases of approved usage. Although the usage of drugs such as salicylates or acetaminophen may have been approved in some instances, most cases involved the self-medication of an underlying condition that would have been disqualifying for flight duties.

LABORATORY TESTS AND INTERPRETATION OF RESULTS

Many laboratory tests are available to assist the investigator, but the correct choice of the methods and careful interpretation of the results are important.

Serologic Studies

Serologic studies, such as the determination of blood type, are often useful in narrowing the possible identities of an unknown body. The investigator must exercise caution in the performance and interpretation of serologic studies, because numerous possibilities exist for error and for the introduction of artifacts.

Perhaps the simplest serologic test is the use of antihuman globulin (Coombs serum) to determine whether a tissue is human or nonhuman. Utilizing proper techniques, this distinction can be made even on dried bones that are more than 100 years old. This test is of particular value in cases where a long time has lapsed from the occurrence of the disaster to the time of discovery and where the possibility exists of commingling with animal remains. The technique is also useful in the investigation of aircraft accidents where a bird strike is suspected.

The detection of A and B blood group substances in blood, tissues, or fluids is helpful in determining the blood type of the deceased. Dried blood in these tests produces the best results, which is advantageous because the investigator cannot always draw blood immediately after death and separate serum and cells. Of the blood group substances, A and B seem more stable than others after death. Many other blood group substances deteriorate rapidly, and even A and B substances may give erratic results to the laboratory tests.

Positive benzidine, orthotoluidine, or phenolphthalein tests may indicate the presence of blood, but interference by many plant, chemical, and other animal sources of peroxidase activity may result in false-positive results. The determination of hemochromogen crystals by procedures such as the Takayama test or of hemin crystals by the Teichmann test also indicates that blood is present.

If blood is present, the investigator may use the absorption-inhibition, absorption-elution, Lattes crust test, or Howard-Martin cellulose acetate sheet test to determine the blood type. The absorption-elution tests are sensitive and accurate, and only small amounts of dried material are needed. Direct agglutination techniques using known antisera give erroneous results because the blood cells are damaged in dried stains, and postmortem changes introduce numerous artifacts.

Several techniques allow the determination of the species of origin of a bloodstain or tissue. The interfacial ring-precipitin test, the Ouchterlony gel double-diffusion test, and the antiglobulin-inhibition technique are three common methods using species-specific antisera.

Toxicologic Studies

The toxicologist has methods to detect many drugs, as well as to determine the levels of substances that occur normally in human tissues. He is especially capable of performing these analyses on postmortem tissues and fluids that would be very difficult for one to perform reliably in the usual hospital laboratory.

Drugs and Volatile Substances

Many toxicology laboratories use solvent-solvent extraction followed by gas chromatographic examination for drugs in the nonvolatile organic acid, basic, and neutral groups. Volatile substances (e.g., alcohol) can be detected by headspace gas chromatography. The investigator should remember that these procedures screen only for classes of compounds; many substances can be detected only by procedures that test for them specifically.

Blood Glucose

Hypoglycemia may be a factor in the cause of aircraft accidents, but the accurate determination of the glucose level in the blood of a fatally injured crewmember at the time of the crash is difficult. The cells continue metabolism for a short time after death, causing the blood glucose level to fall very low. Then, as tissue breakdown occurs, the blood glucose level becomes very elevated. Depending on from where the investigator collects the blood, but especially if he collects it from the inferior vena cava, the glucose level may be greater than 1000 mg/dl. Glucose levels in the vitreous of the eye do not change as rapidly, making the vitreous a good source of fluid for estimating the postmortem glucose level. Rapid chilling further inhibits the postmortem fall in concentrations of vitreous humor glucose.

Brain Lactic Acid

Dominguez and colleagues[24] reported an association of brain lactic acid concentrations greater than 200 mg/100 g with asphyxial deaths. The determination of the lactic concentration in the brain by ultraviolet spectroscopy requires approximately 500 mg of gray matter. The myelinated white matter and peripheral nerves give unreliable results.

Finding elevated concentrations of lactic acid in the brain is helpful in cases of drowning, death occurring in fires, and altitude hypoxia, but the mechanism that produces this elevation is not clear. The reason is probably not that of simply shutting down the aerobic respiratory pathways. Perhaps it results from adrenal hyperactivity causing increased mobilization of lactate precursors during an agonal period of stress. Certainly, the most frequent cause of an elevated postmortem lactic acid level in the brain is resuscitation efforts with intravenous fluids.

Carbon Monoxide, Cyanide, and other Combustion Products

Blood carboxyhemoglobin saturation gives an indication of the magnitude of antemortem exposure to carbon monoxide. More reliable laboratory methods and equipment, such as differential colorimetric spectroscopy and gas chromatography, now allow the accurate determination of carboxyhemoglobin saturations less than 1%, rather than the 10% level generally considered as significant; however, a wise investigator will seek an explanation of even the lowest caboxyhemoglobin saturations.

The ambient concentration of carbon monoxide in the breathed air and the length of exposure determine the level of carboxyhemoglobin saturation. Smokers seldom have carboxyhemoglobin saturations greater than 10%, although higher levels may occur in cigar smokers. One crewmember who smoked more than two packages of cigarettes in less than 30 minutes en route to the hosptial after a crash had a carboxyhemoglobin saturation of 17%. Victims may breathe the products of a postcrash fire for more than 1 minute without reaching a 20% carboxyhemoglobin saturation and for more than 5 minutes without reaching 50% saturation. In rapid conflagration situations, victims who survived the impact forces may be found to have died in the postcrash fire before the carboxyhemoglobin saturation reached even 10%. Thus, the investigator should seek an explanation for even low carboxyhemoglobin saturations.

Carbon monoxide has a great affinity for hemoglobin and competes for its oxygen-carrying capacity. The reduced oxygen-carrying capacity of hemoglobin generally was considered to produce sufficient hypoxia to cause death in fire victims. This may still be the reason for these deaths, but it has been suggested that the true mechanism for carbon monoxide causing deaths in fires is its effect on cellular respiration by binding of intracellular cytochrome a[3] in competition with oxygen. Thus, the carbon monoxide dissolved in plasma, entering the cells, and binding cytochrome a[3] may be more significant than the limitation of the oxygen-carrying capacity of hemoglobin by carboxyhemoglobin. This would explain why some unburned victims die with relatively low carboxyhemoglobin concentrations and some survivors recover even after reaching carboxyhemoglobin saturations greater than 50%.

Fire produces many other products of combustion, depending on the fuels and the composition of the atmosphere in which they burn. Many plastics produce cyanide gas when burned. Cyanide is a potent enzyme poison but may not be any more toxic than carbon monoxide in this regard. Other materials, such as electrical wiring, may produce halogenated hydrocarbon products, and laboratory measurements of chloride and fluoride may be helpful.

Blood Electrolytes

The comparison of electrolyte concentrations in blood from the left and right heart chambers as a diagnostic test for drowning is controversial. Theoretically, freshwater drowning dilutes the electrolytes in the left heart chambers and saltwater drowning concentrates some of the electrolytes in the left heart chambers, and postmortem changes increase the complexity of these interpretations.

The Gettler test relied on finding a difference in chloride concentration of 25 mg/dl between the left and right heart chambers. The interpretation of results is even more complicated when drowning occurs in brackish water, because the chloride concentration of the water may not be very different from the chloride concentration in the blood. The measurement of other electrolytes such as magnesium may be helpful in these cases. Collecting a sample of the water at the drowning site will allow the laboratory to select the electrolytes that might be useful in the comparison.

Artifact and Error

Many factors influence the reliability of various laboratory tests. The investigator should consider carefully the reliability of the test methods used by a particular laboratory, technical ability of the technicians, and quality control procedures in

use when selecting a laboratory to perform toxicology analyses. He must also collect the specimens carefully to avoid contaminating the containers. Indelible ink markers, used to label containers, may be a source of contamination with organic solvents.

Soil, vegetation, and fuel may contaminate the specimens at the crash site, and immersion may dilute the concentrations of the substances being measured. Fire, burning, and putrefaction may change the composition of the tissues or may produce substances that interfere with the test. The duration and temperature of postcrash exposure have significant effects on the rate of the decomposition process.

The postmortem production of alcohol by bacteria causes frequent difficulty in determining whether the ingestion of alcohol may have impaired a crewmember's judgment. The bacterial production of alcohol usually amounts to less than 50 mg/100 g of tissue, but rare instances of the production of more than 100 mg/100 g have occurred.

Aircraft accidents are not new occurrences, but few persons obtain much experience in aircraft accident investigation. As a result, when called on to participate in an accident investigation, the investigators make many mistakes of omission and commission. Investigators can avoid the most serious mistakes by careful planning and by following logical steps such as the six steps recommended by the Joint Committee on Aviation Pathology. Determining the role of the participants and the jurisdiction to conduct the investigation is important.

Identifying the victims is an unpleasant but relatively simple matter. Planning and organization are essential. Someone must obtain sufficient antemortem records before identification can be possible. Once these data are obtained, examination of the bodies and the application of various identification techniques such as fingerprint, dental, and radiologic methods can proceed rapidly.

Injury patterns are determined by the acceleration forces, cockpit configuration, nature of the accident, and occupant kinematics. Investigators can conveniently classify injury patterns by cause: traumatic, environmental, and preexisting disease factors.

The procedures are not difficult, but the investigator must collect and assimilate much information in a short period of time. He must not draw conclusions too quickly lest he make irreparable mistakes. There just may be things out there in the world that he hasn't seen yet.

REFERENCES

1. United States Congress, Senate Committee on Commerce: Safety in Air Hearings (3 parts), before a subcommittee, pursuant to Senate Resolution 146, Seventy-fourth Congress, Second Session, and Seventy-fifth Congress, First Session, 1936–1937. Part 1, Page 1, February 10, 1936 (Copeland Hearings).
2. Armstrong, J.A., Fryer, D.I., Stewart, W.K., and Wittingham, H.E.: Interpretation of injuries in the Comet aircraft disasters. Lancet, 1:1135, June 4, 1955.
3. Joint Committee on Aviation Pathology: Memorandum No. 1: An Autopsy Guide for Aircraft Accident Fatalities. Washington, D.C., Joint Committee on Aviation Pathology, 1957.
4. Fryer, D.I.: The medical investigation of accidents. In A Textbook of Aviation Physiology. Edited by J.A. Gillies. Oxford, Pergamon Press, 1965, p. 1200.
5. Chicago Convention on International Civil Aviation. Article 26, 61 Statute 1180, T.I.A.S. no. 1591, December 7, 1944.
6. Federal Aviation Act of 1958. Section 701, 72 Statute 781, as amended by 76 Statute 921. Forty-ninth Congress. §1441.
7. Lane, J.C., and Brown, T.C.: Probability of casualties in an airport disaster. Aviat. Space Environ. Med., 46:958, 1975.
8. Hays, M.B., Stefanki, J.X., and Cheu, D.H.: Planning an airport disaster drill. Aviat. Space Environ. Med., 47:556, 1976.
9. Lichtenstein, J.D., et al.: Role of radiology in aviation accident investigation. Aviat. Space Environ. Med., 51:1004, 1980.
10. Hill, I.R.: Dental identification in fatal aircraft accidents. Aviat. Space Environ. Med., 51:1021, 1980.
11. Morlang, W.M.: Forensic dentistry. Aviat. Space Environ. Med., 53:27, 1982.
12. Petty, A.E., and McMeekin, R.R.: Laboratory examination of unidentified tissue fragments found at aircraft sites. Aviat. Space Environ. Med., 48:937, 1977.
13. Mason, J.K.: Passenger tie-down failure: Injuries and accident reconstruction. Aerospace Med., 41:781, 1970.
14. Eiband, A.M.: Human tolerance to rapidly applied accelerations. NASA Memo 5-19-59E. Washington, D.C., National Aeronautics and Space Administration, June, 1959.
15. Coltart, W.D.: Aviator's astragalus. J. Bone Joint Surg., 34–B:545, 1952.
16. Dummit, E.S., and Reid, R.L.: Unique tibial shaft fractures resulting from helicopter crashes. Clin. Orthoped., 66:155, 1969.
17. Smelsey, S.O.: Diagnostic patterns of injury and death in USAF aviation accidents. Aerospace Med., 41:790, 1970.
18. Pettyjohn, F.S., and McMeekin, R.R.: Coronary artery disease and preventive cardiology in aviation medicine. Aviat. Space Environ. Med., 46:1299, 1975.
19. Balfour, A.J.C.: Sarcoidosis in aircrew. Aviat. Space Environ. Med., 53:269, 1982.
20. Pettyjohn, F.S., Spoor, D.H., and Buckendorf, W.A.: Sarcoid and the heart—an aeromedical risk. Aviat. Space Environ. Med., 48:955, 1977.
21. Mason, J.D.: Previous disease in aircrew killed in flying accidents. Aviat. Space Environ. Med., 48:944, 1977.
22. Zeller, A.F.: Alcohol and other drugs in aircraft accidents. Aviat. Space Environ. Med., 46:1271, 1975.
23. Smith, P.W., Lacefield, D.J., and Crance, C.R.: Toxicological findings in aircraft accident investigation. Aviat. Space Environ. Med., 41:760, 1970.
24. Dominguez, A.M., et al.: Significance of elevated lactic acid in the postmortem brain. Aerospace Med., 31:897, 1960.

Chapter *28*

Human Factors in Aerospace Medicine

Thomas B. Sheridan and Laurence R. Young

Know then thyself, presume not God to scan, The proper study of mankind is man.

ALEXANDER POPE

Human factors, sometimes called human factors engineering, is the science and art of interfacing man with the machines that he operates. One important interface is with the physical hardware such as displays, controls, and seating. A second interface is soft, in the sense of procedures for doing the task or training, as well as the computer software that the operator may have to use directly. The third interface is with the operational environment such as temperature, vibration, acceleration, radiation, chemical properties, and ambient pressure. The fourth interface of interest is social interaction with other people.

Human factors primarily is identified with the hardware interface, and this chapter will emphasize that interaction. This is certainly the emphasis of the various human factors data books and standards available.[1,2,3] The software interface always has been critical in relation to hardware, and the importance of software is certainly evident as computers become more important in mediating the opera-

tor's relationship to the machine. Problems regarding environmental stressors are dealt with in several other chapters of this text. Social interaction, although too often neglected in the design of complex man-machine systems, is a subject both too large and not sufficiently well codified to treat here.

In contrast to medicine, which is concerned primarily with the health of the individual, human factors engineering is concerned with the performance of the overall system: human performance is of interest as it enhances system performance, and safety is intrinsic to system performance.

The man-machine system is depicted in Figure 28–1. The human operator is subdivided into sensory, control processing/memory, and motor functions. On the machine side of the interface are displays that convert electrical, mechanical, and other signals from the vehicle or system into a form understandable to the human senses of vision, hearing, and touch. Correspondingly, conventional control devices, such

815

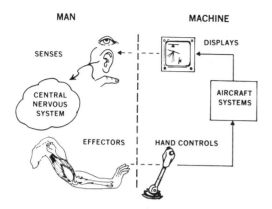

Fig. 28–1. The man-machine system.

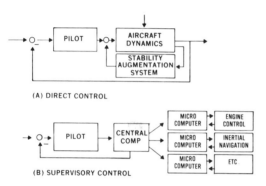

Fig. 28–2. Block diagrams of direct and supervisory control.

as joysticks, push-buttons, or pedals, transduce the operator's voluntary motor responses back to electrical and mechanical signals capable of driving the system. Advanced control devices actuated, for example, by voice, eye position, or brain waves are beyond the scope of this chapter. As shown in Figure 28–2, the information travels in a closed loop. This closed-loop system is essential for the operator to achieve real-time control.

Increasingly, the human operator is removed from the simple task of closing a feedback loop or driving the vehicle and is placed in a supervisory or monitoring role. When the operator's interactions with the vehicle or controlled process are mediated by a computer, the simply closed loop of Figure 28–2A is modified, as shown in Figure 28–2B. The computer

now serves as a direct controller, and the human operator's new role becomes that of supervisor of an otherwise automatic control loop.

HUMAN FACTORS IN AIRCREW TASKS

Human factors considerations are involved intimately with almost every aspect of manned flight, from the initial selection of pilot candidates through test pilot evaluation of vehicle handling qualities to pilot work load evaluation of changes in crew complement. Although a complete discussion of human factors in aviation is not possible in one chapter, a few examples of relevance to aviation can be presented.

When selecting individuals for pilot training by the military or for initial employment by the commercial airlines, it is commonplace to utilize both psychologic and physiologic assessment measures. Although no unanimity exists on the validity of these measurement techniques, the typical characteristics of the traditional pilot have been identified over the years. Continuing study has concerned the desirability of a two-track selection in which the psychologic and physical characteristics of transport pilots are separated from those characteristics appropriate for fighter pilots.

Once a candidate is selected for pilot training, he will be exposed to a variety of training devices, including various types of aircraft systems trainers. The increased reliance on interactive, computer-driven teaching programs will take training beyond the level of the tape-slide or videotape presentation. When properly programmed and appropriately combined with face-to-face instruction, such programs have proven their effectiveness in aircrew training and can provide the motivation, reinforcement, and effectiveness of self-paced study. Cockpit procedures and flying skills may be taught on any of four different devices: a part-task trainer, a cockpit procedures trainer, a flight simulator, or the aircraft itself. These devices are progressively more expensive and of higher fidelity. Although a pilot's first reaction may be to want to do as much as possible of his training in the air, the quest for fidelity often is misplaced. For teaching a sequence of procedures, as in the case of an engine fire, it is neither necessary nor desirable to provide the full fidelity of the aircraft or flight simulator. Furthermore, for crew coordination practice, a part-task trainer in which switches and controls are active but aircraft dynamics are not simulated may be as effective as the aircraft.

For teaching special flying skills, such as engine-out landings or reaction to an engine-out on takeoff, repeated practice in a high-fidelity flight simulator with added visual scenery is more effective, hour for hour, than training in the air. On the other hand, given the current limitations on computer-generated or model-board visual scenes in a simulator, certain skills, such as low-level navigation or treetop flying in a helicopter, are difficult to teach adequately in a simulator. The important human factors considerations in training involve identifying the training goals and providing a device that is capable of meeting these goals rather than one that mimics the aircraft in all respects.

Once a pilot enters the cockpit, the human factors of aviation become readily apparent, particularly as they create problems. Seat adjustments must accommodate the entire range of aircrew anthropometrics, both male and female. Aircraft seat comfort may be limited by the hardness required for the safe use of the ejection seat. Layout of the flight instruments should be in keeping with human factors design rules, grouping the commonly used instruments in the central visual field and placing associated instruments together. All of the important instrument information to be scanned must be readily visible from the pilot's position without interfering with his view outside the cockpit.

Cockpit noise levels should be kept acceptably low to facilitate communication and reduce aircrew fatigue.

The design of cockpit instruments themselves must take human factors principles into account, presenting material in a manner that is easily recognizable and interpretable, with a precision commensurate with their use and in an orientation consistent with the required control action. A devastating example of the results of nonconformity with human factors principles is in altimeter displays. The older, three-pointer altimeter was easily misinterpreted and blamed for numerous fatalities. The newer, drum-type altimeter and particularly the easily read and precise vertical-tape altimeter greatly reduce the likelihood of errors in altitude readings under conditions of stress, poor lighting, or turbulence.

The move from mechanical to electromechanical to electronic displays permits the designer to create almost any form of information display he desires for the pilot. Although the earlier electronic displays tended to mimic their electromechanical predecessors, human factors considerations are moving the field toward the increased use of integrated displays. In a well-designed integrated display, aircraft information is presented in a single, easily interpreted geometric pattern. Any required dynamic compensation or quickening easily can be introduced into the command display or flight director or by quickening the status displays. Finally, information not previously displayed to the pilot, such as malfunction checklists, can now be presented on a cockpit display unit driven by an airborne computer and associated mass storage elements.

Human factors considerations of the appropriate computer-aided checklists and procedures remain to be established. The limitations of the pilot in aircraft or spacecraft control become particularly apparent under stressful conditions, either because of increased work load, fatigue, or environmental disturbances. Communication and display design should leave a sufficient margin so that the additional work required does not lead to an inability to attend to the primary flying objectives. A thorough understanding of pilot work load is necessary, although its measurement remains difficult. Despite significant attempts to develop physiologic measures of work load, subjective rating scales, or side task measurements, the final decision on acceptable work load usually depends on the assessment of pilot performance under stress. Pilots must be made aware of their individual limitations, both psychologic and physical. Aircraft control cannot be expected to be as precise when a pilot is simultaneously loaded with communication, navigation, and checklist tasks. Pilots and designers alike should be made aware of the phenomenon of perceptual narrowing, in which objects in the peripheral visual field are literally not seen while attention is focused on either a visual or nonvisual central task.

The functioning of a pilot or astronaut as a member of a continuous control loop introduces the human factors specialty of manual control. Although the ideal and easiest control task is one in which the vehicle or controlled element is compensated so that the pilot commands its velocity, this situation is not always possible under normal or emergency conditions. Predictable situations leading to pilot-induced oscillations result from excessive delays in a control system, more than two integrations in a control loop, the absence of easily discernible error-rate information, or the need to perform separate parallel tracking tasks. Although one of the major reasons for introducing manual control as opposed to fully automatic piloting is to take advantage of human adaptability, rapidly changing vehicle dynamics can stress the pilot severely. Aerial refueling, for example, involves significant changes in the relationship between control effort and aircraft movement. Similarly, ap-

proaching the runway under instrument landing conditions can easily lead to pilot induced oscillation.

DISPLAYS

Display Function Classification

Displays, meaning any means for communicating information to a pilot or aircrew member, can be categorized as follows:

Primary flight displays
  Attitude indicator/flight director
  Radar/pressure altimeter
  Rate of climb
  Airspeed
  Compass/heading
Navigation displays
  Course
  Way-point
  Radar
  Wind direction and speed
  Moving map
Engineer instruments
  Revolutions per minute (rpm)
  Temperature
  Fuel and flow
  Oil and pressure
Autopilot display
  Settable indicators
  Altitude clearance
  Commanded heading
  Takeoff/landing "speed bugs"
  Decision height
Alarms
  Stall
  Fire
Avoidance
Radio/communications
Status of stores
Other aircraft systems
View out of windscreen
Maps, reports, procedures, other texts and graphics
Auditory information from other crewmembers and miscellaneous sounds of aircraft systems operating

Several of these categories are not usually

thought of as displays, but they are extremely important in complementing the panel instruments.

It is sometimes useful to classify displays by whether they are (1) alarms, discrete attention-getting stimuli; (2) check-reading or status monitoring displays, indicating whether conditions are normal and in some cases a qualitative degree of abnormality; (3) quantitative displays, which provide numeric information in digital or analog form; and (4) tracking displays, to be used in conjunction with controls for nulling out differences.

Alarms such as stall and fire may be auditory, visual, or other. (The "stick shaker" stall warning is an effective way of getting the pilot's attention.) The obvious advantage of an auditory alarm is that the pilot does not have to be looking in any particular place. Traditionally, auditory alarms have been Klaxon horns and buzzers, loud enough to be heard clearly but not so loud as to damage the pilot's hearing or interfere with his control of the aircraft.

Computer-generated speech is now inexpensive and reliable and offers many possibilities for providing alarm and warning signals. Such displays not only can alert the pilot but also can tell him what the condition is, with qualitative or quantitative modifiers, if necessary, to suit the momentary circumstances. Such displays can be presented at a loudness befitting the occasion and are especially valuable when a pilot's eyes must be fixed on a display or out the window, as in the glide-slope voice warning of deviation from an instrument landing system (ILS) during landing. Voice displays sometimes are combined with other sounds, as in the "whoop, whoop, pull-up, pull-up" terrain avoidance warning.

The discriminability of alarms, whether lights or sounds, is an important consideration. Pilots frequently complain that they cannot keep track of what the multiple warning lights and sounds mean, especially during stress. Therefore, the use of synthetic speech is appropriate to tell the pilot the meaning of an alarm after getting his attention, possibly by conventional means. In any case, tonal qualities, location, colors, or other features of alarms should be different from each other and, insofar as possible, should connote their meaning. Flashing lights are useful for attracting the pilot's attention and for discriminating the newly lit alarm or important alarm from status lights. Red lights should be used for emergencies requiring immediate attention, orange lights for warning or change status, and green lights for normal operations. Beyond the few most critical alarms, common practice has been to use master alarms that can tell the pilot that something is wrong within a whole set of functions. The pilot must then visually or manually access some lower-level visual display to find out specifically what is wrong.

Check-reading displays, those to be scanned regularly to check whether the pertinent variable is as expected, conventionally take the form of lights, flags (windows that change color), and linear tapes. Lights are used for discrete on-off information. Flags can indicate several discrete states (e.g., red, green, yellow). Linear or ribbon tapes are used where only qualitative information is necessary and where a quick verification scan is sufficient. The linear tape, depending on its size, can convey quantitative information for a closer second look if that is desired. It can also easily show a variable's rate of change and whether it is above or below some reference. Stacking linear tapes side-by-side (e.g., for engine variables) is useful for making comparisons and checking against normal operating ranges.

True quantitative displays, where numeric information is meaningful, may be analog (long linear tapes or circular dials) or digital. The quick qualitative impression sometimes may be important too (e.g., looking only at the first digit of the numeric display). Thus, the qualitative versus quantitative distinction is seldom a clean one. The altimeter, RPM, compass, and radiofrequency indicators are examples of quantitative displays.

Finally, the tracking or nulling display (for example, the altitude indicator with or without flight director command bars) is necessarily analog. Nulling a digital display is an awkward task; therefore, digital displays are not recommended for this function. Occasionally, displays combine the analog and digital elements, as in a conventional drum altimeter. Figure 28–3 provides some examples.

Cathode Ray Tube (CRT) Displays

The preceding discussion has not emphasized the CRT as a display, although it may serve all four of the above functions and is extremely flexible. Information is limited only by the physical constraints of the CRT and display generation electronics (number of separable picture elements or pixels) in length and width and speed for generating a new picture. The CRT display has drawbacks such as its depth (roughly equal to its width), its high voltage and power requirements, fragility, and problems with legibility in direct sunlight.

A good quality aircraft CRT is from 512 × 515 to 1000 × 1000 pixels. If a raster display generator (left to right sweeps suc-

cessively top to bottom, like an ordinary television) is used, bright colors can be filled in solid. White color line drawings and small objects can be generated quickly, although regeneration of a full screen may take up to several seconds. If a vector, or stroke-writing (calligraphic), display generator is used, new line drawings can be made hundreds of times per second, and thus gradual rotations, zooms, or other presentation formats are easy. To avoid flicker, displays should be refreshed approximately 30 times each second, depending on brightness.

From a human factors viewpoint, perhaps the most important capability of the CRT is permitting the integration of displays. For example, the computer-generated electronic altitude director instrument (EADI) provides the primary flight director display. It can combine pitch and roll, altitude and ground speed, as well as glide slope and localizer deviations. Figure 28–4A shows an example.

The CRT can provide a current list of all variables that either are abnormal or are about to become so. It can provide maps, diagrams, checklists, reminders, and procedural information. The cockpit display of traffic information (CDTI), recently tested by the National Aeronautics and Space Administration (NASA) for com-

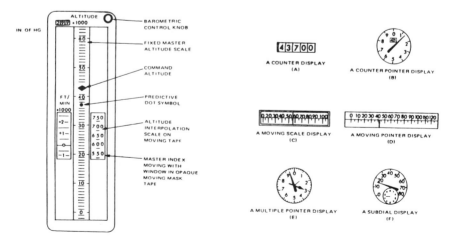

Fig. 28–3. Conventional display formats. (Bioastronautics Data Book, NASA SP-3006, 2nd Ed., 1973.)

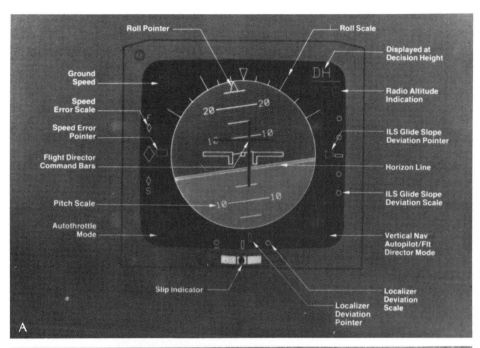

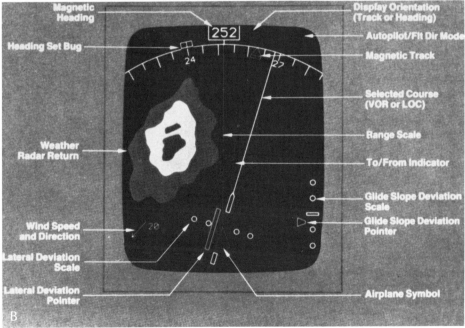

Fig. 28–4A. Electronic attitude director indicator (Courtesy of the Boeing Company). **B.** Electronic horizontal situation indicator VOR/ILS mode (Courtesy of the Boeing Company).

mercial aviation, combines map and waypoint information, weather radar, and position of all aircraft within a slice of airspace, with range adjustment in both altitude and map scale. Figure 28–4b shows the electronic horizontal situation indicator in the Boeing 767, which embodies many of these features. One novel use of CRTs tried in some industrial operations is a cartoon face whose smile represents one variable, direction of gaze a second, openness of eyes a third, furrow of eyebrows a fourth, and so on.

Cathode ray tube displays also can be used to provide different information formats at different times, depending on what the pilot or other operator requests. To have some standardization, it has become common practice to use a hierarchy or tree of pages, where a top-level page may represent the whole aircraft and the principal variables concerning its main subsystems. If more detailed information is wanted about some aspect of the top-level page, one could "page down" and thereby call up a full page concerning a single engine and its variables. This page, in turn, could have lower-level pages associated with it. More than three levels of paging usually is not recommended. Recommended practice for formatting a single page follows the same rules as for designing in general. One generalization is that not more than 20% of the total page area should be taken up with symbols or figures. Further, because lines and edges cannot be drawn as sharply on a CRT display as they can be printed on paper or instrument scales, the designer should be conservative in crowding scales, symbols, and text together. Figure 28–5 shows multiple CRTs in use in a prototype experimental cockpit.

The same CRT display also can be used to call up different types of variables at the same level in the paging tree. For example, one page could be hydraulics, another page electrical power, a third page weapons, and so on. The CRT display can be useful for presenting branching programs for abnormal procedures, troubleshooting, or checklists.

The CRT display can provide trend information on a multitude of variables, scaled on whatever basis is convenient to the user, provided the necessary information has been stored in the computer. Past history, trends, and anticipated future values can be compared. Thus, for failure detection and diagnosis, the CRT display is invaluable.

Other technologies are competing to replace the CRT display, but thus far none has its overall capability. New techniques include gas plasma and light-emitting diode (LED) displays (now in multicolors) and liquid crystal display (LCD) arrays. All of these displays have the advantage of flatness, but either cost, power (plasma), resolution (LED), or the need for adequate incident light (LCD) pose problems.

The head-up display (HUD) commonly is used in conjunction with weapons aiming, landing aids, or the altitude-flight director CRT display. This display is a combining mirror and lens arrangement that superimposes the CRT display image directly on the pilot's frontal view out through the windscreen at optical infinity. Use of the HUD saves the time involved in changing gaze and the time needed to reaccommodate in changing between out-the-window viewing and instrument viewing.

Criteria for Display Location and Design

The location of visual displays is necessarily a trade-off among many criteria such as the following:

1. Function or causal order, that is, mimicking left-to-right or top-to-bottom the cause-and-effect chains
2. Left-to-right or top-to-bottom position in terms of normal procedural sequences
3. Same for emergency procedures
4. General direction of where the corresponding physical system is lo-

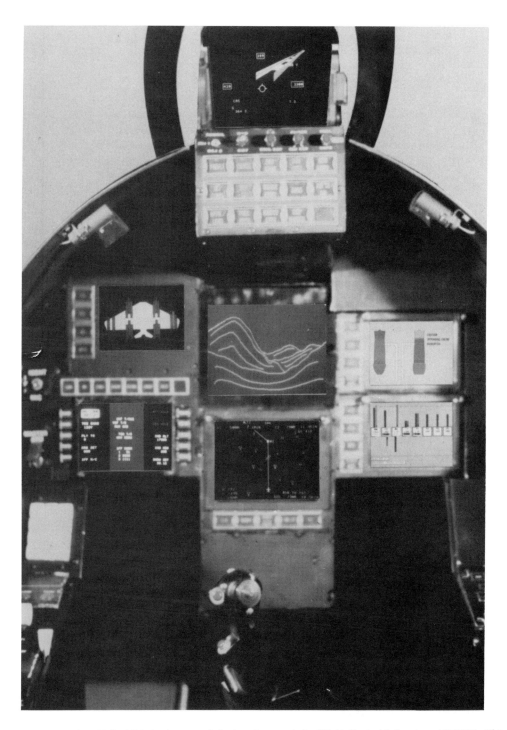

Fig. 28–5. Use of multiple CRTs for integrated displays in a cockpit. (Flight Control Laboratory, W-PAFB, Ohio-USAF PHOTO)

cated (e.g., engines, landing gear, and so on)

5. Front and center position for most important displays for normal use
6. Same for emergency use
7. Subsystem grouping
8. Optimum use of panel space
9. Position where the pilots say they want them and are used to having them

A second set of criteria, not necessarily in conflict with one another, considers the succession of responses the operator must make. The operator first must find the proper display or detect that a display has something to tell him, either because he is looking for it or because it is, in a sense, looking for him. A stereotyped scan pattern combined with easy-to-remember locations, as well as brightness, contrast, and size, help with location and detectability. Next, the pilot must read the details of the display. This reading includes recognizing numbers or symbols, knowing where pointers are pointing, or knowing what the color represents. Finally, the pilot must know what action to take in response to what he has read. The display should suggest the direction to move a control or the numbers to set into the keyboard. By convention, aircraft tracking displays are of the inside-looking-out or fly-to design, in which an error is negated by flying the aircraft toward the deviation indicator. Raising the gear handle to raise the landing gear is an unambiguous situation. Similarly, throttle forward means more thrust. Moving the control level forward to command the wing forward in a swing-wing fighter was rejected by pilots, however, because it had the effect of slowing the aircraft.

Conditions for Good Vision

Good vision is a function of a number of interrelated variables. These empiric relations are well established in the literature of visual psychophysiology[4,5,6] This chapter will examine only the first-order relationships.

The three variables most easily related to visual acuity in terms of ability to resolve two separate points or lines are spatial separation (or size), figure-ground contrast (in percentage of difference relative to the background illumination), and the background illumination. Larger, brighter, higher contrast displays generally can be seen better. The interrelation among the variables has been well established (Figure 28–6). Long parallel lines are easier by an order of magnitude to resolve than dots, other factors remaining the same. One minute of arc is taken visually as a reasonable two-point separation measure of visual acuity for a normal healthy person under good light and contrast.

The retina seems to integrate light intensity over time up to roughly 100 milliseconds (the Bunsen-Roscoe Law), so that a very short but very bright electronic strobe is just as discriminable and even looks the same as a much longer and less bright incandescent flashbulb. Obviously, acuity is much better at the fovea than at the periphery, provided that vision is photoptic, that is, that the light is bright enough to stimulate the cones. Night vision is best about 20° off the optic axis, where rod density is greatest. Other factors, such as vibration of the display or the subject and color of the image, also affect visual acuity.

When exposed to bright light, the visual threshold increases significantly, then falls back slowly when the impact is removed. The impact of flashblindness on display discriminability is significant. Figure 28–7 shows a curve for adaptation to darkness after exposure to bright sunlight. The discontinuity in the curve is the transition from cone to rod vision. Note that only after 30 minutes does the eye reach full sensitivity, becoming most sensitive to violet and least sensitive to dark red (R_1) and reddish-orange (R_{11}).

Because rod sensitivity or night vision

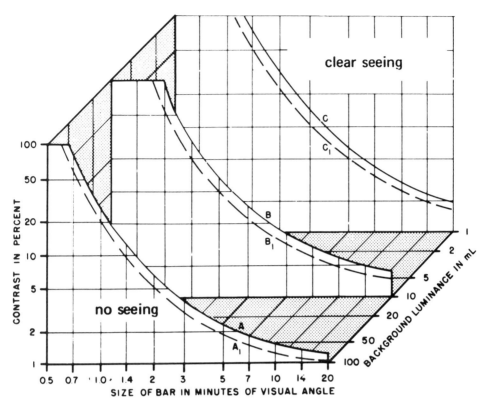

Fig. 28–6. Background luminance and contrast required for subtending various angles to be seen under daylight conditions. (From Chapines, A., et al.: Applied Experimental Psychology: Human Factors in Engineering Design. New York, John Wiley and Sons, Inc. 1955.)

washout depends on sufficient luminant energy within those shorter wavelength colors to which the rods are sensitive, it had been customary in night missions for pilots to wear red glasses and/or to have red filters on cockpit light sources. The light is then kept in a spectral region where cone vision functions but rod vision is minimally affected. After removing the red glasses, rod vision is well adapted to low light levels in the higher frequency, shorter wavelength range. Current practice is to use dim white light for most transport instrument lights.

Design of Instrument Scales and Letters

Based on considerable experimental research, it is clear that some scales are better than others in terms of reading speed and error. Principal number subdivisions of tens or twos (or their multiples) are both fast and accurate, whereas other number subdivisions are not. In the tens case, secondary subdivision by five is appropriate. Fine scale marks at unit intervals are appropriate in both cases if there is room, although a cleaner-looking scale is preferred if fine marks would lie too close together.

Various studies have been conducted on the effects of letter shape and font.[1] A letter height-to-letter width ratio of 1.4:1.7 has been found to be best, with a letter height-to-stroke (line) width ratio of 6:8. Sans serif fonts are not only cleaner but easier to read than fonts with serifs. Mixing capital and lower case letters is quite acceptable and preferred to using all capital letters.

For visibility, the military standard

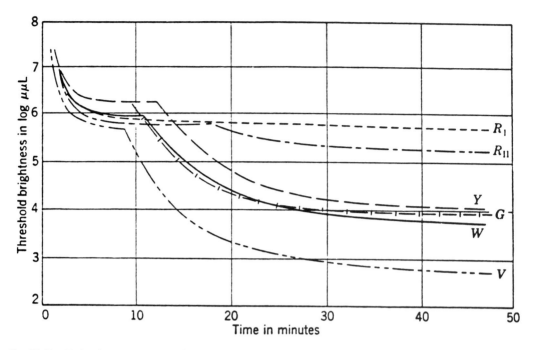

Fig. 28–7. Dark adaptation—Curves show the dominant visible light of different colors seen after various periods of darkness. (After Chapanis) These curves show the dimmest light one can see at various times after going into the dark. It takes about 30 minutes for the eye to reach full sensitivity. Notice that one finally becomes most sensitive to violet (V) and that one is least sensitive to deep red (R_I) and reddish-orange (R_{II}) light. (From Chapines, A., et al.: Applied Experimental Psychology: Human Factors in Engineering Design. New York, John Wiley and Sons, Inc. 1955.)

1472 recommends black letters on white background over white letters on black background or black letters on yellow or other backgrounds (or other combinations). In most situations with good light, the difference is not critical to reading speed or accuracy.

Color often is used for coding displays. Military standard 1472 recommends that red be used for abnormal situations, yellow for warning, green for normal, and blue for background or nonessential lines or for status advisory signals having a neutral quality, all in combination with white and black and observing the requirements for sufficient contrast, size, and illumination. These recommendations also apply to CRTs.

Commonsense Factors in Visual Displays

Certain human factors of critical importance are not so amenable to scientific re-search but must be dealt with using common sense. One such factor is text and abbreviations on labels and warnings. Candidate text should be reviewed by a fair sample of the user-operator community to make sure the text is understandable, unambigous, and not overly complex. Abbreviations should be consistent.

Auditory Signaling and Speech Communication

The first and most important aspect of a sound signal is that it be heard. In Figure 28–8, the standard threshold curve (for no ambient noise) is the 0-dB line. The other curves show equivalent perceived loudness relative to a reference tone at 1000 Hz at various decibel levels. When masking noise (unwanted ambient background sound) is present, however, the desired sound must be at a higher energy level to be heard, depending on its frequency. Typ-

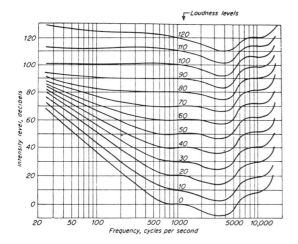

Fig. 28–8. Equivalent perceived loudness relative to a reference tone. (Bioastronautics Data Book, NASA 88-3006, 1964.)

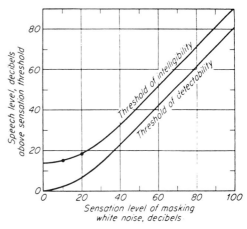

Fig. 28–9. Effect of overall level of white noise on the thresholds of intelligibility and of detectibility of speech. (From Hawkins, J., and Stevens, S.: The masking of pure tones and of speed by white noise. J. Acoust. Soc. Am., 22:6-13, 1964.)

ically, ambient noise is broad-band (energy spread over many frequencies, for example, engine noise, air conditioner noise, or speech). The masking effect on a narrow-band signal is defined as the decibel increase in the signal over the unmasked or no-noise threshold in order to be heard. This increase is roughly proportional to the decibel level of the noise in a "critical band" of frequencies 50 to 100 Hz wide centered on the signal frequency. For noise outside this critical band, the masking effect drops off sharply and becomes negligible as the noise is at a wholly different frequency range than the signal. Military standard 1472 recommends a 20-dB margin for signaling above noise within a one-octave band between 200 and 5000 Hz.

The same general masking rule is operative with speech signal masking by ambient speech or other broad-band noise, where in this case the result is a combined effect of speech or noise components in each critical band. Figure 28–9 shows how speech is masked by white noise. Obviously, the line for detectability (knowing that the speaker is present) is at a lower decibel level than that for intelligibility. The extra bandwidth required for intelligible speech transmission is one of the factors supporting communication of coded data instead of speech.

CONTROLS

Human Control Function Classification

Pilot control tasks are categorized as follows:

Primary flight control
   Attitude
   Speed
   Altitude
   Heading

Autopilot controls
   Flight director
   Turn and climb rate
   Heading/inertial navigation
   Altitude

Engine Controls
Alarm responses
Communications
Operations of stores
Control of other systems
Interpersonal interaction

Primary flight control may be accomplished by pure manual control or by several levels of autopilot use. Autopilot control levels involve increasing equipment sophistication, where each higher level more or less subsumes the previous or lower level.

Controls may be analogic, where their spatial movement or force bears some continuous geometric isomorphism with the control effect. Joysticks, levers, and pedals are examples of analogic controls. Symbolic (normally discrete) controls, on the other hand, are keys or switches whose meaning is understood in terms of a label or coding scheme that is read or learned. An alphanumeric key pad or individual buttons or switches are symbolic controls in this sense.

Analogic and symbolic controls may be combined; for example, the joystick with discrete thumb and finger buttons attached, shown in the lower part of Figure 28–5, is an example of a design problem that has received considerable human factors attention. Finger movements are used to arm and fire weapons, as well as to adjust trim tabs or other control parameters of the aircraft during time-critical periods when the pilot's eyes are busy and reaching forward to a particular location on the control panel would be difficult because of high G forces. To further preclude inadvertent actuation of the joystick during high G maneuvers, a side arm controller may be used, as on the F-16. Such a device senses force rather than displacement. The arm is supported on a shelf, and the wrist is used to provide pitch and roll displacements.

A newer form of analogic control involves the use of the head or the eyes to drive aiming signals, especially when the pilot's hands are occupied or under the stress of high-G turns.[7]

Control may be either direct or supervisory. Supervisory control means the pilot or other human operator supervises a computer while the computer itself is the in-the-loop controller (Fig. 28–2). Once the supervisor has programmed and selected the mode for the computer, unless and until the program runs to its end or some contingency occurs that stops it short, the computer will not need further action by the human supervisor. It may, however, need monitoring by him to check that things are going as expected or to take action if they are not. In the supervisory mode, the human operator performs the following functions:

1. Planning what subgoals the aircraft should achieve over the next time interval in view of given criteria (e.g., nominal schedule) and constraints (e.g., speed, fuel, weather)
2. Programming the computer(s) to control the aircraft or its systems to achieve the subgoal, with suitable contingency plans built into the program
3. Monitoring the (semi) automatic control of the aircraft or other systems by the computer
4. Intervening to stop or modify the program if necessary or to assume direct manual control or do repairs
5. Learning from experience

Control by Cathode Ray Tube Displays and Computer Recognition

It is common to think of CRTs as display devices but less usual to consider them as control devices. When augmented by various types of touch-sensitive overlay devices or cursor drivers, however, they can become virtual control panels (e.g., the display becomes an arrangement of push buttons). When the screen or touch device is pushed with sufficient force at a given button or location, an auditory or visual signal (click or color change) may acknowledge that the computer has received the push information, and the CRT display may then change to provide further feedback or to prepare the operator for the next step in a procedure. This inexpensive and flexible generation of control panels is particularly useful for interactive training programs such as flight control procedures training.

With especially critical actions, it is useful to require a two-step action where the first button press results in an "enabled to do X" state, giving the operator a chance to confirm that X is indeed what he intends. Pressing the second button then initiates the X action.

Computer speech recognition offers many possibilities for the pilot or other crewmember to input signals into the computer, especially when his hands are busy or his body is not likely to be positioned conveniently for a manual response. Computer speech recognition systems depend both on training by a given speaker's voice and on the size of the vocabulary of words or utterances. For a single speaker and limited set of commands, available systems are relatively reliable. Voice changes within a speaker, however (e.g., as he becomes stressed or fatigued), and recognition of connected words can pose difficult problems. Active research and development will lead to more extensive application of this technology in the future.

Criteria for Control

Verification of the accomplishment of the appropriate control requires some feedback. For any discrete response element, the feedback might have one of the following forms:

1. Having the right thoughts about which control to look for
2. Moving the head, eyes, body, and arms in the right direction
3. Grasping the right control
4. Moving the control in the right direction
5. Stopping the control at the right point
6. Achieving the desired response from the aircraft or system

At each stage, it is important to provide feedback cues that are appropriate to correct any error or discrepancy. At the first stage, it might involve a mental model of what the task is or of what procedures and criteria are appropriate, against which the pilot can compare his thoughts. At the second stage, the feedback must be based on familiarity with the aircraft and knowing where to look for needed controls and displays. At the third stage, it involves seeing and feeling the control or reading its associated label. At the fourth stage, feedback is essentially tactile and kinesthetic, and the same is true at the fifth stage, although the final position of a critical control often is visually evident as well, as in the case of flap angle in large aircraft.

Closely associated with the above factors is the criterion of display-control compatibility. Controls should be located adjacent to or below the corresponding display. If there are multiple displays of the same type lined up in left-to-right order, the corresponding controls should be lined up in the same order. Even more important, the direction of movement of the display pointer or indicator should be geometrically the same as the direction of movement of the control that causes that movement.

Earlier, the dilemma of display-control compatibility in aircraft was referred to as the issue of outside-in versus inside-out control display relationships, as illustrated in Figure 28–10, which uses the ex-

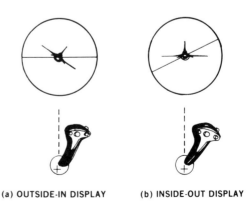

(a) OUTSIDE-IN DISPLAY   (b) INSIDE-OUT DISPLAY

Fig. 28–10. Outside-in and inside-out altitude displays in response to stick deflection.

ample of roll control. Figure 28–10a is the outside-in display, providing the perspective of roll as viewed by an observer fixed relative to the earth. A leftward displacement of the joystick rolls the aircraft symbol counterclockwise with the horizon line fixed. Figure 28–10b shows the inside-out display, providing the perspective of the pilot fixed relative to the aircraft. A leftward displacement of the joystick rolls the horizon line clockwise, with the aircraft symbol fixed. The latter display corresponds to what the pilot sees the actual horizon do and is used commonly in aircraft.

For discrete control-setting, the pilot reaction and movement time varies upward from 0.25 second, depending on several factors:

1. *Accuracy and distance*—the effect on reaction and movement time is given by Fitts' Law, which states that this time increases with the distance the hand must move and with the required accuracy of the movement[8]
2. *Selection from among alternatives*— Hick's Law states that the reaction and movement time is proportional to the logarithm of the number of (equally probable) alternative selections[9]
3. *Anticipation*—this factor can effectively reduce the apparent reaction time to zero as an operator predicts the stimulus
4. *Dynamics*—the mass-elasticity-viscosity characteristics of the control affect movement time. Starting from a resting position, all three characteristics, if present at a significant level, will tend to increase movement time
5. *Display-control compatibility*—controls that are not compatible with displays will take longer to find and use.

Continuous Manual Control

Mathematical models have been developed that are capable of predicting pilot tracking response in aircraft and helicopter flying. The models are functions of the statistical properties of disturbances (wind gusts), the dynamic properties of the controlled process (aircraft), display characteristics, training, and other factors.

The pilot is treated as a control element (servomechanism) in a closed loop, as shown in Figure 28–2A. A large body of experimental literature derived mostly from simulator experiments has shown that when the input-output differential equation of the pilot is lumped together with that of the aircraft, the combined open-loop transfer function from tracking error [e(t)] to aircraft response [y(t)] is quite invariant over task and operator conditions and has the form:

$$y(t) = K\smallint e(t - T_e) \, dt \qquad (1)$$

K is called loop gain and indicates the sensitivity of pilot response to error, and T_e is the effective time delay in operator response due to neural processing, central processing, and muscle response time.[10]

Empirically, parameters K and T_e have been shown to vary systematically but only slightly as a function of both the bandwidth or spectrum of energies in the disturbance signal and the dynamic characteristics of the controlled element, in this case the aircraft and its control system, excluding the pilot. This "crossover model," as it is known in the aircraft industry, says in effect that the pilot tends to shape his own transfer characteristic to compensate for the dynamics of the remainder of the control loop. In doing so, he produces combination open-loop characteristics which approximate that of a simple integrator, with an output rate proportional to the error to be negated. This process, it turns out, is exactly the way a good servomechanism is designed, except for the time delay T_e inherent to the pilot.

To characterize and compare their experimental results and models, manual control researchers tend to use the frequency domain, that is, plots of input-output gain and phase as a function of frequency. The frequency response of the pilot is often characterized in terms of the crossover model, so named because it matches a simple integrator quite well in the region where the forward loop gain line crosses unity. Similar results are obtained with a more general method using a state-space approach to derive the optimal control model of the human operator.[11]

It is common to extract statistically that fraction of the total human response energy which is not determined (perfectly correlated with) the model and call that noise. The noise power can be shown to decrease with training and increase with disturbance and other task difficulty parameters.

Within a disturbance frequency range of up to 1 to 2 Hz and for controlled-element dynamics varying from a pure gain to a double integrator, the human operator can follow reasonably well, and the crossover model fits. When the controlled element increases to third-order (a triple integrator), the human operator can no longer follow; the loop goes unstable. Aircraft are designed with electronic compensation devices to make the net controlled element, from the joystick or control wheel on through to the observed aircraft response, behave well within the stable and easy-to-control range. This includes force-aiding or power steering, making modern aircraft very different from early predecessors that required the pilot to exert considerable stick forces. It is good practice, however, to retain enough force feedback in the control stick to provide tactile feedback cues of the control forces being applied to the aircraft.

The ideal controlled element has dynamics of pure integration, or simply rate control, that permits the operator to merely command a control proportional to observed error and results in an easy task for most tracking.

Figure 28–11 shows that pilot ratings of aircraft handling qualities vary systematically with aircraft dynamics. In assessing the handling qualities of aircraft, test pilots customarily use the Cooper-Harper subjective rating scale, which is described in Figure 28–12. Interestingly, this scale correlates rather well with certain gross parameters of the physical control system, such that ideal systems are neither too sluggish nor too close to instability and are neither overly sensitive nor require excessive control motion.

ANTHROPOMETRY AND GENERAL COCKPIT/WORK PLACE LAYOUT

One aspect of human factors engineering not emphasized thus far in the discussion of displays and controls is whether pilots and operators can see and reach the displays and controls. This criterion must be viewed in terms of the entire population of expected users, a few of whom are bound to be either very large or very small, unless, of course, these individuals are not allowed to operate the equipment. Most operators will be near average. Thus, it is important to use statistics in the specification of cockpit or equipment panels, work places, and seating.

Anthropometric data are available for various military subpopulations, both men and women, and are further specified for flyers and, in some cases, maintenance personnel.[1] Certain key dimensions have been measured for those populations such as overall height, knee height, and reach. From these data, statistical distributions may be estimated and statistical properties, such as means and confidence limits, determined. The 5% and 95% confidence limits are considered reasonable bounds, meaning that it is reasonable not to have to accommodate those who fall outside this range but to accommodate everyone within it. Actually, the range from the 5% confidence limit for females to the 95% confidence limit for males is the operative range if both sexes are being considered

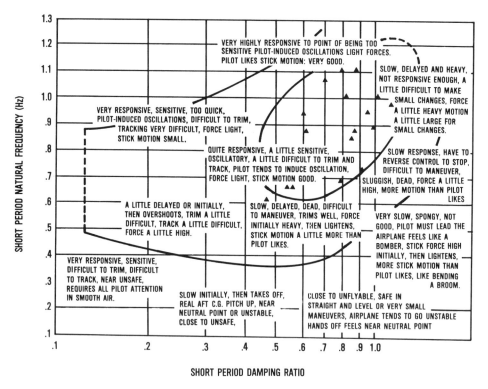

Fig. 28–11. Pilot opinion as a function of vehicle second-order systems dynamics. (Bioastronautics Data Book, NASA 88-3006, 1964.)

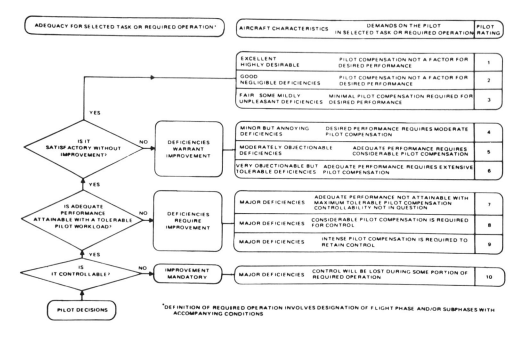

Fig. 28–12. Cooper-Harper Handling qualities rating scale. (Bioastronautics Data Book, NASA 88-3006, 1964.)

and are present in equal numbers. This approach can pose difficulties, however, because if the seat and knee-space arrangements are large enough for the largest man, other dimensions may then be too great for adequate reach for the smallest woman.

One popular fallacy is that the person who falls at 5% on the distribution for one dimension (e.g., overall height) will fall at the same place on the distribution for another dimension (e.g., reach). Although correlation exists between such measures within individuals, it is far from perfect. Thus, by staying between 5% and 95% confidence limits for a number of different dimensions, many more than 10% of the population may be excluded on one or more dimensions.

By making certain assumptions, for example, that a seated operator can conveniently see any display within a 30° cone of vision from a horizontal straight-ahead center line, the range of good vision may then be determined between the 5% confidence limit for females and the 95% confidence limit for males. Figure 28–13 is an example of the kinds of reach and vision anthropometric diagrams available in the literature.

One must be cautious about using some of the available anthropometric data because they were collected in the late 1940s and 1950s. The general population of both males and females has become steadily taller since then, averaging a 2.5 cm increase.

Besides operator body size characteristics, other factors are the forces that can be exerted and the accuracies achieved with controls located in various positions. Large force considerations usually are not critical for pilots and equipment operators in modern aircraft, although they may be for maintenance personnel. Controls should be located where they can be positioned easily and accurately without the inadvertent actuation of other controls.

MENTAL WORK LOAD

During the last decade, interest in mental work load has been increasing.[12] The subject is controversial, not because of disagreement over whether it is important, but because of disagreement over how to define and measure it. Nevertheless, military specifications for mental work load are being prepared, based on the assumption that mental work load measures will predict, either at the design stage or during a flight or other operation, whether the operation can succeed. In other words, it is believed that measurements of mental work load will be more sensitive in anticipating when pilot or operator performance will break down than are conventional measures of performance of the man-machine system.

At the present time, mental work load is a construct similar to intelligence. It must be inferred; it cannot be observed directly like human control response or system performance, although it might be defined operationally in terms of one or several tests. One clear distinction is that between mental and physical work load; the latter is the rate of doing mechanical work and expending calories.

Concern is for situations having long-duration, sustained, mental work load. Many aircraft missions continue to require such efforts by the crew. On the other hand, the introduction of computers and automation in many systems has come to mean that for long periods of time there is nothing to do; the work load may be so low as to result in boredom, complacency, and serious decrement in alertness. Then suddenly the operator may be expected to observe events on a display and make some critical judgments, indeed even to detect an abnormality, diagnose what failed, and take over control from the automatic system. One concern is that the operator, not being in the loop, will not have kept up with the situation and valuable time will be lost as he reacquires the knowledge and orientation needed to make the proper diagnoses or take over control. Of additional concern is that at the beginning of the transient, the computer-based information

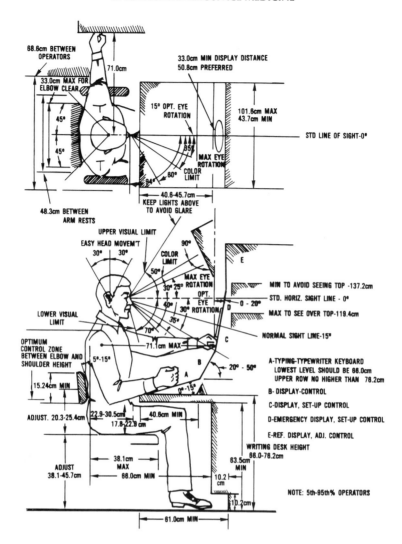

Fig. 28–13. Range of reach and vision for the seated operator. (From Van Cott, H., and Kinkade, R.: Human Engineering Guide to Equipment Design. U.S. Government Printing Office, 1959.)

will be opaque to him and it will take some time even to figure out how to access and retrieve the information he needs from the system.

Four approaches have been used to measure mental work load. One approach, which has been used by the aircraft manufacturers, avoids coping directly with measurements of the operator per se by basing work load on a task time-line analysis: the more tasks the operator has to do per unit of time, the greater the work load. This approach may provide a relative index of work load, other factors being equal, but it does not address the mental work load of any individual relative to his capability, training, or behavior during overload.

The second approach is perhaps the simplest: to use the operator's own subjective judgment rating of his perceived mental work load either during or after the events judged. One form of this approach is a single-category scale similar to the Cooper-Harper scale for rating the handling quality of an aircraft. Perhaps more interesting is a three-attribute scale, there being some consensus that the fraction of total time busy, cognitive complexity, and emotional stress are rather different characteristics of mental work load and that the qualification of one to the others can vary. These scales have been used by the military services and aircraft manufacturers, and the criticism is that people are not always good judges of their own ability to perform in the future. The macho pilot may judge himself to be quite capable of further effort at a higher level when, in fact, he is not.

The third approach is the so-called secondary task or reserve capacity technique. Here, the pilot being tested is asked to allocate whatever attention is left over from the primary task to some unrelated secondary task such as doing arithmetic problems or tracking a dot on a CRT display with a small joystick. Theoretically, the better the performance on the secondary task, the less the time required and, therefore, the less the mental work load associated with the primary task. The criticism of this technique is that it is intrusive; it may itself reduce the attention allocated to the primary task and, therefore, be a self-contaminating measure.

The fourth and final technique is really a whole category of only partially explored possibilities, the use of physiologic measures. Many such measures have been proposed. These include changes in the electroencephalogram (ongoing or steady state), evoked response potential (the best candidate is the attenuation and latency of the so-called P_{300} occurring on average 300 milliseconds after the onset of a challenging stimulus), heart rate variability, galvanic skin response, eye scan pattern, pupillary diameter, integrated muscular activity, and frequency spectrum of the voice. No single physiologic measure, however, has yet been accepted as a valid measure of mental work load.

If mental work load appears to be excessive, several avenues are open for re-ducing or compensating for it. First, one should examine the situation to see if work load causality can be established and if the causal factors can be redesigned to be quicker, easier, or less anxiety-producing. If this approach is not possible, perhaps parts of the task can be reassigned to other individuals who are less loaded or the procedure can be altered so as to stretch out in time the succession of events loading the operator. Finally, one may consider giving all or part of the task to a computer or automatic system.

TASK AND DECISION ANALYSIS

Several types of graphic tools are helpful in analyzing aircrew tasks and decisions for purposes of designing equipment and procedures. Figure 28–14 shows a critical path diagram of tasks that must be done during a nominal mission. The arrows indicate necessary temporal order: A must be done before D, both B and C before E, and all three of D, E, and F before G. Otherwise, these tasks may be done at any time; thus, the precedence of A, B, C, and F is not specified relative to one another. In planning whole missions or detailed procedures for using equipment such as computers, it is important to do this analysis so that design errors will not result from a lack of awareness of priorities.

This approach presupposes that a critical path analysis has been done so that the activities are correctly ordered. The

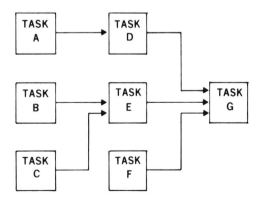

Fig. 28–14. Critical path diagram of tasks.

purpose of this analysis is to establish coordination, fully realizing that in many missions, circumstances will cause one individual to assume an activity normally done by another or force the activities to be done in a somewhat different order. Nevertheless, this has been found to be a useful analysis, especially in a time-critical high-work–load mission.

Figure 28–15 is an event-decision tree. The order of events is from left to right. Following each event, several alternative, mutually exclusive events are usually indicated by lines emanating from the preceding event, with the conditional probability indicated. For example, given that event A occurs, there is a 0.7 probability that event C will then occur and a 0.3 probability that even D will occur. After C, there are three possible events. The sum of probabilities leaving a block must add to 1. In some cases, the succession of events is certain, that is, p = 1. Note that some events may be the result of more than one preceding event. Note also in this case that the sum of probabilities entering a block can be anything; the contingent probabilities need not add to 1. At the right, consequences (dollars, damage)

based on the final column of events are shown. By multiplying through the probabilities for each chain of events that can result in any one consequence and then adding the results for each consequence, one can determine the probability of that consequence occurring. The product of that consequence and its probability is the expected consequence, and the sum of these products is the net expected consequence for the whole situation.

The above discussion takes the viewpoint that the succession of events is determined by nature, that is, it occurs without intervention by a person or machine to manipulate which paths are taken. The other viewpoint may be taken, which assumes that each alternate column is a decision manipulated by a person or machine and the next column is a result (i.e., a decision by nature). In this case, the person or machine is unconstrained in choosing between the alternatives following each result; the probabilities in brackets no longer apply. Now one can work back from the consequences and decide exactly which of the alternative responses maximizes the expected value. Following C, one can choose the greatest of $(.6C_J + .4C_K)$

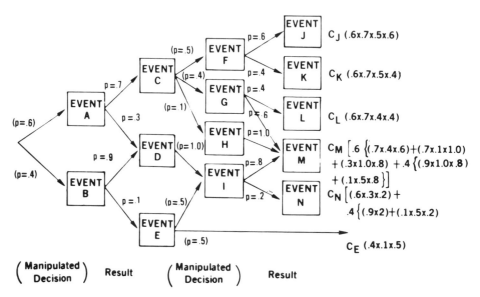

Fig. 28–15. Event-decision tree.

for F, $(.4C_L + .6C_M)$ for G, and C_M for H. This value then becomes the expected consequence of C, assuming one chooses F, G, or H to maximize the expected consequence. Similarly, the expected consequence of D and E can be determined. Finally, a similar analysis can be performed in choosing between alternatives A and B, doing whichever has the greatest expected consequence and expecting that consequence, on the average.

Figure 28–16 shows a fault tree. The purpose of this graph is to show the logical causality of failures. Cause and effect goes from bottom to top, as does time. For example, the AND connecting A, B, and C to J means that all three of the lower failures must occur before the J failure occurs. Either D or E can cause the H failure, but it then takes C and H to cause the K failure. Because there are ORs all the way up the right side, either F or G can make I fail, which is sure to make L fail, which is sure to cause the top event, presumably the failure to which the whole analysis was directed. The same is true for D and E. If probabilities are known for the events along the bottom row and if events are independent, expected failure paths can be traced. The AND means the probabilities must be multiplied for the set of lines com-

ing into the next higher event to determine the probability of that event. In the OR case, the probability of an event is the sum of the two probabilities minus their product. If the convergent events are not independent, some more sophisticated statistical analysis is required. This type of analysis can be applied to a combination of human and machine error, that is, the blocks can represent people or machine failures.

It is common, for example, in the nuclear power industry, to use the fault trees and event trees in combination to do reliability analyses of complex man-machine systems. To do this, failure probabilities must be estimated for both machine and human components. Conservative estimates for machine components are determined from bench-life tests under severe environmental conditions, as well as from operating records. Failure probabilities for the human components are more difficult to obtain. The following considerations enter into such estimates:

1. People tend to make common mode errors. If they learn two responses together or if procedures call for doing them together, if they err on one of the pair, they are likely to err on the other of the pair
2. If there is a well-learned sequence of steps, say A B C, and if a different procedure calls for X B Y, people tend to go off on the wrong track (i.e., do X B C)
3. Both stress and the rate of mental processing demanded increase the tendency to err
4. People tend to persevere and continue to err long after contrary evidence accumulates. On the other hand, people tend to discover their own errors and correct them before serious consequences result

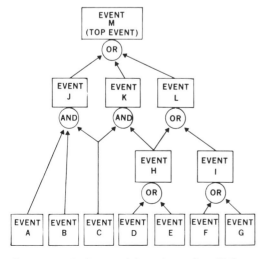

Fig. 28–16. Fault tree with logical causality of failures.

No science of human error is well codified, and these considerations are only a few of the accepted generalities. The best error prevention is good design and good training. Errors may be prevented by not exposing people, that is, not giving them the opportunity to err. This can be done by isolating controls or displays that have particularly critical functions from those with which they might otherwise be confused, by using guards, by recessing push buttons, or by requiring two-step (enable, activate) operation sequences. A final technique is the use of warning labels, but this technique should be used sparingly if at all; more than a few warning labels on a panel can result in clutter and distraction.

The majority of aviation accidents are attributed to operator error. Close examination may reveal that the root cause goes back to a system design in failing to account for human capacity or limitations. The operator errors associated, for example, with misreading a poor altimeter display, mishearing a communication in a high-noise environment, or missing a procedure step during a high-work–load crisis can be reduced by proper attention to human factors considerations. The time to apply human factors is in the design stage rather than as a remedy following aircraft accident investigations.

REFERENCES

1. Parker, J.F., and West, V.R. (eds.): Bioastronautics Data Book. 2nd Ed. Washington, D.C., National Aeronautics and Space Administration, 1973.
2. Van Cott, H.P., and Kinkade, R.G. (eds.): Human Engineering Guide to Equipment Design. Washington, D.C., Government Printing Office, 1972.
3. Military Standard: Human Engineering Design Criteria for Military Systems, Equipment and Facilities. MIL-STD-1472C. U.S. Government Printing Office, Washington, D.C., 1981.
4. Stevens, S.S. (ed.): Handbook of Experimental Psychology. New York, John Wiley and Sons, 1951.
5. McCormick, E.J.: Human Factors Engineering. New York, McGraw-Hill Book Co., 1970.
6. Banks, W.W., Gertman, D.I., and Petersen, R.J.: Human Engineering Design Considerations for Cathode Ray Tube-Generated Displays. Nuclear Regulatory Commission. NUREG/CR-2496. U.S. Government Printing Office, Washington, D.C., 1982.
7. Young, L.R., and Sheena, D.: Eye movement measurement techniques. Am. Psychol., 30(3):315–330, 1975.
8. Fitts, P.M.: The information capacity of the human motor system in controlling the amplitude of movement. J. Exp. Psychol., 47:381–391, 1954.
9. Hick, W.E.: On the rate of gain of information. Q. J. Exp. Psychol., 4:11–26, 1952.
10. McRuer, D., Graham, D., Krendel, E., and Reisener, W.: Human Pilot Dynamics in Compensatory Systems: Theory Models and Experiments with Controlled Element and Forcing Function Variations. AFFDL-TR-65-15. Wright-Patterson Air Force Base, Ohio, 1965.
11. Kleinman, D.L., Baron, S., and Levison, W.: A Control Theoretic Approach to Manual Vehicle Systems Analysis. Institute of Electrical and Electronics Engineers, Transactions, New York, 1971, pp. 824–832.
12. Moray, N.: Mental Workload. New York, Plenum Press, 1979.

Chapter *29*

Biomedical Challenges of Spaceflight

Arnauld E. Nicogossian

Life is short; the art long; opportunity fleeting: Judgment difficult, experience fallacious

HIPPOCRATES

In the past two decades, significant progress has been made in characterizing the biomedical effects of weightlessness on living organisms. Most of this information was derived from actual spaceflight and ground-based simulation studies. These research efforts were justified, considering the novel nature of the space environment and the requirements generated by the technologic achievements necessary to explore the universe beyond the confines of Earth. Until 1971, when the Soviet Union launched the first manned space station (Salyut 1), opportunities for in-flight experimentation were quite limited due to spacecraft size and operational constraints. Thus, prior to 1970, most biomedical studies were conducted before and after flight to determine the net changes undergone during flight and the rate and time-course of the readaptation process to a 1-g environment. With the advent of Skylab (1973 to 1974) and with subsequent Soviet Salyut missions of up to 6 months' duration (1977 to 1982), the time-course of acclimatization to the weightless environment itself could be repeatedly studied through carefully designed in-flight biomedical experiments.

These studies, although mostly observational in nature and often designed to evaluate biomedical changes observed in previous missions, nevertheless have contributed to our general understanding of the gross physiologic changes associated mostly with single exposures to spaceflights of varied duration. As the number of missions increased, with more biomedical data being accrued, as individuals flew repeated missions, and as space endurance records were extended further, a clustering of events began to occur that has allowed scientists to approximate physiologic trends and formulate newer hypotheses.

Despite significant limitations, such as operational constraints, concomitant use of countermeasures, and large intersubject variabilities in a highly select population, the data obtained so far point to the fact that humans do adapt to and can function usefully in the space environment if adequate medical support is provided. Much remains to be learned, however, concerning the true nature of the changes observed to date and the best procedures for providing medical support. It may be instructive to examine these aspects of spaceflight and the support of space missions, beginning with a review of the current knowledge regarding the effects of the spaceflight environment on several key physiologic systems.

PHYSIOLOGIC EFFECTS OF SPACEFLIGHT

Neurovestibular Reactions

One of the primary functions of the neurovestibular system is to provide information about gravity. Previous space missions have shown that when the pull of gravity is neutralized, significant alterations occur in the components of this sensory system and in vestibular interactions with other sensory systems, resulting in numerous side effects. Clinically, the most important vestibular disturbance associated with spaceflight is space motion sickness. Immediately on entry into the weightless environment, most individuals experience the sensation of bodily inversion. This illusion soon passes but may recur with rapid movement or when moving from a small area to a larger space within the space vehicle. More susceptible individuals, however, develop symptoms of space motion sickness. Affecting some 40% of all space travelers, it occurs early in the mission, typically within the first 3 days, and usually lasts for 2 to 4 days. Symptoms range from minimal discomfort (stomach awareness) to nausea and vomiting, in rare cases accompanied by pallor and sweating. Head and body movements tend to worsen the discomfort. When the symptoms are severe, crew performance can be affected and mission efficiency severely compromised. During the Apollo IX mission, for example, certain crew activities were delayed by 24 hours due to space motion sickness. Some work time

was lost in the first 3 days of the Skylab 3 flight for the same reason.

The classic model for the onset of space motion sickness is found in a description provided by the Soviet Cosmonaut Titov.[1] For a brief period after transition into orbit, Titov felt that he was flying upside down. This was followed by dizziness associated with head movements. Some time between the fourth and seventh orbits, or 6 or more hours into the flight, he became nauseated and ill. This was the first recorded instance of space motion sickness.

The medical basis for space motion sickness is not well understood, partly because the phenomenon can be studied effectively only during spaceflight. Dietlein and Johnston[2] noted that direct pressure measurements in animal models and human studies using z-axis recumbent rotation largely discounted the etiologic role of cephalad fluid shifts as a basis for space motion sickness. They concluded that the most plausible explanation was the "sensory conflict" hypothesis, according to which the usual afferent visual and somatosensory inputs to the vestibular receptors and/or the central nervous system were no longer "appropriate" in the weightless environment of space, resulting in aberrant reflexes and/or effector responses. During the adaptation period of several days, new sensory thresholds are established that allow the afferent sensory inputs to once again be correctly interpreted.

In the general population, a number of variables appear to be related to an individual's susceptibility to motion sickness. For example, children below 2 years of age are usually immune to motion sickness; susceptibility increases during childhood and reaches its highest level between the ages of 2 and 12 years. Thereafter, susceptibility declines with age.[3] Reason and Brand[4] found that women report a significantly greater incidence of motion sickness, suggesting that gender may play some role in susceptibility. Personality variables that are positively correlated with increased susceptibility to motion sickness include introversion, neuroticism, and fear, especially fear of flying. Barrett and Thornton[5] reported a relatively strong relationship between measures of discomfort in a car simulator and scores on a test designed to measure a perceptual style called "field of independence." Presumably, subjects who score higher on tests of field independence rely more on vestibular and proprioceptive cues for head and body orientation rather than on external visual cues; they may, therefore, be more susceptible to the conflicting sensory cues associated with motion sickness.

A variety of tests and questionnaires have been devised in an attempt to predict motion sickness susceptibility. Some of these methods measure aspects of vestibular function, and others provide actual exposure to provocative motion stimulation. Although vestibular function tests, particularly the ones that involve actual exposure to Coriolis stimulation, predict susceptibility in 1 g motional environments, they have not successfully predicted space motion sickness susceptibility. Of the potential reasons for the failure of these tests to predict motion sickness susceptibility in space is the variables in individual susceptibility to different motional environments in 1 g.

One approach to reducing susceptibility to space motion sickness has been to subject astronauts to a variety of vestibular loads just prior to flight in an attempt to shorten the required in-flight adaptation period. Astronauts have reported that this "vestibular conditioning" is at least partially effective in reducing the severity and duration of space motion sickness. But time constraints in the immediate preflight period limit the amount of emphasis that can be placed on such conditioning activities.

At present, the accepted method for preventing or treating the symptoms of space motion sickness is the use of medications, usually scopolamine-dextroamphetamine sulfate (Dexedrine) or promethazine-ephedrine combinations. Such drugs, however, have strong central nervous system activity. Thus, it has been suggested that future research should emphasize an in-depth examination of the various psychopharmaceutical agents affecting central neurotransmitter systems. Although such drugs might be of considerable benefit, little progress has been made in their development. Additional approaches, such as the use of biofeedback, mechanical devices to restrain head and neck movements, and adaptation-training techniques, remain under laboratory investigation.

Cardiovascular Deconditioning

To date, all space travelers have evidenced cardiovascular deconditioning upon returning to earth. The cardiovascular system exhibits a decreased ability to function effectively against gravitational stress following exposure to weightlessness. Symptoms of orthostatic intolerance have ranged from an elevated heart rate and inappropriate blood pressure responses to a tendency toward spontaneous syncope during orthostatic stress. Inflight, reduced orthostatic tolerance has been demonstrated by means of the lower-body negative pressure (LBNP) stress test. This condition is primarily attributed to the contraction of effective circulating blood volume resulting from the loss of body fluids and electrolytes during the early period of adaptation to weightlessness.[6]

The deconditioning of the cardiovascular system occurs early in weightlessness but tends to stabilize after about the fifth week of flight. Response to orthostatic stress in flight was measured for the first time during the Skylab program. Figure 29–1 shows the mean heart rates for a Skylab crewmember before, during, and following the 56-day mission. Note that there

SKYLAB 3 - SPT

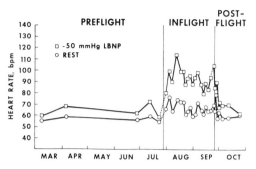

Fig. 29–1. Mean heart rate of Skylab 3 pilot under 50 mm Hg of negative pressure during the lower-body negative-pressure stress test.

is both an increase and variation in heart rate under the −50 mm Hg stress of the LBNP test immediately upon entry into weightlessness. There appears to be a gradual stabilizing of heart rate to a new level of functional efficiency. In even longer Soviet spaceflights (3 to 6 months), a slight increase in heart rate has been noted, particularly toward the end of the mission.[7] Nevertheless, cardiovascular deconditioning appears to be a self-limiting phenomenon that does not continue to worsen with increased flight duration. It represents an adjustment of the cardiovascular system to a new environment in which the load placed on the heart is considerably less than it is on earth.

Cardiovascular deconditioning becomes a medical problem only after a space traveler is subjected to acceleration forces encountered during reentry or upon return to the constant 1 g stress on earth. Depending on the duration of the spaceflight and the amount of exercise performed in flight, the return of cardiovascular function to preflight values might take as long as 1 month. As spaceflight becomes available to a wider population, the problem of adjusting to reentry forces might be of greater consequence. This would be true in the case of a scientist who might be older and not in the same peak physical condition as astronauts tradition-

ally have been in. In such a case, it would be necessary to conduct a careful assessment of the individual's cardiovascular fitness prior to returning to earth and the use of appropriate countermeasures. Cardiovascular deconditioning might present a potentially more serious problem in the space shuttle era because the magnitude of accelerative reentry forces is quite different from that of the earlier missions. For example, the first orbital flight of the space shuttle presented a maximum G reentry profile during descent of approximately 1.6 G (Fig. 29–2).

There are at least two methods for dealing with the problem of cardiovascular deconditioning. The first is through use of antigravity suits. When inflated, an anti-G suit provides a restrictive pressure over the lower half of the body, thus preventing the blood from pooling in the lower extremities during the period of reentry stress. A second approach is through the use of rehydration prior to returning to earth. Dietlein and Johnston[3] referred to simulation studies that have shown that, following 7 and 28 days of bed rest, 1 L of ingested saline solution (156 mEq of sodium) coupled with LBNP (−30 mm Hg pressure for 4 hours) will prevent or greatly lessen the symptoms of cardiovascular deconditioning. The benefits of this relatively simple procedure continue for some 18 to 20 hours and, if used just prior to the end of a mission, should offer protection against the reentry forces. Recent Soviet flights have demonstrated that intensive in-flight physical exercise and an optimal work-rest cycle can have additional prophylactic effects against deconditioning, particularly in long-term missions.[7]

Although all observations to date are optimistic with respect to the ability of the cardiovascular system to acclimate to the space environment, several questions remain unanswered. In particular, it is important to further delineate the effects and time course of the early and substantial in-

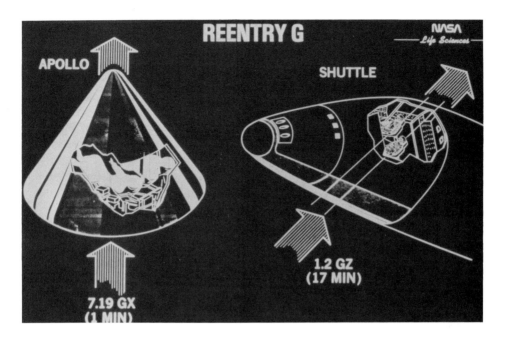

Fig. 29–2. Comparison of Apollo and space shuttle reentry profiles (courtesy of the National Aeronautics and Space Administration).

flight cephalad fluid shifts (up to 1.5 L from lower extremities to the upper part of the body) and the resulting reduction in total blood volume on central venous pressure, stroke volume, and cardiac output. Complete information can only be gained by critical, long-term observations in space.

Motor System Disturbances

Among the most dramatic effects of spaceflight are changes in the musculature of the body and disturbances of the motor regulation system. The former changes are ordinarily indicated in flight by a progressive decrease in total body mass, leg volume, and muscular strength. Substantial muscle atrophy also is suspected to occur, particularly in antigravity muscles, which is usually considered to be responsible for the postflight motor system changes that are observed. Disturbances in postural and motor coordination, loco-

motor function, and equlibrium and also alterations in proprioceptor activity and spinal reflex mechanisms occur. Although all of these changes appear to be dependent, at least to some extent, on flight duration, they nevertheless have been reversible, and no sequelae have been reported so far.

Body Mass

In-flight weight losses of 3 to 4% were seen in association with early, short-duration spaceflights. With the advent of longer missions, it became apparent that most of the weight loss took place during the first 3 to 5 flight days, with a much more gradual decline thereafter. This finding suggested that most of the initial change in body mass was due to the loss of fluids either through diuresis or decreased thirst and fluid intake and that subsequent losses were due to metabolic imbalances and/or muscle atrophy. The changes appear to be self-limiting, with the largest weight losses recorded (6 to 7 kg) being independent of mission duration.

In long-duration space missions, where adequate caloric intake and physical exercise was maintained by some of the crewmembers, actual weight gains have been reported. Such weight gains probably reflect an overall increase in adipose tissue, which was more than sufficient to offset losses of muscle tissue. In any event, body mass lost in flight is rapidly regained in the postflight period.

Muscle Atrophy

Weightlessness and the loss of accustomed gravitational loads produces a number of structural and functional changes in skeletal muscles. These changes are most pronounced in the postural, or antigravity, muscles such as the gastrocnemius and the muscles of the back and neck. There is a gradual atrophy of these muscles along with a decrease in muscle tone. The process is progressive and can be controlled only with a high caloric intake and intensive exercise, especially strength exercises.

Evidence for the deterioration of muscle during spaceflight comes from several sources. In-flight measurements of leg volume show a rapid initial decrease attributable to the headward fluid shift, followed by a gradual recovery. Postflight biostereometric measurements of Skylab astronauts have demonstrated more general losses of volume from the abdomen downward, although losses in the abdomen and buttocks are attributed to the loss of fat.[8] Postflight urinary analyses reveal in-flight increases in the excretion of a number of metabolites associated with muscle breakdown such as nitrogen, potassium, creatinine, and amino acids. Metabolic balance studies, and electromyographic analyses of muscular activity further substantiate the deteriorative effects of zero gravity on muscle function.

Bone and Mineral Changes

It has long been known that removal of muscle forces and weight from bones, as occurs in bed rest or the casting of limbs, causes a loss of mineral, which is known as disuse osteoporosis. Residence in the weightless environment of space, which represents a form of musculoskeletal disuse, also has been found to cause a loss of bone mineral. Early studies of bone mineral changes using x-ray densitometry suggested that large amounts of bone may be lost during relatively brief periods of spaceflight. The 12 crewmembers who participated in Gemini 4, 5, and 7 and Apollo 7 and 8 missions averaged postflight losses of bone density from the os calcis of 3.2% as compared with preflight baseline values. Some losses also were observed from the radius and ulna after these early flights.

For later Apollo missions and Skylab, a more accurate method of photon absorptiometry was developed to assess pre- and postflight bone mineral mass changes. Data from the 84-day Skylab mission showed moderate losses of calcium from the os calcis. In contrast to the earlier flights, increased bone mineral losses were not evident in the radius. These losses are believed to be comparable to those seen in subjects after bed rest. There is no evidence that the in-flight bone losses are self-limiting, and it is the current assumption that calcium losses occur progressively throughout the flight.

The precise mechanisms underlying the loss of bone mineral during spaceflight are still not known. Studies of animals with immobilized limbs indicate that disuse produces a number of time-dependent changes in bone formation and resorption. It may be that a proportionately larger increase in resorption over formation is responsible for the loss of bone mineral mass, at least in immobilized subjects. Whether the skeletal losses in space are due to relatively larger increases in bone resorption over formation is also still conjectural, but autopsies of three Soviet cosmonauts who died after a 21-day Soyuz spaceflight revealed a number of unusually wide osteocytic lacunae, which may have been due to increased bone resorption. Also not known are the underlying physiologic processes, whether hormonal, neural, electrical, or mechanical, that initiate these changes.

In evaluating the loss of bone mineral during spaceflight, investigators have drawn on bed-rest studies as a model. Recently, however, it has been shown that bed rest results are at variance with the composite calcium balance data for all Skylab missions. In bed rest, urinary calcium excretion peaks at about 5 weeks and then gradually decreases almost to its initial level. Fecal calcium excretion increases over a period of 10 to 12 weeks and plateaus at a level of about 120 mg/day. This is far less than the level of 300 mg/day reached on the eighty-fourth day of the Skylab 4 flight. The flight data show a monthly calcium loss for the average skylab crewman of about 8 g, or about 25 g for the 84-day flight. This would mean a total calcium loss in 1 year of over 300 g, or approximately 25% of the total body supply. such a loss is much higher than the 6% per year rate estimated from bed-rest research. The difference appears to lie in the fact that the loss of fecal calcium does not plateau during spaceflight. Dietlein and Johnston[2] speculated that these results might be attributed to a deficiency in 1,25 dihydroxycholecalciferol, a key regulator of calcium absorption in the gastrointestinal tract.

Loss of bone mineral, if allowed to proceed unchecked, could represent a limiting variable for long-duration space missions. At least two countermeasures, however, are considered to be potentially beneficial. The first countermeasure is exercise. Thornton[9] stated that although passive forces may modify the rate of calcium loss, the large forces produced by the activity of large muscle masses appear necessary to prevent or reverse the loss of bone mineral. He considered that 1 to 1.5 hr/day of walking or jogging under a 1 g force applied by elastic straps should be adequate to prevent disuse osteoporosis.

A pharmacologic countermeasure also has been considered. Ground-based studies have shown that drugs such as diphosphonate can control the loss of calcium in subjects undergoing bed rest over a period of many weeks. This approach has not been tried during a space mission but may offer a useful means of reducing bone demineralization during the weightless environment of an extended spaceflight. Other potential measures, such as rotation of spacecrafts to produce artificial gravity, might become a necessity if calcium loss cannot be controlled by any other means. Preliminary data from Soviet missions of 6 months' duration have shown, however, that the mineral loss from weight-bearing bones remains constant and does not exceed 7%. Although these data are encouraging, in view of current hypotheses they do not shed any further light on calcium losses, especially losses from other portions of the skeleton such as vertebral bodies.

Changes in Blood, Fluid, and Electrolytes

The cephalad shift of fluids in weightlessness, with the resulting contraction of circulating blood volume, is responsible for many of the physiologic changes that occur during adaptation to space flight conditions. As has been discussed, it directly affects the functioning of the cardiovascular system. It also has a number of effects on the composition of body fluids, especially blood. The most significant hematologic changes involve a reduction in plasma volume, alterations in red blood cell (RBC) mass, and changes in the distribution of RBC shapes.

Hemotologic Changes

From the time of the early Gemini and Vostok missions, a postflight decrease in total RBC mass has been observed in nearly all United States and Soviet astronauts. There is a gradual decrease, with losses averaging about 9% of the total RBC pool over the first 30 to 60 days in flight and values ranging from 2 to 21%.

The magnitude of the RBC loss does not appear to be related to mission length, except possibly in missions of 30 days or less. Measurements of hemoglobin concentration taken in Skylab astronauts suggested that although RBC mass had declined to the same extent on longer flights as on shorter ones, it had begun to recover before a return to earth in the longer flights. The delay in RBC mass recovery is apparently independent of spaceflight factors because RBC mass in the crew of Skylab 2 did not begin to recover until several weeks after the crew returned; however, recovery followed roughly the same timecourse as in longer missions. A corresponding pattern is seen in the reticulocyte count, which declines initially (26 to 50%) and begins to recover after 30 to 60 days in space.

Accompanying the changes in mass are changes in the shapes of red blood cells. Normally, discocytes predominate by a wide margin. During spaceflight, the proportion of discocytes decreases sharply, whereas the number of echinocytes, spherocytes, and other atypically shaped cells rises. So far, these alterations in erythrocyte shape do not affect crew health or function in flight and are rapidly reversed post flight.

There is still some uncertainty as to the primary mechanism responsible for the reduction in RBC mass. Toward the end of the Apollo program, it was believed that the observed RBC loss was due to mild oxygen toxicity produced by the hyperbaric 100% oxygen atmospheres in use in Gemini and some Apollo spacecraft. Results of missions using different atmospheres, however, did not bear out this hypothesis. A later proposal focused on the increased destruction and removal of cells, but experiments conducted on the Apollo-Soyuz flight demonstrated that this was not the case.

The weight of evidence now suggests that the loss of RBC mass is due, instead, to a suppression of RBC production by the bone marrow. The relatively rapid 4 to 16% decline in plasma volume in flight masks a drop in RBC mass by allowing the ratio of cells to plasma to remain roughly normal. Later, as the level of serum phosphorus rises, the red blood cells increase their release of oxygen. The oxygen-sensitive kidney then counters the increased release of oxygen by further decreasing RBC production. Eventually, additional biochemical changes probably initiate a resumption of normal RBC production. In lengthy missions, this also may be related to the aging of existing cells as their 120-day life span is reached.

Electrolyte Alterations

The weightlessness-induced fluid shift produces at least a transient increase in central blood volume. From ground-based bed-rest studies, it has been suggested that the stretch receptors in the left atrium interpret this as an increase in total circulation blood volume, triggering a compensatory loss of water, sodium, and potassium from the renal tubules. This is the first event in a series of fluid and electrolyte shifts that occur during the adaptation to weightlessness.

So far, the early diuresis has been observed only in bed-rest studies. It has been difficult to demonstrate during spaceflight because of the problems involved in accurately documenting urine volumes early in flight and because water intake is usually reduced during the early stages of flight. Nevertheless, data obtained from Skylab indicate that the nine crewmen decreased their water intake by approximately 700 ml/day during the first 6 days in flight. Their urine volume decreased an average of only 400 ml/day during the same period, indicating a net loss of water.

Additional supporting observations include the observed in-flight increases in the urinary output of sodium, potassium, and chloride, an in-flight decrease in antidiuretic hormone, and a reduced postflight excretion of sodium.[10]

Countermeasures that may prove useful against the effects of spaceflight on fluid and electrolytes include water and electrolyte replenishment and increased exercise. Such measures may partly alleviate the problem of contracted plasma volume and diminish the observed incidence of cardiac arrhythmias in flight, which may be partly due to aberrations in electrolyte balance. Increased exercise appears to have multiple benefits as a countermeasure. Perhaps most importantly, it may diminish the loss of electrolytes and metabolites associated with changes in muscle and bone and in mineral metabolism.

Additional changes observed in conjunction with short- and long-duration space missions are summarized in Table 29–1.

SPACECRAFT ONBOARD LIFE SUPPORT

Most of the physiologic shifts discussed in the preceding sections are either direct or indirect consequences of weightlessness. The space environment, however, includes conditions that are, in themselves, far more hazardous and inhospitable for humans than weightlessness. Prominent among these are temperature extremes and the lack of an atmosphere and atmospheric pressure. Space vehicles provide these environmental conditions at levels that are not only survivable but comfortable. In addition, they provide systems for regenerating air and water, handling wastes, generating necessary power, and even preparing cooked food.

Recent Soviet missions aboard space stations have included experiments directed at the eventual development of a closed ecologic life-support system. Such a system would permit the continuous recycling of organic matter aboard the station, generating food for the crew in the process. It would probably be a prerequisite for very long-term space missions in which resupply was not possible such as manned planetary explorations. For short-term missions in near-earth orbit, the current state of onboard life support is entirely adequate. It is instructive to examine the progressive development of spacecraft environmental control systems that has culminated in the nearly earth-normal environment of a vehicle such as the space shuttle.

Requirements

Pressure Control

For all practical purposes, and particularly in the context of spacecraft, acceptable environmental pressures are determined primarily by the required partial pressures of the component gases and by the necessity for change in pressure in the course of a mission. The important criteria are breathability and the avoidance of physiologic injury from decompression. Too great a rate of decompression can cause the explosive decompression syndrome. Slower rates of decompression may produce decompression sickness if the pressure of dissolved gases in the tissues, particularly nitrogen, exceeds the ambient pressure.

Gas Concentrations

The most important gaseous component of an atmosphere is oxygen. At sea level, the partial pressure of oxygen (Po_2) is 158 mm Hg. Because of the pressure of carbon dioxide and water vapor, the Po_2 at the alveoli of the lung averages 100 mm Hg. Without acclimation, human performance begins to show the debilitating effects of hypoxia at an alveolar Po_2 of about 85 mm Hg. Hyperoxia results when the Po_2 is too high, but a 5-psi (260 mm Hg) 100% oxygen atmosphere has been employed on spacecraft with no adverse effects.

The second gaseous component of con-

Table 29–1.   Physiologic Changes Associated with Short-Term and Long-Term Spaceflight

Physiologic Parameter	Short-Term Spaceflights (1–14 days)*	Long-Term Spaceflights (more than 2 weeks)†	
		Preflight vs In-flight	Preflight vs Post-flight
Cardiopulmonary system			
Heart rate (resting)	Increased post flight; peaks during launch and reentry, normal or decreased during mission; RPB:‡ up to 2 days	Normal or slightly increased	Increased; RPB: 4–5 days
Blood pressure (resting)	Normal or decreased post flight	Diastolic blood pressure reduced	No change
Orthostatic tolerance	Decreased after flights longer than 5 hours. Exaggerated cardiovascular responses to tilt test, stand test, and LBNP post flight; RPB: 3–14 days	Highly exaggerated cardiovascular responses to in-flight LBNP (especially during first 2 weeks), sometimes resulting in presyncope. Last in-flight test comparable to R + 0 (recovery day) test	Exaggerated cardiovascular responses to LBNP; RPB: up to 3 weeks
Cardiac size	Normal or slightly decreased post flight cardiac/thoracic ratio		Decreased post flight cardiac/thoracic ratio
Stroke volume and cardiac output	Decreased post flight; gradual recovery after 5 days post flight	Variable, usually increased during first month (impedance measurements)	Decreased post flight. Gradual recovery 5–21 days, depending on the level of exercise in flight
Electrocardiogram/vectorcardiogram	Moderate rightward shift in QRS and T post flight	Increased PR interval, QT interval, and QRS vector magnitude	Slight increase in QRS duration and magnitude; increase in PR interval duration
Systolic time intervals			Increase in resting and LBNP-stressed PEP/ET ratio/ RPB: 2 weeks
Echocardiography			Decreased stroke volume and left end-diastolic volume. Ventricular function plots indicate no post flight myocardial dysfunction
Arrhythmias	Usually premature atrial and ventricular beats (PABs, PVBs). Isolated cases of nodal tachycardia, ectopic beats, and supraventricular bigeminy in flight	PBVs and occasional PABs; sinus or nodal arrhythmia at release of LBNP in flight	
Exercise capacity	No change or decreased post flight; increased heart rate for same oxygen consumption; no change in efficiency; RPB: 3–8 days	High exercise capacity in flight	Decreased post flight; recovery time inversely related to amount of in-flight exercise rather than mission duration
Lung volume		Vital capacity decreased 10%	No change
Leg volume	Decreased up to 3% post flight. In flight, leg volume decreases exponentially during first 24 hours and plateaus within 3 to 5 days	Same as short missions	Same as short missions
Leg blood flow		Marked increase	Normal or slightly increased
Venous compliance in legs		Increased; continues to increase for 10 days or more; slow decrease later in flight	Normal or slightly decreased
Body fluids			
Total body water	Decreased post flight		Decreased post flight
Plasma volume	Decreased post flight (except Gemini 7 and 8)		Markedly decreased post flight; RPB: 2 weeks
Hematocrit	Normal or slightly decreased post flight		Normal R + 0; decreased R + 2 (hydration effect)

Table 29–1. *Continued*

Physiologic Parameter	Short-Term Spaceflights (1–14 days)*	Long-Term Spaceflights (more than 2 weeks)†	
		Preflight vs In-flight	Preflight vs Post-flight
Hemoglobin	Normal or slightly increased post flight	Increased first in-flight sample; slowly declines later in flight	Decreased post flight; RPB: 1–2 months
Red blood cell (RBC) mass	Decreased post flight; RPB: at least 2 weeks	Decreased ~15% during first 2–3 weeks in flight; begins to recover after about 60 days; recovery of RBC mass is independent of the presence or absence of gravity	Decreased post flight; RPB: 2 weeks to 2 months following landing
Red blood cell half-life (^{51}Cr)	No change		No change
Iron turnover			No change
Mean corpuscular volume (MCV)	Increased post flight; RPB: at least 2 weeks		Variable, but within normal limits
Mean corpuscular hemoglobin (MCH)	Increased post flight; RPB: 2 weeks		Variable, but within normal limits
Mean corpuscular hemoglobin concentration (MCHC)	Increased post flight; RPB: at least 2 weeks		Variable, but within normal limits
Reticulocytes	Decreased post flight; RPB: 1 week		Decreased post flight. In Skylab, RPB: 2–3 weeks for 28-day mission, 1 week for 59-day mission, and 1 day for 84-day mission
White blood cells	Increased post flight, especially neutrophils; lymphocytes decreased; RPB: 1–2 days		Increased, especially neutrophils; post flight reduction in number of T-cells and reduced T-cell function as measured by PHA§ responsiveness; RPB: 3–7 days; transient postflight elevation in B-cells; RPB: 3 days
Red blood cell morphology	No significant changes observed post flight	Increase in percentage of echinocytes; decrease in discocytes	Rapid reversal of in-flight changes in distribution of red blood cell shapes; significantly increased potassium influx; RPB: 3 days
Plasma proteins	Occasional postflight elevations in α_2-globulin due to increases of haptoglobin, ceruloplasmin, and α_2-macroglobulin; elevated IgA and C_3 factor		
Red blood cell enzymes	No consistent postflight changes	Decrease in phosphofructokinase; no evidence of lipid peroxidation and red blood cell damage	No consistent postflight changes
Serum/plasma electrolytes	Decreased potassium and magnesium post flight	Decreased sodium, chloride, and osmolality; slight increase in potassium and phosphate	Postflight decreases in sodium, potassium chloride, and magnesium; increase in phosphate and osmolality
Serum/plasma hormones	Postflight increases in human growth hormone, thyroxine, insulin, angiotensin I, sometimes aldosterone	Increases in cortisol; decreases in adrenocorticotropic hormone and insulin	Postflight increases in angiotensin aldosterone thyroxine, thyroid-stimulating hormone, and growth hormone; decrease in adrenocorticotropic hormone
Serum/plasma metabolites and enzymes	Postflight increases in blood urea nitrogen, creatinine, and glucose; decreases in lactic acid dehydrogenase, creatinine phosphokinase, albumin, triglycerides, cholesterol, and uric acid		Postflight decrease in cholesterol and uric acid

Table 29–1. *Continued*

Physiologic Parameter	Short-Term Spaceflights (1–14 days)*	Long-Term Spaceflights (more than 2 weeks)† Preflight vs In-flight	Preflight vs Post-flight
Urine volume	Decreased post flight	Decreased early in flight	Normal or slightly increased
Urine electrolytes	Postflight increases in calcium, creatinine, phosphate, and osmolality; decreases in sodium, potassium, chloride, and magnesium	Increased osmolality, sodium, potassium, chloride, magnesium, calcium, and phosphate; decrease in uric acid excretion	Increase in calcium excretion; initial postflight decreases in sodium, potassium, chloride, magnesium, phosphate, and uric acid; sodium and chloride excretion increased in second and third week post flight
Urinary hormones	In-flight decreases in 17-hydroxycorticosteroids increase in aldosterone; postflight increases in cortisol, aldosterone, antidiuretic hormone, and pregnanediol; decreases in epinephrine, 17-hydroxycorticosteroids, androsterone, and etiocholanolone	In-flight increases in cortisol, aldosterone, and total 17-ketosteroids; decrease in antidiuretic hormone	Increase in cortisol, aldosterone, norepinephrine; decrease in total 17-hydroxycorticosteroids and antidiuretic hormone
Urinary amino acids	Postflight increases in taurine and β-alanine; decreases in glycine, alanine, and tyrosine	Increased in flight	Increased post flight
Sensory systems			
Audition	No change in auditory thresholds post flight		No change in auditory thresholds post flight
Gustation and olfaction	Subjective and varied human experience. No impairments noted	Same as shorter missions	Same as shorter missions
Somatosensory	Subjective and varied human experience. No impairments noted	Subjective experiences (e.g., tingling of feet)	
Vision	Transitory postflight decrease in intraocular tension; postflight decreases in visual field; constriction of blood vessels in retina observed post flight; dark-adapted crews reported light flashes with eyes open or closed; possible postflight changes in color vision. Decrease in visual motor task performance and contrast discrimination	Light flashes reported by dark-adapted subject; frequency related to latitude (highest in South Atlantic anomaly, lowest over poles)	No significant changes except for transient decreases in intraocular pressures
Vestibular System	Forty to fifty percent of astronauts/cosmonauts exhibit in-flight neurovestibular effects, including immediate reflex motor responses (postural illusions, sensations of tumbling or rotation, nystagmus, dizziness, vertigo) and space motion sickness (pallor, cold sweating, nausea, vomiting). Motion sickness symptoms appear early in flight and subside or disappear in 2–7 days. Postflight difficulties in postural equilibrium with eyes closed or other vestibular disturbances	In-flight vestibular disturbances are same as for shorter missions; markedly decreased susceptibility to provocative motion stimuli (cross-coupled angular acceleration) after 2–7 days adaptation period. Cosmonauts have reported occasional reappearance of illusions during long-duration missions	Immunity to provocative motion continues for several days post flight. Marked postflight disturbances in postural equilibrium with eyes closed. Some cosmonauts exhibited additional vestibular disturbances postflight, including dizziness, nausea, and vomiting

Table 29–1. *Continued*

Physiologic Parameter	Short-Term Spaceflights (1–14 days)*	Long-Term Spaceflights (more than 2 weeks)†	
		Preflight vs In-flight	Preflight vs Post-flight
Musculoskeletal system and anthropometry			
Height	Slight increase during first week in flight (~1.3 cm); RPB: 1 day	Increased during first 2 weeks in flight (maximum 3–6 cm); stabilizes thereafter	Height returns to normal on R + 0
Mass	Postflight weight losses average about 3.4%; about two thirds of the loss is due to water loss; the remainder is due to loss of lean body mass and fat	In-flight weight losses average 3–4% during first 5 days; thereafter, weight gradually declines for the remainder of the mission. Early in-flight losses are probably mainly due to loss of fluids; later losses are metabolic	Rapid weight gain during first 5 days post flight, mainly due to replenishment of fluids. Slower weight gain from R + 5" to R + 2 or 3 weeks. Amount of postflight weight loss is inversely related to in-flight caloric intake
Body composition		Large losses of water, protein, and fat during first month in flight. Fat is probably regained. Muscle mass, depending on exercise regimens, is partially preserved	
Total body volume	Decreased post flight		Decreased post flight. Center of mass has shifted toward head
Limb volume	Inflight leg volume decreases exponentially during first mission day; thereafter, rate of decrease declines until reaching a plateau within 3–5 days. Postflight decrements in leg volume up to 3%; rapid increase immediately post flight, followed by slower RPB	Early in-flight period same as short missions. Leg volume may continue to decrease slightly throughout mission. Arm volume decreases slightly	Rapid increase in leg volume immediately post flight, followed by slower RPB
Muscle strength	Decreased in flight and post flight; RPB: 1–2 weeks		Postflight decrease in leg muscle strength, particularly extensors. Increased use of in-flight exercise appears to reduce postflight strength losses, regardless of mission duration. Arm strength is normal or slightly decreased post flight
Electromyographic analysis	Postflight electromyograms from gastrocnemius suggest increased susceptibility to fatigue and reduced muscular efficiency. Electromyograms, from arm muscles show no change		Postflight electromyograms from gastrocnemius showed shift to higher frequencies, suggesting deterioration of muscle tissue; electromyograms indicated increased susceptibility to fatigue; RPB: about 4 days
Reflexes (Achilles tendon)	Reflex duration decreased post flight		Reflex duration decreased post flight (by 30% or more); reflex magnitude increased; compensatory increase in reflex duration about 2 weeks post flight; RPB: about 1 month
Nitrogen and phosphorus balance		Negative balances early in flight; less negative or slightly positive balances later in flight	Rapid return to markedly positive balances post flight

Table 29–1. *Continued*

Physiologic Parameter	Short-Term Spaceflights (1–14 days)*	Long-Term Spaceflights (more than 2 weeks)†	
		Preflight vs In-flight	Preflight vs Post-flight
Bone density	Os calcis density decreased post flight; radius and ulna show variable changes, depending on method used to measure density		Os calcis density decreased post flight; amount of loss is correlated with mission duration; little or no loss from non-weight–bearing bones; RPB is gradual; recovery time is about the same as mission duration
Calcium balance	Increasing negative calcium balance in flight	Excretion of calcium in urine increases during first month in flight, then plateaus; fecal calcium excretion declines until day 10, then increases continually throughout the flight. Calcium balance is positive before flight, becoming increasingly more negative throughout the flight	Urine calcium content drops below preflight baselines by day 10; fecal calcium content declines but does not reach preflight baseline by day 20. Markedly negative calcium balance post flight, becoming much less negative by day 10. Calcium balance still slightly negative on day 20; RPB: at least several weeks

*Compiled from biomedical data collected during the following space programs: Mercury, Gemini, Apollo, Apollo-Soyuz Test Project, Vostok, Voskhod, and Soyuz.
†Compiled from biomedical data collected during Skylab and Salyut missions.
‡RPB: return to preflight baseline.
§Phytohemagglutination.
‖Recovery day plus postflight days.

cern is carbon dioxide. Normally present on earth at a concentration of 0.04%, carbon dioxide becomes a serious problem at about 20 mm Hg, when hypercapnia can develop. Air regeneration systems include the means for removing carbon dioxide.

Water vapor, or humidity, is a third atmospheric component of physiologic consequence. Low humidity causes drying of mucous membranes, eyes, and skin. Inactivation of protective cilia in the respiratory tract leads to an increased risk of infection. Extremes of humidity also affect heat exchange. To avoid these problems, a water vapor pressure between 6 and 14 mm Hg is desirable.

Temperature Control

As a homeothermic organism, man is able to survive in a range of thermal extremes from subfreezing to tropical—particularly if he is clothed. But in the spacecraft environment, comfort is the primary objective. Thermal discomfort initiates thermoregulatory control responses and subjective sensations that detract from

performance. A practical approach is to provide thermostatic control around an optimum point (usually 22°C) and to permit the modification of individual heat balance through clothing selection or air motion control.

Evolution of Control Systems

Mercury Spacecraft

The Mercury spacecraft had a 5-psi oxygen atmosphere supplied from a store of pressurized oxygen. Carbon dioxide was controlled by a lithium hydroxide absorber in the environmental control loop. Temperature control was accomplished through cooling provided by a sublimator heat exchanger. The sublimator vented water vapor overboard, and cooling resulted from the change of state. The crew stayed in their pressure suits and the onboard environmental control system (ECS) supplied both the pressure suit and the cabin.

Gemini Spacecraft

The Gemini spacecraft retained the 5-psi oxygen atmosphere used in Mercury; however, the primary source of oxygen was now a liquid oxygen tank, with secondary oxygen supplies stored as high-pressure oxygen. Carbon dioxide again was controlled by the use of a lithium hydroxide absorber. The primary means of heat rejection in the Gemini vehicle was a spacecraft radiator that radiated the heat to space. Heat loss was controlled by the flow of coolant to the radiator and the ECS heat exchangers. In the later Gemini flights, extensive periods were spent outside the pressure suit.

Apollo Spacecraft

The Apollo spacecraft atmosphere control systems were similar to the Gemini systems but were improved and more elaborate. The overall ECS included two subsystems: a command module ECS and the lunar landing module ECS. A third module, the service module, carried consumables to support the command module ECS. The atmosphere was 5-psi oxygen, supplied from a cryogenic oxygen supply in the service module. Lithium hydroxide was used to absorb carbon dioxide. Cabin temperature was maintained at 24°C ± 2.8°, with relative humidity limited to the range of 40 to 70%. The primary system for heat rejection was again a space radiator. An evaporator was installed to provide additional cooling, but it was not used after Apollo 11 except for launch, earth orbit, and reentry.

Skylab

The Skylab atmosphere control system incorporated some significant changes. Cabin pressure was 5 psi, but to avoid the minor chronic effects of hyperoxia over a long mission and the possible interference of such effects with medical experiments, a two-gas environment was used. The atmospheric composition was 70% oxygen and 30% nitrogen to provide a P_{O_2} just slightly higher than earth-normal. The two gases could be controlled automatically, but in practice much of the control was accomplished manually to provide constant oxygen pressure during certain medical experiments. Carbon dioxide absorption was accomplished with a regenerable molecular sieve system. A characteristic of this system was that it operated at a nominal carbon dioxide level of about 5 mm Hg, so that although it met the same 7.6 mm Hg carbon dioxide limit as earlier lithium hydroxide systems, the average carbon dioxide level was higher than on earlier spacecraft. The earlier systems had kept carbon dioxide near 1 mm Hg most of the time. The thermal control system for Skylab was primarily a passive one. The vehicle was carefully painted with paints of varying emissivity in specific patterns so that very little active control with radiators or evaporators was necessary.

Space Shuttle

The space shuttle is the first American spacecraft to use a 760 mm Hg (14.6-psi) atmospheric pressure. Gas composition is 80% nitrogen and 20% oxygen, as on earth. Carbon dioxide absorption is accomplished with disposable lithium hydroxide cartridges, as in pre-Skylab flights, and thermal control is accomplished using radiators on the insides of the cargo bay doors.

The space shuttle ECS provides for temperature control within a range of 18°C to 27°C. Under conditions in which a comfortable heat balance is maintained, variations in humidity do not have a strong effect on comfort. When this heat balance can be maintained only at the upper limit of a comfort band or outside a comfort band, however, the humidity becomes very significant. To preserve a strong and effective thermoregulation response to overheating, particularly during the short, transient changes that may be encountered during exercise, an upper value of 0.27 psi P_{H_2O} is a component of the space shuttle orbiter specification.

BIOMEDICAL SUPPORT OF SPACE MISSIONS

Medical Selection Standards

Astronaut Selection

Because of all the unknowns associated with spaceflight when the space program began, early astronaut candidates were subjected to some of the most rigorous selection standards ever employed. To begin with, all candidates were drawn from a highly select pool that consisted of military pilots and test pilots. The selection process involved a detailed review of the individual's biographical and career data, a large array of physical and physiologic tests and examinations, and an extensive physiologic evaluation.

Tables 29–2, 29–3, and 29–4 describe the status and a number of physiologic parameters for astronauts who have been selected during the course of the space program.

The physical and physiologic qualifying criteria remained essentially unchanged from the Mercury program through the Apollo Program. The range and stringency of these standards have been modified for space shuttle astronauts and the screening of civilian scientists and technicians as nonpilot payload specialists in the space lab program. The mental health standards for the selection of pilots, likewise, have undergone an evolution from the early days of spaceflight.

During the Mercury program, psychologic testing and evaluation took 30 hours and resulted in a specific ranking of candidates according to a number of parameters of mental status. After the initial experiences in space demonstrated that the psychologic stresses of speceflight were not extreme, the selection criteria for Gemini and Apollo missions shifted away from a research-oriented approach to proficiency and reliability and toward a determination of adaptability to known spaceflight factors.

After the Apollo program, mental health screenings became even more subjective and were based primarily on unstructured interviews with a psychiatrist. At the present time, no psychologic testing is done; only interviews are employed. The only requirement is that a candidate be free of psychosis, neurosis, and personality disorders. The objective of the screening is no longer to select the best candidate from a psychologic point of view but simply to assure that each candidate is fully qualified to fly space missions.

Table 29–2. Description and Status of United States Astronaut Selections

Selection Year	Selection Group	Number of people selected	Age			Current Status			
			Mean	Standard Deviation	Range	Deceased	Resigned (Never Flown)	Active	Inactive (Flown)
1959	1	7	35.2	2.2	32–37	1	0	1	5
1962	2	9	32.3	1.4	31–34	2	0	1	6
1963	3	14	31.0	2.1	27–33	4	0	1	9
1965	4	6	30.3	3.2	28–34	0	2	3	1
1966	5	19	32.3	2.8	28–36	1	1	7	10
1967	6	11	31.4	5.7	24–40	0	4	7	0
1969	7	7	29.1	3.5	25–35	0	0	7	0
1977	8	35*	32.3	3.3	26–38	0	0	35	0
1980	9	19†	33.5	2.8	28–38	0	0	19	0
Total		127				8	7	81	31

*Six females.
†Two females.

Table 29–3. Selection Results for Astronauts Selected Before 1970

Selection Group	Selection Year	Weight		Systolic Blood Pressure		Diastolic Blood Pressure		Cholesterol		Triglycerides		Glucose		Oxygen (Max)	
		Mean	Standard Deviation	Mean	Standard Deviation	Mean	Standard Deviation	Mean	Standard Deviation	Mean	Standard Deviation	Mean	Standard Deviation	Mean	Standard Deviation
1	1959	166	13	121	8.3	77	1.1	194	26.8	—	—	103	4.6	35.0	3.2
2	1962	162	13	122	11.8	75	8.4	177	33.8	—	—	93	7.1	NA*	
3	1963	161	13	127	12.9	79	11.8	174	16.7	116	36.3	102	9.3	42.2	5.9
4	1965	158	13	123	15.3	77	11.6	151	42.5	117	24.7	84	14.0	46.3	5.5
5	1966	166	15	124	13.4	76	7.6	197	45.7	99	18.5	109	12.3	43.8	4.6
6	1967	164	23	128	10.5	76	9.0	194	72.0	73	28.7	99	8.9	44.4	5.4
7	1969	162	15	127	10.0	68	7.7	194	44.4	93	36.2	112	7.9	43.7	2.7

*Not available.

Table 29–4. Selection Results of Male and Female Crews Selected for Space Shuttle Programs

Selection Group	Selection Year	Sex	Weight		Systolic Blood Pressure		Diastolic Blood Pressure		Cholesterol		Triglycerides		Glucose		Oxygen (Max)	
			Mean	Standard Deviation	Mean	Standard Deviation	Mean	Standard Deviation	Mean	Standard Deviation	Mean	Standard Deviation	Mean	Standard Deviation	Mean	Standard Deviation
8	1977	Males	164	20	122	10.3	78	7.3	192	43.8	82	37.9	95	8.9	46.4	7.7
9	1980	Males	160	14	118	8.8	79	5.1	167	30.6	74	21.0	94	4.5	49.4	5.8
8	1977	Females	131	22	107	11.3	76	3.8	191	47.2	67	24.3	86	6.9	35.0	5.9
9	1980	Females	113	13	118	0.0	75	9.9	150	36.8	54	.7	86	1.4	40.8	2.6

Preflight Health Stabilization

The possibility of crew illness during a space mission—particularly if it involved an infectious disease—was a serious concern from the beginning of the manned space program. A preflight illness could cost the loss of valuable training time and possibly entail the postponement of a mission. In flight, the transient occurrence of space motion sickness was already troublesome; the appearance of infectious diseases could seriously jeopardize crew safety and mission success. For this reason, efforts were made to minimize the risk of such illnesses.

Early Mission Experience

Project Mercury flights were brief, and the risk of developing disease in flight was judged to be low. Even so, efforts were made to restrict the nonessential contact of crewmembers with others during the preflight period. Although some symptoms of upper respiratory tract infection and influenza were manifested post flight, no in-flight illness occurred during Project Mercury.

During the Gemini program, the increase in mission duration also meant an increase in the risk of infectious disease in flight. Medical personnel were able to implement a partial quarantine of crewmembers, screening the personnel with whom the crew came in contact. In particular, access to the crewmembers was closely controlled during the prelaunch period. Again, there were no in-flight illnesses, although there were a number of preflight cases of upper respiratory tract infections and influenza, along with one case of streptococcal pharyngitis and exposure to mumps.

The Apollo Program was not so fortunate. During the first mission, Apollo 7, all three crewmembers were ill with an upper respiratory tract infection throughout most of the flight. After this experience, a medical plan was developed to minimize preflight exposure to infectious diseases in future missions. Conflict with the already-established training schedule reduced the effectiveness of the program, however. During the Apollo 8 preflight period, all crewmembers contracted viral gastroenteritis. Although treatment seemed to be successful, the Commander experienced a recurrence of the disease 18 hours into the flight. In the Apollo 9 preflight period, all three crewmembers came down with the common cold. For the first time, a manned launch was postponed (3 days) for medical reasons.

During this time, stricter health stabilization measures came into use. Crews were restricted to their quarters at the launch site, access to them was controlled, and personnel with whom they came in contact were carefully screened. Nevertheless, a member of the Apollo 13 primary crew was exposed to rubella before flight, necessitating replacement of the command module pilot by a backup crewman. This episode finally led to the development of a detailed and strictly enforced program for minimizing the exposure of flight crews to infectious diseases before launch.

Flight Crew Health Stabilization Program (FCHSP)

First implemented for the Apollo 14 mission, this comprehensive program involved a 3-week preflight isolation of crewmembers and a careful epidemiologic surveillance of hundreds of primary and secondary contacts during the 3 months prior to launch. The program provided for the rapid diagnosis and prompt treatment of any disease event in the crewmembers or their families. An immunization program was carried out, and strict procedures for preventing the exposure of crewmembers to potential disease-carrying persons were enforced.

The success of the FCHSP is evident in that throughout the remainder of the Apollo Program (Apollo 14 to 17), during the three missions of the Skylab program, during the Apollo-Soyuz Test Project, and in the flights of the space shuttle, no infectious diseases have occurred in crewmembers in flight or after flight while the FCHSP has been in effect.

In-Flight Monitoring of Physiologic Status

The spaceflight environment produces a number of changes in the human body, many of which are of considerable physiologic significance. The first, brief manned flights simply confirmed the nature of some of the more dramatic and immediate of these changes such as cephalad shift of body fluids and the vestibular effects. Subsequent biomedical studies have confronted the arduous task of identifying all the physiologic effects of spaceflight. The objective of this research has been to answer the following questions:

1. How long can man stay in space before incurring significant difficulties in performance or long-term health?
2. What are the basic mechanisms of the physiologic changes that occur?
3. What are the most effective preventive countermeasures?

In-flight monitoring of physiologic status provides essential data to support these efforts. It also allows ground control to monitor crew status in real time for purposes of decision making and for ensuring crew safety. As technology has improved, as mission length has increased, and especially as the size and comfort of space cabins has been increased, instrumentation has been added to provide a wider range of functions monitored under a greater variety of conditions. In addition, in-flight biomedical experiments conducted by the crew have added a new dimension to biomedical knowledge derived from spaceflight. Table 29–5 summarizes the illness events observed among United States space crews.

Preflight and Postflight Evaluation

Prior to Skylab, the only source of objective data regarding most of the physiologic changes that occurred in spaceflight was the comparison of measurements taken before launch and after the return to Earth. Although the in-flight medical experiments on Skylab provided a major addition to knowledge in this area, preflight and postflight observations continued to be of great importance.

Mercury flights served primarily to identify some of the changes that occurred in weightlessness. Studies conducted during the Gemini program identified other effects and began to evaluate the extent of these flight-related changes.

Attention was focused to a greater extent on the cardiovascular system. Preflight and postflight studies, however, remained qualitative and were primarily intended to detect gross functional alterations.

Studies were made of blood volume and red blood cell mass, response to lower-body negative pressure, exercise capacity, biochemical changes, bone x-ray densitometry, and microbiologic counts. The results were sufficiently positive to provide reassurance that the long missions of the Apollo series were feasible.

By the time of the Apollo program, the pattern of preflight and postflight examinations was well established and remains essentially the same. Comprehensive examinations are conducted at 30, 15, and 5 days before flight. They include full examinations of internal history and vital signs, ear, nose, and throat, eyes and visual function, skin, lymph nodes, and teeth. In addition, a number of special studies are carried out in the areas of microbiology, hematology and immunology, biochemical analysis of fluids, and cardiopulmonary function. These latter studies in particular form the baseline for comparison with postflight results of the same tests, which are conducted immediately after return to earth and daily thereafter.

Table 29–5. Illness Occurrence in Space Crews*

Illness	Number Involved	Phase	Illness	Number Involved	Phase
Bends	2	In flight	Laceration	1	Preflight
Upper Respiratory Disease	8	Preflight	Serous Otitis	1	In flight
Viral Gastrointestinal Infection	3	Preflight	Eyes and Finger Injury	1	In flight
Eye-skin irritation (Fiberglass)	3	In flight	Sty	1	In flight
Skin infection	2	In flight	Boil	1	In flight
Trauma	1	Landing	Back strain	1	Post flight
Urinary Tract Infection	1	In flight	Rash	1	In flight
Contact dermatitis	2	In flight	Fatigue work-rest cycles	3	In flight
Arrhythmia	2	In flight	Toxic Pneumonia	3	Reentry
Arrhythmia	2	Post flight			

*Does not include isolated premature ventricular beats (PVB) or premature atrial beats (PAB) or motion sickness.

Table 29–6. Ten-Year Trends for Astronauts Selected Before 1970 (N = 57)

Year	Weight Mean	Weight Standard Deviation	Systolic Blood Pressure Mean	Systolic Blood Pressure Standard Deviation	Diastolic Blood Pressure Mean	Diastolic Blood Pressure Standard Deviation	Cholesterol Mean	Cholesterol Standard Deviation	Triglycerides Mean	Triglycerides Standard Deviation	Glucose Mean	Glucose Standard Deviation	Oxygen (max) Mean	Oxygen (max) Standard Deviation
1969	166	16	120	7.4	75	6.5	184	40.6	102	36.3	94	8.3	ND*	
1970	167	16	121	10.2	75	6.7	187	29.7	110	35.5	95	8.2	ND	
1971	168	15	119	9.5	73	7.8	204	36.7	98	32.0	99	6.9	ND	
1972	168	16	116	7.8	74	7.0	202	38.2	103	52.6	99	6.8	ND	
1973	166	16	117	8.6	75	7.9	208	32.5	95	40.8	95	7.1	ND	
1974	167	15	116	9.4	75	7.5	217	32.5	107	47.0	96	8.6	ND	
1975	164	23	119	9.2	71	7.7	220	34.6	103	45.5	97	7.6	ND	
1976	163	25	116	8.7	74	7.5	199	38.9	97	38.4	95	8.5	ND	
1977	168	16	119	10.4	77	9.7	219	40.2	109	51.0	96	7.3	ND	
1978	169	17	117	9.5	77	7.9	224	45.4	108	45.2	96	7.8	43	7.9
1979	165	24	119	9.4	72	7.5	211	39.3	108	46.9	91	7.4	43	7.9

*ND = Not done. N for 1978 = 12; N for 1979 = 29.

Table 29–6 summarizes the major points of the longitudinal health indices obtained from a cohort of 57 individuals after results over a 10-year period. No significant deviations in these data have been noted over this period.

Longitudinal Surveillance

Thus far, the physiologic changes seen to occur in spaceflight have not been debilitating and have been rapidly reversible upon return to earth. Primarily, they consist of a degree of cardiovascular deconditioning and some musculoskeletal deterioration. In flight, space motion sickness is the only remaining medical problem in short-duration missions. But from a strictly epidemiologic point of view, these results are not highly significant. For one thing, the population of space travelers represents a small sample of only a little over 100 individuals. In addition, selection standards and preflight, in-flight, and postflight medical procedures have not been consistent over the data collection period.

Two developments now afford the opportunity to bring space biomedical research into accord with standard public health practices and to give its conclusions the validity of more structured and formalized studies. One factor is the development of formal medical standards by NASA; the other factor is the advent of the space shuttle program, which is expected to expose relatively large numbers of people to spaceflight conditions (400 individuals by 1990). Indeed, a highly efficient system of biomedical record-keeping will be required as part of the biomedical system needed to support the high launch and landing rate and rapid turnaround time of the Space Transportation System (STS).

A major strength of such longitudinal studies would be their specificity for the establishment of a direct or relative measure of risk associated with long-term or repeated exposures to weightlessness.

Space medicine is still in its evolutionary phase; as the number of flights and the length of stay in space increases and as a greater number of individuals are exposed to weightlessness, new problems, both medical and physiologic, will be identified. These problems might require unique solutions, and the practice of space medicine will mature when it is practiced in orbit.

REFERENCES

1. Graybiel, A., Miller, E.F., II, and Homick, J.L.: Equipment M131. Human vestibular function. In Biomedical Results From Skylab. NASA SP-377. Edited by R.S. Johnston and L.F. Dietlein. Washington, D.C., Government Printing Office, 1977.
2. Dietlein, L.F., and Johnston, R.S.: U.S. manned space flight: the first twenty years. A biomedical status report. Acta Astronautica, 8(9–10): 893–906, 1981.
3. Money, K.E.: Motion sickness. Physiol. Rev., 50:1–39, 1970.
4. Reason, J.T., and Brand, J.J.: Motion Sickness. New York, Academic Press, 1975.
5. Barrett, S.V., and Thornton, C.L.: Relationship between perceptual style and simulator sickness. J. Appl. Psychol., 52:304–308, 1968.
6. Nicogossian, A., and Parker, J.: Space Physiology and Medicine. NASA SP-447. Washington, D.C., Government Printing Office, 1983.
7. Gazenko, O.G., Genin, A.M., and Yegorov, A.D.: Summary of medical investigations in the U.S.S.R. Manned space missions. Acta Astronautica, 8(9–10):907–917, 1981.
8. Whittle, M.W., Herron, R., and Cuzzi, J.: Biostereometric analysis of body form. In Biomedical Results From Skylab. NASA SP-377. Edited by R.S. Johnston and L. F. Dietlein. Washington, D.C., Government Printing Office, 1977.
9. Thornton, W.: Rationale for exercise in spaceflight. In Conference Proceedings: Spaceflight Deconditioning and Physical Fitness. Edited by J.F. Parker, Jr., C.S. Lewis, and D.G. Christensen. Prepared under National Aeronautics and Space Administration Contract NASW-3469 by Bio-Technology, Inc., Falls Church, Virginia, U.S. Government Printing Office, Washington, D.C., 1981.
10. Leach, C.S.: An overview of the endocrine and metabolic changes in manned space flight. Acta Astronautica, 8:977–986, 1981.

Chapter *30*

Aircraft Accidents, Survival, and Rescue

Roy L. DeHart and Kenneth N. Beers

One of the greatest maladies of our time is the way sophistication seems to be valued above common sense.

NORMAN COUSINS

Aircraft accidents have been recorded from the earliest days of man's quest for flight. Disregarding the legend of the death of Icarus and the early chronicles of the ill-fated attempts at man-powered flight, the first documented deaths due to flying, as opposed to those due to a failure to remain airborne, were those of Pilatre de Rozier and Romaine near Bologne, France on June 15, 1785. Few of the early aeronauts died from natural causes.

With the advent of heavier-than-air powered flight in 1903, the potential for aviation accidents increased considerably. Because of the inability of the aircraft to remain airborne following power failure, its mode of flying and crashing was inherently less forgiving than either balloons or airships. On September 17, 1908, the first fatal aircraft accident occurred when Lieutenant Selfridge was killed while flying with Orville Wright.

Few records were kept concerning the medical aspects of the early aircraft accidents. Large-scale aviation developments during World War I brought an emergence

of medical concern for the disturbing and often unnecessary injury and loss of life resulting from aircraft accidents. From this interest in the possibilities of protection against crash forces came the development of safety belts, crash helmets, and research on the effects of crash forces on the human body. World War II, with its enormous impetus to aeronautic advances, also stimulated advances in aviation medicine, much of which was oriented toward safety, as well as the prevention and reduction of the effects of accidents. This work resulted in vast improvements in accident rates and the reduction of resultant injuries.

After the war, partly due to new propulsion systems and the demonstration of the possibility of large-scale air transportation, aviation continued its rapid development. Since 1945, flying has become progressively safer. The improvements that have been achieved in the efficiency and safety of aircraft, however, have not excluded the possibilities of crew abandonment of the aircraft in flight or an emergency landing on land or sea and of the survivors having to withstand the rigors of a hostile environment until rescued.

This chapter focuses on the survivability of aircraft incidents and accidents. By definition, to survive is to outlive or to continue to live in spite of adverse circumstances. Traditionally, the period of survival began when it became necessary for the passengers and/or crew to evacuate the aircraft while aloft, on the sea, or on the ground and ended with the successful recovery or unfortunate demise of the survivors.

AIRCRAFT ACCIDENTS

An aircraft accident is defined by the National Transportation Safety Board (NTSB) as "an occurrence associated with the operation of an aircraft which takes place between the time any person boards the aircraft with the intention of flight until such time as all such persons have disembarked, in which any person suffers death or serious injury as a result of being in or upon the aircraft or by direct contact with the aircraft or anything attached thereto, or the aircraft receives substantial damage."[1]

Aircraft accident data can be expressed in several ways. The most frequent expression, although not always the best for comparison purposes, is based on flying hours. The data are expressed as a ratio of accidents per 100,000 flying hours. This method, however, may not allow a reasonable comparison of the risk between commercial flying and general aviation or of military flying in transports with flying fighters. The concern is that flying hours may not reflect an accurate assessment of risk because the most hazardous phases of flight are landings and takeoffs. General aviation and fighter aircraft will have many more takeoffs and landings for a given number of flight hours as compared with airliners or transports.

Flying hours are difficult to compare with other forms of commercial transport; thus, passenger-miles become a factor. The number of takeoffs also may be used. The practitioner should know the type of comparison being used to fully understand the resultant accident data.

Air Carrier Accident Data

United States air carrier accident statistics include (1) certified route air carriers; (2) supplemental or charter air carriers; and (3) commercial operators of large aircraft (included beginning in 1975).

In the period from 1972 to 1982, the number of total accidents occurring on United States certified route air carrier, scheduled domestic passenger services ranged from a high of 37 in 1972 to a low of 8 in 1980. The fatal accidents were reduced from six to one, although the total miles flown increased. Expressed as a passenger fatality rate per 100 million passenger-miles, the worst rate was in 1972 at 0.129 and improved to 0.005 for 1980.[2] For a better perspective of these domestic data, refer to Table 30–1, and for worldwide experience, refer to Figure 30–1.

The data in the accompanying tables make evident the need to understand the associated risk to air travel dependent upon the form such travel takes. The accident rates for commuter air carriers are greater than those for the airlines during the same period (Tables 30–2 and 30–3). The highest accident and fatality rates in commercial aviation are found with the on-demand air taxi services (Table 30–4).

The most significant issue apparent in reviewing conventional aviation accident and fatality data is the continuing downward trend of those rates since the inauguration of passenger airline services. Table 30–5 provides comparative data on passenger fatality rates for the different forms of transportation for the decade ending with 1980.

General Aviation Accident Data

General aviation has maintained the least satisfactory accident record. This cat-

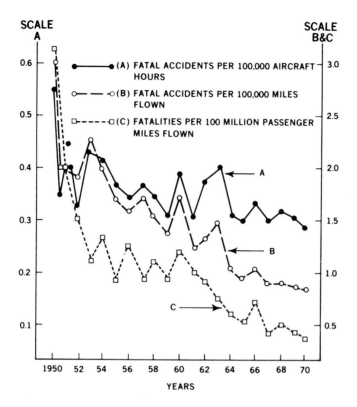

Fig. 30–1. Worldwide air-carrier accident rates for the period 1950–1970.

Table 30–1. Aircraft Accidents, Fatalities and Fatality Rate—United States Certified Route Air Carrier Scheduled Domestic Passenger Service: 1972 to 1980

Year	Aircraft Accidents Total	Aircraft Accidents Fatal	Fatalities Total	Fatalities Passenger	Fatalities Crew/Others	Passengers Carried (Thousands)	Passenger-Miles Flown (Million)	Passenger Fatality Rate Per 100 Million Passenger-Miles
1972	37	6	185	160	25	169,931	123,776	0.129
1973	27	4	138	128	10	183,271	133,733	0.096
1974	31	3	168	158	10	189,724	137,658	0.115
1975	21	2	122	113	9	188,744	140,300	0.081
1976	17	1	1	1	—	206,274	154,323	0.001
1977	15	2	75	64	11	222,284	166,425	0.038
1978	18	4	16	13	3	253,957	218,549	0.006
1979	14	4	279	262	17	292,537	208,856	0.125
1980	8	1	13	11	2	278,600	221,200	0.005

From the Department of Transportation: Federal Aviation Administration Statistical Handbook of Aviation. Washington, D.C., Government Printing Office, 1982.

egory of aviation included commuter and air taxi operations until 1981; however, with the increase in this type of passenger service resulting from airline deregulation, the data have been transferred to the commercial category. These data on general aviation reflect that adjustment (Table 30–6). In the 10-year period from 1972 to 1981, the general trend for both the number of accidents and fatalities has been downward.

For general aviation, the most hazardous phase of flight operations remains landings (40% of accidents). Takeoffs rep-

Table 30–2. Accidents, Fatalities, and Accident Rates for United States Air Carriers—1977 to 1981 (All Scheduled Service)*

	1977	1978	1979	1980	1981
Accidents					
Total	21	21	24	15	24
Fatal	3	5	4	0	4
Fatalities	78	160	351	0	4
Aircraft hours flown (thousands)	5801	6032	6700	6900	6560
Aircraft miles flown (thousands)	2419	2520	2736	2890	2695
Departures	4,934,094	5,015,939	5,379,852	5,479,000	5,235,000
Accident rate per 100,000 hours flown					
Total	0.36	0.35	0.36	0.22	0.37
Fatal	0.05	0.08	0.06	0.00	0.06
Accident rate per million miles flown					
Total	0.01	0.01	0.01	0.01	0.01
Fatal	0.001	0.002	0.001	0.00	0.001
Accident rate per 100,000 departures					
Total	0.43	0.42	0.45	0.27	0.46
Fatal	0.06	0.10	0.07	0.00	0.08

*Operating under 14 CRF 121.
From the Department of Transportation: Federal Aviation Administration Statistical Handbook of Aviation. Washington, D.C., Government Printing Office, 1982.

Table 30–3. Aircraft Accidents, Fatalities, and Accident Rates for United States Commuter Air Carriers—1977 to 1981 (All Scheduled Service)*

	1977	1978	1979	1980	1981
Accidents					
Total	42	55	51	37	28
Fatal	9	13	14	7	9
Fatalities	33	47	65	36	35
Aircraft hours flown (thousands)	1144	1288	1262	1263	1083
Aircraft miles flown (thousands)	194,166	224,228	214,330	202,100	178,500
Departures	1,728,948	1,978,483	2,005,800	1,895,400	1,708,800
Accident rate per 100,000 hours flown					
Total	3.67	4.27	4.04	2.93	2.59
Fatal	0.79	1.01	1.11	0.55	0.83
Accident rate per million miles flown					
Total	0.22	0.25	0.24	0.18	0.16
Fatal	0.05	0.06	0.07	0.03	0.05
Accident rate per 100,000 departures					
Total	2.43	2.78	2.54	1.95	1.64
Fatal	0.52	0.66	0.70	0.37	0.53

*Operating under 14 CFR 135.
From the Department of Transportation: Federal Aviation Administration Statistical Handbook of Aviation. Washington, D.C., Government Printing Office, 1982.

Table 30–4. Accidents, Fatalities, and Accident Rates For United States On-Demand Air Taxis—1977 to 1981 (Nonscheduled Operations)*

Year	Number of Accidents		Fatalities	Aircraft Hours Flown (thousands)	Accident Rate Per 100,00 Aircraft Hours Flown	
	Total	Fatal			Total	Fatal
1977	175	35	122	3064	5.71	1.14
1978	216	57	160	3135	6.89	1.82
1979	173	36	84	3374	5.13	1.07
1980	164	42	88	3535	4.64	1.19
1981	138	34	95	3690	3.74	0.92

*Operating under 14 CFR 135.
From the Department of Transportation: Federal Aviation Administration Statistical Handbook of Aviation. Washington, D.C., Government Printing Office, 1982.

Table 30–5. Comparative Accident Data For Road, Rail, and Airline Travel—1971 to 1980

Year	Passenger Fatalities Per 100 Million Passenger-Miles			
	Automobiles and Taxis	Buses	Passenger Trains	Domestic Scheduled Aircraft
1971	1.90	0.19	0.24	0.15
1972	1.90	0.19	0.53	0.13
1973	1.70	0.24	0.07	0.10
1974	1.50	0.21	0.07	0.12
1975	1.40	0.15	0.08	0.08
1976	1.34	0.17	0.05	0.003
1977	1.33	0.13	0.04	0.04
1978	1.30	0.17	0.13	0.01
1979	1.31	0.15	0.05	0.12
1980	1.32	0.15	0.04	0.01

From the National Safety Council: Accident Facts. U.S. Government Printing Office, Washington, D.C., 1981.

Table 30–6. Aircraft Accidents, Fatalities, and Accident Rates For United States General Aviation Flying—1972 to 1981[2]

Year	Accidents*		Fatalities	Aircraft Hours Flown (thousands)	Accident Rates Per 100,000 Aircraft Hours	
	Total	Fatal			Total	Fatal
1972	4109	653	1305	24,419	16.8	2.67
1973	4090	679	1299	26,908	15.2	2.52
1974	4234	689	1327	27,774	15.2	2.47
1975	4034	638	1247	28,336	14.2	2.24
1976	4005	648	1187	29,975	13.3	2.15
1977	4069	658	1281	31,585	12.9	2.08
1978	4223	723	1562	34,985	12.1	2.07
1979	3800	629	1219	38,767	9.8	1.62
1980	3599	629	1264	37,480	9.6	1.68
1981	3634	662	1265	36,280	10.0	1.82

*As of 1981, general aviation no longer includes air taxi (commuter air carrier and on-demand air taxi) accidents. The number of total accidents, fatal accidents, fatalities, and aircraft hours flown and accident rates for the years 1972 to 1980 have been adjusted to accommodate the exclusion of air taxi accidents and air taxi hours flown.

resent another 20% of accidents, making the combined phases of takeoff and landing by far the riskiest aspects of flight. The in-flight phase accounted for 30% of all accidents but contributed to nearly 70% of all fatal accidents. Most of the in-flight fatal accidents occurred during normal cruise, uncontrolled descent, or initial climb. The major causes of those accidents continue to be pilot judgment and weather. Alcohol as a cause or contributing factor appears less frequently, and this decrease is assumed to be in response to a major educational program on the part of the Federal Aviation Administration (FAA).

No rank-order change has occurred recently for total accident rates by categories of flying. In descending order, these remain pleasure, aerial application, instructional, and corporate-executive flight. The bright spot in the overall statistics is the steady downward trend in the fatal accident rate for aerial application flying. This rate has been below the overall general aviation fatality rate since 1972 and continues a trend that began in 1969 when fatal accidents in aerial application showed a significant drop with the availability of new-generation aircraft. These aircraft were designed with new, built-in crashworthiness features. Analysis of the injury rates in the new aircraft demonstrated a striking 36% reduction.

For the general aviation safety record to improve, the pilot having the most accidents (the pleasure pilot) must be reached. Special emphasis on training is required, especially on subjects pertaining to pre-flight preparation and planning, meteorology and weather evaluation, engine operation and fuel management, instrument flight rule (IFR) procedures and position awareness, and takeoff and landing techniques, particularly under emergency conditions. This same pilot is most likely to find himself in a potential or a real survival situation because of cumulative errors of omission or commission leading to a crash, sometimes with no flight plan, no radio location signal, and with inadequate survival preparation and equipment. The ultimate in search and rescue support and in survival systems are of little value for those pilots who fail to help themselves by planning ahead.

Military Accident Rates

As with the civil aircraft accident rates, the military uses rates based on 100,000 hours of flying. Within the United States, military accident or major mishap rates are similar among the armed forces when similar flying operations are compared. All branches of the armed forces have shown a reduction in the accident rates over the past several decades.

Military aircraft accident rates during 1981 were the lowest for the Navy since 1945 and the second lowest for the United States Air Force in over 50 years. The combined accident rate for the Navy and the Marine Corps was 4.95. This rate compared with an Air Force rate of 2.42. These rates do not include aircraft lost in combat. The Army experienced a combined rate of 2.79 for its helicopter and fixed-wing operations in 1981. The Coast Guard experienced an accident rate of 8.27 during the same period.[3]

All branches of the armed forces have dynamic flying safety programs. These programs have contributed to the exceptionally low accident rates experienced. Figure 30–2 illustrates the Air Force accident rate for the period from 1950 to 1982.

Aircraft Accident Trends

For all forms of aircraft operations, the trend has been for safer flying both for the aircrews and the flying public. Unfortunately, accurate data are not available for some forms of recreational aeronautic activities such as soaring, hot air ballooning, hang-gliding, ultralight flying, and sky diving to permit accident rate comparisons. Such an analysis would be helpful

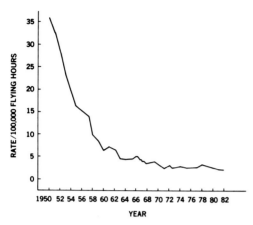

Fig. 30–2. United States Air Force accident rate for the period 1950–1982.

in view of the growing popularity of these sports.

Although the trends have been in the right direction, indicating safer flying, there are spectacular deviations from these trends, as in the case of the ground collision of two jumbo jets at Tenerife, Canary islands on March 27, 1977, resulting in 583 fatalities.

SURVIVAL CONCEPTS

Several concepts that differ from traditional approaches regarding aircraft accidents and survival will be introduced in this section. The first of these is the concept of survivability, which extends the classic survival phase into the actual crash sequence, wherein increased opportunity for occupant survival begins with improved aircraft crashworthiness, including delethalization of the aircraft environment, and ends with improved egress opportunities to avoid the often lethal immediate postcrash environment.

Another innovation described is the total systems approach to search and rescue (SAR), which consists of five SAR stages (awareness, initial action, planning, operations, and mission completion) supported by five functional components (organization, facilities, communications, emergency care, and documentation). The

SAR system may, on occasion, become a part of a more comprehensive emergency system (disaster relief), or parts of another emergency system may merge with the SAR system and become a part of it (emergency medical services).

In the SAR system, survival is defined in terms of time factors with respect to the probability of locating survivors and the probability of their remaining alive until rescue can be effected.

The concept of the survival system as a part of a comprehensive aircraft life-support system will be introduced in this section. The survival subsystem, developed primarily to support military aviation requirements, encompasses packages of equipment, techniques, and methods utilized after escape from a disabled aircraft or a ground or sea landing until successful recovery. Included are communications, locator and signaling devices, flotation gear, clothing and shelter, food and water, tools and weapons, medical/first-aid equipment, recovery enhancement devices, and other miscellaneous, mission-specific equipment. Concentration has been on the development of specific compact packages of varying degrees of sophistication designed to serve from the moment of escape from the disabled aircraft until rescue is effected and configured to avoid encumbering the flyer with excess equipment on the body. The United States survival system concept, which interfaces intimately with the SAR system, assumes short-term survival and early rescue and thereby concentrates on the majority of situations where SAR is rapidly successful rather than the occasional survivable crash in remote, isolated areas.

CRASHWORTHINESS

In October, 1974, the United States General Accounting Office provided the Secretary of Transportation and the Chairman of the National Transportation Safety Board (NTSB) a comprehensive survey that identified the technologies available for increasing the survivability of passengers in civil air transportation accidents and assessed the FAA means for implementing such technologies. The survey recommended that research development and technologic advancement priorities be assigned and controlled relative to their potential for saving lives. It also recommended that the NTSB issue periodic reports on aircraft accidents and fatality and injury data to provide a basis for evaluating the survival problem priorities and to indicate to the FAA the relative significance of particular safety regulations.

In November, 1974, the NTSB published a special study on the safety aspects of emergency evacuation from civil air transport aircraft based on ten United States commercial air accidents in which an emergency evacuation occurred. These ten accidents exemplified the factors most commonly identified as influencing evacuation success. Ten safety recommendations relevant to postfire and postcrash survivability resulted from this study.

In February, 1976, hearings conducted by an investigative subcommittee of the Housing Public Works Transportation Committee, Representative James C. Wright presiding, addressed in detail postcrash survivability measures, examining numerous aircraft accidents in which passengers survived the impact of the crash but died minutes later because of faulty egress procedures, inadequate protection against smoke and fire, poorly trained crewmembers, inferior emergency lighting, and other postcrash factors. The Wright subcommittee identified and examined more than a dozen problem areas in which necessary technology and procedures to make aircraft more survivable after the crash are available for implementation or are awaiting only aggressive action on the part of the FAA, the aircraft industry, and the airlines.

Although the lifesaving and injury-minimizing benefits of crashworthy aircraft design have been recognized for over 50 years, a fundamental change in design philosophy has evolved only in the past 25 years. Whereas all earlier efforts were focused on introducing safety factors or features that would prevent an accident from occurring, it is now recognized that a statistical and socially significant number of accidents are inevitable, and aircraft designers must consider them. Crashworthiness, a technologic concept that deals with the capability of vehicle occupants to survive crash-impact situations with minimal bodily injury, has been introduced into aircraft design. The scientific bases for this technology are manifold, encompassing a spectrum of biomedical and applied mechanical research.

Five factors have been identified as responsible for survivability in aircraft accidents:

1. *Crashworthiness*—the designed ability of the vehicle to withstand crushing or breaking open during crash forces
2. *Restraint*—the tie-down system of structure, floor, seat belts and/or harness that restrains the passengers during the crash
3. *Environment*—the nature of the area surrounding or within striking distance of vital body segments
4. *Energy absorption*—progressive yielding or deformation of structures, restraint systems, and environment, absorbing crash forces and attenuating rather than amplifying loads
5. *Postcrash factors*—those which control or influence the ability of the occupant who survives the dynamic portion of the crash (because of crashworthiness of the structures, adequate restraint, noninjurious environment, and optimum energy absorption capability) to get up and walk away from the "survivable" accident

The factors that control or influence escape are postcrash fire, emergency egress facilities, assistance, instruction, operability and/or function of normal and emergency exits, lighting, smoke and toxic product inhalation, flotation, and survival from the elements after egress but before rescue and recovery.

Exploratory Development

Items in the broad exploratory development category ranged in scope from fundamental studies exploring new systems concepts for the solution of technical problems through improving techniques and methods for advancing the state of the art to the evaluation of sophisticated "breadboard" hardware for assessing the technical and economic feasibility of obtaining the desired system capability. Work on in-flight escape systems represents the concept exploration end of this range; efforts to design crash sensors for passive restraint systems, encompassing diverse designs based on electromechanical, radar, sonar, and inertial guidance components, comprise the other end of the spectrum. In advanced development stages, developmental hardware, techniques, and methods are undergoing evaluation and validation for practical application in experimental or operational testing.

A concentrated effort is under way within the FAA's Flight Standard Service to improve the presentation of safety information to air travelers. This effort is being accomplished by upgrading the safety information card and by applying advanced concepts such as audiovisual techniques. Passengers involved in crashes who had read and understood the safety information cards and who listened to the safety announcements had an increased chance for survival because they were aware of their primary and secondary routes of escape. The percentage of passengers injured during emergency egress is known to be about three times less for those passengers who read the instruction card.

Fire-suppressant isocyanate foam is effective in protecting aircraft interiors from external fuel fire damage. During United States Air Force JP4 fuel fire tests, transport aircraft fuselage sections protected with 6 cm of foam between the outer skin and the cabin interior surface survived the fire with relatively little damage, whereas the unprotected sections were totally destroyed within 2 minutes. The temperatures within the unprotected section rose to a lethal 350° C in less than 2 minutes. Within the foam-protected section, the temperature had changed very little after 6 minutes. Intumescent paint serves as a protective agent against the effects of smoke and flame. During flame tests, the paint retarded the progress of the flames and protected the underlying wood; unprotected wood burned and charred.

Passive restraint systems have undergone considerable development and testing. Unresolved problems relative to aircraft application involve the definition of a crash envelope, that is, accurately distinguishing between crash impact and hard landings or turbulence.

In accidents with sublethal decelerative forces, survival is determined largely by the ability of the injured passenger to make his way from his seat to an exit within the time limits imposed by the thermal-toxic environment (1 to several seconds). With failure to egress, lethality is assured within 3.5 to 5 minutes. As a rule, the passengers do not think in terms of alternate exits; on the contrary, they tend to seek egress through the exit that they entered. Aisle/evacuation path marker systems currently being evaluated or, in some instances, in use are chemoluminescent signs and direction indicators, fluorescent spray, phosphorescent markers, electroluminescent panels, self-luminous (tritium) sources, various electrical light systems, and the use of tactile systems. Because smoke is densest and thickest in the upper portion of the cabin, egress is not infrequently accomplished by literally crawling on the hands and knees. Therefore, regardless of the system ultimately chosen, it must be located at seat arm level or below to achieve maximum effectiveness. Because of this requirement, an other-than-normal postcrash aircraft attitude (e.g., inverted) may invalidate system effectiveness.

A growing need for protection for infants and small children in commercial air transport accidents led to the initiation of a Civil Aeromedical Institute (CAMI) project to develop the criteria for approving future restraint systems for testing prototype designs. This effort has been largely completed.

Research programs are under way in the United States and United Kingdom to modify aviation fuels, using chemical additives to alter volatility, thereby preventing the formation of highly combustible fine fuel mists; rather, the idea is to created coarse spray that inhibits ignition and flame propagation. Thus, the probability and severity of fire following survivable accidents is significantly decreased, and the conditions for occupant evacuation are improved. Although engine and aircraft fuel system compatibility problems exist, efforts under way to resolve these problems show considerable promise. FAA-sponsored, full-scale flammability tests using military twin-jet aircraft to select the best type and concentration of fuel modifier have been accomplished. In 1984 flammable test conducted at Edwards Air Force Base by the FAA involving a four engine commercial type jet was inconclusive. In today's inflationary economy and competitive market, the cost of this safety item may be too much of a burden for the airline to bear and must be realistically balanced against the anticipated benefits in crew and passenger safety.

Engineering Development

Engineering development encompasses tested and qualified hardware destined to become components of major equipments or systems, including the skills and techniques required for support.

Existing emergency lighting systems have proven to be ineffective due to their location high in the cabin and their low light-intensity levels for postcrash fires with dense smoke. Impetus has been generated for the installation of emergency light systems that have significantly improved performance, and such systems are under active development.

The airline industry has shown considerable interest in using flame-retardant materials inside aircraft cabins; nevertheless, most seat cushions, covers, flight attendant uniforms, and other fabrics and yarns, such as found in carpeting, are still flammable. Some materials exhibiting excellent flame retardancy are in quantity production (e.g., Nomex Durette, Kevlar, Kynol, neoprene foams). The unique polymeric chemistry that ensures the initial flame resistance of these materials causes them to undergo thermal-toxic pyrolysis when they do eventually burn. These products of pyrolysis are being investigated to establish their toxicity status. Certain disadvantages, such as high cost, poor dye receptivity, fading, and susceptibility to abrasion, tend to limit the general application of these materials by the airlines. Interest in aircraft fires has gained renewed importance following the 1983 fatal in-flight fire aboard an Air Canada aircraft.

All new United States Army helicopters built since April, 1970 have had crashworthy fuel systems. Despite more than 700 mishaps, no thermal fatalities have occurred. The installation of crashworthy fuel systems resulted in a fivefold decrease in the number of postcrash fires. Due to the incorporation of high-energy–absorption materials and components, the crashworthy fuel system retained its fuel contents both during and after a survivable crash. Crashworthy fuel system design has been validated and requires no scientific breakthroughs for application to the civilian aircraft industry. Advocates of this system indicate that the benefits significantly outweigh the economic costs. It is expected that this technology will become standard equipment in all new-generation aircraft.

The United States Air Force developed an automatic, high-energy egress system for air transport aircraft that was successfully demonstrated in 1973. This system, designated Emergency Lifesaving Instant Exit (ELSIE), provides escape portholes of any predetermined size and shape in the aircraft skin in less than 30 milliseconds by the detonation of a flexible, linear-shaped cutting charge. This charge is usually fitted just inside the perimeter of existing emergency exits to ensure operation even if the exits are deformed in the crash. Although detonation of the charge does not ignite spilled fuel, it does impart momentum to jettison the exit door a sufficient distance to both clear the opening and also deploy an inflatable escape slide/raft. The ELSIE system has been subjected to an extensive test and evaluation program. Having qualified the ELSIE system, the Air Force also has contracted for a Flotation Equipment Deployment System (FEDS) to deploy and inflate two 20-man life rafts from the C-141 cargo aircraft aft fuselage upper deck. It has been estimated that implementation of this feature alone would have saved over 50% of the survivable deaths occurring in C-130, C-135, and C-141 transport aircraft accidents from 1967 through 1974. A recent application for ELSIE provides an emergency escape exit for pilots in the Boeing 747 used to transport the space shuttle. The pilots of the 747 do not have ejection seats as do the pilots in the space shuttle. If an in-flight emergency should occur while transporting the space shuttle in which the 747 is incapable of continued flight to its base landing, an ELSIE system would depressurize the 747, sever a panel in the left forward fuselage under the cockpit area, and extend a telescoped slide/wind baffle

down into the slipstream, thus providing an exit windblast spoiler. The 747 pilots would parachute to safety by simply stepping into the top of the slide, and gravity would expel them from the aircraft.

Operational Applications

Development and engineering work of some items is complete, and all that remains is application in operational systems. The United States Air Force has advocated the protective advantage offered to occupants of aft-facing seats from impact accelerations in the $+G_x$ direction, the predominant force experienced in frontal aircraft crashes. This position permits more optimum distribution of the inertial load, as compared with that provided during $-G_x$ acceleration experienced with forward-facing seats equipped with a harness or lap-belt restraint system. Today, aft-facing air passenger seats and mounting structures are available that are designed to withstand impact forces exerted by the occupant during a frontal crash at no increase in weight over standard seats. Furthermore, improvements in backrest design can significantly decrease the tendency toward "ramping," or traveling upward on impact, even if only a lap belt is worn. Aft-facing seats with a 16-G capability that are now provided in military transport aircraft, such as the Royal Air Force VC-10 and the United States Air Force C-141, offer effective passenger impact protection. A valid reason no longer exists to support the contention that their use would create adverse passenger reaction. Performance characteristics and the configuration of current aircraft, particularly the spaciousness of the wide-body jumbo jets, all but eliminate most cues of motion and direction once airborne. The crashworthy advantages of the rearward-based seats can no longer be ignored in deference to alleged objections on the part of the traveling public.

Over a dozen types of smoke hoods are

available from various manufacturers to offer protection to survivors who now frequently succumb to the inhalation of lethal products of combustion such as smoke, heated gases, and toxic fumes and vapors in the postcrash thermotoxic environment. Passengers could easily pull this lightweight safety hood over their heads after a survivable crash. It would provide them with more than 2.5 minutes of breathable air free from lethal combustion products. Smoke hoods could be utilized on present air carrier and military transport aircraft. In-flight fires aboard commercial transport aircraft have dramatized the need for a simple, safe, effective smoke hood for passengers.

Transport aircraft accident data provide ample evidence that the potential for passenger survival is significantly enhanced in those instances where fully functional, uninjured crewmembers, especially the cabin flight attendants, controlled and assisted evacuation, opened all functional exits, guided and directed all ambulatory occupants, and assisted injured passengers out prior to their own egress. Implementation of measures is necessary to improve survivability and effectiveness of flight attendants, such as (1) stronger, strategically located flight attendant seating, preferably aft-facing and near emergency exits; (2) installation and use of shoulder harness with such seating; (3) readily accessible stowage of portable high-intensity light sources at flight attendants' seat location; (4) availability and use of smoke hoods; (5) use of fire-protective uniforms; and (6) adequate familiarization and frequent hands-on training with all emergency and survival equipment aboard the aircraft.

SEARCH AND RESCUE

Search and rescue (SAR) is defined as the employment of available personnel and facilities in rendering aid to persons and property in distress. SAR is both an art and a science and encompasses or draws on many diverse disciplines. The SAR system is activated when information is received that an emergency exists or may exist and is deactivated when a survivor or endangered craft is delivered to a position of treatment or safety, respectively, when it has been determined that no emergency actually existed, or when there is no longer any hope for rescue.

Historically, the origin of today's worldwide international SAR system can be traced to the beginning of World War II. Early in the war, the German Air Force established a well-organized air/sea rescue service. The British and American forces also recognized the need for an organized air/sea rescue effort, which, once established, saved the lives of thousands of airmen. During the Korean War, air/sea rescue units evacuated approximately 10,000 wounded soldiers from the forward area of battle, and an additional 1000 United Nations personnel were rescued from behind enemy lines. During the Vietnam War, air/sea rescue units of the United States armed forces succeeded in rescuing downed flyers from both friendly and hostile territories. By the end of the conflict, units of the United States Air Force Aerospace Rescue and Recovery Service (ARSS) alone successfully completed nearly 1000 combat recoveries of downed aircrew members.

Initiation of Search and Rescue Activity

Five specific events normally occur sequentially during search operations:

1. Establishing the most probable position of the SAR incident
2. Developing the size of the search area
3. Selecting the appropriate search pattern
4. Determining area coverage
5. Formulating an attainable search plan using available search and rescue units

The amount and type of survival and signaling equipment available to the survivor will influence the urgency of the SAR system's response and the methods and procedures employed in the various SAR stages. For example, if survivors have an emergency position-indicating radio beacon, an immediate, high-altitude electronic search would be conducted.

To provide the high-altitude surveillance needed for a global distress signal monitoring system, a space satellite has been developed. The satellite project is a joint effort on the part of Canada, France, the Soviet Union, and the United States. In the fall of 1982, the Soviet Cospos 1 picked up distress signals from the emergency beacon of a single-engine plane in a remote mountain valley in northern British Columbia. The signal of a capsized trimaran in high seas off the East Coast of the United States was picked up by the satellite and contributed to the safe rescue of the three seamen.

The satellite can pick up the low-power radio distress signal from the emergency locator transmitter. The United States system has the capacity to pinpoint the source of the signal within 5 to 10 miles. With improvements in the locator beam, far better accuracy is possible. With four satellites deployed, an emergency signal from anywhere on earth can be detected within 3 hours. The average detection time should be under 1 hour.

SAR personnel are responsible for taking whatever action they can to save a life at any time and place where facilities are available and can be used effectively. Nevertheless, there is a limit beyond which SAR services are not expected and cannot be justified. Known and inherent risks must be weighed carefully against the mission's chances for success and the gains to be realized. SAR personnel and equipment should not be jeopardized or a mission attempted unless lives are known to be at stake and the chances for saving lives are within the capability of the personnel and equipment available.

All reasonable action shall be taken to locate people in distress, determine their status, and effect their rescue. Prolonged SAR operations are not warranted after all probability of finding survivors has been exhausted. The decision to conduct such an operation must be based on the probability of finding survivors. Studies have shown that the first 12 to 24 hours following the incident are the most critical for the recovery of survivors.

The Search and Rescue Incident

An aircraft SAR incident is considered imminent or actual when any of the following conditions exist:

1. An aircraft has requested assistance
2. An aircraft has transmitted a distress signal
3. It is apparent that an aircraft is in distress
4. An aircraft is reported to have ditched, crashed, made a forced landing, or is about to do so
5. The crew is reported to have abandoned the aircraft or is about to do so
6. Reports indicate that the operating efficiency of the aircraft is so impaired that forced landing or abandonment may be necessary
7. The aircraft is overdue

An aircraft on an instrument flight plan is considered overdue when neither communications nor radar contact can be established with it and 30 minutes have passed after its estimated time over a specified or compulsory reporting point or at clearance limit. An aircraft on a visual flight plan is considered overdue when communication cannot be established with it and it fails to arrive 30 minutes (15 minutes for a jet) after its estimated time of arrival. An aircraft not on a flight plan is considered overdue if a reliable source reports it 1 hour overdue at destination. After the initial report of an incident is received, evaluated, and assigned an emergency phase, three possible actions may be taken: (1) dispatch SAR units immediately and request other facilities to take immediate responsive action; (2) alert SAR facilities to a possible mission but do not dispatch; (3) neither dispatch nor alert other SAR facilities but investigate further to either confirm the reported incident or determine the need for SAR system support.

The Search and Rescue Organization

The International Civil Aviation Organization (ICAO) is a worldwide organization whose primary purpose is administering the Convention on International Civil Aviation designed to promote the safe, orderly, and efficient growth of international civil aviation, including both commercial and general aviation. Over 100 nations are members, including the United States. Of all the various international organizations, ICAO is the most prominent in the SAR, having established comprehensive standards and recommended practices and procedures for the conduct of SAR for international civil aviation. Under the terms of the Convention, each signatory nation undertakes to provide such measures of assistance to aircraft of any nationality in distress within its territory. The Convention also provides that each signatory nation, when searching for missing aircraft, will collaborate and coordinate its activities with other nations as appropriate.

Under the Convention, the United States has an international obligation to furnish SAR services for its own territory. In addition, the United States has accepted international responsibilities for furnishing SAR service over certain international waters, notably large portions of oceanic areas.

The national SAR plan provides for the control and coordination of all available facilities for all types of search and rescue operations. A single federal agency coordinates all federal SAR operations in any one area. The three major groupings of

SAR regions and designated SAR coordinators are inland region, United States Air Force; maritime region, United States Coast Guard; and overseas region, Overseas Unified Commanders.

The regional SAR coordinators are responsible for organizing agencies and their facilities into a basic network for rendering assistance both to military and civilian persons and property in distress and carrying out the United States' ICAO obligations.

Because there is no single requirement for military SAR in support of military operations, each branch of the United States armed services is responsible for providing SAR facilities for its own operations. All Department of Defense facilities are available for use on a noninterference basis to meet civilian needs. Commanders of all military installations are required to establish and maintain a base search and rescue plan designed primarily to provide SAR service for local base equipment and secondarily to assist the national SAR plan.

The ARRS, the designated executive agent for the United States Air Force, serves as SAR coordinator for the inland region, as well as for United States Air Force global and space operations. The latter is accomplished by globally deployed ARRS units. These units are equipped with specifically designed equipment to accomplish precautionary flights, personnel/equipment recovery, and pararescue missions wherever they are needed. ARRS resources include long-range, fixed-wing aircraft, rotary-wing aircraft, and highly trained pararescue personnel.

Other federal organizations involved in supporting the national SAR plan include the Civil Air Patrol, the United States Navy, the Department of the Army, The Defense Civil Preparedness Agency, and the Department of Transportation, which includes the United States Coast Guard, the Coast Guard Auxiliary, the Federal Aviation Administration, the Interagency

Committee on Search and Rescue (a Coast Guard subsidiary), the National Oceanic and Atmospheric Administration, Federal Communications Commission, National Aeronautics and Space Administration, and the NTSB. Other national, state, county, municipal, and private organizations participate in SAR activities. The National Association for Search and Rescue (NASAR) is a national, nonprofit association dedicated to developing increased state, federal, local, and volunteer coordination and improvement in search and rescue services. NASAR also promotes survival education programs. The purpose of NASAR is to ensure the effective utilization of all available resources and facilities in all types of search and rescue activities.

Rapid response to a SAR situation is essential because time remains the key to successful rescue of survivors of an aircraft accident. Within the first 8 hours, the survival rate is more than 50%. Should the rescue be delayed beyond 2 days, however, the survival rate drops to less than 10%.

SURVIVAL

Once the accident has occurred, surviving becomes the major issue. As has been discussed in postcrash events, surviving may begin almost instantaneously with the accident, as in the case of evacuating a burning aircraft. Survival will require a clear head, ingenuity, and a desire to live.

Self

Regardless of how good available survival equipment is or how good the techniques are for its use, the individual faced with a survival situation still must deal with himself. Psychologic reactions to survival stresses often render the individual incapable of using available resources. Although far from complete, information available from actual survival situations provides an understanding of some of the major psychologic factors involved in sur-

vival. Although much appears to be merely common sense, it should be remembered that common sense derives from past experiences that have led to successful adjustments to various situations.

A most significant psychologic requirement for survival is the ability to immediately accept the reality of the new situation and react appropriately to it. Availability of survival information leads to a feeling of confidence in one's ability to survive. Because self-confidence is important in dealing with fear and panic, survival information and training serve to minimize fear and prevent panic. Training for survival must be sufficiently realistic to provide the necessary experience, yet sufficiently safe to avoid casualties. The trainee must feel he has come through a potentially dangerous situation and escaped unharmed.

Fear

Fear is a normal reaction for anyone faced with a threatening emergency situation. Fear influences man's behavior and thus his chances for survival; it may either destroy or improve survival chances. Avoiding fear by denying the existence of danger may prove harmful. Some positive action can be taken to improve the situation. Accepting fear as a natural reaction to a threatening situation is conducive to purposeful rather than random behavior, thereby enhancing the chances for survival. A person's reaction to fear depends more on the individual than on the situation. Timid or anxious persons may respond more coolly and effectively under stress than the physically strong or happy-go-lucky individual. Fear must be acknowledged, coped with, and, if possible, used to advantage. Feelings of helplessness and hopelessness are factors that can inhibit or possibly prevent action.

Attitudes for Survival

Attitudes can actually enhance or greatly endanger survival changes. The mental attitude that "it can't happen to me" obscures the reality of the situation and diminishes the appropriate reaction in the face of real emergency. It is extremely important to have a "preparatory attitude" for whatever emergency may occur. Both mental and physical rehearsal of emergency procedures enhances the preparatory attitudes for survival, encourages automatic action, and tends to counter the "it can't happen to me" attitude that endangers survival and often results in panic, even in persons who appear to be calm under ordinary circumstances. Knowledge and rehearsal of survival and emergency procedures can allow a survivor to function satisfactorily during an emergency, even in a state of semiconsciousness.

Six Enemies of Survival

Within any survival situation, factors in varying combinations compromise the probability of survival even when those components of "self" are adequately controlled. The following is a list of the six enemies of survival:

1. Pain is a natural response directing attention to something that is wrong with the body. Pain may go unnoticed during the intense, concentrated activity shortly following the aircraft crash. In time, however, pain may weaken the will to survive; thus, it is important to take care of those injuries that could produce significant pain.
2. Cold is a significant threat to survival. It not only lowers a person's ability to concentrate but tends to decrease a person's will to accomplish anything but getting warm. Cold is an insidious enemy that numbs the mind, the body, and the will. The urge to sleep must be resisted so that one does not forget that the goal is to survive.
3. Thirst, even if not extreme, can dull

the mind. Nevertheless, it can almost be forgotten if the will to survive is strong enough. Consequently, it is important not to deprive oneself unnecessarily of water, leading to serious dehydration even in the presence of water.
4. Hunger is particularly dangerous because it lessens an individual's ability for rational thought and increases susceptibility to the weakening effects of cold, pain, and fear. This factor becomes significant in the longterm survival situation.
5. Fatigue reduces mental ability. Fatigue can make one careless and reduce motivation. Although a real danger for those who overexert, fatigue and energy expenditure are not necessarily directly related, and fatigue may actually be due to hopelessness, lack of a goal, dissatisfaction, frustration, or boredom. Fatigue may represent an escape from the situation that has become too difficult to deal with. If one recognizes the dangers of such a situation, one also can summon the strength to go on.
6. Boredom and loneliness, two tough enemies of survival, are doubly worse because they are unexpected. When nothing happens and expectations for rescue are high, a sense of abandonment can occur. These feelings can insidiously incapacitate an individual to the point where he cannot contribute toward his own rescue.

Medical Considerations

When survivors are suspected or known to be injured, the delivery of trained medical personnel to the scene can be lifesaving. The seriousness and the urgency of the situation usually define the need for medical support.

Medical personnel may be delivered by helicopters in both inland and maritime missions, provided the victim is within range and the weather cooperates. In the maritime area, a second choice would be to deliver medical personnel by watercraft, and ground vehicles could be used on land, but both methods of transport are relatively slow and subject to indirect routes.

Where helicopters are not available, consideration must be given to deployment of a pararescue team. It is thus desirable that a pararescue team be carried by at least one search aircraft that is suitable and authorized for dropping parachutists when search operations are in remote areas.

The uniqueness of trained pararescue teams gives the search and rescue mission coordinator a valuable resource for placing a land SAR unit at the distress scene with a minimum of delay. By transporting the team to the scene by aircraft and deploying them by parachute, some time delays encountered by ground penetration are eliminated. These teams are also qualified for deployment into the open oceans and have proven more effective in maritime medical missions.

Emergency care components contribute to the SAR system by providing four major capabilities: SAR personnel trained in emergency care, lifesaving and life-sustaining services to survivors after rescue, survivor evacuation and transport facilities, and medical facilities to receive injured survivors.

SAR personnel trained in emergency medical care provide lifesaving services to injured survivors at the accident scene. These personnel provide life-support and life-sustaining services during survivor extraction from wreckage, evacuation from the accident scene, and transport to a receiving medical facility. Search and rescue personnel assigned as crewmen to various SAR units should be qualified to administer basic lifesaving first aid.

When it is known that a rescue craft will be dealing with injured or seriously ill persons, the crew should be supplemented by medically trained personnel. Every effort should be made to send a physician as part of the crew in these circumstances. If a United States Air Force pararescue team is available, excellent emergency stabilizing care can be anticipated for injured survivors.

The ARRS pararescue individuals are highly trained SAR personnel, having completed over 1 year of formal training in such fields as parachuting, mountaineering, survival in all environments, advanced emergency medical care, underwater scuba swimming, and aircraft crash firefighting. Pararescue personnel are stationed at every ARRS squadron location and at some of the ARRS detachments. They are qualified to be deployed from aircraft over any type of terrain or ocean, day or night, to assist survivors of any type of disaster. Pararescue personnel are extremely valuable when there is a need to provide medical assistance without delay to victims beyond the range of an acceptable expected time of arrival of other assistance. The basic ARRS rescue team consists of two pararescue men equipped with emergency medical care kits, survival kits, and either scuba or forest penetration parachute kits.

Time is Critical

The probability of finding survivors and their chances for survival diminish each minute after an incident occurs. It is, therefore, important that all SAR activities occur promptly so as not to jeopardize survivors. The life expectancy of injured survivors decreases by up to 80% after the first 24 hours, whereas the survival of uninjured survivors diminishes rapidly after the first 3 days. Individual survival incidence will vary according to local conditions such as terrain, climatic conditions, abilities and endurance of survivors, and survival equipment available to the survivors.

A review of over 600 SAR incidents is presented in Figure 30–3. This figure dem-

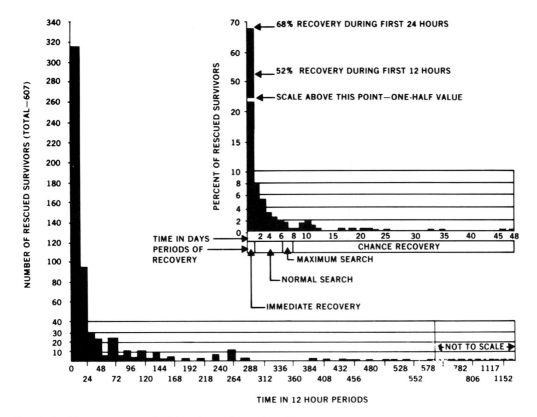

Fig. 30–3. Time at recovery of 607 survivors of aircraft accidents.

onstrates graphically the need for prompt response of the SAR systems if lives are to be saved. Successful recovery of survivors is time-dependent, with 68% recovered in the first 24 hours and 75% recovered within 48 hours.

Adverse weather and darkness are important factors influencing survival recovery time. Survival environment factors further limit the time available to complete survivor rescue and in some cases may prove to be the most critical overall factor. The relationship of the survival time to water temperature, air temperature, humidity, and wind velocity is quite complex; these and other factors often exist in combination to complicate the estimation of the life expectancy of survivors. Individuals will vary in their reactions to cold and heat stresses. Additional factors that affect survivor life expectancy include the type of clothing worn, clothing

wetness, survivor's activity during exposure, initial body temperature, physical condition, thirst, exhaustion from lack of sleep, hunger from lack of food, various psychologic stresses, such as isolation, loneliness, and remoteness, and the all-important individual will to survive.

Heat Loss

Hypothermia is abnormal lowering of the internal body temperature (heat loss) resulting from exposure to the chilling effects of cold air, wind, or water. Death may occur from hypothermia during land survival or water survival situations, although it occurs over four times as often in the latter situation. Internal body temperature is a critical factor in hypothermia.

If body temperatures depress to only 36° C, most persons will survive. At about 34°C, the level of consciousness becomes clouded; unconsciousness occurs at 30° C and below, and the average individual will die, with ventricular fibrillation usually occurring as the final event. In rare cases, however, individuals have survived body temperatures as low as 20° C.

The body will cool when immersed in water having a temperature of less than 34° C. Approximately one third of the earth's oceans have water temperatures of 20° C.

The rate of body heat loss increases as the temperature of air and water decreases. If a survivor is immersed in water, hypothermia will occur rapidly due to the decreased insulating quality of wet clothing and the fact that water will displace the layer of still air that normally surrounds the body (the microclimate). Water allows a rate of heat exchange approximately 25 times greater than that of air at the same temperature.

At water temperatures above 23° C, survival time depends on the fatigue factor of the individual. Individuals have survived over 80 hours at these temperatures. At 16° C, skin temperatures will decrease to near water temperature within 10 minutes of entry, and shivering and discomfort are experienced immediately. From 10 to 16° C, the victim has a reasonably good chance of surviving if rescue is completed within 6 hours. Faintness and disorientation occur at water temperatures of 10° C and below. Violent shivering and muscle cramps will be present almost from the time of entering the water, and intense pain will be experienced in the hands and feet. This excruciatingly painful experience continues until numbness sets in. All skin temperatures decrease to near the water temperature within 10 minutes. In the temperature range from 4 to 10° C, only about 50% of the group can be expected to survive longer than 1 hour. In temperatures of 2° C and below, the survivor suffers a severe shock and severe pain upon entering the water. In some instances, this shock may be fatal, owing to a loss of consciousness and subsequent drowning.

Figure 30–4 depicts the life expectancy of survivors immersed in water wearing typical clothing.[4] The survival times indicated in Figure 30–4 are for uninjured survivors. This graph is a guide for estimating life expectancy, but there will be some deviations. For example, a female will generally survive longer than a male due to the fatty tissue underlying her skin, which acts as an insulator. Also, obese people can survive longer than thin people, and individuals in good physical condition will survive longer than those who are less fit. In addition, the graph is based on data for Caucasians. Orientals may be expected to survive longer, whereas blacks would have a shorter survival time. This spread of time indicated in the marginal portion of the graph is the period in which the survivors usually will lose consciousness and then drown.

Although the body will lose heat approximately 25 times slower in calm air than when immersed in water, the body heat loss will be accelerated with increasing wind velocities. In mountainous, polar, winter, and maritime incidents, this is an additional factor to consider for exposed survivors. Figure 30–5 depicts the effects of various wind speeds and air temperature combinations, with the curves indicating the equivalent temperature as felt on a person's dry skin. For example, suppose a 7-knot wind was blowing and a survivor was walking into the wind at 3 knots. In effect, he would have had 10 knots of wind blowing past him. If the air temperature is only −23° C, his skin would be feeling the equivalent temperature of −38° C.

The wind chill graph (Figure 30-5) is based on studies conducted by the National Science Foundation in Antarctica and is considered to be of greater accuracy than previous wind chill graphs.[4] Wind speeds of over 30 knots will have only a small additional effect on decreasing the equivalent temperatures.

These curves emphasize the necessity for providing shelter for survivors who are

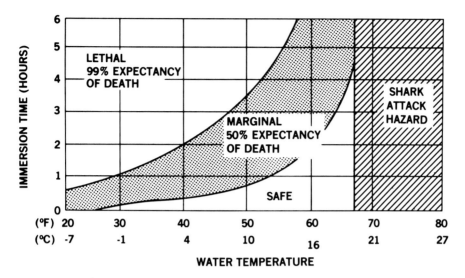

Fig. 30–4. Life expectancy of uninjured survivors immersed in seawater at various temperatures.

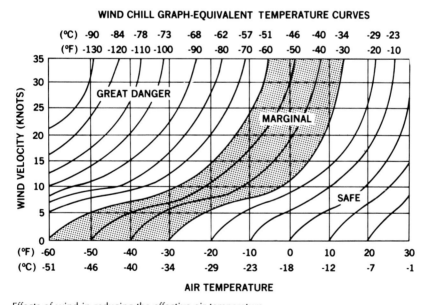

Fig. 30–5. Effects of wind in reducing the effective air temperature.

exposed to severe cold conditions. Dry human flesh freezes when exposed to atmospheric cooling values of between 1300 and 1500 calories/m²/hr. At about an equivalent temperature of − 32° C, exposed flesh will freeze within 60 seconds, whereas at an equivalent temperature of approximately − 56° C, exposed flesh will freeze within 30 seconds. In addition to the problem of freezing flesh at these tem-

peratures, fatigue, clothing, and shelter also become major factors. In temperatures below − 18° C, survivors will easily become fatigued, and establishing a buddy system in which survivors watch each other for frostbite is considered necessary for survival.

Heat Stress

Excess heat and dehydration are dangers in hot climates, particularly in desert areas. The most severe form of heat stress is heat stroke, during which the body temperature rises due to the collapse of the temperature control mechanisms of the body. If the body temperature rises above 42° C, the average person will die. Milder forms of heat stress are heat cramps and heat exhaustion. Another limiting factor both in hot climates and in survival situations at sea is dehydration. Persons totally without water can die within a few days, although some individuals have survived for as long as a week or more.

The combination of high temperatures and lack of water can aggravate the problem of heat stress and lead to dehydration more quickly. The life expectancy of survivors in a desert environment is depicted in Figure 30–6 for stationary, nonwalking

survivors and survivors who walk only at night.[4] Survival time is not appreciably increased until the available water is over 4 L/day. Use of shade or the shading of a few degrees of temperature is as effective and important in increasing survival time as is water. In jungle areas, the water needs of the body are about one-half to one-third that required in the desert at equal temperatures.

SURVIVAL EQUIPMENT

Survival gear encompasses equipment utilized during or after escape or a ground or water landing from a disabled aircraft until successful recovery is accomplished by SAR forces. This equipment includes communication and signaling devices, flotation gear, first-aid supplies, clothing and

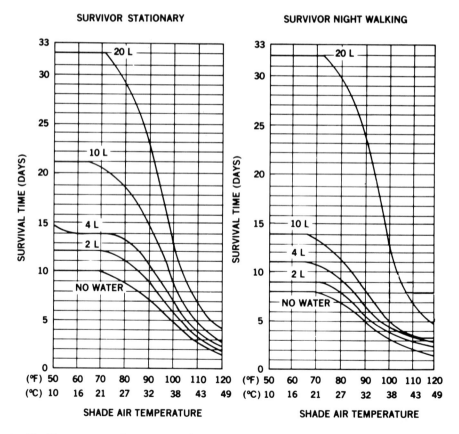

Fig. 30–6. The life expectancy of survivors in a desert environment with various quantities of water while remaining stationary or walking at night.

shelter, food and water, miscellaneous tools, and weapons. The objective of survival is to minimize a downed flyer's probability of injury or death by providing the means to confront the widest possible variety of adverse situations. The degree to which this may be accomplished is defined in part by available technology. Survival equipment, except for a limited resurgence of development during the Vietnam War, has not been significantly advanced since the 1950s. In the noncombat environment, due to low priority, there have been minimal demands for improvements in survival equipment. Combat survival often includes escape and evasion and is inherently more complex than the peacetime survival situation.

The parachute was the first major item developed to safeguard the life of an aircrew member during an in-flight emergency, establishing a precedent for providing life-support equipment that has prevailed until the present time. The escape from an aircraft in flight is fraught with many hazards (e.g., escape path clearance, windblast, cold exposure, and hypoxia at higher altitudes), and is addressed in Chapter 8. Parachute landing, either on land or at sea, may be rough and dangerous, particularly for untrained individuals or those without prior experience.

Although military aviation services have taken the lead in the survival area because of their special requirements, in the past there often was no clear-cut concept or policy for selecting survival equipment or in planning the training to fulfill survival requirements. Rather, survival equipment items were chosen, somewhat arbitrarily, from various sources to provide for long-term survival, changing situations, and, in some instances, the personal preference of the flyers. To clarify this situation, in 1975, the Canadian Forces Defense Civil Institute of Environmental Medicine (DCIEM) conducted a retrospective study of the entire survival scenario as it applies to military flyers for the 10-year period from January, 1965 through December, 1974. Events examined included all ejections, all ditchings, and all crashes or forced landings that occurred outside the perimeters of a recognized landing facility. There were 153 accidents, involving 159 aircraft, that met the established criteria. Some accidents involved multiple aircraft. There were 307 personnel involved in these accidents and 117 fatalities. Of the 190 survivors, 55% were involved in jet accidents, 32% in helicopter accidents, and the remaining 13% in mishaps involving other aircraft. Land survival situations predominated and occurred almost exclusively in the temperate zone. Overall, 69% of the 190 survivors received some degree of injury as a result of the accident; none was injured during the survival period. Of the survivors, 132 were rescued within the first 30 minutes, and an additional 29 victims were rescued by the end of the first hour. A total of 186 survivors (98%) were rescued within 4 hours of the accident. Other survival times were 5.5 hours, 8 hours, and 14.5 hours. The latter was the longest incident recorded during the 10-year period of the study.

Records disclosed that approximately 35% of the survivors did not report using any survival equipment. Among the 124 personnel using equipment, the use of signaling equipment predominated. The frequency of equipment used was 24 flares (27%); 19 survival radios (22%); seven signal panels (8%); and five mirror/heliographs (6%). The sleeping bag was used only once (by the individual who survived for 14.5 hours). First-aid kits, matches, and an axe were each used by four individuals (5%); three persons (4%) used insect repellant. Other available items (mosquito net, sun hat, mitts, gloves, socks, knives, rations, and parachute as shelter) were reported to have been used by two or less survivors. Thus, a total of 17 items from survival kits were used, leaving approximately 80% of available survival kit items unused. The proximity to rescue facilities undoubtedly had an important bearing on survival time and the nature and amount of equipment used by the survivors. Two flyers who survived 5.5 hours were the farthest from help, approximately 720 km from rescue facilities. The majority of survivors were rescued by local base rescue units rather than by SAR units.

The data presented implies that there is a minimal requirement for survival equipment and that the need for training seems to be limited except for basic first aid and instruction in the use of communications and signaling equipment. The data were somewhat misleading, however, because during the study period, the Canadian Forces did not have any survivable accidents in remote regions. Had there been survivors of some of the accidents occurring in remote areas, they could have been stranded for days to weeks during the arctic winter. From this study evolved a philosophy for survival for downed Canadian Forces flyers, which is as follows:

1. Aircrew must be both mentally prepared and trained to face survival situations for an extended period, despite the fact that attempts to rescue will be effected at the earliest possible time, probably within hours
2. Personnel in a survival situation should stay at or near the point of landing
3. The "survival pattern" order of priority (first aid, signal, shelter, heat, water, food, and survival techniques) should be followed in the survival situation in selecting equipment and in survival training
4. Facilities must be provided to expedite rescue in the minimum possible time

During the above mentioned study, inquiries conducted at the Institute of Aviation Medicine (IAM) at Farnborough, England revealed that the Royal Air Force (RAF) had no clear-cut philosophy for sur-

vival and attempted to provide survival equipment to cover all geographic areas and mission roles, resulting in equipment packing problems. The United States military air services have a triservice (Air Force, Army, and Navy) agreement that specifies the areas of responsibility for research, development, and eventual procurement of survival equipment. Considerable research has been accomplished and much is ongoing. Although concentrating on survival packages for specific missions, their concept involves a sophisticated core of survival items that forms the foundation of a survival system. The United States concept assumes short-term survival and early rescue, concentrating on the majority of accident situations.

AIRPORT DISASTER MEDICAL MANAGEMENT

More than 85% of aircraft disasters occur on or in the immediate vicinity of an airport. An analysis of the survival of passengers involved in accidents in the decade from 1970 to 1979 showed approximately three times fewer fatalities in proportion to the number of passengers involved in the wide-body jets than in piston aircraft. Accident data for the period 1970 to 1979, compared with the previous decade, reveal a significant decline in accident rates and an even more significant improvement in survivability of passengers and crews involved in crashes during landing and takeoff phases of flight. According to an NTSB study in 1977 applying both to wide-body and standard-size jet aircraft, several factors have been significant in accounting for this trend: (1) stronger design features; (2) improved occupant seat and restraint systems; (3) improved fuel inerting; (4) improved fire suppression, (5) improved fire extinguishing; (6) diminished toxic products from burning cabin materials; and (7) increased effectiveness of airport firefighting and crash rescue units.

A comparison was made of data for accidents occurring during landing and take-off phases for three categories of air transport aircraft from 1970 until 1979, ICAO designation category III (12,000 to 60,000 pound maximum takeoff weight), ICAO category IV (60,000 to 600,000 pound maximum takeoff weight), and ICAO category V (greater than 600,000 pound maximum takeoff weight). Crashes occurring during the en-route phase were not considered in this study because these are largely impact or disintegration crashes, having little or no bearing on airport disaster medicine. These data revealed that crashes occurring in airports during either landing or takeoff phases of flight resulted in a substantially smaller percentage of persons killed in category V aircraft (wide-body jet) than in crashes of either category IV or smaller, category-III aircraft. This trend is expected to continue as further implementation of the technologic improvements occurs.

Category V aircraft, because of their weight and size, ordinarily utilize only major metropolitan air terminals such as Los Angeles, New York, London, Rome, or Paris. Greater use of high-density seating airbus versions of larger aircraft, such as the A-300B on shorter route segments, however, could introduce operation of these aircraft into any major metropolitan terminal. In the event of a survivable crash of one of these larger jet aircraft during takeoff from or landing at major metropolitan airports, hundreds of casualties could result.

Emergency care for these injured survivors is absolutely essential.[5] How this is accomplished encompasses the concept of airport disaster medical management. The scope of this concept is quite broad, ranging from requirements for a coordinated plan to the on-site provision of medical aid and follow-up medical treatment to the problems of psychologic support for those surviving the disaster. The latter includes friends, family members, and all those individuals who are at or near the airport at the time of the accident.

Medical Planning and Coordination

The goals of an airport disaster medical management plan include care, treatment, and the transportation of the injured, with a quality and quantity of care that minimizes the mortality and morbidity of the survivors. Members of the disaster team must themselves be protected from physical and psychologic harm. Realistic simulation must be carried out to test the plan.[6,7]

The current concept of treating aircraft crash disaster victims begins with their rapid evacuation to a safe site 500 m or more upwind from the crash by a trained crash rescue team for initial care. The victims are then transported to a treatment facility located out of the elements for stabilization and sorting (triage) prior to transport to an appropriate hospital. This triage/treatment center can be fixed or mobile depending on local circumstances and is a place for treatment, stabilization, and holding of survivors. It must have equipment necessary to initiate comprehensive, sophisticated medical care and must have trained medical, nursing, and paramedical personnel in place and ready by the time the first victims arrive. The center must be on standby and ready around the clock, every day of the year, in preparation for an event that actually may never occur.

The triage/treatment center must have a command post, ideally staffed by a physician and a senior nurse trained and experienced in trauma care, a security officer, a hospital administrator, as well as communications and clerical personnel. Both radio communications with the disaster site and ambulances and telephone communications with referral hospitals must be available. The center must be completely stocked with all necessary medical and surgical equipment and supplies and must be functional and ready for instant use. Whether the center is on standby or activated, security still needs to be provided.

The medical personnel who staff the center must be available in a reasonable time when needed by means of a reliable notification and recall system. Ideally, medical personnel other than those from the staff of the designated referral hospital should be used, so that the latter will not be depleted of staff when stabilized victims are transported there for definitive care.

Upon recall, medical personnel will report to the triage/treatment center command post to receive assignments, which are usually prearranged based on their experience and training and can include triage, minor or major surgery, expectant care, burn care, pre- and postoperative care, or emotional crisis intervention.

When shock is reversed, hemorrhage controlled, fluid and electrolyte balance maintained, fractures splinted, thoracocentesis and tracheostomies performed, and burr holes drilled, the transportation of stabilized victims to definitive care referral centers ensues. Transportation needs are critical. Because the normal surface highway congestion around major airports will worsen to almost total impassibility following a major aircraft accident, airlift of medical personnel and accident victims, preferably by helicopter, is an important consideration. The large proportion of survivors in a major aircraft disaster with serious burns requires special consideration; early transfer to a specialized burn care facility is essential for their ultimate survival and recovery. Because the patient census of most burn centers in major metropolitan areas averages 75%, computerized systems have been established and should be utilized to obtain instant reports on the availability of beds in burn centers throughout the region as well as the nation. Since the severely burned survivors are already receiving initial urgent care in the vicinity of an airport, when beds are located by means of this technology, survivors can be expeditiously evacuated aeromedically to wherever beds are available.

Other important factors to consider in airport disaster medical management include liaison with news media, establishment of a temporary morgue, and accommodations for relatives and friends of disaster victims. A disaster drill should be accomplished annually as a vital part of any airport disaster medical management plan. The drill provides an opportunity for all concerned to coordinate their efforts, focuses attention on areas of responsibility, and the efficient deployment of essential services and their needs. The drill is an essential element in the training of personnel and a principal tool whereby the plan can be tested and improved. Management of the remains of those fatally injured is discussed in Chapter 27.

Flying as either a passenger or crewmember is associated with a finite degree of risk. This risk has continued to lessen with the maturing of aviation. When the rare events occur and one must escape from an aircraft accident and survive, a system must be in place to optimize survival. Airframe manufacturers, airline operations, the government, and those associated with flying and the aviation industry are obligated to continue to reduce further the rate of aircraft accidents and enhance the chances of surviving in the event an accident does occur.

REFERENCES

1. National Transportation Safety Board: Annual Review of Aircraft Accident Data. Washington, D.C., Government Printing Office, 1980.
2. Department of Transportation: Federal Aviation Administration Statistical Handbook of Aviation. Washington, D.C., Government Printing Office, 1982.
3. North, D.M.: Military accident rates. Aviat. Week Space Technol., 116:12, 1982.
4. Department of Transportation and United States Coast Guard: National Search and Rescue Manual. Washington, D.C., Government Printing Office, 1973.
5. Abelson, L.C., Star, L.D., and Goldner, A.S.: Twenty years of medical support in aircraft dis-

asters at Kennedy Airport. Aerospace Med., 44:560–566, 1973.

6. Hays, M.B., Stefanki, J.X., and Cheu, D.N.: Planning an airport disaster drill. Aviat. Space Environ. Med., 47:556–560, 1976.

7. Evans, D.: Simulated aircraft instructional exercise at Baltimore-Washington International Airport. Aviat. Space Environ. Med., 47: 445–448, 1976.

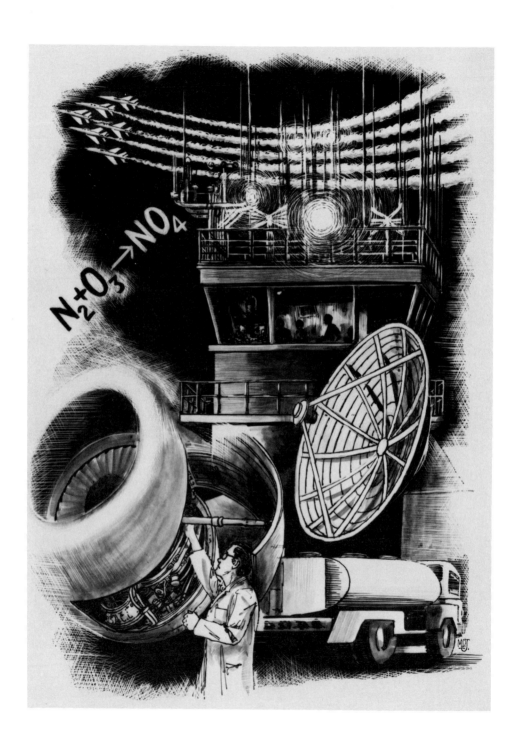

Section V

Impact of the Aerospace Industry on Community Health

With the establishment of the quarantine by the city-state of Venice, Italy, governments began to formalize procedures to protect the public health from the external influences of commerce. The airplane provides an excellent potential vector for the spread of disease worldwide. Disease has been introduced through aircraft operations by passengers who have not had time to develop clinical symptoms from the time of infection, by insects able to survive the short trip in the relative comfort of the aircraft cabin, and by fomites contaminating cargo carried aboard aircraft. Procedures exist to reduce the effectiveness of the aircraft as a disease vector.

Aircraft operations introduces other concerns to the public health. Flight operations generate noise, which is hazardous to those nearby and perhaps injurious to the community health. Air pollution is a concern that has been somewhat alleviated by new jet-engine technology. Ground support to flight operations requires an extensive industrial base and thus introduces the practice of occupational medicine and industrial health.

SUGGESTED READING LIST

1. Committee on Aviation Toxicology, Aero Medical Association: Aviation Toxicology. New York, The Blakiston Co., 1953.
2. Bryan, F.L., et al.: Time-temperature observations of food and equipment in airline catering operations. J. Food Protect., 41(2):80–92, 1978.
3. Cohen, A.: Airport Noise, Sonic Booms, and Public Health. Society of Acoustical Engineers/SAE/ Department of Transportation Conference on Aircraft and the Environment. U.S. Government Printing Office, Washington, D.C., 1971.
4. Galloway, W.: Noise Exposure Forecasts as Indicators of Community Response, Society of Acoustical Engineers/SAE/Department of Transportation Conference on Aircraft and the Environment, Washington, D.C., 1971.
5. McFarland, R.A.: Human Factors in Air Trans-

portation. New York, McGraw-Hill Book Co., Inc., 1953.

6. Moser, M.R., et al.: An outbreak of influenza aboard a commercial airliner. Am. J. Epidemiol., 110(1):1–6, 1979.

7. Naugle, D.F., and Fox, D.L.: Aircraft and air pollution. Environ. Sci. Technol., 15:342, 1981.

8. Occupational Health Surveillance. Department of Defense Manual 6055.5-M, U.S. Government Printing Office, Washington, D.C., 1982.

9. Potter, A.E.: Environmental effects of the space shuttle. Environ. Sci. Technol., 8:173, 1978.

10. Randle, C.J.M., et al.: Cholera: Possible infection from aircraft effluent. J. Hyg. (London), 81(3):361–371, 1978.

11. Tracor, Inc.: Community Reaction to Airport Noise. NASA CR-1761. Washington, D.C., National Aeronautics and Space Administration, 1977.

12. Zenz, C.: Occupational Medicine: Principles and Practical Applications. Chicago, Yearbook Medical Publishers, 1975.

13. Zenz, C.: Developments in Occupational Medicine. Chicago, Yearbook Medical Publishers, 1980.

Chapter *31*

Role of Aircraft in the Transmission of Disease

George D. Lathrop and William H. Wolfe

However secure and well-regulated civilized life may become, bacteria, protozoa, viruses, infected fleas, lice, ticks, mosquitoes, and bedbugs will always lurk in the shadows ready to pounce when neglect, poverty, famine, or war lets down the defenses. . . .About the only genuine sporting proposition that remains. . .is the war against these ferocious fellow creatures, which. . .stalk us in the bodies of rats, mice, and all kinds of domestic animals; which. . .waylay us in our food and drink and even in our love.

HANS ZINSSER

THE HISTORICAL PERSPECTIVE

Transportation of Disease

The idea that disease can be spread by man or his goods in transportation vessels is ancient. Throughout recorded history, military activity and movements of populations have been intimately associated with disease. The aggregation of large numbers of disease-susceptible individuals in military units fostered the spread of disease among the armies, but these same troops, in turn, were often responsible for transmitting diseases to civilian popula-

tions after the outcome of the conflicts had been determined. Likewise, as individuals moved from one area of the world to another, the endemic diseases of one locale were introduced to the susceptible inhabitants of other areas.

The spread of epidemics by military activities and population migrations is not limited to the past. The resurgence of malaria in the United States following the return of troops from southeast Asia and the extension of tourism into endemic areas is a reminder that we must be aware of disease on a global basis.

In 630 A.D., the concept of a sanitary zone was established by the diocese of Cahors by Gallus. Armed guards were placed at all points of entry to prohibit movement. The knight hospitallers of the order of St. John of Jerusalem were the first to adopt

The authors wish to thank John R. Herbold, D.V.M., M.P.H., Ph.D.; Paul H. Grundy, M.D., M.P.H.; and Dennis D. Pinkovsky, Ph.D. of the Epidemiology Division of the United States Air Force School of Aerospace Medicine for their contributions to this Chapter.

the 40-day quarantine because it was the amount of time Christ was in the wilderness. In Venice, Italy in 1348 A.D., vessels, crews, and passengers were detained for 40 days primarily to guard against plague. The idea caught on throughout Europe in the sixteenth and seventeenth centuries, and the word "quarantine" entered our vocabulary from the Italian word "quanta," which means 40.

Major outbreaks of cholera followed the rapid increase in travel brought about by the new technologies of steamships and railroads. The forerunner to our major international health organizations was brought about by the need of governments to cooperate to control cholera. Quarantine was attempted but was largely unsuccessful. This failure led to the First International Sanitary Conference in Paris in 1851, which was attended by one physician and one diplomat from each of the Two Sicilies, Spain, the Papal States, France, Great Britain, Greece, Portugal, Russia, Sardinia, Tuscany, and Turkey. It agreed on rules of international hygiene and sanitation in international commerce and travel. Over the next 56 years, nine more conferences were held, culminating in the formation of the International Office of Public Health at Paris in 1907. This office was the forerunner to the League of Nations Health Office, which later developed into the World Health Organization (WHO). In 1926, 65 countries were represented at the Thirteenth International Sanitary Conference. The treaty signed that year is the basis for our modern international health laws.

Because of the growing importance of aviation, the first sanitary convention for aerial navigation was held in 1933. It used the existing international maritime laws as a model but modified them to suit the 1933 flying environment. The convention addressed such problems as disinfection, medical inspection, and infectious disease control. It formulated a detailed code to prevent the spread of yellow fever, including methods to eliminate the vector, Aedes aegypti. This convention was the forerunner of the WHO Committee on Hygiene and Sanitation in Aviation, which now is responsible for the formulation of guidelines protecting the international community from the importation of disease by military or civilian aircraft. Social and technologic developments have increased the number of people moving from place to place and reduced travel times from weeks to hours, but the population dynamics of disease transmission have remained substantially unchanged.

Impact of Air Travel

Prior to the age of air travel, incubation periods for many diseases were shorter than transit times; thus, epidemic diseases usually were evident during transport or upon arrival at the port of entry, where quarantine measures could be imposed. Unfortunately, with modern high-speed, large-volume air travel, illnesses often develop after rather than during travel, decreasing the probability of a diagnosis being made and of recognizing the epidemic potential. Also, the shorter travel times have reduced the significance of geographic separation as an effective barrier to disease transmission. These factors, combined with the large number of international travelers, make the control of communicable disease a difficult and complex task.

Air travel has been implicated in the transmission of diseases of nearly every etiology. The potential for the transmission of vector-borne diseases is significant because receptive vectors and susceptible populations for many of these diseases are found throughout the temperate zones. Diseases such as malaria, dengue, and yellow fever have been eliminated in many areas, but the reintroduction of these diseases by infected patients or vectors could easily occur. Animal carriers of diseases such as rabies and Marburg virus are also of concern to public health authorities.

Person-to-person transmitted diseases are as great a threat now as ever despite antibiotic therapies. Epidemics of cholera and other highly infectious diseases can be spread far beyond their traditional endemic areas with ease. The movement of refugee populations from southeast Asia, Central America, the Caribbean, and southwestern Asia poses a major disease threat to populations in resettlement areas. The arrival of thousands of Cuban refugees in the United States in the summer of 1980 held the potential for significant disease problems. The refugees were monitored very closely after arrival to identify any significant health problems that might be transmissible. Fortunately, these refugees were in reasonably good health, unlike many of the southeast Asian refugees. If the influx of refugees from Cuba had taken place during 1981, extensive transmissions of dengue fever might have occurred in the southeastern United States because a large outbreak of this disease swept Cuba in that year. Major outbreaks of viral keratoconjunctivitis occurred on the island of Guam in 1975 after the arrival of Asian refugees. Fears of epidemic dengue also stimulated major public health programs on that island, including unnecessary aerial applications of pesticides to control mosquito vectors.

The movement of foodstuffs by airlift presents the very real possibility of transporting contaminated foods that could directly cause illness. Likewise, insect-infested cargo easily could introduce economically significant pests to new areas, thereby severely reducing agricultural productivity and contributing to malnutrition and subsequent disease.

The role of aircraft in disease transmission can be reduced by focusing on three primary factors: people, vectors, and cargo. These elements are addressed in the international health regulations prepared by the WHO and have been endorsed by most nations. These regulations frequently are updated to reflect the changing char-

acter of endemic and epidemic diseases. With the successful eradication of smallpox in 1976, this disease was removed from the list of quarantinable diseases, and by January, 1983, the requirement for vaccination was dropped by all but one country (Chad). The remaining quarantinable diseases are plague, cholera, and yellow fever. Various nations have established immunization requirements against specific diseases. Although many of these restrictions are generated by medical and public health concerns, political and cultural motives often come into play. An annual summary of these requirements and periodic updates are published by the Centers for Disease Control (CDC) in Atlanta, Georgia. It is not our intent in this chapter to review all diseases that have been associated with aircraft transportation, but several illustrative cases will be outlined.

DISEASES SPREAD FROM PERSON TO PERSON

Cholera

Historically, the spread of cholera has followed passenger traffic routes, and major advances in transportation technology have contributed to pandemics. Prior to 1860, transportation over the old land caravan routes was slow enough to allow most epidemics to die out during the trip. The pandemic of the 1860s, however, was due in large part to the advent of the steamship, which allowed an increased number of pilgrims to travel to and from Mecca far more quickly. Similarly, the spread of cholera within the United States in 1866 and later was rapid and geographically followed the newly built railways.

Pandemic cholera continued in the late 1890s with a pattern of spread along the old land routes out of India. An outbreak associated with a pilgrimage to Mecca in 1902 devastated Egypt, with 34,000 deaths in 3 months. The pandemic then spread into most of Europe, following sea lanes. From 1904 until 1923, Europe experienced recurrent waves of cholera. Due to rapid diagnosis, isolation of cases at ports of entry, and improved sanitation, this pandemic failed to spread into Great Britain or the United States.

The next cholera pandemic was the El Tor biotype, which began in Indonesia in 1961. El Tor had been endemic in the Celebes islands of Indonesia since 1937, but from 1961 to 1962, this strain spread into neighboring island groups along traditional sea routes. It became clear that El Tor cholera was being transported by air as well as by sea routes when clusters of cases developed around both airports and seaports throughout much of the western Pacific. By early 1963, the transportation of cholera by air had clearly occurred in Thailand, Vietnam, Cambodia, Japan, and Korea. Air travel also was suspected as a contributing factor in outbreaks of cholera in India, Pakistan, and the Philippines. By 1965, the WHO was concerned enough about the air importation of cholera to publish the numbers of cases occurring in Asian cities serviced by international airlines. In May, 1970, El Tor cholera made a leap from the eastern Mediterranean to Guinea, West Africa. Although the index case was never identified, it was believed that the disease was translocated by aircraft.[1] Guinea was subsequently the focal point for the spread of cholera throughout most of sub-Saharan Africa. Within several months of the Guinea outbreak, the disease spread to the Ivory Coast, either by air or sea route, and inland throughout West Africa. By 1971, 22 countries were infected, with 69,000 cases of cholera reported.

Not only has the airplane been implicated in the transport of passengers who have become the index cases for major outbreaks but aircraft effluent also has been implicated as the possible source of sporadic outbreaks of cholera throughout central and western Europe between 1970 and 1975. When outbreaks were mapped, the areas corresponded to the major air routes

from Calcutta into Europe.[2] Although it has never been proven conclusively that this was the cause of the European outbreaks, this hypothesis has received widespread support and is assumed by some authorities to be the cause of the outbreaks.

Generally, outbreaks of cholera caused by air transportation have occurred in areas with poor sanitary conditions. The outbreaks that occurred in Japan and Europe in the 1960s and 1970s, however, suggest that even communities with good sanitation practices are not totally protected from air-transported cholera if public health policies and standards are relaxed.

Penicillinase-Producing Neisseria Gonorrhoeae

Because of the nature of transmission of gonorrhea and other venereal diseases, exposure has occurred immediately before, during, and immediately after flight. The rapid worldwide spread of penicillinase-producing Neisseria gonorrhoeae (PPNG) underscores the reality of the key role of air transportation in the translocation of a disease. The PPNG represents a new variant of an old disease with clear clinical and laboratory markers that facilitate historical tracing. Throughout its brief existence, PPNG has caused medical, social, and political ramifications on an international scale.

In early 1976, almost simultaneous reports from the United States and Great Britain described the isolation of a PPNG strain. The London variant was traced to air travelers returning from the coast of West Africa, whereas the Far East strain originated from the Philippines. Both strains contained plasmids responsible for the mediation of beta-lactamase, an enzyme that inactivates penicillin. A joint epidemiologic investigation by the United States Air Force School of Aerospace Medicine and CDC authorities quickly established that the prevalence of PPNG among male cases and female hostess cases approached 40% in the areas of Clark Air Base and Subic Bay Naval Air Station, Luzon, Philippines. Concurrent surveys in Manila showed substantially lower prevalence rates, suggesting that the origin of PPNG strain was related to United States military centers. United States Naval personnel did not become involved in the importation cycle because the vast majority of them returned to the United States by ship. A review of the Air Force clinical records suggested that PPNG activity began in December, 1975 and climbed slowly until its discovery. By mid-1976, over 50 PPNG cases had been diagnosed in numerous aerial ports in and around the western Pacific. Information on diagnostic techniques and therapeutic regimens was provided to all national and international health officials. As the PPNG prevalence rate in airmen stationed in the Philippines rose to 70%, stringent control measures were applied to reduce importation to surrounding countries and the United States. Only moderate success was achieved, however, because of the combined factors of inapparent male cases, subclinical female cases, incubating cases, early treatment failures, and late exposures, all of which were transported by military and commercial aircraft to distant points before diagnosis.

From 1977 through 1979, the number of PPNG cases reported in the United States remained relatively constant at 200 to 300 per year. Over half the cases were directly or indirectly linked to an origin in the western Pacific. Case contact tracing procedures and epidemiologic investigations of numerous, small outbreaks revealed that the PPNG strain spontaneously and inexplicably lost its beta-lactamase encoded plasmid early in the communicable chain. In spite of this feature, 1099 cases were reported in the United States in 1980, 2734 cases were reported in 1981, and over 4000 cases were reported in 1982. During 1980 to 1982, specific metropolitan surveillance programs demonstrated a marked decrease in the proportion of cases that could be linked to overseas travel, clearly indicating that indigenous foci had been established in the United States. Plasmid analyses of selected isolates showed that the vast majority were of the Asian profile.

The PPNG experience in Great Britain has paralleled that of the United States. The PPNG strain was a minor problem from 1976 to 1979, but a marked increase in cases was evident from 1980 to 1982. By 1981, imported cases to Great Britain originated not only from West Africa and the western Pacific but also from endemic foci from the Netherlands and the United States. In the Netherlands, the proportion of imported cases rapidly declined from 85% in 1976 to 1977 to 11% in 1979. The corresponding rise in locally acquired PPNG cases implied that prolonged, sustained transmission of PPNG occurred in the Netherlands soon after the strain was first imported.

In Korea, PPNG did not pose a significant problem from 1976 to 1980. Almost all cases were imported by military personnel traveling on military aircraft originating from the Philippines. Vigorous case contact tracing, treatment, and follow-up test of cultures by Korean and United States military public health officials prevented the establishment of endemic foci. In late 1980 and early 1981, however, the number of PPNG cases climbed dramatically. Culture prevalence studies revealed PPNG rates ranging from 20 to 55% in Air Force and Army cases. In 1982, at the recommendation of the CDC, all United States military medical services began using spectinomycin as the primary therapy for acute gonorrhea. By December, 1982, 30 military cases of spectinomycin-resistant gonorrhea had been reported from Korea and the Philippines, presumably as a result of selective pressure exerted by the widespread use of that antibiotic. Laboratory studies indicated that the mechanism of resistance was intrinsic (single-step chromosomal mutation) and not plasmid-mediated. Sustained transmission of the spectinomycin-resistant strain represents a shift in the dynamics of this age-old disease and clearly introduces a new dimension to its proper control.

By 1982, PPNG had been identified in 44 countries and was clearly worldwide in its distribution. The inability to identify PPNG in any country is likely a matter of clinical surveillance and laboratory capability rather than a reflection of the true absence of PPNG. The dilemma of multiple antibiotic resistance patterns generated by two distinct genetic events indicates that the successful control of gonorrhea will pose a significant public health challenge for many years to come. Constantly impacting these public health control efforts will be the rapid worldwide translocation of new gonorrhea strains by modern aircraft.

Influenza

Epidemiologic mapping of recent influenza epidemics points toward the aircraft as being a major factor in the rapid global spread of new viral strains. Although the aircraft is known to be an efficient "vector" of influenza, on rare occasions it has been demonstrated to be the focal environment of a disease outbreak. In 1977, 38 of 53 (72%) interviewed passengers and crewmembers of an Alaskan flight subsequently became ill with influenza A/Texas (H3N2).[3] The index case was identified as a young woman who developed acute respiratory symptoms 15 minutes after boarding the aircraft. The flight aborted because of mechanical difficulty, and most passengers remained on board for more than 3 hours. A nonfunctioning ventilation system, close proximity of the passengers, and low ambient humidity were felt to be contributing factors to the high attack rate. Within 1 week following the incident, a 20% secondary attack rate was discovered among the household contacts of the passengers.

The influenza A/USSR (H1N1) pandemic of 1978 underscored the transmission speed of influenza in contemporary times. In December, 1977, the Soviet Minister of Health notified the WHO that widespread influenza outbreaks had occurred in the Soviet Union. By mid-December, 1977, additional reports of influenza A/USSR activity were made from Hong Kong, Taiwan, and Finland. A later report by the Peoples Republic of China to the WHO suggested that the strain had originated from northern China and had been circulating since May, 1977. In early January, 1978, influenza A/USSR was confirmed in United States Air Force personnel stationed at Royal Air Force Base, Upper Heyford, Great Britain. An Air Force epidemiologic investigation of the Upper Heyford outbreak revealed that all patients were younger than age 25 (consistent with the fact that H1N1 had last circulated during 1947 to 1957) and that the clinical morbidity was sufficient to compromise flying operations. Peculiarly, the outbreak appeared to be initially isolated to the air base at Upper Heyford and surrounding communities. Strongly suspected, but never confirmed, was the transmission of the virus from the Soviet Union to Upper Heyford by means of popular tourist flights by Air Force personnel from Gatwick International Airport to Moscow and Leningrad.

Within 2 weeks of the Upper Heyford outbreak, influenza A/USSR was detected in the United States. A sharp outbreak in a Cheyenne, Wyoming high school reaffirmed the age distribution and morbidity of the H1N1 strain. Almost simultaneous to the Cheyenne episode was an outbreak at F.E. Warren Air Force Base, Wyoming, adjacent to Cheyenne. It is interesting to note that Royal Air Force Base, Upper Heyford, Great Britain and F.E. Warren Air Force Base, Wyoming both contain personnel with common skills and backgrounds and share staff elements that possibly could have been responsible for seeding the H1N1 strain so rapidly into a relatively remote section of the United States. By early February, 1978, influenza A/USSR had spread to other schools and universities in Wyoming and Colorado. At the United States Air Force Academy in Colorado Springs, Colorado, influenza A/USSR caused a particularly severe epidemic that afflicted 76% of the 4300 cadets within 12 days. By March, 1978, 16 other United States Air Force bases had reported substantial influenza activity, and by the end of the influenza season, influenza A/USSR activity had been confirmed in 19 areas of the United States and at least 13 countries in Asia and eastern Europe.

Thus, in less than 12 months, a new antigenic variant of influenza had been distributed throughout the population bulk of the world. Had an H1N1 or an influenza A/USSR-like strain not previously circulated in the 1950s and conferred demonstrable immunity to the now middle-aged and elderly population, the mortality consequences could have been devastating.

The repetitive propagation of influenza A virus in a population rests with its ability to periodically alter its hemagglutinin (H) and neuraminadase (N) genes. These genetic changes, or antigenic "drifts," are largely the result of forced selective pressures exerted by an immune population. Only when the viral antigenicity has changed sufficiently to avert the cancellation effect of conferred immunity will a "new" strain emerge and become clinically and epidemiologically significant. Perhaps a related mechanism for the production of influenza variants is the process of dual infection with a resulting hybrid or recombinant strain. The 1978 influenza season was remarkable in this regard because three distinct influenza strains (A/Victoria, H3N2; A/Texas, H3N2, and A/USSR, H1N1) were circulating simultaneously, causing substantial morbidity in the same regions of the United

States, and documented dual infections occurred with probable hybridization (H3N1).[4] If this process is important in the mutation and survival of influenza, it is clear that the frequency of genetic change may be dependent on the number of active co-circulating strains. Thus, the role of strain translocation by aircraft, when coupled with the improving international communication with the Peoples Republic of China, may have more epidemiologic significance in the future.

Rubella and Rubeola

In recent years, many imported cases of rubella and rubeola have resulted in secondary transmission. During the first 39 weeks of 1982, 96 cases of measles were imported to the United States and resulted in 278 secondary cases. These 374 cases accounted for nearly one third of all measles cases in this country during that time period. In 1978, a 2-year-old child contracted measles in a child-care center in Australia. He arrived in Utah by air while still in the incubation phase and was the index case for six cases of measles in a child-care center outbreak in Salt Lake City. In 1979, a child arriving from Vietnam became ill with rubeola 3 days after arrival and was the index case for nine additional cases.

The spread of rubella and rubeola among recruits has been a major problem for the military. Young adults arrive at centralized training centers from many different areas of the country and often travel by air. Upon arrival, they are placed into an environment that is extremely conducive to the person-to-person transmission of disease: large numbers of susceptible hosts, physical and emotional stress, and close living conditions. Nearly one in five United States Air Force trainees is susceptible to rubella.[5] Prior to 1977, these recruits were exposed to naturally circulating rubella virus in the early weeks of basic training and subsequently developed clinical disease. Secondary trans-

mission occurred among other newly arriving trainees. In the mid-1970s, repeated
outbreaks of rubella also occurred at Air
Force advanced training bases and in surrounding civilian communities after infected trainees arrived by air. In response
to these outbreaks, the Air Force instituted
a program to screen all incoming recruits
for susceptibility to rubella in 1977 and
for susceptibility to rubeola in 1978. All
susceptible males and nonpregnant females were then immunized. Since that
time, no outbreaks of these infections have
been traced to Air Force military recruit
populations.

Lassa Fever

Lassa fever, a disease endemic to the
northern parts of Sierra Leone, Liberia,
and Nigeria, is almost synonymous with
the fear of the international transportation
of highly fatal diseases. The prototype of
the African hemorrhagic fevers, Lassa
fever is highly infectious, pathogenic, and
virulent. Lassa fever is characterized by
high fever, myalgia, weakness, headache,
cough, nausea, vomiting, and chest and
abdominal pains. Although this constellation of symptoms may be unusual and
diagnostic when the symptoms are fully
developed, the complex may be very nonspecific in the early stages of illness and
can be readily confused with many other
infectious and noninfectious diseases.
Hemorrhagic signs occur during the second week of illness and range from petechial skin lesions to severe respiratory and
gastrointestinal hemorrhage. The fatality
rate for this disease varies from 30 to 50%
in hospitalized patients, although serologic surveys in Sierra Leone, West Africa
have found inapparent or mild infections
to be common among the indigenous populations of the endemic areas.

The disease is caused by one of the ar-
enaviruses and was first recognized in
three villagers in Lassa, Nigeria in 1962.[6]
In 1969, a missionary nurse was the index
case for a hospital-based outbreak, which

resulted in a high mortality rate among the
hospital staff in Jos, Nigeria. This episode
captured the attention of the media worldwide. The virus is maintained in a wild
rodent reservoir and is spread to humans
through contact with urine. Endemic
Lassa fever is considered to be a zoonotic
disease, but in epidemic situations its primary mode of transmission is person to
person. Transmission can occur through
contact, droplet, and aerosol exposures to
human blood and other body fluids. The
incubation period is 7 to 21 days, and patients should be considered to be infectious from the febrile period to 8 weeks
after clinical recovery. The public health
impact of Lassa fever is substantial because of its high case-fatality ratio and
transmissibility. These factors and the expanding "adventure" tourist trade make
Lassa fever and the other hemorrhagic fevers significant international health concerns. Five patients with Lassa fever have
been unknowingly transported by air, thus
potentially exposing fellow travelers. A
number of preclinical cases of Lassa fever
have been imported to the United States
on commercial air carriers, and at least two
secondary cases, including one death, also
have occurred as a result of air travel.

The role of air travel in the transmission
of disease has been established, but not as
well appreciated is the lifesaving role of
aircraft in the prompt treatment of infected
individuals. The emergency airlift of medical equipment and personnel to epidemic
sites has been essential in minimizing the
effects of these outbreaks. Patients can be
rapidly transported by air to sophisticated
medical care facilities if strict isolation
precautions are taken. These precautions
include the use of the Vickers isolation
chamber or similar devices that permit full
patient care while affording total protection from environmental contamination.
Such a capability, complete with a medical staff, is available from the CDC in Atlanta, Georgia, the Laboratory Centre for
Disease Control in Ottawa, Canada, and

within the United States Air Force air evacuation system from Scott Air Force Base in Illinois.

FOODBORNE DISEASE

Popular theatrical and literary portrayals of an incapacitating outbreak of "food poisoning" aboard a commercial airliner have suggested that these relatively rare events are common occurrences. Although infrequent, an epidemic of foodborne intoxication or infection on board an in-transit aircraft will present logistic and diagnostic challenges not encountered elsewhere. An etiologic diagnosis is often required to rule out the presence of an exotic or quarantinable disease; however, adequate personnel, supplies, and facilities are rarely available to diagnose and treat large numbers of patients. Epidemiologic investigations are complicated by inadequate passenger manifests and the rapid dispersion of passengers after landing. In actuality, once a major quarantinable disease such as cholera is excluded, extensive follow-up investigations are uncommon.

Although most food preparation practices of airline caterers provide bacteriologically safe foods, improper refrigeration or hot-holding of foods can and has contributed to outbreaks of foodborne disease.[7] Clostridium perfringens was implicated in an outbreak affecting eight separate flights leaving from a southeastern United States air terminal. Although 394 persons were at risk, only 18 passengers and 62 crewmembers could be contacted for follow-up investigation, highlighting the difficulty of identifying the true incidence of food-related disease associated with air transportation. Twenty-two of the 62 crewmembers contacted reported illness characterized by diarrhea, nausea, and abdominal cramps. Turkey dinners prepared earlier from whole turkeys that were precooked, frozen, thawed at room temperature, sliced, and then held at 54° C on board were shown epidemiologically to be the source of the illness.

Food was implicated as the vehicle of a Vibrio cholerae outbreak among aircraft passengers in 1972. The apparent lack of enforcement of accepted international standards for the control and surveillance of foodborne diseases aboard aircraft contributed to the outbreak.[8] In 1973, an outbreak of foodborne staphylococcal intoxication on three separate civilian flights was traced to meals prepared by a single caterer. Illness was experienced by 28 to 84% of the passengers on these flights. First-class passengers and crewmembers had received different meals without the suspect food (custard dessert), and none became ill. In 1975, 197 of 344 passengers (57%) aboard a chartered commercial flight and one of 20 crewmembers experienced symptomatology consistent with staphylococcal food poisoning. This outbreak, the largest reported aboard a single aircraft, was traced to ham contaminated by Staphylococcus aureus from an inflamed finger lesion of a cook. Documented mishandling of the food product over a prolonged period of time permitted growth of the organism and enterotoxin production.[9] A flight from Rio de Janeiro, Brazil to New York in 1976 was diverted to San Juan, Puerto Rico because 16 passengers experienced gastrointestinal illness shown to be caused by chocolate eclairs contaminated with high levels of S. aureus.

Aircraft-related foodborne disease can be classified by the type of flight it will most likely be associated with: in-flight domestic (1- to 4-hour flights), in-flight international (6 to 20 hours), and postflight outbreaks. Two factors usually determine the classification of an etiologic agent: the elapsed time between food preparation and consumption and the incubation period between ingestion and the onset of clinical illness. Chemical and preformed toxin-related illness, such as staphylotoxicosis, usually occur shortly after consumption of the contaminated meal and thus could be observed on short-duration flights. S. aureus, usually linked to ham, meat salads, and custards, has a clinical incubation period of 2 to 4 hours, with a range of 30 minutes to 8 hours. These outbreaks must be differentiated from motion-induced and psychosomatic-related nausea and vomiting. The communicability of vomiting, particularly in enclosed quarters, is well recognized. Longer flights may be associated with both short and intermediate incubation agents, best exemplified by Clostridium perfringens and Bacillus cereus. These intoxication illnesses have incubation ranges of 9 to 16 hours and 2 to 16 hours, respectively. B. cereus is a contaminant of vegetables and grains and is usually associated with boiled or fried rice. C. perfringens intoxication is associated with meat, poultry, and gravy and presents clinically as a complex of abdominal cramps and diarrhea. For extended flights, it is possible that foodborne infections with Vibrio parahaemolyticus, Shigella species, and Salmonella species may be observed on board or at the airport.

The involvement of crewmembers in an outbreak affecting passengers is confounded by several factors. Civilian pilots of domestic flights are paid per diem and usually eat before the flight or "brown bag" lunch; however, meals are available to them on board. Crewmembers on longer international flights are more likely to share the same meals as passengers, but with limits on flight time, crews are charged at intermediate stops, and do not experience the extended flight times and multiple meals of the "Manila to Brussels" passenger. United States military aircrews and passengers commonly share meals from the same source, in-flight kitchens, but the adherence to safe food preparation and storage sanitary standards is considered to be better in this restricted and controlled environment.

The prevention of enteric disease transmission among passengers and crew is best achieved by the strict application of hygiene standards and procedures. Basic principles of food preparation and serving must be followed to ensure that contamination of food does not occur. Similarly, the integrity of the potable water sources and onboard storage and distribution systems must be maintained. Proper handling and disposal of human wastes from aircraft also must be assured, including adequate facilities and supplies for the maintenance of personal hygiene. Although outbreaks on board aircraft can dramatically affect large numbers of passengers and could conceivably incapacitate the aircrew, there are no statutory or policy requirements for the pilot and the copilot to consume different meals or the same meals at different times.

The movement of manufactured food products by aircraft presents the very real possibility of the widespread dispersal of contaminated food. In 1973, raw cocoa beans most likely imported from Ghana arrived in Canada contaminated with Salmonella eastbourne. While the beans were being sorted and cleaned at a Canadian chocolate factory, bean dust cross-contaminated the final product. Christmas chocolate balls from this factory were identified as the source of a major international foodborne outbreak, with cases identified in 23 states in the United States and seven Canadian provinces over 4 months. In addition to inadvertent food contamination, misuse of agricultural products, such as chemically treated seed grains not intended for human consumption, has been documented.[10] It is conceivable that aircraft support of disaster relief operations could contribute to the widespread distribution of inedible products that, owing to misunderstanding, are consumed as food.

VECTOR-BORNE DISEASE

The control of insect-infested cargo and aircraft also is accomplished through international regulation and cooperation. There are numerous documented instances where insect pests or vectors of disease have been introduced by man into new areas. Many insect pests have an indirect effect on health by their adverse impact on the agricultural production of foodstuffs. The Hessian fly, a destructive pest of wheat, was accidently introduced during the American Revolutionary War, and the gypsy moth was purposefully brought to the United States in 1869 to improve silk production. Today, the larvae of the gypsy moth cause significant defoliation over more than 8 million acres of forest in the northeastern United States. Insect vectors of pathogens directly affect the health of man an other animals. Aedes albopictus, and important vector of dengue and chikungunya fevers in the Orient, was found in water in surplus military tires being returned from the western Pacific area to west coast United States surface ports.

Although malaria is normally considered an insect-borne illness, there have been person-to-person cases of this disease introduced into the United States and western Europe. In 1978, a malaria death was reported to the CDC. The individual had received a blood transfusion from a donor who had recently traveled abroad. In the 1960s, a minor outbreak of malaria was reported in Fresno, California among drug abusers. The index case was a soldier who had recently returned from southeast Asia. In an earlier instance in northern California in 1952, a Korean War veteran suffered a relapse of vivax malaria while on a weekend camping trip at a popular outdoor recreation area. He was subsequently responsible for at least 35 cases of malaria among a group of Campfire Girls who camped in the same area some weeks later.[11] This episode serves as a reminder to all medical care providers that a high index of suspicion must be maintained when dealing with individuals who have recently traveled or who have been in contact with other travelers.

A sevenfold increase in the varieties of mosquito species was noted on Guam from 1936 to 1972. Air traffic and seagoing vessels were implicated as the reason for this increase. The history of explosive, nonrepetitive outbreaks of dengue, Japanese B encephalitis, and malaria on Guam may be due to a population of infected individuals or arthropod vectors arriving on the island.[12] Air travel can facilitate the rapid and widespread distribution of vectors and pests. During the 1970s, termite-infested cargo from the Philippines and Thailand frequently was intercepted at McClellan and Travis Air Force Bases in California. The continuing threat to United States agricultural crops posed by the introduction of land snails from Europe and the Far East underscores the necessity to inspect all returning motor vehicles, other cargo, and household goods shipments. Infestations of the devastating stored grain pest, the Khapra beetle, were discovered in at least 19 United States warehouses and burlap bag establishments in 1981. The beetles were traced to commodities imported from the Middle East.

The detection and elimination of exotic pests on or in cargo is paramount in preventing the transfer of pests and disease vectors between geographically separated land masses. A program that includes the maintenance of clean cargo holding areas, preclearance, inspection, and the treatment of cargo prior to shipment is necessary. The surveillance and control of mosquitoes and other vectors around cargo marshalling areas and flight lines and the proper isolation, treatment, and disposal of galley and other wastes are also important aspects of this program. The application of insecticide aerosols or micronized dusts inside aircraft to kill mosquitoes and other insects of public health or economic significance is also a vital aspect of quarantine operations. WHO guidelines specify procedures for the disinsection of passenger and cargo compartments in affected areas, in flight, and upon arrival in unaffected areas. Individual countries and agencies selectively apply these recommendations, however. D-phenothrin (2%) aerosol is currently used in aircraft disinsection by or under the direction of state or federal personnel for the control of public health and agricultural pests. United States Air Force regulations task the military aircraft commander with ensuring that disinsection is accomplished with all passengers and crew on board just before the last takeoff prior to entering the United States or its possessions from a foreign port between 35° N and 35° S latitude and before entering foreign countries with disinsection requirements as specified in the United States Air Force Foreign Clearance Guides. The United States Public Health Service requires disinsection only for international flights arriving from areas where there is active vector-borne transmission in the vicinity of the port of embarkation. When disinsection is required, it is to be accomplished after all passengers and crewmembers have disembarked and prior to the removal of mail, baggage, or other cargo. Proper disinsection prior to departure from endemic areas provides a safe environment for the air evacuation of patients suffering from arboviral or rickettsial diseases as well as malaria.

A complete insect inspection and quarantine program should include trained inspectors with knowledge of agricultural and public health pests of international significance; the conscientious inspection of all freight, baggage, cabins, and holds; appropriate insecticidal or other treatment of infested materials and areas; and proper coordination with national and international regulatory authorities.

The movement of exotic and domestic animals between nations, both developed and developing, is extensive. The introduction of foreign zoonotic diseases compounds the diagnostic and logistic challenges facing public health officials. Quarantine restrictions of varying lengths

are imposed on animals moving from enzootic rabies areas to rabies-free areas, particularly the island nations and states, for example, of Great Britain, Australia, Japan, and Hawaii. Another emerging problem is the transportation of diseased livestock from developed nations to both developed and developing nations. In 1980 and 1981, shipment of United States cattle and sheep to the European Common Market was halted because the United States cattle were infected with blue tongue, an arthropod-borne virus enzootic to North America. The continued expansion of trade between nations and the use of air transport will extend the spectrum of disease entities of concern to agricultural, health, and trade officials.

FUTURE DEVELOPMENTS

Changes in the disease threat can be expected. Epidemic diseases are being eliminated in developed countries. Many of these "obsolete" diseases, however, remain active in less well-developed areas of the world and could reemerge among susceptible individuals and populations at any time. This process is best exemplified by the well-documented reintroduction of smallpox to areas by air prior to its eradication in 1978. In 1947, this scenario caused 12 secondary cases of smallpox that resulted in two deaths and $6 million in public health expenditures in New York. In 1963, a sailor left his ship in Australia and flew home to Stockholm, Sweden through Indonesia, India, and Pakistan. He was mildly ill with smallpox on arrival in Stockholm and was the index case for 26 secondary cases with five deaths. Although the airplane is well documented to have been an instrument in the spread of smallpox, the eradication of smallpox from the world would most likely have been impossible without the aid of air transportation, to move teams rapidly into remote areas when new cases were discovered. In the event that smallpox organisms are released from the laboratory environment or are reintroduced by biologic warfare, air transportation will surely play a role in the rapid transmission of this feared disease to all parts of the world.

New diseases and variants of old diseases also are being recognized. The transmission of influenza, PPNG, Lassa fever, and other diseases can be enhanced by modern air travel. Continued improvements in the technology of air travel are forecast. The speed of travel and the volume of people and cargo will only increase the risk of disease transmission. Tourism to formerly remote and isolated regions will expose greater numbers of susceptible individuals to disease, as will the increasing number of political and economic refugees. As cargo management shifts from the sea-lanes to the air lanes, more ports of entry will be available for the worldwide movement of goods. Thus, the potential for the intermingling of susceptible hosts and agents of disease in a favorable environment will continue to expand.

The effects of space travel and exploration on disease patterns also must be considered. Although the risk of encountering hazardous life forms during foreseeable space explorations may be remote, the effect of the physiologic stresses of prolonged spaceflight on incubating infectious diseases, latent infections, and commensal saprophytic microflora merit particular attention. The long-term effects of prolonged spaceflight on the immunologic system and the response of the human organism to the challenge of even common diseases are not yet fully understood. Just as diseases were transported between the "old world" and the new by the fifteenth- and sixteenth-century explorers, we must be aware of the potential risk of transporting disease-producing organisms with our interplanetary explorations.

REFERENCES

1. Barua, D.: Cholera. Proc. Roy. Soc. Med., 65:423–432, 1972.
2. Randle, C.J.M., et al.: Cholera: Possible infection from aircraft effluent. J. Hyg. (London), 81(3):361–371, 1978.
3. Moser, M.R., et al.: An outbreak of influenza aboard a commercial airliner. Am. J. Epidemiol., 110(1):1–6, 1979.
4. Kendal, A.P., et al.: Laboratory-based surveillance of influenza viruses in the United States during the winter of 1977–1978. Am. J. Epidemiol., 110(4):462–468, 1979.
5. Blouse, L.E., et al.: Rubella screening and vaccination program for United States Air Force trainees: An analysis of findings. Am. J. Public Health, 72(3):280–283, 1982.
6. Frame, J.D., Baldwin, J.M., and Gocke, D.J.: Lassa fever, a new virus disease of man from West Africa. I. Clinical description and pathological findings. Am. J. Trop. Med. Hyg., 19:670, 1970.
7. Bryan, F.L., et al: Time-temperature observations of food and equipment in airline catering operations. J. Food Protect., 41(2):80–92, 1978.
8. Sutton, R.G.A.: An outbreak of cholera in Australia due to food served in flight on an international aircraft. J. Hyg. (London), 72:441–451, 1974.
9. Eisenberg, M.S.: Staphylococcal food poisoning aboard a commercial aircraft. Lancet, II:595–599, 1975.
10. Derban, L.K.A.: Outbreak of food poisoning due to alkyl-mercury fungicide. Arch. Environ. Health, 28:49–52, 1974.
11. Brunetti, R., Fritz, R.F., and Hollister, A.C., Jr.: An outbreak of malaria in California, 1952–1953. Am. J. Trop. Med. Hyg., 3:779–788, 1954.
12. Nowell, W.R.: International quarantine for control of mosquito-borne diseases on Guam. Aviat. Space Environ. Med., 48(1):53–60, 1977.

Chapter *32*

Occupational Medical Support to the Aviation Industry

Robert T.P. deTreville

There are two kinds of certified specialists: Occupational Medicine and Aviation Medicine. Both study man in the environment of his work and the control of that environment for the purpose of the promotion of health, safety and optimum productivity.

ASHE[1]

The work place in the aviation industry incorporates many of the materials, processes, and operations common to manufacturing in general. Airplane repair and maintenance include drilling, riveting, screw fastening, welding, painting, aluminum layout, template work, the subassembly of landing gear, fuselage, wing sections, cowling, and other large units, the placing of motors, engines, propellers, turbines, wing sections, landing gear, electronic and avionic equipment, and the inspection of the plane and equipment and machine tool repair.

The major purposes of this chapter are to help orient those individuals practicing aerospace medicine to the nature and scope of occupational medical responsibilities in the modern aviation industry and to stress the importance of including occupational medicine concepts in providing the aviation industry with cost-effective, high-quality environmental and occupational health services.

It is important for companies of all sizes and types in the aviation industry to keep abreast of and use the latest and best available preventive medical and engineering technology. This technology includes industrial hygiene and occupational medicine, as well as aviation and space physiology and diagnostic clinical sciences. Such assistance is needed to be able to maintain a healthy work force, to satisfy regulations (and the courts), and yet still remain economically viable and able to compete in the international market. In meeting governmental regulations, moving a decimal point one place toward zero often triples the costs of preventive engineering controls. A corporate decision whether to compete often depends on the best possible estimates of toxic hazard control costs, a process requiring considerable skill. To vary on either the high or low side because of error in technique or interpretation becomes costly. Modern industrial management cannot afford to venture into new fields of endeavor and production without the best possible assessment of influences on the work environment, the company's employees, and the entire community. Environmental impact statements may be required prior to governmental approval of major industrial changes and moves. Industrial hygiene consultation to aid management in reaching sound decisions may be available on request from within the company in some cases, but, if not, such assistance can usually be obtained from private consultants in most industrialized states and regions. Specialists in aerospace medicine should develop and maintain sufficient orientation and motivation in the fields of environmental and occupational health to assist their managements in obtaining and using the consultation needed to prevent and solve problems involving potential toxic hazards arising out of planned operations, products, and wastes. In this way, aerospace medicine will better be able to encompass the total program of preventive medicine support to the industry. If not, and this is still far too common, the aviation and occupational medicine programs may exist separately, each concerned only with continuing existing work loads. New health-related problems that are not addressed fully in planning may require much more costly corrective engineering changes at later stages of development. Therefore, it is incumbent on all who intend to be specialists in aerospace medicine to become sufficiently oriented in the preventive aspects of occupational medicine to recognize the need for, and help exercise effective control over, the quality of environmental and occupational health support to their organizations' missions.

The United States Air Force Occupational and Environmental Health Laboratory at Brooks Air Force Base, Texas exemplifies the type of support available on request within a single organization. Although only a few large companies in private industry have developed similar self-sufficiency in as broad an area of coverage, all needs can be satisfied by consulting laboratories and other sources in the private sector.

THE OCCUPATIONAL MEDICINE PROGRAM

With the rise of preventive medicine, occupational medicine has assumed an important role, recognizing as it does that man's health and happiness are affected by many sociologic and environmental influences. Further, the control of the large and ever-increasing list of potential chemical, physical, and biologic hazards of the work place is a matter of growing concern. To the untutored, many of these factors would appear to belong in the field of engineering, but this assumption is invalid. Engineering plans designed to benefit mankind must consider the nature of human anatomy, biochemistry, physiology, and psychology. Likewise, the occupational medicine specialist needs to learn more about the involved engineering principles and control measures before providing professional guidance to management. Such guidance is essential in preventing and controlling problems related to the safety, health, and comfort of the work force, as well as to consumers of the company's products and to the company's neighbors, who may otherwise be adversely affected by industrial wastes finding their way into the air, water, and soil of the surrounding community.

The United States Air Force Preventive Medical Service

The authorization, purpose, and organization of the United States Air Force Preventive Medical Service lists environmental medicine (including public health), occupational medicine, and bioenvironmental engineering (including industrial hygiene), along with flight and missile medicine, as being within the broad field of aerospace medicine. The Directors of Base Medical Services and Chiefs of Flight Medicine at over 100 Air Force bases have all received at least primary training in flight medicine at the United States Air Force School of Aerospace Medicine (USAFSAM). All Air Force bioenvironmental engineers (BEEs) and their assisting technicians also have received formal USAFSAM training in conducting industrial hygiene surveys and environmental quality measurements prior to being assigned to Air Force bases worldwide. The Chiefs of Environmental Medicine who help integrate medical and engineering findings are usually USAFSAM-trained environmental health nurses. At the six largest industrial bases in the Air Force Logistics Command (each having from approximately 12,000 to 25,000 civilian employees), there is a separate Preventive Occupational Medical Service, which is staffed by civilian physicians who are fully qualified in occupational medicine and thoroughly familiar with Civil Service Commission regulations. Thus, within the United States Air Force, there is a full gamut of aviation medical and occupational health specialists.

The United States Air Force Occupational and Environmental Health Laboratory

In support of local capabilities, the United States Air Force Occupational and Environmental Health Laboratory (USAF OEHL) provides professional consultation, specialized laboratory services, and operational field support worldwide to assist the Air Force in meeting its responsibilities in the management of occupational, radiologic, and environmental health programs. To achieve this end, the USAF OEHL is staffed with over 150 military and civilian scientists, chemists, and technicians who are professionally trained and experienced in such diverse fields as agronomy, animal and plant physiology, computer science, all aspects of engineer-

ing, entomology, environmental law, health physics, medicine, medical administration, meteorology, public health, and environmental toxicology. Most of these personnel possess advanced degrees and are recognized and accredited by their respective professional organizations. In addition, the technical assistance of several outside contractors covering many of these areas is utilized to allow needed flexibility in the provision of a wide range of analytic services with minimal delay from backlogs.

With the assistance of the USAF OEHL, physicians and BEEs responsible for providing medical and engineering support to base activities are able to introduce preventive concepts involving the highest level of expertise. Other Department of Defense agencies have their own internal capabilities. The United States Army's Environmental Hygiene Agency is located at Edgewood, Maryland, and the United States Navy's Environmental Health Center is at Norfolk, Virginia.

Industrial Programs

In view of the importance of industrial hygiene measurements and controls to the prevention of potential environmental and occupational hazards in private industry, many larger companies have developed capabilities similar to those that exist in the USAF OEHL, with teams composed of analytic chemists, physicists, engineers, toxicologists, nurses, and industrial physicians, each specialist applying his own skills to combat industrial health problems. Smaller companies may rely chiefly on the comprehensive knowledge of an individual industrial hygienist, who keeps abreast in his specialty and related fields through continuing educational programs conducted by appropriate academic, scientific, and governmental institutions.

Benefits of an Occupational Medicine Program

From management's point of view, the most valuable asset in industry is its trained work force. Hence, when the health of these people is protected by sound occupational medical and industrial hygiene techniques, industry is protecting its own investment. Some other benefits to be derived include:

1. Showing management's concern, hence improving the corporate image
2. Enhancing the productivity and retention of the work force
3. Reducing the costs of workmen's compensation insurance
4. Lowering the costs of health and disability insurance
5. Eliminating environmentally related complaints, thus improving both labor and customer relations
6. Producing "spin-off" state-of-the-art benefits related to improved instrumentation, computerization, and automation of data on environmental contamination and the health of exposed workers
7. Providing internal intelligence on company operations and products, allowing the self-initiated correction of faulty planning and design
8. Assuring a necessary bridge between the medical and safety, personnel, and operating departments, thus helping protect the company from spurious claims
9. Serving as the vital link between management and the myriad of government agencies, competitors, associations, legislators, media, and public relations people involved in such environmental matters as air and water quality conservation
10. Using preventive health and safety for the work force to extend programs of health protection and conservation more widely to benefit the industrial community and the public at large

Organization of an Occupational Medicine Program

The overall organization and functioning of occupational medicine programs in industries of all types and sizes, including aviation, is complex and must be adapted to special needs to satisfy the requirements of a specific corporation. The general scope of such a program is outlined in the Table of Contents suggested by Felton for a *Manual for Physicians* working in an industrial medical department.[2]

Professional Organizations

Occupational Medicine

The American Academy of Occupational Medicine (AAOM), founded in 1946, is the professional association for physicians engaged full time in the field of occupational medicine. Fellowship requires board certification.

The primary objective of AAOM is the maintenance and improvement of the health of the industrial worker, with the improvement of occupational efficiency as a corollary. Some 700 physicians participate as members or fellows, representing over 25 countries. Physicians enrolled in approved residency training programs in occupational medicine may become associates, with all the privileges of membership except the rights to vote and hold office. *The Journal of Occupational Medicine* is the official publication of the AAOM. Annual scientific and business meetings are held every fall jointly with a corresponding academy of industrial hygiene specialists.

Industrial Hygiene

The American Academy of Industrial Hygiene (AAIH) represents those individuals certified in the specialty of industrial hygiene by the American Board of Industrial Hygiene (ABIH). Established in 1960 under the joint sponsorship of the AAIH and the American Conference of Governmental Industrial Hygienists (ACGIH), ABIH had certified over 1000 persons following their specialty examination by 1983. The ABIH is presently composed of

13 members and an executive secretary, none of whom is a physician.

Professional Education

The highest professional goals for career-minded physicians in occupational medicine include:

1. Training in occupational medicine, leading to
2. Certification by the American Board of Preventive Medicine in occupational medicine, with consequent
3. Fellowship in the American Academy of Occupational Medicine, and
4. Continuing educational participation with ABIH-certified industrial hygienists in highly technical, professional, and scientific conferences sponsored jointly between the AAOM and AAIH

Some members and fellows of the Aerospace Medical Association, certified by the American Board of Preventive Medicine in aerospace medicine, who are responsible for supporting and/or supervising programs of industrial hygiene in private industry or governmental agencies have successfully taken their examinations in occupational medicine as well. This option should be carefully considered by every aerospace medicine specialist-in-training. For the preventive medical specialists in aerospace occupational medicine practice to participate at a professional level in industrial hygiene activities, an increasingly sophisticated understanding of how to recognize, measure, control, and communicate effectively on public health aspects of environmental pollution problems is required. Management of employee health problems and documentation of adequacy of compliance with Occupational Safety and Health Administration (OSHA) standards are essential to corporate survival. Responsibility for setting sound industrial hygiene policy resides within corporate management at the highest level. To support prop-

erly and supervise such highly technical services requires motivation and educational background on the part of management, encompassing many of the basic occupational and environmental health disciplines (e.g., bioenvironmental engineering, health physics, and toxicology). Occupational physicians and aerospace medical specialists who are not prepared to work within such a broadly based team effort will be limiting their value in program management.

A CASE STUDY

An excellent illustration of industrial hygiene policy development and implementation in support of the aviation and automotive industries' use of tetraethyl lead (TEL) has been given by Dr. Robert A. Kehoe as a model to guide industrial planners.[3] Although dated, this study has clear implications to both the aviation industry and the national defense. Briefly, herewith are some of the fascinating details. An experimental laboratory in Moraine, Ohio, under the direction of Charles F. ("Boss") Kettering of General Motors (inventor of the self-starter), was attempting to find an "antiknock" additive to gasoline that would slow its detonation in the internal combustion engine, increasing octane rating and power while reducing engine weight. A visitor to the Air Force Museum at Wright-Patterson Air Force Base Ohio, can easily see—even from a distance—the great reduction in the size and weight of aviation engines that resulted from the use of leaded aviation gasoline. The maximum amount of TEL was allowed to range as high as 6 cm^3/gal of aviation gasoline to reach the desired octane rating, in contrast to a limit of 4 cm^3/gal for automotive gasoline. Without the use of TEL, Allied Air Forces would have been unable to compete with the German Luftwaffe during World War II. After several thousands of chemicals had been tested, TEL was the only compound found to be technically suitable. Plans were developed to produce larger quantities of TEL and to begin to add it in concentrated form to gasoline on demand at selected service station pumps. At this stage of development, tragedy struck in the form of a new and unexpected occupational illness. This illness was confined to individuals who worked with the organic lead antiknock concentrate prior to its addition to gasoline and to some of those who entered leaded gas storage tanks without adequate protection. Although TEL had been the subject of technical experimentation since its discovery by Lowig in 1852, no cases of poisoning due to it were reported in the literature until October, 1924, some months after the compound began to be manufactured in commercial quantities. The first such report referred to a series of 138 cases, with a 10% mortality rate.

As a result of the belated recognition of this completely new, unexpected, and potent threat to employee and public health, commercial activities were halted voluntarily in 1924 while the Surgeon General of the Public Health Service conducted an extensive investigation. In 1926, when the industry resumed production, it had instituted all the necessary components of a well-developed industrial hygiene program. Procedures were planned carefully on the basis of the results of preliminary toxicologic investigations. Environmental conditions were monitored, along with clinical surveillance of all personnel involved. Range-finding data obtained by conventional toxicologic procedures were not sufficient. Such information needed to be augmented by means of detection and quantitative measurement of the environmental hazard. Even more important, meaningful biologic monitoring was needed to discover and determine the significance of any physiologic and clinical responses of exposed personnel.

In 1924, Mr. Kettering visited the University of Cincinnati's School of Medicine and discussed the TEL problem with Dr. Kehoe, a young medical research fellow who already was engaged in studying the reversibility of changes in enzymes poisoned by lead. Dr. Kehoe agreed to help guide the new industry's efforts to ensure employee and public health protection. This was done by instituting the most nearly absolute controls of TEL environmental and occupational health hazards practicable—controls that were fully successful then and are still in use today.

Epidemiologic Studies in Support of Continued Operations

By the time Dr. Kehoe became involved, some workers had been engaged for over 2 years in jobs involving potential exposure to TEL already mixed in gasoline without any apparent illness or injury. The stage was well set, therefore, for an epidemiologic investigation of the occupational environment and of the workers who had been and continued to be so engaged. In retrospect, the existing situation in 1924 called for the simplest type of toxicologic experimentation, that is, to determine the order of magnitude of the lethal doses of TEL in various animal species as compared with those for inorganic compounds of lead, which were well known. In addition, it was necessary to discover both the avenues and the speed of absorption of TEL. The remainder of the immediate tasks consisted largely of examining the conditions under which workmen had been poisoned, together with those which had failed to cause illness, and of the appraisal, in clinical terms, of the physiologic and pathologic characteristics of the illness to which several men had succumbed and from which a number of men had not fully recovered. Acquisition of this information enabled the industry to proceed continuously with the operation of its business under close medical surveillance and to develop an effective program of industrial hygiene that was designed to meet certain unusual conditions.

The Design of Commercial Operations

The most important principle in the design of commercial operations was the strict limitation of TEL to its intended use as an antiknock agent at low levels of concentration in gasoline. To justify continued commercial development, large quantities must be manufactured, transported to appropriate sites in proper containers, and introduced into gasoline in exact quantities and under stringent hygienic controls. Human contact with, or hazardous exposure to, this toxic material in concentrated, or "neat," form had to be prevented by the use of reliable, tightly fitted equipment and effective, safe, operating procedures. The feasibility of safe control depended on limiting exposure to as few sites as possible and limiting the number of workers, who would be properly instructed and supervised, both technically and medically. Adequate confidence could not be placed either in "labeling" or in the issuance of technical instructions alone. Instead, careful, detailed planning led to the development of a pattern of commercial operations to which the essential hygienic regimen could be applied. Manufacturing activities were concentrated at sites where expert technical, hygienic, and medical facilities and personnel could join in coordinated activities to examine and improve manufacturing processes and equipment and to develop and test supplementary measures of environmental control, as well as occupational health surveillance procedures. Practically speaking, such support can almost never be completely developed in a new industry in advance of industrial production. The best advanced planning is certain to be found lacking in certain places, requiring modifications in practice. Provision must be made, therefore, to seek and detect such faults and to correct them promptly, effectively documenting the adequacy of control.

Careful consideration was given to the problems involved in transporting the concentrated antiknock additive, reducing accidents in transit to a minimum. Educational programs for concerned workers were conducted in advance so that no one would be exposed inadvertently or without understanding the risks and how to avoid them. This aspect of the program required the use of special containers, distinctive labeling, and special handling adapted to rail, ship, and truck transportation. Particular attention was given to the need to transport the concentrated TEL from consignor to consignee without intermediate handling by untrained personnel. Fully informed employees of the consignor were always available to transport personnel if needed, both for advice and for direct assistance. The acceptance and handling of the shipments at their destinations also were dealt with by informed personnel.

Based on similar strategic considerations, management's decision was made early to limit the sale and distribution of antiknock compounds to gasoline refiners and to make every reasonable attempt to keep the number of sites at which the antiknock preparation was to be mixed with gasoline to a minimum. Model mixing equipment was designed by the manufacturers and further developed subsequently to minimize the exposure of mixing personnel to TEL. A regimen of technical supervision of the mixing plants and the medical selection and supervision of the mixing personnel was devised and carried out by the initial distributors of the product: the Ethyl and DuPont corporations. The authority of the technical and medical staff of the distributors to supervise and regulate these operations was provided by contract. This regimen enabled the distributors to follow their antiknock product to its destination and to regulate its handling in strict accordance with the hygienic recommendations of Ethyl's and Dupont's own medical advisers.

Military/Space Emergency Exposure
Limits

The National Academy of Sciences/National Research Council's (NAS/NRC) Committee on Toxicology has published Emergency Exposure Limits (EELs) for ten chemical contaminants, intended for military and space use (Table 32–3).[9]

The Committee on Toxicology dealt only with situations in which brief exposures to high concentrations are possible but unpredictable. By advance calculations of concentrations that can occur following specific accidents, operating rules can be established to regulate the time an exposed person may work before reducing effectiveness by donning respiratory protection or before retreating to safety. Despite sensory stimulation of sufficient degree to be objectionable and to cause definite effects at these levels, healthy workers will not be incapacitated physically or mentally by performing an essential task and may be expected to return to normal following such exposure without needing medical treatment. No worker, however, should be cleared for possible further exposure without certification of full recovery by a well-qualified physician.

Public Exposure Limits

The possibilities of massive spills of missile propellants on the ground, with the need for emergency escape corridor planning, also caused the Environmental Protection Agency (EPA) to recommend reducing to less than one-fifth some of the NAS/NRC EELs to obtain limiting exposures for the unprotected general public (Table 32–4).[10]

Guidance published by the National Institute for Occupational Safety and Health (NIOSH) and the Occupational Safety and Health Administration (OSHA) makes no mention of emergency exposure limits, nor do Federal Aviation Administration (FAA) standards encompass the emergency exposure concept (e.g., for ozone).

Toxicologic Concepts

The slope of the dose-response curve provides useful information. It suggests the magnitude of the range between a no-effect level and a lethal dose, a concept known as the margin of safety. If the dose-response curve is especially steep, the margin of safety is small. In Figure 32–3, substances A and B both have the same LD_{50}, but substance B has a wider margin of safety than substance A.

The agent may be administered orally or by inhalation at different atmospheric levels for a specific time period. The valves calculated are the LD_{50} and the LC_{50} (i.e., the oral dose and atmospheric concentration expected to be lethal to 50% of a group

Table 32–3. Emergency Exposure Limits Recommended to Military and Space Agencies by the Committee on Toxicology, National Research Council

Chemical Contaminant	Parts Per Million		
	60 Minutes	30 Minutes	10 Minutes
Oxygen difluoride	0.1	0.2	0.5
Fluorine	1	2	3
Monomethyl hydrazine	3	7	10
Hydrogen fluoride	8	10	20
Hydrogen chloride	10	20	30
Nitrogen dioxide	10	20	30
Sulfur dioxide	10	20	30
Unsymmetric dimethyl hydrazine	30	50	100
Carbon disulfide	50	100	200
Hydrogen sulfide	50	100	200
Carbon monoxide	400	800	1500

Modified from Smythe, H.F.: Military and space short term inhalation standards. Arch. Environ. Health, *12*:488, 1966.

Table 32–4.   Public Emergency Limits For Nitrogen Dioxide

Duration of Exposure	Amount
10 minutes	5 ppm
30 minutes	3 ppm
60 minutes	2 ppm

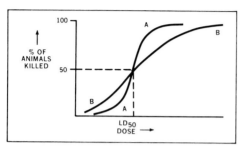

DOSE-RESPONSE CURVE

Fig. 32–3. Dose-response curve. (Reproduced with permission from Proctor, N.H.: Setting health standards: Toxicologic concepts. *In* Chemical Hazards of the Workplace. Edited by N.H. Proctor and J.P. Hughes. Copyright ©1978 by J.B. Lippincott Company, Philadelphia.)

of animals of that species exposed for the specified time period). The LD_{50} or LC_{50} for an agent provides an initial index of comparative toxicity.

During the determination of the LD_{50} or LC_{50}, observation of the animals often provides valuable information concerning the effects that may occur in humans. Autopsy of the animals shows which organs were affected. For many substances, these are the only data available. Until proven otherwise, it is prudent in such cases to suspect that the same effects will occur in humans if exposed to a sufficiently high atmospheric concentration for a sufficient time (Table 32–5).[11]

The regulation of worker exposure to carcinogens is an especially controversial issue. Federal standards were initially promulgated by OSHA in 1974 for 14 carcinogenic substances (Table 32–6). These standards were challenged in 1974 in the United States Court of Appeals. The decision of the court remanded the medical examination provisions of the 14 standards to OSHA for an explanation of why more specific requirements were not adopted. The court also vacated the provisions of the 14 standards regarding laboratory usage, as well as the entire standard governing the chemical agent MOCA on the grounds of invalid promulgation. The court ruling rendered the remanded provisions unenforceable.

In 1977, a generic standard was proposed (Table 32–7), which classifies substances into one of four categories based on the conclusiveness of data on carcinogenicity. The issue of the regulation of carcinogens, however, is still considered a matter of considerable importance. A "weighting system" has been proposed that is designed to lend needed perspective in the interpretation and application of results of epidemiologic studies for the purposes of standards setting. In contrast to the known validity of animal tests and "standard mortality ratios" in epidemiologic studies, "proportional morality ratios" and "risk ratios in case control studies" are reported with no concern for their size or sensitivity. Corroborative or contradictory reports are often ignored, and all case control studies are regarded as

Table 32–5.   Toxicity Classes

Toxicity Rating	Descriptive Term	LD_{50}—weight/kilogram Single Oral Dose Rats	LC_{50}—ppm 4-Hour Inhalation Rats
1	Extremely toxic	1 mg or less	<10
2	Highly toxic	1–50 mg	10–100
3	Moderately toxic	50–500 mg	100–1000
4	Slightly toxic	0.5–5 g	1000–10,000
5	Practically nontoxic	5–15 g	10,000–100,000
6	Relatively harmless	15 g or more	>100,000

From Proctor, N., and Hughes, J.: Chemical Hazards of the Workplace. Philadelphia, J.B. Lippincott Co., 1978.

Table 32–6. Initially Proposed Occupational Safety and Health Administration (OSHA) Carcinogens

Chemical Name	Generic or Trade Name
2-Acetylaminofluorene	2-AAF
4-Aminodiphenyl	4-ADP
Benzidine (and its salts)	—
Bis-chloromethyl ether	BCME
3,3-Dichlorobenzidine (and its salts)	DCB
4-Dimethylaminoazobenzene	Methyl yellow
Beta-naphthylamine	2-NA
4-Nitrobiphenyl	4-NBP
N-Nitrosodimethylamine	Dimethylamine
Betapropiolactone	Betaprone
Methyl chloromethyl ether	CMME
Alpha-naphthylamine	1-NA
4,4-Methylene bis (2-chloroaniline)	MOCA
Ethyleneimine	EI

From Proctor, N., and Hughes, J.: Chemical Hazards of the Workplace. Philadelphia, J.B. Lippincott Co., 1978.

Table 32–7. Generic Standards Proposed by the Occupational Safety and Health Administration (OSHA) in 1977

Category	Definition
Category I	Substances shown to have caused cancer in humans or in two mammalian test species or in one species if the results were replicated
Category II	Suggestive possible results of carcinogenicity in a single species that has not yet been replicated
Category III	All other substances that deserve to be studied further
Category IV	Foreign substances to be regulated if ever introduced into American work places

being of equal importance. A scoring procedure for epidemiologic assessments was proposed by Dinman.[12] Interstudy coherence could be effected by using the mean score of two studies or the geometric mean of three or more studies. Action to regulate would be based on these findings, as shown in Table 32–8. Doubtless, the issue of the regulation of carcinogens will remain unresolved until a systematic method of communicating epidemiologic data can be introduced to aid regulatory decision making.

REGULATORY AGENCY INTEREST

In the western world, rapidly expanding industrial technology and production associated with the preparation for World Wars I and II, in particular, resulted in the increasing exposure of workers in growing numbers to new hazards of the work place. Passage of the Walsh-Healey Act of 1936 for the purpose of regulating wages and hours had added poorly conceived health and safety requirements as an afterthought.[13]

The enactment of the Occupational Safety and Health Act (also commonly abbreviated OSHA, the same as the Administration it created in 1970) translated public concerns into law. Subsequently, regulatory strategies were developed assigning responsibility and accountability for the control of occupational hazards. If these strategies are to succeed, however, the quality and effectiveness of occupational health practice must be improved.

The NIOSH Criteria Documents assembled basic information about chemical, physical, and toxicologic characteristics, diagnostic criteria, including special tests and treatment, and medical control measures on 386 potentially hazardous chemical compounds and elements. These repetitive, rather legalistic publications are not intended primarily to provide a readily available source of guidance to occupational medical practitioners in answering questions and solving problems of the type that arise daily (often by telephone) in the practice of preventive occupational medicine.

OSHA did not automatically adopt as mandatory much of the guidance provided in these Criteria Documents, and this was fortunate in retrospect. From a practical standpoint, for example, it would be naive to expect organotin workers in industry to submit routinely to preplacement and periodic spinal fluid examination.[14]

Three important results of this effort, in addition to the Criteria Documents, have

Table 32–8. Interstudy Coherence in Epidemiologic Studies

Substance	Principal Epidemiologic Investigator	Dinman's Information/ Option Nomogram (Ionogram) Score	Mean Score
Coal tar volatiles	Doll	63	
	Lloyd	135	99*
Coal tar pitch	Rockette	16	
	Selikoff	16	
	Gibbs	63	25*

*Mean score <41 = lowest level of carcinogenic risk; mean score <20 = no action needed to regulate substance as a carcinogen.

From Dinman, B.D.: 1982 Gehrman Lecture. Am. Acad. Occupat. Med.[12]

been (1) a NIOSH/OSHA *Pocket Guide to Chemical Hazards,* which is actually a very cryptic but comprehensive checklist for field use;[15] (2) Proctor and Hughes' *Chemical Hazards of the Workplace,* a well-organized, readable, paperback textbook with pertinent references;[11] and (3) the concept of an effective national occupational health surveillance system. Other guidance, intended to help give occupational medicine specialists improved information and perspective, is contained in two important current textbooks edited by Carl Zenz entitled *Occupational Medicine: Principles and Practical Applications* and *Developments in Occupational Medicine.*[16,17] These texts provide the most detailed and comprehensive coverage available and are indispensable for the fully qualified occupational medical specialists. The failure of NIOSH and OSHA to provide for the use of appropriate biologic monitoring to document the adequacy of personal protection in the presence of above-standard occupational exposure had remained a concern. In 1982, the United States Department of Defense issued the *Occupational Health Surveillance Manual* to help guide occupational medical practices in the military services.[18] It contains a helpful summary of all existing OSHA regulations, along with pertinent policy on special purpose occupational medical examinations and biologic monitoring in Department of Defense components.

BIOLOGIC MONITORING

The chief purpose of the Department of Defense manual is to specify precisely the conditions under which preplacement and periodic special-purpose occupational medical examinations become necessary. Where environmental surveys cannot document adequacy of hazard control below a limiting federal standard (usually one-half the TLV), special-purpose occupational medical examinations and biologic monitoring may be required, even if proper protection is worn. Conversely, where environmental data confirm the adequacy of hazard containment, only a preplacement baseline value may need to be established. With such assistance, occupational medicine practitioners are better able to use and document sound clinical judgment, avoiding the appearance of performing unnecessary tests for regulatory compliance alone. Critically short occupational medicine manpower should be conserved. To accomplish costly biologic monitoring on a routine basis in the absence of potentially hazardous exposures is unjustified. It diverts professional attention and resources from preventive medical activities having greater importance to the health and safety of the work force.

Pre- and postemployment urinary phenol tests on workers in areas of possible benzene overexposure have been used to help recognize and control hazards.[19] The urinary phenol upper tolerable limit for benzene workers is set at 75 mg/

L, which correlates well with findings in workers exposed to the ACGIH TLV of 10 ppm in the working environment.[20] It should be possible to improve controls of possible benzene hazards, documenting adequacy by biologic monitoring results, without the need to remove workers from the job. If exposure is controlled adequately by engineering means or by operational scheduling, it should not be necessary to repeat biologic testing at frequent intervals. If reliance were placed only on personal respiratory and skin protection, however, more frequent sampling might be needed to detect and correct unsafe exposure and thus prevent the chronic toxic effects of benzene (including leukemia).

The industrial hygiene surveys reported in Table 32–9 show environmental levels of benzene measured as a tanker was being unloaded at a refinery's dock. The results suggested the possibility of above-standard exposures and a potentially serious health hazard to any unprotected workers in the area. Biologic monitoring of all workers in the area before and after work (Table 32–10) revealed significant elevations but to less than one-half the NIOSH "harmful" level in all but the industrial hygienist and one inspector.

The plant's medical department report-

Table 32–9. Benzene in Air Concentration

Time	Location	Concentration (ppm)
0830	Manifold hook-up	Nil
1000	Leaky manifold	Trace
1100	Walkway at tank vent	Trace
1200	Ullage port, gauger's breathing zone	125–150
1320	Draining hose to dock pan	60–110
1350	Hooking up to ship's tank	10
1545	Downwind while loading	12
1615	Vent line	1400
1700	Ullage port	600
1706	20 ft downwind of dock manifold	7

From Hammond, J.W.: Living with occupational health legislation. *In* Transactions of the 34th Annual Meeting of the Industrial Hygiene Foundation, Pittsburgh, Pennsylvania, 1969.

Table 32–10. Urinary Phenol Concentrations

Job	Urinary Phenol, mg/L		
	Before	After	Δ
Crane operator	6.6	6.6	0
Pipefitter	5.1	12.8	7.7
Pipefitter	8.6	30.0	21.4
Pipefitter	6.9	10.0	3.1
Pipefitter	7.6	13.0	5.4
Pump operator	4.1	7.9	3.8
Inspector	10.5	44.9	34.4
Inspector	21.9	27.8	5.9
Hygienist	6.0	45.0	39.0

From Hammond, J.W.: Living with occupational health legislation. *In* Transactions of the 34th Annual Meeting of the Industrial Hygiene Foundation, Pittsburgh, Pennsylvania, 1969.

edly repeated these tests weekly until the range of exposures/absorption levels was "normalized." Practically speaking, urinary total phenol levels are most helpful taken on a group basis, after work. A mean level of 45 mg/L (corrected to specific gravity 1.016) indicates a significant benzene exposure, equivalent to the TLV of 10 ppm for an 8 h day.[21] Either supplied air respirator or self-contained breathing apparatus is required until the hazardous exposure can be controlled.[15]

DIAGNOSIS OF OCCUPATIONALLY OR ENVIRONMENTALLY INDUCED DISEASES

The previously mentioned successful preventive medical and engineering program instituted in the TEL industry has controlled toxicity effectively; however, it was to be expected that illness occurring in users of leaded gasoline could become a basis for either a products-liability or compensation claim. An important aspect of Dr. Kehoe's work was to perform a thorough clinical evaluation, attempting to make a definitive diagnosis in each such case. As a result, an approach was developed that is still generally useful as a model in approaching the diagnosis of any illness deemed to be occupationally or environmentally induced.

The following is a list of the occupational medical diagnostic criteria:

1. Was the clinical picture consistent with known human experience and data from experimental toxicology?
2. Was exposure evaluated by an industrial hygiene survey and found to be significant?
3. Were other, equally exposed individuals similarly affected?
4. Did significant and prompt improvement occur after removal from exposure?
5. Were laboratory findings confirmatory and consistent both with the clinical impression and estimated exposure?
6. Are the clinical findings present common to the general public without the need to postulate toxicity, and did they exist prior to the alleged exposure?

The six questions posed, requiring considerable skill in answering, help form the basis for an occupational medicine specialist's opinion concerning environmental etiology. It must be recognized that the largest part of the postdoctorate professional training of an occupational medicine specialist is directed toward understanding the strengths and weaknesses of toxicologic, environmental, epidemiologic, biostatistical, clinicopathologic, and laboratory consultation to exercise the expert assistance required. Aerospace medicine specialists who are not capable of managing such diversified diagnostic consultation personally must appreciate the need for this skill and ensure its availability as a matter of the utmost importance to their preventive medicine programs. The very survival of their corporate employers may be at risk when accidents occur and questions of toxicity arise involving many persons, each of whom is claiming millions of dollars in damages.

Experience in the use of these diagnostic criteria has been extensive. Many examples are evident in the TEL studies: whenever a gasoline service station attendant developed chronic illness, especially if there were neurologic involvement, the question of lead intoxication was raised. After first assuring by proper laboratory and industrial hygiene studies that there was no basis for a diagnosis of environmentally induced lead poisoning, consultations were obtained from clinical specialists who might be able to help in reaching the correct diagnosis. Once established, an accurate diagnosis allowed the proper disposition, treatment, and prognostication of the case.

A similar situation arose at a union's request in connection with the need to determine which recipients of compensation for symptoms of breathlessness actually had pulmonary impairment. A study by the Kettering Laboratory at the University of Cinncinnati, demonstrated that out of over 100 individuals studied, only a third actually had significant impairment on pulmonary function testing.[22]

The importance of the diagnostic criteria is evident in the following examples with nitrogen dioxide. In the development of the Titan II missile propellants system, several contractor employees were engulfed while indoors by a cloud of nitrogen dioxide, to the degree that they thought the lights had gone out. They suffered both acute and subacute classic nitrogen dioxide toxicity. They recovered fairly promptly after removal from exposure and upon receiving proper treatment.[23] A similar situation developed in three astronauts in the Apollo-Soyuz space capsule, with the same outcome.[24]

In a McConnell Air Force Base missile accident near Rock, Kansas, an oxidizer spill acutely overcame and killed two military missile crewmembers.[25] Another crewmember survived miraculously after experiencing cardiac arrest followed by a partial stroke. The remainder of those unprotected individuals who were exposed to visible concentrations of nitrogen dioxide in an enclosed area had classic findings of nitrogen dioxide toxicity. Recovery was prompt after their removal from exposure and the institution of proper therapy. Of those airmen at the accident site who were exposed to nitrogen dioxide without protection for less than 5 minutes, only one had significant respiratory complaints. Two others, however, were found to have significant decreases in arterial oxygen saturation after 2 weeks. They were considered to have early bronchiolitis fibrosa obliterans and were placed on steroid therapy, with good results.

Thirty-two civilians in the neighboring community who did not develop any evidence of classic nitrogen dioxide toxicity were found by environmental survey to have had exposures less than the TLV. They were examined thoroughly by pulmonary disease specialists and found to be essentially free of significant pulmonary impairment, except for asthma in several atopic individuals.

Despite this, claims amounting to over $70 million were made against the United States government and an Air Force contractor on the basis of multiple vague symptoms, common to the general public, which failed to improve with time. The failure to recognize and deal properly with such claims in a timely manner will become increasingly costly to the United States should the present trend continue. There is no question but that improved communication of these occupational medical criteria would help to avoid professional error and misdiagnosis in such cases. It is ironic that no medical student could graduate from medical school without knowing Koch's postulates for the diagnosis of infectious diseases, yet few medical graduates today are prepared to use similar logic in approaching the diagnosis of an illness alleged to have arisen from an environmental exposure, often of such minor degree as to have caused no observable signs or symptoms. Too many doctors do not request expert assistance in evaluating environmental exposures and accept without question their patient's estimate of exposure. As a result, our adversarial judicial system is unduly influenced and rewards many damage claims that are totally lacking in merit.

Sound scientific diagnostic logic similar to that used in deciding on the adverse bioeffects from chemical exposure also should be applied in cases in which the environmental agent is physical.

PHYSICAL HAZARDS IN THE AVIATION INDUSTRY

Physical hazards exist where there is excessive exposure to physical agents. Physical agents are formless and essentially weightless but may produce hazards to exposed workers by the transfer of energy of various types, resulting in rather specific bioeffects, when permissible occupational standards are exceeded. Most important among potentially harmful physical agents are (1) oscillatory motions, including noise and vibration; (2) extreme occupational temperature variations in the ambient environment; and (3) ionizing and nonionizing electromagnetic radiation. As shown in Figure 32–4, other forms of physical hazards on the job involve ergonomics and biomechanics, which also may be important to worker safety and productivity.[16]

Noise

Exposure durations to all continuous and intermittent sound levels above 80 dBA are combined in applying the TLVs shown in Table 32–11. In some cases, it may be possible to rotate personnel or exercise administrative controls to avoid exceeding the permissible exposure standard. The use of hearing protection devices, however, provides immediate and effective protection while the possibility of control by engineering measures is being explored.

Impulsive or impact noise exposure limits, shown in Figure 32–5, involve noise level variations, with maximum noise occurring at intervals of greater than one

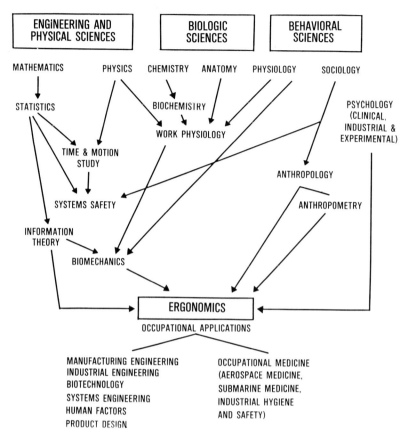

Fig. 32–4.   Disciplines in ergonomics. (Reproduced with permission from Ramsey, J.D.: Occupational vibration. in Zenz, C. (ed.): Occupational Medicine: Principles and Practical Applications. Copyright ©1975 by Yearbook Medical Publishers, Inc., Chicago.)

pulse per second. When intervals are less than this, the variations should be considered continuous for purposes of evaluation and control.

Accrued liability from noise-induced hearing loss in industry is estimated to be in the billions of dollars. Attempts to implement hearing conservation programs in the past have inadvertently precipitated early retirement and compensation claims solely because of high-frequency losses (above speech frequencies). Effective hearing conservation programs are based on proper initial placement, with the establishment of an accurate baseline (or reference) audiogram, as well as follow-up testing in 90 to 120 days, and at least annually thereafter to help insure against un-

protected hazardous exposure and temporary hearing loss. If such temporary losses can be prevented, it has been shown that permanent noise-induced changes are unlikely, except in continuous noise such as constant exposure to a rolling mill or waterfall. Even brief removal from continuous hazardous noise exposure tends to limit the progressive loss of hearing; therefore, rotation out of noise and ear-defender protection are components of an effective preventive program. This is especially important in situations where hazardous noise cannot be controlled by engineering means alone.

The disposition of hearing loss problems encountered and occupational medical involvement in their solution are out-

Gasoline Storage Tanks

After several years, an unanticipated hazard of serious proportions in connection with the handling of leaded gasoline appeared within the refineries and storage plants of the oil companies. Workers engaged in the cleaning and repairing of large storage tanks for leaded gasoline were found to be subjected to hazardous exposure to TEL and its decomposition products. The problem was investigated, and adequate precautionary measures for the control of this hazard were developed and issued to all of the distributors of gasoline soon after the first difficulties occurred. Afterward, to the extent that these precautions were followed faithfully, no further cases of poisoning developed. It was difficult, however, to achieve and maintain a general awareness of this hazard and to ensure the application of the precautions at all outlying points of storage throughout the world, especially in areas controlled by military organizations. Frequent changes in military personnel and the practice of farming out maintenance jobs to contractors with limited understanding of the problem in addition to the difficulties of access to some of these tanks have been responsible for a number of serious casualties. Nevertheless, the distributors of lead-containing antiknock compounds have persevered in their efforts to inform and remind appropriate persons in the military services concerning the safe handling of antiknock compounds. Such difficulties have not been limited strictly to military storage tanks. Because of the geographic scope and complexity of the distribution of leaded gasoline in the United States and Canada, the distributors of antiknock compounds have found it necessary to set up elaborate systems for the exchange of information and on-the-spot consultations between their organizations and those of the oil companies, whereby the cleaning of gasoline storage tanks is supervised by trained personnel throughout the country.

Operating Manuals and Information Exchange

Another feature of the hygienic regimen in the varied operations of the TEL and petroleum industries was the use of detailed operating manuals in which, generally, instructions for all operations included specific guidance with respect to safety and health. These manuals, used regularly both in instructing new personnel and in reminding those more experienced, were reviewed regularly and brought up to date. In this manner, a high degree of uniformity of instruction and performance was developed and maintained. Certain essential operating procedures (such as those concerned with mixing operations, the cleaning of gasoline storage tanks, and the handling of concentrated antiknock compounds in research and testing laboratories) were reproduced onto placards and posted in convenient places for reference by the operators. Familiarity and compliance with the instructions in manuals and placards were reinforced by close supervision and periodic reindoctrination of all operating personnel.

The American TEL industry had, from the beginning, conducted itself responsibly in its operations and in its informal relations with the United States Public Health Service in the absence of specific legal regulations or legislative enactments in the United States. This policy was extended abroad by informing the responsible authorities in various other countries into which the product was to be introduced of all pertinent hygienic facts and considerations. This policy doubtless helped avoid legislative and regulatory constraints that might have complicated international operations and might also have provided serious obstacles to the establishment and maintenance of an essentially uniform program of industrial hygiene. The principal virtue of such a policy in international commercial operations of a hazardous type probably is that of offering full information and cooperation to responsible health authorities and seeking in return their advice and assistance in achieving the best results within their areas.

Distributors of TEL antiknock compounds normally engage the services of competent and reliable medical consultants in each country in which their products are used. They act professionally for the industry in helping to ensure compliance with hygienic regulations and practices of their own country, as well as the requirements of the chief medical advisors of the industry. Through such a professional arrangement, every reasonable provision has been made for the instruction and medical supervision of those to whom exposure to TEL may be hazardous.

From the outset, it had been management's policy in general to sanction the publication of factual medical and hygienic information for the benefit of the medical and hygienic professions. In summary, Dr. Kehoe concluded that, "At a time when full knowledge of the nature and scope of occupational hazards is of great value to students and practitioners of occupational medicine and hygiene, it is important to recognize the soundness of the policy of acquiring the facts as a basis for action, and disseminating the facts as a means of demonstrating the wisdom of such action, if and when it should be questioned."[3]

This case study provides an opportunity to review the complexities involved in resolving but one aviation industrial problem, the safe use of tetraethyl lead.

Aerospace medicine and occupational health share a scientific approach to problem solving. This approach has been vital to the control and prevention of truly life-threatening hazards in space exploration and in atmospheric flight, as well as in industrial and military environments.

TECHNOLOGY DEVELOPMENT

Competing Costs and Benefits

It is essential to national survival that the United States continue to advance competitively in space and undersea exploration, aerospace transportation, and industrial productivity. It is urgent, therefore, that resources be conserved and maximum value obtained for money spent both on engineering controls of public and employee environmental health hazards and on environmental quality conservation, giving higher priority to the former. Occupational medicine support in implementing industrial hygiene programs provides the means of documenting the wisdom and success of programs undertaken to control both real and potential threats to employee safety and health. In most cases, this can be done without the necessity for controlling exposure to "zero level." To be able to afford the expenditures needed to advance our aerospace mission while at the same time protecting our astronauts and aircrews, it will be necessary for the United States to use the best possible judgment, based on competent professional advice and backed by facts (Table 32–1).

Types of occupations encountered in the aviation industry range in sophistication, complexity, injury, and occupational disease potential from ground support crew to astronaut. The per capita costs of environmental controls tend to be inversely proportional to the numbers of workers affected. There also is an inverse relationship between preventive health program costs of protecting aerospace crews versus ground support employees and the public because of the sophistication of the controls needed. Claims of well-meaning consumer and environmental advocates, often sensationalized in the process of reporting of environmental pollution problems having possible adverse health effects, have so sensitized an already anxious public that every "Chicken

Table 32–1. Aerospace Mission Costs

Population		Per Capita Cost of Environmental and Occupational Health Preventive Programs ($)
2×10^9	Consumers/public	2×10^0
2×10^8	Neighbors	2×10
2×10^7	Aviation industry employees	2×10^2
2×10^6	Ground crews	2×10^3
2×10^5	Research and development scientists	2×10^4
2×10^4	Aircrews	2×10^5
2×10^3	Test pilots selection/care	2×10^6
2×10^2	"Space depot" crews	2×10^7
2×10	Astronaut program	2×10^8
2×10^0	Apollo XI/XII (lunar landings)	2×10^9

Little" allegation gets front-page "sky falling" headlines. One purpose of such reporting seems to be to convince the public that there needs to be as nearly absolute protection for the general public as for the astronaut. Because such protection would be neither necessary nor advisable, even if it were economically and technically feasible, the chief intent often appears to be politically inspired rather than related to genuine concern for public and employee safety and health conservation.

Aerospace Occupational and Environmental Health Program Budgeting

The very magnitude of developmental costs makes it essential that provision be made at the earliest possible stage of planning for adequate environmental and occupational health support as an integral part of total research and development, testing, pilot plant, and full-scale industrial production. In this way, occupational medical support and recommendations for employee and consumer health protection from all types of health hazards introduced by new products and processes can be supported as components of the total program budget. Such vital project support is extremely vulnerable. It must not be required to compete for its funding along with general health, safety, maintenance, and fringe benefit programs of the organization. If so, it may be subject to total elimination in the face of a 5 to 10% reduction of project support and/or medical departmental funding.

Vitally important parts of many research and development projects are the supportive technical manuals and information supplied to help ensure their proper and safe use. United States Department of Defense contract performance often misses the opportunity to observe possible health effects on industrial populations of known occupational exposures during early stages of research and development when little is known of potential hazards. With occupational medical and industrial hygiene assistance, some military managers of Department of Defense contracts have performed very effectively, improving the quality of technical publications concerned with protective health and environmental quality. To keep abreast of progress, however, such enlightened implementation of responsibilities will need to be more widely practiced, becoming the rule rather than the exception.

Toxicology Quality Control in Standards Development

At a time when considerable progress is being made in introducing the best current knowledge of computerized assistance to aid clinical and laboratory diagnostic decision making, the situation in the fields of comparative toxicology and toxicokinetics is dangerously inadequate. As in the case of "wars and generals," toxicology research may be too important to leave entirely to toxicologists.

After an accidental or unintentional exposure to chemicals, a 20- to 30-year period of latency may occur before the appearance of any carcinogenic effect. Because the testing of chemicals in humans is ethically unacceptable, the use of animal experimentation has been justified, using high doses to counteract the relative insensitivity of such bioassays. Although in-vitro tests show promise for the future, the carcinogen bioassay is still the standard test, having been used by the National Cancer Institute (NCI) for over 8 years in over 200 bioassays of potential carcinogenic risk to humans.

But even so, the NCI studies do not consider adequately either toxicokinetics or comparative toxicology. This is the view of the Nobel laureate geneticist, Joshua Lederberg, President of Rockefeller University, who commented that the hundreds of millions of dollars a year that are spent on routine animal tests are almost all worthless from the point of view of standard-setting.[4] He recommended that some of our resources, not only money but also time and efforts, be redeployed. The requirment to do such limited kinds of testing has made toxicology tests a less respectable discipline from the standpoint of more fundamental biologic interests. Lederberg concluded that it is simply not possible, with all the animals in the world, to go through new chemicals in the blind way that we have at the present time and reach credible conclusions about the hazards to human health. This impasse, he added, has deep scientific roots, and something had better be done about it.

A major shift of the National Toxicology Program from occupational to environmental health involves the public (and politics). It has diverted national attention from the occupational hazard controls that were the goal of occupational safety and health legislation of the late 1960s. As a result, the great majority of workers, those who work in small plants, are not being reached. These individuals were the ones for whom the Occupational Safety and Health Act (OSHA) was passed in 1970 to help provide preventive programs of safety and health equivalent to those in the largest and most progressive companies in the private sector. Today, such workers are in danger of being ignored.

Of course, attempts to monitor and protect the health and safety of all workers is like trying to control the health of all pilots but on a much larger scale, involving practically the entire adult population of working age. This, ideally, must reach and involve all medical and engineering students and practitioners as a matter of public health with preventive medicine and engineering concepts and practices. Despite attempts to introduce occupational health into undergraduate and graduate medical and technical education at several universities, there is reason to believe that the majority of physicians, scientists, and engineers still receive most of their concepts and information from news media reports, which at best are often sensationalized, if not totally in error. The media constantly must be reminded of its duty to relate environmental health matters accurately, exercising every effort toward improving the quality of its reporting. Aerospace and occupational medical specialists have a responsibility also to share the large and growing body of scientific information in environmental health with all those who need to know the facts. Collectively, this larger group (i.e., the public) has the ability to make and change laws that influence whether and how our nation's industry, and its aerospace program in particular, will survive in an increasingly competitive setting.

AVIATION TOXICOLOGY

A number of potential health hazards from the use of toxic substances in airline maintenance units cited by McFarland[5] are shown in Table 32–2, modified to show the changes in permissible exposure levels under current consensus standards published by the ACGIH (*Documentation of the Threshold Limit Values for Chemical Substances* helps explain the basis for the changes).[6]

Exposure Limits

When, in 1953, an Aeromedical Association Committee published its monograph, *Aviation Toxicology*, 135 chemical compounds were listed, many of which had no established limiting exposure standards.[7] In the three decades since, there have been many changes: twenty-one chemicals have been given a threshold limit value (TLV), the TLVs of 58 chemicals have been lowered, and only 36 chemicals' TLVs remain unchanged. By way of contrast, physical standards (such as melting point, boiling point, and vapor pressure) have remained quite constant, simplifying engineering design.

Threshold Limit Values

The intent of TLVs set by consensus within the ACGIH's Threshold Limit Value Committee was to provide reliable benchmarks to aid plant engineers both in designing new facilities and in renovating old ones, so that the possibility of toxicity occurring in the work force would be minimized. In this way, other protective measures, such as personal protection, limiting exposure time, and special-purpose occupational medical examinations and tests, either could be minimized or, better still, documented as being totally unnecessary. The basic premise involved in industrial hygiene controls below a permissible (safe) exposure level is that repeated exposures 8 hr/day, 5 days/week for a working lifetime could be allowed for the great majority of unprotected employees without harm. Although a few susceptible individuals in the work force might develop evidence of harm, these persons would be detected by close occupational

medical surveillance and removed prior to sustaining irreversible impairment or disability. According to Hatch,[8] this concept, shown in Figure 32–1, involves the most precious information in the field of industrial hygiene, and the time and effort should be taken to confirm and strengthen these standards with reliable, reproducible data based on human experience whenever possible. Otherwise, further efforts to move design standards toward zero will ultimately destroy the concept involved, making designers either disregard them entirely or move increasingly toward reliance on automated, remote operations for general use.

Unfortunately, the facts that would help place matters of environmental and occupational health into proper perspective are not being communicated adequately to new generations of American citizens. As a result, a climate exists today in which the adverse effects on productivity are disregarded while the sensationalistic, science-fiction–type coverage in the media of environmentally induced illness claims are encouraged and even rewarded. The concept of absolute assurance appears to rule, implying absolutely no risk to the individual, the community, or the environment. Just as the Flexnor Report of 1910 directed public attention to failures in medical education as a basis for improving teaching standards, so today there needs to be greater care in environmental and occupational health instruction at all levels, emphasizing the importance of scientific problem solving and encouraging such efforts to the maximum practicable degree.

Emergency Exposure Standards

The monograph *Aviation Toxicology* presented graphs on carbon monoxide, carbon dioxide, carbon tetrachloride, and methyl bromide.[7] One purpose of these graphs was to help aviation physiologists and medical specialists understand certain safety parameters within which air-

Table 32–2.   Major Toxic Hazards Encountered in Airline Maintenance Units

Toxic Substance	Aero Repair	Assembled Engine Cleaning	Battery	Block Test	Carburetor and Ignition	Electroplating	Engine Cleaning	Engine Disassembly	Foundry and Heat-Treating	Hydraulic	Instrument Repair	Minor Repair	Motor Vehicle and Misc. Repair	Paint and Dope	Propeller	Radiator and Tank	Rubber Tank Repair	Spark Plug Cleaning	Spray Painting	Trichloroethylene Degreasing	Welding	1951 ppm	Values mg/m³	TWA	STEL
Gases and vapors																									
Acetone	×											×	×	×					×			500	1000	750	1000
Amyl acetate	×											×	×	×					×			200	1000	100	150
Benzene (benzol)	×	×										×	×	×					×			35	200	10	25
Butyl acetate	×											×	×	×					×			200	1000	150	200
Butyl alcohol	×											×	×	×					×			50	200	50C	—
Carbon monoxide	×			×								×									×	100	100	50	400
Carbon tetrachloride	×						×	×		×	×	×	×			×	×	×				50	500	5	20
Ethyl acetate	×											×	×	×					×			400	1000	400	—
Ethyl alcohol	×											×	×	×					×			1000	2000	1000	—
Ethylene dichloride	×					×	×					×	×									100	400	10	15
Gasoline					×	×	×	×				×										500	2000	300	500
Hydrochloric acid						×	×															10	10	5C	—
Hydrogen cyanide						×																10	20	10C	—
Hydrogen fluoride									×													3	2	3C	6
Naphtha (petroleum)	×											×	×	×		×	×		×	×		500	2000	300	500
Nitrogen dioxide																					×	25	100	3	5
Phosgene	×											×		×								1	5	0.1	—
Sulfur dioxide						×																10	25	2	—
Sulfuric acid			×			×																5	5	1 mg/m³	—
Toluene	×											×	×	×		×			×			200	500	100	150
Trichloroethylene		×					×													×		100	1000	50	200
Turpentine	×											×	×	×	×				×			100	500	100	150
Metallic dusts and fumes																									
Chromic acid						×													×			0.1	0.1	0.05 mg/m³	0.15 mg/m³
Lead	×		×		×	×						×	×	×		×			×			0.15	0.15	0.15 mg/m³	as Cr

*According to the American Conference of Governmental Industrial Hygienists, TLVs refer to airborne concentrations of substances and represent conditions under which it is believed that nearly all workers may be exposed day after day without adverse effect.

†In ppm unless otherwise indicated.

C: denotes ceiling limit.

Modified from McFarland, R.A.: Human Factors in Air Transportation. New York: McGraw-Hill Book Co., 1953.

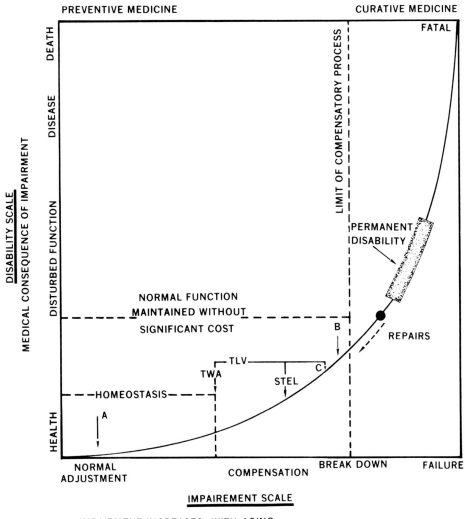

Fig. 32–1. Hatch curve. A healthy individual functioning at point A may respond to environmental stress with a relatively minor and temporary disturbance and will return to point A when the stress is removed. An already impaired individual at point B may find the same kind and degree of stress intolerable and consequently move rapidly up the curve to a position of serious disability and even death. Industrial hygiene engineering controls below a certain level allow the great majority of workers to be exposed safely for up to 8 hr/day, 5 days/week for a working lifetime. This level is known as the Threshold Limit Value-Time Weighted Average (TLV-TWA). The TLV-STEL is defined as the Short-Term Exposure Limit, averaged over a period of 15 minutes, which should not be exceeded at any time during a workday (even if the 8-hour TWA is within TLV). Exposures at the STEL should not be for longer than 15 minutes and should not be repeated more than four times per day. Also, there should be at least 60 minutes between successive exposures at the STEL. The TLV-C is a ceiling concentration that should not be exceeded. If any one of these three TLVs is exceeded, a potential hazard from that substance is presumed to exist.

crews could be exposed briefly, without protection and at altitude, and yet still accomplish essential tasks. Such knowledge helped aircrews make proper decisions regarding the need either for emergency escape or taking the time to don walk-around oxygen bottles. The graph for carbon monoxide is shown in Figure 32–2.

The curves shown in this figure are calculated from the following equations of Henderson and Haggard, in which time is expressed in hours and concentration is expressed in parts per million:

Curve 1.   Time × concentration = 300: no perceptible effect
Curve 2.   Time × concentration = 600: a just perceptible effect
Curve 3.   Time × concentration = 900: headache and nausea
Curve 4.   Time × concentration = 1500: dangerous

The following is a breakdown of the effect of carbon monoxide on health:

Percent carbon monoxide	Degree of danger in relation to exposure time
0.01	Allowable for several hours
0.04 to 0.05	Without appreciable effect in 1 hour
0.06 to 0.07	Just appreciable effect after 1 hour
0.10 to 0.12	Unpleasant but not dangerous after 1 hour
0.15 to 0.20	Dangerous in 1 hour
0.40 and above	Fatal in less than 1 hour

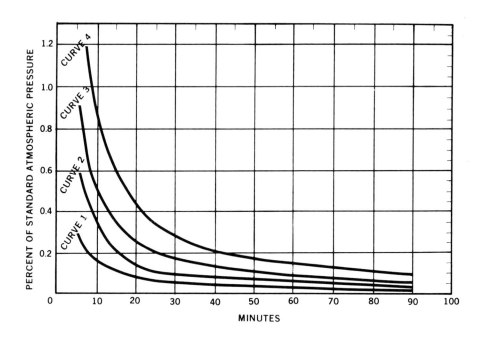

Fig. 32–2. Time-concentration curves for effects from carbon monoxide. See text for discussion. (Modified from Aero Medical Association, Committee on Aviation Toxicology: Aviation Toxicology. New York, The Blakiston Co., 1953.)

from the use of unshielded thoriated glass in night vision devices or lung cancer from the deposition of radioactive dust in the depths of the lungs, in association with epithelial cells lining the bronchioles). Alpha exposure interacting with skin from outside sources is termed external alpha, whereas alpha particles inhaled, ingested, or absorbed and deposited in or near extremely radiosensitive target organs are termed internal alpha. The internal alpha hazard includes bone sarcoma from chronic exposure to radon.

Low LET radiation includes not only external alpha and beta rays or particles but also cosmic, gamma, and x-rays, all of which possess sufficient energy to cause ionization and which share the ability to pass through many substances that are opaque to light. Exposure to a large, single, short-term, whole-body dose of ionizing radiation produces a complex of clinical symptoms, signs, and laboratory changes that correlate well with physical measurements of exposure in a predictable way. An algorithm (Fig. 32–12) explicates a step-wise diagnostic process to help determine the presence and extent of acute radiation syndrome following sufficient exposure, as well as therapeutic requirements and ultimate prognosis in such cases.[16,27] The United States Department of Defense *Occupational Health Surveillance Manual* contains guidance that represents the current consensus of military technical and medical opinion (Table 32–14). It incorporates the mandatory monitoring requirements of the National Council on Radiation Protection and Measurements (NCRP) and protective criteria, which have been accepted in total by the ACGIH as "well established and documented threshold limit values (TLVs) for ionizing radiation."

Nonionizing Radiation (NIR)

Nonionizing radiation (NIR) occupies a major portion of the electromagnetic spectrum, ranging from near-ultraviolet through visible light, infrared, radiofrequency, and microwaves to extremely low-frequency radiation. For purposes of regulating hazard prevention, nonionizing radiation is categorized under several broad headings: (1) laser and high-intensity optical sources; (2) ultraviolet (UV); (3) radiofrequency (RF) and microwave (MW); (4) extremely low-frequency (ELF) radiation; and (5) magnetic fields.

LASER AND HIGH-INTENSITY OPTICAL SOURCES. Laser and high-intensity optical radiation are considered separately from ionizing radiation, although high irradiances have been known to produce ionization in air and other materials because their principal adverse biologic effects (i.e., those requiring preventive measures) are not related to ionization. Depending on the frequencies involved, lasers produce effects of visible, ultraviolet, or infrared radiation but at levels of intensity previously approached only by the sun, nuclear weapons, burning magnesium, or arc-lights. Like light, laser beams are reflected, transmitted, and/or absorbed depending on the nature of the surface encountered. Darker materials such as pigment (melanin) absorb more energy than pale or clear tissues; hence, the eye is particularly susceptible to injury in most hazardous situations.

Absorption of short UV (200 to 315 nm) and far infrared (1400 to 10^6 nm) radiation occurs principally at the cornea, whereas the near UV radiation (315 to 400 nm) is absorbed primarily in the lens of the eye. Light (400 to 700 nm) and near IR (700 to 1400 nm) are transmitted and refracted by the cornea and lens and absorbed at the retina. The TLVs for viewing a diffuse reflection of a laser beam or an extended source laser and for skin exposure from a laser beam have been published by the ACGIH.[6] Where preventive engineering design criteria are met, special-purpose occupational medical examinations are not ordinarily required as part of routine occupational health surveillance.

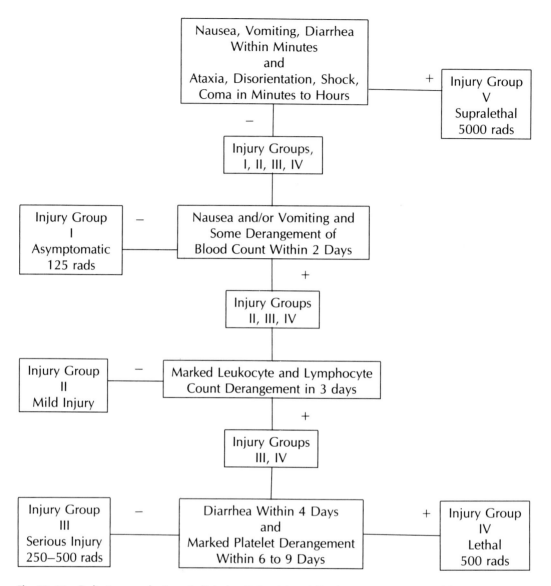

Fig. 32–12. Preliminary evaluation of clinical radiation injury following overexposure. (Modified from Zenz, C. (ed.): Occupational Medicine: Principles and Practical Applications. Copyright ©1975 by Yearbook Medical Publishers, Inc., Chicago.)

In one case, a 65-year-old United States Air Force civil service technician had been tracking magnesium-type flares (dropped from aircraft) with a 24-power telescope using one eye for several hours when he noted he was unable to read with that eye. He was seen by a private ophthalmologist, who agreed that the problem might be related etiologically to exposure at work, stating that the amount of energy required to produce macular degeneration was unknown and thus the possibility that it was due to occupational exposure could not be excluded. A difference in brightness perception also was noted between the left and right eyes.

This claim was discussed with an ophthalmologist experienced in the aviation and military environment who had done considerable experimental research

Table 32–14.   Medical Surveillance Procedures

Physical Agent	Preplacement/Baseline	Periodic	Comments
Low LET radiation (e.g., x-ray, beta particles, gamma ray, external alpha particles)	Work history, especially previous exposure to ionizing radiation	None required routinely	Urine bioassays may be indicated, depending on the previous exposure to radioactive materials and/or the present circumstances of possible exposure. The type of test performed will vary, depending on these circumstances. These tests are usually performed only at certain licensed laboratories
	Complete medical history and physical examination to include vital signs and evaluation of all major organ systems		Periodic analyses and/or examinations may be indicated, depending on potential radiation hazard and circumstances in which the work is performed. The responsible medical authority in conjunction with the radiation protection officer shall determine the necessity. Periodic analyses, if required, shall follow those outlined in the preplacement baseline column
	Clinical laboratory studies to include a complete blood count (white blood cell count, platelet count, and hematocrit) and urinalysis with microscopic		

Modified from the Department of Defense: Occupational Health Surveillance Manual. 6055.5-M. U.S. Government Printing Office, Washington, D.C., 1982.

on retinal burns. He demonstrated that the use of a telescope or binoculars spreads light energy focused on the retina rather than concentrating it. Thus, the use of a telescope would actually reduce the chances of macular damage from a high-intensity light source. The amount of energy needed to produce macular degeneration had been extensively studied, and that involved in flare tracking was far lower than would be required to produce injury. A question of aggravation of an existing problem was considered, but in such a case there would have been some evidence of acute local edema in the macular area with subsequent improvement. No such transient effect was observed. The sudden onset of unilateral visual impairment due to macular degeneration is commonly the result of vascular (arteriosclerotic) disease, especially in individuals over the age of 55 to 60 years. There was no reason to suspect that the alleged relationship to an occupational exposure in this case was other than coincidental.

ULTRAVIOLET (UV). The TLVs for exposure of the eye or the skin to nonlaser UV in the spectral region of 200 to 400 nm published by the ACGIH apply to UV radiation from arcs, gas, and vapor discharges, fluorescent and incandescent sources, as well as solar radiation (Fig. 32–13). For near UV radiation (320 to 400 nm), total irradiance should not exceed 1 mW/cm^2 for periods greater than 16 minutes or 1 J/cm^2 for shorter exposures. Conditioned (tanned) individuals can tolerate skin exposure in excess of the TLV without erythema but may not be protected adequately from actinic UV-induced skin cancers. Also, TLVs do not apply to photosensitized individuals or to those exposed concomitantly to photosensitizing agents.

RADIOFREQUENCY (RF) AND MICROWAVE

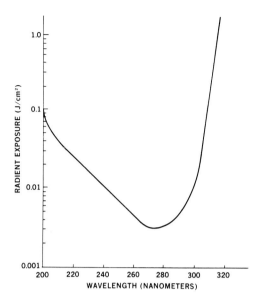

Fig. 32–13. Threshold limit values for ultraviolet radiation.[6]

(MW). These forms of radiation produce biologic effects at varying tissue depths depending on the wavelength/frequency relationship, the higher frequencies/shorter wavelengths having less ability to penetrate, similar to IR exposure from heat lamps. Lower frequency/longer wavelengths reach deeper levels, as with therapeutic microwave devices. The lowest/longest type of RF and MW pass completely through tissues without interact-

ing. This explains the varying TLVs shown in Figure 32–14. The results of extensive bioeffects research performed on RF and MW in recent years have indicated the principal bioeffect to be hyperthermia. Extensive medical studies conducted at the USAFSAM of individuals accidentally exposed above permissible occupational limits have failed to document the cataract formation produced experimentally in animals with acute, high MW radiation exposure or any other adverse bioeffects. Occupational health surveillance procedures required by the Department of Defense appear in Table 32–15.

The contributions of occupational medicine to the aviation industry involve the application of industrial hygiene surveys, analytic measurements, and scientific logic to the recognition, evaluation, and control of environmental hazards. Such hazards, if undetected and uncontrolled, can be expected to produce such adverse effects as illness and impaired efficiency of the aviation industry's employees, neighbors, and customers. Ideally, responsible aerospace medicine specialists will be trained and become fully qualified to direct the occupational medicine function personally. Otherwise, they must recognize the need to provide adequately for its availability and quality, to ensure its ef-

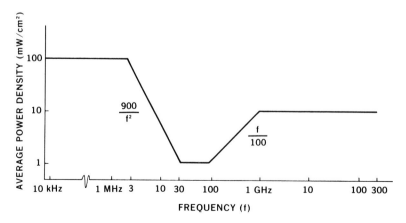

Fig. 32–14. Threshold limit values (TLV) for radiofrequency/microwave radiation in the workplace: whole-body specific absorption rate (SAR) less than 0.4 W/kg. (Between 10 kHz and 3 MHz the average whole-body SAR is still limited to 0.4 W/kg, but the plateau at 100 mW/cm² was set to protect against electrical shock and burn hazards.)[6]

Table 32–15.   Medical Surveillance Procedures

Physical Agent	Preplacement/Baseline	Periodic	Comments
Radiofrequency (RF) and microwave radiation	Preplacement/termination ocular surveillace should be performed on personnel working in research, development, testing, evaluation, and maintenance of equipment capable of free-space radiation of power densities greater than the occupational exposure limit.	None required routinely	When exposures in excess of the occupational exposure limit are suspected or confirmed, the medical history should be reviewed and such test(s) performed as deemed appropriate
	The physical examination should include a comprehensive ocular evaluation, including visual acuity (far and near). If less than 20/20, refractively determine best acuity; funduscopic examination with pupil dilated; slit lamp (biomicroscopic) examination of the cornea and lens with the pupil dilated; and careful description (drawing or photograph) of any abnormalities (see comment 2)		The ocular evaluation shall be performed by an optometrist, ophthalmologist, or physician skilled in biomecroscopy and funduscopy of the eye

Modified from the Department of Defense: Occupational Health Surveillance Manual. 6055.5-M. U.S. Government Printing Office, Washington, D.C., 1982.

fectiveness within the total environmental and occupational health program of their respective organizations and communities.

REFERENCES

1. Ashe, W.F.: Education for industrial (occupational) medical practice. J. Occupat. Med., 2(7):305–311, 1960.
2. Felton, J.S.: Organization and operation of an occupational health program—Part I. J. Occupat. Med., 6(1):26–68, 1964.
3. Kehoe, R.A.: An illustration of industrial hygiene. Arch. Environ. Health, 8(8):378–383, 1964.
4a. Lederberg, J.: Comparative toxicology, environmental health and national productivity. Am. J. Med., 70(1):9–11, 1981.
4b. Lederberg, J.: A challenge for toxicologists. Chem. Eng. News, XI:5, 1981.
5. McFarland, R.A.: Human Factors in Air Transportation. New York, McGraw-Hill Book Co., 1953.
6. Threshold Limit Valves for Chemical Substances and Physical Agents in the Work Environment with intended changes for 1982, and Documentation of the Threshold Limit Valves for Substances in Workroom Air (1971) with Supplements for those substances added since 1971. American Conference of Governmental Industrial Hygienists, Cincinnati, Ohio, 1971.
7. Aviation Medical Association: Aviation Toxicology. New York, The Blakiston Co., 1953.
8. Hatch, T.F.: Changing objectives in occupational health. Am. Indust. Hyg. Assoc. J., 23(1):1–7, 1962.
9. Smythe, H.F.: Military and space short term inhalation standards. Arch. Environ. Health, 12(12):488–490, 1966.
10. Guides for Short-Term Exposures of Public to Air Pollutants. I. Guide for Oxides of Nitrogen. The Committee on Toxicology, National Academy of Sciences, National Research Council. Washington, D.C., Government Printing Office, April 1, 1971.
11. Proctor, N., and Hughes, J.: Chemical Hazards of the Workplace. Philadelphia, J.B. Lippincott Co., 1978.
12. Dinman, B.D., and Sussman, N.: Uncertainty, risk, and the role of epidemiology in public policy development. J. Occup. Med., 25(7):511–516, 1983.
13. The Walsh-Healey Public Contracts Act. Legal Series Bulletin #6. Pittsburgh, Industrial Hygiene Foundation, 1963.
14. Department of Health, Education, and Welfare (NIOSH) Criteria Document: Organotin Compounds. 1977.
15. NIOSH/OSHA Pocket Guide to Chemical Hazards. DHEW (NIOSH) No. 78–210. 1978.
16. Zenz, C.: Occupational Medicine: Principles and Practical Applications. Chicago, Yearbook Medical Publishers, Inc., 1975.
17. Zenz, C.: Developments in Occupational Medi-

cine. Chicago, Yearbook Medical Publishers, Inc., 1980.

18. Department of Defense #6055.5-M: Occupational Health Surveillance. Philadelphia, U.S. Naval Publications and Forms Center, July, 1982.

19. Hammond, J.W.: Living with occupational health legislation. Industrial Hygiene Foundation Transactions Bulletin No. 43:36–41. Industrial Hygiene Foundation of America, Pittsburgh, 1969.

20. Occupational Diseases: A Guide to Their Recognition. Department of Health, Education, and Welfare (NIOSH) No. 77–181.

21. Lauwerys, R.R., Industrial Chemical Exposure: Guidelines for Biological Monitoring. Table 3. Biomedical Publications, Davis, CA. 1983.

22. Ross, W.D., et al.: Emotional aspects of respiratory disorders among coal miners. JAMA, 156(5):484–487, 1954.

23. Clancy, P.J., et al.: Case report: nitrogen tetroxide exposure in the missle industry. J. Occupat. Med., 4(11):691–693, 1962.

24. DeJournette, R.L.: Rocket propellant inhalation in the apollo-soyuz astronauts. Radiology, 125(10):21–24, 1977.

25. Yockey, C.C., et al.: The McConnell missle accident—clinical spectrum of nitrogen dioxide exposure. JAMA, 244(11):1221–1223, 1980.

26. Doyle, H.A., Jr.: Hearings Before a Subcommittee on Government Operations. H.R., 94th congress, Second Session. June 9, 10, 15 and July 23, 1976.

27. Thomas, G.E., and Wald, N.: J. Occupat. Med., 1:421, 1959.

Chapter 33

Impact of Aviation on the Environment

Spurgeon Neel

The end of science is not to prove a theory, but to improve mankind.

MANLY HALL

After almost a century of unparalleled and unrestrained technologic advances in aviation, there is a growing recognition that aerospace operations may contribute considerably to environmental residua. This chapter will discuss some of the more popular notions and assess the impact of aviation on the greater environment.

The effect of aircraft-associated contaminants on crewmembers, passengers, and maintenance personnel has been discussed in Chapter 32, as have the basics of toxicology and physics. This chapter will focus on the impact of the industry on the general community.

ENVIRONMENTAL ASSESSMENT

National Environmental Policy Act

On January 1, 1970, the National Environmental Policy Act of 1969 (NEPA) was signed into law. Within the decade that followed, ecology became a household word and a potent force in contemporary society, influencing everything from international politics to individual lifestyles.[1]

As stated in the law, the purposes of NEPA are fourfold: (1) to declare a national policy that will encourage productive and enjoyable harmony between man and his environment; (2) to promote efforts that will prevent or eliminate damage to the environment and biosphere and stimulate the health and welfare of man; (3) to enrich the understanding of the ecologic systems and natural resources important to the nation; and (4) to establish a Council of Environment Quality.

Further, federal agencies are directed to utilize an integrated, interdisciplinary, and natural and social sciences approach to environmental problems and to develop relevant techniques and methodologies to ensure that unquantifiable amenities receive the same attention given to the more tangible economic and technologic considerations. This twofold approach directive evolved into the environmental assessment process leading to the preparation of detailed environmental impact statements, which indicate the environmental consequences of proposed actions and programs.

Environmental Impact Statements (EISs)

Every federal agency is now required to include in every recommendation or report on proposals for legislation and other major federal actions significantly affecting the quality of human environment a detailed statement, which includes:

1. The environmental impact of the proposed action
2. Any adverse environmental effect that cannot be avoided should the action take place
3. Possible alternatives
4. Discussion of short-term versus long-term advantages of the proposal
5. Any irreversible and irretrievable commitment of resources that would be involved if the proposed action were implemented

Most state and local governments have legislation similar to NEPA to assist in making environmentally related decisions. State, local, and even private-sector actions that require federal licensing or that receive federal funds require the preparation of EISs under NEPA.

The concept is simple, but the process of collecting data, writing, reviewing, debating, and acting on the statement is quite complex and time-consuming. The process involves four major sequential stages. First, the agency must determine whether a statement must be prepared for the proposed project. The law requires a formal statement whenever an agency proposes an action that "significantly affects the environment." This leads to flexibility of interpretation, but each agency has developed guidelines and criteria.

Second, if it is determined that an impact statement is required, a draft statement is prepared. This is a preliminary report of the environmental consequences associated with the project. If a statement is not required, the agency can proceed with the project. In such a case, the agency usually documents the basis for the negative determination.

As a third step, the agency sends the draft statement to all groups having an interest in the proposed action. Depending on the nature of the project, the draft statement is coordinated with other federal agencies, including the Council of Environmental Quality (in the Executive Office of the President), state and local governments, local industry and business, appropriate private citizens, and special-interest groups such as community-level Chambers of Commerce, and conservation groups such as the Sierra Club. Coordinating agencies are provided a reasonable period, usually 6 weeks, to study the draft and submit their comments back to the proponent agency.

The final statement is prepared after review and consideration of the comments of the coordinating agencies. The final impact statement, including the comments and their consideration, accompanies the proposed action throughout the remainder of the agency's decision-making process. The impact to the aerospace industry can be enormous.

AIRPORT-COMMUNITY NOISE PROBLEMS

As a result of advances in aviation technology and increased air travel, aircraft noise has become increasingly prevalent in communities during the last decade or so. Along with the increase in airport noise has been a public awareness of, and irritation with, the noise. Sometimes, this irritation has culminated in complaints and even vigorous opposition to airport operations.

In 1952, Harry Truman convened a President's Airport Commission, the so-called Doolittle Commission, to evaluate the growing airport system. The Commission concluded, among other things, that:

Some excuse may be found for failure to have foreseen the rapid rate of aeronautical progress in designing airports in the past, but it is to be regretted that more consideration was not given to the comfort and welfare of people living on the ground in the vicinity of airports. To be

Table 32–11. Threshold Limit Values For Industrial Noise

Duration Per Day	Sound Level (dBA)*
16 hours	80
8 hours	85
4 hours	90
2 hours	95
1 hour	100
30 minutes	105
15 minutes	110
7.5 minutes	115†

*Sound level in decibels is measured on a sound level meter, conforming as a minimum to the requirements of the American National Standard Specification for Sound Level Meters, S1.4 (1971) type S2A, and set to use the A-weighted network with slow meter response.
†No exposure to continuous or intermittent in excess of 115 dBA.
From Documentation of the Threshold Limit Values and Supplemental Documentations. 4th Ed. With threshold limit values for 1982 with intended changes. American Conference of Governmental Industrial Hygienists of Cincinnati, 1971.

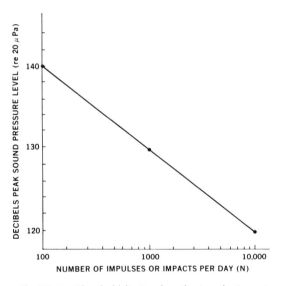

Fig. 32–5. Threshold limit values for impulse/impact noise.[6]

lined in the algorithm shown in Figure 32–6. It should be mentioned that even though 90 dBA is the standard of hazardous noise exposure, the United States Department of Defense uses the level of greater than 84 dBA to require inclusion of its workers in a hearing conservation/audiometric testing program. It provides an example of biologic monitoring within

a program of occupational health surveillance designed to protect the health of all federal employees. The program went well beyond existing OSHA requirements and exemplified enlightened federal leadership in self-regulation as a basis for sound standards setting.

The algorithm requires a 30-day removal from noise in cases of threshold shift (TS) that persist over 30 days. In attempting to implement this guidance, the United States Air Force examined all workers exposed to hazardous noise levels in the early 1970s, some of whom had not had further audiometric testing since initial Air Force employment (dating in some cases back to the time of World War II). Literally hundreds of the Air Force's approximately 100,000 civilian workers were found to have an apparently significant TS. They were recommended for temporary removal from noise for 30 days. Because there were insufficient "noise-free" jobs, many of these workers were sent home on sick or annual leave. Because their absences were job-related, however, compensation was sought by many. The great majority had significant losses only at 3 and 4 kHz. Losses in these frequencies usually do not adversely affect speech comprehension (as would losses in the so-called speech frequencies—0.5, 1, and 2 kHz). For this reason, frequencies above 2 kHz were not included in considering compensability using the formula recommended by the American Academy of Ophthalmology and Otolaryngology. Because of a virtual epidemic of claims, however, the United States Department of Labor's Office of Workers Compensation Programs modified its formula to compensate workers who were "off-the-job" because of noise.[26] Because the hearing losses were permanent, Air Force Hearing Conservation Diagnostic Centers examining such workers frequently gave the cryptic finding, "high-frequency hearing loss, probably noise-induced," often adding, "remove from noise." This placed occu-

DISPOSITION FLOW CHART

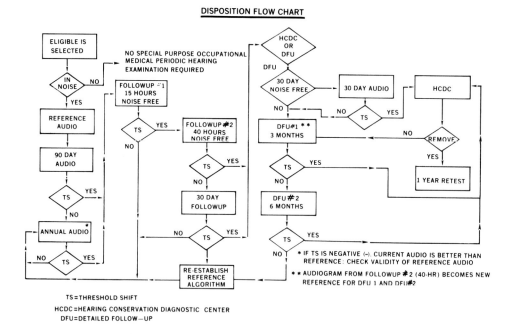

TS = THRESHOLD SHIFT
HCDC = HEARING CONSERVATION DIAGNOSTIC CENTER
DFU = DETAILED FOLLOW—UP

Fig. 32–6. Algorithm for the evaluation and disposition of workers in a noise hazard environment.

pational physicians at several Air Force bases in the difficult position of having to overrule a Hearing Center's recommendations in returning an employee to his skilled job. Some such employees applied for early disability retirement based on having received compensation for noise-induced hearing loss and a medical recommendation for permanent removal from noise.

A special command authority was established by the Air Force Surgeon General in 1976 to review and approve all cases of personnel removed permanently from noise. If careful review of a worker's audiograms over the most recent 3 years revealed stability (as was almost always the case), this became the basis for recommending a return to work with an adjusted (once only) baseline audiogram, allowing reentry into the Air Force hearing conservation program. This experience should alert aerospace medical specialists to the necessity of anticipating difficulties in health conservation programs of all types until sufficient experi-

ence is generated to control troublesome artifacts.

Vibration

Vibratory oscillatory motions, or vibrations, are not presently covered by federal regulations. Adverse effects, however, may result from excessive vibratory exposure of the whole body or its parts.

Whole-Body Vibration

Tolerance levels to different degrees of peak acceleration are a function of the frequency and duration of exposure, as shown in Figure 32–7. A standard proposed by the International Standards Organization (ISO) was unacceptable because it included limits for frequencies up to 90 Hz, but the proposal was based on inadequate data above 30 Hz, and it omitted significant data that would have tended to modify its recommended limits. In the United States, NIOSH is responsible for and is now developing criteria on which OSHA may eventually establish occupational exposure standards.

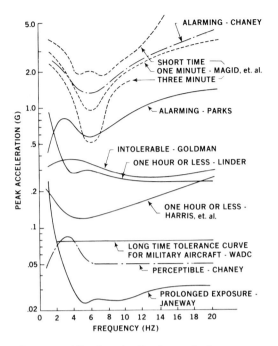

Fig. 32–7. Vibration classification and tolerance; acceleration versus frequency versus exposure time. (Reproduced with permission from Ramsey, J.D.: Occupational Vibration. in Zenz, C. (ed.): Occupational Medicine: Principles and Practical Applications. Copyright ©1975 by Yearbook Medical Publishers, Inc., Chicago.)

Research has established that man's sensitivity to external vibration is highest between 0.5 and 20 Hz because the human system absorbs most of the vibratory energy applied within this range, with maximal amplification between 5 and 11 Hz. Posture can greatly affect tolerance in test subjects. There is also wide variability between and within individuals, depending on such other factors as fatigue, physical conditioning, and perceived risk. Standards for human experimentation and aerospace exploration involve the same careful attention to physical and mental fitness and absence of diseases of all types that characterize the selection of individuals for pilot training. Whole-body vibrational stresses of significance are not commonly encountered outside of such military and space environments, although at least one NIOSH study of the morbidity of heavy

equipment operators caused by vibration exposure was published in 1974, and a NIOSH plan to develop industrial vibration criteria was published in 1972.[16]

Segmental Vibration

Localized bioeffects from the use of oscillatory and rotary tools are most common between 25 and 150 Hz when amplitude is at least 100 μm. For hammer-type tools, the common frequencies for undesirable localized vibration effects are 30 to 50 Hz. In addition to Raynaud's phenomenon, which progressively affects palmar arch and digital arteries, neurologic aspects are being recognized that involve tingling and numbness. Adverse effects tend to vary inversely with the weight of the tool. Reduced exposure time appears to be an important controllable factor in protecting against such adverse bioeffects.

Temperature

Heat Stress

Hot environments are hazardous to life and health because they raise the body's core temperature. Resting deep body temperature is normally about 37.2° C. Variations become intolerable above and below rather narrow physiologic limits, ranging from 35 to 41°C. The TLVs discussed below are based on the assumption that nearly all acclimatized, fully clothed workers with adequate water and salt intake should be able to function effectively under the given working conditions without exceeding a core body temperature of 38° C.

Higher heat exposures than those shown here are permissible under close occupational health surveillance with documentation of workers' tolerance. Workers should not be permitted to continue hot work when their deep body temperature exceeds 38° C.[6,20]

Physicians responsible for the health of workers in hot climates must understand that any prolonged physical activity results in a higher metabolic rate and, hence, an increase in body temperature. Walking in shorts at 80 m/min for 30 to 40 minutes on a cool day may result in a body temperature of 38.3° C for a 70-kg man, whereas a run of 1500 m in less than 8 minutes under similar conditions may boost the body temperature to 39.5° C, based on maximum oxygen uptake. In the general population, anaerobic metabolism sets in when 40 to 50% of the maximum oxygen uptake is reached and results in decreased efficiency and increased heat production, heart rate, and body temperature without leveling off. Intensive physical conditioning improves heat tolerance, as shown in Figure 32-8, but withholding water eliminates the advantage. Heat acclimatization is easily lost after 1 to 3 weeks away from heat stress and must be renewed. The permissible heat exposure TLVs shown in Figure 32-9 are based on the assumption that the environment of the resting place is similar to that in the work place. Where the wet bulb globe temperature (WBGT) of work and rest areas differ, a time-weighted average value

should be calculated for both environmental heat and metabolic heat, as shown in Figure 32-9, using the solid line labeled "continuous." The standard permissible exposure limits for continuous work also assume a work-rest regimen of a 5-day work week and an 8-hour work day with short (15 minutes) midmorning and midafternoon breaks and a longer (30 minutes) lunch break. Where additional resting time is allowed, higher exposure limits are permitted.

On hot jobs, reasonably cool drinking water (10 to 15° C) should be readily available and consumed by workers at a rate of about 150 ml every 15 to 20 minutes. Where workers are unacclimatized and unable to add sufficient salt to their food to replace that lost in sweat, salt should be added to the drinking water at the rate of 1 g of sodium chloride per liter of water, which produces the desired 0.1% concentration.

Permissible heat exposure TLVs are valid only for light-weight, summer-type work clothing. Where insulated or sweat-impervious clothing is required (e.g., fire-

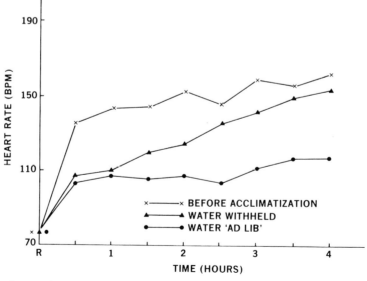

Fig. 32–8. The influence of heat acclimatization and water restriction on heart rate response during 4 hours of heat stress. Water restriction entirely eliminates the beneficial influence of heat acclimatization. (Reproduced with permission from Strydom, N.B.: Physical work and heat stress. In Zenz, C. (ed.): Occupational Medicine: Principles and Practical Applications. Copyright ©1975 by Yearbook Medical Publishers, Inc., Chicago.)

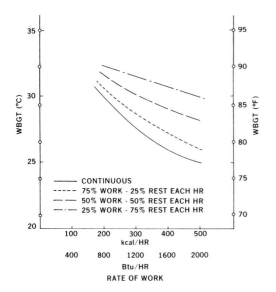

Fig. 32–9. Permissible heat exposure threshold limit value.[6]

fighters' suits, missile propellant handlers' protective clothing), special attention must be given in arriving at safe limits of exposure. It must be emphasized that the TLVs are valid only for heat-acclimatized workers who are fit physically. Extra caution must be used until it can be established both that any unfit workers have been identified and placed in more sheltered work situations and that remaining workers are properly acclimatized and instructed in the avoidance of hazardous heat stress.

Heart rates can exceed 170 beats/min the first day of acclimatization but should stabilize within 3 to 4 days to less than 140 beats/min (Fig. 32–10). Daily hot work periods during the process of full 8-hour acclimatization must last 4 hr/day for 5 to 8 consecutive days. There is no advantage to more than 4 hours, but 2 hours is inadequate for 8-hour acclimatization. Symptoms of thirst and cramps do not give adequate warning of the hazard of heat stress. Attention of all workers should be directed to the following conditions, which have been associated with in-creased susceptibility to serious complications of hazardous heat exposure:

1. Lack of acclimatization
2. Obesity
3. Lack of physical fitness
4. Fatigue
5. Lack of sleep
6. Dehydration
7. Febrile illness
8. Acute and convalescent infections
9. Reactions to immunizations
10. Conditions affecting sweating
11. Skin disorders (e.g., heat rash, sunburn)
12. Drug use (e.g., alcohol, barbiturates)
13. Past history of heat injury
14. Previously living in cooler climate
15. Existing chronic diseases (i.e., diabetes, cardiovascular disease)
16. Central nervous system lesion (e.g., of the hypthalamus, brain stem, and cervical part of the spinal cord)
17. Convalescence from certain surgical operations
18. Recent intake of food
19. Sustained muscular exercise
20. Known intolerance to heat

Cold Stress

Cold stress TLVs have not been published but are under consideration by the ACGIH to prevent hazards of local and generalized injuries and disorders. Low-temperature time limits are shown in Table 32–12.

Local injury from exposure to excessive cold occurs seasonally among the indigent and infirm in northern climates and is also a primary concern of military personnel in the field. It also may occur among civilian workers wherever the predisposing conditions are met such as those outlined in Table 32–13, where exposed flesh is shown to suffer cold injury in the form of freezing (and consequent frostbite) at or below −18° C even at wind velocities as low as 25 kph. Special problems obviously exist in arctic regions, where temperatures

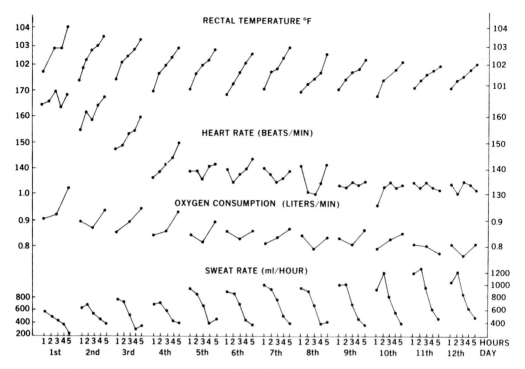

Fig. 32–10. Physiologic responses of men exposed for 5 hours daily to a set work rate in hot, humid heat during an acclimatization experiment. (Reproduced with permission from Strydom, N.B.: Physical work and heat stress. *In* Zenz, C. (ed.): Occupational Medicine: Principles and Practical Applications. Copyright ©1975 by Yearbook Medical Publishers, Inc., Chicago.)

Table 32–12.   Low-Temperature Time Limits

Temperature Range (°C)	Maximal Daily Exposure
−1 to −18	No exposure time limit if properly clothed
−18 to −34	Total cold-room work time: 4 hours (alternate 1 hour in, 1 hour out)
−34 to −57	Two periods of 30 minutes each, at least 4 hours apart. Total cold-room work time allowed: 1 hour
−57 to −73	Maximal permissible cold-room time: 5 minutes over an 8-hour working day, wearing completely enclosed headgear and equipped with a breathing tube running under the clothing and down the leg to preheat the air

Reproduced with permission from Strydom, M.B.: Physical work and heat stress. *In* Occupational Medicine: Principles and Practical Applications. Edited by C. Lenz. Copyright © 1975 by Year Book Medical Publishers, Inc., Chicago.

fall below −40° C and wind speed may reach and maintain hurricane velocities for hours to days at a time.

Hypothermia occurs when the deep body heat falls below 35° C as a result of cold stress. This condition occurs more frequently when body metabolism is reduced as a result of starvation or malnutrition, illness (hypothyroidism), and when certain medications are ingested (alcohol, barbiturates, tranquilizers, narcotics). The normal healthy worker conserves body heat by shivering, but this reflex is diminished in individuals over 40 and may be absent in persons 50 to 60 years of age. Older workers are, therefore, especially susceptible to chronic cold stress at home and en route to work, as well as on the job. In the presence of cold stress, the sudden onset of confusion, agitation, or depression should be noted by fellow workers and reported. Medical facilities

Table 32–13. Cooling Power of the Wind on Exposed Flesh Expressed as an Equivalent Temperature

Estimated Wind Speed (in kph)	Actual Thermometer Reading (°C)											
	10	4	−1	−7	−12	−18	−23	−29	−34	−40	−46	−51
	Equivalent Temperature (°C)											
calm	10	4	−1	−7	−12	−18	−23	−29	−34	−40	−46	−51
8	9	3	−2	−9	−14	−20	−25	−32	−37	−43	−50	−55
16	5	−2	−6	−15	−22	−30	−35	−42	−48	−55	−63	−69
24	2	−7	−12	−21	−28	−34	−43	−51	−57	−63	−71	−81
32	0	−9	−15	−24	−32	−37	−47	−56	−62	−69	−76	−88
40	−1	−10	−18	−26	−34	−40	−51	−60	−65	−73	−85	−93
48	−2	−11	−19	−28	−36	−42	−53	−63	−68	−76	−89	−97
56	−3	−12	−20	−29	−37	−44	−55	−65	−70	−78	−91	−99
64	−4	−13	−21	−30	−38	−46	−56	−67	−71	−80	−92	−101

(wind speeds greater than 64 kph have little additional effect)

Little danger (for properly clothed person)—maximum danger is false sense of security

Increasing danger—danger from freezing of exposed flesh

Great danger

Trenchfoot and immersion foot may occur at any point on this chart may need to procure a means of measuring core body temperatures below 35° C. The usual clinical thermometer is intended to detect fever not hypothermia. It has been shown that bare hands remain warm in −35° C ambient temperatures, but extremities cool rapidly when body heat is reduced by as little as 15%.

Electromagnetic Radiation (EMR) Hazards

The EMR spectrum encompasses an unbroken series of ethereal waves, moving with the velocity of light, which vary widely in wavelength (Fig. 32–11) from cosmic rays as short as 4×10^{-12} cm to hertzian waves (used in radio and power transmission), which extend several miles in length. For purposes of hazard evaluation and control, EMR falls into two distinct categories based on the ability or inability to dissociate a substance in solution into its constituents, or ions.

Ionizing Radiation (IR)

The degree of IR hazard to living tissues is indicated by the average energy imparted in traversing a specified distance.

High linear energy transfer (LET) is characteristic of the particulate emissions of certain elements such as radium. Besides heat and light, radium salts emit three other distinct forms of radiation (alpha, beta, and gamma rays), as well as radon, a radioactive gas. Penetrating power and the range of travel are inversely proportional to LET; hence, high LET radiation (high-energy beta rays or particles, neutrons, and deuterons) would transfer more energy in a specified volume than gamma rays or x-rays of equivalent energy, causing greater damage as a result of secondary ionization induction. Although alpha particles are high LET, their range is so short that a hazard would result only if they were placed in close proximity to a radiosensitive target organ (e.g., cataracts

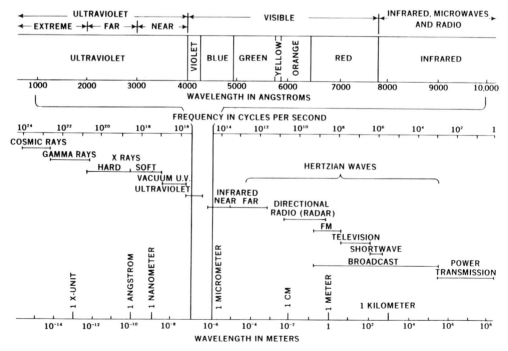

Fig. 32–11. The electromagnetic spectrum. (Modified from Zenz, C. (ed.): Occupational Medicine: Principles and Practical Applications. Copyright ©1975 by Yearbook Medical Publishers, Inc., Chicago.)

sure, many settled near an airport after it was in operation, with little realization of the potential nuisance and hazard. The public cannot be expected, however, to anticipate technical developments and it should be informed and protected by the responsible authorities.[2]

Human Effects of Noise

Temporary or Permanent Hearing Loss

The research basis for the Walsh-Healey Act Hearing Conservation Standards involved industrial situations with a fairly constant noise level during an 8-hour work day and an assumed quiet residential environment for rest and recovery of the auditory system during the other 16 hours of the day. The act now limits an exposure of 106 dBA for a maximum of 1 hr/day and 100 dBA for a maximum of 2 hr/day. This maximum approximates the noise level to which communities closer than 5 to 6 km from airport runways are intermittently exposed.

Physiologic Responses

Noise also can trigger changes in cardiovascular, endocrine, and neurologic functions and is correlated with feelings of distress for sounds above 140 dB. No evidence exists to suggest, however, that noise below 120 dB significantly affects these functions.[3]

Speech Interference

The most disruptive and widespread effect of noise is masking, or interference with the reception of speech. This interference is a major factor in aircraft noise annoyance. Surveys conducted in airport neighborhoods indicate that aircraft noise interference with speech, either in face-to-face conservations, telephone use, or radio and television listening, is more annoying than any other type of noise disturbance.

Interference with Rest, Privacy, and Sleep

Complaints received by airport authorities indicate that interference with sleep causes relatively more intense annoyance and hostility toward aircraft noise than daytime interruptions of communications and social functions. Thus, all composite noise indexes place a greater significance on nighttime operations. The Composite Noise Rating (CNR) index assumes that one nighttime noise exposure is equal to ten daytime exposures. A further concern is that repeated arousal from sleep could generally lead to degradation of health because rest and sleep provide conditions for the restitution of body energy and recovery from fatigue.

Psychologic Annoyance and Irritability

The interruption of speech and sleep and the nonauditory effects of aircraft noise are undesirable, but these interferences do not necessarily produce equal annoyance or hostility among differently predisposed people. Studies such as the one conducted by Tracor, Inc. showed that when noise exposure was the sole predictor, estimation of community annoyance was poor.[4] When other psychologic and social variables were included, the prediction equation was improved. Of the 20 variables investigated, the seven that best explained annoyance were fear of aircraft crashing in the neighborhood, susceptibility to noise, distance from the airport, noise adaptability, city of residence, belief in malfeasance on the part of those able to do something about the noise problem, and the extent to which the airport and air transportation were viewed as important by the respondent. The fear variable contributed more to annoyance and irritability than the other six variables.

Complex Noise Measurement

The methods of measuring single noise exposures have proliferated, each method attempting to integrate the different spectral characteristics of different sounds into simple units of equal noisiness or unpleasantness. These units of noise measurement, however, cannot accurately describe units of environmental annoyance. By definition, noise is unwanted sound, and its "unwantedness" cannot be measured realistically without considering the meaning and emotional content of the noise, as well as its effect in interfering with various desired activities.

Since 1952, techniques have been used to determine how people in the real environment perceived noise and what psychosocial variables influenced their reactions to these noise exposures. The major disadvantages of the survey technique are that data collections are costly and time-consuming and only gross averages of the complex stimulus situations are possible. Engineers and noise abatement officials need to know the independent and interacting contributions of the components of a noise experience to assess the cost-benefits of specific proposals for noise reduction.

More recent research at Columbia University placed human subjects in an acoustic lab, furnished as a typical living room in a middle-class home in which a quadraphonic sound system was employed to produce a realistic aircraft noise experience in which the plane appeared to fly overhead across the room. The subjects rated each randomly allocated experimental noise in terms of the degree of interference with the activity, such as watching television, and the degree of annoyance resulting from the interference. This technique controlled the eight basic variables: the type of plane, operations, slant distance, time of exposure (and by season), rate per hour, position of the subject, ambient noise, and activities.

Research from the past three decades has produced much useful information on noise propagation and the human response to it. Much more, however, still needs to be learned to answer the practical questions posed by noise abatement officials.

According to the Department of Transportation, some 3% of our population,

over 7 million persons, have been exposed to an excessive level of aircraft noise. Older aircraft still in use produce about twice the noise that the Federal Aviation Administration (FAA) rules allow for new airplanes. Present exposures are generally unacceptable and create considerable annoyance in most communities.

Noise has become regulated, as has all other forms of environmental residua. Environmental Protection Agency (EPA) noise control activities are authorized by the Noise Pollution and Abatement Act of 1970 (Title IV of the Clean Air Act) and the Noise Control Act of 1972 (Public Law 92-574). The FAA also is assigned certain responsibilities in the control and abatement of aircraft noise in Section 7 of the latter act.

The EPA Office of Noise Abatement and Control is responsible for identifying and classifying causes and sources of noise, determining their effects on public health and welfare, and proposing any national standards and regulations necessary to protect the public health and welfare. Noise monitoring activities are authorized in the Noise Control Act under Section 14, which deals with research, technical assistance to state and local governments, and public information.

The FAA's responsibilities under the Noise Control Act of 1972 are to provide current and future relief from aircraft noise through appropriate noise control and abatement regulations. It accomplished these goals through the Federal Aviation Regulations (FARs). Of particular interest is FAR Part 36, which prescribes noise standards for aircraft type and airworthiness certification. Part 36 was amended, effective April 3, 1978, and prescribes amended noise limits for new airplane designs, limits the noise level increase of certain older airplanes if their designs are changed, and amends noise-measuring points and noise test conditions. This amendment brings the United States aircraft noise standards into greater conformity with the international standards recently adopted by the International Civil Aviation Organization (ICAO).

Other applicable laws include the Quiet Communities Act (Public Law 95-609), which amends certain portions of the Noise Control Act of 1972, promotes the development of effective state and local noise control programs, and provides for an adequate federal noise control research program. Section 14 of this act also provides for the administrations of a nationwide Quiet Communities Program.

Finally, there is the Aviation Safety and Noise Abatement Act of 1979 (Public Law 96-193). This act specifies noise emission standards and provides for "exemptions from applicable noise standards to permit operation of any non-complying three-engine aircraft, but not beyond January 1, 1985," provided that the operator of the aircraft has a plan for replacement and entered a binding contract by January 1, 1983 for delivery by January 1, 1985. Similarly, two-engine aircraft may be exempted until January 1, 1986.

This act requires that airport operators submit a Noise Compatibility Program to the Secretary of the Department of Transportation. The program will address, but not be limited to, the following:

1. Implementation of any preferential runway system
2. Restriction on the use of the airport by any type or class of aircraft based on noise characteristics.
3. Construction of barriers and acoustic shielding, including soundproofing of public buildings
4. The use of flight procedures to control operations of aircraft to reduce exposure of individuals to noise in areas around the airport
5. Acquisition of land, air rights, easements, and so on to assure the use of property for purposes that are compatible with airport operations

Section 103 of this act provides for the preparation and submission of noise exposure maps for developmental and planning purposes. The objective is to reduce existing noncompatible uses of land around airports and to prevent the introduction of new noncompatible use.

The options available for reducing aircraft noise levels at the source include retrofitting, reengining, and replacement. Retrofitting refers to the placement of sound-absorbent material in the engines and nacelles. The preferred option by most people in the aircraft business appears to be replacement over retrofit.

Coordination

Controlling aircraft noise at the source is difficult because of the expense, the long economic life of the aircraft (approximately 20 years), the limited improvements that technology permits, and the increase in airline operations that occurs as demand for air service increases. Measures to combat aircraft noise at the source may accomplish little more than to prevent us from falling behind.

Although noise source control is necessary, there must also be planning to ensure that land around airports is not used for purposes incompatible with existing and projected noise levels. State and local governments can control the land use through zoning. They also can take other measures such as assuring that noise exposure levels are revealed in real estate transactions. Local governments also have the authority to take noise levels into account in locating and designing schools, hospitals, and other public buildings and in developing highways, sewers, and other basic services that influence local development.

This twofold approach to the solution of the problem of aircraft noise will no doubt contribute to a reduction in the noise experience of persons living in the surrounding airport environs in the future.

SONIC BOOMS

A unique environmental effect of supersonic flight is the sonic boom. Much like the bow wave of a ship, the wave pattern traveling with the aircraft sweeps over the terrain, similar to the advancing shock wave of a mild explosion. Numerous sonic boom studies have been done during the past two decades due to the increased operation of high-performance military aircraft, the proposed United States supersonic transport (SST), and the entry of the British-French Concorde SST into commercial airline service. Documentation of the phenomenon and its effects has been extensively reported.[5]

Effects of Sonic Boom

Figure 33–1 shows the effect of the atmosphere above and below the aircraft on the development of the primary and secondary carpets. It depicts an aircraft at 20 km altitude flying toward the viewer. The downward rays (solid lines) impact the terrain to form the primary boom carpet, extending to 40 km in this example. A secondary carpet region is depicted at about 120 to 170 km from the flight track. The dashed line rays impacting in this carpet may arrive directly as a result of bending in the upper atmosphere, or they may first impact in the primary carpet region, then reflect upward and subsequently bend downward into the secondary region. Between these two carpets there is no boom.

Primary Boom Carpet

The primary boom carpet and its disturbances have been researched intensely and involve only propagation in the lower atmosphere. The disturbances involve high overpressures and steep rise times and have a substantial high-frequency content. Overpressures may reach 700 N/m^2. Levels increase with increasing aircraft size and decrease with increasing altitude. Highest overpressures occur near ground track and are associated with an N-wave–type signature. This is an impact steep rise time followed by straight-line recovery through the negative phase and abrupt cessation. Promulgation distances are typically less than 50 km, and at the lateral cut-off point, the N-wave form is lost and the boom becomes a "rumble." Sonic booms in the primary carpet cause adverse community response.

Secondary Boom Carpet

The secondary boom carpet and its disturbances are not as well defined. Only fragmentary observations and measurements are available. These disturbances involve both the upper and lower levels of the atmosphere during propagation and have low-frequency content. Propagation distances greater than 150 km are common, and relatively large areas are exposed. Secondary carpet booms are generally not audible (0.1 to 1.0 Hz) but can cause building vibrations that are readily observed. These "booms" tend to be more of a curiosity and are not likely to cause serious adverse community response.

Community Response

Human response to impulse noise (such as sonic booms) is most complex, involving not only the physical stimulus but also the immediate environment (ambient noise conditions), the experience, attitudes, and opinions of those exposed, and other factors not directly related to the stimulus. Man's individual and group reactions to sonic booms are summarized by Von Gierke in Figure 33–2.[6]

During the mid-1960s, numerous studies of public reactions to sonic booms were conducted in selected metropolitan areas of the United States and France. In these studies, the number of complaints reported was small. It appears that complaints result only when the respondent is annoyed, feels it is not unpatriotic to complain, knows how to complain effectively, feels that his complaint will do some good,

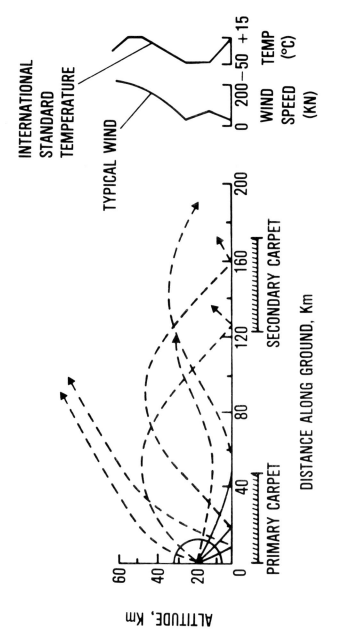

Fig. 33–1. Propagation paths of sonic booms.

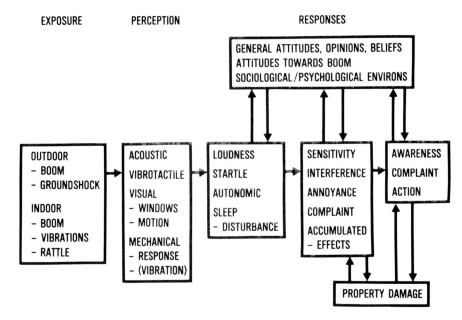

Fig. 33–2.   Reactions to sonic booms.

and believes that the noise is harming his family or house.

Popular notions that sonic booms cause snow avalanches or affect egg-hatching, mink-whelping, and livestock adversely are not supported by scientific data. All these notions and resultant studies produced enough concern over annoyance to cause the FAA to prohibit civil aircraft flights at speeds that create a sonic boom over United States territory. This action effectively ended intensive sonic boom research in 1972.

Prior to this decision, many proposals were advanced to decrease the sonic booms of the SSTs. One of the more imaginative approaches suggested an electromagnetic device to elongate the fuselage signature to modify the shock wave. Thousands of megawatts of electrical power, however, were required to achieve a 10% reduction in boom intensity, and the equipment required exceeded the payload capability of the SST. Another proposal would utilize a second penalty aircraft in formation with the SST so that the shock waves would cancel each other. Neither of these approaches is economically feasible.

RADIOFREQUENCY RADIATION

Characteristics and Sources

Radiofrequency (RF) radiation occupies the lower portion of the electromagnetic spectrum, to the left of infrared radiation. RF wavelengths vary from 10 km to about 1 mm, with frequencies ranging from 30 kHz to 300 GHz. Table 33–1 displays the features of RF and microwave bands.[7]

The growing number of domestic, commercial, and medical applications of RF technology (microwave ovens, materials drying, and diathermy) has resulted in a greater awareness and concern on the part of the public as to potential hazards.

Microwave sources may operate continuously (communication), intermittently (microwave oven), or in a pulsed mode (radar). Natural sources of RF radiation also exist. The movement of a cold front may generate peak field intensities of over 100 V/m at ground level. Solar radiation also includes a relatively small fraction of RF radiation.

Biologic Effects

The photon energy in RF radiation is too low to produce photochemical reactions

Table 33–1. Radiofrequency and Microwave Band Designations

USA	Wavelengths	Frequencies	Typical Uses
Radiofrequency bands			
Low frequency (LF)	10^4–10^3 m	30–300 kHz	Radionavigation, radio beacon
Medium frequency (MF)	10^3–10^2 m	0.3–3 MHz	Marine radiotelephone, loran, AM broadcast
High frequency (HF)	10^2–10 m	3–30 MHz	Amateur radio, worldwide broadcasting, medical diathermy, radio astronomy
Microwave bands			
Very high frequency (VHF)	10–1 m	30–300 MHz	FM broadcast, television, air traffic control, radionavigation
Ultra high frequency (UHF)	1–0.1 m	0.3–3 GHz	Television, citizens band, microwave point-to-point, microwave ovens, telemetry, tropo scatter, and meteorologic radar
Super high frequency (SHF)	10–1 cm	3–30 GHz	Satellite communication, airborne weather radar, altimeters, shipborne navigational radar, microwave point-to-point
Extra high frequency (EHF)	1–0.1 cm	30–300 GHz	Radio astronomy, cloud detection radar, space research, HCN (hydrogen cyanide) emission

Modified from Wilkening, G.M.: Nonionizing radiation. *In* The Industrial Environment—Its Evaluation and Control. National Institute of Occupational Safety and Health, U.S. Government Printing Office, Washington, D.C., 1973, pp. 357–373.

in biologic systems, that is, below 10 eV. Rather, the energy is absorbed by the tissues and ultimately dissipated as heat. At the permissible exposure level (PEL) of 10 MW/cm², approximately 58 W of energy is absorbed, with a body temperature elevation of 1°C, an acceptable value. In comparison, the human basal metabolic rate approximates 80 W at rest and increases to 290 W with moderate work.

Tissue penetration varies with wavelength and frequency. Wavelengths less than 3 cm are absorbed in the outer skin layer; wavelengths of 3 to 10 cm may penetrate up to 1 cm, and wavelengths of 25 to 100 cm may penetrate more deeply and have the potential of damaging internal organs. The human body is thought to be virtually transparent to wavelengths above 200 cm. Above 300 MHz, the depth of penetration declines rapidly with frequency and is only millimeters above 3000 MHz.

Interest has been shown in the potential of microwave radiation to cause cataract formation. In rabbits, lens opacities have

been produced under controlled conditions with power densities of 80 to 40 MW/cm² (well above the PEL). Repeated exposures over time constitute a greater risk, suggesting a cumulative effect, as well as a repair mechanism that limits lens damage if adequate time elapses between exposures.

Research has suggested a possible relationship between Down's syndrome in offspring and previous exposure of the male parent to radar. Of 216 cases of mongolism, 8.7% of the fathers with mongoloid offspring had contact with radar while in military service versus 3.3% of the control fathers. This possible association must be viewed with extreme caution due to many unknowns, including the probability of varied environmental exposures (such as ionizing radiation) while in military service.

Cardiac pacemakers, particularly the demand type, may be seriously compromised by nearby microwave radiation at levels far below those causing detrimental biologic effects. Shielding of pacemakers and appropriate warning signs seem to be the answer. In the medical field, microwave radiation plays a useful and expanding role in therapy. The judicious exposure of humans to diathermy may be as high as 100 MW/cm^2, or ten times the PEL.

Assessment

RF radiation appears to pose no real threat to the general environment or individuals. The PEL is one-tenth the exposure demonstrated to cause biologic effects. Generators and transmitters are inaccessible or airborne. Industrial hygiene and safety monitoring are adequate. Many of the systems are low power (less than 25 MW), most are omnidirectional, and some rotate at 12 rpm, keeping area flux down. Standard tower heights are 10 to 20 m, whereas 12 m away from a generator is generally safe. Navigational radar is directed 2° or more above the horizon, posing no threat to the community. The major danger of significant exposure to microwave and RF radiation is among avionics and maintenance personnel if there is a lapse in safety procedures such as a generator being energized. Particular care must be devoted to the development and operation of tracking radar systems due to the lock-on phenomenon.

ATMOSPHERIC CONTAMINATION

Aircraft Emissions

Aircraft contribute but a small portion of total emissions from all sources on a national scale. Aircraft account for about 1% of hydrocarbons, oxides of nitrogen, and carbon monoxide and an even smaller fraction of particulate matter and oxides of sulfur. Commercial aircraft have lower hydrocarbons but higher emissions of oxides of nitrogen than do military aircraft due to their larger and newer engines. General aviation aircraft contribute the least and have been exempted from emission standards (Table 33–2).

At the regional and local levels, the contributions of aircraft may be greater. Table 33–2 presents information on the Atlanta, Georgia region as well as the Atlanta Airport. At the regional level, aircraft contribute about 3% of total emissions. At the airport, aircraft are the predominant source of emissions, with surface traffic taking second priority. Aircraft emissions are more subject to dispersion and dilution than traffic emissions in congested terminal areas.[8]

In addition to aircraft engine improvements, air pollution at airports can be reduced by changes in ground operations procedures. Among the alternatives available are:

1. Controlling the times of departure to minimize the time spent idling in queue on the taxiway
2. Assigning aircraft to runways to minimize taxi distance/time between gate and runway
3. Shutting down one engine during taxi operations
4. Towing aircraft between runways and gates. (Consider the emissions of towing vehicle in assessing the net reduction)

Controversy continues as to whether aircraft emissions directly endanger public health and welfare and whether federal regulation is actually needed to control aircraft atmospheric pollution. Critics point out that regulations promulgated by the EPA in 1973 under the Clean Air Act are too complex and stringent and have yet to be substantiated by proper air quality studies. Further, significant energy shortages, economic problems, and safety considerations impact on the feasibility of antipollution measures.

Fuel Dumping

Fuel dumping, or fuel jettisoning, is the discharge of unburned fuel directly into the atmosphere by an aircraft while airborne. The basic purpose for jettisoning

Table 33–2.   Aircraft Contribution to Air Pollution

Source	Hydrocarbons (%)	Oxides of Nitrogen (%)	Carbon monoxide (%)
National Level			
All aircraft	1.2	0.6	0.6
Commercial	0.3	0.4	0.2
Military	0.7	0.2	0.2
General aviation	0.2	—	0.2
All sources	30 MT/y	MT/y	116 MT/y
Regional (Atlanta Area)			
Aircraft	3.2	3.1	2.4
Fuel evaporation	0.8	—	—
All sources	89 kt/y	75 kt/y	300 kt/y
Local (Atlanta Airport)			
Aircraft	69	75	58
Fuel evaporation	11	—	—
Traffic, other	20	22	42
All sources	3.9 kt/y	2.9 kt/y	9.5 kt/y

Modified from Naugle, D.F., and Fox, D.L.: Aircraft and air pollution. Environ. Sci. Technol., *15*:342, April, 1981.

fuel is to reduce the aircraft's gross weight to permit a safe landing. To perform their missions, many aircraft must take off with a gross weight much higher than their maximum safe landing weight. An emergency or change in operation plans may require the aircraft to land prematurely, and fuel must be jettisoned to reduce the gross weight to a safe level.

When jettisoned, jet fuel quickly breaks up into small droplets. Within minutes, less than 10% remains in liquid form. When jettisoned 1500 m above ground level at an above-freezing temperature, more than 98% of the fuel will evaporate before reaching the ground.

Atmospheric diffusion processes rapidly disperse and dilute the fuel vapors to levels far below those at which they could be harmful in themselves. The principal environmental problem of these hydrocarbon vapors is their contribution to photochemical oxidant pollution (ozone and smog). This contribution is not important when compared with automobiles, aircraft exhausts, and other sources in the region.

The small fraction of fuel persisting in residual droplets may become seed nuclei for the condensation of water, to the extent of causing precipitation. Usually, they settle directly to the ground and are dispersed over a wide area, reducing ground contamination to low levels.

Hydrocarbons released by fuel dumping continue to be dispersed and scrubbed by natural processes until they reach natural background level. Fuel jettisoning does not appear to have any serious environmental implications.

Alternative Fuels

A continuing and increasing interest exists in developing advanced, improved fuels for aircraft propulsion. The environmental pollution potential of each new candidate fuel receives attention along with essential energy and economic considerations.

The aromatic hydrocarbons, in view of their high carbon content, will continue to produce deposit and smoke problems. In contrast, the liquified hydrocarbon gases are expected to be clean-burning. The alcohols are intermediate as to pollution potential. The nitrogen hydrides, ammonia and hydrazine, are clean-burning in the aviation context.

Liquid hydrogen appears to be the most promising of the alternative fuels evaluated from both the environmental and energy standpoints. The absence of carbon prevents the emission of unburned hydrocarbons, carbon monoxide, carbon dioxide, and most particulates. The only major combustion product is water, which merely returns to the atmosphere. The temperatures involved can give rise to the emission of some oxides of nitrogen but much less than conventional engines.

The major environmental threat in the use of nuclear fuels for aircraft is the potential of a crash landing, with the release of vaporized radioactive materials contaminating a wide area for a long time. Nuclear reactors may be the key to our future expansion into space, however, especially for large satellites on extended missions. Adequate safeguards include maintaining the reactor at a subcritical level until orbit is obtained and boosting the reactor into a higher orbit prior to vehicular reentry. The United States position is that when reactors are the preferred technical choice, they can be used safely and that reactors do not add measurably to the risk associated with the space transportation system.[9]

CONTRAILS

Contrail (condensation trail) formation in the wake of high-flying jet aircraft is a function of the ambient temperature and humidity associated with the excess over the ambient temperature and water content of the exhaust. Whether unburned hydrocarbons and gases in the exhaust make contrails different from regular clouds is not known. It is known that the vapor trails do diffuse laterally, suggesting that they may seed the surrounding atmosphere, spawning adjacent new clouds.

Contrails may be causing subtle weather changes in regions with heavy jet traffic such as the New York to Chicago corridor. Local increases in cloud cover have been associated with expanding jet traffic, with a diminishing average difference between daily high and low temperatures. Heavy jet traffic may be causing climatologic changes affecting crop production and energy use.

Clouds (regular or contrail) have two main effects: shielding the earth from the sun by day and reducing radiation heat loss by night. This contributes to a leveling-off of diurnal temperature extremes. The apparent trend toward increasing cloud cover in jet-traffic corridors could contribute to cooler summer days and warmer winter nights, thereby reducing costly home heating and cooling requirements and lengthening growing seasons in these regions.

Condensation trail formation introduces the possibility of reducing solar radiation at ground level in the order of 1% in regions with low natural lower cloud cover, adding only a trace to the attenuation of natural cloud cover. This effect may increase with increasing jet traffic.

OZONE DEPLETION

Ozone is both foe and friend to man. Its presence in the air that surrounds us has adverse effects as a powerful photochemical oxidant on many of the materials we depend on, greatly speeding their deterioration. Animal studies have shown marked pulmonary changes with exposure to ozone, with evidence of decreased resistance to pulmonary infection. Other studies suggest that ozone is a potent mutagenic and carcinogenic agent. As such, ozone in the troposphere is a potentially dangerous pollutant.

On the other hand, without the ozone layer in the stratosphere, life would not be possible on this planet. The recent development of man's ability to navigate routinely within the stratosphere has caused concerned debate and scientific investigation as to what effect high-flying, air-breathing machines might have on this protective blanket of ozone.

The total amount of ozone in the atmosphere is small. If it were all accumulated at the earth's surface at standard atmospheric pressure, it would form a layer less than 4-mm thick. Ninety-seven percent of this ozone is distributed in the stratosphere between 19 and 50 km altitude in the lower latitudes and 8 to 50 km near the poles. The amount of ozone normally varies up to 30% from season to season, year to year, and decade to decade, complicating the assessment of environmental factors.

This stratospheric ozone layer absorbs solar radiation so thoroughly through a wide range of wavelengths in the ultraviolet (UV) spectrum that none of it reaches the earth. In the so-called UV-B region, longer UV wavelengths from 280 to 320 mm, however, ozone absorbs less perfectly. A decrease of 10% in ozone would lead to a 20% increase in the UV-B waves reaching the earth.

This UV-B radiation causes sunburn and snow blindness, and much evidence suggests that UV-B plays a major etiologic role in skin cancer. Increased UV-B radiation also is associated with decreased agricultural production and with serious damage to certain marine species. In absorbing the energy of UV radiation, ozone causes a warming of the upper stratosphere and a relative cooling of the troposphere. Thus, it is clear that any major decrease in the stratospheric ozone layer could have serious and far-reaching effects on man.

To appreciate the effect, if any, that stratospheric flight will have on the ozone layer, it is helpful to review some basic chemical equations that describe the dynamic equilibrium in the natural formation and breakdown of ozone.

Only a generation ago, the ozone equilibrium was thought to be totally described by the following four photochemical equations (the Chapman Reactions):[10]

$$O_2 + UV \text{ (short-wave)} = O + O \quad (1)$$

$$O + O_2 + M = O_3 + M$$
$$\text{(M is some molecule acting} \quad (2)$$
$$\text{as a catalyst)}$$

$$O_3 + UV \text{ (long-wave)} = O_2 + O \quad (3)$$

$$O_3 + O = 2O_2 \quad (4)$$

Equations 1 and 2 account for the formation of ozone (O_3), which can occur only at high altitudes because short-wave UV does not reach the troposphere. The products of equation 3 immediately recombine to form ozone, so that only equation 4 accounts for its destruction. When measured, however, the amount of ozone was less than predicted by these equations, so other routes of ozone breakdown were sought.

Around 1970, another method, involving oxides of nitrogen, was proposed to explain a more rapid destruction of ozone:

$$NO_3 + O_3 = NO_2 + 2O_2 \quad (5)$$

$$NO_2 + O = NO + O_2 \quad (6)$$

Because the catalyst (NO) remains unchanged, it is available to "attack" other ozone molecules. Thus, a small amount of NO can have a substantial effect in decreasing total ozone. At least 50 other equations are known to involve the ozone layer, but the reactions are judged to be too slow to show any effect.

This information on the link between oxides of nitrogen and ozone depletion coincided with the early SST flights (Concorde and Tupolev 144), which cruise in the low stratosphere (18 to 20 km) and which emit large amounts of oxides of nitrogen. This aroused great concern among many environmentalist groups. Consequently, great public pressure was exerted that threatened the very existence of the SST program. Based on these equations and a proposed SST fleet of 100 aircraft, it was estimated that the ozone layer would decrease by 10% when equilibrium was reached. This led to such alarmist predictions as an FAA Environmental Impact Statement in 1974 that said that ". . . the limited flights to be awarded to Concorde would produce an additional 200 cases of skin cancer per year in the United States."

Two years later, much of this concern was alleviated by new knowledge. Two major changes in the chemistry of high-level flight completely changed the calculations. First, it was shown that the reaction:

$$C/O + NO_2 + M = C/NO_3 + M \quad (7)$$

is fast enough to be important and that C/NO_3 is a fairly stable molecule. Thus, some of the nitrogen oxides are removed from the stratosphere and are unable to destroy ozone. Second, measurement of a reaction constant showed that the reaction proceeds 20 times as fast as originally assumed. This reaction is as follows:

$$HO_2 + NO = OH + NO_2 \quad (8)$$

The additional hydroxyl (OH) added to the stratosphere reacts with oxides of nitrogen to form nitric acid, which does not react with ozone but is eventually removed by rain. The reaction also removes NO so that catalyst reaction becomes less likely.

These latter two equations (7 and 8) reduce the problem of ozone destruction by nitrogen oxides. Results suggest that low-level stratospheric flight (below 20 km) can actually increase ozone; flight at higher altitudes can decrease ozone but by very small percentages. Thus, the SST problem of ozone removal does not appear as important as other difficulties involved in SST operations. Other major threats to the ozone layer still exist, including the use of nitrogen fertilizers and fluorocarbons.

THE SPACE SHUTTLE

The space shuttle is a manned, reusable vehicle, the orbiter, mounted with an expendable external tank containing hydrogen/oxygen propellants and two reusable solid rocket boosters (SRBs). Integral to the orbiter are three main hydrogen/oxygen liquid rocket engines. An environmental impact occurs both during launch and reentry of the vehicle. At launch, toxic gases are produced in the launch area. As the system penetrates the stratosphere, exhaust products are released that can affect the ozone layer. The orbiter produces sonic booms during both launch and reentry. Table 33–3 shows the exhaust products emitted by the space shuttle into selected atmospheric layers.

Tropospheric Effects

The Ground Cloud

Exhaust products from the solid rocket booster (SRB) include the following species in the amounts estimated:[11]

Aluminum oxide—56,100 Kg

Carbon monoxide—240 Kg

Hydrogen chloride—35,200 Kg

Water—65,300 Kg

Nitrogen oxides—2300 Kg

Carbon dioxide—76,800 Kg

Chlorine—4000 Kg

This hot exhaust cloud rises rapidly to altitudes of 0.6 to 3 km, then drifts and disperses with the prevailing wind.

A temporary and localized degradation of air quality occurs in regions over which the cloud passes. Surface contaminations are not expected to exceed the allowable limits for humans, wildlife, or plants. Peak concentrations of ground cloud constituents during a standard launch at Kennedy Space Center are estimated to be the following:

Hydrogen chloride—3.9 ppm

Chlorine—0.4 ppm

Nitric oxide—0.2 ppm

Nitrogen dioxide—0.004 ppm

Carbon monoxide—0.02 ppm

Aluminum oxide—10.0 mg/m^3

Table 33–3. Exhaust Products Emitted by the Space Shuttle Vehicle into Selected Atmospheric Layers

Atmospheric Layer	Altitude Range	Hydrogen Chloride (kg)	Chlorine (kg)	Nitric Oxide (kg)	Carbon Monoxide (kg)	Carbon Dioxide (kg)	Water (kg)	Aluminum Oxide (kg)
Surface boundary layer	0 to 500 m	24,666	2741	1697	131	55,075	45,674	39,284
Troposphere	0.5 to 13 km	78,517	9657	4618	839	172,570	152,677	26,385
Stratosphere	13 to 50 km	59,732	11,727	293	2198	147,684	146,393	110,304
Lower mesosphere	50 to 67 km	0	0	0	0	0	15,542	0
Mesosphere thermosphere	Above 67 km	0	0	0	0	0	149,045	0

Modified from Potter, A.E.: Environmental effects of the Space Shuttle. Environ. Sci. Technol., 12:15–21, March/April, 1978.

Acidic Rain

Raindrops falling through the exhaust cloud will absorb hydrogen chloride and produce acidic rain. The acidity diminishes as hydrogen chloride is washed from the cloud. Near the launch area, the initial rain acidity may reach pH values near 1 and may temporarily damage vegetation. Beyond the immediate launch area, the initial rain is less acidic and damage is less likely. In any case, the effect is highly localized and temporary.

Weather

It is not possible to predict at this point what effects, if any, the shuttle exhaust cloud will have on the weather. Information is insufficient to evaluate this potential effect, but if there is a weather impact, it should be limited in area and duration.

Stratospheric Effects

Ozone Depletion

As the space shuttle penetrates the stratosphere, chlorine compounds are introduced into the ozone layer, decreasing the ozone level. When the space shuttle program is fully operational at 60 launches per year, the mean reduction in ozone level is predicted to be about 0.2%. Further, this 0.2% reduction in ozone is expected to result in about a 0.4% increase in the biologically harmful ultraviolet (BHUV) radiation reaching the surface of the earth.

The consequences of this small increase in BHUV radiation on agriculture, ecology, and climate are believed to be insignificant as compared with larger seasonal and geographic fluctuations. As far as the potential of increasing the incidence of skin cancer among susceptible humans, a 0.4% increase in BHUV radiation corresponds to the increase in BHUV received by an individual who moves 27 km south in the midlatitudes.

Sonic Booms

Sonic booms are produced both during launch and reentry of the space shuttle. The intensity of the launch boom approximates 300 N/m² over a wide area of the ocean, with a narrow carpet a few hundred meters wide where the focused boom may reach 1500 N/m². The launch boom is larger than the orbiter's reentry boom because the total launch vehicle and its exhaust plume are much larger than the orbiter. For launches at Kennedy Space Center, the boom occurs entirely over the Atlantic Ocean and produces no significant environmental impact. The reentry boom of the orbiter is much less, reaching a maximum of 101 N/m². The reentry boom, however, will occur over populated areas of California, New Mexico, and Florida. These low-intensity booms are not expected to cause any effect other than a slight startle reaction in about half of the people who hear the boom.

Environmental Factors

Four basic elements are important in the assessment of the environmental impact of any space system:

1. Propulsion systems exhausts associated with the construction and station-keeping activities of the space segment
2. Transmission and reception of the microwave beam
3. Physical structure and debris associated with the space segment
4. Launch and landing activities with daily launches for 100 plus days, each generating four times the thrust of the Saturn moon rocket, and a similar number of landings

Specific treatment of these environmental concerns is beyond the scope of this chapter. They are presented to provide a perspective of the direction and magnitude of future space exploits and their potential impact on the global, even galactic, environment.

ENVIRONMENTAL CONCERNS IN PERSPECTIVE

Chicken Little is wrong; the sky is not falling in. A review of the environmental consequences of our operations within the atmosphere and in space indicates that we have been prudent and responsible in protecting the ecology as we have ventured higher, faster, and farther in pursuit of our national objectives.

Perspective is the key. Although we have contaminated the air with aircraft emissions, our contribution is but a small fraction of the total anthropogenic pollution activity. The emissions of automobiles bringing observers to space launches exceed the atmospheric contamination of the launches themselves. Continuous efforts are being made to reduce all of these sources of environmental contamination.

Aviation's impact on the weather (from carbon dioxide and contrails) and on increased BHUV radiation reaching the earth through catalytic ozone depletion is likewise insignificant. Any contribution of aviation to these phenomena is lost in the seasonal and geographic perturbations that characterize them.

Noise, particularly adjacent to airports, is the one real significant environmental problem associated with aviation. Its resolution is based on both community and national understanding, cooperation, and action. Sonic booms appear to be novelties more than real problems, with some degree of political overlay.

Statutory provisions and regulatory agencies appear to be adequate to deal with aerospace environmental issues, now and in the future, but we must not become complacent. Research, development, engineering, and operating authorities must remain aware of environmental consequences of their actions and programs. They must receive the full and timely professional advice of biomedical personnel who are also dedicated to mission accomplishment within the constraints of a healthy ecology. We must anticipate and respond to state-of-the-art technologic developments. We always have, and we always will.

REFERENCES

1. Public Law 91–190. 42 U.S. Congress 4321-4347, January 1, 1970. Amended by Public Law 94–83, August 9, 1975.
2. United States Environmental Protection Agency: Aviation Noise: Let's Get on With the Job. Prepared by the Honorable Russell E. Train for delivery before the Inter-Noise 1976 Conference, U.S. Government Printing Office, Washington, D.C., April 5, 1976.
3. Noise, vibration, and thermal problems. In Army Flight Surgeon's Manual. United States Army Aviation School, Fort Rucker, Alabama, August, 1976.
4. Tracor, Inc.: Community Reaction to Airport Noise. NASA CR-1761. U.S. Government Printing Office, Washington, D.C., 1971.
5. Maglier, D.V.: Status of Knowledge of Sonic Booms. NASA TM-80113. U.S. Government Printing Office, Washington, D.C., June, 1979.
6. Von Gierke, H.E.: Effects of sonic boom on people: Review and outlook. Acoust. Soc. Am., 39:543–550, 1966.
7. Wilkening, G.M.: Nonionizing radiation. In The Industrial Environment—Its Evaluation and Control. National Institute of Occupational Safety and Health, U.S. Government Printing Office, Washington, D.C., 1973, pp. 357–373.
8. Naugle, D.F., and Fox, D.L.: Aircraft and air pollution. Environ. Sci. Technol., 15:342, April, 1981.
9. Buden, D.: The Acceptability of Reactors in Space. Report LA-8724-MS, Pl. Los Alamos Scientific Laboratory, Los Alamos, NM. April, 1981.
10. Panofsky, H.A.: A progress report on stratospheric ozone. Weatherwise, 21:61–62, April, 1968.
11. Potter, A.E.: Environmental effects of the Space Shuttle. Environ. Sci. Technol., 21:15–21, March/April, 1978.

Index

Numerals in *italics* indicate a figure, page numbers followed by a "t" indicate tabular matter.